Respiratory Infections

Diagnosis and Management

Third Edition

Respiratory Infections
Diagnosis and Management

Third Edition

Editor

James E. Pennington, M.D.
Clinical Professor of Medicine
University of California, San Francisco
San Francisco, California

Raven Press **New York**

Raven Press, Ltd., 1185 Avenue of the Americas, New York, New York 10036

Made in the United States of America

Library of Congress Cataloging-in-Publication Data

Respiratory infections : diagnosis and management / editor, James E. Pennington. — 3rd.
    p.   cm.
    Includes bibliographical references and index.
    ISBN 0-7817-0173-2
    1. Respiratory infections. I. Pennington, James.
    [DNLM: 1. Respiratory Tract Infections. 2. Pneumonia. WF 140
R43445 1994]
RC740.R46 1994
616.2—dc20
DNLM/DLC
for Library of Congress   93-48578
                                                       CIP

9 8 7 6 5 4 3 2 1

Contents

v

Contributing Authors

Mickael Aoun, M.D.
Infectious Disease Department
Institute Jules Bordet
Rue Heger-Bordet 1
1000 Brussels
Belgium

John G. Bartlett, M.D.
Professor of Medicine
Department of Medicine
Johns Hopkins University School of
  Medicine
720 Rutland Avenue
Baltimore, Maryland 21205

Eugénie Bergogne-Bérézin, M.D.
Professor of Microbiology
Bichat-Claude Bernard Hospital
46 Rue Henri-Huchard
Paris 75877, Cedex 18
France

Scott E. Buchalter, M.D.
Associate Professor
Pulmonary and Critical Care Medicine
University of Nebraska Medical Center
600 South 42nd Street
Omaha, Nebraska 68198-5300

Stephen A. Chartrand, M.D.
Professor and Chairman
Department of Pediatrics
Creighton University School of Medicine
601 North 30th Street
Omaha, Nebraska 68131

Lawrence R. Crane, M.D.
Associate Professor of Medicine
Department of Internal Medicine
Division of Infectious Diseases
Wayne State University School of
  Medicine
4160 John R
Detroit, Michigan 48201

Scott F. Davies, M.D.
Associate Professor
Department of Medicine
University of Minnesota and Hennepin
  County Medical Center
701 Park Avenue South
Minneapolis, Minnesota 55415

Richard D. Diamond, M.D.
Professor of Medicine
Research Professor of Biochemistry
Boston University School of Medicine
88 East Newton Street
Boston, Massachusetts 02118-2393

Jeffrey R. Dichter, M.D.
Department of Critical Care Medicine
National Institutes of Health
Building 10, Room 7D 43
9000 Rockville Pike
Bethesda, Maryland 20892

David J. Drutz, M.D.
Adjunct Professor
Department of Microbiology and
  Immunology
Temple University School of Medicine
Philadelphia, Pennsylvania 19122
and Vice President
Daiichi Pharmaceutical Corporation
1 Parker Plaza
Fort Lee, New Jersey 07024

Paul H. Edelstein, M.D.
Associate Professor
Departments of Pathology and Laboratory
  Medicine
University of Pennsylvania Medical Center
3400 Spruce Street
Philadelphia, Pennsylvania 19104-4283

Janice Eisenstadt, D.O.
Fellow in Infectious Diseases
Department of Clinical Pathology
Microbiology Section
The Cleveland Clinic Foundation
9500 Euclid Avenue
Cleveland, Ohio 44195

Anthony L. Esposito, M.D.
Associate Professor of Medicine
University of Massachusetts School of
* Medicine*
Director, Division of Infectious Diseases
St. Vincent's Hospital
25 Winthrop Street
Worcester, Massachusetts 01604

Hugh E. Evans, M.D.
Professor
Department of Pediatrics
New Jersey Medical School
185 South Orange Avenue
Newark, New Jersey 07103

Christopher H. Fanta, M.D.
Department of Medicine
Brigham and Women's Hospital
Harvard Medical School
25 Shattuck Street
Boston, Massachusetts 02115

Barry M. Farr, M.D.
Wm. S. Jordan Associate Professor of
* Medicine*
Department of Internal Medicine
University of Virginia Health Sciences
* Center*
Charlottesville, Virginia 22908

Sydney M. Finegold, M.D.
Professor
Departments of Medicine and
* Microbiology and Immunology*
UCLA School of Medicine
Wilshire and Sawtelle Boulevards
Los Angeles, California 90073

Anthony A. Floreani, M.D.
Assistant Professor
Pulmonary and Critical Care Medicine
University of Nebraska Medical Center
600 South 42nd Street
Omaha, Nebraska 68198-5300

David E. Griffith, M.D.
Associate Professor of Medicine
Department of Medicine
University of Texas Health Center
P.O. Box 2003
Tyler, Texas 75710

Jack M. Gwaltney, Jr., M.D.
Professor of Medicine
Department of Internal Medicine
University of Virginia Health Sciences
* Center*
Charlottesville, Virginia 22908

Caroline Breese Hall, M.D.
Professor
Department of Pediatrics and Medicine
University of Rochester School of
* Medicine and Dentistry*
601 Elmwood Avenue
Rochester, New York 14642

Howard M. Heller, M.D.
Instructor in Medicine
Harvard Medical School
Massachusetts General Hospital
55 Fruit Street
Boston, Massachusetts 02114

Robert S. Kauffman, M.D.
Assistant Clinical Professor of Medicine
Department of Medicine
Stanford University School of Medicine
Stanford, California 94305

Berndt Kemmerich, M.D.
Practicing Physician
Leopoldstrasse 87
80802 Munich
Germany

Jean Klastersky, M.D.
Professor
Infectious Disease Department
Institut Jules Bordet
Rue Heger-Bordet 1
1000 Brussels
Belgium

Jerome O. Klein, M.D.
Professor
Department of Pediatrics
Boston University School of Medicine
88 East Newton Street
Boston, Massachusetts 02118-2393

Phillip I. Lerner, M.D.
Professor of Medicine
Division of Infectious Diseases
Mount Sinai Medical Center
1 Mount Sinai Drive
Cleveland, Ohio 44106

Stuart M. Levitz, M.D.
Associate Professor of Medicine
Department of Medicine
Boston University School of Medicine
88 Newton Street
Boston, Massachusetts 02118-2393

Hartmut Lode, M.D.
Professor of Medicine
Free University of Berlin
Chief
Chest and Infectious Disease Department
City Hospital Zehlendorf/Hecheshörn
Zum Hecheshom 33
Berlin
Germany

Gerald L. Mandell, M.D.
Professor of Internal Medicine
Chief, Infectious Diseases
Department of Internal Medicine
University of Virginia Health Sciences
  Center
Charlottesville, Virginia 22908

Bonita T. Mangura, M.D.
Associate Professor of Clinical Medicine
Department of Medicine
University of Medicine and Dentistry of
  New Jersey
65 Bergen Street
Newark, New Jersey 07107-3001

Melvin I. Marks, M.D.
Medical Director
Department of Pediatrics
Memorial Miller Children's Hospital
2801 Atlantic Avenue
Long Beach, California 90801-1428

Henry Masur, M.D.
Chief
Department of Critical Care Medicine
Warren G. Magnuson Clinical Center
National Institutes of Health
Building 10, Room 7D43
9000 Rockville Pike
Bethesda, Maryland 20892

John T. McBride, M.D.
Professor of Pediatrics
Department of Pediatrics
University of Rochester School of
  Medicine and Dentistry
601 Elmwood Avenue
Rochester, New York 14642

Richard D. Meyer, M.D.
Professor and Director
Division of Infectious Diseases
Department of Medicine
Cedars-Sinai Medical Center School of
  Medicine
8700 Beverly Boulevard
Los Angeles, California 90048

Henry W. Murray, M.D.
Professor
Department of Medicine
Cornell University Medical College
1300 York Avenue
Chief
Infectious Diseases Division
The New York Hospital
New York, New York 10021

James E. Pennington, M.D.
Clinical Professor of Medicine
University of California, San Francisco
San Francisco, California 94143

Lee B. Reichman, M.D., M.P.H.
Professor of Medicine
Director
New Jersey Medical School
National Tuberculosis Center
University of Medicine and Dentistry of
  New Jersey
65 Bergen Street
Newark, New Jersey 07107-3001

Stephen I. Rennard, M.D.
Larsen Professor and Chief
Pulmonary and Critical Care Medicine
  Section
University of Nebraska Medical Center
600 South 42nd Street
Omaha, Nebraska 68198-5300

Herbert Y. Reynolds, M.D.
Professor and Chairman
Department of Medicine
Milton S. Hershey Medical Center
Pennsylvania State University
P.O. Box 850
Hershey, Pennsylvania 17033

Joseph H. Sisson, M.D.
Assistant Professor
Pulmonary and Critical Care Medicine
University of Nebraska Medical Center
600 South 42nd Street
Omaha, Nebraska 68198-5300

Arnold L. Smith, M.D.
Professor of Pediatrics
Department of Pediatrics
Adjunct Professor of Microbiology
University of Washington
4800 Sand Point Way NE, CH-32
Seattle, Washington 98105

Anthony F. Suffredini, M.D.
Senior Investigator
Department of Critical Care Medicine
Warren G. Magnuson Clinical Center
National Institutes of Health
Building 10, Room 7D43
900 Rockville Pike
Bethesda, Maryland 20892

Austin B. Thompson, M.D.
Associate Professor
Pulmonary and Critical Care Medicine
University of Nebraska Medical Center
600 South 42nd Street
Omaha, Nebraska 68198-5300

Jean-Pierre Thys, M.D.
Associated Professor
Infectious Diseases Clinic
Erasme University Hospital
Route de Lennik 808
B-1070 Brussels
Belgium

Galen B. Toews, M.D.
Division of Pulmonary and Critical Care
  Medicine
Department of Internal Medicine
The University of Michigan Medical
  Center
3916 Taubman Center
Ann Arbor, Michigan 48109-0360

Carmelita U. Tuazon, M.D.
Professor of Medicine
Department of Medicine
George Washington University
2150 Pennsylvania Avenue NW
Washington, DC 20037

Nelson L. Turcios, M.D.
Associate Professor
Department of Pediatrics
New Jersey Medical School
185 South Orange Avenue
Newark, New Jersey 07103-2757

Eric Vallée, Pharm. D.
Department of Microbiology
Bichat-Claude Bernard Hospital
46 Rue Henri-Huchard
75877 Paris, Cedex 18
France

Richard J. Wallace, Jr., M.D.
Professor
Department of Medicine and Microbiology
University of Texas Health Center
P.O. Box 2003
Tyler, Texas 75710

John A. Washington, M.D.
Vice Chairman, Division of Pathology and
  Laboratory Medicine
Chairman, Department of Clinical
  Pathology
Head, Section of Microbiology
The Cleveland Clinic Foundation
9500 Euclid Avenue
Cleveland, Ohio 44195-5140

Arnold N. Weinberg, M.D.
Professor of Medicine
Harvard Medical School
Medical Director
Massachusetts Institute of Technology
77 Massachusetts Avenue
Cambridge, Massachusetts 02139

Peter F. Weller, M.D.
Associate Professor of Medicine
Harvard Medical School
Beth Israel Hospital
330 Brookline Avenue
Boston, Massachusetts 02215

Birgit Winther, M.D.
Professor of Medicine
Department of Internal Medicine
University of Virginia Health Sciences
  Center
Charlottesville, Virginia 22908

Donald E. Woods, Ph.D.
Professor and Chairman
Department of Microbiology and
  Infectious Diseases
University of Calgary
3300 Hospital Drive NW
Calgary, Alberta
Canada T2N 4N1

Lowell S. Young, M.D.
Director, Kuzell Institute for Arthritis and
  Infectious Diseases
Chief, Division of Infectious Diseases
California Pacific Medical Center
Clinical Professor of Medicine
University of California, San Francisco
San Francisco, California 94115

Foreword to the First Edition
Pneumonia:
Past, Present, and Future

Robert G. Petersdorf

Departments of Medicine and Health Sciences, School of Medicine, University of California, San Diego, La Jolla, California 92093

In the first volume of the second edition of the Osler-McCrae textbook, *Modern Medicine* (4), published in 1913, the third longest chapter, nearly 45,000 words in length, was devoted to the topic of lobar pneumonia. Among all the infections, it was surpassed in importance in the text only by typhoid fever and tuberculosis: this despite the fact that much of the information on etiology was lacking or incorrect; the bacteriology of the pneumococcus was incomplete; little was known about the pathogenesis and immunology of the infection; and, of course, there was no treatment. That is not to say that everything written about pneumonia 70 years ago was incorrect or has become obsolete. On the contrary, the presence of pneumococci as part of the oral and respiratory flora in many apparently healthy individuals was well known, but why the organisms set up infection in some people and not in others was not. To my knowledge, this question has not yet been answered. Of course, the pathology of pneumococcal pneumonia was well described; many of the complications had been delineated, and descriptions of the clinical manifestations contained the kind of elegant detail that has since had to be sacrificed to the economy essential in textbook writing. The description of the chill is a case in point:

> Generally a well-marked rigor is promptly followed by a rapid *rise in temperature, cough, pain and dyspnoea.* The chill is often severe, lasting from one to several hours, the patient feeling very cold, shaking from head to foot with teeth chattering, cyanosed lips and icy extremities.

Whereas there is no question that today's textbooks of medicine provide much more factual information in a fraction of the space (the ninth edition of Harrison's chapter on lobar pneumonia is closer to 6,000 words in length), they also lack the clinical detail of their pedagogic forebears.

Of course, the pneumococcus and the infection it causes has been the subject of much important investigation, some of which has turned out to have biological application far beyond pneumonia. But the single most significant event that revolutionized the field was the discovery of penicillin. There is no aspect of pneumonia that has not been subject to the profound impact of this drug. The etiology, ecology, pathogenesis, manifestations, and clinical course and outcome of pneumococcal infection all have undergone marked change, most of which can be attributed in one way or another to penicillin.

In 1964, when I was Chief of Medicine at a busy county hospital, despite a plethora of new antibiotics (in addition to penicillin, we had by that time the tetracyclines, chloramphenicol, erythromycin, vancomycin, and the first of the penicillinase-resistant penicillins, methicillin, and of the extended-spectrum penicillins, ampicillin), my colleagues and I noted that not only were the incidence and prevalence of pneumonia not decreasing, but we were seeing pneumonia under many different guises, and all too often were being badly fooled by its many manifestations. In a paper called "Errors and Hazards in the Diagnosis and Treatment of Bacterial Pneumonias" (5) we made the following points:

The diagnosis of bacterial pneumonia was changing to encompass staphylococci, *Hemophilus influenzae* and gram-negative enteric organisms, in addition to pneumococci. All of these organisms can be suspected on the basis of a gram stain of sputum (it is important to make a smear of sputum not saliva), but they are often missed.

Some organisms are more likely to cause pneumonia than others, depending on the clinical situation. For example, staphylococcal pneumonia in the wake of the influenza should be suspected early, and chronic asthmatics are particularly subject to *H. influenzae* pneumonia. Failure to appreciate these differences often led to delay in the correct diagnosis.

Superinfections are an accompaniment in a small number of patients with pneumonia treated with antibiotics, particularly when broad-spectrum drugs, combinations of several agents, or very large doses are used. Failure to recognize superinfections often led to their tardy treatment.

Although most of the complications of pneumococcal pneumonia had been known for years (most were described in detail in the chapter on pneumonia in the Osler-McCrae textbook), in many instances, meningitis, endocarditis, arthritis, and peritonitis were recognized much later than the patients' signs and symptoms warranted. Perhaps antibiotics lulled the attending physicians and their staffs into a sense of false security. Or perhaps these complications had become sufficiently rare that the newer generations of physicians had not seen them, and hence failed to recognize them.

We were beginning to appreciate that failure of a pneumonia to respond to antibiotics was usually not due to use of an incorrect drug. Rather it was often a consequence of some mechanical factor—a lymph node obstructing a bronchus from without, or a mucus plug from within, or an area of atelectasis that had failed to reexpand, which led to apparent drug failure. We learned that in these and other cases, the answer was not to add more and more antibiotics, but to withdraw the ones the patient was receiving and to reexamine the patient physically, radiographically, or bronchoscopically.

We became aware of the fact that the sputum flora of patients receiving antibiotics changed profoundly. However, we learned that these changes were of little clinical significance unless they were accompanied by changes in signs, symptoms, or clinical course.

Finally, we were surprised how often inflammatory events occurring in association with pneumonia, particularly sterile pleural effusions and slow reexpansion of atelectatic lung, were responsible for prolonged fever and failure to regain well-being.

As I reviewed this paper's clinical homilies, written nearly 20 years ago, it seemed to me to typify the end of an era. Pneumonia had been described, its pathogenetic mechanisms had become better understood, its treatment had been perfected, and some consequences of therapy had come to the fore.

During the next decade, the emphasis shifted to infections in immunocompromised patients, usually those receiving chemo- or radiotherapy in the wake of cancer or organ transplantation. These patients often had pulmonary infections caused by indigenous microorganisms or by hospital bacteria that had become resistant to antibiotics. Fungal pulmonary infections became commonplace in these patients, and supplanted bacteria as a cause of acute pneumonia in many. Many new antimicrobials made their appearance, all presumably aimed at staying one step ahead of the microorganisms that were colonizing and infecting the lungs of immunocompromised, elderly, and debilitated patients, and all to relatively little avail. In fact, with the exception of the efficacy of cephalosporins against Klebsiella and the activity of some third-generation cephalosporins and some of the newer penicillins against Pseudomonas, new antimicrobials have contributed relatively little in the battle against pulmonary pathogens. The many severely ill patients in intensive care units whose coup de grace is a resistant *Serratia* pneumonia attest to that sad fact.

During the past six years, however, three events have occurred that have revitalized the field of pulmonary infections and made it tremendously exciting.

The first was the discovery of *Legionella pneumophila,* a fastidious gram-negative bacterium, as a cause of Legionnaire's disease, and the subsequent identification of several other species of Legionella as human pathogens as well (1). Here was an organism that could cause sometimes lethal pneumonia, that was ubiquitous in the environment (at least on cooling towers and in potable water), and that could produce a spectrum of disease varying from the asymptomatic carrier state to epidemics of pulmonary infections, or rarer manifestations involving the gut, the kidney, and the central nervous system. Legionnaires' disease may occur in epidemics or sporadically and may attack the immunocompetent as well as the immunocompromised. It is characteristically difficult to diagnose, and despite being sensitive to a variety of antibiotics *in vitro,* it is often difficult to treat. Although we have learned a great deal about the Legionella in the 6 years since the Philadelphia epidemic, the answers to many questions remain elusive. Where do these pathogens reside normally? What makes a contaminated site a nidus for spread of the disease? How can decontamination be accomplished? How can the microbiology laboratory identify these organisms more rapidly? How can we arm the host to repel the organism? Clearly there is a lot more we need to learn about this "new" bacterial pneumonia.

Although *Pneumocystis carinii* pneumonia had become all too familiar to oncologists, pulmonary and infectious disease physicians, and transplant surgeons as a cause of a refractory and sometimes terminal, pulmonary infection in patients with compromised immune systems, the reports of *P. carinii* pneumonia occurring in association with Kaposi's sarcoma came as an unexpected surprise (2), particularly since the reports came from widely divergent places geographically, and the disease occurred predominantly in previously healthy, homosexual men. As the experience with this syndrome grew, it became apparent that many patients had infections with other organisms—herpes simplex and cytomegaloviruses, *M. tuberculosis,* fungi, and protozoa. Although much about the pathogenesis of this syndrome remains unknown, a defect in cellular immune defenses appears to be the common denominator. Viewed in this light, the occurrence of pneumocystis infection in this population implies there must be some similarity to patients whose immune systems have been depressed by drugs or irradiation. But it does not explain the cause of this syndrome, its possible relationship to cytomegalovirus, and its possible determination by sexual activity. Indeed, if homosexuality is as old as civilization, why have we not seen the syndrome before?

It has been just over 100 years since the discovery of the pneumococcus, and the first pneumococcal vaccine was tested in 1911, too late to make the second edition of the Osler-McCrae textbook. Work on pneumococcal vaccines, which had reached a reasonable degree of purity by 1940, was relegated to the back burner by the discovery of penicillin. However, Austrian's persistence in calling the high mortality of bacteremic pneumococcal pneumonia to the attention of the infectious disease community led eventually to the development of a pneumococcal vaccine containing 14 capsular polysaccharides (3). This vaccine has been recommended for elderly persons with chronic debilitating disease, including chronic obstructive pulmonary disease, chronic congestive heart failure, cirrhosis, alcoholism, hemoglobinopathies, postsplenectomy, for patients with Hodgkin's disease under chemo- or radiotherapy, or with multiple myeloma, nephrosis, chronic renal failure, and for renal allograft recipients. Most of us have accepted these recommendations with little question, and they made even more sense in the face of discovering an occasional penicillin-resistant pneumococcus. In view of this optimism, reports that the vaccine was of no efficacy in preventing pneumococcal pneumonia, bacteremia, or pneumonia-associated deaths in an elderly institutionalized population, as well as its failure to provide protection in young children, were particularly disappointing (3). On the other hand, there are now a number of studies that credit the vaccine with a high degree of protection. While the vaccine may need continuous fine-tuning, and various studies may be subject to different interpretations, I believe that it represents a very significant advance.

Where do we go from here? What does the future hold in store? Progressively more secure in knowing the causes and pathogenesis of pneumonia; relatively more sophisticated in understanding its epidemiology; somewhat more at home having defined local and systemic host defense mechanisms, and forearmed with a potent armory of antimicrobials, have we reached the millenium? Is the best behind us? I doubt it. While clinicians (this one included) have never won prizes as prognosticators of biologic phenomena (of the three exciting discoveries I described briefly above, only the discovery of polyvalent pneumococcal vaccine seemed predictable), let me venture a few predictions.

We will surely discover more new etiologic agents, not only because of the increasing sophistication of diagnostic microbiology, but because so many bouts of pneumonia remain undiagnosed. I am convinced that in the sputa of patients with pneumonia from whom nothing grows but "normal flora," there lurk a number of putative pathogens. We just have not been smart enough to identify them yet.

As we become more expert at understanding the human immune system, we will almost surely discover, unmask, or induce some new causes of pneumonia. We have learned a great deal about the role of cytomegalovirus pneumonia in the course of bone marrow transplantation. I suspect that similar experiences are in store for us.

The use of new and even more potent antimicrobials will remain a way of life, not necessarily because they are needed but because they are viewed as scientific advances or commercial panaceas. Perhaps because of these new drugs, and perhaps because of spontaneous changes in the genetic makeup of the organism, resistant pathogens will emerge. The timing of such an event is entirely unpredictable; whoever would have thought that any self-respecting pneumococcus would have developed resistance to penicillin 35 years after that drug was introduced? Microbial resistance will inevitably require new therapeutic and prophylactic approaches. We may be closer than we think to a universal gram-negative vaccine that could be administered to patients admitted to intensive care units to prevent them from acquiring gram-negative pneumonia.

We have just scratched the surface of noninvasive diagnostic technology, particularly in infections of the lung. I hope that I am not too irreverent in suggesting that in time even the chest x-ray, innocuous though it may be, will be replaced by a technique that is safer, cheaper, and more reproducible. It has always been one of my pet peeves that in an era when we can send a man to the moon, we still have great difficulty generating chest films that are comparable in the same patient from one occasion to the next.

Finally, we have not scratched the surface at all of some of the therapeutic modalities that are being applied to noninfectious causes of lung disease. Positive end expiratory pressure (PEEP) is a case in point. What is the role of this ventilatory support system in pneumonia? Does it help or does it hurt? What are its indications, and its contraindications? It may well be that some of us old-fashioned infectious disease clinicians will never understand the new pseudophysiology that is bandied about in intensive care units. However we should at least determine what is fact and what is fiction.

This all goes by way of saying that like it or not, pneumonia has a future. If the first 100 years that began with the description of the pneumococcus by Weichselbaum were exciting, the second hundred promise to be even more so.

REFERENCES

1. Cordes, L. G., and Pasculle, A. W. (1982): The Legionellae: newly discovered agents of bacterial pneumonia. In: *Update II: Harrison's Principles of Internal Medicine*, edited by K. J. Isselbacher et al., pp. 111–130. McGraw-Hill, New York.
2. Fishman, A. P., and Pietra, G. G. (1982): The syndrome of *Pneumocystis carinii* pneumonia and/or Kaposi's sarcoma. In: *Update: Pulmonary Diseases and Disorders*, edited by A. P. Fishman, pp. 26–33. McGraw-Hill, New York.
3. Kass, E. H., editor (1981): Assessment of the pneumococcal polysaccharide vaccine. *Rev. Infect. Dis.*, 3 (Suppl):S1-S197.
4. Norris, G. W. (1913): Lobar pneumonia. In: *Modern Medicine*, Vol. I, edited by W. Osler and T. McCrae, pp. 202–286. Lea & Febiger, Philadelphia.
5. Shulman, J. A., Phillips, L. A., and Petersdorf, R. G. (1965): Errors and hazards in the diagnosis and treatment of bacterial pneumonias. *Ann. Int. Med.*, 62:41–58.

Preface to the First Edition

Respiratory tract infection is one of the major afflictions of mankind. This is not surprising considering the vast surface area of respiratory epithelium continuously exposed to potential infectious pathogens. It is a tribute to the effectiveness of the pulmonary host defense apparatus that respiratory infection is not more common.

Pneumonia is an historically important illness, constituting a leading cause of fatality in the preantibiotic era. Yet, at the same time, pneumonia is a timely and rapidly evolving clinical subject. While pneumonia captures the bulk of clinical attention, it should be pointed out that parenchymal infection of the lungs represents a rather small fraction of the total number of respiratory infections, accounting for less than 1% in one clinical survey. Accordingly, this book is not meant to be a "pneumonia" text, rather it is designed to encompass the entire spectrum of respiratory infection from the upper to the lower respiratory tracts.

Every clinician knows that a patient presents not as an "adenoviral pneumonia," or "klebsiella pneumonia," or "Legionnaires' pneumonia," but as a normal host with community-acquired pneumonia, or an elderly patient with pneumonia, or a cystic fibrosis patient with bronchitis, etc. This requires a clinical approach based upon experience in these specific clinical settings. Accordingly, a major section of this book is devoted to the "clinical approach" to respiratory infections.

For those interested in a more in-depth discussion of specific etiologic agents, a section also has been included that offers the traditional etiology-oriented approach to respiratory infection. Finally, this text has not avoided controversy. A number of controversial techniques, both diagnostic (e.g., transtracheal aspiration, microscopic "sputum screening") and therapeutic (e.g., intermittent positive pressure breathing, intrabronchial antibiotics) are discussed in detail.

In summary, we feel that this text is a unique collection of rather detailed yet practical information on this subject. Every effort has been made to incorporate the latest information including the most up-to-date references for the rapidly evolving areas in respiratory infection.

As such this volume will be of interest to a broad-based group of practitioners.

James Pennington
Editor

Preface

It has been over ten years since the publication of the First Edition and five years since the publication of the Second Edition of *Respiratory Infections: Diagnosis and Management*. So what's new in respiratory infection? Some news is good, some not so good. As usual, and as predicted by Dr. Petersdorf in his conceptually timeless Foreword to the First Edition, new agents causing pneumonia have been described. Also as predicted, increasing drug resistance among established pathogens has occurred. The hantavirus, carried in rodent excreta, has finally emerged as a pathogen in the Western Hemisphere, and hantavirus has emerged with a vengeance, causing a frequently fatal form of atypical pnuemonia. It is of no comfort that the TWAR agent, having now been established as a wide-spread human pathogen, has earned itself an official designation within the Chlamydia family (*Chlamydia pneumoniae*). The emergence of rhodococcus as more than a rare pathogen in immunocompromised patients is also worrisome. Even more troubling is the ominous rise in multi-drug resistant tuberculosis cases in the United States, particularly among patients infected with human immunodeficiency virus (HIV).

Good news in respiratory infection is always less abundant, but there are some promising new therapeutic agents available. New macrolides offer the advantages of less frequent dosing and potential expansion of spectrum. Quinolones allow broader-spectrum coverage for gram-negative bacilli, including *Pseudomonas aeruginosa*, using an oral route of administration. Exciting news is developing in methods for suppression or prevention of Mycobacterium avium-intracellulare complex infection of HIV-infected patients. And at last, some promising additions have been made to the antifungal therapeutic armamentarium. Before too much credit is given to development of new therapeutic agents, however, it is noteworthy that virtually no new vaccines or immunotherapeutics have been introduced for use in respiratory infections, despite the boom in biotechnology and molecular genetic research.

Each chapter in the Third Edition has been updated. A few needed only minimal change. In other cases, such as the chapter dealing with HIV-associated respiratory diseases, an almost total redrafting was required. Most chapters fall between these extremes. In all cases, an attempt to provide the most contemporary concepts and citations has been made. The Third Edition should maintain the tradition of this text, namely to serve the dual functions of providing a timely bedside guide to diagnosis and modern therapies, and of serving as a reference text for the latest etiology-oriented information on pathogenesis of respiratory infections.

James E. Pennington

Respiratory Infections

Diagnosis and Management

Third Edition

Respiratory Infections: Diagnosis and Management, 3d ed.,
edited by James E. Pennington.
Raven Press, Ltd., New York © 1994

1

Normal and Defective Respiratory Host Defenses

Herbert Y. Reynolds

*Department of Medicine, The Milton S. Hershey Medical Center, Pennsylvania
State University, P.O. Box 850, Hershey, Pennsylvania 17033*

The respiratory tract has an elaborate array of host defense mechanisms that are coordinated to remove the variety of aspirated microorganisms, dust particles, and inhaled debris that accumulate in the lungs of normal humans and animals (101). Some of these mechanisms are purely mechanical, such as mucociliary clearance and coughing, or anatomical, such as the epiglottis and larynx and the tight-apical junctions of the epithelial cell lining. These have been designated as *surveillance* mechanisms (Table 1-1). Other host defenses that operate in the terminal airways where actual air exchange occurs include phagocytic cells which ingest particulates that reach the alveolar surface. In this milieu, immunoglobulins with opsonic antibody activity, complement components, iron-containing proteins, and chemotactic factors that regulate the influx of inflammatory cells such as polymorphonuclear granulocytes (PMNs) may assist the function of alveolar macrophages. Many of these protein substances, however, are admixed with the mucus lining film and secretions that coat the conducting airways and are, therefore, present along the entire mucosal surface. Thus, the actions of immunoglobulins, for example, are not restricted to the alveolar area but can be important at various points along the respiratory tract.

Unlike surveillance mechanisms, which are in constant action, *augmenting* mechanisms of host defense are used intermittently—perhaps only in times of crisis. The inflammatory reaction is a good example. When alveolar mechanisms are unable to inactivate and contain a virulent bacterial inoculum, inflammation which features a prominent influx of PMNs and fluid components from the intravascular space broadens the host defense response. Elements of systemic immunity are brought in to reinforce local lung mechanisms and to help regain control over a nidus of infection.

When functioning properly, the respiratory host defenses do an exceedingly good job of removing potentially infectious agents from the airways; major respiratory infection is a rarity in healthy people. Considering the constant burden of exposure—inhaling microorganisms expelled by others' coughing and sneezing, aspirating our own bacterial flora in nasooropharyngeal secretions, or transporting viruses (rhinoviruses) on a fingertip to the nasal mucosa—it is a wonder that respiratory infection is not a more common malady. Of course, infection may result if exposure to a particularly virulent microbe or to an excessive inoculum occurs that overwhelms local

TABLE 1–1. *Lung host defenses to airway challenge*

Host defenses	Defect	Potential infection problem
SURVEILLANCE MECHANISMS		
Ciliated and squamous epithelium in nasooropharynx	Poor nutrition, chronic illness	Colonization with pathogenic gram-negative bacteria
Conducting airways		
Mechanical barriers (larynx) and airway angulation	Bypassing barriers with an endotracheal tube or tracheostomy	Aspiration, or direct entry of microorganisms into airway
Mucociliary clearance	Structural defects in cilia	Stagnant secretions, bronchiectasis
Cough	Depressed cough reflex	Poor removal of secretions
Bronchoconstriction	Hyperactive airways, intrinsic asthma	Aspergillus, use of corticosteroids (thrush)
Local immunoglobulin coating-secretory IgA	(a) IgA deficiency	Sinopulmonary infections
	(b) Functional deficiency from breakdown by bacterial IgA$_1$ proteases	Abnormal colonization with certain bacteria (as found with bronchitis)
Alveolar milieu		
Other immunoglobulin classes (opsonic IgG)	Acquired hypogammaglobulinemia, IgG$_4$, IgG$_2$ deficiency	Pneumonia with encapsulated bacteria
Iron-containing proteins (transferrin, lactoferrin)	Iron deficiency	May not inhibit certain bacteria (*Pseudomonas, E. coli, Legionella*)
Alternate complement pathway activation	C$_3$ and C$_5$ deficiency	Trouble with infection but not life-threatening
	Decreased synthesis, acute lung injury	Loss of opsonization activity
Surfactant		Alveolar collapse (atelectasis)
Alveolar macrophages	Subtle effects from immunosuppression, cannot kill intracellular microbes	Certain intracellular m/org *Pneumocystis carinii* and *Legionella* sp infections; poor inactivation of *Mycobacterium*
Polymorphonuclear granulocytes (PMNs)	Absent because of immunosuppression; intrinsic defect in motility or lack of chemotactic stimulus	Poor inflammatory response, propensity for gram-negative bacillary infection and fungus (*Aspergillus*)
AUGMENTING MECHANISMS		
Initiation of immune responses (humoral antibody and cellular)	Part of deficiency syndrome, and to polysaccharides or special antigens	Inadequate S-IgA or IgG antibody (?viral or *Mycoplasma* infection and with encapsulated bacteria)
Generation of an inflammatory response (influx of PMNs, eosinophils, lymphocytes and fluid components)	Generally reflects status and supply of PMNs	Same as for PMNs C$_5$ deficiency might decrease inflammatory response

defenses, but these are not commonly encountered. When repeated respiratory infections occur, however, or particularly severe ones develop, some component of the intricate defense system may be malfunctioning or compromised. The following deficiencies in pulmonary host defense, whether acquired or an inherent genetic problem, are associated with obvious syndromes of respiratory infection and can be correlated with a propensity for infection (Table 1-1). An endotracheal tube, for example, allows direct access to the lung, bypassing the larynx and other upper airway structures; structural defects in cilia on the apical edge of airway epithelial lining cells impair ciliary clearance so that removal of mucus and respiratory secretions is sluggish and ineffective; poor coughing in the postoperative patient with abdominal pain or in the person with depressed consciousness sometimes allows secretions to accumulate in the airways; the absence of opsonic antibody in patients with hypo- or dysgammaglobulinemia can foster infection with encapsulated bacteria; and cytotoxic antineoplastic chemotherapy and other forms of immunosuppression can produce granulocytopenia which prevents mobilization of an inflammatory reaction. The normal person without antecedent lung disease is equally at risk to develop infection under some of the circumstances just posed.

In this review of respiratory infections we attempt to correlate some infections with deficient activity of a specific facet of host defense. These defense mechanisms include elements of the cellular and humoral immune apparatus as well, so a brief description of normal function is included with each topic.

NASOOROPHARYNX

The mucosal surfaces of importance in the upper (extrathoracic) respiratory tract can be considered immunologically as comprising three distinct areas: the salivary glands, the oral cavity, and the nasal mucosa (Fig. 1-1). The fluids bathing these mucosal surfaces differ considerably in their composition of immunoglobulins.

Of these three areas, the nasal mucosa is most like the remainder of the respiratory tract. Although its primary function is as a conduit for inspired gases, it also acts as a mechanical and perhaps immunologic barrier protecting the lower respiratory tract. The histologic appearance is that of a ciliated epithelial layer overlying a submucosa rich in plasma cells (101), which has structural similarity to mucosa in the trachea and conducting airways. The study of nasal proteins is an important part of the analysis of host response to respiratory tract challenge with antigen (Table 1-2), and sampling nasal secretions is a relatively simple procedure.

Whereas the mucosal covering of the nose and airways are similar, the inside surface of the mouth is a squamous epithelium bathed in salivary and parotid gland secretions which are rich in IgA and, to a lesser extent, IgG. The crevicular gum secretions around the roots of the teeth have a somewhat different composition, which is like an ultrafiltrate of plasma. The concentration of IgG is high compared with that in parotid fluid (Fig. 1-1) (106).

Infections in the nose, sinuses, ears, and of the teeth and gums are common and often have ramifications for illness in the lower respiratory tract. Aspiration of anaerobic bacteria in oral secretions contributes to lung abscess formation, whereas

TABLE 1–2. *Proteins in nasal washings from normals*

	Total protein	Albumin	IgG	IgA	FSC[a]
Nonsmokers (n = 31)	220[b]	29	7.9	23	2.2
Cigarette smokers (n = 35)	199	11	3.1	24	2.7

Adapted from Merrill et al. (76).
[a]FSC, free secretory component.
[b]Mean values given in micrograms per milliliter; fluid volume 10 ml of nasal wash.

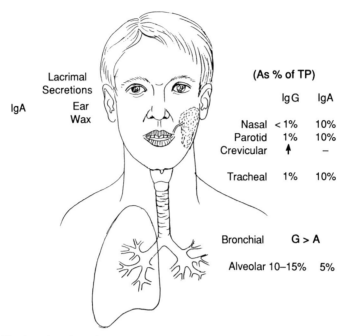

FIG. 1–1. The head and a scheme for the conducting airways and lungs are used to illustrate external secretions in various orifices. IgA is a prominent component in all of those from the upper respiratory tract and in ear wax and lacrimal secretions. Relative proportions of IgG and IgA are given, as a percentage of the total protein in the sample, for airway and bronchoalveolar fluids. Bronchial secretions are the least well characterized.

chronic sinusitis often accompanies such diseases as cystic fibrosis, ciliary dyskinetic syndromes, asthma, and dysgammaglobulinemia. Acute viral infections of the nose may be a prelude to lung infection, and various allergic diseases can simultaneously cause rhinitis and symptoms of hyperactive airways (asthma syndrome). Some of these upper respiratory infections are discussed elsewhere in this volume. One problem that does relate to lower tract infections, however, is the propensity for pathogenic gram-negative bacteria to colonize the nasooropharynx of ill people; and these, then, can be aspirated and initiate pneumonia. Some mechanisms underlying the attachment of bacteria to the mucosa reflect in part the nutritional status of the host and the integrity of the ciliated and squamous epithelia. Thus, abnormal bacterial colonization can be considered an acquired defect in mucosal host defense.

How and why bacteria stick to human mucosal tissues is a fascinating question; the relationship obviously is essential for normal homeostasis. The symbiotic interaction between bacteria and mucosa in the gastrointestinal tract is essential for proper digestion of food, and the presence of bacteria on the dental surfaces and gingiva might be rationalized as necessary, even though caries and pyorrhea can be unpleasant consequences; but why under normal conditions microorganisms need to inhabit other areas of the nasooropharynx (70) or, to a lesser extent, the skin and hair surfaces is unclear. Nonetheless, a healthy mucosa is able to regulate or control the bacterial flora on its surface and is not overrun with microorganisms. In the mouth, chewing motions, abrasive action by the tongue moving over the buccal and dental surfaces, and proteases in saliva (146) and other oral secretions (presumably with local secretory antibodies) combine to limit the ease with which bacteria can attach to the mucosa. Expectoration and swallowing secretions continuously remove microorganisms as well. But what goes awry in the oropharynx of chronically ill people is not known (see Fig. 1-2).

Potential for Colonization with Pathogenic Bacteria

In the nasooropharynx of normal people a variety of aerobic and anaerobic bacteria inhabit the mucosal surfaces (70). Common isolates in cultures include *Neisseria* sp, *Moraxella (Branhamella) catarrhalis* (15), a variety of *Streptococcus* sp, corynebacteria, *Staphylococcus* sp, and often, in people with chronic airways disease (81), *Streptococcus pneumoniae* and *Hemophilus* sp; fungi and protozoa can be

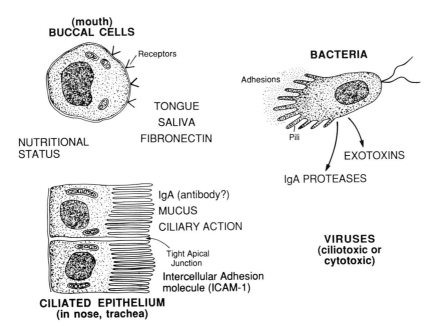

FIG. 1–2. Bacteria have various mechanisms for attaching to mucosal cells which include surface adhesions that fit into cell receptors (various sugar or glycosamine receptors) or special microbial adaptations such as pili (*Neisseria meningitidis* is an example) that promote contact. To reach these receptors, it may be necessary to clear away surface secretions such as IgA, and specific proteases or exotoxins can be produced by some bacteria to accomplish this. Other microbes such as *Mycoplasma* and *Bordetella pertussis* attach specifically to portions of the protruding cilia on the ciliated epithelial cells. In other circumstances, viruses are cytotoxic and infect ciliated cells directly. Counterbalancing the adaptive strategies of microbes, the host has many mechanisms to resist them, and this is part of the defense apparatus of the respiratory tract. Mechanical mechanisms (sneezing, coughing, motion of the tongue, and ciliary action) resist microbial attachment; also, surface secretions are interspersed to impede adherence (salivary proteases, immunoglobulins, fibronectin, and mucus). Undoubtedly, the nutritional status of the host, which may determine the rate of cellular renewal and regeneration, is an important factor, too. Integrity of the tight-apical junctions between the ciliated epithelial cells and the squamous surface in parts of the mouth is important as a mechanical barrier to prevent microbes from penetrating into the submucosa. The whole interaction between host and microbes is very dynamic and constantly changing (from Reynolds [103]).

recovered, too. Quantitatively, anaerobic bacteria around the teeth and gums are most numerous, possibly reaching 10^8 microorganisms/ml of oral secretions, and include a number of various species but usually not *Bacteroides fragilis*. However, the prevalence of aerobic gram-negative bacilli such as Enterobacteriaceae and *Pseudomonas* sp is low and may be isolated from only about 15% of the area swab cultures taken from normals (56,111). Species of Enterobacteriaceae and *Pseudomonas aeruginosa* may be detected in broth cultures, but in all cases the colony counts are low.

Elderly people have a higher prevalence of oropharyngeal colonization with gram-negative bacteria, which is generally correlated with independence of living and dependence on health care facilities (139). The recognition of how quickly hospitalized patients acquire potentially pathogenic gram-negative flora in the oropharynx led to an important study correlating colonization and subsequent nosocomial pneumonia (56). When pharyngeal and sputum cultures become positive for Enterobacteriaceae or *Pseudomonas* and other pathogenic bacteria, it is likely that the respiratory tract is colonized with them. Colonization occurred rapidly in patients in an intensive care unit; within 4 days of admission to the unit it was found in about 40% of them (56). Such colonization of the respiratory tract apparently played a major role in the pathogenesis of nosocomial respiratory infections. Of 95 patients who were colonized with gram-negative bacilli, 22 (23%) developed respiratory infections with these bacteria. In comparison, of 118 patients in whom prior colonization with these bacteria was not shown, only 4 (3.3%) developed infection.

The fact that colonization of the nasooropharynx with potential pathogenic gram-negative rods was a forerunner of subsequent nosocomial pneumonia led Johanson and colleagues (54) to explore mechanisms of bacterial attachment to squamous epithelial cells. This mechanism also contributes to forms of ventilator-associated pneumonia (75). An *in vitro* test, using *P. aeruginosa* and buccal cells that were abraded from the inner cheek of normals and patients, provided a correlation between the amount of bacterial adherence and the occurrence of colonization in postoperative and intensive care–treated patients (55,57). In animal models, the impact of malnutrition or renal failure on increasing the adherence of bacteria to buccal cells was demonstrated (45). Further, they noted that fibronectin, a glycosamine coating buccal epithelial cells, served as a deterrent to bacterial attachment and that cleavage of it by salivary proteases diminished its protective effect (146). In contrast, fibronectin can enhance the adherence of monocytes, perhaps facilitating inflammatory cell response (89).

Our approach was to look at the ciliated cells obtained directly from the nose and trachea and determine their binding characteristics for gram-negative bacteria (87). The actual respiratory lining cells seem to be a more appropriate cell type to study than the buccal ones. Mechanical injury to tracheal cells may promote adherence and growth of *Pseudomonas* also (147).

To explore the relationship between bacterial binding to oral epithelial and ciliated respiratory cells, Niederman et al. (87) measured adherence of *P. aeruginosa* to ciliated cells (from nose and trachea) and compared this to squamous cells (from buccal mucosa). Bacterial binding in this *in vitro* assay was comparable for nasal and tracheal cells (about 4 bacteria per cell), but this adherence was greater than found for buccal cells (mean of about one bacterium per cell). Other factors that influenced adherence were (i) the nutritional status of the host (in patients, an inverse relationship was found between tracheal cell bacterial binding and a prognostic nutritional index [85]) and (ii) the pH of the mucosal surface (92). These interactions between microbes trying to establish adherence or infection on the buccal or ciliated epithelial cell surfaces are summarized in Figure 1-2.

Little work has been done on the kinetics of epithelial cell regeneration or turnover in the respiratory tract in humans, but an interval of at least 7 to 10 days may be needed to replenish ciliated cells. Nonetheless, an *in vitro* cell–bacterial binding assay, perhaps using buccal and nasal mucosal cells, seems to be a surveillance parameter that could help identify high-risk patients. The nutritional status of the host apparently is closely coupled to abnormal bacterial binding, reaffirming what clinicians already know but have had difficulty proving, that the poorly nourished host does not resist infection or illness well.

CENTRAL AIRWAYS

In the nose and conducting airways, the mucociliary transport mechanism is responsible for clearing inhaled particulate material from the respiratory mucosa and for removing the cellular debris that originates in the terminal airways (i.e., senescent alveolar macrophages and epithelial cells). Obviously, there are two components to this mechanism: (i) the tracheobronchial secretions that are composed of globlet cell and bronchial gland mucus fluid admixed with Clara cell secretions, and other fluids and electrolytes that escape across the air–blood barrier from plasma; and (ii) cilia that arise from epithelial lining cells and physically propel secretions up the respiratory tract. Malfunction of this transport may result from intrinsically defective cilia, infections that are ciliolytic *(Mycoplasma pneumoniae)* or actually destroy the cilia-containing epithelial cells (viral agents), microbial products that slow ciliary beating (122), and excessive or abnormal mucus secretion. Tenacious *Pseudomonas* capsular slime-enriched mucus is usually found in cystic fibrosis patients, and excessive secretions are produced by patients with chronic bronchitis, often causally related to cigarette smoking. This increased mucus secretion may cause subtle impairment of ciliary function, although smoking per se may not alter mucus unfavorably in asymptomatic cigarette smokers (114). Thus, a variety of lung infections may arise from specific abnormalities in ciliary function and mucus secretion.

Ciliotoxic Infections: Viruses and *Mycoplasma pneumoniae*

In a subtle way, viral infections can be associated with prolonged airway dysfunction in that they cause peripheral small airway obstruction and hyperreactivity. Mild influenza A infection in the upper airways of young, ostensibly healthy college students was found to cause increased airway resistance and hyperreactivity which persisted for almost 2 months, well beyond the duration of clinical illness (67). Whereas the antiviral agent amantadine appeared to arrest virus proliferation and presumably the associated inflammatory response in peripheral airways, it did not prevent the development of bronchial hyperreactivity. Once infection is established, even early administration of a drug does not appreciably alter the disease's course. Viruses, especially myxoviruses that include influenza, infect and secondarily destroy ciliated epithelial cells along the conducting airways; these infections can lead to denuded areas without functional ciliated cells.

Because certain viruses can infect mucosal epithelial cells and thereby affect ciliary function, the greatest impact of viral infection is often on the lower respiratory tract. When the ciliary apparatus has been disrupted, the accumulated secretions sometimes must be forcefully removed by coughing; the troublesome cough that often accompanies viral respiratory infections may be an attempt of lung host defenses to compensate for the impaired ciliary clearance. However, a viral infection can doubly jeopardize the respiratory tract by causing cytotoxicity among airway lining cells and predisposing to pneumonia. Invading viral droplets or infected epithelial cells that are shed from the mucosa can also reach the alveoli (?aspiration) and infect macrophages. As a consequence, these viral-infected phagocytes may lose some of their bactericidal effectiveness (53). Thus, bacterial superinfection with *Staphylococcus aureus,* for example, is not an infrequent sequela of viral respiratory infection. These bacteria may more easily penetrate the denuded areas of bronchial mucosa or may not be readily killed by alveolar macrophages. *Mycoplasma* can cause a similar problem for the ciliated epithelial cells in the conducting airways. *Mycoplasma* seem to be specifically more ciliolytic than cytotoxic, which characterizes viral infections. Through a sialic acid–binding site on its differentiated terminal organelle, the Mycoplasma organism can attach to cilia and, possibly by liberating H_2O_2 or other toxic substances, shear off cilia from tracheal epithelium (35). The attachment of Mycoplasma is modulated somewhat by the host's availability of S-IgA antibody, so the immune status of the airways is important. Once infection has occurred, antimycoplasmal antibody in sputum in other immunoglobulin classes can be identified (IgM and IgG), attesting to the systemic as well as local immune response this organism can elicit. As with viral infections, persistent cough is a feature of Mycoplasma respiratory infection and, in fact, may be a necessary host compensation for poor ciliary clearance.

Intrinsic Defects in Cilia

Defects in the ultrastructure of respiratory cilia that alter or prevent motility represent a fascinating link between altered airway host defense and a propensity for recurrent or chronic infection at multiple sites along the respiratory tract. A ciliated epithelium covers the nasooropharynx, including the sinuses, the central conducting airways, and the peripheral airways down to the level of the respiratory bronchioles. Cilia are amazing structures, similar to the propulsive flagella found on bacteria and on lower forms of animal life. Sperm tails have a similar construction. Cilia in the respiratory tract can beat at a rate between 300 (144) and 800 beats/minute, but this progressively slows in more distal parts of the tracheobronchial tree (116). The slowest beating rate is found in the midsize conducting airways, and the altered beating at this level may enhance the pooling of secretions and local infection, possibly contributing to the development of bronchiectasis in this portion of the airways (89). Chronic inflammation at various sites along the respiratory tract can result in bronchiectasis, bronchitis, and sinusitis, terms that simply designate the anatomic areas involved with similar processes—stasis and stagnation of mucus secretion produced by globlet and bronchial mucous glands admixed with bacteria and inflammatory cells. Coughing may compensate somewhat for the sluggish removal of mucus and other debris originating from the alveoli, ordinarily cleared by normal ciliary action; but once the cycle of persistent infection and inflammatory exudate in the airways develops, destructive changes in bronchial walls may occur and pooling of secretions is probable.

A number of specific defects in the microtubular structure of cilia have been described (Fig. 1-3). The original abnormality, the absence of dynein arms which causes incoordination of ciliary motility, was implicated as the specific defect in Kartagener's syndrome (1,14,30,59,93,113). The absence of radial spokes connecting the peripherally located doublets of microtubules with the central doublet was the second defect recognized (134). This disease, although causing the usual features of sinusitis and bronchiectasis, was not invariably associated with malrotation of viscera, that is, *situs inversus*. Cilia also can show deletion of the central tubules with the interesting adaptation of transposing one of the peripherally located doublets to the center of the axoneme (133). Whereas the rate of tracheal transport is severely impaired, the cilia are not immotile and activity is retained. This observation along with the fact that dynein-defective cilia retain some motility has prompted some authors to propose that specific congenital abnormalities of cilia that result in defective mucociliary transport should be termed diseases of "ciliary dyskinesis." Thus, the following classification has been proposed (112): type 1: defective dynein, type 2: defective radial spokes, and type 3: microtubular transposition. Another defect, the random orientation of the central tubule in cilia causing uncoordinated beating, can be associated with respiratory tract disease and infection (115).

In addition to congenital defects, cilia can acquire abnormalities in structure, usually as a result of chronic respiratory infection, which can impair beating and hence the propulsive action that clears the airways (2). In this circumstance, variable defects in ultrastructure are often noted.

The detection of abnormal function or structure of cilia is not difficult and can be included in a clinical evaluation. A nuclear medicine department should be prepared to perform a tracheal clearance study. Scraping the nasal mucosa will retrieve a sufficient sample of cilia, which can be fixed in a 3% glutaraldehyde solution for appropriate electron microscopy studies. Interpretation of such a biopsy could be a problem, so it is essential to have an experienced pathologist. Infertility evaluation of men often leads to the recognition of chronic respiratory infections and ultimately

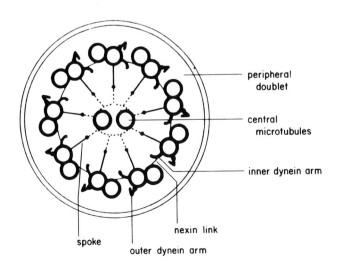

peripheral
doublet

central
microtubules

inner dynein arm

nexin link

spoke

outer dynein arm

FIG. 1-3. Diagram of the cross-section of a cilium. The assembly of the nine outer microtubular doublets and two central microtubules is held together by three kinds of connections: the dynein arms, the nexin links, and the spokes. The dynein arms are generally thought to be responsible for the motility (from Eliasson et al. [30]). Reprinted by permission of the *New England Journal of Medicine* 297(1):1–6, 1977.

to the diagnosis. Diminished ciliary motion is not always the only defect in these diseases, and preliminary evidence indicates that the motility of polymorphonuclear neutrophils is affected in patients with Kartagener's syndrome (72).

Cystic Fibrosis

Cystic fibrosis (CF) in many respects combines several features of poor mucociliary function. CF lung disease does not represent a single or precisely defined defect in respiratory host defenses, but rather is a combination of several impaired ones. A basic problem is with the transport of chloride ions by glandular and ciliated epithelial cells throughout the body of the affected host, contributing to abnormal composition of external secretions (38,65). Inadequate mucociliary clearance, which allows bacteria to excessively colonize and infect the airways and which eventually produces bronchiectasis, has multiple causes. Although there does not seem to be an intrinsic substance in blood or secretions from CF subjects that inhibits ciliary beating (117), it is possible that exotoxins or pigments elaborated by Pseudomonas bacteria could partially paralyze cilia action (122,143). The thick, purulent, and viscous airway secretions themselves probably contribute to sluggish activity of cilia favoring stagnation. No consistent defects have been identified in the ultrastructure of microtubules in CF cilia, as found in the dyskinetic ciliary syndromes.

CF is a common genetic disease, and it is often thought to be a disease of infancy and childhood. However, increasingly, it is recognized at a later age in teenagers and young adults, and occasionally it is first detected in people in their thirties and forties (21,58,68,88,107,124,132). In adults, the disease seems to affect the respiratory tract primarily, and the gastrointestinal signs of malabsorption and poor growth, which often characterize CF in infants and children, are less obvious (29,145).

In adults with CF, decreased exocrine secretions by the pancreas can be compensated for with oral replacement of these enzymes, so liver and gastrointestinal problems may be reasonably controlled; however, recurrent respiratory tract infections, including sinusitis and otitis media, as well as episodes of bronchitis and pneumonia, are the bane of most CF patients. Generalized bronchiectasis, copious and often tenacious mucus secretions, persistent colonization with mucoid strains of *P. aeruginosa* (107,149), exacerbations of bronchitis with Pseudomonas or other microbial pathogens (viruses, bacteria such as staphylococci and *P. cepacia* or mucoid *Escherichia coli* [71], and occasionally a fungus such as *Aspergillus* sp), poorly functioning IgG opsonins in the lung (36), progressive obstructive airways disease, hemoptysis, and usually respiratory failure—all are part of a sequence that plagues the CF patient.

In summary, cystic fibrosis has been recognized in teenagers and adults as a disease that can be limited primarily to the respiratory tract and that is distinguished by a predilection to *P. aeruginosa* infections (99). The mucoid form of the organism is characteristic and, if isolated in culture from sputum, can be a clue to the diagnosis. Once recurrent Pseudomonas lung infections occur in these patients, their management and life expectancy are not unlike those in the younger CF patients. An inexorable cycle of progressively more difficult respiratory infections develops, and all the expertise and ingenuity at the physician's disposal are needed. Judicious use of antibiotics, advice about nutrition, and wise counseling about family, marriage, career, and what to expect with a fatal illness are a few of the things the physician must provide in managing the teenage or young adult CF patient. The prospects of lung transplantation may be factored in (136). And in the near future the possibility of genetic therapy to correct the cellular defect in the chloride channel could become a reality. This illness is still quite a challenge.

Secretory IgA and Infection in Chronic Bronchitis

In the nasal passages, oropharynx, and conducting airways, local secretions that coat the mucosal surface constitute a complex mixture of mucus, bronchial gland secretions, and immunoglobulins, of which IgA is the principal one in the upper airways. Secretory IgA accounts for about 10% of total protein measured in nasal wash fluid and in parotid fluid and for about 5% of the protein content in bronchoalveolar lavage fluid recovered from humans (64).

Approximately 90% of the IgA in external secretions, including those of the respiratory tract, is in dimerous form. In contrast, serum IgA is principally monomeric, and little exists in polymeric form (18). Whereas S-IgA has been thoroughly analyzed in breast secretions (colostrum), parotid fluid, and gastrointestinal fluid, ultrastructural studies of airway S-IgA are few. However, all evidence points to complete similarity of the respective molecules. This 11S-sedimenting IgA seems to be typical S-IgA in that it contains bound SC glycoprotein as well as joining chain (J-chain). Compared with a value of about 2 mg/ml in serum, concentrated BAL fluid (about 25-fold concentration) contained about 150 micrograms/ml; differences between smokers and nonsmokers were not significant (78). Precipitin analysis of purified S-IgA fractionated from bronchoalveolar lavage fluid identified both alpha heavy chain classes. Delacroix and colleagues (26) measured the relative proportions of IgA_1 and IgA_2 in serum and a variety of external secretions. In general, excretory fluids contain mostly A_1, but relatively more A_2 in comparison with serum. In bronchial secretions about 33% of the IgA was the A_2 variety.

However, it is still difficult to document the precise functions of this immunoglobulin, despite the widely held assumption that it is important in protecting external mucosal surfaces throughout the body, especially against infection (11). In reviewing this topic (108), we concluded that the following statements could be made about the function of secretory IgA in the respiratory tract. First, S-IgA is present in high concentration in the upper and large airways but diminishes in relative concentration in distal portions of the lung. It is possible that this reflects its importance in the nasooropharynx and large airways, where it forms part of the mucosal barrier preventing adherence and absorption of foreign substances. Because of its less efficient opsonizing potential and lack of interaction with the complement system (18), it may be less important in the peripheral airways and alveoli. Second, S-IgA has demonstrated antibody activity against certain viruses and bacteria and against common allergens; such activity can be induced either by local respiratory immunization or as a consequence of natural infection or exposure. Once immunity is established and S-IgA antibody has been produced, protection against homologous microbial challenge, especially with viral agents, can be shown. In other words, the most convincing protective role for S-IgA in the host respiratory defense machinery pertains to its antibody activity in the nose and oral cavity. Third, the period of immune protection generally is short, and a booster or anamnestic immune response from later challenge is variable or absent. Frequent reimmunization to maintain good S-IgA antibody levels is probably necessary; unfortunately, it is impractical for mass-population immunoprophylaxis. Fourth, whereas the S-IgA molecule appears to have intrinsic resistance to proteolytic degradation, possibly conferred by its unique glycoprotein moiety-secretory component which gives a favorable tertiary molecular configuration, it seems that a lengthening list of common pathogenic bacteria can elaborate IgA proteases that destroy it (10). It is tempting to speculate about an explanation for the choice of bacteria that colonize the airways of subjects with chronic bronchitis (81). Special properties of these bacteria and some damage to the host's mucosal protective layer (S-IgA?) would be part of the explanation.

Streptococcus pneumoniae and *Hemophilus influenzae* are among the most common bacterial pathogens responsible for respiratory tract infections in otherwise healthy humans and in those with chronic lung disease (81). Mulks and colleagues (80) examined 36 strains of *S. pneumoniae,* 62 strains of *H. influenzae,* 6 hospital-acquired respiratory pathogens, and a strain of *S. pyogenes* for production of IgA protease, a bacterial enzyme whose only known substrate is human IgA. IgA protease was produced by 100% of the isolates of *S. pneumoniae* and 98% of the isolates of *H. influenzae.* The enzyme from both species cleaved human serum and secretory IgA_1 proteins, but not human IgA_2, IgG, or human serum albumin. None of the hospital-acquired pathogens (such as *Staphylococcus aureus, Klebsiella pneumoniae,* and *P. aeruginosa*) had detectable IgA protease activity, a finding indicating that the production of this enzyme can distinguish *S. pneumoniae* and *H. influenzae* from the opportunistic respiratory pathogens.

In another, more technical article, Kilian and colleagues (60) sought the actual cleavage points produced by bacterial-derived IgA_1 proteases in the IgA_1 molecule. Two other bacteria were examined, *Neisseria meningitidis* and *Streptococcus sanguis,* as well as *H. influenzae* and *S. pneumoniae.* In addition to protease activity, *S. pneumoniae* releases an exo- and endoglycosidase that removes a considerable portion of the carbohydrate side chains of IgA, which can impair the immunoglobulin even more (61).

IgA proteases from the above bacteria disrupt the IgA_1 alpha chain in its hinge region, but at different sites: proteases from *S. sanguis* and *S. pneumoniae* cleave the Pro(227)-Thr(228) bond within the hinge region, whereas *H. influenzae*–derived enzyme cleaves a Pro-Ser bond at somewhat different amino acid positions in the same region. The proteases split only the $alpha_1$ chain of the secretory IgA molecule, but had no effect on light chains, or on secretory component and J-chain, which comprise the intact molecule. The metal chelator EDTA–inhibited proteases derived from the two *Streptococcus* sp but not *H. influenzae.* Thus, data demonstrate the existence of at least two types of extracellular bacterial protease specific for IgA_1. The S-IgA form does seem less susceptible to cleavage than does purified myeloma IgA_1 protein. Proteases produced by gram-negative bacteria are not considered to degrade IgA_1. In preliminary experiments we found that a *P. aeruginosa* elastase will fragment IgA in sputum specimens (86); however, the enzyme's specificity for the respective alpha chains was not determined.

In summary, the potential for dynamic interplay between a bacterial enzyme that can partially split and disrupt an important "protective" mucosal protein and one that cannot is interesting because it could give selective advantage to certain bacteria that commonly colonize the airways (Fig. 1-2). The fact that specific protease enzymes have been detected only in *S. pneumoniae* and *S. sanguis; H. influenzae;* two pathogenic strains of Neisseria, *N. meningitidis* and *N. gonorrhea;* and *P. aeruginosa* raises the possibility that these bacteria are frequent inhabitants of the oropharynx (and genital tract) because they can successfully destroy or inactivate mucosal IgA activity. Nonetheless, S-IgA appears to have some intrinsic resistance or possibly antiprotease neutralizing antibody activity, thus providing host balance in the face-off. Moreover, respiratory tract secretions could have other inhibitors that could neutralize the IgA_1 protease activity. The respiratory secretions do contain S-IgA_2, and presumably, although it has not been quantitated, a large proportion of IgA_2 is resistant to protease attack.

INTERACTION OF HUMORAL AND CELLULAR HOST DEFENSE IN THE ALVEOLAR MILIEU

In the upper respiratory tract and large airways, a combination of mechanisms excludes particulate material: (i) anatomic barriers such as the epiglottis; (ii) frequent branching of the pulmonary tree (to affect aerodynamic filtration of inspired air); (iii) mucociliary clearance of particulates that impact on the mucosa, perhaps the phagocytic activity of airway-located macrophages (97); and (iv) cough response. When infectious agents, bacteria in particular, elude the physical or mechanical defenses described above and are deposited in the terminal airways and alveoli (critical size between 0.5 and 3 microns), another group of host factors takes over (Fig. 1-4). These include phospholipid surfactant and proteins (immunoglobulins and complement factors) in the alveolar lining material and phagocytic cells, that is, alveolar macrophages and polymorphonuclear neutrophils (PMNs). Anatomically, lung structure changes at the level of respiratory bronchioles. In the terminal units (alveolar ducts and alveoli), ciliated epithelium and mucus-secreting cells (globlet cells and mucus glands) are no longer present. Therefore, mucociliary clearance does not exist, nor does coughing effectively clear material from the alveoli. Thus, microbial clearance and the removal of other antigenic material from alveoli depends entirely on cellular and humoral factors. Functionally, the portion of the airways from the respiratory bronchioles to the alveoli could be considered the lower respiratory tract.

A more exact accounting of cells recovered from the normal alveolar spaces is given in Table 1-3. As shown in Table 1-3, the usual cell recovery from a healthy, nonsmoking volunteer is about 15 million cells, depending on the volume of lavage fluid used and recovered. The viability of the cells is excellent, and, on a differential cell count (prepared from cytocentrifuged cell specimen and stained with Wright-Giemsa), most of the cells are macrophages. PMNs are rare, as are erythrocytes; the amount of coughing induced by the bronchoscopy influences the number of ciliated epithelial cells found. These cells are often viable in a wet prep mount of the BAL cells, and ciliary motion is visible.

Considerable interest has focused on the identification of lymphocytes, which account for 10% or so of the total cells (25,50,52,63). Aided by the use of T-cell-specific monoclonal antibody staining, most of the lymphocytes have been identified as T-cells. With further T-cell subset identification, about half of these have been identified as helper/inducer cells. A lesser percentage are of the suppressor/cytotoxic variety. The ratio of T H/S cells is about 1.5 in the normal airways, about the same ratio obtained for peripheral blood lymphocytes. Among the T-helper cells, a

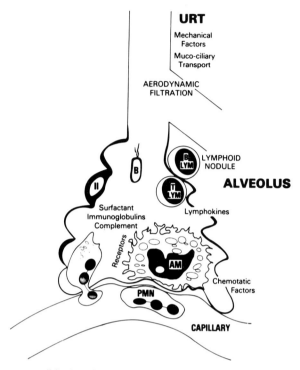

FIG. 1–4. Factors responsible for clearance of bacteria (*B*) inhaled into the lungs are quite different in the upper airway (*URT*) and in the lower respiratory tract, here represented by enlargement of an alveolus. A bacterium of critical size, which escapes mechanical removal from the URT and is deposited in an alveolus, may encounter surfactant and/or immunoglobulins (antibodies) and complement proteins in the epithelial lining fluid which condition it for phagocytosis by a resident alveolar macrophage (*AM*). Antibody with specific opsonizing potential could facilitate attachment of the bacterium to the AM surface membrane through specialized cell receptors. A complement component (C_3) could augment such attachment. At least two alternative mechanisms could be activated to enhance killing and clearance of the microbe. First, the AM can liberate chemotactic factors which attract nearby polymorphonuclear phagocytes (PMNs), marginated in a lung capillary adjacent to the alveolus, and thus initiate an inflammatory response. Second, the bacterium may trigger immune lymphocytes (*T-lym*) to release effector substances (lymphokines), which could activate or stimulate AM phagocytic bactericidal capacity (from Reynolds [101]).

small percentage (about 7% in normals) have an HLA-DR antigen; this subpopulation can increase when a lymphocytic alveolitis develops, as in active sarcoidosis, and is responsible for most of the interleukin-2 produced (119). Approximately 7% of the airway T-cells are killer cells, but these seem dormant in normals (109). In addition, about 5% of the lymphocytes are B-cells, or plasma cells. These cells can release various class-specific immunoglobulins from their surfaces. Finally, a small percentage of lymphocytes are not typeable with the usual immunologic reagents used and could, in fact, be "null" cells. The proportions and activity of lymphocytes will be of significance for several of the lung infections illustrated.

If a bacterium of critical size is deposited in an alveolus (in the absence of edema fluid of either circulatory or inflammatory origin), the microbe could encounter at least three substances that conceivably could inactivate it, exclusive of its eventual inactivation by phagocytosis. First, surfactant, secreted by type II pneumocytes,

TABLE 1–3. *Profile of respiratory cells recovered in BAL fluid*
(for nonsmoker normal subjects after 100 to 300 ml of lavage)

Cell no. total	Differential count (%)				Cytocentrifuge cell stain		
	Viability	Macrophages	PMN	EOS/ BASO[a]	Lymphocytes	Ciliated cells	Erthyrocytes
15×10^6	<90%	85	1 to 2	<1	7 to 12	1 to 5	<5%

Lymphocyte subsets (%)

T-lymphocytes (% of total)	Helper/inducer T-cell[b]	Suppressor/ cytotoxic T-cell	Killer T-lymphocytes	B-lymphocytes (plasma cells)	Untypeable lymphocytes
70	50[c]	30	7	5 to 10	5

Adapted from Reynolds (102).
[a]EOS, eosinophil; BASO, basophil.
[b]As percent of T-cells. The T-helper/suppressor ratio is about 1.5 to 1.8.
[c]Contains about 7% DR antigen-positive cells. Among plasma cells are immunoglobulin-releasing cells with a frequency of: IgG = IgA > IgM > IgE.

could have antibacterial activity against staphylococci and rough colony strains of some gram-negative rod bacteria (22). Second, immunoglobulins, principally of the IgG class, and, in lesser concentration, monomeric and secretory forms of IgA could have specific opsonic antibody activity for the bacterium. Third, complement components, especially properdin Factor B, could interact with the bacterium and trigger the alternative complement pathway. One or all of these possibilities can prepare the bacterium for ingestion by an alveolar macrophage (128), or the activated complement sequence can lyse it directly. Although alveolar macrophages avidly phagocytose some inert particles, they ingest viable bacteria with considerably less enthusiasm. Coating or opsonizing the organisms enhances phagocytosis approximately tenfold. However, immunoglobulin G appears to be the only substance capable of selectively enhancing alveolar macrophage phagocytosis, although there is evidence that complement can function in concert with IgG to enhance or amplify the process. Once phagocytosis has occurred, the alveolar macrophage can inactivate susceptible organisms. Intracellular killing proceeds, but often at a slower rate than that measured in PMNs and along less well studied metabolic pathways. Whereas PMNs may kill ingested bacteria with one or a combination of antimicrobial systems (H_2O_2, superoxide anion [O_2] myeloperoxidase, or halide anion), the process is less certain in alveolar macrophages (128).

Following containment of bacteria, the fate of alveolar macrophages is not certain. They are long-lived tissue cells which can survive at least for several months and presumably are capable of handling repeated bacterial and other microbial challenges. Because they are mobile cells, they can migrate quickly to other alveoli through the "pores of Kohn" or move to more proximal areas of the respiratory tract and get aboard the mucociliary escalator for elimination from the lungs. In addition, macrophages gain entry into lung lymphatics and can be carried to regional lymph nodes. This exit gives access to systemic lymphoid tissue and is important in initiating cellular immune responses. Undoubtedly, macrophages are instrumental in degrading antigenic material and presenting it to appropriate lymphocytes in these nodes. Increasingly, attention is being given to the effector immune role of macro-

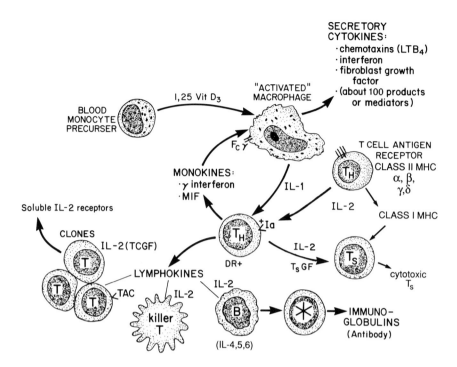

phages, thereby expanding their traditional and limited one of phagocytic function (33,84,128). This interaction between alveolar macrophages and lymphocytes is depicted in Figure 1-5; activation of the macrophages and lymphocytes is essential for them to perform their respective functions.

Alveolar macrophages can usually inactivate microorganisms, and host defense surveillance is successful. Under this happy circumstance, clinical disease and pneumonitis never develop. However, if a sufficiently large bacterial inoculum reaches the lower respiratory tract, or if particularly virulent microorganisms are inhaled, the macrophage system can be overwhelmed. In such a situation, the lung parenchyma mounts an extensive inflammatory response that could be perceived as clinical illness. A chest roentgenogram usually reveals an infiltrate. The development of the inflammatory response and hence pneumonia is a deliberate and controlled reaction in the lungs. The stages of initiation, amplification, and, finally, suppression that occur make this sequence likely and can be reviewed (100,104,128).

The alveolar macrophage is the only resident phagocyte normally present in the alveoli. It is the bona fide first line of cellular defense on the airside of the lower respiratory tract. Reserve phagocytic cells, the PMNs, are close by but located in the intravascular compartment. Even though PMNs are in close proximity to alveolar spaces, they are nonetheless separated by several planes of tissue: capillary endothelium, interstitial space, and alveolar epithelium (Fig. 1-6). Therefore, granulocyte movement into the alveoli must be an orderly reaction initiated from the alveolar side. This is termed *directed migration* or *chemotaxis*. At least two mechanisms for chemotactic activity exist that can set in motion the inflammatory response in the alveoli: direct generation of chemotactic factors by microorganisms entering the alveoli, and release of chemotactic factors from alveolar macrophages following phagocytosis, which might amplify the response (34,51,66,74,77,127,128). These mechanisms permit alveolar macrophages to recruit secondary phagocytes, PMNs, to help contain unruly bacteria in the alveoli. Once PMNs and other components of edema fluid have filled alveolar spaces, an exudative inflammatory reaction exists in lung parenchyma, and, pathologically, pneumonitis is present. Ultimately, lung tissues become consolidated.

After pneumonia has developed, and pending successful containment of the infection, resolution and healing phases eventually occur. At present, however, less is known about the processes that turn off or limit the acute inflammatory reaction of pneumonia and initiate recovery. The identification of such inhibitors and the potential for manipulating them is a part of lung immunophysiology that is still under investigation (23,126).

FIG. 1–5. The complex interaction between lung macrophages and lymphocytes, subtype T-helper/inducer (T_H) and T-suppressor/cytotoxic (T_S), is illustrated. Alveolar macrophages develop from circulating blood monocytes, which undergo further maturation or differentiation in the interstitial spaces before emerging on the alveolar surface. Vitamin D metabolites may be important in this process. The first responsibility of the alveolar macrophage is to be a roving scavenger and phagocyte to clean debris from the alveolar surface. However, it is apparent that the macrophage, especially when activated, can secrete a large array of cellular substances and mediators that affect the function of other cells (cytokines). As an example, macrophage chemotactic factors including interleukin-8 and leukotriene B_4 can attract other inflammatory cells to the alveoli or fibroblast growth factor and fibronectin can influence fibroblast replication. Activated macrophages can secrete interleukin-1 (IL-1), which may attract lymphocytes (127).

The macrophage also serves as an antigen-presenting cell which can process an antigen, display it on its cell membrane where it is taken up by an appropriate T_H lymphocyte, matched with respect to Class II major histocompatibility antigens (18). Antigen is received on the lymphocyte's membrane by a T-cell antigen receptor which has an intricate structure composed of two beta and alpha chains.

Among the populations of T-lymphocytes on the alveolar surface, most are T-helper/inducer cells and a lesser percentage are T-suppressor/cytotoxic lymphocytes; the normal ratio of T H/S cells is about 1.5. T-helper cells when activated are capable of producing two groups of mediators, lymphokines and monokines, which are important in modulating the function of other immune cells. Among the lymphokines, interleukin-2 (IL-2) quantitatively seems most important. This substance has many identified functions. IL-2, formerly known as T-cell growth factor (TCGF), can stimulate other T-cells to proliferate and thereby expand clones of lymphocytes. The responding T-cells must have a TAC surface receptor to respond properly to IL-2. IL-2 can activate killer T-cells. A few killer lymphocytes can be identified among the T-cell population in the alveoli, but these cells seem to be dormant in normals until stimulated to be active. IL-2 (plus IL-4) is needed to stimulate B-lymphocytes to turn into plasma cells which in turn can synthesize various classes of immunoglobulins. This is a mechanism by which local production of immunoglobulins (and antibodies) in the lung can occur.

In a feedback limb toward the macrophage, activated T-helper cells can produce several monokines that affect its function. Such a substance as migration inhibition factor (MIF) may immobilize macrophages and aid phagocytosis. Gamma interferon is a most interesting substance. It seems to induce more Fc receptors on the macrophage cell's membrane, which, in turn, allows for greater phagocytic uptake. Gamma interferon could have other functions as well that aid cellular immunity. It is reported that some macrophages have TAC surface receptors, so that IL-2 could have a role in the proliferation of these cells as well.

The role of the T-suppressor lymphocytes is less well studied, and, as yet, the array of specific mediators attributed to T-helper cells has not been identified for them. Natural inhibitors exist that could neutralize the effect of lymphokines. (Adapted from Reynolds [102].)

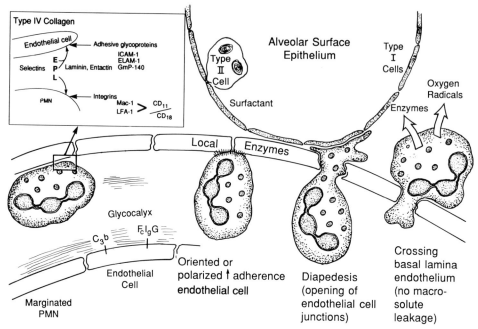

FIG. 1–6. Interaction between polymorphonuclear neutrophils and the endothelial cells of the lung capillaries is a first step initiating the influx of inflammatory cells into the alveoli. Specific attachment (*see inset*), opening of intercellular junctions between endothelial cells, and egress occur in sequence. Presumably a stimulus for chemotaxis comes from the alveolar side. Once the PMN is in the interstitium or alveolus, toxic oxygen radicals and various enzymes can injure alveolar cells or stimulate fibroblasts. Injury to the endothelium, wholesale passage of serum components, and collection of inflammatory cells develop in pneumonia and various other inflammatory diseases (ARDS, alveolitis with interstitial lung diseases, etc.) Reproduced with permission from the *New England Journal of Medicine,* Volume 38, © 1987, by Annual Reviews Inc.

Thus, within the alveolar milieu, alterations in any one of three components of host defense will predictably be associated with pulmonary infection: IgG or opsonic antibody, alveolar macrophages, and polymorphonuclear granulocytes.

IgG Dysfunction

Whereas inactivation of IgA by forms of bacterial proteases is an attractive hypothesis pertaining to bacterial colonization and perhaps to infection in patients with chronic bronchitis, abnormalities in IgG are clearly associated with infection. Common variable immunodeficiency is one of the most frequent forms of immunodeficiency (11) and can represent several different diseases (141). The hallmark is a decreased concentration of some or all of the serum immunoglobulins, especially IgG. Antibody responses and, in some patients, cell-mediated immune responses can be diminished, too. A variety of autoimmune phenomena can be detected in these patients, including overt autoimmune diseases. The disease is not strictly familial or restricted to youth, like x-linked infantile agammaglobulinemia. It may be sporadic in occurrence and is apparently nonfamilial, which raises the probability that it can be acquired.

Respiratory tract infections (pneumonia, sinusitis), as well as otitis media and gastrointestinal infestation with *Giardia lamblia,* are usual manifestations of disease. Bacterial infections with encapsulated organisms that require opsonizing antibody (IgG) for efficient host phagocytosis are common. The disease is peculiar in that its onset can be (i) late in life, occurring in the fourth to seventh decades, (ii) apparently abrupt, and (iii) intermittent or waxing, with spontaneous remissions. Thus, the suspicion that the disease is acquired, especially in the adult, is reinforced.

Immunoglobulin deficiency and propensity for respiratory infections has been shown to be more complex and subtle, with the revelation that selective subclass deficiencies can be responsible (105). With respect to respiratory infections, hypogammaglobulinemia is a well-established cause, and selective IgA deficiency can be associated with a propensity for infection also (11). IgA subclass deficiency has now been coupled to IgG deficiency (91). Recently, abnormalities in IgG subclasses have awakened keen interest in the selective importance of these individual types for lung disease—deficiencies associated with respiratory infections and chronic lung disease and prolonged corticosteroid treatment (62). Elevations of IgG_4 are associated with hypersensitivity lung disease. Representative values for IgG subclasses are given in serum and BAL fluid from normals, nonsmokers, and smokers (Table 1-4).

Serum samples from 37 patients with selective IgA deficiency and associated diseases such as recurrent infections, autoimmune disorders, malabsorption syndromes, and allergic diseases, and from 11 healthy adults with an incidental finding of selective IgA deficiency were analyzed for IgG subclasses G_1, G_2, G_3, and G_4 (91). The striking disease correlation was that in sera showing a combined IgA and IgG_2 (and IgG_4 as well) deficiency, six of seven patients had recurrent upper respiratory infections. However, no details were given about the age of the IgA-IgG_2 deficient patients, about the causative microorganisms, or about the anatomic location of the infections. It is important that no samples of airway secretions were analyzed in this report for secretory IgA or IgG subclasses.

In a similar vein, Oxelius and colleagues (90) studied sera from 22 patients with ataxia-telangiectasia, 10 of whom had concomitant IgA deficiency, which is a common occurrence in this disease. An imbalanced IgG subclass pattern was noted in all, with IgG_2 low in all and IgG_4 undetectable in 19 of 22 patients. The correlation with associated chronic respiratory infections was best with the IgG deficiencies and not with the presence or absence of IgA. IgG_1 was elevated in all subjects. Again, few clinical details were given and no respiratory secretions were analyzed. Finally, the most pertinent example relates to selective IgG_4 deficiency (6). Four subjects suffering from severe, recurrent, sinopulmonary infections and with bronchiectasis

TABLE 1–4. *IgG subclasses in serum and BAL fluid of normal smokers and nonsmokers*

	Nonsmokers (n = 19)		Smokers (n = 12)	
	Serum[a]	BAL	Serum[a]	BAL
IgG_1	67 ± 2.4	65 ± 2.4	80 ± 2.4	79 ± 2.0
IgG_2	31 ± 0.1	28 ± 0.9	18 ± 0.6	13 ± 0.5
IgG_3	0.4 ± 0.01	1.8 ± 0.2	0.5 ± 0.2	3.7 ± 0.3
IgG_4	1.3 ± 0.02	5.2 ± 0.6	1.0 ± 0.03	4.6 ± 0.1

Adapted from Merrill et al. (78).
[a]As percent of total IgG, presented as mean ± SEM.

were found to have virtually absent levels of IgG_4 in serum and no striking abnormalities in other IgG subclasses or other immunoglobulins. This is the purest example of an IgG subclass deficiency alone being associated with recurrent bacterial respiratory infections. The IgG_2 subclass contains antibodies made in response to polysaccharide antigens, as found in *Streptococcus* and *Hemophilus* species, and to teichoic acid, as present in staphylococci (125,138). Antibodies to lipopolysaccharides, as found in the cell wall of gram-negative bacilli such as *P. aeruginosa,* can be of this subclass also (37). As IgG_2 contains a particularly important group of antibodies to some common bacteria that are frequent respiratory pathogens, this subclass will be emphasized.

Antibodies to Polysaccharide Antigens from Strains of Streptococcus pneumoniae

Pneumonia caused by *S. pneumoniae* (or pneumococci) remains one of the most frequent respiratory infections in adults, especially as a form of community-acquired pneumonia in healthy people without lung disease. All of the 84 serotypes of pneumococci can cause illness, but a group of 23 serotypes is the etiology of about 95% of the bacteremias and/or pneumonias caused by these bacteria. It has therefore been feasible to develop a polyvalent-23 antigen polysaccharide vaccine for prophylactic immunization of potentially susceptible people. Pneumococci can be isolated as normal flora from the nasopharyngeal areas of some people (estimated to be about 10%) (70), and certainly most people at some point in life have had an infection caused by one of the strains. Yet it is unlikely that many people have a very broad battery of antibodies against many of the strains, so natural immunity can be supplemented logically by vaccine use. This is indicated for people who may not effectively raise antibodies (asplenic or functionally asplenic people) or who are at increased risk for infection, such as with HIV infection (110).

The availability of specific antibody is an important ingredient in resisting these bacteria, and antibodies developed against their polysaccharide antigens are found largely in IgG_2. As pneumococci are encapsulated bacteria, coating the microbes with IgG opsonic antibody and perhaps the union with C_3 will facilitate phagocytosis by inflammatory cells and macrophages which handle the infecting inoculum in the lungs and elsewhere.

The effectiveness of immunizing susceptible patients, especially older people with chronic lung disease and other illnesses such as renal or liver insufficiency, has now been questioned (8,123,129). Although various points are debated about the design of the Veterans Administration Cooperative Study (24) and its impact, still, important facts emerge about the immune response in older people. Most vaccine recipients who developed infection had not responded with antibody to a broad range of pneumococcal capsular polysaccharides (response was to only 5 of 12 immunizing antigens), nor was the elevated titer of antibody, achieved initially, sustained after a month or so (129). It appeared that a serum antibody concentration of at least 400 ng of antibody per millimeter was needed for a protective effect. The factor of age as it relates to immune reactivity continues to be relevant in advising use of this vaccine. The very young (less than 2 years of age) cannot process polysaccharide antigens effectively to mount a good antibody response, and the elderly could have lost immune vigor, or a sufficient number of T-helper/inducer lymphocytes, so that their humoral response no longer generates a sufficient amount of antibody. Thus, for the very susceptible or elderly patient for whom pneumococcal infection is perceived to be a significant risk, passive immunization will have to be reconsidered and evaluated (43). Continued flexibility and new approaches to immunization need to be considered (32). As an example, HIV-infected persons with CD_4 blood cell counts of less than 500 did not respond with antibody as well to *S. pneumoniae* capsular polysaccharides as did those with >500 CD_4 cells/mm^3; therefore, for this immunization to be more effective, pneumococcal vaccine should be given when HIV infection is first diagnosed (110).

Absence of IgG Antibody Response to Polysaccharide Antigens

A frank deficiency of IgG_2 and IgG_4 subclasses can be associated with recurrent sinopulmonary infections, but an inability to develop specific antibody in a subclass despite a normal amount and profile of IgG subclasses in serum was a novel presentation for an immunodeficiency and was described as a report (3). In brief, a 30-year-old man, who had had repeated episodes of otitis media and bronchitis in childhood and multiple episodes of pneumonia in various areas of his lungs, was evaluated for his propensity to develop pneumococcal and *H. influenzae* lung infections. Pneumococcal pneumonias continued to occur despite two immunization attempts with pneumococcal vaccine. A diagnosis of cystic fibrosis or dyskinetic cilia disease was excluded, and serum immunoglobulin levels were normal (IgG of 917 mg/dl) except for an increased IgM value. IgG subclass values were also normal.

Upon immunization with polysaccharide antigens (*H. influenzae* type B, meningococcal and pneumococcal antigens), no specific serum IgG antibodies were detected; a small amount of IgM antibodies did develop. However, antibody to tetanus toxoid was present and in the IgG_2 subclass. This interesting patient had a selectively impaired antibody response to polysaccharides yet could respond to a protein antigen in the IgG_2 subclass appropriately. Lack of a polysaccharide-specific antibody response seemed to be the cause of this recurrent sinopulmonary infection with encapsulated bacteria. In this report, actual respiratory secretions were not analyzed for immunoglobulins or antibody activity.

Alveolar Macrophage

Traditionally, alveolar macrophages have been considered only efficient phagocytes that scavenge the alveolar surface, creating an important front line of lung host defense against inhaled particles and microbes, but recently this role has been expanded to include important effector cell functions (83,84,128). It is now apparent that macrophages can modulate the activity of other inflammatory and immune responses through presentation of antigen to T-lymphocytes and secretion of lymphokines (18,27) and cytokine mediators. These effector cell functions can be summarized by noting that macrophages can secrete an incredible array of substances (over 60 in one count [83]), which can include complement fragments, chemotactic factors that promote directed PMN movement (66,74,77,127), lymphocyte chemotaxis, platelet activating factor, fibroblast growth factor, and leukotrienes from the lipoxygenase pathway of arachidonic acid metabolism that constitute the mediator–slow reacting substance of anaphylaxis (96). Therefore, it seems plausible that alveolar macrophages may be pivotal cells that have a dual function as phagocyte and immune effector cells.

It is difficult to find specific defects in alveolar macrophage function to account for the frequency and number of respiratory infections immunocompromised people have. The cells are long lived (perhaps existing months to several years), and they are reusable phagocytes in that they can withstand repeated challenges of particulates that must be ingested and intracellularly degraded, in contrast to short-lived PMNs. Prolonged periods of monocytopenia in patients treated for monocytic leukemia did not decrease the number of alveolar macrophages retrieved from the lungs by lung lavage, showing that the absence of circulating blood precursors for alveolar macrophages (and other tissue macrophages) did not cause depletion of the lung supply (41). In fact, a low level of macrophage replication was detected, suggesting that a form of *in situ* cell proliferation could occur in order to maintain the macrophage population (40). The functional activity of these macrophages, once removed from the leukemic host, was normal *in vitro*.

The pulmonary disease alveolar proteinosis features an exudation of lipid- and protein-containing fluid into the terminal airspaces of the lungs; patients may have pulmonary infection with unusual microorganisms such as *Nocardia*. Defects in mucociliary clearance and in lung phagocytic cell defense have been postulated. When alveolar macrophages are lavaged from the lungs of patients with alveolar proteinosis, it is noted that they are filled with large lipid inclusions, adhere poorly to a glass surface, and have diminished chemotactic movement. Moreover, these macrophages can ingest fungi normally (*Candida pseudotropicalis* were used) but are markedly defective in killing the organisms (42,44). However, it is thought that the macrophages are intrinsically normal (blood monocytes from patients with this disease are), but they ingest the lipid material from the abnormal alveolar environment, which crowds their cytoplasm so there is not room for adequate lysozymes. Thus, decreased lysosomal enzyme killing is an acquired defect. Similarly, the cellular burden of lipid also affects the macrophages' adherence and mobility.

As mentioned, patients with cystic fibrosis have a difficult problem with lung infection, especially *P. aeruginosa*. The question of defective phagocytic function in the lung has been debated extensively. Perhaps the only study to investigate the integrity of alveolar macrophages recovered from the lungs of CF patients (135), all with prior *Pseudomonas* respiratory infection, found that these macrophages were morphologically similar to normal macrophages and could phagocytose *Pseudomonas* and staphylococcal bacteria normally. There are probably external factors in the lungs of CF subjects (defective opsonins or other inhibitory factors [36,95,122,143]) that inhibit optimal function of the alveolar macrophages, but from this limited study no evidence of an intrinsic defect could be found.

Two other facets of phagocytic and microbial function of alveolar and interstitially located lung macrophage can be explored: (i) certain microorganisms have an affinity for monocyte-macrophage cells, and (ii) there exists the possibility of acquired defects in macrophage function.

There is a small group of microbes that seem to be adapted to survive in macrophages, and containment or eradication can be difficult for this phagocyte (Table 1-5). Obviously, some of these microbes are not involved in lung infections, but they do afflict tissue macrophages in other organ systems. The network of tissue macrophages within the reticuloendothelial system of the body is extensive and represents specialized macrophages in numerous locations: Kupffer's cells in the liver, Langer-

TABLE 1–5. *Some intracellular microbes that can be resident in human monocytes and macrophages and require cell-mediated activation to be killed or contained*

Chlamydia psittici
Cytomegalovirus
Legionella pneumophila
Leishmania donovani
Listeria monocytogenes
Mycobacterium leprae murium
Mycobacterium tuberculosis and other species
Pneumocystis carinii
Salmonella typhi
Toxoplasma gondii

hans' cells in the skin, peritoneal macrophages, alveolar macrophages, and osteoclasts in bone. The common precursor cell is the blood monocyte. Macrophages are generally considered to be the first line of defense against facultative and obligate intracellular parasites such as *Mycobacterium tuberculosis* and *M. leprae*. Although macrophages can ingest and contain these organisms, if delayed hypersensitivity and cell-mediated immune functions of the host are operating well, the microbes are not killed but can survive within the cell.

Pneumonias Reflecting Inadequate Cellular Immunity

Two important causes of respiratory infection are apparent when the macrophage-lymphocyte axis, as illustrated in Figure 1-5, cannot properly generate cell-mediated immune effector function. This is particularly evident when the microorganism is one that can reside inside a macrophage, referred to as facultative intracellular organism. A number of important infectious agents have this ability and can be a problem for macrophages located in other parts of the reticuloendothelial system, not just for lung macrophages (Table 1-5). Infection with Legionella bacteria illustrates a host defense problem that can exist until macrophages are activated to contain the microorganism. The other example, *Pneumocystis carinii* in patients with the acquired immunodeficiency syndrome, reflects the absence of part of the immune apparatus, T-helper cells, and an overbalance of T-suppressor cells, with the net effect that macrophages could not be sufficiently activated (12).

Legionella is an important cause of community-acquired pneumonia (CAP) in patients with underlying illness. It was identified as the single pathogen in about 16% of cases (13/79 patients) in which a microbial etiology was established (5). It might be added that the cause of CAP was found in only 51% of patients (79/154 patients) in this thorough Veterans Hospital study. After an infection with *L. pneumophila*, which causes the majority of lung infections among this genus of bacteria, the host develops specific IgM and IgG serum antibodies (Fig. 1-7). However, subjecting the organisms to a mixture of specific antibody plus complement *in vitro* does not create a lytic state that is sufficient to kill the bacteria (48). However, the availability of these opsonins does ensure that the Legionella organisms can attach and be ingested by various phagocytic cells, including PMNs, blood monocytes, and alveolar macrophages (47,49), but once inside the phagocytes, *Legionella* multiply without impedance and eventually kill and disrupt the host cells (82). However, immune lymphocytes can be taken from a subject who has successfully recovered from a

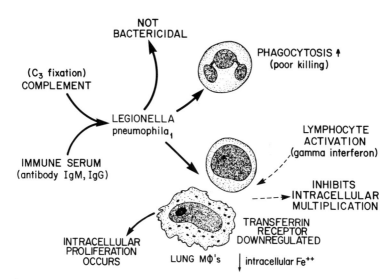

FIG. 1–7. Cellular mechanisms involved in host defense against *Legionella*. Although specific antibody (IgM and IgG) and complement are not bactericidal for the bacteria, these opsonins do increase phagocytic uptake by PMNs, monocytes, and lung macrophages; but, once inside these cells the Legionella bacteria proliferate. However, if products from activated immune T-cells (gamma interferon) are incubated with the phagocytes, especially alveolar macrophages, some cellular activation develops; then the intracellular *Legionella* can be contained at least within the phagocytes. The gamma interferon appears to down-regulate the number of transferrin receptors on the surface of the macrophages, thus decreasing the transport of iron which is an essential nutritional factor for this microbe (7, 130; from Reynolds [102]).

Legionella infection, and these can be stimulated to produce lymphokines in their cell-culture medium. These lymphokine mediators when reacted with virgin phagocytes will energize them, activating the cells through cellular immunity (82). Now such stimulated phagocytes after ingesting the Legionella inoculum will contain the growth of the bacteria within themselves, although they are not actually able to kill the bacteria. Gamma interferon is the lymphocyte mediator that accomplishes this function (7,130). Interferon-gamma down-regulates the transferrin receptors on monocytes and macrophages, thus diminishing the amount of intracellular iron. Without this essential metabolite, the Legionella organisms do not thrive (13). Cell-mediated immunity would seem to be an important factor in optimizing lung host defense by macrophages and PMNs and perhaps in preventing recurrent infection. These mechanisms are similar in concept to other situations involving facultative intracellular microbes, such as myobacterial species.

Another contemporary example is the acquired immunodeficiency syndrome (AIDS) in which the human host is infected with a lymphotropic retrovirus (HTLV$_3$ or HIV) that has a propensity to destroy certain subpopulations of T-lymphocytes, namely, T-cells belonging to the inducer/helper subset (120). AIDS patients may have a variety of respiratory infections, involving organisms such as viruses (cytomegalovirus or herpes simplex), *Pneumocystis carinii* (16,17), *Mycobacterium tuberculosis* and *M. avium–intracellulari,* common gram-positive (110) and gram-negative bacteria, and, less frequently, *Cryptococcus neoformans, Toxoplasma gondii,* or, rarely, *Legionella.* Monocytes and alveolar macrophages also can be infected with HIV (46,118), and transport of the virus in mobile phagocytes may be a means of spreading the virus to the lung and brain. As mentioned, most of these infectious agents have the common requirement of residing in a macrophage or similar cell as a facultative intracellular organism. Just why the AIDS victim should have so much trouble with this group of infections is not certain, but a possible explanation may involve the relative imbalance of lymphocytes found in the alveoli, as sampled by bronchoalveolar lavage of the lung.

As the immunologic milieu of the AIDS-involved lung is being described, several facts now give insight into the cause of recurrent infections and the ineffectiveness of alveolar host defenses. Bronchoalveolar lavage (BAL) studies (63) have been reported from several groups of AIDS patients with opportunistic pulmonary infections, those with risk factors for AIDS, and subjects with a preliminary stage of illness described as AIDS-related complex (ARC) or with chronic generalized lymphadenopathy (CGL) (98,140,142,148). Results emphasizing lymphocyte values in BAL are summarized. Results in lung lavage stand in contrast to the usual lymphocyte pattern in blood and other tissue of AIDS patients (31), for peripheral blood lymphocyte counts are decreased and a paucity of T-helper lymphocytes are characteristic in blood and in nodal tissue. As these cells are infected with HIV and destroyed, blood lymphocyte counts, although low, show a relative increase in T-suppressor/cytotoxic lymphocytes giving a low T-helper/T-suppressor ratio.

In contrast to blood counts that reflected lymphopenia, the alveolar spaces and peripheral airways sampled by BAL had increased numbers of lymphocytes. Although T_4 and Leu_3 staining lymphocytes, phenotypically identifying T-helper cells, might be low in blood, some were present in the lung. Actually, based on absolute lymphocyte counts, T-helper cells in AIDS lavage fluid approximated the number of these cells usually found in the alveoli of normals. Uniformly, the proportion of T_8 or Leu_2 staining cells that identify T-suppressor cells was increased, usually to a marked degree. Alveolar macrophages were recovered in proportionally smaller numbers, reflecting the greater percentage of lymphocytes (ranging from 19.4 to 26.1% of BAL cells in AIDS versus 5.1 to 10.2% in normals). Polymorphonuclear neutrophils were increased (2.1–18.8% in AIDS); this suggests that factors including PMN chemotaxis into the alveoli were in operation.

An explanation for this increase of phenotypically T-suppressor cells in the alveoli of AIDS patients infected with an opportunistic microorganism is intriguing but not proven. Venet et al. (140) evaluated cytomegalovirus (CMV) infection in 48 of their 63 AIDS patients; of these 48, 30 had a positive CMV culture in BAL fluid (62%). Wallace et al. (142) noted CMV cultures in 5 of 12 and Young et al. (148) in 3 of 15 patients. Certainly prior or concomitant viral infection in the lungs is a frequent finding in AIDS. Infection with viruses such as CMV and Epstein-Barr typically induces or stimulates a response of T-suppressor lymphocytes and could be a reason why an excess of these cells accumulates in AIDS.

As the intracellular opportunistic microbial agents causing respiratory infection in AIDS patients are those that are envisioned to be difficult for macrophages to contain and kill, it is probable that tissue or alveolar macrophages are defective because of prior infection with a viral agent, or cannot be adequately activated with exogenous stimuli such as gamma interferon or monokines. The later stimuli arising from T-lymphocytes may be lacking because of a paucity of T-helper cells or their dysfunction. Alveolar macrophages probably exist in an environment where they cannot be activated sufficiently, that is, induction of cell-mediated immunity, to contain or kill organisms such as pneumocystis or mycobacteria (Fig. 1-8). This is not the sit-

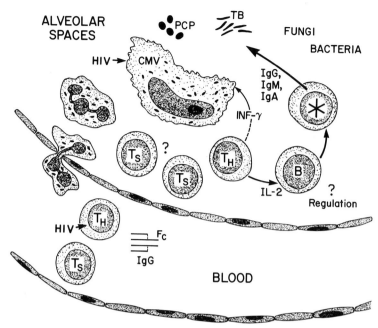

FIG. 1–8. Cellular interactions that can occur in the lungs of AIDS patients with infection. Macrophages already infected with viruses (CMV, and possibly HIV) are confronted with a variety of microbes that traditionally are difficult for them to control. *Pneumocystis carinii* (PCP) is the most frequently encountered infection. Aside from infection with virus, the macrophage might not be energized with gamma interferon to become "activated." Although T-helper lymphocytes are decreased (but not absent in the lung), it is possible that they do not secrete their mediators in amounts needed for cells with the CD_4 receptor, which could also be infected with HIV. Moreover, the increased number of T-suppressor cells present could contribute other unknown mediators that depress macrophage function. Other arms of the immune response seem intact in that PMNs are found, indicating that chemotaxins are available, and immunoglobulin production is high. However, immunoglobulin responses are not well regulated, and the specific antibody could not be developed. Again, a lack of lymphokine (IL-2) from T-helper cells could be part of the poor B-cell and plasma cell response. Alternatively, B-cell infection with HIV could disorder the response, also (from Reynolds [102]).

uation for asymptomatic subjects with HIV infection (12)—a sort of double suppressor effect. Usually, macrophages themselves have suppressive function, because they are not especially good accessory cells for producing or sustaining proliferative responses by lymphocytes when co-cultured with them under cell-culture conditions. However, HIV-infected alveolar macrophages may secrete more T-cell stimulatory factors, such as Il-1B and Il-6, than normal macrophages, which can enhance T-cell proliferation and therefore increase these lymphocytes to HIV (137). Thus, in AIDS, there is a decrease in T-helper lymphocytes that ordinarily could help active macrophages through various monokines (Fig. 1-4) such as gamma interferon, migration inhibition factor, or interleukin-1 (28). This is coupled with a relative increase in T-suppressor lymphocytes which probably dampens down further macrophage function. The net effect may be macrophages that cannot be activated nor respond appropriately to cellular stimuli which are needed to optimize intracellular antimicrobial processes.

PMNs and the Lung Inflammatory Response

The complex nature of altered lung host defenses in the heavily immunosuppressed patient is not known completely, especially the function of perhaps minor and inconspicuous components. The effects of granulocytopenia, and hence an impaired inflammatory cell response in the lungs, have been well correlated with susceptibility to a variety of aerobic gram-negative bacteria and fungi. In contrast, little is known about the impact of cytotoxic chemotherapy on the regeneration of airway ciliated epithelial cells or on the function of their cilia; similarly, local secretion along the airways of such immunoglobulins as IgA could be diminished because of sluggishly synthesizing submucosal plasma cells. Damage to other populations of lymphoid cells in the lungs that are involved with cell-mediated immunity has not been systemically assessed, either.

The capability of mounting an appropriate inflammatory response in lung tissue is an important component of host defense (104) (see Table 1-1). This mechanism is a complex biologic reaction requiring specific initiation, containing steps for amplification that allow systemic elements of immunity to be recruited into the lung, and, finally, terminating the reaction and allowing subsequent tissue repair. Although several kinds of phagocytic cells participate, PMNs are the most numerous, and perhaps the most important host factor once the full-blown inflammatory response has begun.

Normal lungs contain PMNs sequestered in interstitial areas and marginated in capillaries (20,94). The lungs also have ready access to the circulating granulocyte pool. Previously, in considering various stimuli and chemotactic factors that might attract PMNs to alveoli and airways, we assumed that an ample supply of PMNs existed to support the requirements of a local inflammatory reaction. This might not be the case, for either a deficient number of cells or abnormal function can result in an insufficient migration of PMNs into lung tissue and a blunted response.

An absolute deficiency of PMNs is not uncommon. The leukopenic patient, often granulocytopenic from antineoplastic chemotherapy or other forms of immunosuppression, basically has insufficient reserve bone marrow function to support a peripheral white count and an adequate marginated pool. Infection, particularly bacterial or fungal pneumonia, is frequent in these patients and is a common cause of death. The offending organisms are usually *Pseudomonas* or gram-negative bacilli that inhabit the normal gut but commonly colonize the oropharynx of debilitated hospitalized patients. Having an inadequate number of circulating PMNs in the blood is one of the best predictors of susceptibility to gram-negative bacillary infection.

In lung vasculature, PMNs arrive in the blood and either pass through the capillaries or linger and stick to the endothelium, thus becoming marginated and temporarily stored (Fig. 1-6). Margination is a resting stage for this short-lived phagocytic cell. However, marginated cells remain in dynamic equilibrium with circulating cells, so margination could represent only a temporary removal from the intravascular circuit. Recently, a number of interesting observations have been made regarding PMN adherence to vascular endothelium (121,131). Adherence involved in margination is equivalent to the "activated" sticking preliminary to the PMNs leaving the vascular space and migrating to an extravascular site.

Mechanisms that cause PMNs to marginate and stick to vascular endothelium will not be reviewed extensively, but a number of conditions do alter adherence. Because sticking seems necessary before PMN diapedesis, or egress into tissue can occur, it is a vulnerable step which can interfere with the inflammatory response. A variety of agents and conditions can decrease PMN sticking, including ethanol, corticosteroids, and other antiinflammatory drugs such as aspirin (4,69). Exocytosis of an appreciable portion of the PMN granule–associated enzymes can affect *in vitro* adherence and motility (39). With secretion of 30% or more of the lysozyme content, cell adhesiveness was increased and chemotaxis was inhibited, whereas with more limited exocytosis of the intracellular granules' contents, chemotactic responses were increased. Thus, events that interfere with the adherence of PMNs to capillary endothelial surfaces could functionally limit the number of phagocytic cells that can be mobilized to an inflamed site.

The direct application of such reasoning to clinical problems is tempting but is not yet well substantiated. For example, the inebriated alcoholic who loses consciousness and aspirates oropharyngeal bacteria in the process could develop a pneumococcal or *Klebsiella* pneumonia. Stupor, stasis, and pooling of respiratory secretions, poor cough response, and other depressed host factors all contribute to establishing the infection. In addition, poor PMN sticking, also attributed to acute ethanol intake, could impair the local inflammatory process in the lung and allow bacteria to proliferate.

Occasionally, intrinsic defects in the PMNs can account for poor extravascular migration and susceptibility to infection. PMNs from subjects with Chediak-Higashi syndrome, who have large, abnormally fused lysosomes, do not deform well mechanically and therefore respond sluggishly to chemotactic stimuli (19). A patient was found with a deficiency in actin, part of the actin-myosin filamentous structure that propels PMN cytoplasm; the deficiency resulted in poor granulocyte movement (9). Finally, some PMNs exhibit poor spontaneous motility *in vitro;* they are termed *lazy leukocytes* (79).

To review further the multitude of metabolic and biochemical abnormalities that can affect PMNs is not our intention. This has been done thoroughly (73). Although these deficiencies cause general problems with phagocytic intracellular killing and inflammation, they probably do not produce specific disorders in the lungs. However, the point to emphasize is that a variety of things can impair the response of PMNs in the inflammatory reaction. External factors are important because there could be insufficient chemotactic stimuli to direct migration. The role of other external factors, such as drugs that impair PMN adherence, is obvious. However, appropriate stimuli might not interact with an appropriately responsive PMN cell, one that is compromised by poor intrinsic mobility or excessive granular enzyme depletion, for example. The net effect is an inadequate influx or concentration of PMN phagocytes in alveoli and parenchyma and an inability of the lung to cope with an infectious inoculum or other troublesome particulate substances or antigens.

References

1. Afzelius, B.A. (1976): A human syndrome caused by immotile cilia. *Science,* 193:317–319.
2. Afzelius, B.A. (1981): Immotile-cilia syndrome and ciliary abnormalities induced by infection and injury. *Am. Rev. Respir. Dis.,* 124:107–109.
3. Ambrosino, D.M., Siber, G.R., Chilmonczyk, B.A., Jernberg, J.B., and Finberg, R.W. (1987): An immunodeficiency characterized by impaired antibody responses to polysaccharides. *N. Engl. J. Med.,* 316:790–793.
4. Atkinson, J.P., Sullivan, T.J., Kelly, J.P., and Parker, C.W. (1977): Stimulation by alcohols of

cyclic AMP metabolism in human leukocytes—possible role of cyclic AMP in the inflammatory effects of ethanol. *J. Clin. Invest.*, 60:284–294.

5. Bates, J.H., Campbell, G.D., Barron, A.L., McCracken, G.A., Morgan, P.N., Moses, E.B., and Davis, M. (1992): Microbial etiology of acute pneumonia in hospitalized patients. *Chest*, 101:1005–1012.

6. Beck, C.A., and Heiner, D.C. (1981): Selective immunoglobulin G_4 deficiency and recurrent infections of the respiratory tract. *Am. Rev. Respir. Dis.*, 124:94–96.

7. Bhardwaj, N., Nash, T.W., and Horwitz, M.A. (1986): Interferon-gamma activated human monocytes inhibit the intracellular multiplication of *Legionella pneumophila*. *J. Immunol.*, 137: 2662–2669.

8. Bolan, G., Broome, C.V., Facklam, R.R., et al. (1986): Pneumococcal vaccine efficacy in selected populations in the United States. *Ann. Intern. Med.*, 104:1–6.

9. Boxer, L.A., Hedley-Whyte, E.T., and Stossel, T.P. (1974): Neutrophil actin dysfunction and abnormal neutrophil behavior. *N. Engl. J. Med.*, 291:1093–1099.

10. Brooks, G.F., Lammel, C.J., Blake, M.S., Kuseck, B., and Achtman, M. (1992): Antibodies against IgA_1 protease are stimulated both by clinical disease and asymptomatic carriage of serogroup A *Neisseria meningitidis*. *J. Infect. Dis.*, 166:1316–1321.

11. Buckley, R.H. (1992): Immunodeficiency diseases. *J.A.M.A.*, 268:2797–2806.

12. Buhl, R., Jaffe, H.A., Holroyd, K.J., et al. (1993): Activation of alveolar macrophages in asymptomatic HIV-infected individuals. *J. Immunol.*, 150:1019–1028.

13. Byrd, T.F., and Horwitz, M.A. (1989): Interferon-gamma activated human monocytes down regulate transferrin receptors and inhibit the intracellular multiplication of *Legionella pneumophila* by limiting the availability of iron. *J. Clin. Invest.*, 83:1457–1465.

14. Camner, P., Mossberg, B., and Afzelius, B.A. (1975): Evidence for congenitally nonfunctioning cilia in the tracheobronchial tract in two subjects. *Am. Rev. Respir. Dis.*, 112:807–809.

15. Catlin, B.W. (1990): *Branhamella catarrhalis:* an organism gaining respect as a pathogen. *Clin. Microbiol. Rev.*, 3:293–320.

16. Centers for disease control. (1981): *Pneumocystis* pneumonia. Los Angeles. *Morbid. Mortal. Weekly Rep.*, 30:250–252.

17. Centers for disease control. (1981): Kaposi's sarcoma and pneumocystis pneumonia among homosexual men. New York City and California. *Morbid. Mortal. Weekly Rep.*, 30:305–308.

18. Claman, H.N. (1992): The biology of the immune response. *J.A.M.A.*, 268:2790–2806.

19. Clark, R.A., and Kimball, H.R. (1971): Defective granulocyte chemotaxis in the Chediak-Higashi syndrome. *J. Clin. Invest.*, 50:2645–2652.

20. Cohen, A.B., Batra, G., Petersen, R., Podany, J., and Nguyen, D. (1979): Size of the pool of alveolar neutrophils in normal rabbit lungs. *J. Appl. Physiol.*, 47:440–444.

21. Colton, H.R. (1981): Case records of Massachusetts General Hospital. *N. Engl. J. Med.*, 304: 831–836.

22. Coonrod, J.D. (1986): The role of extracellular bactericidal factors in pulmonary host defense. *Sem. Respir. Infect.*, 1:118–129.

23. Cooper, J.A.D., Sibille, Y., Zitnik, R.J., Bayles, G., Buck, M.G., and Merrill, W.W. (1991): Isolation of an inhibitor of neutrophil function from bronchial lavage of normal volunteers. *Amer. J. Physiol.*, 260:L501–L509.

24. Correspondence (to the Editor). (1978): *N. Engl. J. Med.*, 316:1272–1273.

25. Daniele, R.P., Altose, M.D., and Rowland, D.R., Jr. (1975): Immunocompetent cells from the lower respiratory tract of normal human lungs. *J. Clin. Invest.*, 59:986–996.

26. Delacroix, D.L., Dive, C., Rambaud, J.C., and Vaerman, J.P. (1982): IgA subclasses in various secretions and in serum. *J. Immunol.*, 44:383–385.

27. Dinarello, C.A., and Mier, J.W. (1987): Current concepts: lymphokines. *N. Engl. J. Med.*, 317:940–945.

28. Dinarello, C.A., and Wolff, S.M. (1993): The role of interleukin-1 in disease—review. *N. Engl. J. Med.* 328:106–113.

29. DiSant'Agnese, P.A., and Davis, P.B. (1976): Research in cystic fibrosis. *N. Engl. J. Med.*, 295:481–485, 534–541, 597–602.

30. Eliasson, R., Mossberg, B., Camner, P., and Afzelius, B.A. (1977): The immotile cilia syndrome: a congenital ciliary abnormality as an etiologic factor in chronic airway infections and male sterility. *N. Engl. J. Med.*, 297:1–6.

31. Fauci, A.S. (1987): AIDS: immunopathogenic mechanisms and research strategies. *Clin. Res.*, 35:503–510.

32. Fedson, D.A. (1987): Influenza and pneumococcal immunization strategies for physicians. *Chest*, 91:436–443.

33. Fels, A.O.S., and Cohn, Z.A. (1986): The alveolar macrophage. *J. Appl. Physiol.*, 60:353–369.

34. Fels, A.O.S., Pawloski, N.A., Cramer, E.B., King, T.K.C., Cohn, Z.A., and Scott, W.A. (1982): Human alveolar macrophages produce leukotriene B_4. *Proc. Natl. Acad. Sci.*, USA, 79:7866–7870.

35. Fernald, G.W., and Clyde, W.A., Jr. (1976): Pulmonary immune mechanisms in *Mycoplasma pneumonia disease*. In: *Immunologic and Infectious Reactions in the Lung*, edited by C.H. Kirkpatrick and H.Y. Reynolds, pp. 101–130. Marcel Dekker, New York.

36. Fick, R.B., Naegel, G.P., Squier, S.U., Wood, R.E., Gee, J.B.L., and Reynolds, H.Y. (1984): Proteins of the cystic fibrosis respiratory tract: fragmented IgG opsonic antibody causing defective opsonophagocytosis. *J. Clin. Invest.*, 74:236–248.

37. Fick, R.B., Olchowski, J., Squier, S.U., Merrill, W.W., and Reynolds, H.Y. (1986): Immunoglobulin G-subclasses in cystic fibrosis: IgG$_2$ response to *Pseudomonas aeruginosa* lipopolysaccharide. *Am. Rev. Respir. Dis.*, 133:418–422.

38. Frizzell, R.A., Rechkemmer, G., and Shoemaker, R.L. (1986): Altered regulation of airway epithelial cell chloride channels in cystic fibrosis. *Science*, 233:558–560.

39. Gallin, J.I., Wright, D.G., and Schiffman, E. (1978): Role of secretory events in modulating human neutrophil chemotaxis. *J. Clin. Invest.*, 62:1364–1374.

40. Golde, D.W., Byers, L.A., and Finley, T.N. (1974): Proliferative capacity of human alveolar macrophage. *Nature*, 247:373–375.

41. Golde, D.W., Finley, T.N., and Cline, M.J. (1974): The pulmonary macrophage in acute leukemia. *N. Engl. J. Med.*, 290:875–878.

42. Golde, D.W., Territo, M., Finley, T.N., and Cline, M.J. (1976): Defective lung macrophages in pulmonary alveolar proteinosis. *Ann. Intern. Med.*, 85:304–309.

43. Hamill, R.J., Musher, D.M., Groover, J.E., Zavell, P.J., and Watson, D.A. (1992): IgG antibody reactive with five serotypes of *Streptococcus pneumoniae* in commercial intravenous immunoglobulin preparations. *J. Infect. Dis.*, 166:38–42.

44. Harris, J.O. (1979): Pulmonary alveolar proteinosis: abnormal *in vitro* function of alveolar macrophages. *Chest*, 76:156–159.

45. Higuchi, J.G., and Johanson, W.G. (1980): The relationship between adherence of *Pseudomonas aeruginosa* to upper respiratory cells *in vitro* and susceptibility to colonization *in vivo*. *J. Lab. Clin. Med.*, 95:698–705.

46. Ho, D.D., Rota, T.R., and Hirsch, M.S. (1986): Infection of monocyte/macrophages by human T lymphotropic virus type III. *J. Clin. Invest.*, 77:1712–1715.

47. Horwitz, M.A., and Silverstein, S.C. (1980): Legionnaires' disease bacterium multiplies intracellularly in human monocytes. *J. Clin. Invest.*, 66:441–450.

48. Horwitz, M.A., and Silverstein, S.C. (1981): Interaction of Legionnaires' disease bacterium *(Legionella pneumophila)* with human phagocytes. I. Resists killing by polymorphonuclear leukocytes, antibody and complement. *J. Exp. Med.*, 153:386–397.

49. Horwitz, M.A., and Silverstein, S.C. (1981): Interaction of Legionnaires' disease bacterium *(Legionella pneumophila)* with human phagocytes. II. Antibody promotes binding of *L. pneumophila* to monocytes but does not inhibit intracellular multiplication. *J. Exp. Med.*, 153:398–406.

50. Hunninghake, G.W., and Crystal, R.G. (1981): Pulmonary sarcoidosis: a disorder mediated by excess helper T-lymphocyte activity at sites of disease activity. *N. Engl. J. Med.*, 305:429–434.

51. Hunninghake, G.W., Gadek, J.E., Fales, H.M., and Crystal, R.G. (1980): Human alveolar macrophage-derived chemotactic factor for neutrophils. *J. Clin. Invest.*, 66:473–483.

52. Hunninghake, G.W., Gadek, J.E., Kawanami, O., Ferrans, V.J., and Crystal, R.G. (1979): Inflammatory and immune processes in the human lung in health and disease: evaluation by bronchoalveolar lavage. *Amer. J. Pathol.*, 97:149–206.

53. Jakab, G.J. (1981): Mechanisms of virus-induced bacterial superinfections of the lung. *Clin. Chest Med.*, 2:59–66.

54. Johanson, W.G., Jr. (1986): Microbial adherence as a pathogenic factor in respiratory infections. In: *Respiratory Infections—Contemporary Issues in Infectious Diseases*, Vol. 5, edited by M.A. Sande, L.D. Hudson, and R.K. Root, pp. 13–23. Churchill Livingstone, New York.

55. Johanson, W.G., Jr., Higuchi, J.H., Chaudhuri, T.R., and Woods, D.E. (1980): Bacterial adherence to epithelial cells in bacillary colonization of the respiratory tract. *Am. Rev. Respir. Dis.*, 121:55–63.

56. Johanson, W.G., Jr., Pierce, A.K., and Sanford, J.P. (1969): Changing pharyngeal bacterial flora of hospitalized patients—emergence of gram-negative bacilli. *N. Engl. J. Med.*, 281:1137–1140.

57. Johanson, W.G., Jr., Woods, D.E., and Chaudhuri, T. (1979): Association of respiratory tract colonization with adherence of gram-negative bacilli to epithelial cells. *J. Infect. Dis.*, 139:667–673.

58. Karlish, A.J., and Tarnoky, A.L. (1960): Mucoviscidosis as a factor in chronic lung disease in adults. *Lancet*, 2:514–515.

59. Kartagener, M. (1983): Zur pathogenese der bronchiektasien. *Bietr. Klin. Tuberk.*, 83:489–501.

60. Kilian, M., Mestecky, J., Kulhavy, R., Tomana, M., and Butler, W.T. (1980): IgA$_1$ proteases from *Hemophilus influenzae*, *Streptococcus pneumonia*, *Neisseria meningitidis* and *Streptococcus sanguis:* comparative immunochemical studies. *J. Immunol.*, 124:2596–2600.

61. Kilian, M., Mestecky, J., and Russell, M.W. (1988): Defense mechanisms involving Fc-depen-

dent functions of immunoglobulin A and their subversion by bacterial immunoglobulin A proteases. *Clin Microbiol. Rev.,* 52:296–303.

62. Klaustermeyer, W.B., Gianos, M.E., Kurohara, M.L., Dao, H.T., and Heiner, D.C. (1992): IgG subclass deficiency associated with corticosteroids in obstructive lung disease. *Chest,* 102:1137–1142.

63. Klech, H., and Hutter, C. (1990): Clinical guidelines and indications for bronchoalveolar lavage (BAL). Report of the European Society of Pneumology Task Group on BAL. *Eur. Respir. J.,* 3:937–974.

64. Klech, H., and Pohl, W. (Editors). (1989): Technical recommendation and guidelines for bronchoalveolar lavage. Report of the European Society of Pneumology Task Group on BAL. *Eur. Respir. J.,* 2:561–585.

65. Knowles, M., Gatzy, J., and Boucher, R. (1983): Relative ion permeability of normal and cystic fibrosis nasal epithelium. *J. Clin. Invest.,* 71:1410–1417.

66. Leonard, E.J., and Yoshimura, T. (1990): Neutrophil attractant/activation protein-1 (NAP-1 [Interleukin-8]). *Am. J. Respir. Cell. Mole. Biol.,* 2:479–486.

67. Little, J.W., Hall, W.J., Douglas, R.G., Jr., Mudholkar, G.S., Speer, D.M., and Patel, K. (1978): Airway hyperreactivity and peripheral airway dysfunction in influenza A infection. *Am. Rev. Respir. Dis.,* 118:295–303.

68. Lober, C., Wood, R.E., DiSant'Agnese, P.A., Rourk, M.H., and Spock, A. (1974): Patterns of presentation of cystic fibrosis of the pancreas seen in patients over age twenty. *Chest,* 66:332.

69. MacGregor, R.R., Macarak, E.J., and Kefalides, N.A. (1978): Comparative adherence of granulocytes to endothelial monolayers and nylon fiber. *J. Clin. Invest.,* 61:697–702.

70. Machowiak, P.A. (1982): The normal microbial flora. *N. Engl. J. Med.,* 307:83–93.

71. Macons, G.G., Pier, G.E., Pennington, J.E., Matthews, W.J., and Goldman, D.A. (1981): Mucoid *Escherichia coli* in cystic fibrosis. *N. Engl. J. Med.,* 304:1445–1499.

72. Malech, H.L. (1980): Abnormal neutrophil migration in Kartagener's syndrome. *Ann. Intern. Med.,* 92:520–538.

73. Malech, H.L., and Gallin, J.I. (1987): Current concepts: immunology: neutrophils in human diseases. *N. Engl. J. Med.,* 317:687–694.

74. Martin, T.R., Raugi, G., Merritt, T.L., and Henderson, W.R., Jr. (1987): Relative contribution of leukotriene B_4 to the neutrophil chemotactic activity produced by the resident human alveolar macrophage. *J. Clin. Invest.,* 80:1114–1124.

75. Meduri, G.U., and Johanson, W.G. (1992): Introduction to international consensus conference on clinical investigation of ventilator-associated pneumonia. *Chest* (Suppl. 1), 102:551S–552S.

76. Merrill, W.W., Hyun, H., Strober, W., Rankin, J., Fick, R.B., and Reynolds, H.Y. (1982): Correlation between respiratory tract proteins obtained from upper (nasal) and lower (bronchial lavage) sites. *Am. Rev. Respir. Dis.,* 125S:268.

77. Merrill, W.W., Naegel, G.P., Matthay, R.A., and Reynolds, H.Y. (1980): Alveolar macrophage-derived chemotactic factor. *J. Clin. Invest.,* 65:268–276.

78. Merrill, W.W., Naegel, G.P., Olchowski, J.J., and Reynolds, H.Y. (1985): Immunoglobulin G subclass proteins in serum and lavage fluid of normal subjects: quantitation and comparison with immunoglobulins A and E. *Am. Rev. Respir. Dis.,* 131:584–591.

79. Miller, M.E., Oski, F.A., and Harris, H.B. (1971): Lazy leukocyte syndrome. *Lancet,* 1:665–669.

80. Mulks, M.H., Kornfeld, S.W., and Plaut, A.G. (1980): Specific proteolysis of human IgA by *Streptococcus pneumoniae* and *Hemophilus influenzae. J. Infect. Dis.,* 141:450–456.

81. Murphy, T.F., and Sethi, S. (1992): Bacterial infection in chronic obstructive pulmonary disease: state of the art. *Am. Rev. Respir. Dis.,* 146:1067–1083.

82. Nash, T.W., Libby, D.M., and Horwitz, M.A. (1984): Interaction between the Legionnaires' disease bacterium *(Legionella pneumophila)* and human alveolar macrophages. *J. Clin. Invest.,* 74:771–782.

83. Nathan, C.F. (1987): Secretory products of macrophages. *J. Clin. Invest.,* 79:319–326.

84. Nathan, C.F., Murray, H.W., and Cohn, Z.A. (1980): The macrophage as an effector cell. *N. Engl. J. Med.,* 303:622–626.

85. Niederman, M.S., Merrill, W.W., Ferranti, R.D., Pagno, K.M., Palmer, L.B., and Reynolds, H.Y. (1984): Nutritional status and bacterial binding in the lower respiratory tract in patients with chronic tracheostomy. *Ann. Intern. Med.,* 100:795–800.

86. Niederman, M.S., Merrill, W.W., Polomski, L.M., Reynolds, H.Y., and Gee, J.B.L. (1986): Influences of sputum IgA and elastase on tracheal cell bacterial adherence. *Am. Rev. Respir. Dis.,* 133:255–260.

87. Niederman, M.S., Rafferty, T.D., Sasaki, C.T., Merrill, W.W., Matthay, R.A., and Reynolds, H.Y. (1983): Comparison of bacterial adherence to ciliated and squamous epithelial cells obtained from the human respiratory tract. *Am. Rev. Respir. Dis.,* 127:85–90.

88. Nolan, A.J. (1976): Cystic fibrosis in adults: the unsuspected pulmonary diagnosis. *Can. Med. Assoc. J.,* 114:142–145.

89. Owen, C.A., Campbell, E.J., Hill, S.L., and Stockley, R.A. (1992): Increased adherence of monocytes to fibronectin in bronchiectasis. *Am. Rev. Respir. Dis.*, 146:626–631.
90. Oxelius, V.A., Berkel, A.I., and Hanson, L.A. (1982): IgG$_2$ deficiency in ataxia-telangiectasia. *N. Engl. J. Med.*, 306:515–517.
91. Oxelius, V.A., Laurall, A.B., Lindquist, B., Golebiowski, H., Axelson, U., Björkander, J., and Hanson, L.A. (1981): IgG subclasses in selective IgA deficiency—importance of IgG$_2$-IgA deficiency. *N. Engl. J. Med.*, 304:1476–1477.
92. Palmer, L.B., Merrill, W.W., Niederman, M.S., Ferranti, R.D., and Reynolds, H.Y. (1986): Bacterial adherence to respiratory tract cells—relationship between *in vivo* and *in vitro* pH and bacterial attachment. *Am. Rev. Respir. Dis.*, 133:784–788.
93. Pedersen, H., and Mygind, N. (1976): Absence of azonemal arms in nasal mucosa cilia in Kartagener's syndrome. *Nature*, 262:494–495.
94. Perlo, S., Jalowayski, A.A., Durand, C.M., and West, J.B. (1975): Distribution of red and white blood cells in alveolar walls. *J. Appl. Physiol.*, 38:117–124.
95. Pier, G.B., Saunders, J.M., Ames, P., Edwards, M.S., Auerbach, H., Goldfarb, J., Speert, D.P., and Hurwitch, S. (1987): Opsonophagocytic-killing antibody to *Pseudomonas aeruginosa* mucoid exopolysaccharide in older noncolonized patients with cystic fibrosis. *N. Engl. J. Med.*, 317:793–798.
96. Rankin, J.A., Hitchcock, M., Merrill, W., Bach, M.K., Brashler, J.R., and Askenase, P.W. (1982): IgE-dependent release of leukotriene C$_4$ from alveolar macrophages. *Nature*, 297:329–331.
97. Rankin, J.A., Marcy, T., Rochester, C.L., Sussman, J., Smith, S., Buckley, P., and Lee, D. (1992): Human airway macrophages—a technique for their retrieval and a descriptive comparison with alveolar macrophages. *Am. Rev. Respir. Dis.*, 145:928–933.
98. Rankin, J.A., Walzer, P.D., Dwyer, J.M., et al. (1983): Immunologic alterations in bronchoalveolar lavage fluid in the acquired immunodeficiency syndrome. *Am. Rev. Respir. Dis.*, 128:189–194.
99. Reynolds, H.Y. (1981): Could a defect in host-immunity be the cause of respiratory infections? *Clin. Chest Med.*, 2:102–110.
100. Reynolds, H.Y. (1983): Lung inflammation: role of endogenous chemotactic factors in attracting polymorphonuclear granulocytes. *Am. Rev. Respir. Dis.*, 127:S16–S25.
101. Reynolds, H.Y. (1985): Respiratory infections may reflect deficiencies in host defense mechanisms. *Disease-A-Month*, 31:1–98.
102. Reynolds, H.Y. (1986): Lung immunology and its contribution to the immunopathogenesis of certain respiratory diseases. *J. Allergy & Clin. Immunol.*, 78:833–847.
103. Reynolds, H.Y. (1987): Bacterial adherence to respiratory tract mucosa—a dynamic interaction leading to colonization. *Sem. Respir. Infect.*, 2:8–19.
104. Reynolds, H.Y. (1987): Lung inflammation: normal host defense or a complication of some diseases? *Ann. Rev. Med.*, 38:295–323.
105. Reynolds, H.Y. (1988): Immunoglobulin G and its function in the human respiratory tract. *Mayo Clin. Proc.*, 63:161–174.
106. Reynolds, H.Y. (1991): Immunologic system in the respiratory tract. *Physiol. Rev.*, 71:1117–1133.
107. Reynolds, H.Y., DiSant'Agnese, P.A., and Zierdt, C.H. (1976): Mucoid *Pseudomonas aeruginosa*. A sign of cystic fibrosis in young adults with chronic pulmonary disease? *J.A.M.A.*, 236:2190–2192.
108. Reynolds, H.Y., and Merrill, W.W. (1981): Pulmonary immunology: humoral and cellular immune responsiveness of the respiratory tract. In: *Current Pulmonology*, Vol. 3, edited by D.H. Simmons, pp. 381–422. John Wiley and Sons, New York.
109. Robinson, B.W.S., Pinkston, P., and Crystal, R.G. (1984): Natural killer cells are present in the normal human lung but are functionally impotent. *J. Clin. Invest.*, 74:942–950.
110. Rodriquez-Barradas, M.C., Musher, D.M., Lahart, C., Lacke, C., Groover, J., Watson, D., Baughn, R., Cate, T., and Crofoot, G. (1992): Antibody to capsular polysaccharides of *Streptococcus pneumoniae* after vaccination of human immunodeficiency virus-infected subjects with 23-valent pneumococcal vaccine. *J. Infect. Dis.*, 165:553–556.
111. Rosenthal, S., and Tager, I.B. (1975): Prevalence of gram-negative rods in the normal pharyngeal flora. *Ann. Intern. Med.*, 83:355–357.
112. Rossman, C.M., Forrest, J.B., Lee, R.M.K.W., and Newhouse, M.T. (1980): The dyskinetic cilia syndrome—ciliary motility in immotile cilia syndrome. *Chest*, 78:580–582.
113. Rossman, C.M., Forrest, J.B., Ruffin, R.E., and Newhouse, M.T. (1980): Immotile cilia syndrome in persons with and without Kartagener's syndrome. *Am. Rev. Respir. Dis.*, 121:1011–1016.
114. Rubin, B.K., Ramirez, O., Zayas, J.G., Finegan, B., and King, M. (1992): Respiratory mucus from asymptomatic smokers is better hydrated and more easily cleared by mucociliary action. *Am. Rev. Respir. Dis.*, 145:545–547.

115. Rutland, J., and de Iongh, R.U. (1990): Random ciliary orientation—a cause of respiratory tract disease. *N. Engl. J. Med.*, 323:1681–1684.
116. Rutland, J., Griffin, W.M., and Cole, P.J. (1982): Human ciliary beat frequency in epithelium from intrathoracic and extrathoracic airways. *Am. Rev. Respir. Dis.*, 125:100–105.
117. Rutland, J., Penketh, A., Griffin, W.M., Hodson, M.E., Batten, J.C., and Cole, P.J. (1983): Cystic fibrosis serum does not inhibit human ciliary beat frequency. *Am. Rev. Respir. Dis.*, 128:1030–1034.
118. Salahuddin, S.Z., Rose, R.M., Groopman, J.E., Markham, P.D., and Gallo, R.C. (1986): Human T-lymphotropic virus type III infection of human alveolar macrophages. *Blood*, 68:281–284.
119. Saltini, C., Spurzem, J.R., Lee, J.J., Pinkston, P., and Crystal, R.G. (1986): Spontaneous release of interleukin-2 by lung T-lymphocytes in active pulmonary sarcoidosis is primarily from the Leu 3+DR+T cell subset. *J. Clin. Invest.*, 77:1962–1970.
120. Seligmann, M., Pinching, A.J., Rosen, F.S., et al. (1987): Immunology of human immunodeficiency virus infection and the acquired immunodeficiency syndrome—an update. *Ann. Intern. Med.*, 107:234–242.
121. Senior, R.M., Gresham, H.D., Griffin, G.L., Brown, J.E., and Chung, A.E. (1992): Entactin stimulates neutrophil adhesion and chemotaxis through interactions between its Arg-Gly-Asp (RDG) domain and the leukocyte response integrin. *J. Clin. Invest.*, 90:2251–2257.
122. Seybold, Z.V., Abraham, W.M., Gazeroglu, H., and A. Wanner. (1992): Impairment of airway mucociliary transport by *Pseudomonas aeruginosa* products. *Am. Rev. Respir. Dis.*, 146:1173–1176.
123. Shapiro, E.D., and Clemens, J.D. (1984): A controlled evaluation of the protective efficacy of pneumococcal vaccine for patients at high risk of serious pneumococcal infections. *Ann. Intern. Med.*, 101:325–330.
124. Shwachman, H. (1977): Case records of Massachusetts General Hospital. *N. Engl. J. Med.*, 296:1519–1526.
125. Siber, G.R., Schur, P.H., Aisenberg, A.C., Weitzman, S.A., and Schiffman, G. (1980): Correlation between serum IgG_2 concentrations and the antibody response to bacterial polysaccharide antigens. *N. Engl. J. Med.*, 303:178–182.
126. Sibille, Y., Merrill, W.W., Naegel, G.P., Care, S.B., Cooper, J.A.D., and Reynolds, H.Y. (1989): Human alveolar macrophages release a factor that inhibits phagocyte function. *Am. J. Respir. Cell. Mole. Biol.*, 1:407–416.
127. Sibille, Y., Naegel, G.P., Merrill, W.W., Young, K.R., Care, S.B., and Reynolds, H.Y. (1987): Neutrophil chemotactic activity produced by normal and activated human bronchoalveolar lavage cells. *J. Lab. Clin. Med.*, 110:624–633.
128. Sibille, Y., and Reynolds, H.Y. (1990): Macrophages and polymorphonuclear neutrophils in lung defense and injury: state of the art. *Am. Rev. Respir. Dis.*, 141:471–501.
129. Simberkoff, M.S., Cross, A.P., Al-Ibrahim, M., et al. (1986): Efficacy of pneumococcal vaccine in high-risk patients: results of a Veterans Administration Cooperative Study. *N. Engl. J. Med.*, 315:1318–1327.
130. Skerrett, S.J., and Martin, T.R. (1992): Recombinant murine interferon-gamma reversibly activates rat alveolar macrophages to kill *Legionella pneumophila*. *J. Infect. Dis.*, 166:1354–1361.
131. Smith, C.W. (1990): Molecular determinants of neutrophil adhesion. *Am. J. Respir. Cell. Mole. Biol.*, 2:487–489.
132. Stern, R.C., Boat, T.F., Doershuk, C.F., Tucker, A.S., Miller, R.B., and Matthelos, L.W. (1977): Cystic fibrosis diagnosed after age 13: twenty-five teenage and adult patients including three asymptomatic men. *Ann. Intern. Med.*, 87:188–191.
133. Sturgess, J.M., Chao, J., and Turner, J.A.P. (1980): Transposition of ciliary microtubules: another cause of impaired ciliary motility. *N. Engl. J. Med.*, 303:318–322.
134. Sturgess, J.M., Chao, J., Wong, J., Aspin, N., and Turner, J.A.P. (1979): Cilia with defective radial spokes. *N. Engl. J. Med.*, 300:53–56.
135. Thomassen, M.J., Demko, C.A., Wood, R.E., Tandler, B., Dearborn, D.G., Boxerbaum, B., and Kuchenbrod, P.J. (1980): Ultrastructure and function of alveolar macrophages from cystic fibrosis patients. *Pediatr. Res.*, 14:715–721.
136. Trulock, E.P., Cooper, J.D., Kaiser, L.R., Pasque, M.K., Ettinger, N.A., and Dresler, C.M. (1991): The Washington University–Barnes Hospital experience with lung transplantation. *J.A.M.A.*, 266:1943–1946.
137. Twigg, H.L., Iwamoto, G.K., and Soliman, D.M. (1992): Role of cytokines in alveolar macrophage accessory cell function in HIV-infected individuals. *J. Immunol.*, 149:1462–1469.
138. Umetsu, D.T., Ambrosio, D.M., Quinti, I., Siberg, G.R., and Gena, R.S. (1985): Recurrent sinopulmonary infection and impaired antibody response to bacterial capsular polysaccharide antigen in children with selective IgG-subclass deficiency. *N. Engl. J. Med.*, 313:1247–1251.
139. Valenti, W.M., Trudell, R.G., and Bentley, D.W. (1978): Factors predisposing to oropharyngeal colonization with gram-negative bacilli in the aged. *N. Engl. J. Med.*, 298:1108–1111.
140. Venet, A., Clavel, F., Israel-Biet, D., et al. (1985): Lung in acquired immune deficiency syn-

drome: infectious and immunological status assessed by bronchoalveolar lavage. *Bull. Eur. Physiopathol. Respir.,* 21:535–543.

141. Waldmann, T.A., Blaese, R.M., Broder, S., and Krakauer, R.S. (1978): Disorders of suppressor immunoregulatory cells in the pathogenesis of immunodeficiency and autoimmunity. *Ann. Intern. Med.,* 88:226–238.

142. Wallace, J.M., Barbers, R.G., Oishi, J., and Prince, H. (1984): Cellular and T-lymphocyte subpopulation profiles in bronchoalveolar lavage fluid from patients with acquired immunodeficiency syndrome and pneumonitis. *Am. Rev. Respir. Dis.,* 130:786–790.

143. Wilson, R., Pitt, T., Taylor, G., Watson, D., MacDermot, J., Sykes, D., Roberts, D., and Cole, P. (1987): Pyocyanin and 1-hydroxyphenazine produced by *Pseudomonas aeruginosa* inhibit the heating of human respiratory cilia *in vitro. J. Clin. Invest.,* 79:221–229.

144. Wong, L.B., Miller, I.F., and Yeates, D.B. (1988): Stimulation of ciliary beat frequency by automatic agonists: *in vitro. J. Appl. Physiol.,* 65:971–981.

145. Wood, R.E., Boat, T.F., and Doershuk, C.F. (1976): Cystic fibrosis: state of the art. *Am. Rev. Respir. Dis.,* 113:833–878.

146. Woods, D.E., Strauss, D.C., Johanson, W.G., Jr., and Bass, J.A. (1981): Role of salivary protease activity in adherence of gram-negative bacilli to mammalian buccal epithelial cells *in vitro. J. Clin. Invest.,* 68:1435–1440.

147. Yamaguchi, T., and Yamada, H. (1991): Role of mechanical injury on airway surface in the pathogenesis of *Pseudomonas aeruginosa. Am. Rev. Respir. Dis.,* 144:1147–1152.

148. Young, K.R., Rankin, J.A., Naegel, G.P., Paul, E.S., and Reynolds, H.Y. (1985): Bronchoalveolar lavage cells and proteins in patients with the acquired immunodeficiency syndrome: an immunologic analysis. *Ann. Intern. Med.,* 103:522–533.

149. Zierdt, C.H., and Williams, R.L. (1975): Serotyping of *Pseudomonas aeruginosa* isolates from patients with cystic fibrosis of the pancreas. *J. Clin. Microb.,* 1:521–526.

Respiratory Infections: Diagnosis and Management, 3d ed.,
edited by James E. Pennington.
Raven Press, Ltd., New York © 1994

2

Bacterial Colonization of the Respiratory Tract: Clinical Significance

Donald E. Woods

*Department of Microbiology and Infectious Diseases, University of Calgary,
3330 Hospital Drive, N.W., Calgary, Alberta, Canada T2N 4N1*

It is probable that the initiating event in the pathogenesis of most bacterial pulmonary infections is the establishment of the organisms in the upper respiratory tract (17). If the organisms are successful in avoiding elimination at this stage, their numbers increase and can reach sufficiently high concentrations to subsequently gain access to the lungs. Here, a failure of lung clearance mechanisms results in disease (39).

Evidence has accumulated to suggest that the initial event in colonization and invasion is the adherence of microorganisms to epithelial cells of mucosal surfaces (9,12). Organisms that are unable to adhere to mucosal surfaces are removed by secretions which bathe these surfaces and thus fail to colonize (24). The adherence process is dependent upon specific recognition systems between bacteria and epithelial cells. In this chapter we examine specific examples of adherence of bacterial pulmonary pathogens to upper respiratory tract cell surfaces and attempt to correlate adherence with subsequent infection.

THE COLONIZATION PROCESS

Bacteria may gain access to the pulmonary parenchyma by at least three routes. Organisms may enter the lung via the blood from an extrapulmonary source. They may also enter by inhalation of aerosolized bacterial particles (27,38). However, the majority of bacterial pulmonary infections are thought to follow endogenous aspiration of oropharyngeal bacteria. A variety of evidence supports this hypothesis. Instillation of bacteria intranasally into unanesthetized rabbits results in the appearance of the microorganisms in the lung within minutes (5). Also, occlusion of dog bronchii with sterile cotton plugs leading to atelectasis is associated with the recovery of pharyngeal organisms distant to the occlusion (20). Huxley et al. (14) investigated a proposal made originally by Amberson (2) that nocturnal aspiration of oropharyngeal secretions is a common event. They found that approximately 50% of normal subjects and 70% of subjects with impaired consciousness aspirate during sleep. As nonaspirating subjects were noted to sleep poorly during the study, the investigators proposed that everyone probably aspirates during deep sleep (14).

Inhaled bacteria are cleared by the lung much more efficiently than those introduced by aspiration. Aerosol deposition of 10^6 *Streptococcus pneumoniae* into the lungs of experimental animals causes no evident illness and the organisms are cleared rapidly. In contrast, intratracheal instillation of 10^3 of the same organism reproducibly causes pneumonia (3). It should be noted that oropharyngeal secretions contain over 10^7 organisms per ml, a significantly large challenge if presented to the lung by aspiration.

Thus, aspiration of oropharyngeal secretions occurs in normal individuals as well as those with impaired consciousness; large numbers of bacteria are introduced by aspiration, and the lung deals with bacteria presented in this manner poorly. Therefore, the bacterial composition of aspirated oropharyngeal secretions could be an important determinant of the etiology of pneumonia.

The factors that regulate the bacterial flora of the upper respiratory tract have been intensively studied. The neonate acquires oropharyngeal commensal organisms shortly after birth (6,13,25). It is believed that most of these indigenous oral organisms are acquired from the parents or attendants of the infants (35), because few of these organisms are free-living in nature (12). The resident pharyngeal flora remains constant over time in a given individual but differs among individuals (19). Exchange of flora between adult family contacts has been demonstrated (7), but it has not been shown to be of significance in the pathogenesis of bacterial pneumonia.

Gibbons (12) has reviewed factors that have been postulated to account for the selection of the resident bacterial flora of the mouth. Many of these factors, including pH, redox potential, temperature, nutrient supply, inhibitory substances such as lysozyme, and bacterial products such as bacteriocins, might be expected to influence the outcome of the selection process. However, because of the large variety of species in the oral cavity which coexist with each other in high proportions, Gibbons concluded that both the physical and the chemical conditions existing in the mouth most probably exert relatively weak selective influences. Although the upper respiratory tract is bathed with secretions which are in constant motion toward the pharynx, the resident bacterial flora of this region is not uniformly distributed. Rather, certain bacterial species exhibit a definite predilection for specific sites. The oral streptococci *S. sanguis* and *S. mutans* are found in highest proportion on the tooth surfaces, whereas *S. salivarius* favors the dorsal surface of the tongue, and *S. mitis* the buccal mucosa (10,21,22). It has been found that the microbial composition of a region is proportional to the relative abilities of the individual species to attach to the epithelial cells of that region (11,12,22). Thus, selective bacterial adherence to mucosal surfaces of the respiratory tract seems to be a major determinant of the indigenous bacterial flora. Organisms that are unable to attach to surfaces are removed by secretions and thus fail to maintain colonization (24).

Colonization of mucosal surfaces by newly acquired pathogenic bacteria can also be mediated by bacterial adherence and appear to involve both host and microbial factors. Aside from the nonspecific cleansing mechanisms operating to remove bacteria from mucosal surfaces, certain specific factors could influence the adherence of particular organisms to these surfaces. Oral secretions contain IgA antibodies which have been shown to coat various bacteria and prevent their adherence (40). Glycoproteins in saliva, which function as receptor analogues, specifically inhibit the adherence of certain bacteria (9). In conjunction with the aforementioned selective pressures, the availability of specific binding sites in a particular environment serve to select a certain population for any given mucosal surface.

The surface of eucaryotic cells plays an important and perhaps the central role in diverse biological phenomena including cell–cell recognition and intercellular adhesion. Although the precise chemical structure of the surface of any given cell type is largely undefined, there are some data available from immunological, histological, and chemical studies that greatly enhance our knowledge of cell surface interactions. These studies, reviewed by Roseman (29), show that cell surfaces are rich in carbohydrates, that is, the so-called glycocalyx. In general, the major carbohydrate fraction of eucaryotic cell surfaces consists of mixtures of glycoproteins and glycolipids. In mammalian cells, the glycolipids are primarily glycosphingolipids which may be divided into two groups, one containing sialic acid (the gangliosides) and the other (neutral glycolipids) containing uncharged sugars. The glycoproteins can be divided into two major classes, the serum-type glycoproteins and the mucins. The serum-type glycoproteins contain from one to three branched oligosaccharide chains attached to the protein core. The first sugar in the oligosaccharide chain is N-acetylglucosamine, glycosidically bound via the amide nitrogen atom of an asparagine residue in the protein. The second major class of glycoproteins are the mucins. Here, numerous short oligosaccharide chains, perhaps as many as 800, are found linked to an unusual polypeptide chain, via 0-glycoside bonds, to the hydroxyl groups in serine and threonine, whereas the major amino acids in the mucin polypeptide are serine, threonine, glycine, and proline. Thus, the cell surface can be visualized as a complex array of variously charged molecules, all of which presumably contribute to various cell surface functions, including those related to the process of heterologous intracellular adhesion, and, in particular, the interaction of eucaryotic cell surfaces with bacteria.

Long and Swenson (23) found a selective adherence of oral streptococci over *Escherichia coli* in studies of oral epithelial cells obtained from normal newborn infants. Other investigators have demonstrated that *Streptococcus pyogenes* adhere more readily to oral epithelial cells *in vitro* than enteropathogenic *E. coli* (8). In an earlier era, Bloomfield (4) found that viable gram-negative bacilli were rapidly removed from the upper respiratory tract of humans following experimental inoculation. These observations suggest that highly efficient mechanisms exist that serve to prevent colonization of the respiratory tract with enteric bacilli. Because the resistance of normal respiratory epithelial cells to colonization has been shown to persist *in vitro,* the mechanisms that exclude gram-negative bacilli appear to involve cell-associated factors. Discussion of these cell-associated factors must include the possibility of receptors on normal cells that are unavailable for the binding of gram-negative bacilli. It is therefore likely that persistence of gram-negative bacilli among the respiratory tract flora of seriously ill patients is due to their ability to adhere to epithelial cell surfaces that have been altered in some manner, allowing the microorganisms to escape mechanical removal.

We have demonstrated that colonization of the respiratory tract of seriously ill patients by gram-negative bacilli is, in every case, accompanied by *in vivo* adherence of the colonizing species to epithelial cells of the upper respiratory tract (18). Using a radioimmunoassay employing purified antibody to fibronectin (^{125}I-labeled), we demonstrated that there is, in fact, a decreased amount of fibronectin present on the surface of buccal cells from colonized patients relative to controls (42). In addition, using an ^{125}I-labeled fibrin plate assay, we demonstrated increased protease levels in the secretions from colonized patients over controls (42). Thus, an absolute correlation can be demonstrated between increased *P. aeruginosa* adherence, decreased cell surface fibronectin, and increased protease levels in secretions.

Although the loss of fibronectin is probably not the only *in vivo* alteration that leads to increased *P. aeruginosa* adherence, the correlation of fibronectin loss with increased adherence and increased salivary protease levels makes this hypothesis an attractive one. Further support for this was obtained from the results of a prospective study of patients undergoing elective coronary artery bypass surgery (44). The status of these patients shifts suddenly from relatively good health, to seriously ill, and back again to a healthy state in a relatively short time span averaging 5 days. In coronary artery bypass patients we have demonstrated a sequential departure from and return to normal values for *P. aeruginosa* adherence, buccal cell surface fibronectin, and salivary protease levels. *P. aeruginosa* adherence in these patients varied directly with salivary protease levels, whereas cell surface fibronectin varied inversely with adherence and protease levels (44).

In later studies, Simpson and colleagues (31,33) showed that fibronectin on the surface of oral epithelial cells blocks the binding of gram-negative bacilli including *E. coli* and *P. aeruginosa*. Ramphal (28) has also demonstrated that fibronectin blocks the binding of *P. aeruginosa* to tracheal epithelium. Furthermore, a number of studies have confirmed that gram-negative bacilli do not, in general, bind to fibronectin (26,34,36,37). Thus, it seems clear that cell surface fibronectin may serve, as Simpson (31) has stated, to "modulate" the composition of the oral flora.

The source of the fibronectin that resides on the surface of oral epithelial cells remains unclear; however, Simpson et al. (32) have demonstrated that salivary fibronectin or plasma fibronectin added exogenously to saliva can bind to buccal epithelial cells in the presence of whole saliva. Zetter et al. (46) have demonstrated that the fibronectin in the mucosa is confined to the surface of the epithelium exposed to the oral cavity, indicating that exogenous acquisition of fibronectin from saliva is a plausible hypothesis.

Our view of the process of gram-negative bacillary colonization of the upper respiratory tract states that there is an inverse relationship between cell surface fibronectin and gram-negative bacterial adherence to these cells (43). Although the source of the fibronectin that acts to block binding sites for gram-negative bacilli is an important concept, a more immediate problem is to define the source of the proteolytic activity that acts to remove fibronectin from the cell surface or to prevent its deposition thereon. We have demonstrated that *P. aeruginosa* proteases are able to degrade fibronectin (42); others have demonstrated that host proteases can also accomplish this (45). Subsequently, Wikström and Linde (41) examined the ability of a variety of oral bacteria to degrade fibronectin. In an examination of 116 strains for the ability to degrade fibronectin, the investigators concluded that fibronectin-degrading ability is a quality of bacterial species closely associated with soft tissue destruction (41). As a number of anaerobic bacteria were found to be positive in these studies, this might explain the strong association between anaerobic bacteria and aerobic gram-negative bacilli as etiologic agents of aspiration pneumonia.

Colonization of the upper respiratory tract by gram-negative bacilli is correlated with adherence of gram-negative bacilli to epithelial cells. Increased adherence is associated with a loss of fibronectin from the surface of oral epithelial cells. Thus, fibronectin has been described as a modulator of the composition of the oral flora. In fact, the "real" modulator of the oral flora is most likely the pathogenic determinant(s) that control the levels of protease activity in the oral secretions. It seems unlikely that this would be a single determinant, but would involve a series of complex interactive phenomena between host and oral bacterial flora components. The delineation of these interactions should, however, lead to a greater understanding of the pathogenesis of gram-negative bacillary pneumonia.

COLONIZATION VERSUS INFECTION

The distinction between a "colonizing" and an "infecting" organism cultured from a specimen obtained from the respiratory tract is often a difficult problem for the clinician. In most cases of community-acquired pneumonia, however, it is not a serious one. In cases of hospital-acquired pneumonia due to gram-negative bacilli, on the other hand, the presence of several different species of gram-negative bacilli in a single specimen makes the identification of the etiologic agent(s) of pneumonia difficult, to say the least. In cases of definite clinical symptoms of pneumonia (fever, purulent sputum, radiologic changes, etc.) the isolation and identification of the causative agent is normally accomplished with proper diagnostic procedures, discussed in later chapters. In the absence of clinical signs of infection, the presence of gram-negative bacilli in respiratory secretions should signal the clinician to vigilance.

Because the pharyngeal flora could be an important determinant of the etiology of pneumonia, the presence of gram-negative bacilli in the oropharynx might be expected to serve as a prelude to pneumonia by these organisms. Several studies have shown that gram-negative bacilli are not routinely present in the oropharynx of normal subjects. Only 2–18% of this population have been reported to harbor gram-negative bacilli at any given time, and such colonization has been documented to be transient, although its duration has not been defined (30). Studies by Johanson et al. (16) confirm these observations but demonstrate a striking increase in the prevalence of gram-negative bacilli isolated from oropharyngeal cultures obtained from seriously ill patients. Further, the authors conclude that the occurrence of colonization with gram-negative bacilli constitutes a definite hazard to the seriously ill patient, increasing the likelihood of subsequent pneumonia nearly tenfold over that of noncolonized but seriously ill patients (16). Suppression of the normal bacterial flora by antibiotics, with the subsequent emergence of a gram-negative flora, could not account entirely for these observations because many of the patients were colonized with gram-negative bacilli upon initial contact with medical services, and others had not received antibiotics in the hospital (16). Likewise, exogenous exposure through inhalation therapy could not be implicated in many of these patients. Thus, gram-negative bacillary pneumonia can develop in a group of patients whose pharyngeal flora has been modified as a result of illness per se, and under these circumstances can be independent of the usually incriminated exogenous sources.

CONCLUSIONS

Increasing emphasis has recently been placed on the role of adherence as a major factor in the infectious process. Evidence suggests that adherence is necessary for bacterial colonization and that, in many bacterial diseases, including pulmonary infections, it is the requisite initial event. Thus, bacterial colonization of the respiratory tract must be defined in terms of bacterial adherence to the mucosal surfaces of the respiratory tract. As only those organisms that adhere to the mucosal surfaces of this region will maintain colonization, perhaps it would be profitable to examine the "adherent" bacterial population of the oropharynx. If, indeed, the primary mode of bacterial entry into the lung is by aspiration of oropharyngeal contents, then a knowledge of the resident bacteria adherent to upper respiratory epithelium should allow a prediction of the etiologic agent of pneumonia.

ACKNOWLEDGMENTS

This work was supported in part by grants from the Medical Research Council of Canada and the Canadian Cystic Fibrosis Foundation.

REFERENCES

1. Abraham, S.M., Beachey, E.H., and Simpson, W.A. (1983): Adherence of *Streptococcus pyogenes, Escherichia coli,* and *Pseudomonas aeruginosa* to fibronectin-coated and uncoated epithelial cells. *Infect. Immun.,* 41:1261–1268.
2. Amberson, J.B., Jr. (1937): Aspiration bronchopneumonia. *Int. Anesthesiol. Clin.,* 3:126–138.
3. Ansfield, M.J., Woods, D.E., and Johanson, W.G., Jr. (1977): Lung bacterial clearance in murine pneumococcal pneumonia. *Infect. Immun.,* 17:195–201.
4. Bloomfield, A.L. (1920): The fate of bacteria introduced into the upper air passages, Vol. 5, The Friedländer bacillus. *Bull. Johns Hopkins Hosp.,* 31:203–206.
5. Cannon, P.R., and Walsh, T.E. (1937): Studies on the fate of living bacteria introduced into the upper respiratory tract of normal and intranasally vaccinated rabbits. *J. Immunol.,* 32:49–62.
6. Carlsson, J., Grahnen, H., Jonsson, G., and Wikner, S. (1970): Early establishment of *Streptococcus salivarius* in the mouths of infants. *J. Dent. Res.,* 49:415–481.
7. Dunlap, M.B., and Harvey, H.S. (1956): Host influence on upper respiratory flora. *N. Engl. J. Med.,* 255:640–646.
8. Ellen, R.P., and Gibbons, R.J. (1974): Parameters affecting the adherence and tissue tropisms of *Streptococcus pyogenes. Infect. Immun.,* 9:85–91.
9. Gibbons, R.J. (1977): Adherence of bacteria to host tissues. In: *Microbiology,* edited by D. Schlessinger, pp. 127–131. American Society for Microbiology, Washington, D.C.
10. Gibbons, R.J., Kapsimalis, B., and Socransky, S.S. (1964): The source of salivary bacteria. *Arch. Oral Biol.,* 9:101–103.
11. Gibbons, R.J., Spinell, D.M., and Skobe, Z. (1976): Selective adherence as a determinant of the host tropisms of certain indigenous and pathogenic bacteria. *Infect. Immun.,* 13:238–246.
12. Gibbons, R.J., and van Houte, J. (1975): Bacterial adherence in oral microbial ecology. *Ann. Rev. Microbiol.,* 29:19–44.
13. Hurst, U. (1957): Fusiforms in the infant mouth. *J. Dent. Res.,* 36:513–515.
14. Huxley, E.J., Viroslav, J., and Gray, W.R. (1978): Pharyngeal aspiration in normal adults and patients with depressed consciousness. *Am. J. Med.,* 64:564–568.
15. Johanson, W.G., Jr., Higuchi, J.H., Chaudhuri, T.R., and Woods, D.E. (1980): Bacterial adherence to epithelial cells in bacillary colonization of the respiratory tract. *Am. Rev. Respir. Dis.,* 121:55–63.
16. Johanson, W.G., Jr., Pierce, A.K., and Sanford, J.P. (1969): Changing pharyngeal bacterial flora of hospitalized patients. Emergence of gram-negative bacilli. *N. Engl. J. Med.,* 281:1137–1140.
17. Johanson, W.G., Jr., Pierce, A.K., and Sanford, J.P. (1972): Nosocomial respiratory infections with gram-negative bacilli. The significance of colonization of the respiratory tract. *Ann. Intern. Med.,* 77:701–706.
18. Johanson, W.G., Jr., Woods, D.E., and Chaudhuri, T. (1979): Association of respiratory tract colonization with adherence of gram-negative bacilli to epithelial cells. *J. Infect. Dis.,* 139:667–673.
19. Kraus, F.N., and Gaston, C.J. (1956): Individual constancy of numbers among the oral flora. *J. Bacteriol.,* 71:703–707.
20. Lansing, A.M., and Jamieson, W.G. (1976): Determinants of the developing oral flora in normal newborns. *Appl. Environ. Microbiol.,* 32:494–497.
21. Liljemark, W.F., and Gibbons, R.J. (1971): Ability of *Veillonella* and *Neisseria* species to attach to oral surfaces and their proportions present indigenously. *Infect. Immun.,* 4:264–268.

22. Liljemark, W.F., and Gibbons, R.J. (1972): Proportional distribution and relative adherence of *Streptococcus miteor (mitis)* on various surfaces in the human oral cavity. *Infect. Immun.*, 6:852–859.

23. Long, S.M., and Swenson, R.M. (1976): Determinants of the developing oral flora in normal newborns. *Appl. Environ. Microbiol.*, 32:494–497.

24. Mandel, I.D. (1976): Oral secretions and fluid flow. *J. Dent. Res.*, 55(Suppl.):22–37.

25. McCarthy, C., Snyder, M.K., and Parker, R. (1965): The indigenous oral flora of man. I. The newborn to the 1-year-old infant. *Arch. Oral Biol.*, 10:61–70.

26. Myhre, E.B., and Kuusela, P. (1983): Binding of human fibronectin to group A, C and G streptococci. *Infect. Immun.*, 40:29–34.

27. Pierce, A.K., and Sanford, J.P. (1973): Bacterial contamination of aerosols. *Arch. Intern. Med.*, 131:156–159.

28. Ramphal, R., and Pyle, M. (1985): Further characterization of the tracheal receptor for *Pseudomonas aeruginosa*. *Eur. J. Clin. Microbiol.*, 4:160–162.

29. Roseman, S. (1974): In: *The Cell Surface in Development*, edited by A. Moscona, pp. 255–271. John Wiley and Sons, New York.

30. Rosenthal, S., and Tager, I. (1975): Prevalence of gram-negative rods in the normal pharyngeal flora. *Ann. Intern. Med.*, 83:355–357.

31. Simpson, W.A., Courtney, H.S., and Beachey, E.H. (1982): Fibronectin—a modulator of the oropharyngeal bacterial flora. In: *Microbiology*, edited by D. Schlessinger, pp. 346–347. American Society for Microbiology, Washington, D.C.

32. Simpson, W.A., Courtney, H.S., and Beachey, E.H. (1985): Inhibition of the adhesion of *Escherichia coli* to oral epithelial cells by fibronectin. In: *Molecular Basis of Oral Microbial Adhesion*, edited by S.E. Mergenhagen and B. Rosen, pp. 40–44. American Society for Microbiology, Washington, D.C.

33. Simpson, W.A., Hasty, D.L., and Beachey, E.H. (1985): Binding of fibronectin to human buccal epithelial cells inhibits the binding of type 1 fimbriated *Escherichia coli*. *Infect. Immun.*, 48:318–323.

34. Stanislawski, L., Simpson, W.A., Hasty, D., Sharon, N., Beachey, E.H., and Ofek, I. (1985): Role of fibronectin in attachment of *Streptococcus pyogenes* and *Escherichia coli* to human cell lines and isolated oral epithelial cells. *Infect. Immun.*, 48:257–259.

35. Torrey, J.L., and Reese, M.K. (1944): Initial aerobic flora of newborn (premature) infants. *Am. J. Dis. Child.*, 67:89–99.

36. van de Water, L., Destree, A.T., and Hynes, R.O. (1983): Fibronectin binds to some bacteria but does not promote their uptake by phagocytic cells. *Science*, 220:201–204.

37. Vercellotti, G.M., Lussenhop, D., Peterson, P.K., Furcht, L.T., McCarthy, J.B., Jacob, H.S., and Moldow, C.F. (1984): Bacterial adherence to fibronectin and endothelial cells: a possible mechanism for bacterial tissue tropism. *J. Lab. Clin. Med.*, 103:34–43.

38. Wells, W.F. (1955): *Airborne Contagion and Air Hygiene.* Harvard University Press, Cambridge, Massachusetts.

39. Williams, D.M., Krick, J.A., and Remington, J.S. (1976): Pulmonary infection in the compromised host. *Am. Rev. Respir. Dis.*, 114:359–364.

40. Williams, R.C., and Gibbons, R.J. (1972): Inhibition of bacterial adherence by secretory immunoglobulin A: a mechanism for antigen dispersal. *Science*, 177:697–699.

41. Wikström, M., and Linde, A. (1986): Ability of oral bacteria to degrade fibronectin. *Infect. Immun.*, 51:707–711.

42. Woods, D.E., Bass, J.A., Johanson, W.G., Jr., and Straus, D.C. (1980): Role of adherence in the pathogenesis of *Pseudomonas aeruginosa* lung infection in cystic fibrosis patients. *Infect. Immun.*, 30:694–699.

43. Woods, D.E., Straus, D.C:, Johanson, W.G., Jr., and Bass, J.A. (1981): Role of fibronectin in the prevention of adherence of *Pseudomonas aeruginosa* to buccal cells. *J. Infect. Dis.*, 143:784–790.

44. Woods, D.E., Straus, D.C., Johanson, W.G., Jr., and Bass, J.A. (1981): Role of salivary protease activity in adherence of gram-negative bacilli to mammalian buccal epithelial cells *in vivo*. *J. Clin. Invest.*, 68:1435–1440.

45. Yamada, K.M. (1983): Cell surface interactions with extra-cellular materials. *Ann. Rev. Biochem.*, 52:761–799.

46. Zetter, B.R., Daniels, T.E., Quadra-White, C., and Greenspan, J.S. (1979): LETS protein in normal and pathologic human and oral epithelium. *J. Dent. Res.*, 58:484–488.

Respiratory Infections: Diagnosis and Management, 3d ed.,
edited by James E. Pennington.
Raven Press, Ltd., New York © 1994

3

Pulmonary Clearance of Infectious Agents

Galen B. Toews

*Division of Pulmonary and Critical Care Medicine, Department of Internal Medicine,
3916 Taubman Center, University of Michigan Medical Center,
Ann Arbor, Michigan 48109-0360*

The lungs are repeatedly inoculated with microorganisms from the upper airway and from inhaled aerosols and yet pneumonia rarely occurs. This fact implies the existence of efficient mechanisms of defense that are capable of eliminating microorganisms before their multiplication leads to clinical disease. Several comprehensive reviews have detailed the existence of a complex array of defense mechanisms spread throughout the entire respiratory tract from the nares to the alveolar surface (10,35). Defense of the lungs against harmful agents involves responses ranging from neural reflexes such as cough and bronchoconstriction to the initiation of inflammatory and humoral immune responses. This review will concentrate on the mechanisms involved in defense against microbes that reach the distal portion of the lung.

MODELS OF PULMONARY ANTIBACTERIAL DEFENSE

Experimental infections of the lower respiratory tract have been studied extensively since the turn of the century. The concept of an antibacterial defense mechanism intrinsic to the lung that was dependent on phagocytosis by macrophages was established by the early 1900s (1). From the 1920s through the 1950s this concept was extended and amplified as a consequence of a series of elegant studies of the pathogenesis of bacterial pneumonia (31,50,51,66–70). These studies clearly defined the histopathology of bacterial pneumonia; but the great majority of these studies, with the notable exception of those dealing with surface phagocytosis and heat labile opsonins, were descriptive rather than mechanistic. With the development of quantitative bacteriologic methods, it became possible to quantify the number of bacteria deposited in the respiratory tract and to follow changes with time (28). A rapid decrease in viable bacteria recovered from the lungs of challenged animals was noted at various time intervals after inoculation, and the term *pulmonary bacterial clearance* was coined to describe this process.

The entire sequence of events involved in bacterial clearance can be studied *in vivo*. Various routes of inoculation have been utilized. Intranasal inoculation of bacteria supposes that an upper respiratory inoculum will be aspirated into the lower respiratory tract and is seldom utilized. Aerosol deposition of bacteria allows exposure of a large number of small animals to a relatively uniform bacterial inoculum. An aerosol exposure deposits a large number of bacteria in the lung, but the bacteria are widely and uniformly dispersed resulting in a small bacterial burden in each anatomic focus. Deposition at the alveolar level is maximized and a physiologic analogue to droplet infection is achieved. Aerosol inoculation rarely leads to sufficient bacterial replication to cause pneumonia in normal animals even if the rate of bacterial clearance is decreased by experimental manipulations. Organisms may also be instilled directly into a localized area of lung through an endobronchial tube in a lightly anesthetized animal. The number of bacteria inoculated into a single anatomical location can be more accurately controlled than with the aerosol model. By appropriate manipulation of inoculum, it is possible to produce a high ratio of infectious agents to potential phagocytes. Since studies of normal animals and sleeping normal and comatose humans suggest that pharyngeal contents are commonly aspirated into focal areas of the lung, this technique may simulate the genesis of bacterial pneumonia in humans (18).

The percentage of an initial inoculum remaining at a subsequent time is quantified utilizing one of the following methods. Groups of animals are sacrificed immediately after inoculation and at various time intervals thereafter. The lungs are excised and homogenized to ensure the rupture of all phagocytic cells but not bacteria. Bacterial clearance is determined by dividing the number of organisms present at the later intervals by the mean number present at the time of inoculation (0 hour). An alternate method for computing bacterial clearance involves the use of radiolabeled bacteria. Animals are sacrificed at some interval after inoculation; the amount of radio-

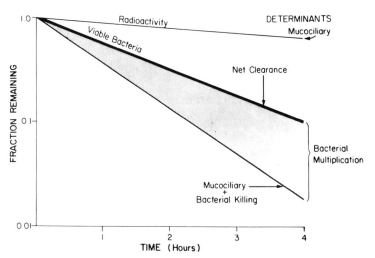

FIG. 3–1. The determinants of bacterial clearance are shown as the fraction of original counts (radioactivity and viable organisms) remaining in the lung at various post exposure times. Net bacterial clearance is depicted by the heavy black line. This is the variable measured in standard bacterial clearance experiments. In this example, viable bacteria have decreased to 10% of the initial inoculum by 4 hours. A small portion of this decrease is due to physical removal of bacteria by the mucociliary system as shown by the decrease in radioactivity. The lower line represents the combined effects of mucociliary clearance and *in situ* killing in the absence of bacterial multiplication. The decrease in viable bacteria is more pronounced if bacterial multiplication is prevented. The slower clearance rate shown by the heavy line is due to the effect of bacterial multiplication shown as a shaded area. Bacterial clearance can be altered by changes in the rates of any of these processes.

activity provides an index of the number of bacteria originally deposited in the lungs and bacterial cultures determine the number of viable organisms remaining at the chosen time period. These values are then utilized to calculate bacterial clearance as previously described.

PROCESSES INVOLVED IN BACTERIAL CLEARANCE

The term *bacterial clearance* has led to some confusion. The term *net bacterial clearance* is perhaps a more accurate term since this process is the net result of three independent processes (Fig. 3-1). These are physical transport out of the lung, phagocytosis and *in situ* killing, and bacterial multiplication (23). Analysis of the various processes involved in bacterial clearance allows determination of the rate-limiting factor for clearance of individual bacterial species under different circumstances. Different species of bacteria are cleared from the lung at markedly different rates. Disappearance of radiolabeled organisms is similar for all species studied, and the rate of bacterial killing greatly exceeds the rate of mucociliary transport. Species differences are likely due to different rates of bacterial multiplication and killing. Intracellular killing appears to be the rate-limiting factor in the inactivation of staphylococci in the normal lung. Some organisms are particularly resistant to phagocytosis and killing. In the case of *Klebsiella pneumoniae* or *Pseudomonas aeruginosa*, a net increase rather than clearance may occur, since intrapulmonary killing is slow and is exceeded by multiplication of this organism within the lung.

DETERMINANTS OF BACTERIAL CLEARANCE

Inoculum size, bacterial virulence, and the state of the host defenses determine the pathogenic potential of a bacterial challenge. Each of these determinants has been studied in animal models of bacterial clearance.

Inoculum Size

The magnitude of bacterial deposition which results in the development of pneumonia in man is not known. Early animal studies reported initial deposition values from 10^2 to 10^5 bacteria and concluded that the antibacterial defenses of the lung could not be overwhelmed by increasing the deposition of bacteria (29,65). However, inoculum size is clearly an important determinant of not only the rate of bacterial clearance but also of the cell type and magnitude of the phagocytic defense against bacteria (36,55). Pulmonary clearance of *Staphylococcus aureus* was clearly inoculum dependent; an inoculum of 10^5 organisms was rapidly and efficiently cleared by 4 hours, while clearance of an inoculum of 10^6 organisms was delayed but effective by 8 hours. However, an inoculum of 10^8 organisms was not cleared. Bacterial multiplication occurred within the lungs and eventually led to death of the animal. Thus, it is clear that inoculum size is an important determinant of the pathogenicity of a pulmonary bacterial challenge.

In addition, both the cell type and the magnitude of the phagocytic defense of the lung against bacteria are dependent on inoculum size. Small inocula of *S. aureus*

($<10^5$) appear to be rapidly cleared by the resident alveolar macrophages; however, larger inocula of *S. aureus* as well as gram-negative organisms require granulocytes for effective, although delayed, clearance. It appears that there are sufficient numbers of alveolar macrophages on alveolar surfaces to successfully ingest and kill certain inocula of bacteria but that larger inocula overwhelm the resident alveolar macrophages. The mechanism whereby alveolar macrophages sense that they are overwhelmed and need additional phagocytic help is unknown. These studies suggest that a critical bacteria–phagocyte ratio may have been exceeded, a factor of known importance in phagocytic studies *in vitro*. In addition, bacterial virulence factors may play some role in this process.

Bacterial Virulence

Bacterial species differ in their capacity for growth in the lung and in their capacity to cause parenchymal damage. These different degrees of pathogenicity are believed to be related to the presence or absence of microbial virulence factors.

The best characterized and probably most important virulence factor is a mucopolysaccharide capsule. The capsule prevents phagocytosis by macrophages and neutrophils in the absence of an effective opsonin. Pneumococci with large capsules (type III) tend to be more virulent than those with small capsules (9). The presence of a polysaccharide capsule is believed to be the most important virulence factor in *K. pneumoniae* pulmonary infection as well. However, the presence of a capsule was not important in clearance of *Hemophilus influenzae* from the lung: unencapsulated *H. influenzae* were cleared at the same rate as encapsulated *H. influenzae* (60).

A number of extracellular products may also play a role in bacterial virulence. *P. aeruginosa* produces a variety of extracellular enzymes and toxins (30); however, the importance of these substances in determining rates of bacterial clearance has not been systematically examined or firmly established. When different strains of *P. aeruginosa* were compared with respect to their *in vitro* production of these substances in an attempt to assess virulence factors, only strains producing extracellular lecithinase increased in numbers in the mouse lung (47). Recent studies have suggested that bacterial proteases may be responsible for the extensive destruction of alveolar walls, bronchial and arterial walls, hemorrhage, infarction, and abscess formation which occurs following inoculation of *P. aeruginosa* and high doses of *S. aureus*. Pneumococci also produce extracellular products, including pneumoloysin (a hemolytic enzyme), neuraminidase, and purpura producing principle (which causes dermal hemorrhage). It is unclear whether these toxins play a significant role in the pathogenesis of pneumococcal pneumonia.

The fact that some bacterial strains do not generate an effective opsonin may also be an important factor. Effective opsonization of many pneumococcal types is mediated nonspecifically by the alternative complement pathway which allows rapid phagocytosis and killing of these organisms. Certain pneumococcal types (types III, IV, and VIII) do not activate the alternative pathway unless specific antibody is present, and other types (type I) do not activate complement even in the presence of antibody (7). It is intriguing to speculate that the lack of nonspecific opsonization of these capsular types might underlie their propensity to cause pneumonia in humans.

STATUS OF THE HOST DEFENSES

Components of the pulmonary antibacterial defense system are present from the point of air entry in the upper respiratory tract to the point of gas exchange in the lower respiratory tract. This system includes the mucociliary apparatus, alveolar macrophages, and humoral factors such as complement, immunoglobin, and surfactant. Each of these components is present within normal pulmonary parenchyma and together constitute the resident antibacterial host defenses. The resident defenses inactivate day to day bacterial challenges (small inocula, avirulent organisms) very efficiently, but under certain circumstances bacteria overwhelm these defenses. Under these circumstances, resident defenses can be augmented by the development of an alveolar inflammatory response and the development of a humoral immune response.

Resident Pulmonary Antibacterial Defenses

Mucociliary clearance is of importance for particulates that are deposited in the airways but accounts for little clearance of organisms deposited on alveolar surfaces. Following aerosols of radiolabeled bacteria, greater than 90% of bacteria are present in the lungs after 4 hours even though only 10% are viable (28). The relative contribution of this mechanism to bacterial clearance following other routes of inoculation has not been studied.

The alveolar macrophage is the first line of phagocytic cellular defense against infectious agents that reach the alveolar surface. Components of the complement system are present in normal pulmonary secretions and are an important resident defense mechanism (11). Normal human lavage fluids contain a functional alternative complement pathway (43). C5 has been shown to be present in both rabbit and baboon lavage fluids (15,26). The concentrations of C4 and C6 in alveolar fluids suggest they are passively transudated from serum to respiratory secretions, whereas concentrations of C5 and Factor B suggest active local secretion of these later factors, perhaps by alveolar macrophages. Complement components are involved in pulmonary bacterial defenses by contributing opsonic and chemotactic fragments (14).

Alterations of any of these resident host defenses would be expected to alter pulmonary bacterial clearance. Alveolar hypoxia, pulmonary edema, acidosis, ethanol intoxication, and azotemia have all been shown to decrease net bacterial clearance. Environmental manipulations including exposure to cold, noxious gases, pollutants, and cigarette smoke also alter host defenses (24). Each of the above experimental manipulations is associated with increased susceptibility to lung infections in clinical medicine.

Viral infections have been shown to induce a variety of defects in alveolar macrophage bactericidal activity. Pulmonary viral infection suppressed *in vivo* pulmonary bactericidal activity by causing a defect in intracellular killing of *S. aureus* by alveolar macrophages (20,21). The host antiviral immune response may also play a role in the virus-induced defect in bacterial clearance. Addition of antiviral immune serum to virus-infected macrophages decreased the binding of *Candida,* decreased the ingestion of antibody-coated erythrocytes, and reduced the ingestion of *S. aureus* by alveolar macrophages (22). The exact role that each defect plays in the observed suppression of pulmonary antibacterial defenses is uncertain.

Immunosuppressive drugs also adversely affect pulmonary bacterial clearance by inducing local defects in host defenses (39,41). A combined regimen of cyclophosphamide plus cortisone inhibited clearance of Pseudomonas. A major component of the drug-induced defect was related to decreased number and function of local phagocytic cell populations (38). In addition to lowering the numbers of alveolar macrophages, immunosuppressive drugs decreased the bactericidal capabilities of alveolar macrophages. At relative high doses of cyclophosphamide, *in vitro* alveolar macrophage anti-*Pseudomonas* activity was decreased by 50% (37).

Alveolar Inflammatory Response

Effective early bacterial clearance depends on an intact capacity to develop an alveolar inflammatory response. The functional significance of polymorphonuclear neutrophils (PMNs) in early bacterial clearance has been shown by selectively depleting experimental animals of PMNs. Neutropenic animals were unable to clear inocula of *P. aeruginosa, K. pneumoniae, H. influenzae,* and *Streptococcus pneumoniae* as efficiently as normal animals (3,42,59). Although small inocula of some organisms may be cleared exclusively by alveolar macrophages, larger inocula of the same species, or inocula of gram-negative organisms, usually require recruitment of granulocytes to supplement the action of alveolar macrophages.

The mechanisms of granulocyte recruitment to alveolar spaces are being dissected. Because the development of a pulmonary inflammatory response after bacterial inoculation is dependent on bacterial species and inoculum size, it seems likely that the initiation of the response is dependent on the interaction of the bacterium and some component of the humoral or cellular resident defenses.

The initiation of an inflammatory response after bacterial entry into the lower respiratory tract involves the generation of intraalveolar chemotaxins (57,58,59,63). The specific chemotactic factors responsible for PMN recruitment have not been completely characterized. The C5 molecule and its fragments have been shown to be important chemotaxins in lung exposed to *S. aureus, S. pneumonia, H. influenza,* and *P. aeruginosa* (27,58,59). The mechanisms responsible for the cleavage of C5 into its chemotactic fragments in the lung is unknown. Bacteria might generate chemotactic fragments of C5 by activating the alternative pathway. Alternatively, the C5 may be cleaved by proteinases derived from alveolar macrophages (46).

Non–complement-derived chemotactic factor(s) are also involved in PMN recruitment following bacterial challenges (17,57,58,59). Numerous studies have demonstrated that alveolar macrophages produce inflammatory response modifiers (8,16,25,34) and generate products of arachidonic acid such as 5- or 11-monohydroxyeicosatetraenoic acid and leukotriene B4 (6,61).

Recently, studies have also defined a supergene family of small inducible protein mediators of inflammation. This group of cytokines, referred to as chemokines, are related by primary structural similarities and by the conservation of a four cysteine motif. The superfamily has two branches, classified according to the position of the first two cysteines in the conserved motif. The C-X-C branch, which includes IL-8, is characterized by the separation of the first two cysteines by an intervening amino acid (5,13,62). In the C-C branch, which contains RANTES, monocyte chemoattractant protein-1, and macrophage inflammatory protein-1, these two cysteines are directly adjacent (45). C-X-C molecules generally affect neutrophils while C-C cytokines affect monocytes (45).

These chemokines are produced by a variety of immune and nonimmune cells including blood mononuclear cells, macrophages, endothelial cells, fibroblasts, smooth muscle cells, and epithelial cells (2,32,44,48,49,52–54). Stimulus specificity for the elaboration of these chemokines has been demonstrated using exogenous and endogenous stimuli. Mononuclear phagocytes and endothelial cells have the ability to generate chemokines in response to microbial products such as lipopolysaccharides (LPS). In contrast, an endogenous host-derived stimulus, such as tumor necrosis factor (TNF) or interleukin-1 (IL-1), is required for the production of fibroblast or epithelial cell derived chemokines. This requirement for host-derived stimuli is demonstrative of cytokine networking where one cell population is dependent on mediators synthesized by neighboring cells (2,44,48,49,52–54).

The entry of microbes or microbial products into the lower respiratory tract likely initiates a complex series of events that result in the generation of an inflammatory response. Multiple chemotaxins are probably generated sequentially with some contributing to early inflammation, whereas others are involved at later times. The complement pathway is likely activated by the arrival of the microbes in the lower respiratory tract. Complement activation could occur via the alternative pathway or via the classical pathway if specific IgG antibody is present, generating the important early chemotaxin C5a. The microbe is also recognized by alveolar macrophages (AMs) which are anatomically positioned to provide a communication link between cells in the alveolus and the parenchyma of the lung. AMs probably play a central role in inflammatory cell recruitment by responding to microbial signals such as LPS which stimulates AMs to produce chemokines (52). In addition, LPS induces AM synthesis of TNF and IL-1, which act in a paracrine fashion to induce the synthesis of chemokines by cells of the alveolar wall. An interaction between AMs, alveolar epithelial cells, fibroblasts, and endothelial cells likely generate the chemotactic gradient which results in the directed movement of inflammatory cells from the vascular space into the interstitium and eventually into the alveolar spaces.

Humoral Immune Response

The role of antibody in resident bacterial defenses is uncertain, but immunization can clearly enhance antibacterial defenses in the lower respiratory tract. Immunization enhanced the clearance of aerosols of *P. aeruginosa* and *Proteus mirabilis* but did not augment the clearance of *S. pneumoniae* or *H. influenzae* (19). Systemic immunization enhanced pulmonary clearance of bolus inoculated *P. aeruginosa* and *H. influenzae* (4,12,40,56). Both IgG and IgM have been proposed as the class of immunoglobulin in alveolar fluids that enhances clearance. Since antibody specificities of serum and alveolar antibodies (determined by Western analysis) were identical, it is likely that alveolar antibodies were derived at least in part from serum (56). Passive immunization with opsonic IgG monoclonal antibody directed against nontypeable *H. influenzae* lipooligosaccharide results in both the appearance of this antibody in the alveolar spaces of unperturbed lungs and enhanced pulmonary clearance of nontypeable *H. influenzae,* which demonstrates an important role for serum antibody in the immunodefense of the lower respiratory tract (33).

SUMMARY

The appearance of a clinical infectious disease in the lung is largely determined by the success or failure of pulmonary defense mechanisms. This complex system is remarkably efficient, considering the probable frequency of challenge with microorganisms. Although a combination of mechanical barriers and the alveolar macrophage system effectively deal with many insults to the lung, if the burden of microorganisms is large or virulent, an inflammatory response is required for effective clearance. For optimal clearance in these circumstances, all components of the response need to be functional and coordinated. Not only must effector cells, responder cells, and mediators be present, but their action must be integrated. In addition, the development of a humoral immune response can augment the clearance of bacteria from the lower respiratory tract.

Studies of bacterial clearance have provided a framework for evaluating host–bacterial interactions in the lung. As this response is studied further, it is likely that increasing attention will be directed at the amplifying and inhibitory factors of cell–cell and cell–bacterial interactions, since characterization of these regulatory factors should offer possibilities for clinical control of infectious diseases in the future.

ACKNOWLEDGMENTS

This work was supported in part by NIH Grant P50-HL-46487 and funds from the Research Office of the Veterans Administration through funding of a Merit Review Grant.

REFERENCES

1. Briscoe, J.C. (1908): An experimental investigation of the phagocytic action of the alveolar cells of the lung. *J. Pathol. Bacteriol.,* 12:66–100.
2. Colotta, F., Borre, A., Ming Wamg, J., Tattanelli, M., Maddalena, F., Polentarutti, N., Peri, G., and Mantovani, A. (1992): Expression of a monocyte chemotactic cytokine by human mononuclear phagocytes. *J. Immunol.,* 148:760–765.
3. Dale, D.C., Reynolds, H.Y., Pennington, J.E., Pitts, T.W., and Graw, R.G. (1974): Granulocyte transfusion therapy of experimental *Pseudomonas pneumonia. J. Clin. Invest.* 54:664–671.
4. Dunn, M.M., Toews, G.B., Hart, D., and Pierce, A.K. (1985): The effects of systemic immunization on pulmonary clearance of *Pseudomonas aeruginosa. Am. Rev. Respir. Dis.,* 131:426–431.
5. Farber, J.M. (1990): A macrophage mRNA selectively induced by γ-interferon encodes a member of the platelet factor 4 family of cytokines. *Proc. Natl. Acad. Sci.,* USA, 87:5238–5242.
6. Fels, A.O.S., Pawlowski, N.A., Cramer, E.G., King, T.K.C., Cohn, Z.A., and Scott, W.A. (1982): Human alveolar macrophages produce leukotriene B₄. *Proc. Natl. Acad. Sci.,* USA, 79:7866–7870.
7. Fine, D.B. (1975): Pneumococcal type-associated variability in alternate complement pathway activation. *Infect. Immun.,* 12:772–778.
8. Gadek, J.E., Hunninghake, G.W., Zimmerman, R.L., and Crystal, R.G. (1980): Regulation of the release of alveolar macrophage-derived neutrophil chemotactic factor. *Am. Rev. Respir. Dis.,* 121:723–733.
9. Gaskel, J.F. (1927): Pathology of the lung. *Lancet,* 2:951–957.
10. Green, G.M., Jakab, G.J., Low, R.B., and Davis, G.S. (1977): Defense mechanisms of the respiratory membrane. *Am. Rev. Respir. Dis.,* 115:479–519.
11. Gross, G.N., Rehm, S.R., and Pierce, A.K. (1978): The effect of complement depletion on lung clearance of bacteria. *J. Clin. Invest.,* 62:373–378.
12. Hansen, E.J., Hart, D.A., McGehee, J.L., and Toews, G.B. (1988): Immune enhancement of pulmonary clearance of nontypable *Haemophilus influenzae. Infect. Immun.,* 56:182–190.

13. Haskil, S., Peace, A., Morris, J., Sporn, S.A., Anisowicz, A., Lee, S.W., Smith, T., Martin, G., Ralph, P., and Sager, R. (1990): Identification of three related human GRO genes encoding cytokine functions. *Proc. Natl. Acad. Sci., USA*, 87:7732–7736.
14. Heidbrink, P.J., Toews, G.B., Gross, G.N., and Pierce, A.K. (1982): Mechanisms of complement-mediated clearance of bacteria from the murine lung. *Am. Rev. Respir. Dis.*, 124:517–520.
15. Henson, P.M., McCarthy, K., Larsen, G.L., Webster, R.O., Giclas, P.C., Dreisen, R.B., King, T.E., and Shaw, J.O. (1979): Complement fragments, alveolar macrophages and alveolitis. *Am. J. Pathol.*, 97:93–110.
16. Hunninghake, G.W., Gadek, J.E., Fales, H.M., and Crystal, R.G. (1980): Human alveolar macrophage-derived chemotactic factor for neutrophils: stimuli and partial characterization. *J. Clin. Invest.*, 66:473–483.
17. Hunninghake, G.W., Gallin, J.I., and Fauci, A.S. (1978): Immunologic reactivity of the lung: the *in vivo* and *in vitro* generation of a neutrophil chemotactic factor by alveolar macrophages. *Am. Rev. Respir. Dis.*, 117:15–23.
18. Huxley, E.J., Viroslav, J., Gray, W.R., and Pierce, A.K. (1978): Pharyngeal aspiration in normal adults and patients with depressed consciousness. *Am. J. Med.*, 64:564–568.
19. Jakab, G.J. (1976): Factors influencing the immune enhancement of intrapulmonary bactericidal mechanisms. *Infect. Immun.*, 14:389–398.
20. Jakob, G.J., and Dick, E.C. (1973): Synergistic effect in viral-bacterial infection: combined infection of the murine respiratory tract with Sendai virus and *Pasteurella pneumotropia*. *Infect. Immun.*, 8:762–768.
21. Jakab, G.J., and Green, G.M. (1976): Defect in intracellular killing of *Staphylococcus aureus* within alveolar macrophage in Sendai virus-infected murine lungs. *J. Clin. Invest.*, 57:1535–1539.
22. Jakab, G.J., and Warr, G.A. (1981): Immune-enhanced phagocytic dysfunction in pulmonary macrophages infected with Parainfluenza I (Sendai) virus. *Am. Rev. Respir. Dis.*, 124:575–581.
23. Jay, S.J., Johanson, W.G., Jr., Pierce, A.K., and Reisch, J.S. (1976): Determinants of lung bacterial clearance in normal mice. *J. Clin. Invest.*, 57:811–817.
24. Kass, E.H., Green, G.M., and Goldstein, E. (1966): Mechanisms of antibacterial action in the respiratory system. *Bact. Rev.*, 30:488–497.
25. Kazmierowski, J.A., Gallin, J.I., and Reynolds, H.Y. (1977): Mechanism for the inflammatory response in primate lungs, demonstration and partial characterization of an alveolar macrophage-derived chemotactic factor with preferential activity for polymorphonuclear leukocytes. *J. Clin. Invest.*, 59:273–281.
26. Kolb, W.P., Kolb, L.M., Wetzel, R.A., Rogers, W.R., and Shaw, J.O. (1981): Quantitation and stability of the fifth component of complement (C5) in bronchoalveolar lavage fluids obtained from nonhuman primates. *Am. Rev. Respir. Dis.*, 123:226–231.
27. Larsen, G.L., Mitchel, B.C., Harper, T.B., and Henson, P.M. (1982): The pulmonary response of C5 sufficient and deficient mice to *Pseudomonas aeruginosa*. *Am. Rev. Respir. Dis.*, 126:306–311.
28. Laurenzi, G.A., Berman, L., First, M., and Kass, E.H. (1964): A quantitative study of the deposition and clearance of bacteria in the murine lung. *J. Clin. Invest.*, 43:759–768.
29. Libertoff, J., and Huber, G. (1973): The *in situ* inactivation of inhaled bacteria by the pulmonary alveolar macrophage. *J Cell Biol.*, 59:194A.
30. Liu, P.V. (1974): Extracellular toxins of *Pseudomonas aeruginosa*. *J. Infect. Dis.*, 130:594–599.
31. Loosli, C.G. (1942): The histogenesis of cells in experimental pneumonia in the dog. *J. Exp. Med.*, 75:657–672.
32. Matsusshima, K., and Oppenheim, J.J. (1989): Interleukin 8 and MCAF: novel inflammatory cytokines inducible by IL-1 and TNF. *Cytokine*, 1:2–13.
33. McGehee, J.L., Radlof, J.D., Toews, G.B., and Hansen, E.J. (1989): Effect of primary immunization on pulmonary clearance of nontypable *Haemophilus influenzae*. *Am. J. Respir. Cell Mol. Biol.*, 1:201–210.
34. Merrill, W.W., Naegel, G.P., Matthay, R.A., and Reynolds, H.Y. (1980): Alveolar macrophage derived chemotactic factor, kinetics of *in vitro* production and partial characterization. *J. Clin. Invest.*, 65:268–276.
35. Newhouse, M., Sanchis, J., and Bienenstock, J. (1976): Lung defense mechanisms. *N. Engl. J. Med.*, 295:990–998 and 1045–1052.
36. Onofrio, J.M., Toews, G.B., Lipscomb, M.F., and Pierce, A.K. (1983): Granulocyte-alveolar macrophage interactions in the pulmonary clearance of *Staphylococcus aureus*. *Am. Rev. Respir. Dis.*, 127:335–341.
37. Pennington, J.E. (1977): Bronchoalveolar cell response to bacterial challenge in the immunosuppressed lung. *Am. Rev. Respir. Dis.*, 116:885–893.
38. Pennington, J.E. (1977): Quantitative effects of immunosuppression on bronchoalveolar cells. *J. Infect. Dis.*, 136:127–131.
39. Pennington, J.E., and Harris, E.A. (1981): Influence of immunosuppression on alveolar macrophage chemotactic activities in guinea pigs. *Am. Rev. Respir. Dis.*, 123:299–304.

40. Pennington, J.E., Hickey, W.F., Blackwood, L.O., and Arnaut, M.A. (1981): Active immunization with lipopolysaccharide Pseudomonas antigen for chronic Pseudomonas bronchopneumonia in guinea pigs. *J. Clin. Invest*, 68:1140–1148.

41. Pennington, J.E., Matthews, W.J., Jr., Marino, J.T., Jr., and Colten, H.R. (1979): Cyclophosphamide and cortisone acetate inhibit complement biosynthesis by guinea pig bronchoalveolar macrophages. *J. Immunol.*, 123:1318–1321.

42. Rehm, S.R., Gross, G.N., and Pierce, A.K. (1980): Early bacterial clearance from murine lungs: species-dependent phagocyte response. *J. Clin. Invest.*, 66:194–199.

43. Robertson, J., Coldwell, J.R., Castle, J.R., and Waldman, R.H. (1976): Evidence for the presence of components of the alternative (properdin) pathway of complement activation in respiratory secretions. *J. Immunol.*, 117:900–903.

44. Rolfe, M.W., Kunkel, S.L., Standiford, T.J., Phan, S., Burdick, M.D., and Strieter, R.M. (1992): Expression and regulation of human pulmonary fibroblast-derived monocyte chemotactic peptide (MCP-1). *Am. J. Physiol. (Lung Cell. Mol. Physiol. 7)*, 263:L536–L545.

45. Schall, T.J. (1991): Biology of the RANTES/SIS cytokine family. *Cytokine*, 3(3):165–183.

46. Snyderman, R., Skin, H.S., and Dannenberg, A.M. (1977): Macrophage proteinase and inflammation: the production of chemotactic activity from the fifth component of complement by macrophage proteinase. *J. Immunol.*, 109:896–898.

47. Southern, P.M., Mays, B.B., Pierce, A.K., and Sanford, J.P. (1970): Pulmonary clearance of *Pseudomonas aeruginosa*. *J. Lab. Clin. Med.*, 76:548–559.

48. Standiford, T.J., Kunkel, S.L., Basha, M.A., Chensue, S.W., Lynch, J.P., Toews, G.B., and Strieter, R.M. (1990): Interleukin-8 gene expression by a pulmonary epithelial cell line: a model for cytokine networks in the lung. *J. Clin. Invest.*, 86:1945–1953.

49. Standiford, T.J., Kunkel, S.L., Phan, S.H., Rollins, B.J., and Strieter, R.M. (1991): Alveolar macrophage-derived cytokines induce monocyte chemoattractant protein-1 expression from human pulmonary type II like epithelial cells. *J. Biol. Chem.*, 266:9912–9918.

50. Stillman, E.G. (1923): The presence of bacteria in the lungs of mice following inhalation. *J. Exp. Med.*, 38:117–126.

51. Stillman, E.G., and Branch, A. (1924): Experimental production of pneumococcus pneumonia in mice by the inhalation method. *J. Exp. Med.*, 40:733–742.

52. Strieter, R.M., Chensue, S.W., Basha, M.A., Standiford, T.J., Lynch, J.P., and Kunkel, S.L. (1990): Human alveolar macrophage gene expression of interleukin-8 by TNF-α, LPS and IL-1β. *Am. J. Respir. Cell Mol. Biol.*, 2:321–326.

53. Strieter, R.M., Kunkel, S.L., Showell, H., Remick, D.G., Phan, S.H., Ward, P.A., and Marks, R.M. (1989): Endothelial cell gene expression of a neutrophil chemotactic factor by TNF-α, LPS, and IL-1β. *Science*, 243:1467–1469.

54. Strieter, R.M., Phan, S.H., Showell, H.J., Remick, D.G., Lynch, J.P., Genard, M., Raiford, C., Eskandari, M., Marks, R.M., and Kunkel, S.L. (1989): Monokine-induced neutrophil chemotactic factor gene expression in human fibroblasts. *J Biol. Chem.*, 264:10621–10626.

55. Toews, G.B., Gross, G.N., and Pierce, A.K. (1979): The relationship of inoculum size to lung bacterial clearance and phagocytic cell response in mice. *Am. Rev. Respir. Dis.*, 120:559–566.

56. Toews, G.B., Hart, D.A., and Hansen, E.J. (1985): Effect of systemic immunization on pulmonary clearance of *Haemophilus influenzae* type b. *Infect. Immun.*, 48:343–349.

57. Toews, G.B., and Pierce, A.K. (1984): The fifth component of complement is not required for the clearance of *Staphylococcus aureus*. *Am. Rev. Respir. Dis.*, 129:82–86.

58. Toews, G.B., and Vial, W.C. (1984): The role of C5 in polymorphonuclear leukocyte recruitment in response to *Streptococcus pneumoniae*. *Am. Rev. Respir. Dis.*, 129:82–86.

59. Toews, G.B., Vial, W.C., and Hansen, E.J. (1985): Role of C5 and recruited neutrophils in early clearance of nontypable *Haemophilus influenzae* from murine lungs. *Infect. Immun.*, 50:207–212.

60. Toews, G.B., Viroslav, S., Hart, D.A., and Hansen, E.J. (1984): Pulmonary clearance of encapsulated and unencapsulated *Haemophilus influenzae* strains. *Infect. Immun.*, 45:437–442.

61. Valone, F.H., Franklin, M., Sun, G.G., and Goetzl, E.J. (1985): Alveolar macrophage lipoxygenase products of arachidonic acid: isolation and recognition as the predominant constituents of the neutrophil chemotactic activity elaborated by alveolar macrophages. *Cell Immunol.*, 54:390–401.

62. Vanguri, P., and Farber, J.M. (1990): Identification of CRG-2. *J. Biol. Chem.*, 265:15049–15057.

63. Vial, W.C., Toews, G.B., and Pierce, A.K. (1984): Early pulmonary granulocyte recruitment in response to *Streptococcus pneumoniae*. *Am. Rev. Respir. Dis.*, 129:87–91.

64. Ward, P.A., Lepow, I.H., and Newman, L.J. (1968): Bacterial factors chemotactic for polymorphonuclear leukocytes. *Am. J. Path.*, 52:725–736.

65. Warshauer, D., Goldstein, E., Hoeprich, P.D., and Lippert, W. (1974): Effect of vitamin E and ozone on the pulmonary antibacterial defense mechanisms. *J. Lab. Clin. Med.*, 83:228–240.

66. Wood, W.B., Jr. (1941): Studies on the mechanism of recovery in pneumococcal pneumonia. I. The action of type specific antibody upon the pulmonary lesion of experimental pneumonia. *J. Exp. Med.*, 73:201–222.

67. Wood, W.B., Jr., and Irons, E.N. (1946): Studies on the mechanisms of recovery in pneumococcal pneumonia. II. The effect of sulfonamide therapy upon the pulmonary lesion of experimental pneumonia. *J. Exp. Med.*, 84:365–376.
68. Wood, W.B., Jr., McLeod, C., and Iron, E.B. (1946): Studies on the mechanism of recovery in pneumococcal pneumonia. III. Factors influencing the phagocytosis of pneumococci in the lung during sulfonamide therapy. *J. Exp. Med.*, 84:377–386.
69. Wood, W.B., Jr., and Smith, M.R. (1950): Host–parasite relationships in experimental pneumonia due to pneumococcus Type III. *J. Exp. Med.*, 92:85–90.
70. Wood, W.B., Jr., Smith, M.R., and Watson, B. (1946): Studies on the mechanism of recovery in pneumococcal pneumonia. IV. The mechanism of phagocytosis in the absence of antibody. *J. Exp. Med.*, 84:387–402.

Respiratory Infections: Diagnosis and Management, 3d ed.,
edited by James E. Pennington.
Raven Press, Ltd., New York © 1994

4

Noninvasive Diagnostic Techniques for Lower Respiratory Infections

John A. Washington

Department of Microbiology, The Cleveland Clinic Foundation, 9500 Euclid Avenue, Cleveland, Ohio 44195-5140

The laboratory diagnosis of lower respiratory infection is complicated by the diversity of etiologic agents involved, the large number and multiple species of indigenous microorganisms in the mouth and pharynx, and the difficulty of obtaining suitable specimens by noninvasive techniques for microbiologic examination. Diagnosis is often suggested by the patient's age, clinical presentation, underlying disease, environmental factors, and other laboratory results. Therefore, special attention must be given to the selection of an appropriate specimen and the proper procedures for its examination. Listed in Table 4-1 are the specimens for isolation and tests for detection of lower respiratory tract pathogens. As shown in Table 4-1, expectorated sputum may be helpful in the diagnosis of pneumonias due to aerobic and facultatively anaerobic bacteria, *Legionella,* mycobacteria, *Nocardia, Mycoplasma,* and fungi. Because of the magnitude and diversity of anaerobic bacteria normally present in the mouth, expectorated sputum is not suitable for the diagnosis of anaerobic pulmonary infections. In contrast to the situation with bacterial, mycobacterial, and fungal pneumonias, upper respiratory specimens are preferred for the diagnosis of chlamydial and viral pneumonias. In some instances, the only reliable means of determining the etiologic agent is by invasive means or serologic tests (Table 4-1). The laboratory can be most helpful when a tentative diagnosis is provided on the test order form and tests to detect specific microorganisms or their antigens or antibodies are requested.

SPECIMEN COLLECTION AND TRANSPORT

Microbiological examination of sputum can yield valuable diagnostic information rapidly and accurately, provided certain guidelines and precautions are followed. The most important guideline is that given to the patient concerning specimen collection. The simplistic directive to "spit in the jar" is often rewarded with a specimen consisting solely or predominantly of saliva, the microscopic and microbiologic characteristics of which need no further documentation in the literature or on the patient's chart and contribute nothing—and, often, misleading information—for the patient's care. It is imperative, therefore, for the patient to be instructed properly and to be supervised by a physician, nurse, or respiratory therapist to obtain secre-

TABLE 4–1. *Specimens for isolation and tests for detection of lower respiratory tract pathogens[a]*

Organism	Specimen	Microscopy	Culture	Serology	Other
Bacteria					
Aerobic and facultatively anaerobic	Expectorated sputum, blood, TTA, PSB, BAL, empyema fluid, lung biopsy	Gram stain	X		
Anaerobic	TTA, empyema fluid, tissue, abscess, PSB	Gram stain	X		
Legionella	Sputum, lung biopsy, pleural fluid, TTA, serum	IFA	X	IFA	Gene probe; IA (urine)
Nocardia	Expectorated sputum, TTA, bronchial washings, tissue, abscess	Gram and/or modified carbol fuchsin stain	X		
Chlamydia	Nasopharyngeal or throat swab, lung aspirate or biopsy, serum	IFA	X	IFA for *C. trachomatis* and *C. pneumoniae* and CF for *C. psittaci*	PCR for *C. trachomatis*
Mycoplasma	Expectorated sputum, nasopharyngeal swab, serum		X	CF, IFA, or MI; cold agglutinins	
Mycobacteria	Expectorated or induced sputum, tissue, gastric washings	Carbol fuchsin or fluorochrome stain	X		PPD
Fungi					
Deep-seated					
Blastomyces	Expectorated or	KOH with	X	CF, ID	
Coccidioides	induced sputum,	phase-		CF, ID, LA	
Histoplasma	TTA, bronchial washing or biopsy, tissue, serum	contrast, GMS stain		CF, ID	
Opportunistic					
Aspergillus	Lung biopsy, serum	H & E, GMS stain	X	ID	
Candida	Lung biopsy, serum	H & E, GMS stain	X	ID, LA	
Cryptococcus	Expectorated sputum, serum	H & E, GMS stain	X	LA	
Zygomycetes	Expectorated sputum, tissue	H & E, GMS stain	X		
Viruses	Nasopharyngeal washings (respiratory syncytial), pharyngeal swab (adenovirus, influenza, parainfluenza), lung biopsy, serum	IFA	X	CF, HI, neutralization, IA	
Pneumocystis	Lung biopsy, TTA, bronchial brushings or washings induced sputum	Toluidine blue, Giemsa, or GMS stain, IFA			

Adapted from Bartlett et al. (6) and Washington (37).

[a]Abbreviations: PSB, protected specimen brush; BAL, bronchoalveolar lavage; TTA, transtracheal aspirate; KOH, potassium hydroxide; GMS, Gomori methenamine silver; H & E, hematoxylin and eosin; IFA, immunofluorescent antibody; CF, complement fixation; HI, hemagglutination inhibition; ID, immunodiffusion; LA, latex agglutination; MI, metabolic inhibition; EM, electron microscopy; IA, immunoassay; PCR, polymerase chain reaction.

tions resulting from a deep cough. The patient should be told specifically that naso-pharyngeal secretions and saliva or spit are not sputum. An essential ingredient of this procedure is an alert and cooperative patient who is able to follow instructions. Seriously ill and debilitated patients are often unable to follow instructions and are therefore unable to provide anything other than their copious oropharyngeal secretions which may include small and often imperceptible amounts of lower respiratory secretions. It is a daily occurrence for laboratory personnel calling about an unacceptable sputum specimen to be told by nursing personnel that collection of another specimen would be difficult because the patient is comatose or has a nonproductive cough. The requirement for good specimens is not unique to sputum collected for bacterial culture and was recognized over 70 years ago by Laird (22), who correlated the gross and microscopic appearance of sputum with the rate of recovery of tubercle bacilli from cases with tuberculosis (Table 4-2).

In patients with suspected mycobacterial or fungal pulmonary infections, a series of three successive, single, early-morning specimens should be collected. Pooled 12- to 24-hour sputum collections are subject to bacterial overgrowth and therefore are not recommended.

Although most patients with pneumonia have productive coughs, some may require aerosol induction of sputum with hypertonic (3 to 10%) salt solution or, if this procedure is unproductive, gastric aspiration (1) or an invasive procedure (see Chapter 5).

Sputum specimens must be collected in a sterile, leakproof, screw-capped jar. Since the exterior of the jar may become contaminated, jars with specimens from patients with suspected tuberculosis should be placed in a water-tight plastic bag for transport to the laboratory (1).

Sputum can seldom be collected from children under the age of 10 years. Because of the high upper respiratory carrier rates of potential bacterial pathogens in infants and children, neither nasopharyngeal nor tracheal (unless obtained under direct laryngoscopic visualization) aspirates are reliable for determining the bacterial etiology of pneumonia in this age group (25). For these reasons, thoracenteses, lung punctures, or taps, have been suggested in critically ill children from whom isolation of the etiologic agent is required for proper management, in those who have deteriorated during therapy, and in immunocompromised children (21). Blood cultures may also be helpful in these cases.

In suspected viral respiratory infections, throat swabs are probably adequate for recovering adenoviruses; however, nasopharyngeal swabs or even washings are probably superior for recovering respiratory syncytial, influenza, and parainfluenza viruses (7). Neither the composition of the swab nor that of the transport medium

TABLE 4–2. *Correlation between character of sputum and recovery of tubercle bacilli from 541 cases*

Group	Appearance	Predominant cells	Patients	
			No.	No. positive (%)
1	Watery or mucoid	Squamous epithelial	94	2 (2.1)
2	Purulomucoid	Squamous epithelial	147	13 (8.8)
3	Purulomucoid	Leukocytes	91	54 (59.3)
4	Mucopurulent	Leukocytes	144	110 (76.3)

Adapted from Laird (22).

appears critical for the survival of respiratory viruses. In suspected *Chlamydia trachomatis* pneumonitis, a throat swab or nasopharyngeal or tracheal aspirate in sucrose-phosphate (2 SP) transport medium is necessary for recovery of this organism. The isolation of *C. pneumoniae* (TWAR) has proven to be difficult in tissue culture so that the diagnosis of pneumonia due to this agent is more accurately made by the microimmunoflourescence antibody test, particularly with the use of IgM- and IgG-specific conjugates (14). Compared with the microimmunoflourescence antibody test, the sensitivity of culture is in the range of 55 to 75%. It also appears that the use of the polymerase chain reaction (PCR) technique provides a level of sensitivity that exceeds that of culture by 25% (14).

As a general rule, sputum specimens should be transported promptly to the laboratory for processing. Transportation delays of lower respiratory secretions for 2 to 5 hours at room temperature result in reduced isolation rates of pneumococci, staphylococci, and gram-negative bacilli and increased numbers of microorganisms which are indigenous to the upper respiratory tract (19). Specimens for mycobacterial culture which cannot be processed immediately or must be transported to another laboratory for processing should be refrigerated, while those which must be shipped to a reference laboratory should be treated with a solution of cetylpyridinium chloride and sodium chloride (32). Although it is desirable to perform fungal cultures with freshly collected sputum specimens, most clinically significant fungi do appear to tolerate 4 to 5 days of transport and storage (16). Specimens for viral culture should be transported in the cold using cold packs or wet ice but should *not* be frozen. Sucrose-phosphate (2 SP) transport medium for *C. trachomatis* should be shipped on dry ice or frozen at $-70°C$ when the specimen cannot be processed within 24 hours.

When shipping specimens by mail, it is mandatory to comply with federal regulations governing the shipment of etiologic agents and specifying minimum packaging requirements. These include sealing the specimen in a screw-capped tube or jar, placing the tube or jar in a metal can with absorbent material, packing the can in an approved mailing or shipping container, and affixing to the container a label designating the package as containing etiologic agents. These regulations are not designed to discourage shipment of specimens or cultures, but rather to protect the shippers and those receiving the specimen for processing.

DIRECT EXAMINATION OF SPUTUM

Microscopic

Cytology

The cytologic characteristics of inflammatory cells in sputum were thoroughly reviewed and beautifully illustrated by von Hoesslin (36) in 1926 but were generally neglected by those interested in nonmalignant pulmonary disease for nearly half a century. Although helpful in differentiating chronic bronchial diseases (8), the major value of microscopic examination of sputum is to determine that the specimen collected for examination is from the lung. This procedure should be performed routinely with any sputum specimen that has been submitted to the laboratory for bacterial culture. The procedure is basically that described by Chodosh (8), in which a strand or fleck of dense purulent material is transferred from the specimen container

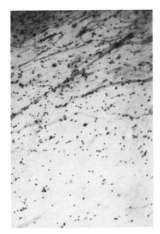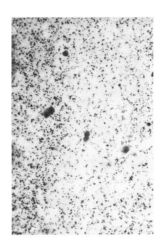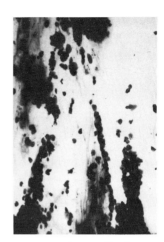

FIG. 4–1. Smears of representative sputum specimens (gram stain; original magnification, ×
100). Leukocytes >25/lpf, squamous epithelial cells <10/lfp (*left*); leukocytes >25/lpf, squamous epithelial cells <25 lpf (*middle*); leukocytes <10/lpf, squamous epithelial cells >25 lpf
(*right*). Specimens represented on the left and in the center are acceptable for bacterial culture,
while that on the right is not. (Reproduced with permission from Murray and Washington [27].)

to a petri dish using the frayed ends of a splintered applicator stick or a wire needle
or loop. A drop-sized portion of this material is applied to a glass microscope slide
and examined microscopically under low-power magnification (× 100), either as a
wet preparation under reduced illumination or stained with buffered aqueous crystal
violet or as a fixed gram-stained preparation. Initially, it may be helpful to the microbiologist to review a number of slides with a cytopathologist to gain familiarity
with the various cell types seen in sputum; however, with some practice, squamous
epithelial cells, which have exfoliated from the oral cavity and pharynx, can be readily differentiated from bronchiolar-alveolar and inflammatory cells, which have exfoliated from the tracheobronchial tree (Fig. 4-1).

Various criteria based on cytologic characteristics have been suggested for scoring
the quality of sputum specimens. Most criteria are based on those recommended by
Bartlett (Table 4-3) wherein only those specimens with scores of 1 to 3 are cultured
(4). Murray and Washington (27) found that specimens with more than 10 squamous
epithelial cells (SEC) per low-power field (lpf) yielded similar numbers of species
(4.2 to 4.4), regardless of the number of leukocytes and alveolar macrophages present, in contrast to the 2.4 to 2.7 species found in specimens with less than 10 SEC/
lpf and in transtracheal aspirates. The researchers concluded that such specimens

TABLE 4–3. *Criteria for scoring the quality of lower respiratory secretions*

Cells or characteristics per low-power field	Score
10–25 neutrophils	+1
>25 neutrophils	+2
Mucus	+1
10–25 squamous cells	−1
>25 squamous cells	−2

Adapted from Bartlett (4).

should be considered unacceptable for culture. Although this rejection criterion was challenged by one of my colleagues (35), the dilemma as to what constitutes reasonable objective evidence of excessive oropharyngeal contamination appears to have been resolved by Geckler et al. (13), who performed a parallel cytologic and microbiologic analysis of sputa and transtracheal aspirates from patients with clinical and radiographic evidence of pneumonia and found that the results of cultures of sputum containing >25 SEC/lpf showed poor agreement with those of transtracheal aspiration, regardless of the number of leukocytes that were present.

Based on the findings of Geckler et al. (13), it seems reasonable to recommend that a gram-stained smear be prepared from a selected portion of all sputum specimens submitted to the laboratory for bacteriologic examination, that several fields be examined microscopically under low-power magnification (10× objective; ×100 magnification), and that another specimen be requested when there are >25 SEC/lpf, regardless of the number of leukocytes present. Similar criteria should be applied to tracheal aspirates. Because of the clinical importance of the isolation of *Mycobacterium tuberculosis* and the majority of other mycobacterial species, and because of the selective nature of decontaminating specimens and culturing for mycobacteria, cytologic screening of sputum specimens submitted for this purpose is not generally indicated (9). It must, however, still be emphasized that there is a significantly higher probability of recovery of tubercle bacilli from specimens with a predominance of leukocytes (Table 4-2) (22). It is probably safe to assume that the same principles are true of specimens submitted for fungal culture.

Stained and Unstained Preparations for Microbial Detection

Direct microscopic examination of fixed stained or of stained or unstained wet mount preparations can often provide the earliest and, in some instances, the only etiologic diagnosis of lower respiratory infection. For most purposes, it is adequate to have a compound binocular microscope with low-power (10×), high dry (40×), and oil immersion (100×) objectives; 8 or 10× widefield oculars; a mechanical stage; and a good light source. Phase contrast microscopy is desirable for examining wet mount preparations. Fluorescence microscopy can be used to identify the presence of certain microorganisms in specimens (e.g., *Legionella* and certain viruses) but it requires special equipment and training.

The reagents and techniques required for performing stains and wet mount preparations are described elsewhere (37) in detail and will not be considered in this chapter.

Gram-Stained Smear

The gram-stained smear can be used for cytologic examination of sputum, as described above. Gram-stained smears of acceptable specimens should then be examined under oil immersion (×1000 magnification) to determine whether bacteria of a specific or characteristic morphologic type are present. Neither the fields being examined nor any of the immediately adjacent fields should contain any squamous epithelial cells, but there should be present at least several inflammatory cells or other cells originating in the tracheobronchial tree (3). Examples of characteristic gram-stained morphologies of *Streptococcus pneumoniae, Hemophilus influenzae, Moraxella catarrhalis,* and enteric bacilli in sputum are illustrated in Figure 4-2.

Baigelman et al. (3) quantitated the number of morphologic types of bacteria in sputa from patients with bronchial disease and found, by using the mean number of organisms per oil immersion field ($\times$ 1000) plus 3 standard deviations, that $\geq$12 organisms resembling *H. influenzae,* $\geq$8 resembling *S. pneumoniae,* or $\geq$18 resembling *Neisseria (Moraxella)* clearly separated patients with acute bacterial exacerbations from those in three other groups: recovery from acute bacterial exacerbations, acute allergic exacerbations, and stable states. Similarly, in a study of patients with community-acquired pneumonia, Rein et al. (29) found that $\geq$10 gram-positive lancet-shaped diplococci per oil immersion field predicted the isolation of pneumonococci in sputum cultures in about 90% of cases (Table 4-4). It appears, therefore, that the gram-stained smear of sputum is a useful test in the evaluation of patients with community-acquired pneumonia.

Although it has been stated that the importance of the initial gram-stained smear of sputum cannot be overemphasized in the evaluation of gram-negative pneumonias (34), there have been few reports of the sensitivity, specificity, or predictive (positive or negative) values of the gram-stained smear of sputum in such patients. Tillotson and Lerner (34) noted that gram-negative bacilli were seen in smears of all sputum specimens and empyema fluids from 20 cases of *Escherichia coli* pneumonia. Noone and Rogers (28) noted that 19 of 20 patients with gram-negative pneumonia had pus

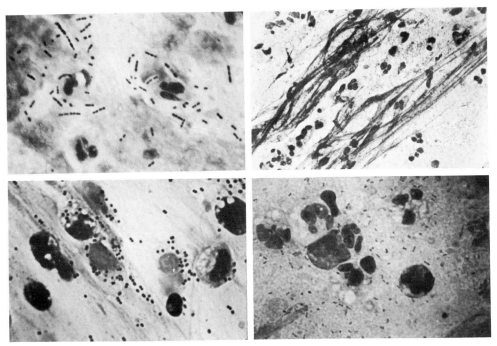

FIG. 4–2. Gram-stained smears of sputum (original magnification, $\times$ 1000), demonstrating organisms with morphology characteristic of *Streptococcus pneumoniae* (*upper left*), *Hemophilus influenzae* (*upper right*), *Moraxella catarrhalis* (*lower left*), and enteric bacilli (*lower right*).

TABLE 4–4. *Accuracy of gram-stained smear in identifying pneumococci in sputum*

Criteria	Sensitivity	Specificity	Posterior probability[a]
Gram-positive, lancet-shaped diplococci:		%	
any field	83	38	75
>10/o.i.f.[b]	55	85	89
preponderant or > 10/o.i.f.[b]	62	85	90
preponderant	48	100	100

Adapted from Rein et al. (29).
[a]Probability that patient with pneumonia and positive gram-stained smear has pneumococci in sputum.
[b]o.i.f., oil immersion field ($\times$ 1,000).

cells and profuse numbers of gram-negative bacilli in sputum smears. The interpretation of these findings, however, is complicated by studies demonstrating approximately 10^7 colony-forming units (cfu) per milliliter of gram-negative bacilli in saline gargles from aspiration-prone patients (i.e., chronic alcoholics, diabetics) (23) and up to 10^8 cfu/ml of gram-negative bacilli in sputum from intensive care unit patients without evidence of infection (20).

Acid-Fast Smear

The acid-fast smear provides the first evidence of the presence of mycobacteria in approximately half of culture-positive specimens for *Mycobacterium tuberculosis* (15). A higher correlation between smears and cultures occurs in specimens from patients with extensive disease and in those with far advanced cavitary disease. False-positive acid-fast smears are rare in experienced hands (15). Carbol fuchsin (e.g., Kinyoun, Ziehl-Neelsen) and fluorochrome (i.e., auramine-rhodamine) stains have equivalent sensitivity and specificity (37); however, since carbol fuchsin–stained smears must be examined under oil immersion (95 $\times$ objective), and fluorochrome-stained smears can be examined under lower power magnification (25 $\times$ objective), it is possible to scan a much larger area more rapidly with the fluorochrome method. *Nocardia* can be seen in auramine-rhodamine-stained smears but may not be seen in carbol fuchsin–stained smears unless the decolorizer is modified (37).

Potassium Hydroxide Wet Mount Preparation

Examination of a potassium hydroxide (KOH) wet mount preparation by a trained observer may allow definitive diagnosis of blastomycosis, cryptococcosis, and coccidioidomycosis within a few minutes of the specimen's arrival in the laboratory (Fig. 4-3) (30). Filamentous fungi may also be detected.

Immunologic

Quellung Reaction

The quellung reaction, resulting from an interaction between bacterial capsular polysaccharide and homologous capsular antibody, has been used to identify the

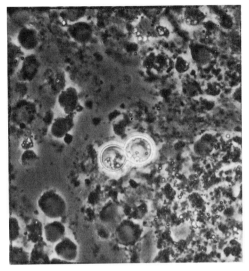
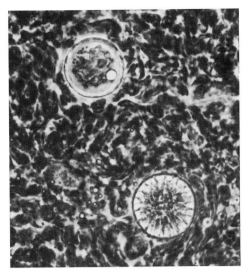
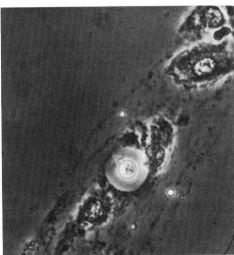

FIG. 4–3. Potassium hydroxide (KOH) wet mount preparations (phase contrast; original magnification, × 2000) of sputum. *Blastomyces dermatitidis* (*top left*), demonstrating characteristic yeast form with budding cell attached by broad base and "double contoured" cell wall. *Cryptococcus neoformans* (*bottom left*), demonstrating spherical cell surrounded by large capsule with small bud arising from parent cell. *Coccidioides immitis* (*top right*), demonstrating large thick-walled spherules with few endospores scattered within interior of upper spherule and cleavage furrows developing along periphery of lower spherule to form endospores. (Reproduced with permission from Roberts [30].)

presence of pneumococci in sputum specimens from patients with pneumonia. The test is performed by applying a drop of polyvalent pneumococcal antiserum (Omniserum, Statens Seruminstitut, Copenhagen, Denmark) to an air-dried loopful of sputum spread over an area 0.5–1 cm in diameter on a glass slide and an equal amount of 1% aqueous methylene blue onto a coverslip which is inverted over the preparation and blotted lightly (2). The preparation is then examined with reduced illumination under oil immersion (× 1000 magnification) for the quellung or capsular swelling process. The procedure is simple and rapid and was found to correlate with the results of culture in 89% of cases by Merrill et al. (24).

Counterimmunoelectrophoresis and Coagglutination

Counterimmunoelectrophoresis (CIE) has been used to detect microbial antigens because of its speed. In pneumococcal pneumonia, antigen is detected frequently in sputum, less often in urine, and infrequently in serum. Pneumococcal antigen is also frequently detected in patients with chronic bronchitis but without pneumonia (12). Edwards and Coonrod (12) found that the results of CIE and coagglutination of sputum were similar in patients with pneumococcal pneumonia prior to antibiotic therapy but that coagglutination was significantly more sensitive (and technically simpler) than CIE during antibiotic therapy. Coagglutination may, therefore, be useful diagnostically in patients who have already begun antibiotic therapy and from whom, as a consequence, pneumococci are unlikely to be cultured (33). Because of its greater technical complexity and lower sensitivity, CIE has been largely abandoned in clinical laboratories. CIE has been less satisfactory in the detection of other microbial antigens in sputum.

Direct Immunofluorescence

The most frequent application of direct immunofluorescence (IF) to the examination of sputum is in the detection of *Legionella* sp. Using positive cultures or antibody titers to define Legionnaires' disease, Edelstein et al. (11) found that the sensitivity of direct IF of respiratory tract secretions was 50% but that the test's specificity was 94%. Moreover, it was found that sputum consistently contained more bacilli per smear than specimens collected transtracheally or bronchoscopically, perhaps because of the smaller or more diluted amounts of specimens obtained by these procedures. Direct immunofluorescence using monoclonal, instead of polyclonal, antibody provides greater sensitivity and less background fluorescence in examining specimens for *Legionella pneumophila*.

Direct IF may also be used to detect *Chlamydia trachomatis* influenza A and B viruses; parainfluenza 1, 2, and 3 viruses; adenovirus; and respiratory syncytial virus in nasopharyngeal and throat swab specimens (7). Strict criteria for interpretation of IF patterns are required to ensure maximum specificity (7).

Radioimmunoassay and Enzyme-Linked Immunosorbent Assay

Solid-phase radioimmunoassay (RIA) and a sandwich-type enzyme-linked immunosorbent assay (ELISA) to detect antigen in urine have been found to be specific and sensitive methods for diagnosing Legionnaires' disease (31). The ELISA technique is not as rapid as RIA but is a technically simpler and less expensive test to perform than RIA.

Gene Probes and Amplification

Gene probes have become commercially available for the detection or identification of *Legionella, Mycobacterium avium complex, M. tuberculosis, M. gordonae, Mycoplasma pneumoniae, Blastomyces dermatitidis,* and *Histoplasma capsulatum.* Although there are ample data establishing the accuracy of the mycobacterial probes for the rapid identification of these species, in cultures, data are more limited on the use of the *Legionella* and *Mycoplasma pneumoniae* probes for detection of these organisms in respiratory specimens and on the use of the *Blastomyces* and *Histoplasma* probes for the identification of these organisms in cultures.

The use of gene probes is becoming rapidly affected by the advent of gene ampli-fication technology, such as polymerase chain or ligase reaction, which provides rapid amplification of a small amount of genetic material that may be present in a specimen to a sufficient quantity that the nucleic acid sequence characteristic of a specific microorganism can be readily detected. This technology is evolving ex-tremely rapidly and encompasses virtually the entire spectrum of microbial diseases. Its most obvious application is in the detection of microorganisms for which existing methodologies of detection do not exist, are very labor intensive, or are very slow. The price of this technology will force careful consideration of its application and careful analysis of its cost-efficiency. Gene amplification, for example, for the de-tection of *Mycoplasma pneumoniae* might be of limited benefit in young, previously healthy patients who present with signs and symptoms characteristic of atypical pneumonia and who are then treated empirically. On the other hand, with the rising incidence of *Mycobacterium tuberculosis* and the risk posed, particularly by multi-ple drug-resistant strains, to other patients and to health care workers the sensitivity and speed of detection of this organism may justify the added expense of the use of gene amplification technology for early detection, despite the fact that culture would still be necessary for the isolation of colonies of *M. tuberculosis* to determine their drug susceptibilities.

CULTURAL EXAMINATION OF SPUTUM

The diagnosis and treatment of lower respiratory infections depends in most in-stances on cultural examination of respiratory tract secretions or tissue. Isolation of the etiologic agent permits its definitive identification and, in many instances, deter-mination of its susceptibility to antibiotic and chemotherapeutic agents. As a general rule, the approaches selected are those that offer maximum sensitivity for isolation of the microorganisms most likely to be causing respiratory infection. Whereas the procedures for bacterial cultures are usually quite nonspecific, those for mycobac-terial, fungal, and viral cultures are usually highly specific. The diagnostic value of all of these procedures, however, remains directly related to the quality of the spec-imen examined.

The discussion that follows on the cultural examination of respiratory secretions will be limited to essential principles. A detailed description of methods for an ex-amination of cultures is given elsewhere (37).

Bacteria

Because of the variety of potentially pathogenic bacteria and general lack of se-lective media for separating pathogenic from nonpathogenic species in cultures, the single most important step in the process of bacterial culture of sputum is proper specimen collection. Attempts have been made to differentiate between pathogenic and nonpathogenic bacteria in sputum on the basis of quantitative cultures or reduc-ing the amount of indigenous flora by washing or freeze-cracking. Conclusions have been reached and recommendations made in the majority of such studies without validation by cultures of concurrently obtained transtracheal aspirates. Bartlett and Finegold (5) did, however, compare the results of quantitative cultures of washed and unwashed liquefied sputum with those of transtracheal aspiration and found that the washing procedure decreased the concentrations of contaminants in purulent sputum 1000-fold to a mean of $10^{2.1}$ cfu/ml and that the mean numbers of potential pathogens isolated concurrently from transtracheal aspirates and sputum specimens were $10^{6.5}$ and $10^{6.6}$ cfu/ml, respectively. The number of unwashed sputum specimens yielding contaminants in concentrations exceeding 10^6 cfu/ml was 70%, in contrast to 26% for washed sputum specimens. Bartlett and Finegold (5) concluded, however, that their wash-quantitative culture technique would be impractical for routine use in the clinical laboratory but might be reserved as an alternative to transtracheal aspiration for difficult cases.

Since Bartlett and Finegold (5) found that potential pathogens were present in sputum at mean concentrations of $10^{6.6}$ cfu/ml, which would correspond approximately to the growth of at least five colonies in the third streak area on a conventionally inoculated agar plate, grading of growth, as shown in Table 4-5, is generally advised in conventionally plated cultures (6). By using such a grading system, identification can be restricted to predominant colonies (3 to 4 +), assuming, of course, that the culture was of a microscopically acceptable specimen in the first place (6). Identification of organisms present in smaller numbers can then be limited to circumstances in which clinical information or gram-stained smear findings suggest it would be useful. Some may still prefer to report diphtheroids, coagulase-negative staphylococci, and neisseriae as usual or normal oral flora, regardless of their numbers, unless their predominance in the gram-stained smear of the specimen suggests an etiologic role. The predominance, for example, of gram-negative diplococci in a sputum smear (Fig. 4-2) strongly suggests the possibility of respiratory infection due to *Neisseria meningitidis* or *Moraxella* (formerly *Branhamella*) *catarrhalis*. Similarly, the predominance of small, gram-negative coccobacilli (Fig. 4-2) is strongly suggestive of the diagnosis of *Hemophilus* pneumonia. In these instances, the gram-stained smear findings greatly assist in the interpretation of the culture results.

The accuracy of identifying isolates in sputum cultures is markedly improved when organisms which are present in predominance in the smear and have characteristic morphology (e.g., pneumococci) are specifically sought in cultures. In other words, gram-stained smear results should be used to direct the efforts of the technologist examining the culture (17).

Procedures that are not recommended in sputum bacteriology include the use of highly sensitive procedures, such as broth cultures, or of highly selective media. Anaerobic cultures are never indicated because of the large number and variety of gram-positive and gram-negative anaerobic bacteria which are normally present in the oropharynx; however, anaerobic incubation has been reported to increase the yield of pneumococci from sputum cultures (16).

TABLE 4–5. *Semiquantitative grading of growth on streaked agar plates*

Grade	Colonies in consecutive streak areas		
	First	Second	Third
1 +	<10	—	—
2 +	>10	<5	—
3 +	>10	>5	—
4 +	>10	>5	>5

Adapted from Bartlett (6).

Isolates of *Staphylococcus aureus,* the Enterobacteriaceae, and *Pseudomonas aeruginosa* would ordinarily be subjected to antimicrobial susceptibility testing. In cases of suspected *Moraxella* or *Hemophilus* pneumonia, isolates should be tested for β-lactamase production.

Blood cultures should not be overlooked as a means of identifying the bacterial etiology of pneumonia.

Legionella

The diagnosis of legionellosis is usually made, as discussed earlier in this chapter, by the direct or indirect immunofluorescent antibody (IFA) test; however, it is also possible to isolate the organism from sputum with a selective buffered charcoal yeast extract medium containing vancomycin or cefamandole, polymyxin B and anisomycin (10). Growth appears in an average of 3 days on this medium and may be confirmed as being *Legionella* by the direct IFA test. Despite the incorporation of inhibitors in the medium, growth of resistant organisms other than *Legionella* may occur.

Because of the variable sensitivity of the direct fluorescent antibody stain and the time lag required for development of antibody, it is mandatory that cultures for *Legionella* be performed whenever the diagnosis is clinically suspected. More specifically, cultures should be part of the routine protocol for examining respiratory secretions for the presence of *Legionella.*

Mycobacteria

Sputum inevitably contains a multitude of non-acid-fast contaminants which can rapidly overgrow the usually slower growing mycobacteria on culture media (20 to 22 hour generation time). Because of the high lipid content of their cell walls, mycobacteria are more resistant to strong acid or alkaline solutions than are the non-acid-fast contaminants. Hence, sputum submitted for mycobacterial culture is ordinarily treated (digested) with a chemical (e.g., N-acetyl-L-cysteine or dithriothreitol plus 2% NaOH) to reduce the numbers of non-acid-fast contaminants and to liquefy mucus to expedite concentration of the remaining mycobacteria by centrifugation.

Concentrates are inoculated on either an egg- or agar-based solid medium and, increasingly throughout the United States, into a radiometric detection system (BACTEC 460, Becton Dickinson Diagnostic Instrument Systems, Sparks, MD) in which growth of mycobacteria is detected by the evolution of $^{14}CO_2$ from radiolabeled substrates in the medium. The major advantage of the radiometric system is the faster detection of mycobacterial growth. If sufficient growth is present, it is possible to use one of the commercially available gene probes for rapid identification; however, growth on solid agar often provides distinctive morphologic features that are characteristic of certain species. As a result, use of a solid medium in conjunction with the radiometric system is generally advisable.

It is estimated that a minimum of 10,000 acid-fast bacilli must be present per milliliter of sputum to be detected microscopically, whereas cultures will detect as few as 10 acid-fast bacilli per milliliter of digested and concentrated sputum. All specimens from patients with suspected mycobacterial infection should, therefore, be cultured. Susceptibility studies are indicated for isolates of *M. tuberculosis* because of the appearance of multidrug-resistant isolates. Testing is expedited by use of the BACTEC 460. Susceptibility testing of mycobacteria other than *M. tuberculosis* remains unstandardized, and the results are of uncertain clinical relevance.

It should be noted that not all clinical laboratories perform mycobacteriology and that, among those that do, various levels of mycobacteriologic services are performed, depending upon the workload and proficiency of the laboratory. Services may, therefore, extend from those of collection and transportation of specimens to those performing definitive mycobacterial identification and susceptibility testing.

Fungi

A variety of commercially prepared media are available for fungal cultures. Antibiotics, such as chloramphenicol and gentamicin, are usually incorporated in the medium to inhibit bacterial overgrowth. Cycloheximide is another useful additive to media when culturing contaminated specimens such as sputum for *Blastomyces dermatitidis, Coccidioides inmitis,* and *Histoplasma capsulatum;* however, it is inhibitory to most saprophytic and opportunistic filamentous fungi, as well as to *Cryptococcus neoformans* and some *Candida* species. Respiratory secretions should, therefore, be inoculated onto media with and without cycloheximide. All cultures should be incubated at 22° to 30°C for 4 weeks before being discarded as negative.

All isolates of filamentous fungi should be considered potential pathogens and identified with extreme caution in biological safety cabinets. The major identifying feature of filamentous fungi is the characteristic arrangement of spores. Definitive identification of *B. dermatitidis, C. immitis,* and *H. capsulatum,* however, usually entails the use of the exoantigen test by which antigen is extracted from the mold form of the fungus and tested by the immunodiffusion technique for lines of identity with the homologous antibody. Alternatively, a commercially available gene probe may be used for the identification of *Blastomyces* and *Histoplasma.* Although the clinical importance of isolates of *B. dermatitidis, C. immitis,* and *H. capsulatum* is seldom in doubt, that of other filamentous fungi is often uncertain and may only be established by demonstration of the fungus in tissue. Moreover, negative sputum cultures are notoriously unreliable in excluding the diagnosis of opportunistic pulmonary aspergillosis. The only reliable methods of diagnosis in such cases are invasive.

The frequency of isolation of yeasts from respiratory secretions is directly related to the extent of oropharyngeal contamination, on which basis Murray et al. (26) concluded that yeasts other than *C. neoformans* represent normal respiratory tract flora and do not merit further identification. They may be reported simply as "yeast present, not *Cryptococcus.*"

The diagnosis of deep mycotic infection due to *B. dermatitidis, C. immitis,* or *H. capsulatum* may be suggested by serologic testing of paired acute and convalescent samples. Single complement-fixing antibody titers of ≥1 : 64 to the yeast and mycelial phases of *H. capsulatum* and the presence of H and M precipitin bands are highly suggestive of histoplasmosis. Tests for antibody to *B. dermatitidis* have less sensitivity and specificity; however, complement-fixing titers of ≥1 : 8 are suggestive of recent or active disease and are highly suggestive of active disease when A or B precipitin bands are present.

Chlamydiae

Both *Chlamydia psittaci* and *Chlamydia trachomatis* can be readily isolated in tissue culture; however, because of its relative rarity in causing human infections, slow growth rate (7 to 10 days), and significant risk in causing laboratory-acquired infections, *C. psittaci* is not isolated from clinical specimens in most laboratories, and infection due to this agent is usually diagnosed serologically with a complement-fixation test. In contrast, *C. trachomatis* is a common cause of infection, is rapidly detected in tissue culture (2 to 3 days), and poses no special risk to laboratory workers. Cultures of nasopharyngeal secretions or nasotracheal aspirates are, therefore, useful in establishing the diagnosis of *C. trachomatis* pneumonia. Infants with *C. trachomatis* pneumonia rapidly develop high levels ($\geq 1 : 128$) of IgM antibody which can be readily detected by a microimmunofluorescent antibody test. Serology, therefore, is a suitable alternative to culture for the diagnosis of this respiratory tract infection.

As previously mentioned, the isolation of *Chlamydia pneumoniae* in tissue culture remains problematic, and the diagnosis is most accurately made by the microimmunofluorescence antibody test (14). Additional diagnostic sensitivity may become available in the future by the use of gene amplification technology.

Mycoplasma pneumoniae

Culture is not particularly useful as the primary method for diagnosing *M. pneumoniae* pneumonia because isolation of the organism requires a minimum of 4 to 6 days but may take up to 30 days. Hence, the diagnosis is usually established serologically. Approximately 50% of patients with *M. pneumoniae* pneumonia develop cold agglutinins, as do many patients with a variety of other infections; therefore, more sensitive and specific serology, such as immunoassay, is advised.

Viruses

The isolation of influenza, parainfluenza, respiratory syncytial, rhinoviruses, and coronaviruses from respiratory secretions has a high (90 to 100%) probability of association with respiratory tract disease (7). Moreover, provided there has been proper communication with the laboratory before initiating studies, collection of specimens early in the acute phase of illness, careful attention to specimen collection and transport, and avoidance of bacterial and fungal contamination of cultures, negative virological results can also be interpreted with a high degree of confidence (7).

Serology is not particularly useful as the primary method for diagnosing viral infections since definitive diagnosis must be based on conversion from sero-negativity to positivity, or a fourfold or greater antibody rise between acute and convalescent sera that have been collected 2 to 3 weeks apart. For retrospective diagnostic or epidemiologic purposes, however, paired (acute and convalescent) sera may be tested for antibodies to influenza A and B, respiratory syncytial, parainfluenza 1–3 and adenoviruses.

REFERENCES

1. American Thoracic Society. (1981): Diagnostic standards and classification of tuberculosis and other mycobacterial diseases, 14th edition. *Am. Rev. Respir. Dis.*, 123:343–358.
2. Austrian, R. (1976): The quellung reaction, a neglected microbiologic technique. *Mt. Sinai J. Med.*, 43:699–709.
3. Baigelman, W., Chodosh, S., Pizzuto, D., and Sadow, T. (1979): Quantitative sputum Gram stains in chronic bronchial disease. *Lung*, 156:265–270.
4. Bartlett, R.C. (1974): *Medical Microbiology: Quality Cost and Clinical Relevance*, p. 27. John Wiley and Sons, New York.
5. Bartlett J.G., and Finegold, S.M. (1978): Bacteriology of expectorated sputum with quantitative culture and wash technique compared to transtracheal aspirates. *Am. Rev. Respir. Dis.*, 117:1019–1027.
6. Bartlett, J.G., Ryan, K.J., Smith, T.F., and Wilson, W.R. (1987): *Cumitech 7A:* Laboratory diagnosis of lower respiratory tract infections. Coordinating editor, J.A. Washington II, pp. 1–18. American Society for Microbiology, Washington, D.C.
7. Chernesky, M.A., Ray, C.G., and Smith, T.F. (1982): *Cumitech 15:* Laboratory diagnosis of viral infections. Coordinating editor, W.L. Drew, pp. 1–17. American Society for Microbiology, Washington, D.C.
8. Chodosh, S. (1970): Examination of sputum cells. *N. Engl. J. Med.*, 282:854–857.
9. Curione, C.J., Kaneko, G.S., Voss, J.L., Hesse, F., and Smith, R.F. (1977): Gram stain evaluation of the quality of sputum specimens for mycobacterial culture. *J. Clin. Microbiol.*, 5:381–382.
10. Edelstein, P.H. (1987): The laboratory diagnosis of Legionnaires' disease. *Seminars in Respiratory Infections*, 2:235–241.
11. Edelstein, P.H., Meyer, R.D., and Finegold, S.M. (1980): Laboratory diagnosis of Legionnaires' disease. *Am. Rev. Respir. Dis.*, 121:317–327.
12. Edwards, E.A., and Coonrod, J.D. (1980): Coagglutination and counterimmunoelectrophoresis for detection of pneumococcal antigens in the sputum of pneumonia patients. *J. Clin. Microbiol.*, 11:488–491.
13. Geckler, R.W., Gremillion, D.H., McAllister, C.K., and Ellenbogen, C. (1977): Microscopic and bacteriological comparison of paired sputa and transtracheal aspirates. *J. Clin. Microbiol.*, 6:396–399.
14. Grayston, J.T. (1992): Infections caused by *Chlamydia pneumoniae* strain TWAR. *Clin. Infect. Dis.*, 15:757–763.
15. Greenbaum, M., Beyt, B.E., and Murray, P.R. (1980): The accuracy of diagnosing pulmonary tuberculosis at a teaching hospital. *Am. Rev. Respir. Dis.*, 121:477–481.
16. Hariri, A.R., Hempel, H.O., Kimberlin, C.L., and Goodman, N.L. (1982): Effects of time lapse between sputum collection and culturing on isolation of clinically significant fungi. *J. Clin. Microbiol.*, 15:425–428.
17. Heineman, H.S., and DiAntonio, R.R. (1982): Bacteriology of sputum—purpose, significance, problems, and role in diagnosis. In: *Significance of Medical Microbiology in the Care of Patients*, 2nd edition, edited by V. Lorian, pp. 169–196. Williams and Wilkins, Baltimore, MD.
18. Howden, R. (1976): Use of anaerobic culture for the improved isolation of *Streptococcus pneumoniae. J. Clin. Pathol.*, 29:50–53.
19. Jefferson, H., Dalton, H.P., Escobar, M.R., and Allison, M.J. (1975): Transportation delay and the microbiological quality of clinical specimens. *Am. J. Clin. Pathol.*, 64:689–693.
20. Johanson, W.G., Jr., Pierce, A.K., Sanford, J.P., and Thomas, G.D. (1972): Nosocomial respiratory infections with gram-negative bacilli: the significance of colonization of the respiratory tract. *Ann. Intern. Med.*, 77:701–706.
21. Klein, J.O. (1992): Bacterial pneumonias. In: *Textbook of Pediatric Infectious Diseases*, edited by R.D. Feigin and J.D. Cherry, pp. 299–309. W.B. Saunders, Philadelphia.
22. Laird, A.T. (1909): A method for increasing the diagnostic value of sputum reports. *J.A.M.A.*, 52:294–296.
23. Mackowiak, P.A., Martin, R.M., Jones, S.R., and Smith, J.W. (1978): Pharyngeal colonization by gram-negative bacilli in aspiration-prone persons. *Arch. Intern. Med.* 138:1224–1227.
24. Merrill, C.W., Gwaltney, J.M., Hendley, J.O., and Sande, M.A. (1973): Rapid identification of pneumococci: gram stain vs. the quellung reaction, *N. Engl J. Med.*, 288:510–512.
25. Mimica, I., Donoso, E., Howard, J.E., and Ledermann, G.W. (1971): Lung puncture in the etiological diagnosis of pneumonia; a study of 543 infants and children. *Am. J. Dis. Child.*, 122:278–282.
26. Murray, P.R., Van Scoy, R.E., and Roberts, G.D. (1977): Should yeasts in respiratory secretions be identified? *Mayo Clin. Proc.*, 52:42–45.
27. Murray, P.R., and Washington, J.A., II (1975): Microscopic and bacteriologic analysis of expectorated sputum. *Mayo Clin. Proc.*, 50:339–344.

28. Noone, P., and Rogers, B.T. (1976): Pneumonia caused by coliforms and *Pseudomonas aeruginosa. J. Clin. Pathol.,* 29:652–656.
29. Rein, M.F., Gwaltney, J.M., Jr., O'Brien, W.M., Jennings, R.H., and Mandell, G.L. (1978): Accuracy of Gram's stain in identifying pneumococci in sputum. *J.A.M.A.,* 239:2671–2673.
30. Roberts, G.D. (1975): Detection of fungi in clinical specimens by phase-contrast microscopy. *J. Clin. Microbiol.,* 2:261–265.
31. Sathapatayavongs, B., Kohler, R.B., Wheat, L.J., White, A., Winn, W.C., Jr., Ginod, J.C., and Edelstein, P.H. (1982): Rapid diagnosis of Legionnaires' disease by urinary antigen detection. Comparison of ELISA and radioimmunoassay. *Am. J. Med.,* 72:576–582.
32. Smithwick, R.W., Stratigos, C.B., and David, H.L. (1975): Use of cetylpyridinium chloride and sodium chloride for the decontamination of sputum specimens that are transported to the laboratory for the isolation of *Mycobacterium tuberculosis. J. Clin. Microbiol.,* 1:411–413.
33. Spencer, R.C., and Philp, J.R. (1973): Effect of previous antimicrobial therapy on bacteriological findings in patients with primary pneumonia. *Lancet,* ii:349–351.
34. Tillotson, J.R., and Lerner, A.M. (1967): Characteristic of pneumonias caused by *Escherichia coli. N. Engl. J. Med.,* 277:115–122.
35. Van Scoy, R.E. (1977): Bacterial sputum cultures: a clinician's viewpoint. *Mayo Clin. Proc.,* 52:39–41.
36. von Hoesslin, H. (1926): *Das Sputum,* 2nd edition. J. Springer, Berlin.
37. Washington, J.A., II (Editor). (1985): *Laboratory Procedures in Clinical Microbiology,* 2nd edition. Springer-Verlag, New York.

Respiratory Infections: Diagnosis and Management, 3d ed.,
edited by James E. Pennington.
Raven Press, Ltd., New York © 1994

5

Invasive Diagnostic Techniques in Pulmonary Infections

John G. Bartlett

*Department of Medicine, Johns Hopkins University School of Medicine,
720 Rutland Avenue, Baltimore, Maryland 21205*

A consensus impression is that the management of pulmonary infections is simplified and optimal when an etiologic agent is defined. There is, however, considerable controversy regarding the utilization of diagnostic resources to establish this goal, especially with invasive techniques which are performed at some risk to the patient. The purpose of this chapter is to review the relative merits of transtracheal aspiration, fiberoptic bronchoscopy, transthoracic needle aspiration, and lung biopsy in the diagnostic evaluation of pulmonary infections. There are several unifying factors which require emphasis at the outset:

1. An assumption is made that techniques described are reserved for patients in whom appropriate studies with alternative noninvasive and more simply performed methods to obtain specimens fail to provide conclusive results.

2. It is intuitively obvious that the diagnostic yield is markedly influenced by the quality of microbiological studies in terms of both stains and cultures. Nevertheless, this is a critical factor which deserves emphasis and represents a major source of erroneous results regardless of the specimen source. Our recommendation is that preprocedure planning for invasive tests include a tabular listing of possible or likely etiological agents with a clear definition of the desired microbiological studies. In addition, specimens obtained by invasive techniques are regarded as "precious" and should be immediately delivered to the laboratory with specific instructions for processing.

3. A major factor in the decision regarding various invasive methods concerns availability of resources. This applies to laboratory experience as well as to technical competence for obtaining the specimen.

4. A common mistake with bacterial infections of the lung concerns failure to appreciate the importance of the concentrations of bacteria according to quantitative or semiquantitative evaluation. Repeated studies have shown that bacterial infections of the lung, as well as infection at other anatomical sites, contain 10^5 or more bacteria/ml of exudate. Lower concentrations, especially with bacteria that are recovered only in broth, must be interpreted with cautious skepticism. The pathogenic potential of isolates and clinical correlations also deserve emphasis. In addition, repeated studies have shown that antimicrobial agents rapidly alter the cultivable flora

in the lower respiratory tract so that prior treatment markedly modifies the results of conventional bacterial cultures.

5. An important factor in the selection of an invasive technique concerns diagnostic considerations. In many instances, the differential diagnosis includes diseases that require tissue for histologic section, necessitating the use of procedures that might be quite different from those that yield simply exudate.

6. A critical factor in the assessment are the microorganisms recovered. Some agents are regarded as pathogens regardless of the specimen source. *Legionella, Mycoplasma pneumonia, M. tuberculosis,* pathogenic fungi, and most viruses are examples. Other organisms can colonize the oropharynx or even the lower airways without causing disease. Examples in this category include most "conventional" bacteria and some appropriate fungi.

TRANSTRACHEAL ASPIRATION

Transtracheal aspiration (TTA) was originally described by Pecora and Yegian (117) in 1959 as a means to obtain specimens from the lower respiratory tract that are free of contamination by the normal flora of the upper airways. This procedure has proved useful in studying the microbiology of pulmonary infections, primarily in patients with suspected bacterial infections. It is also an invasive technique that requires an experienced technician and careful patient selection. Major controversies concern risk–benefit ratio and the relative merits of this technique compared to alternative methods.

Contraindications

Contraindications include severe hemoptysis, bleeding diathesis, and inability to cooperate with severe hypoxemia. All are relative contraindications, but for general guidelines we arbitrarily require a platelet count exceeding 100,000/ml, a prothrombin time exceeding 60% of the control value, no other serious disturbance in bleeding parameters, and a po_2 exceeding 60 mm Hg with supplemented oxygen. There has been an understandable reluctance to do this procedure in pediatric patients due to the small caliber of the airway and the inability of these patients to cooperate. Nevertheless, there are two large series in which TTAs were performed in pediatric patients as young as 6 weeks of age without incident (8,22).

Technique

The technique of transtracheal aspiration includes placing the patient in the supine position with the neck hyperextended (11). Patients who require oxygen should continue to receive it throughout the procedure. The palpable notch between the lower border of the thyroid cartilage and the cricoid cartilage is prepped and infiltrated with 1–2% lidocaine containing epinephrine (to facilitate hemostasis). The 14-gauge needle of an intermediate-sized intracath is inserted through the cricoid membrane with the open bevel facing anteriorly; the needle is advanced only a few mm into the trachea to avoid injury to the posterior pharynx and then angulated to ensure that the catheter is directed caudad into the trachea. The catheter is passed to its full extent and the covering needle is withdrawn leaving the catheter in place. Aspiration is performed with a 20–30 cc syringe with a tight Luer lok attachment or, preferably, by suction aspiration into Luken's trap with a Y connector. Saline without bacteriostatic additive may be injected to facilitate aspiration, but this should be avoided because it will dilute the specimen making semiquantitative bacteriological analysis less meaningful. The only requirement is for a few drops of secretions, and these should be transported immediately to the laboratory for processing. Firm pressure is applied to the needle puncture site for several minutes following catheter withdrawal. Subsequent expectorations induced by the procedure are analogous to the "postbronchoscopy specimen" and can prove valuable for cytologic examinations or mycobacterial culture.

Complications

Transtracheal aspiration is a noxious procedure for the patient, due primarily to the unpleasant sensation of a foreign body in the lower airways. Nevertheless, most patients appear to tolerate the procedure well providing it is done expeditiously by an experienced person. Complications can be divided into three categories: (i) side effects at the needle puncture site, (ii) complications due to the catheter placement in the lower airways, and (iii) vasovagal reactions (11,39,89,113,123,126,143,149, 163,176). Major complications at the needle puncture site include bleeding, puncture of the posterior tracheal wall, and cutaneous or paratracheal abscess and subcutaneous emphysema which can dissect to the face or mediastinum or cause a pneumothorax. Catheter placement in the lower airways produces a profound irritant effect which often results in a severe cough paroxysm. This can be complicated by poor air exchange with hypoxemia or can precipitate severe hypoxemia or cause cardiac arrhythmias, hypotension, or myocardial ischemia; atropine should be readily available. Serious complications, including fatalities, have been reported. These concern anecdotal cases; the overall incidence of serious complications shows most of the patients had contraindications to the procedure (126). Our experience with over 800 transtracheal aspirations showed only a single serious complication in one patient with severe hemoptysis at the needle puncture site which resolved spontaneously without therapy. However, the special precautions taken at our institution deserve emphasis. TTA trays comparable to lumbar puncture (LP) trays were available on all wards. They were almost always used because they contained all necessary supplies. These trays had a cover sheet with two admonitions: the procedure was to be performed or overseen by someone designated as the "TTA" person on call, and TTA specimens had to be hand-delivered to the microbiology laboratory for immediate processing.

Accuracy

The theoretical basis for transtracheal aspiration is that the oropharyngeal flora stops abruptly at the level of the larynx and that samples obtained from the carina will reflect the bacteria present in the pulmonary parenchyma. There is considerable evidence that this is correct within certain limitations, enumerated below.

The greatest published experience with TTA concerns patients with suspected bacterial infections of the lower airways, and here the results have been almost uniformly favorable (10,17,58,67,73,115,131,144,147). The procedure has also been used to recover Nocardia (166), *Pneumocystis carinii* (83,166), *Legionella* (44,77,166), and mycobacteria (156). Transtracheal aspirates cultured on appropriate media yielded *Legionella pneumophila* in 9 of 14 patients with Legionnaires' disease reported by Edelstein et al. (44). Lau et al. (83) noted *P. carinii* cysts with methenamine silver stains of transtracheal aspirates in 8 of 9 patients with pneumocystis pneumonia. Thadepalli et al. (156) noted positive smears for acid-fast bacilli (AFB) in transtracheal aspirates from 34 of 35 patients with pulmonary tuberculosis who had negative AFB smears of expectorated sputa. These studies demonstrate the potential utility of transtracheal aspiration for detecting certain relatively unusual pulmonary pathogens. However, the greatest experience with the procedure is to detect bacteria that are recovered with conventional aerobic and anaerobic microbiological techniques.

The usual method to evaluate the diagnostic accuracy of TTA in bacterial infections of the lower airways is with clinical correlations. The largest review concerns 488 patients. These included 383 patients who satisfied clinical criteria for bacterial pneumonia as evidenced by fever, a pulmonary infiltrate on chest x-ray, and clinical response to antimicrobial therapy or autopsy evidence of bacterial pneumonia (Table 5-1) (10). Likely pulmonary pathogens were recovered from 235, but 44 of the 48 "false-negative" cultures were from patients who had received antimicrobial treatment prior to the procedure. Restricting analysis to untreated patients, the incidence of false-negative cultures was only 1%. The diagnostic accuracy of the procedure was further documented by showing the same organism recovered from blood cultures in 23 pneumonia patients with bacteremia was also present in the companion transtracheal aspirate. Analogous results have been reported by numerous other observers (10,17,58,67,73,115,131,144,147). An exception is the report by de Vivo (166) et al. who noted 17 of 82 (20%) false-negative TTAs, but the status of prior antibiotic treatment was not treated.

Occasional discrepancies have been noted with transtracheal aspiration bacteriology compared to results using alternative invasive diagnostic techniques such as transthoracic aspiration, with the assumption that the latter method provides a more accurate reflection of the infecting flora due to sampling from the pulmonary parenchyma (38,69,166). However, scrutiny of the comparative data shows that the dif-

TABLE 5–1. *Results of 488 transtracheal aspirates*

Clinical criteria for bacterial pneumonia[a]	383
Culture yielded pulmonary pathogen	335
Culture yielded no pulmonary pathogen	48
Antimicrobials given prior to TTA	44
No prior antimicrobials	4[b]
No clinical evidence for bacterial pneumonia[a]	105
Culture yielded pulmonary pathogen	34
Exacerbation of chronic bronchitis	16
No exacerbation	18[b]
No potential pathogen isolated	71

[a]Clinical observation based on usual symptoms of a pulmonary infection; x-ray evidence of an infiltrate and either response to antibacterial agents or autopsy evidence of bacterial pneumonia.
[b]Figures used to determine false-negative culture rate of 1% and false-positive culture rate of ~20%.

ferences were modes and unlikely to modify therapeutic decisions. Furthermore, this type of analysis presupposes the diagnostic accuracy of the transthoracic aspirate, which may be an erroneous assumption, to be discussed below. The usual discrepancy is organisms recovered in the TTA that were not present in the transthoracic aspirate, e.g., false-positive cultures. Some have expressed concern that microorganisms in the peripheral lung may not be detected in the trachea (38), but this has not been an apparent problem according to most in clinical studies. Furthermore, Pecora showed that TTA specimens yielded *Serratia marcescens* in each of 20 dogs 15 minutes after injection of the strain into the peripheral lung (116). A conclusion from these studies is that false-negative cultures are unusual in bacterial infections of the lower airways providing the procedure has been properly performed, the specimen has been collected before antibiotic therapy, and the specimen has been processed using appropriate microbiological techniques.

False-positive cultures occur in occasional patients according to results of a concurrent transthoracic aspiration (38,69,166). Further information on this point is available from studies of TTA bacteriology in persons with no apparent active pulmonary infection (Table 5-2). Studies in volunteers have shown positive cultures in 0–16%, but in most instances the organisms recovered were present in low concentrations (18,73). Our studies with quantitative cultures of transtracheal aspirations in patients with pneumonia have shown pathogens in concentrations averaging 10^7/ml and almost always present in concentrations of 10^6/ml (14). Benner et al. (17) performed TTAs in 85 patients with suspected pneumococcal pneumonia and found all had counts of *Streptococcus pneumoniae* that exceeded 10^5/ml. This experience suggests that healthy persons occasionally harbor bacteria in the lower airways, but they are usually present in relatively low concentrations. The importance of semiquantitative analysis deserves particular emphasis in distinguishing colonization or the transient presence of bacteria from infecting pathogens. The pathogenic potential of the isolate and results of direct gram stain are critical components of the assessment as well. Interpretation using these guidelines, however, may be more difficult

TABLE 5–2. *Incidence of false-positive transtracheal aspiration cultures: results of microbiology studies in patients sampled when there was no evidence for bacterial infection*

Source (ref.)	Population studied	No.	No. with bacteria	Concentration "3" + or 10^5/ml
Hoeprich (67)	Healthy medical students	13	0	0
Berman et al. (18)	Asthmatics with exacerbation	27	15 (56%)	1 (4%)[a]
Berman et al. (18)	Volunteers aged 25–50 years	15	10 (67%)	1 (7%)[a]
Berman et al. (18)	Comatose patients without pneumonia	8	6 (75%)	0[a]
Benner et al. (17)	Posttherapy for pneumococcal pneumonia	85	11 (13%)	0[b]
Bjerkestrand et al. (20)	Chronic bronchitis	36	30 (83%)	14 (40%)[b]
Lober and Swenson (87)	Bronchogenic neoplasm	45	26 (58%)	10 (22%)[b]

[a]Indicates 3 + (moderate) or greater growth on primary isolation plates according to semiquantitative anlaysis.
[b]Indicates 10^5/ml with quantitative analysis.

in patients with chronic diseases of the lower airways, and this especially applies to patients with chronic lung disease. Patients with chronic bronchitis usually harbor organisms in the lower airways in concentrations that generally exceed 10^6/ml, and the bacteria recovered often include potentially pathogenic strains such as *S. pneumoniae* or *Hemophilus influenzae* (20). Patients who are comatose may also pose a problem for interpretation of TTA, due presumably to repeated aspiration, although bacterial concentrations are generally low (87). Similarly, patients with bronchogenic neoplasms often harbor bacteria in the lower airways (51).

Indications

The major use of the TTA is to identify accurately bacterial pathogens in the lower airways in a setting where contamination by organisms in the oral cavity pose a problem with more conventional specimen sources. TTA has proved highly successful in anaerobic pulmonary infections, it appears to be the preferred pulmonary specimen for anaerobic culture in patients without empyema (15,22,51,87,131), and it is sometimes used in the compromised host with enigmata pneumonia (166). It should be noted that the previously cited problem of contaminants or colonizing bacteria in occasional healthy persons—and most persons with chronic bronchitis—concerns aerobic bacteria. This does not appear to pose a problem with respect to anaerobes with the occasional exception of bronchiectasis (20). The necessity to perform a TTA seems doubtful when the diagnosis of anaerobic infection is readily apparent on the basis of clinical observations, especially in the presence of putrid discharge. In this instance, the importance of identifying specific bacterial pathogens must be weighed against the risk of the procedure and the reasonably good results with empiric selection of drugs directed against presumed pathogens. There is also little point in performing a TTA to detect anaerobic bacteria if the available laboratory resources have not established expertise for the bacteriology studies required.

It is difficult to describe specific indications for TTA in the general population of patients with pulmonary infections in which aerobic bacteria are suspect due to the multiple variables that must be considered. A general guideline is that this technique is best justified in clinical situations where:

1. Bacterial pathogens are suspected,
2. Alternative specimens utilizing less invasive techniques are inconclusive or not available,
3. The severity of the illness justifies the risk incurred,
4. Technical expertise is available,
5. Patient contraindications do not apply.

Previous or recent antibiotic exposure represents a relative contraindication since results are often misleading. Our experience, summarized above, showed nearly all false-negative cultures occurred in this setting (10). There may also be false-positive cultures. For example, Benner (17) noted new bacterial pathogens in TTAs in 11 of 85 patients during treatment for pneumococcal pneumonia, although concentrations were low and none of these patients had evidence for superinfection.

Settings that appear to satisfy the specified guidelines include hospital-acquired pneumonia, pneumonia in the compromised host, and necrotizing pneumonia characterized by multiple small abscesses within a pulmonary segment or lobe. The procedure may also prove especially useful in the patient with unusual pulmonary diseases in which there are multiple diagnostic considerations, including noninfectious diseases such as heart failure, pulmonary embolism, bronchogenic neoplasm, and so forth. A properly processed TTA specimen obtained before antibiotic therapy that fails to yield a likely bacterial pathogen in this setting virtually excludes bacterial pneumonia. This finding may avoid unnecessary exposure to antibiotics and expedite the diagnostic evaluation to detect alternative diagnoses.

TTA has been used to detect mycobacteria on direct stain when more conventional culture sources failed (156). However, the major advantage of the procedure is avoidance of oropharyngeal contamination which should not be a problem with mycobacteria. Expectorated sputa, induced sputa, or bronchoscopy aspirates would be preferred so that TTA is warranted only when these specimens are negative or when concurrent bacterial infection is suspect.

BRONCHOSCOPY SPECIMENS

Bronchoscopy was developed in the 1930s when it was used primarily for investigations of noninfectious pulmonary diseases. During the last 20 years there has been extensive use of fiberoptic bronchoscopy for detection of unusual microbes in the immunocompromised host, and, more recently, fiberoptic bronchoscopy has found a special niche in the detection of *P. carinii* and other opportunists in patients with AIDS. A major problem with the usual specimens obtained at bronchoscopy is contamination by the normal flora of the upper airways, but specialized methods are now available to improve the quality of bronchoscopy specimens even for the recovery of "conventional" bacterial pathogens. It should be noted that the techniques used for the immunocompromised host to detect unusual pathogens and those used for the recovery of conventional bacterial agents of pneumonia are quite different and will be discussed separately, although obviously both may be used in a single patient.

Technique for Recovering Opportunistic Pathogens

This refers to studies designed to detect microbes that do not pose a problem for interpretation despite contamination by the flora of the upper airways including parasites, most viruses, Legionella, mycobacteria, and pathogenic fungi. The yield is magnified by the use of multiple specimens including fixed-tissue specimens, touch imprints of tissue from transbronchial biopsy, bronchial lavage, and brush biopsies. A bleeding diathesis or the requirement for mechanical ventilation represents relative contraindications to transbronchial biopsy.

For bronchoalveolar lavage (BAL) the tracheobronchial tree is inspected; the instrument is removed for clearing of secretions and then reinserted and wedged into the lingular or right middle lobe bronchus. Twenty ml of isotonic saline is added to the suction apparatus with a 3-way stopcock which is instilled and then aspirated using a vacuum of 50–100 mm of mercury to collect the lavage fluid. This is repeated 5 times for a total instillation of 100 ml and an expected return of 40–70 ml. The lavage fluid is then inoculated into appropriate media for bacteria, Legionella, fungi, Nocardia, and mycobacteria using a total of approximately 15 ml of BAL fluid. The remaining fluid is useful for cytocentrifuge preparations using the gram stain for bacteria, the DFA stain for Legionella, acid-fast for mycobacteria and Nocardia, Gomori methenamine silver stains for fungi and *P. carinii,* and monoclonal antibodies to detect cytomegalovirus, herpes simplex viruses, or other viruses.

Accuracy

The high diagnostic yield of bronchoscopy as it applies to patients with AIDS was the subject of extensive review at a workshop sponsored by the Division of Lung Diseases, National Heart, Lung and Blood Institute, in 1983 (105), and repeated for an "update" in 1986 (106). The combined experience of multiple centers reviewing 348 AIDS patients with pulmonary infections is summarized in Table 5-3. This, along with multiple other reports (9,26,33,34,109,134,151), shows an extraordinarily high diagnostic yield of approximately 95% for patients with *P. carinii* and a high yield for other treatable pathogens as well. The report of the second workshop (106) showed four developments that occurred during the intervening three years as applied to AIDS patients: (i) increased frequency of serious pulmonary infections caused by pyogenic bacteria; (ii) increased recognition of the importance of *M. tuberculosis;* (iii) in contrast to the early report, Legionnaires' disease was infrequently encountered; and (iv) increased recognition of lymphocytic interstitial pneumonia in adults. Two other subsequent developments for the detection of Pneumocystis pneumonia included the potential utility of nonbronchoscopic methods using induced sputum and nonbronchoscopic lavage. Induced sputum is now commonly recommended as the initial step in the evaluation, since it is less expensive, less invasive, and shows a sensitivity averaging 60% (19,27,132). Induced sputa may also be used for detection of other pathogenic organisms in the lower airways such as *M. tuberculosis* and pathogenic fungi, but utility with culture for conventional bacteria is questioned. Nonbronchoscopic lavage utilizes modified suction catheters for intubated patients or a fiberoptic catheter for nonintubated patients. This approach has been suggested as a safe, effective, inexpensive bedside technique that could be used as an alternative to bronchoscopy, but it has not received widespread acceptance (27,92).

The second workshop participants concluded that fiberoptic bronchoscopy was the procedure of choice for diagnosing opportunistic pulmonary infections following negative induced sputa exams (106). Transbronchial biopsies are considered complementary but are often restricted to selected patients. Three options were suggested for patients with nondiagnostic procedures: (i) repeated bronchoscopy, (ii) open lung biopsy, or (iii) observation. The former two are recommended when the patient's clinical condition deteriorates.

TABLE 5–3. *Diagnostic yield with fiberoptic bronchoscopy in patients with AIDS*

Condition	No.	Diagnostic yield
Pneumocystis pneumonia	368	348 (95%)
Mycobacterium avium	74	58 (78%)
Cytomegalovirus	74	63 (85%)
Legionella	19	18 (95%)
Fungi	17	14 (82%)
Kaposi's sarcoma	25	2 (8%)

Adapted from Murray et al. (105).

Other relevant issues concerning AIDS patients are the following: Biopsy specimens are required to detect lymphocytic interstitial pneumonitis; the sensitivity of biopsies for detecting Kaposi's sarcoma in the lung is poor, but detection of typical raised, cherry red endobronchial lesions is nearly diagnostic. Patients with established Pneumocystis pneumonia often have persistence of demonstrable *P. carinii* cysts on repeat examination for at least one month despite appropriate therapy and good clinical response (145). There appears to be no correlation between clinical response and either histologic resolution on follow-up biopsy or detection of the putative agent, thus negating the utility of repeat bronchoscopy as a method to monitor therapeutic response; cytomegalovirus (CMV) may be detected by immunofluorescence using monoclonal antibodies on smears prepared from resuspended cells of sedimented BAL fluid, but the sensitivity reported has ranged from only 33% (94) to 100% (46,65); the yield for *Mycobacterium avium* with culture (Table 5-3) is high, although the AFB stain is often negative so that definitive results are not available for 2 to 3 weeks (106).

Technique for Detecting Conventional Bacteria

Specimens collected by suction aspiration through the inner channel and processed in the usual fashion represent no clear advantage over expectorated sputum or endotracheal tube aspiration due to contamination of the instrument by upper airway flora during passage.

Alternative methods that are now being used extensively for detection of conventional bacteria in the lower airways are (i) the protected double lumen brush catheter combined with quantitative culture (PBC) (ii) bronchoalveolar lavage with quantitative culture, and (iii) a single brush catheter with quantitative culture. All three require quantitative culture based on the assumption that pathogenic bacteria are present in concentrations exceeding 10^5/ml at the infected site, whereas contaminate or colonizing bacteria are found in lower concentration. It should be acknowledged that this application of quantitative bacteriology to detect pathogens in a fashion analogous to urine cultures has also been used successfully with expectorated sputum (14[p. 1019],41,55,76) and endotracheal tube aspirates (111). Some investigators have also used immunofluorescence to detect antibody-coated bacteria in respiratory secretions, once popular with urinary tract infections (172). However, Vereen et al. (164) noted antibody-coated bacteria in 17 of 18 patients with stable chronic bronchitis, and the procedure has not found widespread acceptance.

A major question posed by these studies concerns the necessity for specialized techniques to reduce the level of contamination of upper airway secretions; the concentrations of bacteria in saliva exceed the usual cut-point for "significant concentrations" at infected sites by 4 logs or more, so that salivary contamination even in minute quantities poses an ominous potential concern. Also important are obvious issues such as cost, technical ease of performance, demands on the microbiology laboratory, and the need for coordinated activities. The first description of techniques that have now become commonplace by bronchoscopists for evaluating pneumonia in selected populations was by Wimberly et al. (171). The technique described requires a commitment by the bronchoscopist to follow precise methodology in obtaining the specimen and the microbiologist for performing quantitative cultures as described (171). The patient is premedicated with atropine 30 to 60 minutes before the procedure to inhibit nasovagal response, decrease oropharyngeal secretions, and minimize aspiration of upper airway flora. Topical anesthesia is provided by inhalation of nebulized lidocaine without preservation due to its undesired antibacterial properties. The nostril is then sprayed with 5% cocaine solution and the patient then sniffs approximately 10 ml of lidocaine jelly. The bronchoscope is then introduced into the trachea and the catheter is placed through the channel to the bronchoscope tip. The inner cannula is advanced to discharge the distal polyethylene glycol plug. The inner cannula is then advanced into the area of purulent collections or the appropriate bronchial orifice under direct observation. The brush is then advanced to obtain secretions either from the central airways or from the bronchial segment of involvement according to the chest x-ray findings. Once the specimen is collected, the brush is retracted into the inner cannula and the entire catheter system is then removed. Lidocaine is then injected through the suction catheter for completion of the bronchoscopic exam.

Once the catheter system has been removed, the outer surface is cleansed with alcohol and then transacted distal to the brush. The brush is advanced for preparation of slides for gram stain and any special stains such as DFA for Legionella. The brush is then severed and placed into a transport vial containing one ml of sterile lactated Ringer's solution. Nutrient broth should not be used as transport media if there is to be any significant delay in microbiologic processing. In the laboratory, the vial is vortexed, and then a 0.1 ml aliquot is inoculated into appropriate media for the recovery of aerobic bacteria, anaerobic bacteria, and Legionella. Two successive 100-fold dilutions are also made, so that the final dilutions are 10^{-1}, 10^{-3}, and 10^{-5}. Studies of the brush specimens indicate that the amount of secretions obtained vary from 0.01 to 0.001 ml, so that growth at the 10^{-3} dilution represents 10^5 and 10^6 bacteria/ml which is considered "significant."

Accuracy

The most extensive studies have been done by the group from the University of South Alabama. These include the original reports of *in vitro* studies by Wimberly et al. (171) and subsequent clinical reports by others (78,125,170). The first clinical report included 53 patients with clinical evidence for a bacterial infection involving the lower airways and 12 patients with a final diagnosis of nonbacterial pulmonary disease (170). Significant concentrations of likely bacterial pathogens were recovered in all but one of patients in the former category except for seven who had received previous antibiotic treatment (Table 5-4). Cultures were uniformly negative or yielded only low concentrations of bacteria in all 12 patients who had alternative diagnoses. This report emphasizes the fact that previous antibiotic treatment negates to a large extent the potential utility of this specimen source (as well as virtually all other specimen sources including expectorated sputum and transtracheal aspirates). The sequel report from this group provided more details regarding microbiology and an updated review of the series which now included 172 patients (125). The overall results were similar to those previously reported, in that 75 of 78 (96%) of patients with a clinical diagnosis of bacterial infection of the lower airways had a likely pulmonary pathogen in significant concentration, whereas high counts were recovered

TABLE 5–4. *Quantitative cultures of protected brush catheter bronchoscopy specimens*

Patient category	>10³/ml	<10³/ml
Bacteremic pneumonia	10	0
Nonbacteremic pneumonia	23	1
Lung abscess	12	0
Pneumonia with prior antibiotic treatment	0	7
Nonbacterial pulmonary disease	0	12

Adapted from Wimberly et al. (171).

in only 2 of 35 control patients. There were 13 patients with bacteremic pneumonia, and 12 of these had the blood culture isolate recovered in the bronchoscopy specimen in significant concentrations. The predominant isolates were *S. pneumoniae* (38 patients), *H. influenzae* (17 patients), and a mixed aerobic-anaerobic flora (16 patients). The most common anaerobic isolate was *Prevotella melaninogenicus*. Gram stains revealed the organism isolated in significant numbers for 47 of 68 specimens. The only discrepancy beyond the problem of false-negative cultures in patients with prior antibiotic therapy was high counts of bacteria found in presumably uninfected patients who had endobronchial structural disease.

Subsequent investigators have confirmed the favorable results (29,31,43,47,61, 72,78,88,103,159). Diagnostic accuracy has been supported by clinical correlations (29,47,125,170), negative cultures in healthy controls (78,171), reproducibility with duplicate samplings (93), analysis of borderline quantitative results (43), comparison with needle aspiration (88), comparison of results in moribund patients with autopsy findings (88), and in a primate model (66). Nevertheless, some investigators have found relatively poor results that are either unexplained (48,158) or presumably represent marked departures from the standardized methods (59). An additional problem that needs reiteration is false-negative cultures with prior antibiotic treatment (78,125,170).

Alternative techniques include quantitative culture of a standard brush-catheter system with a distal plus (120) and blind bronchial sampling in mechanically ventilated patients (103,112,127,160) including use of a telescoping plugged catheter (160). Results of these methods appear to compare favorably with the double-lumen plugged catheter system, or with clinical correlations, but the database supporting their use is far less extensive. One technique that does appear to have an extensive experience is quantitative culture of bronchoalveolar lavage fluid (28,30,52,56,62, 100,102,138,157,161). This includes evidence that gram stains of centrifuged BAL fluid showing under one bacterium/oil emersion field or intracellular bacteria in >2% alveolar cells have a good predictive power for culture results and for a diagnosis of bacterial pneumonia by clinical criteria (30,100,102,157,161). The concentration of bacteria that is considered significant in these studies is 10^3/ml, 10^4/ml, or 10^5/ml. Techniques used include both bronchoscopic and nonbronchoscopic BAL. There is also considerable variation in catheters used, including the standard bronchoscopic catheter, the Swan-Ganz catheter, the double lumen plugged catheter, and a protected transbronchoscopic balloon-tipped catheter. Results with these studies show substantial variation in terms of sensitivity and specificity (Table 5-5). Some conclude that the contradicting results in comparing studies combined with the lack of a consensus on procedural issues indicate that additional studies are required before

TABLE 5–5. *Bronchoalveolar lavage in the diagnosis of pneumonia*

Source (ref.)	No.	Bacterial threshold	Technique	Reference test	Sensitivity	Specificity
Gaussorges et al. (52)	13	NS	Cuffed catheter	Lung biopsy	93%	89%
Chastre et al. (30)	21	10^4/ml	Fiberoptic bronchoscopy	Protected brush catheter	NS	69%
Torres et al. (161)	25	10^3/ml	Fiberoptic bronchoscopy	Protected brush catheter	72%	71%
Guerra and Baughman (56)	60	10^4/ml	Fiberoptic bronchoscopy	Clinical correlations	60%	100%
Rouby et al. (138)	59	NS	Protected catheter	Lung biopsy	80%	66%
Meduri et al. (102)	25	10^4/ml	Protected catheter	Lung biopsy	100%	100%
Thorpe et al. (157)	92	10^5/ml	Fiberoptic bronchoscopy	Clinical correlations	86%	100%
Meduri et al. (100)	49	10^4/ml	Protected catheter	Clinical correlations	97%	92%
Papazian et al. (112)	64	10^4/ml	Fiberoptic bronchoscopy	Protected brush catheter; clinical correlation	98%	31%
Kirkpatrick and Bass (78)	8	10^4/ml	Fiberoptic bronchoscopy	Healthy controls; protected brush catheter	NS	100%

specific recommendations can be given (159). There does appear to be increasing enthusiasm for results of direct stains as a guide to both diagnosis and initial antibiotic decisions.

Risks

Bronchoscopy is regarded as a noninvasive diagnostic test which has been associated with few serious complications. Retrospective surveys of over 72,000 procedures (99,100) showed 13 deaths (.015%), the major risk factor being severe cardiovascular disease. There are also 41 life-threatening reactions to anesthesia and just two deaths due to hemorrhage following forceps biopsy. Transbronchial biopsy magnifies the risk substantially with a 5% risk of pneumothorax and a 2–3% risk of bleeding. Pereira et al. (119) reported a more careful prospective analysis of 100 procedures in which there was a 16% incidence of transient fever, 6% of patients had new pulmonary infiltrates after bronchoscopy, and postprocedure pneumonia resulted in one death. Burham (24) also recorded a 46% incidence of fever and a 15% incidence of bacteremia during bronchoscopy with a rigid bronchoscope. Others have noted essentially no cases of pneumonia following fiberoptic bronchoscopy (153), and bacteremia, although reported, appears to be very rare (3,74). The American Heart Association no longer recommends prophylaxis for patients with valvular heart disease undergoing bronchoscopy. Contamination instruments may lead to outbreaks of pneumonia or pseudo-outbreaks due to contaminated respiratory specimens (75,168). There is also a 1–20 mm Hg decrease in $_pO^2$ which could pose difficulty for some patients with severe hypoxemia (2). This work collectively indicates some risk, although the incidence of serious complications is extremely low.

Indications

Fiberoptic bronchoscopy is advocated to detect selected pathogens from the lower airways when less invasive procedures are unsuccessful. The specific pathogens are microbes that are indicative of an etiologic diagnosis, often in a clinical setting that specifically suggests their role. Specific pathogens of greatest interest are the following:

1. Tuberculosis: Bronchoscopy is commonly advocated for the diagnosis of tuberculosis when expectorated or induced sputum samples fail to reveal AFB. Studies from the Mayo Clinic in the pre-AIDS era showed bronchoscopy specimens yielded *M. tuberculosis* in 32 of 34 patients with tuberculosis and positive cultures in 38 of 40 patients with lung infections involving atypical organisms (70). In AIDS patients, Broaddus et al. (21) reported positive BAL cultures from 4 of 5 patients with tuberculosis and 22 of 29 (76%) patients with *M. avium* pulmonary infections. Others have found similar results (140). With regard to AFB smear, the yield in bronchoscopy specimens from patients with positive cultures for *M. tuberculosis* was 15 of 31 (48%) and only 4 of 40 (10%) from patients with positive cultures for *M. avium*.

2. *P. carinii:* The diagnostic yield in AIDS patients from multiple studies shows an average sensitivity of 60% for induced sputa and 95% for bronchoscopic specimens (105,146). The yield is somewhat lower in other patient populations (42,130).

3. Cytomegalovirus: The major clinical setting for CMV pneumonitis is organ or marrow transplantation where CMV accounts for about 50% of all cases associated

with bilateral interstitial infiltrates. An important distinction is CMV infection versus CMV disease; many asymptomatic patients excrete CMV in various body fluids including saliva. CMV pneumonia is usually diagnosed by fluids or tissues from the lower airways, although caution is necessary when salivary contamination is present. BAL is particularly useful since the site of infection is alveolar lining cells. Studies from Memorial Sloan-Kettering Cancer Center showed 100% sensitivity using immunofluorescent stains of BAL specimens, although some false-positives were present according to other data (46[p. 476]). Interpretation when culture or histology studies are negative is problematic. Cultures are relatively sensitive, but will require 2 to 4 weeks. The shell viral method gives results in one day and shows a sensitivity of 80–100% compared to culture.

The host settings in which bronchoscopy is commonly advocated are the following:

1. The immunocompromised host (42,46,48,49,108,130,146,152): The yield according to aggregate data from multiple studies shows the following (146):

Procedure	No.	Diagnosis	False-negative
Transbronchial biopsy	584	264 (45%)	65 (21%)
Bronchial brushing	328	98 (30%)	63 (35%)
BAL	327	173 (55%)	47 (22%)

2. Nosocomial pneumonia and ICU pneumonia in patients, with or without mechanical ventilation (2,3,9,12,14,19,21,24,26,27,29–31,33–35,41,46,47,52,55,56,59,61, 65,66,70,72,74–76,78,88,92–94,100–103,106,109,111,112,119,120,125,127,132,134,138, 145,151,153–155,158–161,164,168,170–172): Bronchoscopy with specimens obtained by the protected brush catheter or BAL using quantitative cultures is being used with increasing frequency to define the presence and cause of bacterial infection. Of particular interest is a convincing study using these techniques to show that only 31% of patients with common clinical and roentgenographic evidence for pneumonia actually had supporting evidence from cultures obtained by quantitative cultures of protected brush catheter specimens (47). Major questions in patients with mechanical ventilation is the need for bronchoscopy versus suction aspiration or "blind" BAL specimens (29,30,103,127,159,160), the need for quantitative versus semiquantitative cultures, and the relative merits of direct gram stains.

3. Chronic or enigmatic pneumonia in the immunocompetent host.

TRANSTHORACIC NEEDLE ASPIRATION

Transthoracic needle aspiration permits collection of uncontaminated specimens directly from the pulmonary parenchyma for cytologic and microbiological study. This procedure was initially introduced in 1982 (84) and has been used with variable enthusiasm since that time. The most extensive experience was in the prechemotherapeutic era when the major indication was to recover *S. pneumoniae* to provide appropriate type-specific antisera which was the only therapy available at that time (23). More recently the procedure has been used primarily for cytologic evaluation of suspected pulmonary malignancies in which the diagnostic yield has been reported as high as 96% (139). Transthoracic aspiration has also been attractive for microbiological studies of suspected pulmonary infections in pediatric patients due to the difficulty encountered in obtaining specimens from alternative sources, and in unusual pulmonary infections in adults. Problems with the procedure include a relatively high rate of false-negative cultures and potentially serious complications which are most common in patients with severe underlying diseases.

Technique

The area of involvement is determined by chest x-ray and the site for needle insertion is identified by physical examination, cutaneous markers, or direct fluoroscopic visualization (37). Fluoroscopy is preferred for small nodular lesions or infiltrates that are located adjacent to the heart or major vessels. The mid-axillary line is the usual site of aspiration in patients with diffuse pulmonary lesions. Focal lesions are preferably sampled with imaging guidance to assure needle placement. This may be done with biplane fluoroscopy, ultrasound, or computerized tomography (CT) guidance. Premedication is generally necessary, although diazepam, meperidine, or similar agents may be used for patients who are extremely apprehensive. The area of needle insertion is prepared with topical antiseptics and the use of local anesthesia is optimal. The procedure may be performed with an 18–22-gauge, thin-walled spinal needle attached to a tight fitting 10–30 ml locking syringe or the "skinny" 25-gauge needle which some prefer due to reduced trauma. The needle is inserted into the appropriate site during suspended respiration. Many use a dry syringe and obtain the specimen by continuous negative pressure during slow withdrawal of the needle. Alternative techniques include suction during entry as fluids, such as saline or broth medium. In many instances, especially when using a dry syringe, there are only a few drops of aspirate, requiring arbitrary decisions for cytology preparations and microbiological stains and cultures. Assuming an adequate volume and depending on the clinical setting, stains and cultures using appropriate media should be employed for the recovery of aerobic and anaerobic bacteria, fungi, mycobacteria, and Legionella. An expiration chest x-ray should be obtained several hours after the procedure to detect evidence of pneumothorax.

Contraindications

Major contraindications to the procedure include bullous pulmonary disease in the region to be aspirated, the requirement for mechanical ventilatory assistance, vascular lesions, and severe bleeding diathesis which cannot be corrected. Relative contraindications include localized lesions adjacent to major vessels, uncontrollable coughing, inability of the patient to cooperate, pulmonary hypertension, suspected Echinococcus cyst, and hypoxemia. Pneumothorax is the most frequent complication, and patients who had inadequate pulmonary reserve to tolerate a significant pneumothorax should not have this procedure except for urgent indications.

Complications

The incidence of complication depends to a large extent on the experience of the person performing transthoracic aspiration and on associated diseases in the host. The most frequent complication is pneumothorax which is generally noted in 20–

30%, but these are sufficiently severe to require chest tube drainage in only 1–19% (Table 5-6). Approximately 3–10% of patients have hemoptysis following the procedure. This is usually transient and self-limited, although fatal hemorrhage has been reported in at least six patients including some with no defined bleeding diathesis (114). Another rare, but potentially serious complication is air embolism which results from the entry of air from the atmosphere, bronchus, or lung into the pulmonary vein (169). Predisposing risk factors include needle puncture into areas of consolidation or abscesses, failure to maintain needle closure, inability of the patient to suspend respiration, a rigid lung, and intractable cough. The relative safety of transthoracic needle aspiration in uncomplicated patients with pneumonia was emphasized by Sappington and Favorite (142). These investigators noted only a single death with over 2,000 reported cases, and the exception actually was a case in which the lung was accidentally punctured in an attempted thoracentesis. The procedure appears to be especially benign in previously healthy pediatric patients with pneumonia. However, the complication rate increases substantially when transthoracic puncture is performed in patients with serious associated diseases. For example, Davidson et al. (38) noted no major complications among 25 Navajo Indians with acute pneumonia, but this same group reported major complications in 11 of 39 patients who had serious concurrent diseases (110). Extension of infection to the pleural space with empyema has been notably rare (142). Herman and Hessel (64) reported their results of a survey of 105 institutions with transthoracic needle aspiration in 1,562 patients which showed the following complication rates: death, 0.1%; major hemorrhage, 0.2%; and pneumothorax requiring a chest tube, 7%.

Accuracy

The diagnostic accuracy of transthoracic needle aspiration in 19 reported series is summarized in Table 5-6. The yield of microbial agents is somewhat variable, in part reflecting the enormous variation in the patient population sampled. However, it should be noted that this analysis is restricted to series in which the procedure was performed to detect etiologic agents in patients with suspected infections. Studies in the prechemotherapeutic era were conducted primarily in patients with lobar or bronchopneumonia, especially for the detection of *S. pneumoniae*. Sappington and Favorite (142) summarized the experience with transthoracic aspirates in seven series reported prior to 1936 and found that a bacterial pathogen was recovered in approximately 50%. The largest experience was reported by Bullowa (23) who examined lung aspirates in 1,467 patients with suspected pneumococcal pneumonia and found positive cultures for this organism in 510 for a diagnostic yield of 35%. Perhaps the most accurate definition of the incidence of false-negative cultures from this or any other series concerns 211 patients with bacteremic pneumonitis in whom lung aspirates yielded *S. pneumoniae* in 165 (78%) (23). Theoretical explanations include improper placement of the needle or nonviable organisms, the latter apparently occurring more frequently in later stages of the disease (136). More recent studies in pediatric patients have shown a somewhat lower yield which generally ranges from 40 to 60% (40,71,81,90,104,128). This presumably reflects the inclusion of patients with infections involving organisms which cannot be cultured with routine techniques such as viruses, Mycoplasma, and Chlamydia. Unfortunately, no etiologic diagnosis was established in the majority of these cases so that the true incidence of false-negative cultures cannot be determined.

TABLE 5–6. *Reported experience with transthoracic needle aspiration*

Source (ref.)	Population studied	Needle gauge	No. studied	Microbial agent	False neg.	Contaminant	Pneumothorax	Chest tube
Lyon, 1922 (90)	Children <12 yrs; pneumonia	NS	38	19 (50%)	NS	1 (35)	NS	NS
Disney, 1956 (40)	Children <2; S. aureus pneumonia	16, 18	17	14 (82%)	NS	NS	3/17 (18%)	0
Klein, 1969 (81)	Children 6 day–2 yrs; pneumonia	20	28	20 (36%)	NS	5 (18%)	3/17 (18%)	0
Johnson, 1970 (71)	Children 1–10 yrs; malignancy + pneumonia	22	35	20 (57%)	NS	NS	NS	2/35 (6%)
Mimica, 1971 (104)	Children <2 yrs; pneumonia	18, 20	505	187 (37%)	NS	51 (10%)	9/530 (2%)	2/530 (0.4%)
Rapkin, 1975 (128)	Children–pneumonia	20, 21	27	3 (11%)	NS	3 (11%)	3/27 (11%)	0
Chaudhary, 1977 (32)	Children 4 mo–21 yrs; suspected P. carinii	20	228	121 (53%)	16	9 (4%)	74/228 (32%)	29/228 (13%)
Bullowa, 1935 (23)	Bacteremic pneumococcal pneumonia	22	211	165 (78%)	46	NS	NS	NS
Sappington, 1936 (142)	Lobar pneumonia	18	68	54 (79%)	5	NS	1/68 (1%)	0
Gherman, 1965 (53)	Compromised host–pneumonia	22	11	9 (82%)	NS	2 (20%)	4/11 (36%)	1/11 (1%)
Beerens, 1965 (16)	Pyogenic lung abscess	NS	33	26 (79%)	NS	NS	NS	NS
Bandt, 1972 (7)	Compromised host–pneumonia	18	21	16 (76%)	NS	NS	NS	1/21 (5%)
Greenman, 1975 (54)	Compromised host–pneumonia	18	15	9 (60%)	6	NS	NS	3/34 (9%)
Davidson, 1976 (38)	Pneumonia	20	25	17 (68%)	5	4 (16%)	4/25 (16%)	0
Sagel, 1978 (139)	Compromised host-focal infiltrate	18	31	24 (77%)	NS	NS	292/1211 (26%)	167/1211 (14%)
Castellino, 1979 (25)	Compromised host-focal infiltrate	18	108	79 (73%)	NS	NS	28/108 (26%)	14/108 (13%)
Palmer, 1980 (110)	Complex pneumonia	20	39	22 (56%)	6	1 (2%)	12/39 (31%)	8/39 (21%)
Wallace, 1985 (167)	AIDS patients	22	16	14 (87%)	1	NS	7/16 (44%)	3/16 (19%)
Yang, 1991 (174)	Lung abscess	18, 20	33	31 (94%)	0	NS	2/33 (6%)	0/33

No. studied indicates number of lung aspirates performed in patients with suspected pulmonary infection. *False neg.* indicates number in which a likely pulmonary pathogen was recovered with a repeat aspirate in patients with initial negative culture or recovered from alternative, uncontaminated source. *Contaminant* refers to organisms interpreted by author as contaminants, usually *S. epidermitidus*. *Pneumothorax* and *pneumothorax requiring chest tube* are complications.

Most of the more recent experience with this procedure in adults concerns the immunologically compromised host with focal or diffuse pulmonary infiltrates. Numerous pathogens have been recovered in such patients including opportunistic fungi, Nocardia, mycobacteria, Legionella, and *P. carinii*. The overall diagnostic yield in this population is reported at 53–82% (7,25,32,53,54,110,139,167). However, the true incidence of false-negative cultures is difficult to decipher because no diagnosis was established in a major portion of patients with negative studies. Some information along these lines is available on the basis of repeat aspirates or the use of alternative specimen sources which are not subject to contamination, such as open lung biopsy, autopsy findings, or transtracheal aspirates. These methods showed organisms that were not recovered with the initial transthoracic lung aspirate in 6 of 15 patients studied by Greenman et al. (54), 6 of 17 cases studied by Palmer et al. (110), and 16 of 38 reported by Chaudhary et al. (32). Compared to transtracheal aspiration, Davidson et al. (38) considered transthoracic lung aspiration to be more accurate due to a reduced number of cases with multiple pathogens. However, transtracheal aspiration does appear to have the benefit of fewer false-negative cultures. These data suggest that negative microbiological studies of transthoracic lung aspirates do not necessarily exclude infection, and a repeat procedure or an alternative specimen source may be required in some cases. False-positive cultures are a limited problem as might be expected from the site of sampling. Nevertheless, many reports indicate the recovery of nonpulmonary pathogens in 5–20% of specimens (Table 5-6). Most of the isolates are *S. epidermitidus* or other likely skin contaminants.

Indications

The major indications for transthoracic needle aspiration or biopsy according to the American Thoracic Society are for the diagnosis of (i) solitary nodules and masses, (ii) mediastinal and hilar masses, (iii) mastitic disease, (iv) chest wall invasion in lung cancer, and (v) pulmonary infections in pulmonary nodules or airspace consolidation (57,141). This procedure has been particularly attractive in children since respiratory secretions may be difficult to obtain and transtracheal aspiration is infrequently performed. For adults with infections, the major use has been in the immunologically compromised host or unusual pneumonia in which the usual (less invasive) diagnostic specimen sources are either contraindicated or unrewarding. Data summarized in Table 6 indicate that transthoracic needle aspiration is a reasonable diagnostic test in selected patients with complex pneumonias, although the incidence of false-negative cultures appears to be substantially larger compared with transtracheal aspiration for bacterial infection, and fiberoptic bronchoscopy is often preferred to detect unusual pathogens in the compromised host.

LUNG BIOPSY

The first lung biopsy was reported in 1883 by Leyden (84) who used a closed procedure, but no large series were recorded prior to 1949. Since that time there has been increasing interest in lung biopsy for patients with pulmonary lesions which require tissue for histologic study. The usual indications are localized lesions in which malignancy is suspected or diffuse pulmonary disease ascribed to a variety of noninfection conditions. The major use of microbial diagnoses is for the immunocompromised host in whom a variety of opportunistic pathogens as well as noninfectious conditions are major diagnostic considerations. Three methods to obtain lung biopsies are transbronchial biopsy, core biopsy using a cutting needle or trephine drill, and open lung biopsy. It should be emphasized that tissue for cytologic and microbiological studies may also be obtained by transthoracic needle aspiration or bronchial brushings, but these do not yield intact tissue sections which may be required for some diagnoses. This especially applies to the immunocompromised host in whom the differential diagnosis often includes noninfectious diseases such as radiation pneumonitis, lung injury due to cytotoxic drugs, pulmonary hemorrhage, and tumor invasion.

Transbronchial Biopsy

Transbronchial biopsy was initially used in 1965 with a rigid bronchoscope (5). A subsequent report of the experience in 939 patients provides testimony to the relatively high diagnostic yield in a variety of conditions (4). Preprocedure evaluation should include blood gas determination and coagulation studies. Relative contraindications include a bleeding diathesis, severe respiratory insufficiency, pulmonary hypertension, severe cardiovascular disease, and uremia (60,68,178). Patients with hypoxemia (pO_2 less than 60 mm Hg on room air) should receive supplemental oxygen. Different authorities require minimal platelet counts of 50,000 to 100,000/ml. Patients with active bleeding or thrombocytopenia refractory to platelet transfusion should not undergo transbronchial biopsy.

The procedure is performed in the usual fashion including complete inspection of the tracheobronchial tree. The types of specimens that may be obtained with bronchoscopy include BAL, endobronchial brushings, and forceps biopsy. Biplane fluoroscopy may prove useful for positioning the instrument for biopsy. This probably reduces the possibility of inadvertent pleural biopsy as well. The forceps are advanced into the appropriate location and several specimens are obtained to ensure adequate tissue for histologic study.

The diagnostic accuracy of transbronchial biopsy varies considerably depending on the nature of the pulmonary lesion, technical expertise of the bronchoscopist, method of handling the specimen, and experience of the pathologist (177). The major experience with detecting possible microbial agents concerns studies in immunocompromised patients with diffuse or localized infiltrates. The overall results with this group show a microbial diagnosis is achieved in 15–34% of the patients and the average diagnostic yield is 29% (108,124,146,162). Definitive information is somewhat greater with diffuse infiltrates compared to local lesions, but the difference is modest. The diagnostic yield in the compromised host category is somewhat better for transbronchial biopsy compared to bronchial brushings or bronchoalveolar washings as might be expected (108,121,146). Nevertheless, the total diagnostic yield appears to be improved when BAL and brush specimens are added to the biopsy. In general, approximately 30–50% of the biopsy specimens in immunocompromised patients with diffuse pulmonary infiltrates show nonspecific inflammation (36,108, 121,146).

The most common complications with transbronchial biopsy are pneumothorax or hemorrhage in 3–5% (108,121,124,146,162,177). Restricting analyses to studies of immunocompromised hosts, the incidence of pneumothorax ranges from 0 (36) to 19% (124) with an average of 8%, and the incidence of "significant" hemoptysis is about 7% (95,108,118,162). ("Significant" is arbitrarily defined as 25 ml or more of grossly bloody sputum.) Fatal hemorrhage has been reported (50) and severe bleeding is most common in the presence of uremia or a bleeding diathesis due to leukemia or cancer chemotherapy. A 10–20 mm Hg decrease in arterial oxygen tension is frequently noted during bronchoscopy which emphasizes the importance of supplemental oxygen in patients who are hypoxemic (2).

Advantages of the transbronchial biopsy include relatively low cost, minimal patient discomfort, a low incidence of complications, a relatively high diagnostic yield, and ability to visualize the lower airways. Especially attractive is the ability to avoid general anesthesia and the chest tube required with open lung biopsies. Limitations to the procedure largely concern the tissue samples obtained which are small and subject to considerable crush artifact. The procedure has proved to be the most successful in sarcoidosis, granulomatous diseases, and malignancy. Infectious agents commonly detected with this technique include *P. carinii,* Legionella, H. simplex, cytomegalovirus, Nocardia, mycobacteria, and fungi. "Conventional" bacteria, such as Staphylococci or gram-negative bacilli, may be recovered with transbronchial biopsy. However, interpretation of cultures is complicated due to contamination of the specimen during passage of the instrument through the upper airways, as noted previously. Furthermore, most patients who undergo transbronchial biopsy have already received antibiotics directed against likely pathogens. As a result of these observations, transbronchial biopsy is recommended for the immunocompromised host with localized or diffuse pulmonary infiltrates, especially if (i) alternative diagnostic specimens are negative; (ii) diagnostic possibilities suggest tissue will be required, and (iii) bacterial infection is unlikely due to negative cultures or failure to respond to antibacterial agents. A distinct disadvantage is that open lung biopsy may be required if tissue obtained transbronchially shows only "nonspecific" changes.

Percutaneous Puncture

Pulmonary tissue may be obtained by transthoracic puncture using a cutting instrument such as the Vim Silverman or Cope needle, or trephine drill biopsy (1,6,36,54,82,86,91,107,150,165,175,179). These procedures provide a small sample which is subject to significant crush artifact. The diagnostic yield according to prior reports varies from 30 to 31% in various types of pulmonary conditions with an average of approximately 40% in patients with diffuse pulmonary infiltrates. The major complications are pneumothorax and bleeding which have been noted in 20–60% of patients. The rate of serious complications including mortality is similar to that of open lung biopsy which also provides a higher diagnostic yield. For this reason, cutting needle biopsy of the lung has been largely abandoned (63).

Open Lung Biopsy

Open surgical biopsy provides the optimal specimens for histopathic diagnosis and is regarded as the most definitive method to obtain lung tissue. The first large series was reported in 1949 by Klassen et al. (80) in 1949. Use of this procedure in more recent years for detection of infectious diseases has been primarily for the immunocompromised host. The original procedure, as described by Klassen et al. (79,80), utilizes a posterolateral thoracotomy which permits extensive evaluation of the lung with the potential for biopsying the hilar, peribronchial, or mediastinal lymph nodes as well as the lung and pleura. This procedure is now generally reserved for patients in relatively good clinical condition when lymph nodes examination is desirable. A more common procedure is a small anterior thoracotomy of 4–8 cm, usually through the fourth intercostal space when there is a diffuse disease. The accessible thoracic cavity is inspected and palpated, and biopsies are obtained from appropriate lesions for permanent sections, touch preparations, and cultures.

The principal advantage of open lung biopsy are the availability of larger specimens, the opportunity to biopsy multiple segments from different anatomical sites, and the ability to control bleeding or airleak. Major disadvantages include the use of general anesthesia and time delays inherent in preparing the patient for the procedure. Complication rates are 8–20% with 3% being major complications (79,98,129). The incidence of death ascribed to open biopsy was six of a combined total of 866 patients in three large series (79,98,129). The most common complication was delayed pneumothorax followed by bleeding complications.

The diagnostic yield in patients undergoing open lung biopsy varies from 34 to 91% (54,85,96–99,135,137,146,148,173). Combining data from multiple series, Matthay and Moritz (96) found an overall yield in the immunocompromised host of 69% for patients undergoing open lung biopsy and 52% for patients undergoing transbronchial biopsy. The more recent NIH experience is a diagnostic yield of 81% in 180 patients compared to 45% with transbronchial biopsy in 584 patients (98,146). Clinical circumstances in individual cases as well as available resources dictate the relative advantage for the possibly higher diagnostic yield versus the disadvantage of intubation and general anesthesia. One of the major limitations in recommending this procedure is that the clinical outcome is more often related to the primary disease than to the secondary pulmonary infection (97). Furthermore, multiple investigators have noted that the biopsy often either shows no treatable lesion or a diagnosis that merits no important changes in treatment. The conclusion by some is that mortality rates are often not notably altered by the knowledge gained.

REFERENCES

1. Adamson, J.S., Jr., and Bates, J.H. (1967): Percutaneous needle biopsy of the lung. *Arch. Intern. Med.*, 119:164.
2. Albertini, R.E., Harrell, J.H., Kurihara, N., et al. (1974): Arterial hypoxemia induced by fiberoptic bronchoscopy. *J.A.M.A.*, 230:1666–1667.
3. Alexander, W.J., Baker, G.L., and Hunker, F.D. (1981): Bacteremia and meningitis following fiberoptic bronchoscopy. *Arch. Intern. Med.*, 139:580–582.
4. Andersen, H.A. (1978): Transbronchial lung biopsy for diffuse pulmonary disease. *Chest*, 73(Suppl.):734–736.
5. Andersen, H.A., Fontana, R.S., and Harrison, E.G. (1965): Transbronchial lung biopsy in diffuse pulmonary disease. *Dis. Chest*, 48:187–192.
6. Aronovitch, M., Chartier, J., Kahana, L.M., et al. (1963): Needle biopsy as an aid to precise diagnosis of intrathoracic disease. *Can. Med. Assoc. J.*, 88:120.
7. Brandt, P.O., Bank, N., and Castellino, R.A. (1972): Needle diagnosis of pneumonia: value in high risk patients. *J.A.M.A.*, 220:1578–1580.
8. Baran, D., and Cordier, N. (1973): Usefulness of transtracheal puncture in the bacteriological diagnosis of lung infections in children. *Helv. Paediatr. Acta.*, 28:391–399.
9. Barrio, J.L., Harcup, C., Baier, H.J., et al. Value of repeat fiberoptic bronchoscopies and significance of nondiagnostic bronchoscopic results in patients with the acquired immunodeficiency syndrome.
10. Bartlett, J. (1977): Diagnostic accuracy of transtracheal aspiration bacteriologic studies. *Am. Rev. Respir. Dis.*, 115:777–782.
11. Bartlett, J.G. (1986): The technique of transtracheal aspiration. *J. Crit. Ill*, 1(1):43–49.

12. Bartlett, J.G., Alexander, J., Mayhew, J., et al. (1976): Should fiberoptic bronchoscopy aspirates be cultured? *Am. Rev. Respir. Dis.*, 114:73–78.

13. Bartlett, J.B., and Finegold, S.M. (1974): Anaerobic infections of the lung and pleural space. *Am. Rev. Respir. Dis.*, 110:56–77.

14 Bartlett, J.G., and Finegold, S.M. (1978): Bacteriology of expectorated sputum with quantitative culture and wash technique compared to transtracheal aspirates. *Am. Rev. Resp. Dis.*, 117:1010–1027.

15. Bartlett, J.G., Rosenblatt, S.M., and Finegold, S.M. (1973): Percutaneous transtracheal aspiration in the diagnosis of anaerobic pulmonary infection. *Ann. Intern. Med.*, 79:535–540.

16. Beerens, H., and Tahon-Castel, M. (1965): *Infections humaines a bacteries anaerobies non toxigenes*, pp. 92–107. Presses Academiques Europeennes, Bruxelles.

17. Benner, E.J., Munzinger, J.P., and Chan, R. (1974): Superinfection of the lungs: an evaluation by serial transtracheal aspiration. *West. J. Med.*, 121:173–178.

18. Berman, S.Z., Mathison, D.A., Stevenson, D.D., et al. (1975): Transtracheal aspiration studies in asthmatic patients in relapse with "infective" asthma and in subjects without respiratory disease. *J. Allergy. Clin. Immunol.*, 56:206–214.

19. Bigby, T.D., Margolskee, D., Curtis, J.L., et al. (1986): The usefulness of induced sputum in the diagnosis of *Pneumocystis carinii* pneumonia in patients with the acquired immunodeficiency syndrome. *Am. Rev. Respir. Dis.*, 133:515–518.

20. Bjerkestrand, G., Digranes, A., and Schreiner, A. (1975): Bacteriological findings in transtracheal aspirates from patients with chronic bronchitis and bronchiectasis. *Scand. J. Resp. Dis.*, 56:201–207.

21. Broaddus, C., Dake, M.D., Stulbarg, M.S., et al. (1985): Bronchoalveolar lavage and transbronchial biopsy for the diagnosis of pulmonary infections in the acquired immunodeficiency syndrome. *Ann. Intern. Med.*, 102:747–752.

22. Brook, I., and Finegold, S.M. (1980): Bacteriology of aspiration pneumonia. *Pediatrics, 54:*1115–1120.

23. Bullowa, J.G.M. (1935): The reliability of sputum typing and its relation to serum therapy. *J.A.M.A.*, 105:1512–1523.

24. Burham, S.O. (1960): Bronchoscopy and bacteremia. *J. Thorac. Cardiovasc. Surg.*, 40:635.

25. Castellino, R.A., and Blank, N. (1979): Etiologic diagnosis of focal pulmonary infection in immunocompromised patients by fluoroscopy guided percutaneous needle aspiration. *Radiol.*, 132:563–576.

26. Catterall, J.R., Potasman, I., and Remington, J.S. (1985): *Pneumocystis carinii* pneumonia in the patient with AIDS. *Chest, 85:*758–762.

27. Caughey, G., Wong, H., Gamsu, G., et al. (1985): Nonbronchoscopic bronchoalveolar lavage for the diagnosis of *Pneumocystis carinii* pneumonia in the acquired immunodeficiency syndrome. *Chest, 88:*659–662.

28. Chastre, J., Fagon, J.Y., Domart, Y., and Gilbert, C. (1989): Diagnosis of nosocomial pneumonia in intensive care unit patients. *Eur. J. Clin. Microbiol. Infect. Dis.*, 8:35–39.

29. Chastre, J., Fagon, J.Y., and Lamer, C.H. (1992): Procedures for the diagnosis of pneumonia in ICU patients. *Intensive Care Med.*, 18:S10–S17.

30. Chastre, J., Fagon, J.Y., Soler, P., et al. (1988): Diagnosis of nosocomial bacterial pneumonia in intubated patients undergoing ventilation. *Amer. J. Med.*, 85:499–506.

31. Chastre, J., Viau, F., Brun, P., et al. (1984): Prospective evaluation of the protected specimen brush for the diagnosis of pulmonary infections in ventilated patients. *Am. Rev. Respir. Dis.*, 130:924–929.

32. Chaudhary, S., Hughes, W.T., Feldman, S., et al. (1977): Percutaneous transthoracic needle aspiration of the lung. *Amer. J. Dis. Child.*, 131:902–907.

33. Coleman, D.L., Dodek, R.M., Luce, J.M., et al. (1983). Diagnostic utility of fiberoptic bronchoscopy in patients with *Pneumocystis carinii* pneumonia and the acquired immune deficiency syndrome. *Amer. Rev. Resp. Dis.* 128:795–799.

34. Coleman, D.L., Hattner, R.S., Luce, J.M., et al. (1984): Correlation between gallium lung scans and fiberoptic bronchoscopy in patients with suspected *Pneumocystis carinii* pneumonia and the acquired immunodeficiency syndrome. *Am. Rev. Respir. Dis.*, 130:1166–1169.

35. Credle, W.F., Jr., Smiddy, J.F., and Elliott, R.C. (1974): Complications of fiberoptic bronchoscopy. *Am. Rev. Respir. Dis.*, 109:67–72.

36. Cunningham, J.H., Zavala, D.C., Corry, R.J., et al. (1977): Trephine air drill bronchial brush and fiberoptic transbronchial lung biopsies in immunosuppressed patients. *Am. Rev. Respir. Dis.*, 115:213–220.

37. Dahlgren, S., and Nordenstrom, B. (1966): *Transthoracic Needle Biopsy*. Chicago Year Book Medical Publishers, Chicago.

38. Davidson, M., Tempest, B., and Palmer, D.L. (1976): Bacteriologic diagnosis of acute pneumonia: comparison of sputum, transtracheal aspirates and lung aspirates. *J. Amer. Med. Assoc.*, 235:158–163.

39. Deresinski, S.C., and Stevens, D.A. (1974): Anterior cervical infections. Complications of transtracheal aspiration. *Am. Rev. Respir. Dis.*, 110:354–356.
40. Disney, M.E., Wolff, J., and Wood, B.S.B. (1956): Staphylococcal pneumonia in infants. *Lancet*, 1:767–771.
41. Dixon, J.M.S., and Miller, D.C. (1965): Value of dilute inocula in cultural examination of sputum. *Lancet*, ii:1046–1048.
42. Drew, W.L., Finley, T.N., Mintz, L., and Klein, H.Z. (1974): Diagnosis of *Pneumocystis carinii* pneumonia by bronchopulmonary lavage. *J. Amer. Med. Assoc.*, 230:713–715.
43. Dreyfuss, D., Mier, L., Bolurdelles, G., et al. (1993): Clinical significance of borderline quantitative protected brush specimen culture results. *Am. Rev. Respir. Dis.*, 147:946–951.
44. Edelstein, P.H., Meyer, R.D., and Finegold, S.M. (1980): Laboratory diagnosis of Legionnaires' disease. *Am. Rev. Respir. Dis.*, 12:317–327.
45. Editorial: Transtracheal aspiration. (1963): *N. Engl. J. Med.*, 269:703.
46. Emanuel, D., Peppard, J., Stover, D., et al. (1986): Rapid immunodiagnosis of cytomegalovirus pneumonia by bronchoalveolar lavage using human and murine monoclonal antibodies. *Ann. Intern. Med.*, 104:476–481.
47. Fagon, J.Y. Chastre, J., Hance, A.J. (1988): Detection of nosocomial lung infection in ventilated patients. *Am. Rev. Respir. Dis.*, 138:110–116.
48. Ferrer, M., Torres, A., Xaubet, A., et al. (1992): Diagnostic value of telescoping plugged catheters in HIV-infected patients with pulmonary infiltrates. *Chest*, 102:76–83.
49. Finley, R., Klieff, E., and Thomsen, S. (1974): Bronchial brushing in the diagnosis of pulmonary disease in patients at risk for opportunistic infection. *Am. Rev. Respir. Dis.*, 109:379–387.
50. Flick, M.R., Wasson, K., Dunn, L.J., and Block, J. (1975): Fatal pulmonary hemorrhage after transbronchial lung biopsy through the fiberoptic bronchoscope. *Am. Rev. Respir. Dis.*, 111:853–856.
51. Fossieck, B.E., Parker, R.H., Cohen, M.H., et al. (1977): Fiberoptic bronchoscopy and culture of bacteria from the lower respiratory tree. *Chest*, 73:5–9.
52. Gaussorges, P., Piporno, D., Bachman, P., et al. (1989): Comparison of nonbronchoscopic bronchoalveolar lavage to open living biopsy for the diagnosis of pulmonary infections in mechanically ventilated patients. *Intensive Care Med.*, 15:94–98.
53. Gherman, C.R., and Simon, H.J. (1965): Pneumonia complicating severe underlying disease. *Dis. Chest*, 48:297–310.
54. Greenman, R.L., Goodall, P.T., and King, D. (1975): Lung biopsy in immunocompromised hosts. *Am. J. Med.*, 59:488–496.
55. Guckian, J.C., and Christensen, W.D. (1968): Quantitative culture and gram stain of sputum in pneumonia. *Am. Rev. Respir. Dis.*, 118:997–1005.
56. Guerra, L.F., and Baughman, R.P. (1990): Use of bronchoalveolar lavage to diagnose bacterial pneumonia in mechanically ventilated patients. *Crit. Care Med.*, 18:169–173.
57. Guidelines for percutaneous transthoracic needle aspiration (1989): *Am. Rev. Respir. Dis.*, 140:255–256.
58. Hahn, H.H., and Beaty, H.N. (1970): Transtracheal aspiration in the evaluation of patients with pneumonia. *Ann. Intern. Med.*, 72:183–187.
59. Halperin, S.A., Suratt, P.M., Gwaltney, J.M., Jr., et al. (1982): Bacterial cultures of the lower respiratory tract in normal volunteers with and without experimental rhinovirus infection using a plugged double catheter system. *Am. Rev. Respir. Dis.*, 125:678–680.
60. Hanson, R.R., Zavala, D.C., Rhodes, M.L., et al. (1976): Transbronchial biopsy via flexible fiberoptic bronchoscope: results in 164 patients. *Am. Rev. Respir. Dis.*, 114:67–72.
61. Hayes, D.A., McCarthy, L.C., and Friedman, M. (1980): Evaluation of two bronchoscopic methods of culturing the lower respiratory tract. *Am. Rev. Respir. Dis.*, 122:319–323.
62. Henriquez, A.H., Mendoza, J., and Gonzalez, P.C. (1991): Quantitative culture of bronchoalveolar lavage from patients with anaerobic lung abscesses. *J. Infect. Dis.*, 164:414–417.
63. Herman, P.G. (1978): Needle biopsy of the lung (Editorial). *Ann. Thorac. Surg.*, 26:396.
64. Herman, P.G., and Hessel, S.J. (1977): The diagnostic accuracy and complications of closed lung biopsies. *Radiol.*, 125:11–14.
65. Heurlin, N., Brattstrom, C., Tyden, G., et al. (1989): Cytomegalovirus the predominant cause of pneumonia in renal transplant patients. *Scand. J. Infect. Dis.*, 21:245–253.
66. Higuchi, J.H., Coalson, J.J., and Johanson, W.G., Jr. (1982): Bacteriological diagnosis of nosocomial pneumonia in primates. *Am. Rev. Respir. Dis.*, 125:53–57.
67. Hoeprich, P.D. (1970): Etiologic diagnosis of lower respiratory tract infections. *Calif. Med.*, 112:1–8.
68. Ikeda, S. (1970): Flexible bronchoscope. *Ann. Otol. Rhinol. Laryngol.*, 79:915.
69. Irwin, R.S., Garrity, F.L., Erickson, A.D., et al. (1981): Sampling lower respiratory tract secretions in primary lung abscess. *Chest*, 79:559–565.
70. Jett, J.R., Cortese, D.A., and Dines, D.E. (1981): The value of bronchoscopy in the diagnosis of mycobacterial disease. *Chest*, 80:575–578.

71. Johnson, H.D., and Johnson, W.W. (1970): *Pneumocystis carinii* pneumonia in children with cancer. *J. Amer. Med. Assoc.*, 214:1067–1073.
72. Joshi, J.H., Wang, K.-P., De Jongh, C.A., et al. (1982): A comparative evaluation of two fiberoptic bronchoscopy catheters: the plugged telescoping catheter versus the single sheathed non-plugged catheter. *Am. Rev. Respir. Dis.*, 126:860–863.
73. Kalinske, R.W., Parker, R.H., and Brandt, E. (1970): Diagnostic usefulness and safety of transtracheal aspiration. *N. Engl. J. Med.*, 276:604–608.
74. Kane, R.C., Cohen, M.H., and Fossieck, B.E., Jr. (1975): Absence of bacteremia after fiberoptic bronchoscopy. *Am. Rev. Respir. Dis.*, 111:102–104.
75. Kellerhals, S. (1978): A pseudo-outbreak of *Serratia marcescens* from a contaminated fiber-bronchoscope. *Assoc. Pract. Infect. Control J.*, 6:5–9.
76. Kilborn, J.P., Campbell, R.A., Grach, J.L., and Willis, M.D. (1968): Quantitative bacteriology of sputum. *Am. Rev. Respir. Dis.*, 98:810–818.
77. Kirby, B.D., Snyder, K.M., Meyer, R.D., et al. (1980): Legionnaires' disease: report of sixty-five nosocomially acquired cases and review of the literature. *Medicine*, 59:188–205.
78. Kirkpatrick, M.B., and Bass, J.B. (1989): Quantitative bacterial cultures of bronchoalveolar lavage fluids and protected brush catheter specimens from normal subjects. *Am. Rev. Respir. Dis.*, 139:546–548.
79. Klassen, K.P., and Andrews, N.C. (1967): Biopsy of diffuse pulmonary lesions: a seventeen-year experience. *Ann. Thorac. Surg.*, 4:117–124.
80. Klassen, K.P., Aniyan, A.J., and Curtis, G.M. (1949): Biopsy of diffuse pulmonary lesions. *Arch. Surg.*, 59:694–704.
81. Klein, J.O. (1969): Diagnostic lung puncture in the pneumonias of infants and children. *Pediatr.*, 44:486–492.
82. Krumholz, R.A., Manfredi, F., Weg, J.G., and Rosenbaum, D. (1975): Needle biopsy through the bronchoscope. *Chest*, 67:532–535.
83. Lau, W.L., Young, L.S., and Remington, J.S. (1976): *Pneumocystis carinii* pneumonia. *J. Amer. Med. Assoc.*, 236:2399–2402.
84. Leyden, I. (1883): VII. Verhandlungen des Vereins fur innere Medicin: Ueber infectiose pneumonie. *Deutsch Med. Wschr.*, 9:52–54.
85. Light, G.S., and Michaelis, L.L. (1978): Open lung biopsy for the diagnosis of acute, diffuse pulmonary infiltrates in the immunosuppressed patients. *Chest*, 73:477–482.
86. Lincoln, C.P., Grover, F.L., and Trinkle, J.K. (1975): Open versus needle biopsy of the lung. *J. Thorac. Cardiovasc. Surg.*, 69:507–509.
87. Lober, B., and Swenson, R.M. (1974): Bacteriology of aspiration pneumonia. *Ann. Intern. Med.*, 81:329–331.
88. Lorch, D.G., John, J.F., Tomlinson, J.R., et al. (1987): Protected transbronchial needle aspiration and protected specimen brush in the diagnosis of pneumonia. *Am. Rev. Respir. Dis.*, 136:565–569.
89. Lourie, B., McKinnon, B., and Libler, L. (1974): Transtracheal aspiration and anaerobic abscess. *Ann. Intern. Med.*, 80:417–418.
90. Lyon, A.B. (1922): Bacteriologic studies of one hundred and sixty-five cases of pneumonia and postpneumonic empyema in infants and children. *Amer. J. Dis. Child.*, 23:72–89.
91. Manfredi, F., and Krumholz, R. (1966): Percutaneous needle biopsy of the lung in evaluation of pulmonary disorders. *J.A.M.A.*, 198:1198–1202.
92. Mann, J.M., Altus, C.S., Webber, C.A., et al. (1987): Nonbronchoscopic lung lavage for diagnosis of opportunistic infection in AIDS. *Chest*, 91:319–322.
93. Marquette, C.H., Herengt, F., Mathieu, D., et al. (1993): Diagnosis of pneumonia in mechanically ventilated patients. *Am. Rev. Respir. Dis.*, 147:211–214.
94. Martin, W.J., II and Smith, T.F. (1986): Rapid detection of cytomegalovirus in bronchoalveolar lavage specimens by a monoclonal antibody method. *J. Clin. Microbiol.*, 23:1006–1008.
95. Matthay, R.A., Farmer, W.C., and Odero, D. (1977): Diagnostic fiberoptic bronchoscopy in the immunosuppressed host with pulmonary infiltrates. *Thorax*, 32:539–545.
96. Matthay, R.A., and Moritz, E.D. (1981): Invasive procedures for diagnosing pulmonary infections: a critical review. In: *Clinics in Chest Medicine*, Vol. 2, no. 1, edited by H.Y. Reynolds, pp. 3–18. W.B. Saunders, Philadelphia.
97. McCabe, R.E., Brooks, R.G., Mark, J.B.D., et al. (1985): Open lung biopsy in patients with acute leukemia. *Amer. J. Med.*, 78:609–616.
98. McCabe, R.E., and Remington, J.S. Lung biopsy. (1991): In: *Respiratory Diseases in the Immunosuppressed Host*, edited by J. Shelhamer, P. Pizza, J.E. Parillo, and E. Masur, pp. 105–117. J.B. Lippincott, Philadelphia.
99. McKenna, R.J., Mountain, C.F., and McMurtrey, M.J. (1984): Open lung biopsy in immunocompromised patients. *Chest*, 86:671–674.
100. Meduri, G.U., Beals, D.H., Maijub, A.G., and Baselski, V. (1991): Protected bronchoalveolar lavage. *Am. Rev. Respir. Dis.*, 143:855–864.

101. Meduri, G.U., Stover, D.E., Lee, M., et al. (1986): Pulmonary Kaposi's sarcoma in the acquired immune deficiency syndrome: clinical, radiographic and pathologic manifestations. *Am. J. Med.* 81:11–18.
102. Meduri, G.U., Wunderink, R.G., Leeper, K.V., and Beals, D.H. (1992): Clinical investigations in critical care: management of bacterial pneumonia in ventilated patients. *Chest,* 101: 500–508.
103. Middleton, R., Broughton, W.A., and Kirkpatrick, M.B. (1992): Comparison of four methods for assessing airway bacteriology in intubated mechanically ventilated patients. *Am. J. Med. Sci.,* 304(4):239–245.
104. Mimica, I., Donoso, E., Howard, J.E., and Ledermann, G.W. (1971): Lung puncture in the etiologic diagnosis of pneumonia. *Am. J. Dis. Child.,* 122:278–282.
105. Murray, J.F., Felton, C.P., Garay, S.M., et al. (1984): Pulmonary complications of the acquired immunodeficiency syndrome. *N. Engl. J. Med.,* 310:1682–1688.
106. Murray, J.F., Garay, S.M., Hopewell, P.C., et al. (1987): Pulmonary complications of the acquired immunodeficiency syndrome: an update. *Am. Rev. Respir. Dis.,* 135:504–509.
107. Neff, T.A. (1972): Percutaneous trephine biopsy of the lung. *Chest,* 61:18.
108. Nishio, J.N., and Lynch, J.P., III. (1980): Fiberoptic bronchoscopy in the immunocompromised host: the significance of a "nonspecific" transbronchial biopsy. *Am. Rev. Respir. Dis.,* 121:307–312.
109. Ognibene, F.P., Shelhamer, J., Gill, V., et al. The diagnosis of *Pneumocystis carinii* pneumonia in patients with the acquired immunodeficiency syndrome using subsegmental bronchoalveolar lavage.
110. Palmer, D.L., Davidson, M., and Lusk, R. (1980): Needle aspiration of the lung in complex pneumonias. *Chest,* 78:16–21.
111. Papazian, L., Martin, C., Albanese, J., et al. (1989): Comparison of two methods of bacteriologic sampling of the lower respiratory tract: a study in ventilated patients with nosocomial bronchopneumonia. *Crit. Care Med.,* 17:461–464.
112. Papazian, L., Martin, C., Meric, B., et al. (1993): A reappraisal of blind bronchial sampling in the microbiologic diagnosis of nosocomial bronchopneumonia. *Chest,* 103:236–242.
113. Parsons, G.H., Price, J.E., and Auston, P.W. (1976): Bilateral pneumothorax complicating transtracheal aspirations. *West. J. Med.,* 125:73–76.
114. Pearce, J.G., and Patt, N.L. (1974): Fatal pulmonary hemorrhage after percutaneous aspiration lung biopsy. *Am. Rev. Respir. Dis.,* 110:346–349.
115. Pecora, D.V. (1963): A comparison of transtracheal aspiration with other methods of determining the bacterial flora of the lower respiratory tract. *N. Engl. J. Med.,* 296:664–666.
116. Pecora, D.V. (1974): How well does transtracheal aspiration reflect pulmonary infection? *Chest,* 66:220.
117. Pecora, D.V., and Yegian, D. (1958): Bacteriology of lower respiratory tract in health and chronic disease. *N. Engl. J. Med.,* 258:71–74.
118. Pennington, J.E., and Feldman, N.T. (1977): Pulmonary infiltrates and fever in patients with hematologic malignancy. Assessment of transbronchial biopsy. *Amer. J. Med.,* 62:581–587.
119. Pereira, W., Kovnat, D.M., Khan, M.A., et al. (1975): Fever and pneumonia after flexible bronchoscopy. *Am. Rev. Respir. Dis.,* 112:59–69.
120. Pham, L.H., Brun-Buisson, C., Legrand, P., et al. (1991): Diagnosis of nosocomial pneumonia in mechanically ventilated patients. *Am. Rev. Respir. Dis.,* 143:1055–1061.
121. Phillips, M.J., Knight, R.K., and Green, M. (1980): Fiberoptic bronchoscopy and diagnosis of pulmonary lesions in lymphoma and leukemia. *Thorax,* 35:19–25.
122. Pinkhas, J., Oliver, I., de Vrjies, A., et al. Pulmonary nocardiosis complicating malignant lymphoma successfully treated with chemotherapy.
123. Pitts, J.C., Brantigan, C.O., and Hopeman, A.R. (1977): Mycocardial ischemia associated with transtracheal aspiration. *J.A.M.A.,* 237:2526–2527.
124. Poe, R.H., Utel, M.J., Israel, R.H., et al. (1979): Sensitivity and specificity of the nonspecific transbronchial lung biopsy. *Am. Rev. Respir. Dis.* 119:25–31.
125. Pollock, H.M., Hawkins, E.L., Bonner, J.R., et al. (1983): Diagnosis of bacterial pulmonary infections during quantitative protected catheter cultures obtained during bronchoscopy. *J. Clin. Microbiol.,* 17:255–259.
126. Pratter, M.R., and Irwin, R.S. (1979): Transtracheal aspiration: guidelines for safety. *Chest,* 76:518–520.
127. Pugin, J., Auckenthaler, R., Mili, N., et al. (1991): Diagnosis of ventilator-associated pneumonia by bacteriologic analysis of bronchoscopic and nonbronchoscopic "blind" bronchoalveolar lavage fluid. *Am. Rev. Respir. Dis.* 143:1121–1129.
128. Rapkin, R.H. (1975): Bacteriologic and clinical findings in acute pneumonia of childhood. *Clin. Pediatr.,* 14:130–133.
129. Ray, J.F., Lawton, B.R., Myers, W.O., et al. (1976): Open pulmonary biopsy: nineteen-year experience with 416 consecutive operations. *Chest,* 59:43–47.

130. Repsher, L.H., Schroter, G., and Hammon, W.S. (1972): Diagnosis of *Pneumocystis carinii* pneumonitis by means of endobronchial brush biopsy. *N. Eng. J. Med.*, 287:340–341.
131. Ries, K., Levison, M.E., and Kaye, D. (1974): Transtracheal aspiration in pulmonary infection. *Arch. Intern. Med.*, 133:453–458.
132. Ritchenik, A.E., Ganjeri, P., Torres, A., et al. (1986): Sputum examination of the diagnosis of *Pneumocystis carinii* pneumonia in the acquired immunodeficiency syndrome. *Am. Rev. Respir. Dis.*, 133:119, 226.
133. Robin, E.D., and Burke, C.M. (1986): Lung biopsy in immunosuppressed patients. *Chest*, 89:276–277.
134. Rorat, E., Garcia, R.L., and Skolom, J. (1985): Diagnosis of *Pneumocystis carinii* pneumonia by cytologic examination of bronchial washings. *J.A.M.A.*, 254:1950–1951.
135. Rosen, P.P., Martini, N., and Armstrong, D. (1975): *Pneumocystis carinii* pneumonia: diagnosis by lung biopsy. *Amer. J. Med.*, 58:794–802.
136. Rosenow, E.C. (1911): A bacteriological and cellular study of the lung exudate during life in lobar pneumonia. *J. Infect. Dis.*, 8:500–503.
137. Rossiter, S.S., Miller, D.C., Churg, A.M., et al. (1979): Open lung biopsy in the immunosuppressed patient. Is it really beneficial? *J. Thorac. Cardiovasc. Surg.*, 77:338–356.
138. Rouby, J.J., Rossignon, M.D., Nicolas, M.H., et al. (1989): A prospective study of protected bronchoalveolar lavage in the diagnosis of nosocomial pneumonia. *Anesthesiology*, 71:679–685.
139. Sagel, S.S., Ferguson, T.B., Forrest, J.V., et al. (1978): Percutaneous transthoracic aspiration needle biopsy. *Ann. Thorac. Surg.*, 26:399–405.
140. Salzman, S.H., Schindel, M.L., Aranda, C.P., et al. (1992): The role of bronchoscopy in the diagnosis of pulmonary tuberculosis in patients at risk for HIV infection. *Chest*, 102:143–146.
141. Sanders, C. (1992): Transthoracic needle aspiration. *Clin. Chest Med.*, 13:11–16.
142. Sappington, S.W., and Favorite, G.O. (1936): Lung puncture in lobar pneumonia. *Amer. J. Med. Sci.*, 191:225–234.
143. Schillaci, R.F., Locovoni, V.E., and Conte, R.S.A. (1976): Transtracheal aspiration complicated by fatal endotracheal hemorrhage. *N. Engl. J. Med.*, 295:488–490.
144. Schreiner, A., Digranes, A., and Myking, O. (1972): Transtracheal aspiration in the diagnosis of lower respiratory tract infections. *Scand. J. Infect. Dis.*, 4:49–52.
145. Shelhamer, J.H., Ogniebene, F.P., Macher, A.M., et al. (1984): Persistence of *Pneumocystis carinii* in lung tissue of acquired immunodeficiency syndrome patients treated for *Pneumocystis* pneumonia. *Am. Rev. Respir. Dis.*, 130:1161–1165.
146. Shelhamer, J.H., Toews, G.B., Masur, H., et al. (1992): Respiratory disease in the immunosuppressed patients. *Ann. Intern. Med.*, 117:415–431.
147. Shoutens, E., De Koster, J.P., Vereerstraetes, J., et al. (1973): Use of transtracheal aspiration in the bacteriological diagnosis of bronchopulmonary infection. *Biomedicine*, 19:160–163.
148. Singer, C., Armstrong, D., Rosen, P.P., et al. (1979): Diffuse pulmonary infiltrates in immunocompromised patients. *Amer. J. Med.*, 66:110–120.
149. Spencer, C.D., and Beaty, H.N. (1972): Complications of transtracheal aspiration. *N. Engl. J. Med.*, 286:304–306.
150. Steel, S.J., and Winstanley, D.P. (1969): Trephine biopsy of the lung and pleura. *Thorax*, 24:576.
151. Stover, D.E., White, D.A., Romano, P.A., et al. (1984): Diagnosis of pulmonary disease in acquired immune deficiency syndrome (AIDS). *Am. Rev. Respir. Dis.*, 130:659–662.
152. Stover, D.E., Zaman, M.B., Hajdu, S.I., et al. (1984): Bronchoalveolar lavage in the diagnosis of diffuse pulmonary infiltrates in the immunosuppressed host. *Ann. Intern. Med.*, 101:1–7.
153. Suratt, P.M., Gruber, B., Wellons, H.A., and Wenzel, R.P. (1977): Absence of clinical pneumonia following bronchoscopy with contaminated and clean bronchofiberscopes. *Chest*, 7: 52–59.
154. Suratt, P.M., Smiddy, J.F., and Gruber, B. (1976): Deaths and complications associated with fiberoptic bronchoscopy. *Chest*, 747–751.
155. Teague, R.B., Wallace, R.J., Jr., and Awe, R.J. (1981): The use of quantitative sterile brush culture and gram stain analysis in the diagnosis of lower respiratory tract infection. *Chest*, 79:157–161.
156. Thadepalli, H., Rambhatla, K., and Niden, A.H. (1977): Transtracheal aspiration in diagnosis of sputum-smear-negative tuberculosis. *J. Amer. Med. Assoc.*, 238:1037–1040.
157. Thorpe, J.E., Baughman, R.P., Frame, P.T., et al. (1989): Bronchoalveolar lavage for diagnosing acute bacterial pneumonia. *J. Infect. Dis.*, 155:855–861.
158. Timsit, J.F., Misset, B., Francoual, S., et al. (1993): Is protected specimen brush a reproducible method to diagnose ICU-acquired pneumonia. *Chest*, 104:104–108.
159. Torres, A. (1991): Accuracy of diagnostic tools for the management of nosocomial respiratory infections in mechanically ventilated patients. *Eur. Respir. J.*, 4:1010–1019.
160. Torres, A., Bellacasa, J., Rodriguez-Roisin, R., et al. (1988): Diagnostic value of telescoping plugged catheters in mechanically ventilated patients with bacterial pneumonia using the metras catheter. *Am. Rev. Respir. Dis.*, 138:117–120.

161. Torres, A., Puig de la Bellacasa, J., Xaubet, A., et al. (1989): Diagnostic value of quantitative cultures of bronchoalveolar lavage and telescoping plugged catheters in mechanically ventilated patients with bacterial pneumonia. *Am. Rev. Respir. Dis.*, 140:306–310.

162. Travis, W.D., and Roth, D.B. (1991): Histopathologic evaluation of lung biopsy specimens. In: *Respiratory Diseases in the Immunosuppressed Host*, edited by J. Shelhamer, P. Pizza, J.E. Parillo, and E. Masur, pp. 182–217. J.B. Lippincott, Philadelphia.

163. Unger, K.M., and Moser, K.M. (1973): Fatal complication of transtracheal aspiration. *Arch. Intern. Med.*, 132:437–439.

164. Vereen, L., Smart, L.M., and George, R.B. (1986): Antibody coating and quantitative cultures of bacteria in sputum and bronchial brush specimens for patients with stable chronic bronchitis. *Chest*, 90:534–551.

165. Vitims, V.C. (1972): Percutaneous needle biopsy of the lung with a new disposable needle. *Chest*, 62:717–719.

166. deVivo, F., Pond, G.D., Rhenman, B., et al. (1988): Transtracheal aspiration and fine needle aspiration biopsy for the diagnosis of pulmonary infection in heart transplant patients. *J. Thorac. Cardiovasc. Surg.*, 96:696–699.

167. Wallace, J.M., Batra, P., Gong, H., Jr., et al. (1985): Percutaneous needle lung aspiration for diagnosing pneumonitis in the patient with acquired immunodeficiency syndrome (AIDS). *Am. Rev. Respir. Dis.*, 131:389–392.

168. Webb, S.F., and Vall-Spinosa, A. (1975): Outbreak of *Serratia marcescens* associated with the flexible fiberbronchoscope. *Chest*, 68:703–708.

169. Westcott, J.L. (1973): Air embolism complicating percutaneous needle biopsy of the lung. *Chest*, 63:108–110.

170. Wimberly, N.W., Bass, J.B., Boyd, B.W., et al. (1982): Use of a bronchoscopic protected catheter brush for the diagnosis of pulmonary infections. *Chest*, 81:556–562.

171. Wimberly, N., Faling, J., and Bartlett, J.G. (1979): A fiberoptic bronchoscopy technique to obtain uncontaminated lower airway secretions for bacterial culture. *Am. Rev. Respir. Dis.*, 119:337–343.

172. Winterbauer, R.H., Hutchinson, J.F., Reinhardt, G.N., et al. (1983): The use of quantitative cultures and antibody coating of bacteria to diagnose bacterial pneumonia by fiberoptic bronchoscopy. *Am. Rev. Respir. Dis.*, 138:98–103.

173. Wolff, L.J., Bartlett, M.S., Baehner, R.L., et al. (1977): The causes of interstitial pneumonitis in immunocompromised children: an aggressive systematic approach to diagnosis. *Pediatrics*, 60:41–45.

174. Yang, P.C., Luh, K.T., Lee, Y.C., et al. (1991): Lung abscesses: US examination and US-guided transthoracic aspiration. *Radiol.*, 180:171–175.

175. Yomans, R.C., Jr., Middleton, J.M., Derrick, J.R., et al. (1968): Percutaneous needle biopsy of the lung for diffuse parenchymal disease. *Dis. Chest*, 54:105–111.

176. Yoshikawa, K.T.T., Chow, A.W., Montgomerie, J.Z., and Guze, L.B. (1974): Paratracheal abscess: an unusual complication of transtracheal aspiration. *Chest*, 65:105–106.

177. Zavala, D.C. (1975): Diagnostic fiberoptic bronchoscopy: techniques and results of biopsy in 60 patients. *Chest*, 68:12–19.

178. Zavala, D.C. (1978): Transbronchial biopsy in diffuse lung disease. *Chest* 74(Suppl.):727–733.

179. Zavala, D.C., and Bedel, G.N. (1972): Percutaneous lung biopsy with a cutting needle. *Am. Rev. Respir. Dis.*, 106:186193.

Respiratory Infections: Diagnosis and Management, 3d ed.,
edited by James E. Pennington.
Raven Press, Ltd., New York © 1994

6

Upper Respiratory Tract Infections: The Common Cold, Pharyngitis, Croup, Bacterial Tracheitis and Epiglottitis

Caroline Breese Hall and John T. McBride

Department of Pediatrics and Medicine, University of Rochester School of Medicine and Dentistry, 601 Elmwood Avenue, Rochester, New York 14642

THE COMMON COLD

The one thing man's not leashed despite the strides today—
The "common cold," maligned to have no noble aim.
Yet it respects not class, but finds all equal prey;
And makes each man afflicted woefully the same.

For who has seen a royal cold, befitting kings?
When sneezing makes the eyes red flags above the sea
Of mucous tides that flow through crimson rings
To tunes of foghorn blows . . . Then, jesters all are we![*]

The scourge of a cold is well known to everyone. It is the leading acute illness in the United States today, and major cause to visit a physician or be absent from work or school. Although a "cold" may have a variety of connotations, it is usually defined as an acute illness involving nasopharyngitis and catarrh with little or no fever and minor systemic symptoms.

Colds have long been recognized as highly contagious. In 1914 Kruse (97) demonstrated the transmission of a cold to healthy subjects via filtered nasal secretions from people suffering from an upper respiratory tract infection. The agent was thus proved to be smaller than a bacterium. However, it was some 40 years later before the first common cold viruses were isolated and associated with respiratory disease in humans (21,123,126).

Etiology

Rhinoviruses lead the list as the most common group of viruses that cause colds in both children and adults (Table 6-1). Coronaviruses are also responsible for an appreciable proportion of colds. However, their contribution cannot be closely de-

---

[*]Reprinted from C.B. Hall (1976): The Great Commoner Cold. *Perspec. Biol. Med.*, 10:170, by permission of the University of Chicago Press.

TABLE 6–1. *Viruses associated with the common cold*

Virus	Types	Predominant seasons
Most common:		
Rhinoviruses	1–100+	Fall, mid-spring to summer
Coronaviruses	3	Winter
Common:		
Parainfluenza viruses	4	Fall, spring
Respiratory syncytial virus	1	Winter to early spring
Influenza viruses	3	Winter
Less Common:		
Adenoviruses	33	All seasons
Enteroviruses	60+	Summer, fall
Reoviruses	3	All seasons

fined because of the difficulty in identifying and isolating these agents. The parainfluenza viruses, respiratory syncytial virus, and influenza are all epidemic viruses associated with colds, but these viruses also cause more serious forms of respiratory illness which may overshadow the milder colds. The other viruses listed in Table 6-1 frequently cause upper respiratory tract infections, but not the infections predominantly associated with rhinorrhea and signs typical of a cold.

Incidence

A glance at the number of types of viruses causing colds and anecdotal experience testify to the ubiquitous nature of these infections. In general, the number of colds acquired per year decreases with age (7,15,34,44,61). Infants and preschool children have the highest incidence, four to eight colds per year. That rate may even double when children are in day care or nursery school. In school-aged children the incidence is two to six colds per year (7,15,34,44). Adults generally acquire two to five colds per year, but in households with children, adults suffer even more colds per year (61).

The frequency with which the common cold is acquired throughout life is related not only to the 200 or more types of viruses that produce colds (Table 6-1), but also to the transient immunity produced by some respiratory viruses (23,108). Reinfections are common with the coronaviruses, respiratory syncytial virus, and parainfluenza viruses.

Pathophysiology

Transmission of these viruses may occur by (i) suspension of viral particles in large droplets produced by a cough or sneeze with direct inoculation into the eyes or onto the upper respiratory passages (large-particle droplets can only travel short distances), (ii) virus suspended in the small-particle aerosol of a sneeze or cough, both of which are capable of traversing greater distances, or (iii) spread of contaminated secretions on fomites and hands with self-inoculation. For most of the respiratory viruses it is not known which of these modes of spread are important. In part, it depends on the ability of the virus to survive in the environment under different conditions of humidity and temperature, as well as on the number of virus particles present and their stability in aerosols. Most exhaled large droplets sediment rapidly and, therefore, require close personal contact for spread to occur. In contrast, small particles, one to 20 or more microns in diameter, may remain airborne for prolonged periods with wide and rapid dissemination (94).

For rhinovirus and respiratory syncytial virus close contact with an infected person or infected secretions is necessary. The careful studies of Gwaltney and Hendley (58,60,79) on rhinovirus transmission have shown that people infected with rhinovirus colds have recoverable infectious virus on their hands. Furthermore, these researchers have shown that rhinovirus may be readily transferred from the contaminated hands of one person to the hands of another, who, if susceptible, may acquire infection by touching his nasal or conjunctival mucosa. However, transmission by air over long or short distances is not a major means of transmission for rhinoviruses.

Similar modes of transmission appear to pertain for respiratory syncytial virus (64,66). Respiratory syncytial virus may be spread by close contact or by fomites and self-inoculation via the eye or nose, but not by mouth.

Coxsackievirus A-21 has been shown by experimental infection to be transmitted by small particle aerosols (27). It has been suggested, but not proved, that influenza and adenovirus are transmitted by small-particle aerosols. Nasal secretions are most contagious because of the large quantities of virus they contain. Therefore, nose blowing, and especially the aerosols produced by sneezing, is a highly effective means of spreading virus (94). Coughing, exhaling, and talking result in much less viral spread.

For most respiratory viruses the peak amount of viral shedding correlates with the period of clinical symptoms. Rhinoviruses are usually shed for a week or less by young adults and coronaviruses may be shed for slightly shorter periods (12,36). Other viruses, however, such as respiratory syncytial virus, parainfluenza, and influenza viruses, may be shed for longer periods, particularly in young children (46,65).

After an incubation period of 2 or 3 days (or occasionally up to 7 days for some viruses) infection develops in the epithelium of the upper respiratory tract. Contiguous spread occurs, resulting in local inflammation and submucosal edema with sloughing of ciliated epithelial cells (78,80,108). Nasal secretions containing large amounts of protein become abundant. During the initial couple of days the nasal discharge appears watery and clear, but subsequently contains greater numbers of sloughed epithelial and polymorphonuclear cells to become mucopurulent in appearance.

The pathophysiology of the production of the typical signs and symptoms of a cold recently has had heightened interest and research. The belief that signs such as rhinorrhea and nasal congestion resulted from the direct cytolytic effect of viral replication on the tissue of the upper respiratory tract has been challenged. Winther and colleagues (156,157) some time ago noted that the histology of the nasal mucosa obtained on biopsy in patients with upper respiratory tract infections was unchanged from the periods before and after the cold when they were healthy. Subsequent studies, which showed that symptoms correlated with an increase in the nasal secretions of albumin, polymorphonuclear cells, and bradykinin, suggested that kinins rather than viral cytopathology were the instigators of the typical clinical signs (116,127). Bradykinin may be activated in nasal mucosa following leakage of plasma kininogen into the submucosa and along with other kinins produce the signs of a cold. Rhinorrhea and congestion can result from kinin-induced increased vascular permeability and stimulation of mucus secretion. Indeed, bradykinin sprayed into one nostril of volunteers has been shown to produce unilateral signs and symptoms classically associated with a cold (128).

Abnormal ciliary function may also contribute to the pathogenesis of a cold. Focal areas of nasal mucosa dysmorphic ciliary forms with microtubular aberrations have been identified during viral respiratory infections (21). These findings, which can persist for 2 to 10 weeks, may compromise mucociliary clearance.

Psychological stress also appears to play a role in enhancing susceptibility to colds. Recent studies in volunteers inoculated with rhinovirus 2, 9, or 14, respiratory syncytial virus, or coronavirus type 229E demonstrated that psychological stress increased in a dose-response manner the rate of acquiring both respiratory infections and clinical colds (23). These observations suggest that because the increased rates of infection occurred with all five viruses, stress can lead to a general suppression of resistance to infections.

Clinical Characteristics

The signs and symptoms of the common cold are so universally experienced that all become expert diagnosticians. In most adults and older children the onset is marked by a dry, "scratchy," or sore throat. The usual progression leads to a watery nasal discharge associated with the feeling of an irritated nasal mucosa and sneezing. Systemic symptoms are variable, but commonly the initial couple of days are associated with some general malaise and myalgia. Fever is commonly absent or low grade. The throat may have a burning sensation and pain on swallowing, but the pharynx is generally only minimally injected. After one to three days the nasal secretions thicken and become mucopurulent, causing nasal obstruction. In the infant and young child the common cold viruses can follow a more acute course and lead to lower respiratory tract involvement. Fever and other systemic signs are more common in infants with colds and can be associated with anorexia, vomiting, and diarrhea. Involvement of the eustachian tubes causing obstruction and ear pain is also common in young children.

In neonates these viruses can cause atypical disease with minimal respiratory signs and symptoms (67,149). Outbreaks of infection with respiratory syncytial virus and rhinovirus in neonatal intensive care units have produced a spectrum of illness ranging from mostly nonspecific signs, such as poor feeding and lethargy, to the unexpected onset of apnea.

The severity of the common cold in an individual is related in part to that person's experience with the agent or with a related agent, but, for the most part, the factors associated with the variable degrees of illness in different individuals remain arcane. Smoking, however, has been shown to aggravate the signs and symptoms of a cold, but not to increase the attack rate (61,62). In contradiction to the sacred dictum of many grandmothers, chilling or exposure to cold does not increase the chance of acquiring or aggravating a cold (37).

Treatment

Despite the multitudinous remedies available, advertised, and accepted, no remedy for the common cold exists. Symptomatic treatment is also steeped with ancient folklore and anecdotes, but probably narrows to only analgesics and decongestants (108). Acetaminophen, aspirin, and ibuprophen can ameliorate some of the miseries of the common cold. In two double-blind trials young adults were challenged with rhinovirus and treated with either aspirin or placebo (101). Aspirin therapy was associated with some decrease in the number and severity of cold symptoms, although not significantly so. In addition, however, aspirin treatment was associated with a significant increase in the rate of shedding of rhinovirus from the nasal secretions (142).

In a more recent placebo-controlled study of aspirin, acetaminophen, and ibuprofen in experimental rhinovirus infection, aspirin and acetaminophen treatments were associated with a suppression of the serum-neutralizing antibody response and increased nasal symptoms (55). A trend toward prolonged viral shedding also occurred in those treated with aspirin and acetaminophen. Ibuprofen, however, was not significantly associated with these effects. Analgesics, therefore, can increase the contagion of a cold, not only by making the cold sufferer feel well enough to go to work or school, but also by enhancing the actual shedding of the virus.

Local nasal decongestants can be helpful for sleeping and eating, particularly in young children. However, use of these decongestants should be limited to short periods of time, as excessive use can be irritative and can result in "rebound" nasal congestion. In young infants saline nosedrops are usually beneficial and safe in relieving nasal congestion. Orally administered decongestants are often associated with side effects and are of questionable benefit (85,101,144).

Antihistamines and antibiotics are frequently prescribed for the common cold, not only to treat the acute symptoms but to prophylax against the complication of otitis media and sinusitis. However, in controlled studies these therapies are shown to be of no benefit and should be discouraged (20,54,108,138,154). Linus Pauling (122) noted that early man and his ape relatives had consumed barrels of leaves, ingesting far greater quantities of natural vitamin C than we currently do, and suggested that ascorbic acid could be beneficial in preventing colds. Vitamin C as a therapy has been surrounded with interest and controversy.

Controlled double-blind studies have shown variable results (5,28,76,91,112). The attack rate of colds has not consistently been shown to be diminished despite daily prophylactic intake of vitamin C. However, both the duration and severity of cold symptoms have consistently been ameliorated. The doses of vitamin C administered both for prophylaxis and for treatment in these studies generally have been large, and the therapeutic benefit could correlate with increased doses. A possible explanation for the beneficial effect of ascorbic acid on the symptoms of a cold is that vitamin C reacts with the detrimental oxidants released by neutrophils during an infection (76).

Zinc gluconate in the form of lozenges was initially reported to reduce cold symptoms (40), but subsequent controlled studies in experimental rhinovirus colds have failed to show benefit (43,152).

Specific methods to control the common cold have met with frustration. Hundreds of viral agents produce this common ailment, so prevention by vaccination seems farfetched. Research has thus focused on other means for control and treatment. Prevention of viral attachment in the upper respiratory tract has been considered, such as by blockading the receptors of rhinoviruses with monoclonal antibodies or with soluble receptors artificially produced (75,145). Specific treatment against rhinoviruses with several antiviral agents has been tried in volunteers, but none has produced appreciable clinical benefit (3,73,74,139,140).

Theory suggests that the symptoms of a cold are produced mainly by mediators; therefore, antiinflammatory agents could produce a better therapeutic response. Ipratropium bromide, a compound with parasympatholytic activity, and naproxen, a prostaglandin inhibitor, have both been shown to have beneficial effect on some of the symptoms of colds (47,141). Recent studies by Gwaltney (59) suggest that combining an antiviral agent with antiinflammatory agents could have greater benefit. In blinded, placebo-controlled studies of experimental rhinovirus colds, volunteers who received an antiviral compound, interferon-α 2b, combined with ipratropium bromide and naproxen, had significantly reduced symptoms.

Topical interferon has been explored with variable results. Intranasal alpha interferon has been used most successfully in short-term prophylaxis against rhinovirus and coronavirus colds (26,38,72,95,115,148). However, local side effects and toxicity are frequently a problem, limiting the use and dose range of topically administered interferon.

Interferon inducers, also tried as topical antiviral agents, have shown limited efficacy against some rhinovirus serotypes (26). Aerosolized ribavirin has been shown to be effective against influenza A and B viral infections in college students and against lower respiratory tract infections caused by respiratory syncytial virus infections (68,95); however, mode of administration makes it impractical for treatment of usual upper respiratory tract infections. Zinc gluconate in the form of lozenges has also been reported, in a double-blind study, to reduce the duration of the symptoms of the common cold by an average of 7 days (40).

Complications

Most common colds resolve in 1 to 2 weeks. Inconvenience is usually the only complication. However, a cold can occasionally contribute to the development of more important medical consequences, including bacterial infections, especially otitis media in the young child, apnea or disordered breathing during sleep, and airway hyperreactivity (69,108,131,151). Mechanical obstruction of the nasal passages can lead to bacterial sinusitis. The relationship between viral colds and otitis media, although real, remains unclear (77,132). However, in the first 3 years of life, colds may be complicated by otitis media in 29% (151).

Colds are suspected of contributing to apnea in infancy because up to 90% of children dying with the sudden infant death syndrome have clinical or pathologic evidence of a mild upper respiratory tract infection (11). Respiratory syncytial virus infection has been associated with recurrent nonobstructive periods of apnea in infants (4,17). Cold may exacerbate or precipitate obstructive sleep apneas in adults when nasal obstruction is prominent. In healthy adults complete nasal obstruction frequently leads to disturbed sleep patterns and an increase in respiratory pauses (161). Airway reactivity is also increased during and for a period following colds (6,41). Viral respiratory infections frequently precipitate exacerbations of bronchospasm in asthmatic patients (110). This phenomenon may be related to mucosal inflammation with increased mucosal permeability or to direct effects of the viral infection on immune mechanisms (19).

PHARYNGITIS

Most all of the agents associated with the common cold can also cause pharyngitis, which is commonly overshadowed by the more prominent rhinitis or nasopharyngitis. The agents that can produce an illness with pharyngitis as the major sign, not associated with rhinitis, are listed in Table 6-2. The proportion of pharyngitis caused by beta-hemolytic streptococci group A—in comparison to that caused by viruses—changes according to age. In the first 3 years of life most cases of pharyngitis are caused by nonbacterial agents (49,129). According to the study by Glezen and colleagues (49) of pharyngitis in children from a pediatric practice, group A streptococci were identified in only 3% of children in the first 2 years of life, whereas viruses were identified as the cause of 50%. During the school years, group A streptococci are the most frequently identified agents of pharyngitis, with a peak incidence at 5 to 10 years of age (14,111). In this age group viral pharyngitis can be just as frequent, but identification and therefore quantitation are difficult. In college-aged students, viruses are the predominant pathogens, but streptococcal pharyngitis remains frequent. In the Evans and Dick (42) study of pharyngitis in university students, 26% of the cases were associated with streptococci and 38% with viruses. The rest were of unknown cause.

Although *Mycoplasma pneumoniae* is a major respiratory pathogen, frequently producing bronchitis and pneumonia in school-aged children and young adults, its role in producing illness characterized mainly by pharyngitis is less well-defined.

TABLE 6–2. *Agents producing illness with pharyngitis as major sign*

Children	Adults
COMMONLY ASSOCIATED AGENTS IN:	
Streptococci, Group A	Streptococci, Group A
Adenoviruses	Influenza A and B
Enteroviruses	Epstein-Barr virus
Influenza A and B	*Herpesvirus hominis*
Parainfluenza, types 1–4	Adenoviruses
Epstein-Barr virus	Enteroviruses
Herpesvirus hominis	
LESS FREQUENTLY ASSOCIATED AGENTS:	
Respiratory syncytial virus[a]	Streptococci (Groups C, G)
Rhinovirus[a]	*Corynebacterium diphtheriae*
Coronaviruses[a]	Anaerobic bacteria
Reoviruses	*Neisseria gonorrhoeae*
Cytomegalovirus	*Neisseria meningitidis*
Rubeola	*Hemophilus influenzae*
Rubella	*Salmonella typhi*
Toxoplasma gondii	*Yersinia pseudotuberculosis*
Candida sp	*Treponema pallidum*

[a]Commonly causes rhinitis or nasopharyngitis; less commonly pharyngitis alone.

In a study of pharyngitis in pediatric practice by MacMillan and colleagues (111), *M. pneumoniae* was cultured from 15.8% of pharyngitis patients, but also from 17.6% of controls.

Chlamydia trachomatis has also been implicated as a pharyngitis-producing pathogen, but its etiologic role has not been proved. In a study of adults with pharyngitis seen in private practice, serologic evidence of infection with *C. trachomatis* was obtained in 20.5% and with *M. pneumoniae* in 10.6% (96). However, Gerber et al. (48), in their study of 95 college students with acute pharyngitis, did not find any pharyngeal cultures with *C. trachomatis,* nor did MacMillan et al. (111) in their study of 627 children.

The characteristic clinical findings and clues associated with the various agents of pharyngitis are shown in Table 6-3. Group A streptococcal pharyngitis can be mimicked by a number of viral agents, most commonly Epstein-Barr virus, herpes simplex, and sometimes adenoviruses and enteroviruses. With all of these agents the onset may be abrupt and the fever high. However, in streptococcal pharyngitis, the elevated and shifted peripheral white blood cell count can be helpful, along with the appearance of the pharynx in a florid infection (14). The uvula can be intensely inflamed and edematous. In contrast to viral pharyngitis, the exudate is yellowish, which is best observed on the culture swab. Raised, red follicular lesions with yellowish centers, the so-called doughnut lesions, if present on the soft palate, are highly diagnostic of streptococcal disease (14).

Herpesvirus hominis can produce an exudative tonsillitis that closely mimics streptococcal pharyngitis in university students (51). In university students herpes pharyngitis was accompanied by an exudate in 43% of the cases, whereas the classical anterior lesions on the buccal mucosa and lips were present in only 11%. The exucate covering the posterior pharynx and tonsils was grayish in color, and anterior cervical and submandibular lymphadenopathy were present in about half the cases.

The clinical diagnosis of the cause of the pharyngitis can be aided by associated findings such as a rash or conjunctivitis, as noted in Table 6-4. However, in many cases of pharyngitis, differentiation from streptococcal disease requires a throat culture; therefore, antibiotic therapy should not be initiated first.

CROUP (ACUTE LARYNGOTRACHEOBRONCHITIS)

The disease generally comes on in the evening, after the little patient has been exposed to the weather during the day and after a slight catarrh of some days standing. At first his voice is observed to be hoarse and pulling; . . . he awakes with a most unusual cough, rough and stridulous. And now his breathing is laborious, each inspiration being accompanied by a harsh, shrill noise.

—John Cheyne (*Essays on the Diseases of Children,* 1814)

Croup, or laryngotracheobronchitis, is a striking syndrome of the first few years of life. It is marked by the acute onset of dyspnea and the characteristic inspiratory notes of stridor. The sobriquet *croup* derives from the old Scottish word "roup," meaning "to cry out in a shrill voice." It was introduced by the 18th century treatise of Francis Home, "An Inquiry Into the Nature, Cause and Cure of the Croup" (83).

Epidemiology and Etiology

Croup is primarily a disease of children 3 months to 3 years of age, with the peak attack rate in toddlers during the second year of life, which in a Chapel Hill practice

TABLE 6–3. *Characteristic clinical features associated with agents producing pharyngitis*

	Streptococci Group A (14)	Adenoviruses (113,124,143)	Influenza A and B (120,134)	Parainfluenza Type 1–4 (119)	Epstein-Barr virus (42,82)	Enteroviruses (22,93,113)	Herpes hominis (51,113)	Mycoplasma pneumoniae (32)
Peak season	Nov–April	All seasons	Winter	Fall, spring	All seasons	Summer, fall	All seasons	All seasons
Pharyngeal: Erythema	4+ "Beefy red" uvula	3–4+	3+	2+	3+	2–3+	2–3+	1–2+
Exudate	4+ Yellowish, membranous	2+ Follicular, occasionally membranous	—	—	4+ Gray-white, membranous	1+ Usually follicular	2+ Gray-white	—
Ulcers	—	—	—	—	—	3+ Posterior lesions of Herpangina, hand-foot-mouth syndrome	4+ Large, anterior and posterior	—
Petechiae	3+ Soft palate, "doughnut" lesions	—	±	—	2+ Hard palate	±	—	—
Cervical nodes	4+ Tender, submandibular	2+	—	+	2–3+	1–2+	2+ Anterior submandibular	±
Findings sometimes associated	Voice "thick sounding," scarlet fever, rash, strawberry tongue	Conjunctivitis	Cough, myositis	Laryngitis, otitis	Splenomegaly, generalized lymphadenopathy	Rash	Stomatitis	Cough, pneumonia

TABLE 6–4. *Percent of croup cases associated with various agents*

Agent	Reported series							
	Cramblett 1960 (29) (%)	Parrott et al. 1962 (121) (%)	Loda et al. 1968 (105) (%)	Glezen et al. 1971 (52) (%)	Foy et al. 1973 (45) (%)	Buchan et al. 1974 (18) (%)	Downham et al. 1974 (39) (%)	Denny et al. 1983 (33) (%)
Parainfluenza								
Type 1	8	21	39	21	13[a] 6.4[b]	25	26	18.0
Type 2	6	8	1.6	4	1.4 7.3	1.7	6	3.2
Type 3	14	10	1.6	9	3 13	8	10	6.6
Influenza A	6			2	1 3.7	10	6	1.4
Influenza B		8		1	1 2			1.2
Respiratory syncytial		8	11.4	6	1 9	1.7	6	3.8
Adenovirus	4	9	3	1	4 4.6	1.7	3	
Rhinovirus				0.6	2	1	6	2
Enterovirus	12			1	1	1		
Other viruses						5		
Mycoplasma pneumoniae			5	1.4	0.5 2		1	1.4
Total % of cases with identified agent	50	64	62	47	56	54	64	37.6

Adapted from C.B. Hall (1990): Acute laryngotracheobronchitis. In: *Principles and Practice of Infectious Diseases*, edited by G.L. Mandell, R.G. Douglas, Jr., and J.E. Bennett, p. 499. With permission from John Wiley and Sons, Inc.

[a] Identified by isolation of agent.
[b] Identified by serology.

was 4.7/100 children per year (33). The annual incidence of croup in a Seattle prepaid group practice was 7 per 1,000 children under 6 years of age (45). The peak incidence of approximately double that figure was observed during the second year of life. In studies of both hospitalized and ambulatory patients (18,33,45,50,52), boys are more commonly affected.

Croup now generally refers to an acute laryngotracheobronchitis of viral etiology. Many children experience only a single episode of croup, usually when an associated virus is prevalent in the community. Certain children, however, are subject to recurrent episodes of croup, most of which are associated with viral infections that would otherwise be considered minor. In these children the illness is often termed *spasmodic croup*. Possibly allergy or airway reactivity contributes to spasmodic croup. Positive intradermal skin test reactivity and a family history of allergy are more common in children with recurrent croup compared with those with single episodes, and their serum IgA tends to be lower (159,160). The distinction between "spasmodic" and "regular" croup is important in studies of therapy and outcome, but clinically the two cannot be differentiated. Furthermore, each episode of croup, whether spasmodic or regular, is probably initiated by a viral infection.

Welliver and colleagues (153) have suggested that an abnormal immune response to parainfluenza virus may occur in children with both recurrent and primary croup. Elevated lymphoproliferative responses and diminished histamine-induced suppression of lymphocyte transformation to the parainfluenza viral antigen were noted in children whose parainfluenza viral infection was manifest by croup, in comparison with those with infection limited to the upper respiratory tract.

The cast of viruses causing croup is considerable, as noted in Table 6-4 (63). Only a few, however, play lead parts, and their role is influenced by the season and locale. Parainfluenza virus type 1 is the most frequent cause of acute laryngotracheobronchitis at all ages and evokes the major outbreaks of croup (18,33,50,52). Respiratory syncytial virus generally causes croup only in children under 5 years of age, whereas influenza viruses and *Mycoplasma pneumoniae* cause croup in children over 5 (33). Parainfluenza virus type 1 generally displays its epidemic nature during the autumn, which, in Rochester, New York, for the last 10 years, has occurred in the fall of the odd-numbered years. Well-defined swells of croup cases are also observed during influenza outbreaks. Although the proportion of influenza infections that are manifest as croup is less than that associated with parainfluenza type 1 virus, the disease may be more severe and protracted with influenza (16,84,120). Thus, croup cases occurring during the fall are most likely associated with parainfluenza type 1 virus and to a lesser extent with parainfluenza type 2 virus. Winter cases are most frequently associated with influenza or respiratory syncytial virus. In the spring parainfluenza type 3 may be the prominent pathogen.

Clinical Features

John Cheyne's description of croup remains fitting for most cases of viral laryngotracheobronchitis. Several days of catarrh or upper respiratory tract symptoms commonly precede the acute onset of dyspnea. Heralding the stridor are a deepening, often spasmodic, cough and hoarseness. The distinctive cough has elicited a number of picturesque descriptions. Its hollow, metallic sound has been described as a "seal's bark," a "crowing cock," a "braying ass," or the percussion note of a "brazen tube" or "brass bell."

With increasing stridor and progression of the dyspnea, chest wall retractions may become evident, especially in the supraclavicular and suprasternal areas. In some children auscultation of the chest reveals rales or rhonchi. In severely affected children, expiratory as well as inspiratory stridor, diminished breath sounds, and poor air exchanges can be evident. Fever is frequently present, but somewhat dependent on the viral agent and the age of the child.

Croup characteristically has a fluctuating course. Some children appear to improve during the day and worsen again at night. For most children the course is 3 to 4 days, although other upper respiratory tract signs may persist for longer periods. In a few children the disease can be protracted, or associated with appreciable pneumonitis and hypoxemia, and lead to respiratory failure.

The associated laboratory findings are usually not distinctive or helpful in the diagnosis of croup. The total white blood cell count may initially show some elevation and, particularly in the child who is stressed and hypoxemic, a shift to the left. Subsequently, the white blood cell count can fall and show a predominance of lymphocytes. Blood gas determinations usually show hypoxemia with or without hypercapnia (118).

Pathophysiology

Critical upper airway obstruction in children with croup is explained in part by the small cross-sectional area of the subglottic airway early in childhood and in part because the young child's airway is particularly subject to forces that narrow the extrathoracic airway during inspiration. The subglottic trachea, the narrowest portion of the child's airway, is relatively smaller in children than in adults and is further narrowed in croup by mucosal edema and secretions. During inspiration, the extrathoracic airway normally narrows slightly as the intraluminal pressure falls below atmospheric pressure. This dynamic narrowing, which gives rise to the characteristic inspiratory stridor, is exaggerated in croup for a number of reasons: (i) the pressure collapsing the trachea is greatest when the cross-sectional area is smallest, and thus the narrowed subglottic airway is particularly vulnerable to further collapse with inspiration; (ii) the collapsing force is greater if obstruction is present in the airway above the site of collapse (nasal congestion or laryngeal edema, therefore, will also increase dynamic narrowing); and (iii) rapid, short inspirations associated with anxiety or crying increase the degree of collapse and compromise ventilation while increasing the metabolic demand for gas exchange. Furthermore, the cartilage rings which support the airway are less rigid in childhood than later in life and therefore allow a greater degree of dynamic inspiratory collapse. As airway narrowing increases, the child with croup attempts to maximize airflow by widely opening the glottis with inspiration and by dilating the pharyngeal airway, but can do little to directly increase the diameter of the subglottic airway. With further narrowing, expiratory airflow obstruction becomes audible, in addition to inspiratory stridor. Recent data suggest that narrowing of the upper airway in some children with recurrent episodes of croup is related to airway hyperreactivity and can be reproduced by a bronchoconstrictor challenge (160). Whether this represents reactive mucosal edema or active constriction of the pharyngeal, laryngeal, or subglottic airway, and the extent to which such mechanisms might play a role in the majority of croup episodes, is not clear.

Precipitous respiratory failure is less common in croup than in epiglottitis, probably because the airway edema is less extensive or rapidly progressive, and the child is less toxic. The nature of the obstruction in croup is such that as the child tires and inspires less forcefully, the dynamic narrowing is less severe, and the metabolic demand may fall nearly in proportion to the fall in ventilation. Nevertheless, in a few children, especially those with high levels of obstruction for several days or longer, respiratory muscle fatigue and respiratory failure may appear.

Although hypoxemia is an expected finding when CO_2 retention occurs in croup, low pO_2 values are commonly observed even when pCO_2 values are normal or low (118). This observation suggests that croup could be associated with lower airway (parenchymal) lung involvement. Possible pathophysiologic mechanisms might include spread of the viral infection to the lower respiratory tract, which is common in this age group; transient airway hyperreactivity; or pulmonary edema from the very negative intrathoracic pressures exerted during inspiration in the face of acute upper airway obstruction (146).

Diagnosis

The diagnosis of acute laryngotracheobronchitis is usually made on the characteristic clinical picture. However, confirmation can be obtained by a roentgenogram of the posterior-anterior neck. Typically, in acute viral laryngotracheobronchitis, a narrowing of the trachea shadow occurs in the subglottic area due to the area's characteristic inflammation. The resulting configuration of the airway has been described as an "hourglass."

The etiologic diagnosis of croup requires viral isolation or one of the newer, rapid viral diagnostic techniques detecting viral antigen in the respiratory secretions. Serologic diagnosis is rarely helpful, not only because of the weeks required for acute and convalescent sera to be obtained, but also because the serologic response of young children to some of these viral agents, such as the parainfluenza viruses, is not always detectable or is heterotypic.

Treatment

The efficacy of various therapies is difficult to study objectively. The degree of airway obstruction fluctuates from hour to hour, the course from day to day is unpredictable, and differentiation of spasmodic croup from regular croup may be impossible. Children with croup are anxious, and maneuvers designed to obtain physiologic measurements can increase anxiety and exacerbate the airway obstruction. For these reasons, nearly all forms of treatment for croup are controversial and will remain so until further, objective clinical and laboratory studies are available.

The primary treatment for croup has long been the administration of cold and/or moist air. Many children improve dramatically when taken outside to breathe the cold (and very dry) winter air. One of the few animal studies of croup supports the efficacy of airway cooling (158). In that study, cold-dry, cold-moist, and warm-dry air (all of which would cool the airway because of their low moisture content) were effective in the dog model in decreasing upper airway resistance after the development of mucosal edema. Warm, moist air, with its high water content, was ineffective.

The value of moisture or mist is not well established. If the child has difficulty with inspissated secretions in the upper respiratory tract, humidification can help. If the mist is cold, it can improve the efficacy of airway cooling. However, there have been no studies that clearly demonstrate the value of mist therapy in the treatment of croup.

The administration of nebulized racemic epinephrine, either by IPPB or by mask, has become a popular approach to the treatment of severe croup (1). Racemic epinephrine probably works by inducing local vasoconstriction, in that nebulized phenylephrine has been shown to be similarly effective (111). Clinical improvement is transient, however, lasting only a couple of hours. Vaponephrine treatment does not alter the arterial pO_2 or the duration of the illness, but can result in fewer children requiring tracheostomy or intubation (2,98,155). Rebound mucosal vasodilation, similar to that occurring with the prolonged use of topical nasal vasoconstrictors, has not been reported, but is, theoretically, a drawback to the use of this agent. Children treated with vaponephrine aerosols should be watched closely for at least 2 hours after treatment.

Systemic corticosteroids in the treatment of croup have been evaluated over the last 30 years in at least 15 controlled studies (90,136,147). The long-time controversy over their use has been diminished, with the recent demonstration that much of the variability in results among the studies could be related to different dosages of steroids utilized. Analysis of these studies indicate that larger doses are needed to produce clinical benefit. In the studies, 0.3 mg/kg to 0.6 mg/kg of dexamethasone (or its equivalent), given once or repeated every 6 hours for two to four doses, resulted in clinical benefit (90,136) and could diminish the need for intubation in hospitalized children.

Complications

Croup has long been considered a self-limited illness of childhood. However, two studies indicate that viral croup could have long-term sequelae. Loughlin and Taussig (107) demonstrated increased bronchial reactivity in children 6 to 15 years after an episode of croup. Gurwitz and colleagues (57) also documented increased bronchial reactivity and signs of possible small airway dysfunction in another group of children who had had croup an average of 8 years earlier. It is not clear from these studies whether the episode of croup caused the observed abnormalities or whether underlying abnormalities of airway function contribute to the severity or susceptibility to croup. Nevertheless, viral croup and other respiratory viral infections occurring in early childhood appear capable of distorting lung development and of contributing to permanent lung dysfunction (92).

BACTERIAL TRACHEITIS

Bacterial tracheitis is an unusual, atypical croup-like syndrome that should be differentiated from acute viral laryngotracheobronchitis (31,35,87,103,104,106,117). This clinical entity affects older children with an acute onset of high fever, respiratory stridor, and production of abundant, purulent sputum. The course can be severe and protracted, often requiring endotracheal intubation or tracheotomy. The subglottic area appears acutely inflamed and covered with a thick exudate. The severity and degree of airway obstruction is similar to that observed with epiglottitis. However, in bacterial tracheitis, the epiglottis and supraglottic structures are usually minimally involved. Also, children with bacterial tracheitis are not apt to sit forward and drool, as is characteristic in epiglottitis.

The pathophysiology of the entity is not entirely clear. However, the organisms most commonly involved are *Staphylococcus aureus* Group A beta-hemolytic streptococci, and *Hemophilus influenzae* type b (31,35,103,104,106). The entity often appears to occur in children intubated for other reasons, in those who have had trauma to that area, or as secondary bacterial invaders of a viral infection, especially parainfluenza infection. The diagnosis is suspected by the acute, epiglottitis-like onset, a peripheral white blood cell count that is shifted to the left, and a lateral soft tissue roentgenogram of the neck showing a normal epiglottis and usually subglottic narrowing. The diagnosis can be confirmed by direct laryngoscopy revealing the localized exudate and inflammation in the subglottic area. This infection requires a specific diagnosis because of its severe course, and the need for prompt antibiotic treatment. It does not respond to racemic epinephrine. It is, however, an unusual entity, and the greater majority of cases of croup are viral and should not be treated with antibiotics in an attempt to cover or prevent bacterial tracheitis. Secondary bacterial infection after viral laryngotracheobronchitis is unusual.

EPIGLOTTITIS

The first reported case of acute epiglottis was a 49-year-old French woman described by LaMierre in 1936 (100). This woman developed the classical findings of fever, dysphagia, dyspnea, and pharyngeal obstruction, along with a cervical abscess. *H. influenzae* type b was recovered from the abscess and blood. After a protracted course of one month she recovered.

Etiology

Epiglottitis, which might more appropriately be called supraglottitis, involves not only the epiglottis but also the aryepiglottic folds and the arytenoids. This acute and often severe infection is almost always caused by *H. influenzae* type b. On rare occasion reports implicate other organisms, including streptococci, pneumococci, staphylococci, *H. paraphrophilus,* and even respiratory viruses (8,10,56,89,99). The recent widespread use of the new conjugated *H. influenzae* type b vaccines in infants, starting at 2 months of age, has markedly diminished the occurrence of this and other invasive infections from *H. influenzae* type b (24).

Incidence and Epidemiology

The epidemiology of *H. influenzae* epiglottitis is being dramatically changed by the conjugate vaccines. However, prior to the use of these new vaccines, and in countries not using them, the incidence of epiglottitis appears to vary in different climates and populations. Temperate climates and Caucasian populations appear to have higher incidences (8,114). In Denver over a 17-year period the number of children admitted with epiglottitis varied from none to 12 per year. In Alaska epiglottitis accounted for one of every 600 admissions (8). Cases occur throughout the year, but clustering or an increased incidence has been reported to occur in the spring and warmer months in some areas (9,30,150), whereas a winter seasonal predominance has occurred in other locales (87,114).

Despite LaMierre's initial report of epiglottitis, the usual age range of patients is 1 to 6 years (10,30,114). For unexplained reasons the peak age of 2 to 4 years is older than that of meningitis caused by the same organism, *H. influenzae* type b (30,137). Nevertheless, epiglottitis can occur at both ends of the age spectrum from newborns to the elderly (9,70,71,81,86,109,133). In Rochester, New York, during a 9-year period, prior to immunization, 21% of the 47 patients admitted to the hospital with acute epiglottitis were adults (133). In some series the proportion of patients with epiglottitis who were adults is even higher (13,70). In Rhode Island, the annual incidence of acute epiglottitis in adults was estimated to be 9.7 cases per million adults (109).

Clinical Features

The abrupt onset and rapidly progressive course are striking, but characteristic of epiglottitis. Typically the child is a preschooler, more commonly a boy, who presents with an acutely sore throat and fever of only hours duration. Dysphagia and respiratory distress usually rapidly ensue and the child appears anxious. In contrast to the child with viral croup, the child with epiglottitis will sit up, lean forward, and drool. Inspiratory stridor may be evident, but the harsh, spasmodic cough or seal's bark characteristic of viral croup is usually absent. Tachycardia, associated with the often high fever, is common, but the respiratory rate is usually not markedly elevated. The child generally appears toxic with physical findings related to the respiratory distress. Auscultation of the chest can reveal rhonchi and sometimes decreased breath sounds. The diagnostic physical finding is the "beefy" red, stiff, and swollen epiglottis which on direct visualization appears as a "red cherry." Thick secretions also coat the epiglottis and surrounding tissues.

In adults, the clinical picture can be similar, with the abrupt onset of sore throat, dysphagia, fever, and progression to respiratory distress. However, in Hawkins and colleagues' (71) description of epiglottitis in 17 adults, the course was not as rapidly progressive. Sore throat and dysphagia were the most common symptoms, but the onset occurred over an average of 2 to 3 days, before medical attention was required. The average temperature was only 38.2°C, and a few patients remained afebrile. Ten of the 17 went on to develop respiratory distress.

Pathophysiology

In epiglottitis, edema and inflammation of the epiglottis and aryepiglottic folds rapidly progress to narrow the supraglottic airway. Dynamic airway narrowing on inspiration produces inspiratory stridor early in the course, and with further progression expiratory obstruction is audible as well. The major difference between epiglottitis and viral croup is the very rapid progression of obstruction in epiglottis and the risk of abrupt apnea and death. Sudden apnea was previously thought to represent complete occlusion of the airway by the swollen epiglottis. It is possible, however, to ventilate an individual with epiglottitis who has ceased to breathe with positive pressure and a face mask (2,53). This argues against total airway occlusion, and suggests that a combination of secretion, airway obstruction, and extreme toxicity precipitate the apnea. Patients with epiglottitis are systemically ill, and can reach a point at which they precipitiously fail to compensate for the increased work of breathing. Appreciation of the fact that such patients do not have total mechanical obstruction is important for appropriate management. An appreciable number of children with epiglottitis often have hypoxemia, similar to children with viral croup (25). In a recent study by Costigan and Newth (25), 77% of their patients with acute epiglottitis had hypoxemia that was not explained by alveolar hypoventilation and that occurred irrespective of the presence of an artificial airway or infiltrates on the chest roentgenogram, but could be corrected by oxygen administration. This suggests the hypoxemia results from a ventilation to perfusion mismatch and indicates an abnormality of the lung parenchyma in addition to upper airway obstruction.

Diagnosis

The initial diagnosis of epiglottitis must be made on the characteristic, often striking, clinical findings, and should be accompanied by immediate hospitalization. Although direct visualization of the epiglottis may be diagnostic, the required manipulation may initiate sudden and fatal airway obstruction. Even examination of the posterior pharynx with a tongue blade has triggered fatal obstruction of the inflamed airway. Visualization, therefore, should not be attempted without trained personnel and equipment present to establish an artificial airway if necessary.

Posterior-anterior and lateral neck roentgenograms have been shown to be a reliable and noninvasive means of differentiating epiglottitis from viral croup (130). The lateral film of the neck with the patient upright shows a dilated hypopharynx with a swollen epiglottis, aryepiglottic folds and arytenoids, and edema of the prevertebral soft tissues. Narrowing or obliteration of the valleculae is also commonly present. The swollen epiglottis has been termed the "thumb sign" from its similar appearance to a thumb viewed anteriorally, whereas the normal epiglottis appears as a lateral view of the "little finger" (125). Generally the subglottic tissues appear normal. However, in one series, 25% of the children with acute epiglottitis also had localized subglottic edema similar to that seen in viral croup (135).

The etiologic diagnosis can be made by cultures of *H. influenzae* type b, obtained from upper respiratory tract specimens and blood. The blood culture, if correctly obtained, is almost always positive in *H. influenzae* type b epiglottitis.

Treatment

The best treatment for acute epiglottitis is prevention, a goal recently made possible with the licensure of the new *H. influenzae* type b conjugated vaccines (24). These vaccines are recommended in the United States for all children beginning at 2 months of age, with the result that *H. influenzae* type b epiglottitis and other forms of invasive disease are now rarely encountered on our pediatric wards.

The acute management of a patient suspected to have epiglottitis is dictated by two facts: (i) the ever-present risk of sudden deterioration and apnea, which may be precipitated by an attempt to manipulate the patient; and (ii) the difficulty of emergency intubation in face of supraglottic inflammation. If epiglottitis is suspected, the patient should be attended constantly by a physician skilled in managing airway emergencies. In many centers, when the diagnosis is confirmed (or before, if the patient is critically ill), an endotracheal tube is inserted under direct laryngoscopy in the operating room with a surgeon on hand, prepared to perform a tracheostomy. After the airway is secured and appropriate cultures are obtained, intravenous antibiotic therapy is initiated, and the patient is transferred to an intensive care unit or other facility where constant monitoring is available. Initial antibiotic therapy should be with a drug, as chloramphenicol, that is effective against ampicillin-resistant *H. influenzae* type b, today an appreciable problem throughout much of the United States. A few isolates of *H. influenzae* type b resistant to chloramphenicol have also been reported. In such areas initial therapy should also include ampicillin or one of the newer cephalosporins effective against both types of organisms. Accidental extubation can be avoided by constant observation and the use of adequate restraints and seuatic¬ if necessary. The patient should be extubated when the edema and inflammation appear to be resolving, usually within 1 to 3 days of admission. Parenteral antibiotics are continued for 7 to 10 days.

For patients who become apneic prior to reaching the operating room, previous recommendations were that an airway be established immediately by intubation, tracheostomy, or puncture of the cricothyroid membrane. However, these procedures require skill and time, and can be associated with morbidity in an emergency situation. It is now recognized that most patients with epiglottitis can be ventilated adequately by mask and bag, and the positive pressure ventilation should be the immediate first step in resuscitation of the apneic patient (2).

Treatment of epiglottitis is different in different centers. In some, tracheostomy is preferred to intubation; in others, systemic steroids are used in an attempt to decrease airway inflammation. In a few places, patients are managed without an artificial airway but with aggressive medical treatment and bag and mask ventilation when necessary (53). The standard approach, however, is to secure the airway in all patients with epiglottitis. The possible exception is children who are not toxic, have no inspiratory stridor, and can be observed continuously while medical therapy is begun. Whatever the plan, it is important that all personnel in each institution be familiar and comfortable with the protocol for managing these patients.

Complications

Foci of infection with *H. influenzae* beyond the epiglottis can complicate the course. Pneumonia and cervical lymphadentitis have been the most frequent complications, occurring in 25 to 33% of patients (25,114). Exudative tonsillitis, otitis media, and epiglottic abscess are occasionally present (80,114). Despite the frequent presence of bacteremia in epiglottitis other septic foci are rare. Meningitis has been rarely reported in combination with epiglottitis (114).

The major and most feared complication of epiglottitis is sudden airway obstruction. However, with prompt recognition and management, including elective intubation, this complication should be rare.

REFERENCES

1. Adair, J.C., Ring, W.H., and Jordan, W.S. (1971): Ten-year experience with IPPB in the treatment of acute laryngotracheobronchitis. *Anesth. Analg.,* 50:649–655.
2. Adair, J.C., and Ring W.H. (1975): Management of epiglottitis in children. *Anesth. Analg.,* 54:622–625.
3. Al-Nakib, W., Higgins, P.G., Barrow, G.I., et al. (1989): Suppression of colds in human volunteers challenged with rhinovirus by a new synthetic drug (R61837). *Antimicrob. Agents Chemother.,* 33:522–525.
4. Anas, N., Boettrich, C., Hall, C.B., and Brooks, J.G. (1982): The association of apnea and respiratory syncytial virus infection in infants. *J. Pediatr.,* 101:65–68.
5. Anderson, T.W., Beaton, G.H., Corey, P.N., and Spero, L. (1975): Winter illness and vitamin C: the effect of relatively low doses. *Can. Med. Assoc. J.,* 112:823–826.
6. Aquilina, A.T., Hall, W.J., Douglas, R.G., and Utell, M.J. (1980): Airway reactivity in subjects with viral upper respiratory tract infections: the effects of exercise and cold air. *Am. Rev. Respir. Dis.,* 122:3–10.
7. Badger, G.F., Dingle, J.H., and Feller, A.E. (1953): A study of illness in a group of Cleveland families. II. Incidence of common respiratory diseases. *Am. J. Hyg.,* 41–46.
8. Bass, J.W., Steele, R.W., and Wiebe, R.A. (1974): Acute epiglottitis: a surgical emergency. *J.A.M.A.* 229:671–675.
9. Baxter, J.D. (1967): Acute epiglottitis in children. *Laryngoscope,* 77:1358–1367.
10. Berenberg, W., and Kevy, S. (1958): Acute epiglottitis in childhood. *N. Engl. J. Med.,* 258:870–874.
11. Bergman, A.B., Rax, C.G., Pomeroy, M.A., Wahl, P.W., and Beckwith, J.B. (1972): Studies of the sudden infant death syndrome in King County, Washington. III. Epidemiology. *Pediatrics,* 49:860–870.
12. Bradburne, A.F., Bynue, M.L., and Tyrrell, D.A.J. (1967): Effects of a "new" human respiratory virus in volunteers. *Br. Med. J.,* 3:767–769.
13. Branefors-Helander, P., and Jeppson, P.H. (1975): Acute epiglottitis: a clinical, bacteriological and serological study. *Scand. J. Infect. Dis.,* 7:103–111.
14. Breese, B.B. (1978): *Pharyngitis and Scarlet Fever in Beta-Hemolytic Streptococcal Diseases,* edited by B.B. Breese and C.B. Hall, pp. 65–78. Houghton Mifflin, Boston.
15. Brimblecombe, F.S.W., Cruickshank, R., Masters, P.L., and Reid, D.D. (1958): Family studies of respiratory infections. *Br. Med. J.,* 1:119–128.
16. Brocklebank, J.T., Court, S.D.M., McQuillin, J., and Gardner, P.S. (1972): Influenza-A infection in children. *Lancet* 2:497–500.
17. Bruhn, F.W., Mokrohisky, S.T., and McIntosh, K. (1977): Apnea associated with respiratory syncytial virus in young infants. *J. Pediatr.,* 90:382–386.
18. Buchan, K.A., Marten, K.W., and Kennedy, D.H. (1974): Aetiology and epidemiology of viral croup in Glasgow 1966–72. *J. Hyg. Camb.,* 73:143–150.
19. Busse, W.W., Anderson, C.L., Dick, E.C., and Warshauer, D. (1980): Reduced granulocyte response to isoproterenol histamine, and prostaglandin E, after *in vivo* incubation with rhinovirus 16. *Am. Rev. Respir. Dis.,* 122:641–646.
20. Cantekin, E.I., Mandel, E.M., Bluestone, C.O., Rockette, H.E., Paradise, J.L., Stool, S.E., Fria, T.J., and Rogers, K.D. (1983): Lack of efficacy of decongestant: antihistamine combination for otitis media in children. *N. Engl. J. Med.,* 308:297–301.
21. Carson, J.L., Collier, A.M., and Hu, S.S. (1985): Acquired ciliary defects in nasal epithelium of children with acute viral upper respiratory infections. *N. Engl. J. Med.,* 312:463–468.
22. Cherry, J.D., and Jahn, C.L. (1965): Herpangina. The etiologic spectrum. *Pediatrics,* 36:632–634.
23. Cohen, S., Tyrrell, D.A.J., and Smith, A.P. (1991): Psychological stress and susceptibility to the common cold. *N. Engl. J. Med.,* 325:606–612.
24. Committee on Infectious Diseases, American Academy of Pediatrics. (1993): *Hemophilus influenzae* type b conjugate vaccines: recommendations for immunization with recently and previously licensed vaccines. *Pediatrics,* 92:480–488.
25. Costigan, D.C., and Newth, C.J.L. (1983): Respiratory status of children with epiglottitis with and without an artificial airway. *Am. J. Dis. Child.,* 137:139–141.
26. Couch, R.B. (1984): The common cold: control? *J. Infect. Dis.,* 150:167–173.
27. Couch, R.B., Cate, T.R., Douglas, R.G., Jr., Gerone, P.J., and Knight, V. (1966): Effect of route of inoculation on experimental respiratory viral disease in volunteers and evidence for airborne transmission. *Bacteriol. Rev.,* 30:517–531.
28. Coulehan, J.J., Eberhard, S., Kapner, L., Taylor, F., Rogers, K., and Garry, P. (1976): Vitamin C and acute illness in Navajo school children. *N. Engl. J. Med.,* 18:973–977.

29. Cramblett, H.G. (1977): Croup (epiglottitis, laryngitis, laryngotracheobronchitis). In *Disorders of the Respiratory Tract in Children,* 3rd edition, edited by E.L. Kendig, Jr., pp. 353–360. W.B. Saunders, Philadelphia.

30. Dajani, A.S., Asmar, B.I., and Thirumoorthi, M.C. (1979): Systemic *Haemophilus influenzae* disease: an overview. *J. Pediatr.,* 94:355–364.

31. Davidson, S., Barzilay, Z., Yahav, J., and Rubenstein, E. (1982): Bacterial tracheitis—a true entity? *J. Laryngol. Otolaryn.,* 96:173–175.

32. Denny, F.W., Clyde, W.A., Jr., and Glezen, W.P. (1971): *Mycoplasma pneumoniae* disease: clinical spectrum, pathophysiology, epidemiology and control. *J. Infect. Dis.,* 123:74–92.

33. Denny, F.W., Murphy, T.F., Clyde, W.A., Jr., Collier, A.M., and Henderson, F.W. (1983): Croup: A 11-year study in a pediatric practice. *Pediatr.,* 71:871–876.

34. Dingle, J.H., Badger, G.F., and Jordan, W.S., Jr. (1964): Illness in the home: study of 25,000 illnesses in a group of Cleveland families, Chapter 1, pp. 1–3. The Press of Western Reserve University, Cleveland.

35. Donnelly, B.W., McMillan, J.A., and Weiner, L.B. (1990): Bacterial tracheitis: report of eight new cases and review. *Rev. Infect. Dis.,* 12:729–735.

36. Douglas, R.G., Jr., Cate, T.R., Gerone, P.J., and Couch, R.B. (1966): Quantitative rhinovirus shedding patterns in volunteers, *Amer. Rev. Resp. Dis.,* 94:159–167.

37. Douglas, R.G., Jr., Lindgren, K.M., and Couch, R.B. (1968): Exposure to cold environment and rhinovirus common cold: failure to demonstrate effect. *N. Engl. J. Med.* 279:743–747.

38. Douglas, R.M., Moore, B.W., Miles, H.B., Davies, L.M., Graham, N.M.H., et al. (1986): Prophylactic efficacy of intranasal alpha$_2$ interferon against rhinovirus infections in the family setting. *N. Engl. J. Med.,* 314:65–70.

39. Downham, M.A.P.S., McQuillan, J., and Gardner, P.S. (1974): Diagnosis and clinical significance of parainfluenza virus infections in children. *Arch. Dis. Child.,* 49:8–15.

40. Eby, G.A., Davis, D.R., and Halcomb, W.W. (1984): Reduction in duration of common colds by zinc gluconate lozenges in a double-blind study. *Antimicrob. Agents Chemother.,* 25:20–24.

41. Empey, D.W., Laitinen, L.A., Jacobs, L., Gold, W.M., and Nadel, J.A. (1976): Mechanisms of bronchial hyperreactivity in normal subjects after upper respiratory tract infection. *Am. Rev. Respir. Dis.,* 113:131–139.

42. Evans, A.S., and Dick, E.C. (1964): Acute pharyngitis and tonsillitis in University of Wisconsin students. *J.A.M.A.,* 190:699–708.

43. Farr, B.M., Conner, E.M., Betts, R.F., Oleske, J., Minnefor, A., and Gwaltney, J.M. (1987): Two randomized controlled trials of zinc gluconate lozenge therapy of experimentally induced rhinovirus colds. *Antimicrob. Agents Chemother.,* 31:1183–1187.

44. Fox, J.P., Hall, C.E., Cooney, M.K., Luce, R.E., and Kronmal, R.A. (1972): The Seattle virus watch. II. Objectives. Study population and its observation data processing and summary of illnesses. *Am. J. Epidemiol.,* 96:270–285.

45. Foy, H.M., Cooney, M.K., Maletzky, A.J., and Grayston, J.T. (1973): Incidence and etiology of pneumonia, croup and bronchiolitis in preschool belonging to a prepaid medical care group over a four-year period. *Am. J. Epidemiol.,* 97:80–92.

46. Frank, A., Taber, L.H., Wells, C.R., Wells, J.M., Glezen, W.P., and Paredes, A. (1981): Patterns of shedding of myxoviruses and paramyxoviruses in children. *J. Infect. Dis.,* 144:433–441.

47. Gaffey, M.J., Hayden, F.G., Boyd, J.C., and Gwaltney, J.M., Jr. (1988): Ipratropium bromide treatment of experimental rhinovirus infection. *Antimicrob. Agents Chemother.,* 32:1644–1647.

48. Gerber, M.A., Ryan, R.W., Tilton, R.C., et al. (1984): Role of *Chlamydia trachomatis* in acute pharyngitis in young adults. *J. Clin. Microbiol.,* 20:993–994.

49. Glezen, W.P., Clyde, W.A., Jr., Senior, R.J., Sheaffer, C.I., and Denny, F.W. (1967): Group A streptococci, mycoplasms, and viruses associated with acute pharyngitis. *J.A.M.A.,* 202:455–460.

50. Glezen, W.P., and Denny, F.W. (1973): Epidemiology of acute lower respiratory disease in children. *N. Engl. J. Med.,* 288:498–505.

51. Glezen, W.P., Fernald, G.W., and Lohr, J.A. (1975): Acute respiratory disease of university students with special reference to the etiologic role of *Herpesvirus hominis. Am. J. Epidemiol.,* 101:111–112.

52. Glezen, W.P., Loda, F.A., Clyde, W.A., Jr., Senior, R.J., Sheaffer, C.I., Conley, W.G., and Denny, F.W. (1971): Epidemiological patterns of acute lower respiratory disease of children in a pediatric group practice. *J. Pediatr.,* 78:397–406.

53. Glicklich, M., Cohen, R.D., and Jona, J.Z. (1979): Steroids and bag and mask ventilation in the treatment of acute epiglottitis. *J. Pediatr. Surg.,* 14:247–251.

54. Gordon, M., Lovell, S., and Dugdale, A.E. (1974): The value of antibiotics in minor respiratory illness in children. A controlled trial. *Med. J. Aust.,* 1:304–306.

55. Graham, N.M.H., Burrell, C.J., Douglas, R.M., Debelle, P., and Davies, L. (1990): Adverse effects of aspirin, acetaminophen, and ibuprofen on immune function, viral shedding, and clinical status in rhinovirus-infected volunteers. *J. Infect. Dis.,* 162:1277–1282.

56. Grattan-Smith, T., Forer, M., Kilham, H., and Gillis, J. (1987): Viral supraglottitis. *J. Pediatr.*, 110:437–442.
57. Gurwitz, D., Corey, M., and Levison, H. (1980): Pulmonary function and bronchial reactivity in children after croup. *Am. Rev. Respir. Dis.*, 122:95–99.
58. Gwaltney, J.M. (1983): Rhinovirus colds: epidemiology, clinical characteristics and transmission. *Eur. J. Respir. Dis.*, 64 (suppl. 128):336–339.
59. Gwaltney, J.M., Jr. (1992): Combined antiviral and antimediator treatment of rhinovirus colds. *J. Infect. Dis.*, 166:776–782.
60. Gwaltney, J.M., Jr., and Hendley, J.O. (1978): Rhinovirus transmission, one if by air, two if by hand. *Amer. J. Epidemiol.*, 107:357–361.
61. Gwaltney, J.M., Jr., Hendley, J.O., Simon, G., and Jordan, W.S., Jr. (1966): Rhinovirus infections in an industrial population. I. The occurrence of illness. *N. Engl. J. Med.*, 275:1261–1268.
62. Gwaltney, J.M., Jr., Hendley, J.O., Simon, G., and Jordan, W.S., Jr. (1967): Rhinovirus infections in an industrial population. II. Characteristics of illness and antibody response. *J.A.M.A.*, 202:494–500.
63. Hall, C.B. (1990): Acute laryngotracheobronchitis. In *Principles and Practice of Infectious Diseases*, edited by G.L. Mandell, R.G. Douglas, Jr., and J.E. Bennett, p. 499, John Wiley and Sons, New York.
64. Hall, C.B., and Douglas, R.G., Jr. (1981): Modes of transmission of respiratory syncytial virus. *J. Pediatr.*, 99:100–103.
65. Hall, C.B., Douglas, R.G., Jr., and Geiman, J.M. (1976): Respiratory syncytial virus infections in infants: quantitation and duration of shedding. *J. Pediatr.*, 89:11–15.
66. Hall, C.B., Geiman, J.M., and Douglas, R.G., Jr. (1980): Possible transmission by fomites of respiratory syncytial virus. *J. Infect. Dis.*, 141:98–107.
67. Hall, C.B., Kopelman, A.E., Douglas, R.G., Jr., Geiman, J.M., and Meagher, M.P. (1979): Neonatal respiratory syncytial virus infection. *N. Engl J. Med.*, 300:393–396.
68. Hall, C.B., McBride, J.T., Walsh, E.E., Bell, D.M., Gala, C.L., Hildreth, S.W., Ten Eyck, L.G., and Hall, W.J. (1983): Aerosolized treatment of infants with respiratory syncytial viral infection: a randomized double-blind study. *N. Engl. J. Med.*, 308:1443–1447.
69. Hall, W.J., and Douglas R.G., Jr. (1980): Pulmonary function during and after common respiratory infections. *Ann. Rev. Med.*, 31:233–238.
70. Harris, R.D., Berdon, W.E., and Baker, D.H. (1970): Roentgen diagnosis of acute epiglottitis in the adult. *J. Can. Assoc. Radiol.*, 21:270–272.
71. Hawkins, D.G., Miller, A.H., Sachs, G.B., and Benz, R.T. (1973): Acute epiglottitis in adults. *Laryngoscope*, 83:1211–1220.
72. Hayden, F.B., Albrecht, J.K., Kaiser, D.L., and Gwaltney, J.M. (1986): Prevention of natural colds by contact prophylaxis with intranasal alpha$_2$-interferon. *N. Engl. J. Med.*, 314:71–75.
73. Hayden, F.G., Andries, K., and Janseen, P.A.J. (1992): Safety and efficacy of intranasal pirodavir (R77975) in experimental rhinovirus infection. *Antimicrob. Agents Chemother.*, 36:727–732.
74. Hayden, F.G., and Gwaltney, J.M., Jr. (1984): Intranasal interferon-α$_2$ treatment of experimental rhinovirus colds. *J. Infect. Dis.*, 150:174–180.
75. Hayden, F., Gwaltney, J., Jr., and Colonno, R. (1988): Modification of experimental rhinovirus colds by receptor blockade. *Antiviral Res.*, 9:233–247.
76. Hemilä, H. (1992): Vitamin C and the common cold. *Brit. J. Nutr.*, 67:3–16.
77. Henderson, F.W., Collier, A.M., Sanyal, M.A., Watkins, J.M., Fairclough, D.L., Clyde, W.A., Jr., and Denny, F.W. (1982): Longitudinal study of respiratory viruses and bacteria in the etiology of acute otitis media with effusion. *N. Engl. J. Med.*, 306:1377–1383.
78. Hendley, J.O. (1983): Rhinvirus· colds: immunology and pathogenesis. *Eur. J. Respir. Dis.*, 64(suppl. 128):340–343.
79. Hendley, J.O., Wentzel, R.P., and Gwaltney, J.M., Jr. (1973): Transmission of rhinovirus colds by self-inoculation. *N. Engl. J. Med.*, 288:1361–1364.
80. Hilding, A. (1930): The common cold. *Arch. Otolaryngol.*, 12:133–150.
81. Hirschmann, J.V., and Everett, E.D. (1979): *Haemophilus influenzae* infections in adults: report of nine cases and review of the literature. *Medicine*, 58:80–94.
82. Hoagland, R.J. (1960): Clinical manifestations of infectious mononucleosis: a report of two hundred cases. *Am. J. Med. Sci.*, 240:21–28.
83. Home, F. (1965): *An inquiry into the nature, cause and cure of the croup.* Edinburgh.
84. Howard, J.B., McCracken, G.H., Jr., and Luby, J.P. (1972): Influenza A-2 virus as a cause of croup requiring tracheostomy. *J. Pediatr.*, 81:1148–1150.
85. Hutton, N., Wilson, M.H., Mellits, E.D., Baumgardner, R., Wissow, L.S., Bonuccelli, C., Holtzman, N.A., and DeAngelis, C. (1991): Effectiveness of an antihistamine-decongestant combination for young children with the common cold: a randomized, controlled clinical trial. *J. Pediatr.*, 118:125–130.

86. Johnstone, J.M., and Lawy, H.S. (1967): Acute epiglottitis in adults due to infection with *Haemophilus influenzae* type b. *Lancet*, 2:134–136.
87. Jones, H.M., and Camps, F.E. (1957): Acute epiglottitis. *Practitioner*, 178:223–229.
88. Jones, R., Santos, J.I., and Overall, J.C. (1979): Bacterial tracheitis. *J.A.M.A.*, 242:721–726.
89. Jones, R.N., Slepack, J., and Bigelow, J. (1976): Ampicillin-resistant *Hemophilus paraphrophilus* laryngoepiglottitis. *J. Clin. Microbiol.*, 4:405–407.
90. Kairys, S.W., Olmstead, E.M., and O'Connor, G.T. (1989): Steroid treatment of laryngotracheitis: a meta-analysis of the evidence from randomized trials. *Pediatrics*, 83:683–693.
91. Karlowski, T.R., Chalmers, T.C., Frenkel, L.D., Kapikian, A.Z., Lewis, T.L., and Lynch, J.M. (1975): Ascorbic acid for the common cold. A prophylactic and therapeutic trial. *J.A.M.A.*, 231:1038–1042.
92. Kattan, M. (1979): Long-term sequelae of respiratory illness in infancy and childhood. *Ped. Clin. Nor. Amer.*, 26:525–535.
93. Kibrick, S. (1964): Current status of Coxsackie and ECHO viruses in human disease. *Prog. Med. Virol.*, 6:27–70.
94. Knight, V. (1973): Airborne transmission and pulmonary deposition of respiratory viruses. In: *Viral and Mycoplasmal Infections of the Respiratory Tract*, edited by V. Knight, pp. 1–9. Lea and Febiger, Philadelphia.
95. Knight, V., and Gilbert, B.E. (1986): Chemotherapy of respiratory viruses. *Adv. Intern. Med.*, 31:95–118.
96. Komaroff, A.L., Aronson, M.D., Pass, C.T., et al. (1983): Serologic evidence of chlamydial and mycoplasmal pharyngitis in adults. *Science*, 222:927–928.
97. Kruse, W. (1914): Eie erreger von husten und schnupten. *Munchen. Med. Wchschr.*, 61:1547.
98. Kuusela, A.-L., and Vesikari, T. (1988): A randomized double-blind, placebo-controlled trial of dexamethasone and racemic epinephrine in the treatment of croup. *Acta Paediatr. Scand.*, 77:99–104.
99. LaCroix, J., Ahronheim, G., Arcand, P., Gauthier, M., Rousseau, E., Girouard, G., and Lamarre, A. (1986): Group A streptococcal supraglottitis. *J. Pediatr.*, 109:20–24.
100. LaMierre, A., Meyer, A., and Laplane, R. (1936): Les septicemies a bacille de pfe¹ffer. *Ann. Med.*, 39:94.
101. Lampert, R.P., Robinson, D.S., and Soyka, L.F. (1975): A critical look at oral decongestants. *Pediatrics*, 55:550–552.
102. Lenney, W., and Milner, A.D. (1978): Treatment of acute viral croup. *Archiv. Dis. Child.*, 53:704–706.
103. Liston, S.L., Gehrz, R.C., and Jarvis, C.W. (1981): Bacterial tracheitis. *Arch. Otolaryngol.*, 107:581–584.
104. Liston, S.L., Gehrz, R.C., Siegel, L.G., and Tilelli, J. (1983): Bacterial tracheitis. *Am. J. Dis. Child.*, 137:764–767.
105. Loda, J.A., Clyde, W.A., Jr., Glezen, W.P., Senior, R.J., Sheaffer, C.I., and Denny, F.W., Jr. (1968): Studies on the role of viruses, bacteria and *M. pneumoniae* as causes of lower respiratory tract infections in children. *J. Pediatr.* 72:161–176.
106. Long, S.S. (1992): Bacterial tracheitis. *Report on Pediatric Infectious Diseases*, 2(8):29–31.
107. Loughlin, G., and Taussig, L.M. (1979): Pulmonary function in children with a history of laryngotracheobronchitis. *J. Pediatr.*, 94:365–369.
108. Lowenstein, S.R., and Parrino, T.A. (1987): Management of the common cold. *Adv. Intern. Med.* 32:207–234.
109. Mayo-Smith, M.F., Hirsch, P.J., Wodzinski, S.F., and Schiffman, F.J. (1986): Acute epiglottitis in adults: an eight-year experience in the state of Rhode Island. *N. Engl. J. Med.*, 314:1133–1139.
110. McIntosh, K., Ellis, E.F., Hoffman, L.S., Tillinghast, G.L., Eller, J.J., and Fulginiti, V.A. (1973): The association of viral and bacterial respiratory infections with exacerbations of wheezing in young asthmatic children. *J. Pediatr.*, 82:578–590.
111. McMillan, J.A., Sandstrom, C., Weiner, L.B., Forbes, B.A., Woods, M., Howard, T., Poe, L., Keller, K., Corwin, R.M., and Winkelman, J.W. (1986): Viral and bacterial organisms associated with acute pharyngitis in a school-aged population. *J. Pediatr.*, 109:747–752.
112. Miller, J.Z., Nance, W.E., Norton, J.A., Wolen, R.L., Griffith, R.S., and Rose, R.J. (1977): Therapeutic effect of vitamin C: a co-twin control study. *J.A.M.A.* 237:248–251.
113. Moffet, H.L., Siegel, A.C., and Doyle, H.K. (1968): Nonstreptococcal pharyngitis. *J. Pediatr.*, 73:51–60.
114. Molteni, R.A. (1976): Epiglottitis: incidence of extraepiglottic infection: report of 72 cases and review of the literature. *Pediatrics*, 58:526–531.
115. Monto, A.S., Shope, T.C., Schwartz, S.A., and Albrecht, J.K. (1986): Intranasal interferon-α2b for seasonal prophylaxis of respiratory infection. *J. Infect. Dis.*, 154:128–133.
116. Naclerio, R.M., Proud, D., Lichtenstein, L.M., et al. (1988): Kinins are generated during experimental rhinovirus cold. *J. Infect. Dis.*, 157:133–142.

117. Nelson, W.E. (1984): Bacterial croup: a historical perspective. *J. Pediatr.*, 105:52–55.
118. Newth, C.J.L., Levison, H., and Bryan, A.C. (1972): Respiratory status of children with croup. *J. Pediatr.*, 81:1068–1073.
119. Parrott, R.J., Vargosko, A., Luckey, A., Kim, W.H., Cumming, C., and Chanock, R. (1959): Clinical features of infection with hemadsorption viruses. *N. Engl. J. Med.*, 260:731–738.
120. Parrott, R.H., Kim, H.W., Vargosko, A.J., and Chanock, R.M. (1962): Serious respiratory tract illness as a result of Asian influenza and influenza B infections in children. *J. Pediatr.*, 61:205–213.
121. Parrott, R.H., Vargosko, A.J., Kim, H.W., Bell, J.A., and Chanock, R.M. (1962): Acute respiratory diseases of viral etiology. III. Myxoviruses: parainfluenza. *Am. J. Public Health*, 52:907–917.
122. Pauling, L.C. (1970): *Vitamin C and the Common Cold*, pp. 26–38. W.H. Freeman, San Francisco.
123. Pelon, W., Mogabgab, W.J., Phillips, I.A., Pierce, W.E., and Roth, L.W. (1957): A cytopathogenic agent isolated from naval recruits with mild respiratory illness. *Proc. Soc. Exper. Med.*, 94:262–267.
124. Pereira, M.S. (1973): Adenovirus infections. *Postgrad. Med. J.*, 49:798–801.
125. Podgore, J.K., and Bass, J.W. (1976): The "thumbsign" and "little finger" sign in acute epiglottitis. *J. Pediatr.*, 88:154–155.
126. Price, W.H. (1956): The isolation of a new virus associated with respiratory clinical disease in humans. *Proc. Natl. Acad. Sci.*, 43:892.
127. Proud, D., Naclerio, R.M., Gwaltney, J.M., Jr., and Hendley, J.O. (1990): Kinins are generated in nasal secretions during natural rhinovirus colds. *J. Infect. Dis.*, 161:120–123.
128. Proud, D., Reynolds, C.J., Lacapra, S., Kagey-Sobotka, A., Lichtenstein, L.M., and Naclerio, R.M. (1988): Nasal provocation with bradykinin induces symptoms of rhinitis and a sore throat. *Am. Rev. Respir. Dis.*, 137:613–616.
129. Putto, A. (1987): Febrile exudative tonsillitis: viral or streptococcal? *Pediatr.*, 80:6–12.
130. Rapkin, R.H. (1972): The diagnosis of epiglottitis: simplicity and reliability of radiographs of the neck in the differential diagnosis of the croup syndrome. *J. Pediatr.*, 80:96–98.
131. Reed, S.E. (1981): The aetiology and epidemiology of common colds, and the possibilities of prevention. *Clin. Otolaryngol.*, 6:379–387.
132. Sanyal, M.A., Henderson, F.W., Stempel, E.C., Collier, A.M., and Denny, F.W. (1980): Effect of upper respiratory tract infection on eustachian tube ventilatory function in the preschool child. *J. Pediatr.*, 97:11–15.
133. Schabel, S.I., Katzberg, R.W., and Burgener, F.A. (1977): Acute inflammation of epiglottis and supraglottic structures in adults. *Radiology*, 122:601–604.
134. Schmidt, J.P., Metcalf, T.G., and Miltenberger, F.W. (1962): An epidemic of Asian influenza in children at Ladd Air Force Base, Alaska, 1960. *J. Pediatr.*, 61:214–220.
135. Shakelford, G.D., Siegel, M.J., and McAlister, W.H. (1978): Subglottic edema in acute epiglottitis in children. *Am. J. Roentgenol.*, 131:603–605.
136. Skolnik, N.S. (1989): Treatment of croup. *Am. J. Dis. Child.*, 143:1045–1049.
137. Smith, D.H., Ingram, D.L., Smith, A.L., Gilles, F., and Breshan, M.J. (1973): Bacterial meningitis. *Pediatrics*, 52:586–600.
138. Soyka, L.F., Robinson, D.S., Lachant, N., and Monaco, J. (1975): The misuse of antibiotics for treatment of upper respiratory tract infections in children. *Pediatrics*, 55:552–556.
139. Sperber, S.J., Doyle, W.J., McBride, T.P., Sorrentino, J.V., Riker, D.K., and Hayden, F.G. (1992): Otologic effects of interferon-β_{serine} in experimental rhinovirus colds. *Arch. Otolaryngol. Head Neck Surg*, 118:933–936.
140. Sperber, S.J., and Hayden, F.G. (1988): Chemotherapy of rhinovirus colds. *Antimicrob. Agents Chemother.*, 32:409–419.
141. Sperber, S.J., Hendley, J.O., Hayden, F.G., Riker, D.K., Sorrentino, J.V., and Gwaltney, J.M., Jr. (1992): Effects of naproxen on experimental rhinovirus colds. *Ann. Intern. Med.*, 117:37–41.
142. Stanley, E.D., Jackson, G.G., Panusarn, C., Rubenis, M., and Dirda, V. (1975): Increased virus shedding with aspirin treatment of rhinovirus infection. *J.A.M.A.*, 231:1248–1251.
143. Sterner, G. (1962): Adenovirus infection in childhood. An epidemiologic and clinical survey among Swedish children. *Acta Paediatr.*, 142:5–30.
144. Szilagyi, P.G. (1990): What can we do about the common cold? *Contemp. Pediatr.*, 7:23–49.
145. Tomassini, J.E., Graham, D., DeWitt, C.M., Lineberger, D.W., Rodkey, J.A., and Colonno, R.J. (1989): cDNA cloning reveals that the major group rhinovirus receptor on HeLa cells is intercellular adhesion molecule 1. *Proc. Natl. Acad. Sci.* (USA), 86:4907–4911.
146. Travis, K.W., Todres, I.D., and Shannon, D.C. (1977): Pulmonary edema associated with croup and epiglottitis. *Pediatrics*, 59:695–698.
147. Tunnessen, W.W., and Feinstein, A.R. (1980): The steroid-croup controversy: an analytic review of methodologic problems. *J. Pediatr.*, 96:751–756.

148. Turner, R.B., Felton, A., Kosak, K., Kelsey, D.K., and Meschievitz, C.K. (1986): Prevention of experimental coronavirus colds with intranasal α-2b interferon. *J. Infect. Dis.*, 154:443–447.
149. Valenti, W.M., Clarke, T.A., Hall, C.B., Menegus, M.A., and Shapiro, D.L. (1982): Concurrent outbreaks of rhinovirus and respiratory syncytial virus in an intensive care nursery: epidemiology and associated risk factors. *J. Pediatr.*, 100:722–726.
150. Vetto, R.R. (1960): Epiglottitis: a report of 37 cases. *J.A.M.A.*, 173:990–994.
151. Wald, E.R., Guerra, N., and Byers, C. (1991): Upper respiratory tract infections in young children: duration of and frequency of complications. *Pediatrics*, 87:129–133.
152. Weismann, K., Jakobsen, J.P., Weismann, J.E., Hammer, U.M., Nyholm, S.M., Hansen, B., Lomholt, K.E., and Schmidt, K. (1990): Zinc gluconate lozenges for common cold. *Dan. Med. Bull.*, 37:279–281.
153. Welliver, R.C., Sun, M., and Rinaldo, D. (1985): Defective regulation of immune responses in croup due to parainfluenza virus. *Pediatr. Res.*, 19:716–720.
154. West, S., Brandon, B., Stolley, P., and Rumrill, R. (1975): A review of antihistamines and the common cold. *Pediatrics*, 56:100–107.
155. Westley, C.R., Cotton, E.K., and Brooks, J.G. (1978): Nebulized racemic epinephrine by IPPB for the treatment of croup. *Am. J. Dis. Child.*, 132:484–487.
156. Winther, B., Brofeldt, S., Christensen, B., Mygind, N. (1984): Light and scanning electron microscopy of nasal biopsy material from patients with naturally acquired common colds. *Acta Otolaryngol.* (Stockholm) 97:309–318.
157. Winther, B., Farr, B., Turner, R.B., Hendley, J.O., Gwaltney, J.M., and Mygind, N. (1984): Histopathologic examination and enumeration of polymorphonuclear leukocytes in the nasal mucosa during experimental rhinovirus colds. *Acta Otolaryngol.* (Stockholm), 413(Suppl.):19–24.
158. Wolfsdorf, J., and Swift, D.L. (1978): An animal model simulating acute infective upper airway obstruction of childhood and its use in the investigation of croup therapy. *Pediatr. Res.*, 12:1062–1065.
159. Zach, M., Erban, A., and Olinsky, A. (1981): Croup, recurrent croup, allergy, and airways hyperreactivity. *Archiv. Dis. Child.*, 56:336–341.
160. Zach, M., and Messner, H. (1983): Serum IgA in recurrent croup. *Am. J. Dis. Child.*, 137:184–185.
161. Zwillich, C.W., Pickett, C., Hanson, F.N., and Weil, J.V. (1981): Disturbed sleep and prolonged apnea during nasal obstruction in normal man. *Am. Rev. Resp. Dis.*, 124:158–160.

Respiratory Infections: Diagnosis and Management, 3d ed.,
edited by James E. Pennington.
Raven Press, Ltd., New York © 1994

7

Acute and Chronic Sinusitis

Birgit Winther and Jack M. Gwaltney, Jr.

*Department of Internal Medicine, University of Virginia Health Sciences Center,
Charlottesville, Virginia 22908*

ACUTE SINUSITIS

Acute sinusitis is an infectious process that involves the paranasal sinuses. The majority of cases are due to bacterial infection and last 1 to 3 weeks. Most of these infections follow a common cold or other upper respiratory infection, although some are secondary to other processes that impair mucociliary clearance or to dental infection. The majority of cases represent self-limited disease, but serious complications may ensue by local extension of the infection into the orbit, skull, meninges, or brain. Also, untreated sinus infection may irreparably damage the mucosa, leading to chronic sinus disease.

Epidemiology

A small percentage of colds, estimated at 0.5 (4) to 5% (58), results in sinus infection. The incidence of acute sinusitis parallels the incidence of upper respiratory tract infections, being highest in the fall, winter, and spring. Children acquire six to eight colds per year, as opposed to two or three for the average adult.

Pathogenesis

Viral infection of the nose appears to be the first step in most cases of acute sinusitis. In one small study, a third of volunteers with experimental rhinovirus colds developed MRI abnormalities of the ethmoid or antral sinuses (55). The sinuses, which are normally sterile (15,47,60), can be invaded through the sinus ostia by a respiratory virus or be secondarily affected by inflammatory events in the nasal passages. The severity of damage to the respiratory epithelium from viral infection varies. Influenza leads to the erosion of the epithelium, whereas rhinovirus causes minimal cellular damage (64) but impedes mucociliary clearance. Inflammatory edema of the mucosa leads to obstruction of sinus ostia. Respiratory viruses have been cultured from sinus puncture aspirates obtained in the early phase of sinus infection, and an inflammatory exudate containing a predominance of polymorphonuclear neutrophils has been found (15,23). At this stage of the disease, when the normal clearance mechanisms of the sinus have been impaired, resistance to bacterial invasion is reduced and bacterial superinfection occurs. Titers of the bacteria usually range from 10^5 to 10^8 cfu/ml in sinus puncture aspirates obtained from patients with acute sinusitis. Polymorphonuclear neutrophils are predominant in the sinus contents, usually numbering at least 5,000/mm^3 and occasionally exceeding 100,000/mm^3 (15).

Bacterial sinusitis may also occur in patients with other predisposing conditions that alter mucociliary clearance, such as cystic fibrosis, immotile cilia syndromes (e.g., Kartagener's syndrome) (11), allergic rhinitis, nasal polyposis, septal deviation, choanal atresia, the presence of foreign bodies, and intranasal tumors. Intranasal cocaine abuse has also been reported as a possible risk factor for sinusitis (46). Nasotracheal intubation, nasogastric intubation, and nasal packing have been recognized as risk factors for the development of nosocomial sinusitis (9,12,13,28,41). Penetrating injuries and surgery involving the sinuses may also be complicated by sinusitis.

The maxillary and ethmoid sinuses are pneumatized shortly after birth and thus may be infected as early as infancy. The sphenoid sinuses are pneumatized at the age of 2 to 3 years and the frontal sinuses by approximately 6 years of age (50).

Microbial Etiology

Although viral infection appears to be the usual initial event in cases of acute sinusitis, viruses have been isolated in only about 15% of patients who have been studied with sinus puncture at the time of presentation (15,23). Most of these cases already had bacteria present in the aspirate at the time of the initial sinus puncture. Rhinoviruses account for the largest proportion of viral isolates from sinus aspirates (Table 7-1), followed by influenza and parainfluenza viruses.

Most studies of the microbial etiology of sinusitis have dealt with the maxillary antrum which is the most commonly infected sinus and also the one most accessible for puncture and aspiration (3,6,15,22,23,33,56). When other sinuses are involved, maxillary sinusitis is also usually present. Bacterial cultures are positive in about two-thirds of patients studied by sinus aspiration after a clinical diagnosis of acute sinusitis. Approximately half of the bacterial isolates are accounted for by *Streptococcus pneumoniae*, unencapsulated strains of *Hemophilus influenzae*, or both of

TABLE 7–1. *Etiology of acute community-acquired maxillary sinusitis*

	Mean percent of cases (range)
Bacterial	
Streptococcus pneumoniae	30 (20–35%)
Hemophilus influenzae	20 (6–26%)
Anaerobic bacteria	10 (0–23%)
Staphylococcus pyogenes	4 (0–8%)
Moraxella catarrhalis	2 (up to 25% of pediatric cases)
Streptococcal species	2
Aerobic gram-negative bacilli	9 (up to 75% of nosocomial cases)
Viral	
Rhinovirus	15
Influenza	5
Parainfluenza	3
Adenovirus	<1

these organisms combined. These are followed in prevalence by anaerobes, *Staphylococcus aureus, Streptococcus pyogenes, Moraxella catarrhalis,* and other streptococcal species (21). Both *H. influenzae* and *M. catarrhalis* have shown a rising prevalence of beta-lactamase production. Aerobic gram-negative bacilli, especially *Pseudomonas aeruginosa,* are a prominent cause of nosocomial sinusitis resulting from nasal intubation (9). Anaerobic infection is often related to prior dental infection. *Legionella pneumophila* has been reported as the cause of one case of maxillary sinusitis in a patient with AIDS (45).

Fungi have been increasingly recognized as causing community-acquired sinusitis (2,38,39,42). These include strains of *Phaeohyphomycosis, Pseudallescheria,* and *Hyalohyphomycis.* Zygomycosis (mucormycosis) is a cause of acute necrotizing sinusitis, most commonly associated with diabetic ketoacidosis (44). Invasive *Aspergillus sinusitis* has been reported in immunocompromized patients including those undergoing chemotherapy for leukemia (38,57).

Clinical Manifestations

The symptoms of sinusitis are similar to those of a protracted but uncomplicated common cold. Because most cases of sinusitis appear to follow a cold, a history of exacerbation of certain symptoms is helpful. These include worsening nasal obstruction, purulent nasal or postnasal discharge, and facial pain over the involved sinus which can be exacerbated by bending forward. Pain in the maxillary teeth could be present with maxillary sinusitis. Fever is usually not prominent and is absent in one-half of adult patients (15). Fever is seen more commonly in nosocomial sinusitis (9) and perhaps in childhood disease (59). Patients with sphenoid sinusitis characteristically complain of headache which can be frontal, temporal, or retro-orbital and can radiate to the occiput or into one or more branches of the trigeminal nerve distribution (31). Patients with ethmoid sinusitis often complain of pain medial to the eye.

The chief complaint in children with sinusitis is usually persistent cough and nasal discharge. Fever, facial pain and swelling, and fetid breath are additional symptoms noted by the parents of children with sinusitis (48,59).

Physical examination can reveal tenderness to palpation or percussion over an involved maxillary or frontal sinus, and, rarely, erythema or swelling of the overlying skin. When transillumination of the maxillary and frontal sinuses reveals opacity or dullness over a previously normal sinus, infection is usually present, as determined by sinus puncture (15). Conversely, normal transillumination militates against a diagnosis of acute sinusitis. Sinus transillumination is much less helpful in the presence of chronic sinus disease where abnormalities can persist and obscure changes associated with intercurrent disease. Normal variations in bone thickness can influence the results of transillumination in normal individuals, making it desirable to obtain baseline evaluations when examining new patients.

Complications

Longitudinal follow-up studies of patients with acute sinusitis are not available, but it is believed that untreated acute sinusitis can occasionally cause permanent damage to the sinus mucosa, leading to chronic sinus disease. Bacterial sinusitis can be complicated by local extension of the infection into the orbit, skull, meninges, or brain (17,29,34,37,65). Such patients can present with periorbital cellulitis, orbital cellulitis, or retro-orbital abscess; orbital complications occur most commonly with ethmoid or maxillary sinusitis but can also follow frontal or sphenoidal sinusitis. Osteomyelitis of the frontal bone can cause visible soft tissue swelling (Pott's puffy tumor), usually of the mid-forehead but sometimes involving the scalp (62,66). Brain abscess complicating frontal sinusitis involves the frontal lobe and can be present with the signs of a systemic infection, a frontal lobe mass, or both. A bacteria commonly associated with this complication is a microaerophilic organism, *Streptococcus milleri* (7). Meningitis is a dramatic complication, resulting in the sudden onset of fever, rigor, headache, and meningismus. Epidural and subdural abscess can occur with dull, persistent headache and less prominent signs of infection. Cavernous sinus thrombosis is a catastrophic sudden illness with rigor, fever, retro-orbital pain, and bilateral ocular palsy (53). Persistent fever and bacteremia have been reported with nosocomial sinusitis (12,13,28,41).

Diagnosis

Sinusitis is difficult to diagnose accurately from the history alone or from examination of the nose. Diagnostic criteria have recently been proposed which incorporate clinical and imaging results (Table 7-2) (49). These consensus criteria are helpful in evaluating the results of a diagnostic evaluation, but have not been compared with pathologic or microbiological findings which constitute the "gold standard." Also,

TABLE 7–2. *Clinical diagnosis of sinusitis*

Signs and Symptoms
  Major criteria:
    Purulent nasal discharge
    Purulent pharyngeal drainage
    Cough
  Minor criteria:
    Periorbital edema[b]
    Headache[c]
    Facial pain[c]
    Tooth pain[c]
    Earache
    Sore throat
    Foul breath
    Increased wheeze
    Fever
Diagnostic Tests
  Major criteria:
    Waters' radiograph with opacification, air fluid level, or thickened mucosa filling ≥50% of antrum
    Coronal CT[a] scan with thickening of mucosa or opacfication of sinus
  Minor criteria:
    Nasal cytologic study (smear) with neurophils and bacteremia
    Ultrasound studies

Probable Sinusitis
  Signs and symptoms: 2 major criteria or 1 major and ≥2 minor criteria
  Diagnostic tests: 1 major = confirmatory, 1 minor = supportive

Adapted from Shapiro and Rachelefsky (49).
[a]CT, computerized tomographic.
[b]More common in children.
[c]More common in adults.

recent study has identified five independent predictors of acute sinusitis using sinus radiography as the diagnostic standard (63). These predictors were maxillary toothache, abnormal transillumination, poor response to decongestants, purulent secretions, and colored nasal discharge by history. Unfortunately, no single predictor was both sensitive and specific. However, the presence of the predictors was cumulative in usefulness, and when all five were present there was a 92% probability of the sinus radiographs showing mucosal thickening of ≥6 mm, complete opacity, or an air-fluid level.

Sinus radiography is a sensitive diagnostic technique for detecting acute sinus infection of the maxillary antrum (15,48). Patients with a history compatible with acute maxillary sinusitis but whose radiographs are normal rarely have bacteria recovered from sinus aspiration. On the contrary, similar patients with opacity, air-fluid level, or mucosal thickening of greater than 6 mm of the maxillary sinus have a high probability of having an infectious agent isolated (15). Radiography has not been compared with culture results for the frontal and sphenoid sinuses but is regarded as a sensitive test there as well. Radiographic abnormalities can persist in patients with chronic sinus disease making interpretation of sinus films for intercurrent, acute sinusitis more difficult and dependent upon comparisons with baseline films.

Standard radiography is not sensitive for ethmoid sinusitis, and computerized tomography (CT) demonstrates disease of the ethmoid sinuses better and reveals the anatomy of all diseased sinuses with great precision. Limited sinus CT exam is now priced at cost-effective levels at some medical facilities and is used for diagnosing and evaluating routine causes of sinusitis, especially when response to treatment is not satisfactory. For cases complicated by extension into the orbit or brain, CT is essential (10,51).

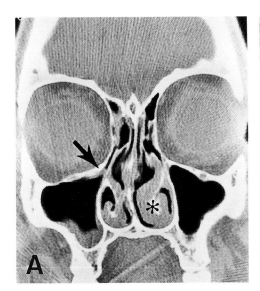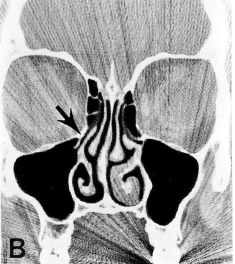

FIG. 7–1. Coronal CT image of the nasal cavity and paranasal sinus from a patient with a common cold. (*A*) The ethmoid infundibulum (*arrow*) is occluded during the acute illness and there is retained mucus/mucosal swelling of the right maxillary sinus cavity. The left inferior turbinate is engorged (*asterisk*). (*B*) Fourteen days later the ethmoid infundibulum is patent and the maxillary sinus cavity has returned to normal.

Sinus aspiration with quantitative culture is required to determine specific microbial etiology. It requires otolaryngologic consultation and is unnecessary in the majority of cases of community-acquired sinusitis. Aspiration may be required to guide the antibiotic therapy of extremely ill, hospitalized patients. Nosocomial sinusitis can also be an indication for sinus puncture because of the high incidence of gram-negative organisms with possible antibiotic resistance (9,13). Patients not responding to empiric therapy and those suspected of having the serious complications described above should also undergo aspiration. Cultures of nasal pus or sinus washings obtained through the natural ostium do not correlate well with cultures of sinus aspirates and are not recommended for use in the management of acute sinus infection (3,15).

Sinus aspirates are obtained after antiseptic disinfection of the puncture site with povidone-iodine. A needle is then placed into the maxillary antrum beneath the inferior turbinate or into the frontal sinus beneath the supraorbital rim of the eye. If free fluid is absent, one ml of nonbacteristatic saline may be instilled into the sinus and aspirated to provide a specimen. The specimen should be transported to the laboratory in the capped syringe where gram stain and aerobic and anaerobic bacterial cultures are performed. Because such aspirates may yield low titers of contaminating normal flora, quantitative cultures are recommended. Pathogens are usually present in titers of $\geq 10^5$ cfu/ml (15).

Treatment

Most cases of acute sinusitis are treated empirically with antibiotics selected to cover the usual bacterial causes. Antibiotics shown to be effective in studies employing quantitative cultures of sinus aspirates before and after treatment include amoxicillin, amoxicillin-clavulanic acid, trimethoprim-sulfamethoxazole, cefuroxime axetil, loracarbef, and cefixime (21) (Table 7-3).

Amoxicillin has been successfully used for treating acute sinusitis in the past because it provides excellent coverage against *S. pneumoniae* and *H. influenzae* but should not be used in areas with a high prevalence of lactamase-producing *H. influenzae* or *M. catarrhalis*. Treatment is recommended for 10 to 14 days. Trimethoprim-sulfamethoxazole provides an alternative which is also inexpensive and is active against beta-lactamase positive *H. influenzae* or *M. catarrhalis*. However, trimethoprim-sulfamethoxazole is associated with frequent allergic reactions, some of which are rare but serious. In addition, it should not be used to treat cases known or suspected to be due to *S. pyogenes*. Amoxicillin-clavulanic acid and cefuroxime axetil

TABLE 7–3. *Antimicrobial treatment of acute bacterial sinusitis*

Recommended agents	Daily dose (adult)
Amoxicillin	500 mg tid
Trimethoprim-sulfamethoxazole	80 mg/40 mg bid
Amoxicillin/clavulanate	500/125 mg tid
Cefuroxime axetil	250 mg bid
Loracarbef	400 mg bid
Cefixime	200 mg bid

bid, 2 times daily; tid, 3 times daily.

provide more expensive alternatives which are effective against beta-lactamase-producing organisms.

In cases not responding to empiric therapy and in patients thought to have severe life-threatening complications, sinus aspiration should be performed to provide a specimen for gram stain and quantitative culture to guide further therapy. Staphylococcal infection may require treatment with a penicillinase-resistant penicillin, alternatives being a first generation cephalosporin or vancomycin, the latter being the drug of choice for methicillin-resistant *S. aureus.* Hospitalized, intubated patients often have gram-negative infection requiring an aminoglycoside, and/or an advanced generation beta-lactam. Immunoincompetent patients may have fungal infection requiring surgical debridement and treatment with amphotericin B.

In addition to antibiotic therapy, ancillary treatment including local drainage using nasal decongestants such as topical neosynephrine (0.25% or 0.5% for a 3-day course) is usually recommended despite the lack of data confirming efficacy in randomized, controlled trials (67). Codeine may be required for pain. Although most patients can be treated as outpatients, those with severe illness or with suspected serious complications should be hospitalized for evaluation and therapy. Immediate surgical decompression and drainage is required in patients with intracranial extensions.

Prevention

There are no proven methods for preventing acute sinusitis. The majority of cases complicate acute respiratory infections, which are themselves largely unpreventable at present. Influenza vaccine and amantadine are both effective as prophylaxis for influenza infections. It has been suggested that prompt and regular use of vasoconstricting nasal drops or sprays during a cold might prevent this complication, but no data are available regarding this claim. Dental hygiene and prompt treatment of periodontal infection may prevent progression to sinus involvement. Medical control of allergic rhinitis and surgical correction of obstructive nasal abnormalities may also obviate some cases of sinus infection.

CHRONIC SINUS DISEASE

Epidemiology

Most cases of acute sinusitis are either self-limited or effectively treated so that only a small proportion of patients continue to have symptoms beyond three weeks. The continuing symptoms are usually minor, such as nasal stuffiness and discharge, change in voice quality, a vague sinus ache, and cough. This continuing symptom complex constitutes subacute sinusitis, which may progress to irreversible mucosal damage and permanent narrowing or occlusion of the osteomeatal complex resulting in the longer-lasting clinical entity: chronic sinus disease. Host defense deficits such as agammaglobulinemia may impair normal healing of acute sinusitis, leading to an increased incidence of the chronic disease. This is also true of allergy and conditions altering mucociliary clearance, such as cystic fibrosis and immotile cilia syndrome.

Chronic sinus disease was found in 0.02% of the general population in one study with a dental cause being evident in 40% of cases and nasal polyps in 16% (36).

Pathogenesis

The pathogenesis of chronic sinus disease has become better understood in recent years, but much about the process is still unknown. It usually follows an acute infection or series of infections in the sinuses. Narrowing of the passages from the sinuses to the nose with, most importantly, obstruction of the osteomeatal complex are often demonstrated in chronic sinus disease by modern imaging techniques and nasal endoscopy. Anatomic abnormalities such as concha bullosa and Haller cells as well as recurrent acute mucosal swelling may predispose to obstruction of the osteomeatal complex. Obstruction of the osteomeatal complex and impaired mucociliary clearance in turn interrupts drainage from the sinuses and results in stagnation of mucus in the sinus cavity.

Although bacteria, especially anaerobes, appear to be continuously present in chronic sinus disease, their pathologic role remains unclear (5,8,18,25,54). Most of the bacteria that have been recovered from the sinus cavity of patients with chronic sinus disease are of the type that would be expected to colonize a functionally impaired sinus. This is probably why data regarding the efficacy of antibiotic treatment of chronic sinus disease have been contradictory (35,43), except in the treatment of intercurrent acute sinusitis, when treatment is usually effective. Cases of chronic fungal and mycobacterial sinusitis appear to have a more clearly infectious etiology (14,16,19,39). Chronic fungal infections have been caused by such organisms as *Pseudoallescheria boydii* (62), Alternania sp (38), *Curvularia lunata* (40), Aspergillus sp, and *Sporothrix schenkii* in normal hosts. Pathologic specimens may show a dense mat of hyphae without inflammatory cells, or signs of tissue invasion.

Another condition has been termed allergic aspergillus sinusitis. The pathogenesis of this condition is thought to be an allergic response to colonizing Aspergillus sp analogous to that of allergic bronchopulmonary aspergillosis. Pathology shows an allergic mucin with many eosinophils, Charcot-Leyden crystals, and occasional branching, septate hyphae (26,27).

Clinical Manifestations

Symptoms of chronic sinus disease are usually similar to those of subacute sinusitis with nasal discharge, stuffiness, and perhaps some mild sinus discomfort. These symptoms may continue unchanged for years. Some patients complain of persistent cough with nocturnal exacerbations or asthma (52). Patients with allergic aspergillus sinusitis typically give a history of asthma, nasal polyps, and chronic sinusitis (26,27). Patients regularly abusing cocaine intranasally may suffer chronic nasal symptoms and may develop sinusitis as well (46).

Complications

Infectious complications similar to those following acute sinusitis may occur as discussed above (24). It has been suggested that infectious complications occur more often following acute than chronic sinus disease, but firm epidemiological data are lacking.

Diagnosis and Treatment

Subacute sinusitis may be diagnosed in a patient with symptoms continuing for more than three weeks and with abnormal sinus transillumination or sinus imaging. In such patients who do not respond to empiric antibiotic therapy as discussed above, sinus aspiration and quantitative culture should be undertaken to determine if there is a causative organism and its antibiotic sensitivity. After the sinus aspiration a therapeutic sinus lavage may be performed. Topical and short-course oral steroid therapy may also be beneficial at this stage.

Chronic sinus disease can be diagnosed by the same historical, physical, and laboratory maneuvers as discussed above when the disease has been present for more than three months. Some cases may respond to appropriate antibiotic therapy and treatment of nasal allergies. In many cases surgical treatment is required, depending upon the severity of symptoms.

The Caldwell-Luc operation with resection of the sinus mucosa and creation of an artificial ostia below the interior turbinates (1,20) is being replaced by endonasal endoscopic surgery where the natural ostia are enlarged to reestablish the sinus drainage (30,32). The new approach seems more physiological as it removes obstruction in the osteomeatal area. Comparative studies of the effect of Caldwell-Luc and endoscopic surgery are not available. Nonrandomized case series of patients treated with the Caldwell-Luc procedure suggest a higher long-term response rate than patients treated with antibiotics and sinus lavage (35), but the utility of surgical therapy has never been tested in a randomized controlled trial. Surgical debridement and specific antifungal chemotherapy with amphotericin B may be required for fungal sinusitis (19). Allergic aspergillus sinusitis may be suspected clinically and confirmed by pathologic examination of allergic mucin removed from the sinus. A majority of these patients exhibit total IgE elevation and serum precipitins to Aspergillus. A small series of patients have been successfully treated with debridement and postoperative systemic steroids (61).

In cases of chronic sinusitis with associated pulmonary and renal disease, Wegener's granulomatosis should be considered. In this disease cytotoxic therapy is indicated after a histologic diagnosis. Cases with local erosion of facial bones should suggest a diagnosis of midline granuloma.

Prevention

Chronic sinus disease may be prevented by prompt and effective antimicrobial therapy of acute and subacute sinusitis although proof of this is lacking. Ancillary measures such as steroid therapy and treatment of nasal allergies are also used to prevent the development of chronic disease. In some cases, surgery to correct obstruction of the osteomeatal complex has been associated with reversal of chronic changes (13).

REFERENCES

1. Alusi, H.S. (1980): A new approach to the surgical treatment of chronic maxillary sinusitis. *J. Laryngol. Otol.*, 94:1145–1149.
2. Aviv, J., Lawson, W., Bottone, E., Sachdev, V., Som, P., and Biller, H. (1990): Multiple intracra-

nial mucoceles associated with *Phaeohyphomycosis* of the paranasal sinuses. *Arch. Otolaryngol. Head Neck Surg.*, 116:210–213.

3. Axelsson, A., and Brorson, J.E. (1983): The correlation between bacteriological findings in the nose and maxillary sinus in acute maxillary sinusitis. *Laryngoscope*, 82:2003–2011.

4. Badger, G.F., Dingle, J.H., and Jordan, W.S., Jr. (1964): *Illness in the Home: A Study of 25,000 Illnesses in a Group of Cleveland Families.* The Press of Western Reserve University, Cleveland, Ohio.

5. Balantyne, J.C., and Row, A.R. (1947): Some points in the pathology, diagnosis and treatment of chronic maxillary sinusitis, *J. Laryngol. Otol.*, 68:337–341.

6. Bjorkwall, T. (1950): Bacteriological examinations in maxillary sinusitis. Bacterial flora of the maxillary sinusitis. Bacterial flora of the maxillary antrum, I. Bacterial findings in the normal (healthy) maxillary antrum. *Acta Otolaryngol.*, 83(Suppl.):33–58.

7. Blayney, A.W., Frootko, N.J., and Mitchell, R.G. (1984): Complications of sinusitis caused by *Streptococcus milleri. J. Laryngol. Otol.*, 98:895–899.

8. Brook, I. (1981): Bacteriologic features of chronic sinusitis in children. *J.A.M.A.*, 246:967–969.

9. Caplan, E.S., and Hoyt, N.J. (1982): Nosocomial sinusitis. *J.A.M.A.*, 247:639–641.

10. Carter, B.L., Bankoff, M.S., and Fisk, J.D. (1983): Computed tomographic detection of sinusitis responsible for intracranial and extracranial infections. *Radiology,* 147:739–742.

11. Corkey, C.W.B., Levison, H., and Turner, J.A.P. (1981): The immotile cilia syndrome: a longitudinal survey. *Am. Rev. Resp. Dis.*, 124:544–548.

12. Deutschman, C.S., Wilton, P.B., Sinow, J., Thienprasit, P., Konstantinides, F.N., and Cerra, F.B. (1985): Paranasal sinusitis: a common complication of nasotracheal intubation in neurosurgical patients. *Neurosurgery,* 17:296–299.

13. Deutschman, C.S., Wilton, P.B., Sinow, J., Thienprasit, P., Konstantinides, F.N., and Cerra, F.B. (1985): Paranasal sinusitis associated with nasotracheal intubation: a frequently unrecognized and treatable source of sepsis. *Crit. Care Med.*, 14:111–114.

14. Eron, L.J., Huckins, C., Park, G.H., et al. (1981): *Mycobacterium chelonei* infects the maxillary sinus: a rare case. *Va. Med. Monthly,* 108:335–338.

15. Evans, F.O., Sydnor, J.B., Moore, W.E.C., Moore, G.R., Manwaring, J.L., Brill, A.H., Jackson, R.T., Hanna, S., Skaar, J.S., Holdeman, L.V., Fitzhugh, G.S., Sande, M.A., and Gwaltney, J.M., Jr. (1975): Sinusitis of the maxillary antrum. *N. Engl. J. Med.*, 293:735–739.

16. Finby, N., and Begg, C.F. (1972): Aspergilloma of sinus. *New York State J. Med.*, 72:493–494.

17. Finkelstein, R., Honigman, S., Doron, Y., and Braun, Y. (1986): Sphenoid sinusitis presenting as chronic meningitis. *Eur. Neurol.*, 25:183–187.

18. Frederick, J., and Braude, A.I. (1974): Anaerobic infection of the paranasal sinuses. *N. Engl. J. Med.*, 290:135–137.

19. Gluckman, S.J., Ries, K., and Abrutyn, E. (1977): *Allescheria (Petriellidium) boydii* in a compromised host. *J. Cl. Microbiol.*, 5:481–484.

20. Goode, R.L., Strelzow, V., and Fee, W.E. (1980): Frontal sinus septectomy for chronic unilateral sinusitis. *Otolaryngol. Head Neck Surg.*, 88:18–21.

21. Gwaltney, J.M., Jr., Scheld, W.M., Sande, M.A., and Sydnor, A. (1992): The microbial etiology and antimicrobial therapy of adults with acute community-acquired sinusitis: a fifteen-year experience at the University of Virginia and review of other selected studies. *J. Allergy Clin. Immunol.*, 90:457–462.

22. Gwaltney, J.M., Jr., Sydnor, A., Jr., and Sande, M.A. (1981): Etiology and antimicrobial treatment of acute sinusitis. *Ann. Otol., Rhinol., and Laryngol.*, 84:68–71.

23. Hamory, B.H., Sande, M.A., Sydnor, A., Jr., Seale, D.L., and Gwaltney, J.M., Jr. (1979): Etiology and antimicrobial treatment of acute maxillary sinusitis. *J. Infect. Dis.*, 139:197–202.

24. Ichino, Y., Masahide, N., and Ishikawa, T. (1985): Subpenosteal orbital hemorrhage associated with chronic sinusitis. *Auris Nasus Larynx* (Tokyo), 12:27–30.

25. Karma, P., Jokipii, L., Sipila, P., Luotonen, J., and Jokippi, A.M.M. (1979): Bacteria in chronic maxillary sinusitis. *J. Arch. Otolaryngol.*, 105:386–390.

26. Katzenstein, A.L.A., Sale, S.R., and Greenberger, P.A. (1983): Allergic aspergillus sinusitis: a newly recognized form of sinusitis. *J. Allergy Clin. Immunol.*, 72:89–93.

27. Katzenstein, A.L.A., Sale, S.R., and Greenberger, P.A. (1983): Pathologic findings in allergic aspergillus sinusitis. *Am. J. Surg. Pathol.*, 7:439–443.

28. Kronberg, F.G., and Goodwin, W.J. (1985): Sinusitis in intensive care unit patients. *Laryngolscope,* 95:936–938.

29. Kutnick, S.L., and Kerth, J.D. (1976): Acute sinusitis and otitis: their complications and surgical treatment. *Otolaryngol. Clin. of No. Amer.* 9:689–701.

30. Lanza, D.C., and Kennedy, D.W. (1992): Current concepts in the surgical management of chronic and recurrent acute sinusitis. *J. Allergy Clin. Immunol.*, 90:505–511.

31. Lew, D., Southwick, F.S., Montgomery, W.W., Weber, A.L., and Baker, A.S. (1983): Sphenoid sinusitis: a review of 30 cases. *N. Engl. J. Med.*, 309:1149–1154.

32. Lusk, R.P. (1992): Endoscopic approach to sinus disease. *J. Allergy Clin. Immunol.*, 90:496–505.

33. Lystad, A., Berdal, P., and Lund-Iverson, I. (1964): The bacterial flora of sinusitis with an *in vitro* study of the bacterial resistance to antibiotics. *Acta Otolaryngol.*, 188(Suppl.):390–400.
34. Manigalia, A.J., Van Buren, J.M., Bruce, W.B., Bellucci, R.J., and Hoffman, S.R. (1980): Intracranial abscesses secondary to ear and paranasal sinus infections. *Otolaryngol. Head Neck Surg.*, 88:670–680.
35. Melen, I., Lindahl, L., and Andreasson, L. (1986): Short and long-term treatment results in chronic maxillary sinusitis. *Acta Otolaryngol.*, 102:282–290.
36. Melen, I., Lindahl, L. Andreasson, L., and Rundcrantz, H. (1986): Chronic maxillary sinusitis. *Acta Otolaryngol.*, 101:320–327.
37. Moon, T., Lin, R.Y., and John, A.F. (1986): Fatal frontal sinusitis due to *Neisseria sicca* and *Eubacterium lentum*. *J. Otolaryngol.*, 15:193–195.
38. Morgan, M.A., Wilson, W.R., Neel, H.B., and Roberts, G.D. (1984): Fungal sinusitis in healthy and immunocompromised individuals. *Am. J. Clin. Pathol.*, 82:597–601.
39. Morriss, F.H., and Spock, A. (1970): Intracranial aneurysm secondary to mycotic orbital and sinus infection. *Am. J. Dis. Child.*, 119:357–362.
40. Nishioka, G., Schwartz, J.G., Rinaldi, M.G., Aufdemorte, T.B., and Mackie, E. (1987): Fungal maxillary sinusitis caused by *Curvulernia lunata*. *Arch. Otolaryngol. Head Neck Surg.*, 113:665–666.
41. Oreilly, M.J., Reddick, E.J., Black, W., Carter, P.L., Erhardt, J., Fill, W., Maughn, D., Sado, A., and Klatt, G.R. (1984): Sepsis from sinusitis in nasotracheally intubated patients: a diagnostic dilemma. *Am. J. Surg.*, 147:601–604.
42. Padhye, A., Ajello, L., Wieden, M., and Steinbronn, K. (1986): *Phaeohyphomycosis* of the nasal sinuses caused by a new species of *Exserohilum*. *J. Clin. Microbiol.*, 24:245–248.
43. Rachelefsky, G.S., Katz, R.M., and Siegel, S.C. (1982): Chronic sinusitis in children with respiratory allergy: the role of antimicrobials. *J. Allergy Clin. Immunol.*, 69:382–387.
44. Sandler, R., Tallman, C.B., Keamy, D.G., and Irving, W.R. (1971): Successfully treated rhinocerebral phycomycosis in well controlled diabetes. *N. Engl. J. Med.*, 285:1180–1182.
45. Schlanger, G., Lutwick, L.I., Kurzman, M., Hoch, B., and Chandler, F.W. (1984): Sinusitis caused by *Legionella pneumophila* in a patient with the acquired immune deficiency syndrome. *Am. J. Med.*, 77:957–960.
46. Schweitzer, V.G. (1986): Osteolytic sinusitis and pneumomediastinum: deceptive otolaryngologic complications of cocaine abuse. *Laryngoscope*, 96:206–210.
47. Shapiro, E.D., Wald, E.R., Doyle, W., and Rohn, D. (1982): Bacteriology of the maxillary sinus of rhesus monkeys. *Ann. Otol.*, 91:150–151.
48. Shapiro, G.G., Furukawa, C.T., Pierson, W.E., Gilbertson, E., and Bierman, C.W. (1986): Blinded comparison of maxillary sinus radiography and ultrasound for diagnosis of sinusitis. *J. All. Clin. Immun.* 77:59–64.
49. Shapiro, G.G., Rachelefsky, G.S. (1992): Introduction and definition of sinusitis. *J. Allergy Clin. Immunol.*, 90:417–418.
50. Siegel, J.D. (1987): Diagnosis and management of acute sinusitis in children. *Pediatr. Infect. Dis. J.*, 6:95–99.
51. Silver, A.J., Baredes, S., Bello, J.A., Blitzer, A., and Hilal, S.K. (1987): The opacified maxillary sinus: CT findings in chronic sinusitis and malignant tumors. *Radiology*, 163:205–210.
52. Slavin, R.G. (1984): Sinusitis. *J. Allergy Clin. Immunol.*, 73:712–716.
53. Sofferman, R.A. (1983): Cavernous sinus thrombophlebitis secondary to sphenoid sinusitis. *Laryngoscope*, 93:797–800.
54. Su, W.Y., Liu, C., Hung, S.Y., and Tsai, W.F. (1983): Bacteriological study in chronic maxillary sinusitis. *Laryngoscope*, 93:931–934.
55. Turner, B.W., Cail, W.S., Hendley, J.O., Hayden, F.G., Doyle, W.J., Sorrentino, J.V., and Gwaltney, J.M., Jr. (1992): Physiologic abnormalities in the paranasal sinuses during experimental rhinovirus colds. *J. Allergy Clin. Immunol.*, 90:474–478.
56. Urdal, K., and Berdal, P. (1949): The microbial flora in 81 cases of maxillary sinusitis. *Acta Otolaryngol.*, 37:22–25.
57. Viollier, A.F., Peterson, D.E., DeJongh, C.A., Newman, K.A., Gray, W.C., Sutherland, J.C., Moody, M.A., and Schimpff, S.C. (1986): Aspergillus sinusitis in cancer patients. *Cancer*, 58:366–371.
58. Wald, E.R., Guerra, N., and Byers, C. (1991): Upper respiratory tract infections in young children: duration of and frequency of complications. *Pediatrics*, 87:129–133.
59. Wald, E.R., Milmoe, G.J., Bowen, A., Ledesma-Median, J., Salamon, N., and Bluestone, C.D. (1981): Acute maxillary sinusitis in children. *N. Engl. J. Med.*, 304:749–754.
60. Wald, E.R., Reilly, J.S., Casselbrant, M., Ledesma-Median, J., Milmoe, G.J., Bluestone, C.D., and Chiponis, D. (1984): Treatment of maxillary sinusitis in childhood: a comparative study of amoxicillin and cefaclor. *J. Pediatr.*, 104:297–302.
61. Waxman, J.E., Spector, J.G., Sale, S.R., and Katzenstein, A.L. (1987): Allergic aspergillus sinusitis: concepts in diagnosis and treatment of a new clinical entity. *Laryngoscope*, 97:261–266.

62. Wells, R.G., Sty, J.R., and Landers, A.D. (1986): Radiologic evaluation of Pott puffy tumor. *J.A.M.A.,* 255:1331–1333.
63. Williams, J.W., Jr., Simel, D.L., Roberts, L., and Samsa, G.P. (1992): Clinical evaluation for sinusitis: making the diagnosis by history and physical examination. *Ann. Intern. Med.,* 117:705–710.
64. Winther, B., Gwaltney, J.M., Jr., Mygind, N., Turner, R.B., and Hendley, J.O. (1986): Intranasal spread of rhinovirus during point-inoculation of the nasal mucosa. *J.A.M.A.,* 256:1763–1767.
65. Yarington, C.T. (1979): Sinusitis as an emergency. *Otolaryngol. Clin. of No. Amer.,* 12:447–454.
66. Young, L.W. (1986): Radiologic imaging of Pott puffy tumor and other frontal sinusitis complications. Editorial. *Am. J. Dis. Child.,* 140:197.
67. Zeiger, R.S. (1992): Prospects for ancillary treatment of sinusitis in the 1990s. *J. Allergy Clin. Immunol.,* 90:478–495.

Respiratory Infections: Diagnosis and Management, 3d ed.,
edited by James E. Pennington.
Raven Press, Ltd., New York © 1994

8

Otitis Media

Jerome O. Klein

*Department of Pediatrics, Boston University School of Medicine,
Boston, Massachusetts 02118*

Otitis media, or inflammation of the middle ear, is the most frequent diagnosis recorded for children under 3 years of age who visit physicians because of illness.
Otitis media also occurs in older children, adolescents, and adults, although less
commonly. Acute otitis media (AOM) is defined by the presence of fluid in the middle ear accompanied by signs or symptoms of acute illness. Suppurative complications of middle ear infection such as mastoiditis, labyrinthitis, and brain abscess are
now uncommon but there is increasing concern for the morbidity of otitis media
associated with persistence of middle ear fluid and accompanying hearing loss. Fluid
persists in the middle ear for weeks to months after onset of infection even when
appropriate antimicrobial therapy has reduced the acute signs. Hearing is impaired
to some degree in most individuals who have fluid present in the middle ear. Thus,
there is particular concern about the effects of recurrent episodes of otitis media
during the first years of life when perception of language is critical to the development of speech and the learning processes. Adults suffer from the sequelae of otitis
media of childhood including hearing loss, chronic perforation of the tympanic membrane, cholesteatoma, and adhesive otitis media. Further information about otitis
media is contained in a 1988 monograph by C. D. Bluestone and J. O. Klein (6).

EPIDEMIOLOGY

Children may be categorized into three groups relative to the incidence of AOM:
one group is free of ear infections; a second group may have occasional episodes of
otitis media usually associated with infections of the upper respiratory tract; and a
third group is "otitis prone" with repeated episodes of acute middle ear infections.
By 3 years of age more than two-thirds of children have had one or more episodes
of AOM and one-third of children have had three or more episodes (51). The highest
incidence of AOM occurs in infants between 6 and 24 months of age. Subsequently,
the incidence of otitis media declines with age except for a limited reversal of the
downward trend between 5 and 6 years of age, the time of entrance into school.
Although the incidence of AOM is limited in adults, a survey by the National Disease
and Therapeutic Index found that there are almost 4 million visits by adults each
year to private physicians for middle ear infection (36).

Some racial groups such as American Indians and Canadian and Alaskan Eskimo
children have high rates of infection and severe middle ear disease (23,43). Poverty,

with its accompanying factors of crowding, poor sanitation, and inadequate medical facilities, is common to these children. Studies of urban children suggest that the incidence of ear pathology is lower among black children than among white children of similar socioeconomic status (24). Black children have fewer episodes of acute otitis media, as well as a shorter duration of middle ear effusion after an episode of acute otitis media (39).

Other features important in the epidemiology of the disease include the fact that males are affected more frequently than females (51), increased incidence during periods of viral infections in winter and spring when compared with summer and fall (17), and clustering in families with problems with ear infections in siblings and parents (51).

Age at the time of the first episode of AOM appears to be among the most powerful predictors of recurrent AOM. Most children who have severe and recurrent AOM have episodes early in life. This epidemiological feature of middle ear disease is analogous to infections of the urinary tract in infants; early onset of infection indicates a risk for an underlying anatomical or physiological disability.

Breast feeding for 3 or fewer months was associated with a decreased risk for AOM in the first year of life (51). As the duration of breast feeding during the first year was not associated directly with protection, and as little as 3 months was equivalent to a year of protection, the role of an immune factor in breast milk, rather than the infant's position or the act of suckling in itself, was the likely protective mode. The results of a feeding study of children with cleft palate suggests that one or more immunological factors in breast milk protected these infants in spite of their severe anatomical disability (38).

Introduction of infants into large day care groups increases the incidence of respiratory infections, including otitis media. A Pittsburgh study identified more episodes of AOM in children in day care than children in home care; as a reflection of the increased experience with middle ear disease, 21% of children in day care had received a myringotomy and tube placement by the second year compared with 3% of children in home care (54).

Passive smoking affects pulmonary function in children and increases the incidence of new episodes of otitis media with effusion and the duration of effusion. In a recent study by Etzel and colleagues (10), exposure to tobacco smoke was identified by use of a biochemical marker, serum cotinine concentrations.

Most children have no obvious defect responsible for severe and recurrent AOM, but a small number manifest anatomical changes (cleft palate, cleft uvula, submucous cleft), alteration of normal physiological defenses (patulous eustachian tube), or congenital or acquired immunological deficiencies. Some children with recurrent AOM have subtle differences in immune function. Children with acquired immunodeficiency syndrome (AIDS) have a higher age-specific incidence of AOM, beginning at 6 months of age, compared with uninfected children or children who initially were positive for human immunodeficiency virus (HIV) antibody, but who seroreverted (3).

MICROBIOLOGY

Bacteriology

The microbiology of otitis media has been documented by appropriate cultures of middle ear effusions obtained by needle aspiration (tympanocentesis). Many studies of the bacteriology of acute otitis media have been performed, and the results are remarkably consistent in demonstrating the importance of *Streptococcus pneumoniae* and *Hemophilus influenzae* (Table 8-1) (5). Recent studies of asymptomatic children with middle ear effusion indicate that bacterial pathogens are also present in these fluids, suggesting that bacteria may be a factor in the development and persistence of the effusion.

S. pneumoniae is responsible for one-quarter to one-half of episodes of acute infection in the middle ear in all age groups. Relatively few types are responsible for most disease. The most common types in order of decreasing frequency are 19, 23, 6, 14, 3, and 18 (2,13,22). All of these types are included in the currently available 23-type pneumococcal vaccine.

The incidence of pneumococci with intermediate resistance to penicillins is increasing in the United States. In a survey conducted by the Centers for Disease Control for the years 1979 to 1987 (50), 9.2% of pneumococci isolated from middle ear fluids had minimum inhibitory concentrations in excess of 0.1 ug/ml. In Spain, the incidence of resistant pneumococci rose from 6% in 1979 to 44% in 1989 (11).

H. influenzae is the etiologic agent for about one-fifth to one-third of cases of otitis media. Nontypeable strains are responsible in most patients. In approximately 10%, the otitis is due to type b; some of these children are very toxic, and about one-quarter have concomitant bacteremia or meningitis (16). Until recently, *H. influenzae* appeared to be limited in importance to preschool children; however, new information suggests that this organism is also a significant cause of otitis media in older children, adolescents, and adults (18,46). Approximately 15 to 30% of nontypeable strains of *H. influenzae* isolated from middle ear effusions of children with acute otitis media produce β-lactamase (7).

Reports from Pittsburgh and Cleveland (27,47) note a marked increase in isolation of *Moraxella catarrhalis* from purulent middle ear fluids of children with acute otitis media; the organism was isolated from middle ear fluids of 22 and 27%, respectively, of a consecutive series of children with acute otitis media. Prior to 1970 almost all strains of *M. catarrhalis* were sensitive to penicillin. Today, a majority of strains of *M. catarrhalis* produce beta-lactamase (7).

Group A *Streptococcus* has been a significant pathogen in some studies from Scandinavia, but this has not been the case in most studies from the United States. During the preantibiotic era, middle ear suppuration, often of a very destructive form, was frequently associated with scarlet fever (9). But otitis media due to this organism is

TABLE 8–1. *Bacterial pathogens isolated from middle ear fluid*
in 4,675 children with acute otitis media

Microorganism	% of children with pathogen	
	Mean	Range
Streptococcus pneumoniae	39	27–52
Hemophilus influenzae	27	16–52
Moraxella catarrhalis	10	2–15
Streptococcus, group A	3	0–11
Staphylococcus aureus	2	0–16
Miscellaneous bacteria	8	0–24
None or nonpathogens	28	12–35

Nine reports from centers in the United States, Finland, and Sweden, 1980–1987 (5).

now less frequent and rarely severe. Group B *Streptococcus* has been isolated from various body fluids including middle ear fluid in neonates and young infants.

Gram-negative enteric bacilli are responsible for about 20% of otitis media in young infants, but these organisms are rarely present in the middle ear fluids of older children and adults with acute otitis media. However, patients with diabetes mellitus, malignancy, or other diseases that diminish immune response and patients with chronic suppurative otitis media with perforation may encounter middle ear infection due to gram-negative enteric bacilli.

Anaerobic bacteria often in association with aerobic organisms were isolated from 2 of 20 children with acute otitis media (8). More data are needed to identify the importance of anaerobic bacteria in acute and chronic infections of the middle ear.

Disparate results of middle ear cultures occur frequently in children with bilateral otitis media (15,40). Disparate results occur when the cultures of the two ears yield different results: effusion from one ear is sterile but a bacterial pathogen is isolated from the other ear; or a different pathogen is isolated from each of the two ears. In some cases, mixed cultures, two types or two species of bacteria, are found in the same middle ear fluid. Disparate results occur in from one-fifth to one-third of children with acute otitis media. Different serotypes of *S. pneumoniae* were identified in 1.5% of cases of bilateral pneumococcal otitis media (2). These data indicate that investigative studies of the microbiology of bilateral otitis media must include aspiration of both ears to determine the efficacy of methods of treatment (i.e., trials of antimicrobial agents) or prevention (i.e., evaluation of vaccines or drugs) or when the bacteriology of the middle ear fluid is necessary to guide choices of antibiotics.

In all studies of acute otitis media a significant proportion (approximately one-third) of middle ear fluids are sterile after appropriate cultures for bacteria (5). The etiology of these cases may be one or more of the following: presence of a nonbacterial organism such as a virus, chlamydia, or mycoplasma; presence of fastidious bacterial organisms, such as anaerobic bacteria, that are not isolated by usual laboratory techniques; prior administration of an antimicrobial agent that would suppress growth of a bacterial pathogen; or an acute illness in a child who has persistent middle ear effusion from an episode of otitis media that occurred sometime in the past.

Viruses

Epidemiologic data suggest that viral infection is frequently associated with acute otitis media. In a longitudinal study of respiratory illness and complications in children attending a day care and school program, Henderson and colleagues demonstrated a correlation between isolation of viruses from the upper respiratory tract and the clinical diagnosis of otitis media (17). Virus outbreaks coincided with epidemics of otitis media. Adenoviruses, respiratory syncytial viruses, and enteroviruses accounted for the majority of isolates from the upper respiratory tract.

Virus isolations from middle ear fluids indicate an important role for respiratory syncytial virus, adenoviruses, and influenza viruses.

Studies of viral antigens yield more information about their role in otitis media (25); Klein and colleagues found evidence of viral antigens (most frequently respiratory syncytial virus) in approximately one-quarter of children with acute otitis media. Infections with concurrent isolation from middle ear fluids of respiratory viruses and bacteria may be more severe or prolonged than when virus or bacteria is present alone.

Mycoplasma pneumoniae

Myringitis, inflammation of the tympanic membrane, associated with hemorrhage and bleb formation in the more severe cases, was observed in nonimmune volunteers inoculated with *Mycoplasma pneumoniae* (42). However, the middle ear fluids of a large number of patients (771) have been cultured using appropriate methods, and *M. pneumoniae* was isolated in only one case (49). Thus, mycoplasms do not appear to play a significant role in acute otitis media. However, it does appear likely that some patients with lower respiratory tract disease due to *M. pneumoniae* may have concomitant otitis media.

Chlamydia trachomatis

Chlamydia trachomatis causes a mild but prolonged pneumonitis in infants. Many of these infants have otitis media. *C. trachomatis* has been isolated from ear aspirates of some infants with chlamydial pneumonitis (53).

PATHOGENESIS

Otitis media is a disease involving contiguous structures: the nares, nasopharynx, eustachian tube, middle ear, and the mastoid. Whatever affects one element affects the others as well. These structures are lined with a respiratory epithelium that contains ciliated cells, mucus-secreting goblet cells, and cells capable of secreting local immunoglobulins.

The middle ear resembles a flattened box that is approximately 15 mm from top to bottom, 10 mm wide, and only 2 to 6 mm deep. The superior wall lies over the jugular bulb; the lateral wall includes the tympanic membranes; the medial wall includes the oval and sound windows; the mastoid air cells lie behind; and the orifice of the eustachian tube is in the superior portion of the front wall.

The eustachian tube connects the middle ear with the posterior nasopharynx. The lateral one-third of the tube lies in bone and is open. The medial two-thirds is in cartilage, and the walls are in apposition except during swallowing or yawning. In the young child the eustachian tube is shorter and proportionately wider than in the older child, and the cartilaginous and osseous portions of the tube form a relatively straight line. In the older child the angle of the tube is more acute, and the tube is longer and narrower. These anatomic differences may be one reason why most infections of the middle ear occur in early childhood.

Anatomic or physiologic dysfunction of the eustachian tube appears to play a critical role in the development of infection of the middle ear. The eustachian tube has at least three physiologic functions with respect to the middle ear: (i) protection of the ear from nasopharyngeal secretions; (ii) drainage into the nasopharynx of secretions produced within the middle ear; and (iii) ventilation of the middle ear to equilibrate air pressure inside the ear cavity with pressure in the environment (as represented by pressure in the external ear canal). When one or more of these functions is compromised, the result may be development of fluid and infection in the middle ear. Congestion of the mucosa by infection or allergy may result in obstruction of the isthmus, the narrowest portion of the eustachian tube between the bony and cartilaginous sections. Secretions that are constantly formed by the mucosa of the middle ear accumulate behind the obstruction, and if a bacterial pathogen is present, a suppurative infection may result.

CLINICAL MANIFESTATIONS

Acute otitis media is defined by the presence of middle ear fluid accompanied by a sign or symptom of acute illness such as ear pain, ear drainage, or fever. Infants may have only general signs of disease such as lethargy, irritability, feeding problems (anorexia or vomiting), and diarrhea. Vertigo, nystagmus, and tinnitus may occur. Hyperemia of the tympanic membrane is an early sign of otitis media, but redness of the tympanic membrane may be caused by inflammation of the mucosa throughout the upper respiratory tract. Thus "red ear" alone does not establish the diagnosis of otitis media; the diagnosis requires the presence of fluid in the middle ear.

DIAGNOSIS

The presence of fluid in the middle ear is best determined by use of pneumatic otoscopy, a technique that permits assessment of mobility of the tympanic membrane. The motion of the tympanic membrane is proportional to the pressure applied by gently squeezing and then releasing the rubber bulb attached to the head of the otoscope. Normal mobility is apparent when positive pressure is applied and the membrane moves rapidly inward; with release of the bulb and the resulting negative pressure, the membrane moves outward. The presence of fluid in the middle ear (or high negative pressure) dampens the mobility of the tympanic membrane. Tympanometry uses an electroacoustic impedance bridge to record compliance of the tympanic membrane and middle ear pressure. Acoustic reflectometry is based on the fact that a sound wave in a closed tube will be reflected when it strikes the end of the tube. These techniques provide objective evidence of the status of the middle ear and the presence or absence of fluid.

The correlation between bacterial cultures of the nasopharynx and the oropharynx and cultures of the middle ear fluids is poor. Thus, cultures of the upper respiratory tract are of limited value in specific bacteriologic diagnosis of otitis media. In contrast, the consistent results of the microbiologic studies of middle ear fluid of children with acute otitis media provide an accurate guide to the most likely pathogens. If the patient is toxic or has a localized infection elsewhere, culture of the blood and of the focus of infection should be performed.

Needle aspiration of middle ear effusion of patients with acute otitis provides immediate and specific information about bacterial pathogens and should be considered in special circumstances: if the patient is critically ill when first seen, if the patient fails to respond appropriately to initial therapy for acute otitis media, or if the patient has altered host defenses. The latter group includes the newborn infant and the patient with malignancy or immunologic disease since these patients may be infected with unusual agents.

MANAGEMENT OF ACUTE OTITIS MEDIA

The antimicrobial agent prescribed for the patient with otitis media must be active against *S. pneumoniae, H. influenzae,* and *M. catarrhalis.* Clinical trials indicate that many antimicrobial agents are effective in resolving acute signs and symptoms of otitis media. Antimicrobial agents approved for therapy of AOM in the United States include amoxicillin and amoxicillin clavulanate, five cephalosporins (cefaclor, cefixime, cefprozil, cefpodoxime, and cefuroxime axetil) and two sulfonamide-containing agents (trimethoprim-sulfamethoxazole and erythromycin-sulfisoxazole). Although similar in clinical efficacy for all children with AOM, there are microbiological and administrative advantages for some.

Aspirates of middle ear fluids before and following administration of the drug document microbiological efficacy. In general, the results corroborate data based on the *in vitro* susceptibility of organisms and concentrations of drug achieved in the middle ear. Thus, amoxicillin is very effective in sterilizing the middle ear fluids when pneumococcus or beta-lactamase negative *H. influenzae* are isolated but fails to eradicate beta-lactamase positive *H. influenzae* (19–21,30–32,34,35). In addition to knowledge of the results of studies of clinical and microbiological efficacy of available antimicrobial agents, physicians must also consider the incidence of side effects, palatability, convenience of storage, dosage schedule, and cost.

The usual duration of therapy for AOM is 10 to 14 days in the United States, but shorter schedules have been suggested. A prospective, randomized double-blind study of a single dose of intramuscular ceftriaxone and 10 days of oral amoxicillin indicated equivalent clinical efficacy (14). As it is likely that concentrations of ceftriaxone that are effective against the major bacterial pathogens of AOM are present in the middle ear for only 3 to 4 days, the data showing comparability of the clinical results suggest that shorter courses of oral antimicrobial agents could be effective for many patients with AOM.

Recommendations for Initial Choice of Antimicrobial Therapy

Amoxicillin is the currently preferred drug for initial treatment of otitis media, since it is active both *in vitro* and *in vivo* against *S. pneumoniae* and *H. influenzae.* If recent clinical failures suggest increased incidence of beta-lactamase-producing *H. influenzae* or *M. catarrhalis,* alternative agents including amoxicillin-clavulanate, a cephalosporin, or a sulfonamide-containing agent should be considered. The cephalosporins may be used in patients who have ambiguous skin reactions associated with administration of a penicillin but should be avoided if the patient has had an immediate or accelerated allergic reaction due to a penicillin. Trimethoprim-sulfamethoxazole or erythromycin and sulfisoxazole are appropriate for the patient with a significant reaction to a penicillin or cephalosporin.

With appropriate antimicrobial therapy, most patients with acute bacterial otitis media are significantly improved within 48 to 72 hours. The physician should be in contact with the patient (or the patient's parents) to ascertain that improvement has occurred. If the patient remains toxic or the condition worsens, he or she must be reevaluated and a change in antimicrobial therapy, myringotomy for drainage, or needle aspiration for diagnosis should be considered.

MANAGEMENT OF CHRONIC OTITIS MEDIA

The term *chronic otitis media* includes recurrent episodes of acute infection and prolonged effusion of the middle ear resulting from acute infection. For prevention of recurrent episodes of acute otitis media, management should include consideration of chemoprophylaxis (use of antimicrobial agents for prolonged periods) or immunoprophylaxis (use of pneumococcal vaccine). For management of persistent middle ear effusions, three methods are considered: myringotomy, adenoidectomy, and placement of tympanostomy tubes. Although there is evidence for the support of each method for management of chronic otitis media, the data are at present incomplete.

Management of Recurrent Episodes of Otitis Media

Chemoprophylaxis

Controlled clinical trials (4,28,33,41,44,45) suggest the value of chemoprophylaxis in children with recurrent episodes of acute otitis media. Reduction in number of new episodes of acute infection in children in the prophylaxis group, when compared with results for the controls, varied from 47 to 90%. Although the available studies do not provide conclusive evidence of the validity of chemoprophylaxis, the data are persuasive that children who are prone to recurrent episodes of acute infection of the middle ear are benefited. It is reasonable to consider the following program:

1. Who? Children who have had three episodes of acute otitis media in 6 months or four episodes in 12 months.
2. Which drugs? Sulfisoxazole and amoxicillin were the agents used in published studies.
3. What dosage? Half the therapeutic dosage should be administered once a day.
4. How long? During the winter and spring, when respiratory infections are most frequent, up to a period of 6 months.

Decongestants and Antihistamines

Nasal and oral decongestants, alone or in combination with an antihistamine, are popular medications for the treatment of otitis media with effusion. These agents may provide symptomatic relief for the patient with rhinorrhea or congestion of the nasal mucosa but have no documented beneficial effect for acute otitis media or otitis media with effusion.

Pneumococcal Vaccine

Randomized trials of use of the vaccine for prevention of recurrence of acute otitis media in children were begun in Boston (52) and Huntsville, Alabama (48), in 1975 and in Oulu and Tampere, Finland, in 1977 (29). *S. pneumoniae* due to types present in the vaccine were isolated significantly less frequently from children in the vaccine groups than from children in the control groups. However, the clinical experience of immunized children was not significantly different in children who received the vaccine when compared with the experience of children who received the control materials. The number of children who had one or more episodes of otitis media and the mean number of episodes of acute otitis media after immunization were similar in the vaccine and control groups. The lack of clinical efficacy was due to the poor immunogenicity of the polysaccharide vaccines in infants. Current experimental conjugate vaccines combining pneumococcal polysaccharides with proteins are immunogenic in children as young as 2 months of age and suggest efficacy in prevention of type-specific pneumococcal otitis media.

Management of Persistent Middle Ear Effusion

Myringotomy

Myringotomy, or incision of the tympanic membrane, is a method of draining middle ear fluid. Before the introduction of antimicrobial agents, myrinogotomy was the main mode of management of acute otitis media. Today, it is used only under selected circumstances. Current usage of myringotomy includes relief of intractable ear pain, hastening resolution of mastoid infection, drainage of persistent middle ear effusion that is unresponsive to medical therapy, and management of acute otitis media that is accompanied by signs of cranial nerve (IV or VII) involvement.

Adenoidectomy

Enlarged adenoids may obstruct the orifice of the eustachian tube in the posterior nasopharynx and interfere with adequate ventilation and drainage of the middle ear. The preliminary results indicate that adenoidectomy does not prevent recurrent otitis media, but it remains uncertain whether the procedure reduces the rate, severity, or duration of recurrent episodes.

Results of studies in San Antonio (12) and Pittsburgh (37) suggest benefit of adenoidectomy in some children with persistent middle ear effusion or recurrent episodes of AOM. Although obstruction of the orifice of the eustachian tube may play a role in chronic and recurrent middle ear infection, it is also possible that a chronically infected adenoid serves as a reservoir for microorganisms and antigens with frequent seeding of the middle ear and the sinuses.

Tympanostomy Tubes

Tympanostomy tubes that resemble small collar buttons are placed through an incision in the tympanic membrane to avoid drainage of fluid and ventilation of the middle ear. The criteria for placement of the tubes include persistent middle ear effusions that are unresponsive to adequate medical treatment over a period of 3 months, persistent tympanic membrane retraction pockets with impending cholesteatoma, persistent negative pressure, and any of the above in lesser degrees when accompanied by impairment of hearing. Hearing improves dramatically after placement of the ventilating tubes. The tubes also have been of value in patients who have difficulty maintaining ambient pressure in the middle ear. Thus, barotrauma occurring in airline personnel frequently resolves when tubes are placed in the tympanic membrane.

REFERENCES

1. Arola, M., Ziegler, T., and Ruuskanen, O. (1990): Respiratory virus infection as a cause of prolonged symptoms in acute otitis media. *J. Pediatr.*, 116:697–701.
2. Austrian, R., Howie, V.M., and Ploussard, J.H. (1977): The bacteriology of pneumococcal otitis media. *Johns Hopkins Med. J.*, 141:104–111.
3. Barnett, E.D., Klein, J.O., Pelton, S.I., and Luginbuhl, L.M. (1992): Otitis media in children born to human immunodeficiency virus–infected mothers. *Pediatr. Inf. Dis. J.*, 11:360–364.
4. Biedel, C.W. (1978): Modification of recurrent otitis media by short-term sulfonamide therapy. *Am. J. Dis. Child.*, 132:681–683.
5. Bluestone, C.D., and Klein, J.O. (1983): Otitis media with effusion, atelectasis and eustachian tube dysfunction. In: *Pediatric Otolaryngology*, edited by C.D. Bluestone and S.E. Stool, p. 403. W.B. Saunders, Philadelphia.
6. Bluestone, C.D., and Klein, J.O. (Editors) (1988): *Otitis Media in Infants and Children*. W.B. Saunders, Philadelphia.
7. Bluestone, C.D., Stephenson, J.S., and Martin, L.M. (1992): Ten-year review of otitis media pathogens. *Pediatr. Infect. Dis. J.*, 11:S7–S11.
8. Brook, I., and Schwartz, R. (1981): Anaerobic bacteria in acute otitis media. *Acta Otolaryngol.*, 91:111–114.
9. Clarke, T.A. (1962): Deafness in children: otitis media and other causes; a selective survey of prevention and treatment and of educational problems. *Proc. R. Soc. Med.*, 55:61–70.
10. Etzel, R.A., Pattishall, E.N., Haley, N.J., et al. (1992): Passive smoking and middle ear effusion among children in day care. *Pediatrics*, 90(2):228–232.
11. Fenell, A., Beargon, D.M., Munoz, R., Nicioso, D., and Casal, J. (1991): Serotype distribution and antimicrobial resistance of *Streptococcus pneumoniae* isolates causing systemic infections in Spain, 1979–1989. *Rev. Infect. Dis.*, 13:56–60.
12. Gates, G.A., Avery, C.S., Phihooa, T.J., et al. (1987): Effectiveness of adenoidectomy and tympanostomy tubes in the treatment of chronic otitis media with effusion. *N. Engl. J. Med.*, 317:1444.
13. Gray, B.M., Converse, G.M., and Dillon, H.C., Jr. (1979): Serotypes of *Streptococcus pneumoniae* causing disease. *J. Infect. Dis.*, 140:979–983.
14. Green, S.M., and Rothrock, S.G. (1993): Single-dose intramuscular ceftriaxone for acute otitis media in children. *Pediatrics*, 91:23–30.
15. Gronroos, J.A., Kortekangas, A.E., Ojala, L., and Vuori, M. (1964): The aetiology of acute middle ear infection. *Acta Otolaryngol.* (Stockholm), 58:149–158.
16. Harding, A.L., Anderson, P., Howie, V.M., Ploussard, J.H., and Smith, D.H. (1973): *Haemophilus influenzae* isolated from children with otitis media. In: *Haemophilus influenzae*, edited by S.H.W. Sell and D.T. Karzon, pp. 21–28. Vanderbilt University Press, Nashville, Tenn.
17. Henderson, F.W., Collier, A.M., Sanyal, M.A., et al. (1982): A longitudinal study of respiratory viruses and bacteria in the etiology of acute otitis media with effusion. *N. Engl. J. Med.*, 306:1377–1383.
18. Herberts, G., Jeppson, P.H., Nylen, O., and Branefors-Helander, P. (1971): Acute otitis media: etiological and therapeutic aspects of acute otitis media. *Prac. Otol. Rhinol. Laryngol.* 33:191–202.
19. Howie, V.M. (1992): Discussion: antibiotic efficacy studies. *CID*, 14:209–210.
20. Howie, V.M., Dillard, R., and Lawrence, B. (1985): *In vivo* sensitivity test in otitis media: efficacy of antibiotics. *Pediatrics*, 75:8–13.
21. Howie, V.M., and Ploussard, J.H. (1969): The "in vivo sensitivity test": Bacteriology of middle ear exudate during antimicrobial therapy in otitis media. *Pediatrics*, 44:940–944.

22. Kamme, C., Ageberg, M., and Lundgren, K. (1970): Distribution of *Diplococcus pneumoniae* types in acute otitis media in children and influence of the types on the clinical course in penicillin V therapy. *Scand. J. Infect. Dis.*, 2:183–190.
23. Kaplan, G.J., Fleshman, J.K., Bender, T.R., Baum, C., and Clark, P.S. (1973): Long-term effects of otitis media: a ten-year cohort study of Alaskan Eskimo children. *Pediatrics*, 52: 577–585.
24. Kessner, D.M., Snow, C.K., and Singer, J. (1974): *Assessment of Medical Care for Children*, Vol. 3. Institute of Medicine, National Academy of Sciences, Washington, D.C.
25. Klein, B.S., Dollette, F.R., and Yolken, R.H. (1982): The role of respiratory syncytial virus and other viral pathogens in acute otitis media. *J. Pediatr.*, 101:16–20.
26. Klein, J.O., Teele, D.W., and Pelton, S.I. (1992): New concepts in otitis media: results of investigations of the Greater Boston Otitis Media Study Group. *Advances in Pediatric*, 39:127–156.
27. Kovatch, A., Wald, E.R., and Michaels, R.H. (1983): β-lactamase-producing *Branhamella catarrhalis* causing otitis media in children. *J. Pediatr.*, 102:261–264.
28. Liston, T.E., Foshee, W.S., and Pierson, W.D. (1983): Sulfisoxazole chemoprophylaxis for frequent otitis media. *Pediatrics*, 71:524–530.
29. Makelä, P.H., Leinonen, M., Pukander, J., and Karma, P. (1981): A study of the pneumococcal vaccine prevention of clinically acute attacks of recurrent otitis media. *Rev. Infect. Dis.*, 3:S124–S130.
30. Marchant, C.D., Shurin, P.A., Johnson, C.E., et al. (1986): A randomized controlled trial of amoxicillin plus clavulanate compared with cefaclor for treatment of acute otitis media. *J. Pediatr.*, 109:891–896.
31. Marchant, C.D., Shurin, P.A., Turczyk, V.A., et al. (1984): Course and outcome of otitis media in early infancy: a prospective study. *J. Pediatr.*, 104:826–831.
32. Marchant, C.D., Shurin, P.A., Turcyzk, V.A., et al. (1984): A randomized controlled trial of cefaclor compared with trimethoprim-sulfamethoxazole for treatment of acute otitis media. *J. Pediatr.*, 105:633–638.
33. Maynard, J.E., Fleshman, J.K., and Tschopp, C.F. (1972): Otitis media in Alaskan Eskimo children: prospective evaluation of chemoprophylaxis. *J.A.M.A.*, 219:597–599.
34. McLinn, S.E. (1980): Cefaclor in treatment of otitis media and pharyngitis in children. *Am. J. Dis. Child.*, 134:560–563.
35. McLinn, S.E., and Serlin, S. (1983): Cyclacillin versus amoxicillin as treatment for acute otitis media. *Pediatrics*, 71:196–199.
36. NDTI Review. (1970): Leading diagnoses and reasons for patient visits. 1:18–23.
37. Paradise, J.L., Bluestone, C.D., Rogers, K.D., and Taylor, F.H. (1980): Efficacy of adenoidectomy in recurrent otitis media: historical overview and preliminary results from a randomized, controlled trial. *Ann. Otol. Rhinol. Laryngol.*, 89(68):319–321.
38. Paradise, J.L., and Elster, B.A. (1984): Breast milk protects against otitis media with effusion. *Pediatr. Res.*, 18:283A.
39. Pelton, S.I., Shurn, P.A., and Klein, J.O. (1977): Persistence of middle ear effusion after otitis media. *Pediatr. Res.*, 11:504.
40. Pelton, S.I., Teele, D.W., Shurin, P.A., and Klein, J.O. (1980): Disparate cultures of middle ear fluids. *Am. J. Dis. Child.*, 134:951–953.
41. Perrin, J.M., Charney, E., MacWhinney, J.B., Jr., et al. (1974): Sulfisoxazole as chemoprophylaxis for recurrent otitis media: a double-blind crossover study in pediatric practice. *N. Engl. J. Med.*, 291:664–667.
42. Rifkind, D.R., Chanock, R.M., Kravetz, H., Johnson, K., and Knight, V. (1962): Ear involvement (myringitis) and primary atypical pneumonia following inoculation of volunteers with Eaton agent. *Am. Rev. Respir. Dis.*, 85:479–489.
43. Schaefer, O. (1971): Otitis media and bottle-feeding. An epidemiological study of infant feeding habits and incidence of recurrent and chronic middle ear disease in Canadian Eskimos. *Can. J. Public Health*, 62:478–489.
44. Schuller, D.E. (1983): Prophylaxis of otitis media in asthmatic children. *Pediatr. Infect. Dis.*, 2:280–283.
45. Schwartz, R.H., Puglese, J., and Rodriguez, W. (1982): Sulfamethoxazole prophylaxis in the otitis-prone child. *Arch. Dis. Child.*, 57:590–593.
46. Schwartz, R.H., and Rodriguez, W.J. (1981): Acute otitis media in children eight years old and older: a reappraisal of the role of *Hemophilus influenzae*. *Am. J. Otolaryngol.*, 2:19–21.
47. Shurin, P.A., Marchant, C.D., Kim, C.H., et al. (1983): Emergence of beta-lactamase-producing strains of *Branhamella catarrhalis* as important agents of acute otitis media. *Pediatr. Infect. Dis.*, 2:34–38.
48. Sloyer, J.L., Jr., Ploussard, J.H., and Howie, V.M. (1981): Efficacy of pneumococcal polysaccharide vaccine in preventing acute otitis media in infants in Huntsville, Alabama. *Rev. Infect. Dis.*, 3:S119–S123.

49. Sobeslavsky, O., Syrucek, L., Bruckoya, M., and Abrahamovic, M. (1965): The etiological role of *Mycoplasma pneumoniae* in otitis media in children. *Pediatrics,* 35:652–657.
50. Spika, J.S., Facklan, R.R., Plikoytis, B.O., and Oxtoby, M.J. (1991): Pneumococcal Working Group. Antimicrobial resistance of *Streptococcus pneumoniae* in the United States 1979–1987. *J. Infect. Dis.,* 163:1273–1278.
51. Teele, D.W., Klein, J.O., and Rosner, B. (1989): Epidemiology of otitis media during the first seven years of life in children in greater Boston: a prospective, cohort study. *J. Infect. Dis.,* 160:83–94.
52. Teele, D.W., Klein, J.O., and The Greater Boston Collaborative Otitis Media Group. (1981): Use of pneumococcal for prevention of recurrent acute otitis media in infants in Boston. *Rev. Infect. Dis.,* 3:S113–S118.
53. Tipple, M.A., Beem, M.O., and Saxon, E.M. (1979): Clinical characteristics of the afebrile pneumonia associated with *Chlamydia trachomatis* infection in infants less than six months of age. *Pediatrics,* 63:192–197.
54. Wald, E.R., Dashefsky, B., Byers, C., et al. (1988): Frequency and severity of infections in day care. *J. Pediatr.,* 112:540–546.

Respiratory Infections: Diagnosis and Management, 3d ed.,
edited by James E. Pennington.
Raven Press, Ltd., New York © 1994

9

Chronic Bronchitis

Anthony A. Floreani, Scott E. Buchalter, Joseph H. Sisson,
Austin B. Thompson, and Stephen I. Rennard

Pulmonary and Critical Care Medicine Section, Department of Internal Medicine,
University of Nebraska Medical Center,
600 South 42nd Street, Omaha, Nebraska 68198-5300

Chronic bronchitis is a clinical disorder characterized by the presence of cough with sputum production over an extended period of time. Arbitrarily, chronic bronchitis has been defined as a productive cough for 3 months per year for at least 2 years, and sputum production not due to other causes such as tuberculosis or bronchiectasis (83). Chronic bronchitis and emphysema are traditionally described as comprising the larger syndrome of chronic obstructive pulmonary disease (COPD) (363). Many agree that COPD presents a heterogeneous spectrum of clinical conditions with features that overlap to a variable extent in different patients. Compatible with this view is that COPD also encompasses disorders that share common features, the way asthmatic bronchitis and adult bronchiolitis do with chronic bronchitis and emphysema (182,303,313,361).

In the 1980s, COPD was the fifth leading cause of death in the United States (278). Chronic bronchitis and other forms of COPD are responsible for the increases seen in morbidity, health care expenditure, and mortality trends in the United States and other areas of the world (214[p.S35],393). Thus, chronic bronchitis has had a tremendous impact on society and on the health care profession. In the following sections we discuss the etiology, pathogenesis, diagnosis, and management of patients with chronic bronchitis, focusing on the stable patient with COPD.

ETIOLOGY AND PATHOGENESIS

Host Factors

A genetic basis for COPD is supported by familial aggregations of pulmonary function, or familial aggregation of COPD (161,193,365,384,387). Laurell and Ericksson (114,212) provided the first clear evidence for a genetic basis for COPD with their description of severe alpha-1 globulin deficiency in the serum of patients with chronic bronchitis, emphysema, and bronchiectasis.

Chronic bronchitis, bronchiolitis, and bronchiectasis are common airway disorders observed in patients with cystic fibrosis (CF). This genetic disorder is characterized by the development of bronchial and bronchiolar inflammation, mucous hypersecretion, and progressive airflow obstruction. There are a number of other non-cigarette-related causes of chronic bronchitis. In some individuals with a history of asthma there is concurrent mucous hypersecretion. This syndrome has been termed *chronic asthmatic bronchitis* (67,68,288,291,293). Reversibility of airflow obstruction and bronchial hyperreactivity, features consistent with asthma, have been hypothesized as etiologic factors for the development of chronic airflow obstruction, the so-called Dutch hypothesis (288,310,311,313).

Both immunoglobulin deficiencies and "primary ciliary dyskinesia" are associated with the sinopulmonary or bronchopulmonary symptoms. The former can be acquired or congenital and affect specific immunoglobulin subtypes. Cilia dyskinesias are a heterogeneous group of structural and functional cilia disorders. Kartagener's syndrome, which includes the triad of rhinosinusitis with nasal polyps, *situs inversus*, and bronchiectasis, is probably the best-known example of primary ciliary dyskinesia (3,262,297,328,332,354,409,438). Epidemiologic studies have examined other factors in the development of chronic obstructive pulmonary disease. Prevalence rates for respiratory symptoms increase with age and are higher for men, particularly Caucasian men (61,160,163,214,215,349,413).

Extrinsic Factors

Tobacco

In his historical review of emphysema, Gordon Snider (363) reported that as far back as 1604 James I of England regaled against the use of tobacco as "hateful to the nose, harmful to the braine and dangerous to the lungs." In the United States, cigarette smoking increased in popularity after the Civil War. The average annual per-capita consumption of cigarettes rose alarmingly in the United States after the 1920s, reaching a peak in the 5-year period studied, 1960–1964 (363). Comparable increases in cigarette smoking were seen in Europe in the 20th century (329). Presently, about 25% of the population continues to smoke cigarettes (122). Unfortunately, each year, one million individuals begin, and, of those, 90% become addicted before they reach the age of 18.

A number of longitudinal studies have described the association between the inhalation of tobacco smoke and the subsequent development of respiratory symptoms and, specifically, chronic bronchitis (126,128,289,349,361,381). Epidemiologic studies have also examined the effects of tobacco smoke on lung function. In their landmark studies, Fletcher et al. and Fletcher and Peto reported that cigarette smoking was the most important factor associated with the accelerated decline of FEV_1 in adult men in London (125,126; Fig. 9-1). Other investigators have also reported the effects of cigarette smoking on increased respiratory symptoms and diminished lung function, while Tager and colleagues described how normal adult decline in FEV_1 was significantly delayed in male nonsmokers, as compared to their smoking counterparts (38,162,385,441).

Effects of Cigarette Smoking on Airway Inflammation

Bronchoalveolar lavage (BAL) has been useful in assessing the effects of cigarette smoke on airway inflammation (8). Smoking alters a number of noncellular constituents found in BAL fluid, and increased numbers of macrophages and neutrophils

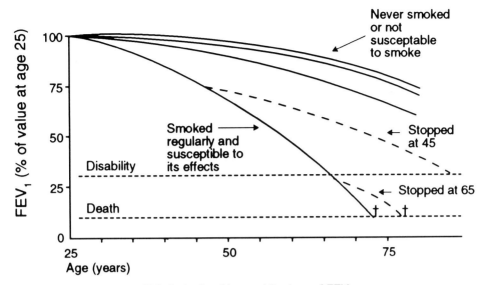

FIG. 9–1. Smoking and the loss of FEV₁.

are found in BAL fluid recovered from smokers, suggesting intraluminal evidence for inflammation (176,222,230,321,322,351,396,411). In patients with chronic bronchitis, increased numbers of macrophages and a more striking increase in the number of neutrophils are observed in BAL fluid (230,394). Thompson and colleagues (69,71) demonstrated that bronchial neutrophilia ($\geq$20% neutrophils) directly correlated with the number of pack years of cigarette smoking and the degree of airflow obstruction exhibited by patients with chronic bronchitis.

Alveolar macrophages recovered from the lavage fluid of smokers display a number of function alterations. These include decreased accessory cell function, decreased expression of the CD11/CD18 adhesion molecule complex on the macrophage surface, enhanced motility, increased metabolic activity, enhanced chemoactivity, and increased amount and release of lysosomal enzymes including proteases (12,90,117,123,171,172,188,241,401). Although the cause of the increased accumulation of alveolar macrophages in smokers and patients with chronic bronchitis is unknown, there are a number of molecules that exhibit chemotactic activity for monocytes, including BAL fluid obtained from smokers (177,199,309,419).

There are several proposed mechanisms responsible for the intraluminal accumulation of neutrophils in smokers and patients with chronic bronchitis. Alveolar macrophages are capable of elaborating such neutrophil chemoattractants as interleukin-8 (IL-8), leukotriene B4 (LTB4), tumor necrosis factor (TNF), and platelet activating factor (PAF) (9,205,231,277,317,370). There is also evidence that macrophage-derived products prime neutrophils for antibacterial and other proinflammatory functions (216,290,299). Chemotactic activity is also released from human tracheal and endobronchial epithelial cells and lung fibroblasts (276,326). Tobacco smoke can increase the amount of neutrophil co-chemotaxins, such as GC globulin, or reduce the functional activity of neutrophil chemotactic inactivator. These factors could then lead to an accumulation of airway neutrophils (247,324).

In addition to the intraluminal recruitment of neutrophils and airway macrophages examined by BAL studies, autopsy studies in young smokers have demonstrated inflammation in peripheral airways. This respiratory bronchiolitis, consisting primarily of pigmented macrophages in respiratory bronchioles, could be an inciting lesion for the development of chronic airflow obstruction in susceptible smokers (88,283,440).

Mucociliary Clearance in Chronic Bronchitis

Airway mucus is composed of water, electrolytes, proteins, lipids, and nucleic acids. The most prominent molecules found in mucus are mucous glycoproteins, referred to as *mucins*. Mucins are a heterogeneous and complex group of polyanionic glycoproteins released by exocytosis from airway epithelial cells and mucous glands (197,347,412). Carbohydrate chains of these glycoproteins are expressed on the surface of tracheobronchial epithelial cells, and are potential sites of attachment by bacterial and viral ligands or adhesions (209,383). Mucin size and composition varies considerably in patients with chronic bronchitis, cystic fibrosis, and bronchiectasis (93,116,196,207–209,397,439). The airway mucus that bathes airway epithelium is composed of the hypophase (sol) layer, the thickness of which should be approximately equal to the length of the cilia for sufficient coupling to occur between the cilia and the overlying mucous epiphase (gel) layer (49,220,319,368; Fig. 9-2). The effectiveness of mucociliary clearance depends on several interrelated factors: (i) the integrity of the ciliated epithelium; (ii) ciliary beating; (iii) thickness and consistency of the sol layer; (iv) visoelastic, electrolyte, and biochemical properties of mucus; and (v) thickness of the epiphase, or gel layer (368). The excessive accumulation of mucus in the airways of cigarette smokers and patients with chronic bronchitis occurs as a result of excessive production of mucus by airway epithelial cells and submucosal glands, and impaired clearance of this mucus present in conducting airways (422).

Cigarette smoke is composed of both a gas and particulate phase in which is suspended over 4,000 different chemicals. Hydrocarbons, oxidants and free radicals,

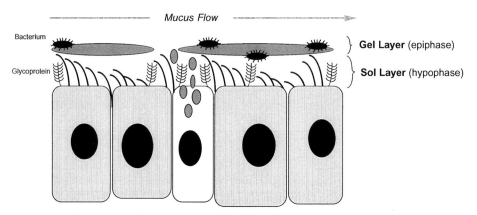

FIG. 9–2. Simplified schematic illustration of ciliated epithelial cells with overlying sol and gel layers of airways mucus. Also depicted are respiratory glycoproteins on the cell surface of epithelial cells which are potential sites of attachment by bacterial ligands or adhesion molecules, including fimbriae or pili.

acrolein, tars, and aldehydes are major components of cigarette smoke (404; Table 9-1). A number of structural and functional alterations rendered by the effects of cigarette smoke have been observed in airway cilia and the underlying mucosal epithelial cells (28,132,238,353,422; Fig. 9-3). Slowing of ciliary beat frequency in animals exposed to cigarette smoke has been described. One possible mechanism suggested by *in vitro* studies is cigarette smoke–induced formation of aldehyde adducts to cilia dynein and tubulin (179,353). *In vivo* studies utilizing aerosol clearance in humans have reported altered mucociliary transport in cigarette smokers, individuals with chronic bronchitis, and in bronchiectasis (44,73,144,198,221,235,422). Even in otherwise healthy individuals, cigarette smoking alters mucociliary clearance and increases the risk for pulmonary infection (44). Improvement in mucociliary clearance is reported to occur within just 3 months of smoking cessation in otherwise healthy smokers (73,422).

Some investigators have been able to show that cigarette smoke oxidizes alpha-1 antitrypsin (α-1 AT) (78,135,172). However, the relevance of these findings *in vivo* is unclear; other investigators have been unable to confirm the presence of reduced α-1 AT activity in smokers, whereas inactive α-1 AT has been reported in BAL fluid of healthy nonsmokers (2,50,377). In addition, it is now clear that other elastase inhibitors are present in the lower respiratory tract. Antileukoprotease inhibitor (ALP), also referred to as secretory leukocyte proteinase inhibitor (SLPI), most likely confers significant airway antiproteinase protection (50,60,200,260). Nevertheless, because neutrophil elastase has been implicated in the pathogenesis of chronic bronchitis and emphysema, the effects of cigarette smoke on protease inhibitors may contribute to airway elastase/antielastase imbalances and the development of chronic lung disease in susceptible cigarette smokers (84,181,362,364). Along with neutrophil elastase, other proteinases such as cathepsin G and the cystine proteinases cathepsin B and L have been identified in the bronchial secretions obtained

TABLE 9–1. *Major toxic and carcinogenic components present in cigarette smoke*

Phase	Component	Amount
Gas	Carbon dioxide (CO_2)	10–80 mg
	Carbon monoxide (CO)	0.5–26 mg
	Hydrogen cyanide	280–550 μg
	Nitrogen oxides (NO_x)	16–600 μg
	Ammonia (NH_3)	10–130 μg
	Formaldehyde	20–90 μg
	Acrolein	10–140 μg
	Acetone	100–940 μg
	Nitrosamines	0–180 μg
	Peroxyl radical (R-00)$^\bullet$	—
	Hydroxyl radical (OH)$^\bullet$	—
Particulate	Nicotine	0.06–2.3 mg
	Toluene	108 μg
	Benzenes	1.7–90 μg
	Quinolines	1.1–6.7 μg
	Phenol	20–150 μg
	Naphthalenes	1.0–2.8 μg
	Pyrenes	8–90 ng
	Superoxide anion (O_2)$^\bullet$	—
	Hydroxyl radical (OH)$^\bullet$	—

From U.S. Department of Health and Human Services. A Report of the Surgeon General, U.S. Government Printing Office, Washington, D.C., 1979, 1982.

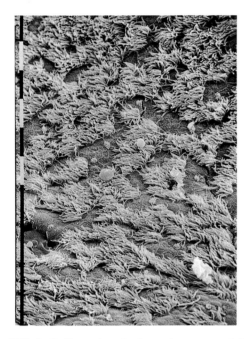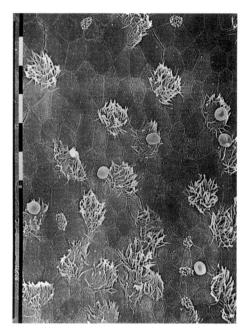

FIG. 9–3. Scanning electron microscopy of the luminal surface of bovine bronchi taken from air- and smoke-exposed lungs. These sections are representative of changes seen in three separate experiments (Bar = 10 μM). Air-exposed bronchus (*left*). Normal ciliated epithelium is seen across the entire luminal surface of the airway. Smoke-exposed bronchus (*right*). The ciliated epithelium of the bronchus is disrupted with nonciliated "bare" areas visible over a large portion of the luminal surface. (Courtesy of Joseph H. Sisson, M.D., University of Nebraska Medical Center.)

from patients with chronic bronchitis and bronchiectasis (57–59,141,373,376). Features of bronchitis are also present in habitual marijuana smokers. Increased recovery of neutrophils in BAL fluid, histologic changes consisting of squamous metaplasia, goblet cell hyperplasia, and intraepithelial inflammation have been demonstrated in marijuana smokers with or without concurrent use of tobacco (31,143).

Effects of Air Pollution and Occupational Exposure

Both ambient and indoor air pollution can contribute to chronic bronchitis (202,389,392). Cooking stoves are a known source of nitrous oxide (NO_2) and carbon monoxide (CO), and wood smoke is a potent source of carbon monoxide, particulates, and aromatic hydrocarbons. Acute respiratory symptoms have been described in patients with chronic lung disease who have been exposed to NO_2 or CO, although no conclusive statements regarding these molecules as etiologic factors in the development of chronic bronchitis can be made at present (101,261,338,345). Indoor air pollution from coal-burning stoves is a significant risk factor for chronic bronchitis and lung cancer (134,157,389).

Industrial bronchitis is a term coined for those with high levels of occupational exposure to dust, gas, or fumes (250,258,367). Chronic exposure to dust is an independent risk factor for decline in lung function, and a 50% increase in chronic bronchitis was observed in those occupationally exposed to dust(s) or chemical fumes, even when adjustments were made for age, smoking habits, socioeconomic status, and air pollution (14,39,131,192,202,203,248). Experimental inhalation of ozone has resulted in mucous hypersecretion, and this phenomenon has been associated with a significantly increased recovery of airway neutrophils by bronchoalveolar lavage (146). Farmers exposed to grain dust during harvest or individuals working in hog confinement areas develop respiratory symptoms such as cough, sputum production, and dyspnea (343,415–417). The above studies suggest that exposure to air pollutants and occupational exposure to airborne or volatile compounds can contribute to the etiology of chronic bronchitis.

The Role of Infection in Chronic Bronchitis

Infection is the most common identifiable cause of death for those with COPD (63). Controversy still remains, however, over whether or not infectious episodes are associated with an accelerated loss of lung function over the clinical course of those with chronic bronchitis or emphysema (34). It could be that acute infection promotes the loss of lung function in selected patients. Unfortunately, there are no practical methods to identify such patients.

Bacterial Infection and Colonization in Chronic Bronchitis

Since the 1950s, evidence has suggested bacterial infection as a cause of acute exacerbations of chronic bronchitis (55,236,386). Bacteria can be the primary invaders of the airways, resulting in initial colonization and subsequent infection; or, alternatively, bacteria can invade after initial viral or microplasmal infection (69,272,358). Patients hospitalized with purulent exacerbations of chronic bronchitis have been shown to have greater numbers of *Hemophilus influenzae* and pneumococcal organisms recovered from tracheal aspirates than do normal individuals (217). However, demonstration of bacteria in the sputum of patients with chronic bronchitis does not necessarily imply a pathologic role for such organisms; similar bacteria can be cultured from the sputum of patients with chronic bronchitis during stable periods of their disease as well as from the upper respiratory tract of normal individuals (159,213,386). Similarly, a documented serologic response to a particular bacterial antigen could reflect a prior acute infection by that organism. It is often difficult, then, to clearly differentiate between bacterial colonization of the airways and an acute bacterial infection in those with chronic bronchitis (139,213,217,273, 357,386). In some cases the precipitating factors for patients' acute respiratory symptoms are unclear: they could be related to primary bacterial infection or bacterial superinfection following viral or microplasmal infection; or they could be unidentified (69,357,386).

In addition to the possible role of bacteria in acute exacerbations of chronic bronchitis, the presence of bacteria in the airways can further enhance airway mucosal inflammation as conceptualized by the "vicious circle hypothesis." This theory implies that bacterial infection plays a role in the chronic inflammation and injury observed in those with bronchiectasis (85,87,115,374). The release of microbial product(s) damages respiratory mucosal cells leading to recruitment of inflammatory cells to involved airways (346,437). These cells amplify the inflammatory response by the elaboration of cytokines, oxidants, and proteolytic enzymes, which further damages airway epithelial cells and the extracellular matrix. Injury to the airway architecture may then predispose to future infections. Thus, a vicious circle of infection, inflammation, injury, and subsequent infection ensues in such individuals (85,86,221,435,437; Fig. 9-4). Support for this concept can be seen in studies of sputum samples obtained from those with chronic bronchitis. Such sputum specimens frequently contain increased numbers of neutrophils, particularly during purulent exacerbations, and increased amounts of neutrophil-derived myeloperoxidase (70,373). Neutrophil chemoattractants, such as interleukin-8 and leukotriene B4, are detectable in sputum samples from chronic bronchitis (323,442). Elastolytic activity increases with acute infection, and sputum concentrations of antiproteinases, including alpha-1 antitrypsin and antileukoprotease, can also be elevated during purulent exacerbations of chronic bronchitis.

Serologic and bacteriologic data have confirmed that the three most common bacterial pathogens involved in patients with chronic bronchitis are *Streptococcus pneumoniae*, nontypeable (unencapsulated) *Hemophilus influenzae*, and *Moraxella*

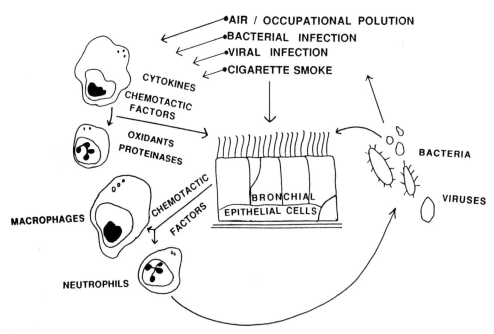

FIG. 9–4. Schematic representation of possible interrelated mechanisms involved in airway inflammation and injury. Cigarette smoke, air pollution, and occupational exposure result in mucus hypersecretion, depressed cilia function, and epithelial cell injury. Viral infection also results in cellular injury, with above factors predisposing epithelial cells to bacterial adherence, colonization, and infection. The above mechanisms draw increased numbers of PMNs and macrophages into airways, with release of their cellular products (such as proteinases and inflammatory cytokines), which results in further epithelial cell damage. The respiratory mucosa is then more prone to bacterial colonization and infection. Such a paradigm is consistent with the vicious circle hypothesis envisioned for those with bronchiectasis.

catarrhalis (55,139,150,152,154,213,236,237,239,267,281,282,408,431). Other gram-negative bacteria, *Staphylococcus aureus,* and, rarely, Pseudomonas sp, are recovered from bronchial secretions from those with chronic bronchitis (150,213,281).

Streptococcus pneumoniae

S. pneumoniae is a normal inhabitant of the upper respiratory tract of both children and adults, with pharyngeal carrier rates in adults ranging from 15 to 50%. Carrier rates for *S. pneumoniae* are commonly higher in winter months (81,159,217,249). Patients with chronic bronchitis have higher colonization rates in the upper respiratory tract than normal individuals. In contrast to the normally sterile lower respiratory tract present in patients without chronic lung disease, *S. pneumoniae* can be retrieved by transtracheal aspiration or bronchoscopic protected brush catheters in patients with chronic bronchitis (152). Colonization of airway epithelial cells by *S. pneumoniae* and other streptococcal species can occur through linking of bacterial cell surface proteins or adhesions with epithelial cell glycoconjugant receptors (10,11,36,37,155,156,382). The capsular polysaccharide component of the *S. pneumoniae* cell wall has been shown to confer antigenicity and is related to bacterial virulence (423).

Hemophilus influenzae

Nontypeable *H. influenzae* is the most common pathogen implicated in acute, purulent exacerbations of chronic bronchitis. Nontypeable *H. influenzae* is commonly found in the nares of children, whereas nasal carrier rates in adults have been reported as high as 80% (386). *H. influenzae* also colonizes the lower respiratory tract of patients with chronic bronchitis, with virtually all strains of *H. influenzae* recovered in these individuals being the nontypeable or unencapsulated strain of the bacteria (249,267). Mechanisms responsible for adherence and colonization of *H. influenzae* to airway epithelial cells are not fully known, but most likely involve both bacterial and host factors. Mucins present in bronchial mucus also provide multiple attachment sites for airway bacteria, thereby trapping bacteria in a mucous blanket and facilitating their removal by mucociliary clearance mechanisms (208,209, 316,414). However, just as airway mucus can enhance bacterial clearance, it also appears that organisms such as *H. influenzae* adhere to mucus present in luminal airways; this adherence could then precede binding of the bacteria to bronchial epithelial cells. Mucous hypersecretion and impaired clearance mechanisms could then predispose individuals with chronic bronchitis to bacterial adherence and colonization. Fimbriae, or pili, the hairlike, extracellular appendages on gram-negative bacteria, are known to mediate bacterial attachment to epithelial cells (175,187,204). Pili proteins and nonfimbriated ligands or adhesions of *H. influenzae* and other gram-negative bacteria bind the digalactoside Gal-Nac-B(1-4)-Gal and related galactoside sequences that have been isolated as the epithelial cell surface receptors. Adhesion-mediated binding to epithelial cell receptors appears to be a critical step in bacterial adherence to tracheobronchial mucosa (30,169,187,201,204,218,223,308,379,380, 407).

A number of pathogenic bacteria, including *H. influenzae,* release bacterial cell products such as lipooligosaccharide, which directly depress ciliary beat frequency and damage epithelial cells (185,435–437). *In vitro* studies have revealed that nontypeable *H. influenzae* preferentially adhere to damaged respiratory epithelium (318).

The above observations could thus have important implications for the bacterial adherence and colonization observed in patients with chronic lung disease. Excessive airway mucus can impair bacterial clearance, predispose to bacterial adherence and colonization, and ultimately lead to the release of bacterial cell products injurious to respiratory mucosal cells. This concept is consistent with the well-known observation that mucociliary clearance is significantly depressed during acute respiratory infections (295). It is also consistent with the altered mucociliary transport characteristic of patients with chronic bronchitis, bronchiectasis, and cystic fibrosis (198,368,371).

The cell envelope of *H. influenzae* is comprised of a cytoplasmic membrane, an overlying peptidoglycan layer, and a complex outer membrane bi-layer, which has important antigenic properties (32,269; Fig. 9-5). Lipooligosaccharide (LOS) is a surface antigen component of the outer membrane which displays diverse heterogenicity among various strains of the bacteria (19,74,270). LOS is comparable to lipooligosaccharide of enteric gram-negative bacteria, is an endotoxin, and a potent proinflammatory mediator. LOS is one of the bacterial products of *H. influenzae* that have been shown *in vitro* to directly damage respiratory epithelium and depress ciliary function (185,437). Thus, it is likely that LOS is an important factor in the pathogenesis of nontypeable *H. influenzae* infection in patients with chronic bronchitis. Two other constituents of the outer membrane bi-layer are proteins referred

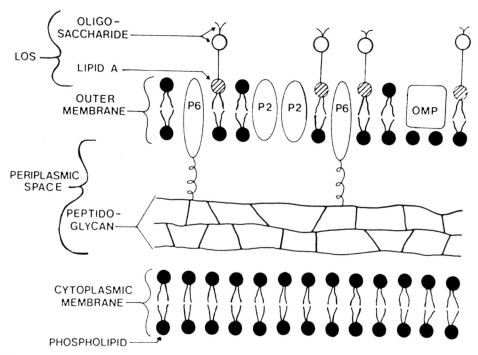

FIG. 9–5. Schematic diagram of the cell envelope of nontypeable *Hemophilus influenzae*. (Reproduced with permission from Murphy and Sethi [272].)

to as P2 and P6. Both of these proteins express epitopes on the bacterial cell surface (153,279). Studies indicate that antibodies to the P6 protein are protective against infection from nontypeable *H. influenzae* (147,271).

Moraxella catarrhalis

A normal inhabitant of the oral pharynx, *M. catarrhalis* was for many years cast as a harmless commensal that contaminated gram stain smears and cultures of sputum. Since 1976, an increasing number of bronchopulmonary infections implicating *M. catarrhalis* as the offending organism have been reported (226,239,240,284,369).

Serologic and bacteriologic evidence has accumulated to indicate that *M. catarrhalis* is a lower respiratory tract pathogen in patients with acute purulent exacerbations of chronic bronchitis (5,100,108,154,239,284,420,421). Transtracheal aspirates have retrieved pure cultures of *M. catarrhalis* in chronic bronchitics with lower respiratory tract infections, and clinical improvement of these patients occurred with antimicrobial agents active against *M. catarrhalis* (5,154,239).

Viral and Mycoplasmal Infection in Acute Exacerbations of Chronic Bronchitis

A number of investigators have examined the role of viruses and mycoplasmal organisms in acute exacerbations of chronic bronchitis (69,76,107,150,210,242, 255,256,357). The reported association of viral respiratory infection with acute exacerbations of chronic bronchitis ranges from 7 to 64% (107,150,210,242,372). Smith and colleagues (357) were able to associate respiratory viruses and *M. pneumoniae* in approximately 20% of acute respiratory illness in patients with chronic bronchitis. This was in contrast to recovery of only 6% of the time of these organisms during clinically stable disease periods. The data were similar to that of Gump et al. (150) who found the incidence of viral infections to be 32% per patient week of exacerbation, but only 0.9% per patient week spent in remission. Buscho et al. (69) found comparable rates of viral or *M. pneumoniae* infection (30%) in 166 acute exacerbations of chronic bronchitis, but, unlike the previous two studies, they found no significant difference in the rates of infection with these organisms between acute illness and remission periods (27.5%). These authors concluded that although viruses and *M. pneumoniae* were a frequent cause of acute respiratory infections in patients with chronic bronchitis, such infectious episodes were not associated with acute worsening of respiratory status.

Data from the above investigations imply that viral and mycoplasmal infections are responsible for up to a third of the acute exacerbations of patients with chronic obstructive pulmonary disease, and that viral infection appears to be more clinically significant than mycoplasmal infection (69,107,242,327). Viruses more commonly isolated or detected serologically include influenza A, parainfluenza virus, coronavirus, rhinovirus, and herpes simplex virus (69,76,150,242,357). Some studies report increased susceptibility to viral infection in smokers and those with COPD, although such increased risk has not been clearly substantiated by others (44,190,255–257,357). However, several reports describe lower respiratory tract sequelae such as pneumococcal and staphylococcal pneumonia following influenza epidemics (120,180,211,357,359). Such outbreaks of bacterial pneumonia are associated with increased morbidity and mortality, particularly in those with COPD and marginal pulmonary function.

Childhood Respiratory Illness and the Pathogenesis of COPD

Lower respiratory tract infections in infancy and childhood have been hypothesized as an etiologic factor for the development of chronic bronchitis and airflow obstruction, independent of smoking history (289,339). An extensive body of epidemiologic data has been collected examining the role of childhood respiratory illness in adult chronic lung disease. Methodologic differences between these studies make comparison of data difficult, and retrospective collection of data through questionnaires tends to introduce bias into the methodology (339). Children hospitalized with bronchiolitis can develop long-term impairment of pulmonary function, and biopsy evidence for epithelial inflammation and damage is found in children with chronic cough following lower respiratory tract infection (151,158,191). In summary, there is some evidence to link childhood illness with the later development of chronic airflow limitation.

CLINICAL FEATURES IN PATIENTS WITH CHRONIC BRONCHITIS

COPD is a heterogeneous syndrome in which clinical features and symptoms overlap to a variable extent in affected individuals. Physicians encounter the "blue bloater" of classic chronic bronchitis, or the "pink puffer" typical of emphysema, although it is also common for chronic bronchitics to have features associated with emphysema. Alternatively, symptoms consistent with asthma can be present, in addition to the chronic productive cough observed in patients with chronic bronchitis; hence the term *asthmatic bronchitis* has been used to characterize patients who display features of both asthma and chronic bronchitis (15,62,303). Not all individuals with chronic bronchitis have associated airflow obstruction (34,301). Those chronic bronchitics without associated airflow limitation usually have better preservation of lung function and a better prognosis than do those individuals who do develop chronic airflow obstruction. In fact, the majority of chronic bronchitics who have progressive airflow limitation also have fixed small airways disease and acinar destruction characteristic of emphysema (252,275,361,364,399).

Chronic cough and sputum production are usually what bring the patient with chronic bronchitis to seek medical attention. Sputum production is often insidious, and usually more prominent in the mornings after awakening, although it can be present throughout the day (360). Sputum can be sufficiently viscous that it is difficult to expectorate, and, in such cases, this further aggravates patients' respiratory symptoms. Hemoptysis can occur, usually as part of a purulent exacerbation. The most common cause attributed to episodes of hemoptysis in the United States is chronic bronchitis (360). Dyspnea with exercise is a common feature of patients with chronic bronchitis, and, in severe cases, dyspnea can be observed at rest.

Physical exam in patients with chronic bronchitis can be unremarkable early in the course of the disease. The presence of rhonchi and wheezes can be heard with auscultation of the chest. A prolonged, forced expiratory time could also be observed with auscultation. In more advanced cases, the "blue bloater" appearance of chronic bronchitics can be observed on physical exam, indicating the presence of chronic hypoxemia with cor pulmonale (64,252). Physical exam findings in such individuals can include jugular venous distention, hepatojugular reflux or a tender liver on abdominal palpation, a right ventricular gallup, and peripheral edema (164).

Pulmonary function abnormalities reveal an obstructive pattern with a decline in FEV_1, and a decrease in the ratio of FEV_1 to forced vital capacity (FVC) (62,66,301). In general, mucus hypersecretion has not been independently correlated with the development of airflow obstruction by pulmonary function testing (24,34,275,366). Reductions in mid-expiratory flow rates are more controversial, although such reduced mid-flow rates are commonly observed in patients with chronic bronchitis and airflow obstruction. Diffusion capacity is normal or only mildly reduced in "pure" chronic bronchitis, but is generally reduced in those with more severe airflow obstruction and emphysema. Radiographic evidence of chronic bronchitis includes thickened bronchial walls or peribronchial cuffing and nonspecific reticulonodular densities on plain film radiography (77,133).

HISTOPATHOLOGIC FEATURES IN CHRONIC BRONCHITIS

Morphologic abnormalities in the airway wall of patients with COPD are observed in the large- and medium-sized airways (bronchitis). They can also be seen in smaller airways of less than 2–3 mm in diameter (bronchiolitis). Table 9-2 summarizes these features. Hypertrophy and hyperplasia of goblet cells and submucosal gland hypertrophy are the correlates of mucus hypersecretion in chronic bronchitis, whereas bronchiolar mucous cell hyperplasia and metaplasia are characteristic of small airways (bronchiolar) findings (89,106,140,182,283).

Alterations in the airway epithelium in chronic bronchitis most likely reflect complex repair response to chronic airway inflammation and injury. There is variable loss of squamous epithelial cells reflecting mucosal damage, with replacement of surface epithelium often displaying features of stratified squamous metaplasia (104,105,182). Damage to cilia and loss of ciliated cells can be variably present in biopsies from those with chronic bronchitis, although no uniform changes of cilia structure or density have been described (130,183).

Mononuclear cells predominate in the mucosa and submucosa of biopsy specimens from chronic bronchitis (106,140,337). Increased mucosal, mural, and glan-

TABLE 9–2. *Histopathologic features of COPD*

Feature	COPD
Areas involved	Large bronchi (chronic bronchitis), small bronchi/bronchioles <2 mm in diameter (bronchiolitis). Alveoli involved.
BAL findings	Increased numbers of macrophages, PMNs.
Biopsy findings mucosa	Variable loss of surface cells, loss of ciliated cells. Stratified squamous cell metaplasia. Hypertrophy and hyperplasia of goblet cells, shift to increased numbers of mucous over serous cells. Bronchiolar goblet cell hyperplasia. Mucosal infiltration of mononuclear cells, PMNs.
Basement membrane	Not consistently thickened (focal, patchy). Thickening of BM.
Submucosa	Mononuclear cells, macrophages (respiratory bronchiolitis), important early lesion. PMNs, lymphocytes, variable edema.
Smooth muscle	Smooth muscle hypertrophy in small bronchi and bronchiolar airways (<2 mm).
Supporting tissue (bronchioles, alveoli)	Degradation of elastin, destruction of supporting elastic tissue and alveolar wall attachments. Peribronchiolar fibrosis.

dular inflammation has been observed in the cartilaginous airways ≥2 mm in diameter from those with chronic bronchitis, in contrast to those with only a history of cigarette smoking (264). Increased numbers of macrophages and both helper (CD4+) and suppressor (CD8+) lymphocytes have been shown in the central airway walls of patients with chronic bronchitis compared to normal volunteers (129,335).

Small airways (<2 mm in diameter) appear to be the site primarily responsible for airflow obstruction and airway resistance in patients with COPD (48,88,89,170,274, 275,283,440). Inflammation of bronchioles consists primarily of pigmented macrophages with occasional lymphocytes and neutrophils. Mural inflammation, bronchiolar smooth muscle hypertrophy, and peribronchiolar fibrosis are thought to be responsible for this small airway airflow obstruction. Mucus is present in both large and small airways, and mucus plugging of bronchioles most likely adds to the airway resistance and limitation to airflow seen in peripheral airways of patients with COPD (388).

The above histopathologic studies support the hypothesis that chronic bronchitis, small airways disease, and limitation to airflow are most likely separate, although interrelated, clinical and pathologic entities (1,48,125,264,301,440).

COMPLICATIONS OF CHRONIC BRONCHITIS

Cor Pulmonale

Progressive airflow obstruction characteristic of individuals with severe COPD causes air trapping, hyperinflation, and focal ventilation/perfusion (V/Q) abnormalities of both low and high V/Q ratios. The end-result of these processes is the insidious onset of hypoxemia and later hypercapnia in patients with severe chronic bronchitis, leading to chronic hypoxic vasoconstriction (124,228,418). Second, those bronchitics with an emphysematous component to their disease will have alveolar/capillary membrane destruction and loss of cross-sectional pulmonary capillary bed area. These two factors appear to be primarily responsible for the pulmonary hypertension seen in severe chronic bronchitis. Other contributory factors could be an increase in pulmonary blood volume and viscosity, increased intrathoracic pressures, and elevated cardiac output (4,430,440). Cor pulmonale can be viewed as right ventricular dysfunction imposed by pulmonary hypertension, and reflects preload, ventricular contractility, and afterload. Right ventricular ejection fraction is inversely correlated with determinants of afterload, those being pulmonary artery pressure and pulmonary vascular resistance (54). Increases in pulmonary vascular resistance, or afterload, would then impose an increased burden on right ventricular function and could have potential consequences as to cardiac output, oxygen delivery, tissue oxygenation, and mixed venous saturation (41,54,121).

Pulmonary hypertension is related to chronic hypoxemia and is supported by studies demonstrating that the degree of pulmonary arterial hypertension is most closely related to awake resting arterial oxygenation. Indeed, deterioration of arterial blood gasses appears to separate those patients with COPD who have stable pulmonary hypertension from those individuals with progressive pulmonary vascular disease (42,427). The pathophysiological consequences of disabling airflow limitation are a decline in arterial oxygen and mixed venous oxygen, with a compensatory polycythemia to increase oxygen capacity (391). Patients with COPD and cor pulmonale typically have normal cardiac outputs until the terminal phase of their disease. However, some individuals with progressive disease may be unable to sufficiently augment their cardiac output to maintain oxygen delivery and adequate mixed venous oxygen saturation. This inability to increase cardiac output still further as a compensatory response to worsening oxygenation has been proposed to adversely affect survival in such individuals (41,391,430).

Even in less extreme cases, patients with COPD and cor pulmonale often demonstrate normal right ventricular systolic performance at rest, but decreased right ventricular ejection fraction in response to exercise (224,259,287). Impaired right ventricular function, then, can contribute to the diminished exercise capacity observed in many patients with chronic bronchitis and airflow limitation (287).

Acute Respiratory Failure in Chronic Bronchitis with Airflow Obstruction

Acute respiratory failure is the most feared complication of COPD. Epidemiologic data suggest that COPD is both one of the most frequent causes of admissions to intensive care units and a major complicating problem which produces significant co-morbidity in many other medical and surgical patients who are critically ill (23,56,94,145,263,344,355,356). The majority of patients with COPD die as a result of the development of respiratory failure or its complications.

In general, the greater severity of baseline, fixed airflow obstruction, the worse the prognosis for those who develop acute respiratory failure. Similar comments can also be made for associated factors of older age, right ventricular dysfunction, elevated carbon dioxide, and malnutrition (92,138). It appears that patients with COPD who develop respiratory failure and require mechanical ventilation rarely die simply because of inability to maintain gas exchange. More often, their mortality is increased because of underlying organ system disease, development of multiorgan failure, sepsis, and complications of critical illness in an intensive care setting (Table 9-3).

Clinical Profile and Pathogenesis of Acute Respiratory Failure in COPD

Current thinking suggests that the typical patient with chronic bronchitis who develops acute respiratory failure will be older, also have emphysema, and demonstrate significant irreversible baseline airflow obstruction (FEV_1 less than 1 liter). Physiologically, then, these individuals operate with very little pulmonary reserve.

TABLE 9–3. *Factors associated with mortality in COPD*

Stable patient	Acute respiratory failure
• Age > 70	• Age > 70
• FEV_1 < 1.0L	• FEV_1 < 1.0L
• RV dysfunction	• RV dysfunction
• Elevated pCO_2	• Elevated pCO_2
• Malnutrition	• Malnutrition
• CXR hyperinflation	• Lifestyle score
• Reduced MVV	• History of CAD or LVD
• Increased HR	• Unknown precipitating event
• Rate FEV_1 decline	• Reduced LOC
• Hypoxemia	• MOF

RV = Residual volume; CXR = Chest x-ray; MVV = Maximal voluntary ventilation; CAD = Coronary artery disease; LVD = Left ventricular dysfunction; LOC = Level of consciousness; MOF = Multiorgan failure.

TABLE 9–4. *Parameters of ventilatory function and metabolic requirements in three groups of patients and as factors involved in the pathogenesis of acute respiratory failure (ARF) in patients with COPD*

	V_E (min)	MVV	V_E/MVV	Respiratory O_2 uptake	% Total VO_2
Normals	7	150	4%	2.5 ml/min	2
Severe COPD	10	35	28%	30 ml/min	15
COPD with ARF	15	35	43%	100 ml/min	40

Baseline airflow obstruction creates hyperinflation, air trapping, and significant V/Q mismatching, which leads to gas exchange abnormalities (hypoxemia and hypercarbia) (43,119,124,228,243,418,428,429). In the majority of cases, the diaphragm is placed at a mechanical disadvantage from inspiratory muscle loading, which predisposes individuals to diaphragmatic dysfunction and increased work of breathing. The stable patient with severe COPD operates with an increased dead space to tidal volume ratio (V_D/V_t) and therefore has a requirement for an increased resting minute ventilation (V_E), which results in increased resting oxygen consumption (VO_2) (Table 9-4). Maximal ventilation (MVV) is markedly reduced in these patients with an increased proportion of V_E to MVV, and which is close to the known limit for the V_E/MVV ratio of 50–60% that typically results in diaphragmatic fatigue and respiratory failure (243,254,330,331). Contrary to past belief, central respiratory drive is probably normal to increased in these individuals (26,98,331).

The precarious balance in the chronic state is dependent upon function of the respiratory muscles and the load applied to them as a result of resistance to airflow and increased airway obstruction. As the primary site of airflow limitation in stable

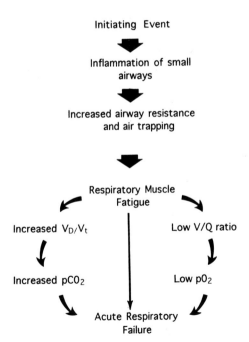

FIG. 9–6. Pathogenesis of acute respiratory failure in COPD.

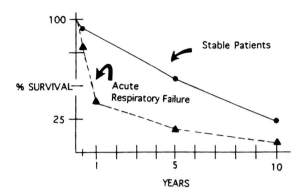

FIG. 9–7. Mortality in moderate to severe COPD.

patients with COPD is the peripheral airways, it follows that this is likely a critical area for acute events that precipitate acute respiratory failure. More often, some initiating event is associated with small airways inflammation, which leads to further air trapping and hyperinflation (Fig. 9-6). Under these circumstances, the required minute ventilation markedly increases and may become almost 50% of MVV, resulting in respiratory muscle fatigue (Table 9-4). V/Q mismatching produces severe hypercarbia and/or hypoxemia, despite an elevated respiratory drive. Patients are usually breathless, tachypneic, and breathe with reduced tidal volumes. They are likely to be anxious and often cyanotic. Paradoxical diaphragmatic movement is also often present, suggestive of diaphragmatic fatigue. Work of breathing may be so high, in fact, that inadequate blood flow to support the respiratory muscles results in lactic acidosis, which often necessitates intubation and mechanical ventilation.

It is likely that events that increase airway inflammation and obstruction (i.e., infection) are the most common precipitants of acute respiratory failure. However, anything that imposes an inordinate load upon the respiratory muscles, depresses respiratory drive, or reduces oxygen delivery to the respiratory muscles might also be expected to cause respiratory failure in these patients.

Survival of patients with moderate to severe COPD who develop acute respiratory failure has improved over the past 30 years (46,138,229). Unfortunately, long-term prognosis after an episode of acute respiratory failure in those with COPD is still quite poor, with prognosis being much worse than in the same group without respiratory failure (95,136,296; Fig. 9-7).

MANAGEMENT OF PATIENTS WITH CHRONIC BRONCHITIS

Smoking Cessation

Table 9-5 lists the various management strategies employed in patients with chronic bronchitis. Smoking cessation is one long-term intervention that has been shown to impact on the natural history of chronic bronchitics with progressive air-flow obstruction. Individuals with COPD who discontinue smoking clearly demonstrate a less rapid decline in FEV_1 than do those who continue smoking (72,126). Even smoking reduction has a positive influence on mitigating respiratory symptoms when compared to failure to modify smoking behavior (320).

TABLE 9–5. *Treatment strategies in stable patients with chronic bronchitis*

Smoking cessation
Oxygen therapy
Bronchodilators
    Anticholinergics
    B_2-agonists
    Theophyllines
Antiinflammatory agents
    Corticosteroids
    Antibiotics
Preventive therapy (immunizations)
Pulmonary rehabilitation/respiratory muscle training
Mechanical ventilation
Mucolytics/antitussives
Anxiolytics

The benefits derived from smoking cessation should compel physicians to initiate a formal cessation program for patients who continue to smoke. Even in individuals with moderate to advanced chronic bronchitis and airflow obstruction, abstinence from smoking results in a less accelerated decline in lung function and an overall attenuation of respiratory symptoms experienced by these individuals (122,125, 126,405). Unfortunately, long-term abstinence from cigarette smoking has had variable success in studies in which therapeutic interventions range from minimal intervention to behavioral programs and nicotine replacement therapy (91,96,333,402). It is beyond the scope of this chapter to discuss in detail the different methods used by physicians and other health professionals to aid patients to stop smoking. Table 9-6 classifies a number of these strategies for smoking cessation. Factors that influence success rates include increasing age, desire to quit, marriage, higher socioeconomic status, and the patient's own perception of how successful they are in stopping smoking (298). Comparison of multiple trials with one-year follow-ups has revealed

TABLE 9–6. *Classification of smoking cessation methods*

Unassisted	Assisted
Quit "cold turkey"	Program/course for a fee
Gradually decreased the number of cigarettes smoked per day	Program/course free
Used low-tar/nicotine cigarettes	Psychiatrist/psychologist counseling
Quit with friends, relatives, or acquaintances	Nicotine gum and counseling
Used special filters or holders	Hypnosis
Used other nonprescription product	Acupuncture
Substituted another tobacco product (snuff, chewing tobacco, pipes, cigars)	Other[a]
Other[a]	

From Fiore, M.C., Novotny, T.E., Pierce, J.P., et al., Methods used to quit smoking in the United States: do cessation programs help? Reproduced with permission from *J.A.M.A.*, 263:20;2760–2765. Copyright 1990, American Medical Association.

[a]Some survey respondents reported methods of cessation other than those listed. These "other" responses were reviewed and, if clearly appropriate, reclassified as one of the listed methods of cessation. No single "other" method was reported by more than 1% of the population.

one-year abstinence rates ranging from 5 to 88%. Two-thirds of these trials achieved at least 33% success rates (342).

Pharmacologic intervention includes nicotine replacement with either nicotine polacrilex chewing gum or nicotine transdermal patches. Nicotine transdermal replacement therapy appears promising compared to placebo groups (96,334,403). Other forms of replacement, including nicotine nasal spray and vapor inhaler, are being investigated. Although nicotine replacement is a valuable adjunct to smoking cessation, the physiological effects of nicotine and symptoms related to its withdrawal are but one component of the complex and interrelated properties that comprise smoking addiction. Social and psychological factors also appear to play a major role in the addictive process to tobacco. Thus, the clinician who simply prescribes nicotine replacement for his or her patients without other interactive measures will most likely not achieve as high a success rate as with more aggressive, combined interventions for smoking cessation (334).

Antibiotics

Antibiotics are widely used to treat acute, purulent exacerbations of chronic bronchitis, but their benefit has been controversial. In addition to antimicrobial therapy for acute respiratory symptoms, antibiotic prophylaxis has in some cases reduced the number of acute exacerbations in those with chronic bronchitis. Reviews by Rodnick and Gude (325), and more recently by Murphy and Sethi (272), have examined prior placebo-controlled prospective studies of antibiotics in acute exacerbations of COPD (16,111,112,281,306). Collectively, these trials suggest equivocal benefit from antibiotic therapy for acute exacerbations; although the most significant benefit derived from antibiotics may be in patients with more severe respiratory symptoms (16,305,306). In a double-blind, placebo-controlled study by Anthonison and co-workers (16), 173 patients with 362 exacerbations of COPD were followed for three and a half years as to the beneficial effect of antibiotic therapy for acute exacerbations. Clinical recovery from symptoms was significantly accelerated (68%) in those individuals who received antibiotics compared to the placebo group (55%). Antibiotic therapy was also associated with significantly less deterioration in clinical symptoms.

Who, then, should be prescribed antibiotics during the course of exacerbations? Advocates recommend that patients with moderate or severe symptoms of cough and sputum production, increased sputum purulence, and dyspnea be given antibiotic therapy in the hope of shortening the duration of symptoms and to lessen the likelihood of acute deterioration in lung function. This may be particularly important for those individuals with severe COPD and limited pulmonary reserve in whom antibiotic treatment of bacterial-induced airway inflammation could prevent further deterioration of lung function and need for hospitalization (16,35,272).

Antibiotics traditionally used are trimethoprim/sulfamethoxazole, ampicillin or amoxicillin, and the tetracyclines. Table 9-7 lists a number of antibiotics reported as efficacious in the treatment of bacterial infections associated with chronic bronchitis. In choosing an antibiotic, consideration should be given whenever possible to determining the least expensive agent with the narrowest spectrum of activity. Use of sputum gram stains and culture during acute exacerbations of chronic bronchitis

TABLE 9–7. *Antibiotics frequently employed in the treatment of acute exacerbations of chronic bronchitis*

Antibiotic	Advantages	Disadvantages
Ampicillin/ amoxicillin	Cost	Majority of *M. catarrhalis*-resistant, some (20–25%) of nontypeable *H. influenzae*-resistant
Amoxicillin/ clavulanate	Extended spectrum including B-lactamase, *Hemophilus, M. catarrhalis*	Cost, GI side effects
Trimethoprim/ sulfamethoxazole	Cost, BID dosing	Some strains of *S. pneumoniae*-resistant
Tetracyclines	Doxycycline, minocycline have convenient dosing, B-lactamase resistance	Gastric and drug side effects
Erythromycin	Cost, activity against *S. pneumoniae, Mycoplasma*	GI side effects, activity against *Hemophilus* and *M. catarrhalis*
Macrolides (clarithromycin, azithromycin)	Extended spectrum, 5-day course (azithromycin)	Cost
Fluoroquinolones	Gram-negative including *P. aeruginosa,* (ciprofloxacin, ofloxacin), B-lactamase resistance	Cost, drug side effects
First-generation cephalosporins	Good streptococcal coverage, *M. catarrhalis*	Some *H. influenzae*-resistant
Cefuroxime axetil	Extended spectrum over first-generation cephalosporins	Cost
Cefactor	Extended spectrum	Cost
Cefixime	Increased gram-negative coverage, B-lactamase-resistant stains of *H. influenzae*	Cost, less effective gram (+) coverage compared to first generation cephalosporins
Cefprozil	Extended spectrum BID dosing	Cost
Loracarbef (carbacephem class)	B-lactamase stains of *H. influenzae* and *M. catarrhalis*	Cost
Cefpodoxime proxetil	Extended spectrum, B-lactamase-resistant *H. influenzae* and *M. catarrhalis*. BID dosing	Diarrhea (dose-related)

is controversial (444). However, when properly performed, gram stain analysis may provide valuable information, narrow the search for likely pathogens, and, in turn, enable appropriate selection of antibiotic therapy. Comparison of sputum samples obtained during an acute exacerbation, as opposed to stable clinical periods, will frequently demonstrate increased numbers of neutrophils and bacteria, findings that are consistent with acute lower respiratory tract infection (249). Recovery of gram-negative coccobacillary rods is consistent with *Hemophilus* species, whereas gram-negative diplococci and gram-positive diplococci imply *Moraxella* and *S. pneumoniae,* respectively. In antibiotic selection, it is important to identify Moraxella-like organisms which frequently are resistant to the penicillins, except for amoxicillin/ clavulanic acid (108,154,249,272). Sputum cultures may be useful when gram stain analysis suggests gram-negative bacilli or staphylococcal-like organisms, or if there is reason to suspect antimicrobial resistance (249). Antibiotic therapy for acute bacterial bronchitis in patients with COPD is associated with a shorter duration of clinical symptoms, prevents further determination of symptoms, and increases the infection-free interval (16,35,189).

Antimicrobial therapy in stable patients with chronic bronchitis and bronchiectasis can also ameliorate markers of chronic airway inflammation, such as decreased sputum ciliotoxicity, decreased neutrophil activation and chemotaxis, and reduced free elastase activity (167,373,375,376). Moreover, several classes of antibiotics possess antiinflammatory as well as antibacterial properties. Erythromycin is capable of suppressing neutrophil chemotaxis and chemiluminescence, and in asthmatics, erythromycin has been reported to reduce bronchial hyperresponsiveness (6,168,253). Aminoglycosides have been shown to protect epithelial cells *in vitro* from myeloperoxidase-dependent cytotoxocity, whereas thioether-containing antibiotics such as ticarcillin and ceftazidime are hypochlorous acid (HOCL) scavengers *in vitro* and protect epithelial cells against oxidant-induced cytotoxicity (75). Such intriguing studies suggest that antiinflammatory effects of various antibiotics play a role in suppressing the chronic airway inflammation implicated in the pathogenesis of disorders such as bronchiectasis and chronic bronchitis.

In most cases, outpatient management with oral antibiotics is indicated, although in severe exacerbations requiring hospitalization initial parental therapy is generally preferred. Duration of oral therapy is usually 10 to 14 days; in some individuals longer courses may be necessary.

Antibiotic Prophylaxis

Patients with more severe chronic bronchitis could experience numerous exacerbations over the course of a year. In some individuals, the frequency of acute symptoms makes it difficult to delineate exacerbations and periods of remission. A number of trials have examined the use of antibiotic prophylaxis in an attempt to reduce the number of exacerbations in such individuals (97,186,245,304,315). The greatest benefit from antibiotic prophylaxis appears to be observed in those individuals who have numerous exacerbations of respiratory symptoms during the course of a year (186,272,304).

Treatment of Influenza and Immunotherapy

Patients with chronic bronchitis who appear to be a high risk for influenza or who have typical symptoms suggestive of acute influenza infection can benefit from amantadine if this medication is started in the first 48 hours of infection. Because chronic bronchitics suffer greater morbidity and potential mortality from acute influenza infection, influenza vaccine is recommended on a yearly basis for patients with chronic bronchitis and other forms of COPD (118,405,444).

The use of bacterial vaccines has, so far, achieved equivocal results in terms of reducing the frequency of bacterial pneumonia in patients with COPD (352,431). Despite the mixed results observed in clinical trials, consensus has emerged for the use of pneumococcal vaccine in patients with COPD. Revaccination should probably occur every 6 years in individuals at risk for severely depressed immune function (79). Molecular determination of the P6 outer membrane protein of *H. influenzae* has caused enthusiasm over the potential development of a vaccine to nontypeable *H. influenzae*. Preliminary results indicate that antibody to the P6 protein protects from *H. influenzae* infection (147,268,271,280).

Bronchodilator Therapy

The management of patients with COPD has traditionally included bronchodilators, even in those individuals who demonstrate with only partially reversible, or so-called fixed airflow obstruction by pulmonary function testing. Bronchodilators include the xanthene derivatives (theophylline), oral and inhaled beta$_2$ (B$_2$) sympathomimetics, and inhaled anticholinergics.

Theophylline appears to have a number of pharmacologic actions, the most important of which could be its effect on calcium influx into muscles or the transfer of calcium from the sarcoplasmic reticulum of muscle cells. The dose effects of theophylline on bronchial smooth muscle relaxation appear to be dose related, the greater effect seen in asthmatics rather than in those with COPD (294,444). However, despite even mild bronchodilatory effects from theophylline, other benefits have been exhibited: improved mucociliary clearance, increased tidal volume and vital capacity, improvement in blood gasses, increased hypoxic respiratory drive, and a decrease in the subjective sense of dyspnea by patients (82,225,266,340). These improvements could be related to increased diaphragmatic blood flow and augmented diaphragmatic contractility. Along these lines, it has been proposed that theophylline mitigates against diaphragmatic fatigue in COPD (25,266). In some studies, but not others, the use of theophylline combined with either a beta-sympathomimetic or anticholinergic drug has been more effective than either agent alone in patients with COPD (227,292).

Theophylline may also have favorable cardiovascular effects in patients with COPD with and without cor pulmonale. Mean pulmonary artery pressure has been shown to decrease with theophylline, and an increase in both right and left ventricular ejection fraction has been demonstrated, independent of significant improvement in arterial oxygen tension or FEV$_1$ (232,233). Thus, even in those patients with chronic bronchitis who exhibit little reversibility in spirometric testing, or theophyllines that attain serum levels in the range of 10–15 µg/ml may well improve respiratory and cardiovascular function (165,444). Furthermore, one should consider the parental administration of theophylline in acute respiratory failure complicating COPD, given this agent's potential beneficial effect on respiratory muscle function. Disadvantages of utilizing theophylline derivatives in patients with congestive heart failure or liver disease are variable drug clearance and potential for toxic accumulation of the medication. Caution should be exercised in such patients, with long-term monitoring of blood levels to reduce the likelihood of deleterious side effects. Another disadvantage of theophylline derivatives is that a number of other factors can affect clearance, including other medications, hypoxia, and fever (444).

Sympathomimetics

Sympathomimetics act by stimulation of beta-2 adrenoceptors on bronchial smooth muscle, with the net effect of muscular relaxation and bronchodilation. Beta-2 agonists can also improve mucociliary clearance (18,285,443). In the management of COPD, beta-sympathomimetics are usually delivered by metered dose inhaler, although oral preparations and nebulized delivery of the drug are also commonly employed. Relief of bronchospasm can be improved with increasing doses of beta$_2$-agonists. In some studies (albuterol), dose-related bronchodilation was accomplished without significant side effects (184,350). However, when only patients with chronic bronchitis were examined, albuterol achieved dose-related increases in FEV$_1$, vital capacity, and peak flow rates, but was associated with a dose-dependent increase in patient symptoms, heart rate, tremor, and a mild decrease in arterial oxygen saturation (410).

Anticholinergics

Increased cholinergic bronchomotor tone is a feature of the large and medium-sized airways of patients with COPD (148,149). This enhanced cholinergic tone has led to the use of anticholinergic bronchodilators in acute exacerbations of COPD (80,148,149,390). In stable chronic bronchitics, the anticholinergic ipratropium bromide has been shown to be a more effective bronchodilator than beta-2 agonists, and an equivalent dose of ipratropium may have a longer duration of effect than beta-2 agonists (148,390).

Ipratropium bromide induces bronchodilation with significantly fewer side effects than beta-sympathomimetics. In therapeutic doses, it does not appear to alter mucous clearance or viscosity, although in one study ipratropium was associated with decreased sputum volume (80,137,234). In the United States, delivery of ipratropium has been confined to metered dose inhalers. Nebulized forms of the medication are available elsewhere in the world and are soon expected to be approved in this country as well.

Antiinflammatory Therapy

Corticosteroids have been included in the management of chronic bronchitis, particularly in patients with acute deterioration of lung function and worsening of respiratory symptoms (110,336). Some have recommended a short-term trial of corticosteroids in chronic bronchitics whose symptoms and spirometry have not been optimally improved despite maximal therapy with bronchodilators in theophylline. Two uncontrolled, retrospective studies have suggested that oral prednisolone in doses greater than 7.5 mg/day may slow the progression of airflow obstruction in patients with COPD (312,314). Beneficial effects associated with oral steroids were not appreciated until after a period of at least 6 months of steroid administration. Although this suggests a potential benefit of long-term steroid therapy, such an approach is also fraught with possible side effects stemming from long-term steroid use. The rationale for the use of either oral or inhaled corticosteroids is to ameliorate airway inflammation present in patients with chronic bronchitis. A short course of oral corticosteroids in chronic bronchitis has shown to attenuate several markers of airway inflammation present in expectorated sputum (59,373,374). Corticosteroids may also facilitate airway adrenergic function (336). In asthmatics, inhaled corticosteroids have clearly been associated with improved symptoms, improved airway function by spirometry, and reduced bronchial hyperresponsiveness. It has been suggested that such improvements are predominantly due to the antiinflammatory effects of corticosteroids (33,52,99).

Recent studies provide intriguing evidence that inhaled steroids are beneficial in patients with chronic bronchitis. A 6-week course of inhaled beclomethasone resulted in improved spirometric values, decreased bronchial cell counts, and decreased markers of inflammation in airway lavage such as albumin, lysozyme, and lactoferrin (395). Other investigators have also reported either a significant improvement in lung function (FEV_1) or a less accelerated decline in FEV_1 with inhaled beclomethasone in patients with COPD (102,195,424,425). Patients who may derive the greatest benefit from inhaled corticosteroids are those with asthmatic bronchitis or those with more accelerated loss of lung function (102,195).

The time course of treatment with corticosteroids in stable patients has not been established. Inhaled corticosteroids can produce improvements in peak flow rates earlier than oral prednisolone, an effect that could last more than 14 days after cessation of steroid therapy (422). In some cases, a beneficial effect with oral steroids is not observed until more than 14 days of treatment has elapsed, suggesting that a trial with corticosteroids be extended beyond this period of time in patients with COPD (426).

Oxygen Therapy

In addition to smoking cessation, oxygen therapy has been shown to significantly affect survival in hypoxic patients with chronic bronchitis (245,286). In addition to improved survival, oxygen therapy has been associated with improved quality of life, improved sleep, and enhanced exercise performance (71,127,142). Oxygen therapy can be delivered by a number of different devices, for which reviews may be found elsewhere (400). Table 9-8 lists conditions for which reimbursement for oxygen therapy has been provided by Medicare.

Nutritional Support

Undernutrition, defined as less than 90% of ideal body weight, has been reported in up to 25% of patients with COPD, and has been shown to adversely affect mortality in this group of patients (434). Malnourished patients with COPD have decreased total body muscle mass, and body weight correlates with respiratory muscle mass. These individuals also demonstrate reduced respiratory muscle strength and

TABLE 9–8. *Medicare criteria for reimbursement of supplemental oxygen therapy*

Meets criteria and is reimbursable
  $PaO_2 \leq 55$ mmHg or $SaO_2 \leq 88\%$ at rest or with low-level exercise.
Meets criteria and is reimbursable with cor pulmonale
  PaO_2 of 56–59 mmHg or SaO_2 of 89% *and* evidence for: congestive heart failure, polycythemia, or "p" pulmonale on ECG.
Does not meet criteria
  $PaO_2 \geq 60$ mmHg or $SaO_2 \geq 90\%$ *unless*: documentation of additional clinical condition, such as nocturnal desaturation from sleep-disordered breathing is provided.
Does not meet criteria
  PaO_2 60 mmHg or $SaO_2 \geq 90\%$ *but* clinically justified: conditions as terminal nonrespiratory illness, angina pectoris, peripheral vascular disease.

endurance, including the diaphragm and expiratory muscles (20–22,219,398). In addition, malnourished patients frequently demonstrate impaired delayed cutaneous hypersensitivity and reduced total lymphocyte counts. Both humoral and T-cell function may be altered in these individuals (103,178). These nutritionally related abnormalities may then be factors in the development of chronic respiratory failure and respiratory infections that afflict those with severe, progressive COPD. Refeeding malnourished patients has been shown to improve the above abnormalities (109,348,433).

Patients with severe COPD can have difficulty with high carbohydrate loads secondary to the increased CO_2 production that results from carbohydrate metabolism. Significantly elevated CO_2 production necessitates an increased minute ventilation which, in turn, may increase work of breathing and make COPD patients prone to respiratory muscle fatigue (13,206). Diets or supplemental feedings with lower carbohydrate and higher fat percentages could be more suitable in these at-risk individuals.

Management of Acute Respiratory Failure

Management strategies in ARF should include clinical consideration and search for possible precipitating factors. These factors could be oversedation, infection, inhalation of noxious agents, pulmonary emboli, pneumothorax, or dehydration with excessive drying of airway secretions (47,98,173; Fig. 9-8). Supplemental oxygen is of paramount importance in the hypoxemic patient to improve oxygen delivery to tissues, including respiratory muscles. Oxygen should be carefully titrated to achieve

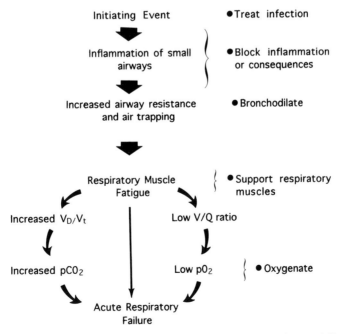

FIG. 9–8. Treatment strategies for COPD with acute respiratory failure.

minimum arterial oxygen saturations of 88–90% or a PO_2 of 58–60, with careful observation for development of worsening hypercapnia and respiratory acidosis following initiation of supplemental oxygen (27,29,378). Failure to adequately oxygenate the patient in ARF without the worsening of respiratory acidosis is an indication for either noninvasive or invasive (endotracheal intubation) means of mechanical ventilation (45,173).

Management of ARF and chronic bronchitis also encompasses treatment of airway inflammation which may be the cause of increased airway resistance and work of breathing. Frequently, this involves the parental administration of corticosteroids. In one randomized trial of ARF in chronic bronchitis, the use of corticosteroids was associated with improved pulmonary function within 12 hours of their initiation, although these results have not been substantiated elsewhere (7,113). Data on the efficacy of corticosteroids in this setting is limited, although it has been recommended that a short course of corticosteroids be administered in acute respiratory failure complicating chronic bronchitis (174). The definitive role of antibiotics in ARF is unclear as in patients with stable COPD, except where there is a known source of infection, such as pneumonia. However, many clinicians traditionally choose to administer intravenous antibiotics in cases where infection is uncertain. Proving that an infection exists is sometimes not possible, and bacterial infection is a known cause of acute respiratory failure (16,98,386).

Other management strategies include removal of offending noxious stimuli, regular use of inhaled bronchodilators, parental theophylline for improved diaphragmatic contractility, nutritional support, and, if needed, support of the respiratory muscles by noninvasive or invasive means of mechanical ventilation (25,173,265,307,432,433).

Assisted Ventilation

Several methods employing invasive and noninvasive methods for assisted ventilation have been used to rest respiratory muscles and improve gas exchange in patients with hypercapnic respiratory failure (53). Alternatives to tracheostomy and positive pressure ventilation have included negative pressure devices such as the body Cuirass ventilator and positive pressure ventilation via nasal masks (40,166,194,246,300,341). The use of positive airway pressure with assisted mechanical support (PEEP), or without mechanical support (CPAP), have both been examined in COPD patients suffering from acute hypercapnic respiratory failure. These studies have shown that both CPAP and PEEP may reduce the work of breathing in patients with severe airflow limitation. Proposed mechanisms for accomplishing this are pneumatically splinting the airway to prevent dynamic collapse during exhalation, recruiting expiratory muscles to affect end-expiratory lung volume, and increasing transpulmonary pressures and lung inflation to overcome the inspiratory threshold imposed by auto PEEP (251,302).

PROGNOSIS

Work by a number of investigators has identified risk factors that adversely affect prognosis in patients with chronic bronchitis and airflow obstruction. Although a greater number of individuals will develop chronic bronchitis, only about 15% of smokers will develop disabling airflow obstruction (361,406). It is clear that uncor-

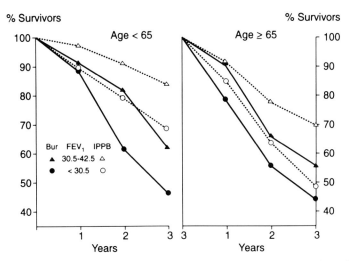

FIG. 9–9. Comparison of survival in the IPPB trial (*open symbols*) with that of patients reported by the Burrows Group (*closed symbols*). Data for patients are segregated by age and FEV₁. (Reproduced with permission from Anthonisen [15].)

rected hypoxemia portends a grave prognosis in patients with chronic bronchitis and severe airflow obstruction (244,287). The classic studies by Fletcher and colleagues (65,125) demonstrated that the initial "level" of FEV_1 was predictive of subsequent decline in FEV_1 over time (i.e., slope of FEV_1), the so-called horse-racing effect. Clearly, baseline FEV_1 and patient age are the two best predictors of mortality in patients with COPD (15; Figs. 9-9, and 9-10). Other variables have been examined, including a reduced diffusion capacity, an increased total lung capacity, and resting

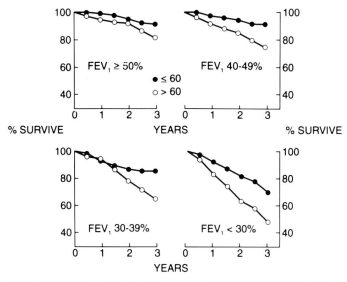

FIG. 9–10. Survival among patients in the IPPB trial, segregated according to baseline FEV_1 and the median age of 60 years. (Reproduced with permission from Anthonisen [15].)

heart rate (17,51,63). A history of respiratory trouble before the age of 16 appears to correlate with adverse effects of cigarette smoking. Patients with asthmatic features to their disease did better over time than those with fixed airflow obstruction (62,67).

SUMMARY

Chronic bronchitis is an important cause of morbidity and mortality in the United States and worldwide. It is a clinical diagnosis characterized by mucus hypersecretion, although patients can have features in common with asthma and emphysema, including morphologic abnormalities of peripheral airways and increases in small airway resistance. Cigarette smoking is the most important etiologic factor in the pathogenesis of chronic bronchitis. A number of other conditions and factors have also been implicated in the development of this disorder, including immunologic factors, occupational exposure, air pollution, and childhood respiratory illnesses. Viral infections and bacterial colonization can also influence natural history and clinical course of patients with chronic bronchitis. At present, the only two interventions that have clearly been shown to affect the natural history and survival of patients with chronic bronchitis and other forms of COPD are smoking cessation and appropriate oxygen therapy. However, other management strategies can be viewed as preventive, such as influenza vaccine and, in some cases, antibiotic therapy. Antibiotic therapy has been controversial, although it appears appropriate in moderate to severe acute exacerbations of chronic bronchitis and, for some, as prophylactic therapy. Bronchodilators are effective in the symptomatic therapy of those who have airflow obstruction, and there is promising evidence for the use of corticosteroids in curbing airway inflammation of chronic bronchitis. Further research is needed on the role of infection and airway injury, the airway repair process following injury, and the bronchiolitis that, in smokers, appears to be the crucial early lesion for the development of fixed airflow obstruction in those with chronic bronchitis.

REFERENCES

1. Adesina, A.M., Vallyathan, V., McQuillen, E.N., Weaver, S.O., and Craighead, J.E. (1991): Bronchiolar inflammation and fibrosis assoicated with smoking. *Am. Rev. Respir. Dis.*, 143:144–149.
2. Afford, S.C., Burnett, D., Campbell, E.J., Cury, D., and Stockley, R.A. (1988): The assessment of α_1-proteinase inhibitor form and function in lung fluid from healthy subjects. *Biol. Chem. Hoppe Seyler*, 369:1065–1074.
3. Afzelius, B.A. (1976): A human syndrome caused by immotile cilia. *Science*, 19:317–319.
4. Agarwal, J.B., Paltoo, R., and Palmer, W.H. (1970): Relative viscosity of blood at varying hematocrits in pulmonary circulation. *J. Appl. Physiol.*, 29:866–871.
5. Aitken, J.M., and Thornby, P.E., (1983): Isolation of *Branhamella catarrhalis* from sputum and tracheal aspirate. *J. Clin. Microbiol.*, 18:1262–1263.
6. Akamatsu, H., Kurokawa, I., Nishijima, S., and Asada, Y. (1992): Inhibition of neutrophil chemotactic factor production in comedonal bacteria by subminimal inhibitory concentrations of erythromycin. *Dermatology*, 185:41–43.
7. Albert, R.K., Martin, T.R., and Lewis, S.W. (1980): Controlled clinical trial of methylprednisolone in patients with chronic bronchitis and acute respiratory insufficiency. *Ann. Int. Med.*, 92:753–758.
8. American Thoracic Society (1990): Clinical role of bronchoalveolar lavage in adults with pulmonary disease. *Am. Rev. Respir. Dis.*, 142:481–486.
9. Amoux, B., Duval, D., and Benveniste, J. (1980): Release of platelet-activating factor (PAF-acether) from alveolar macrophages by the calcium inophore A23187 and phagocytosis. *Eur. J. Clin. Invest.*, 10:437–441.

10. Anderson, B., Beachey, E.H., Tomasz, A., Tuomanen, E., and Svanborg-Eden, C. (1988): A sandwich adhesin on *Streptococcus pneumoniae* attaching to human oropharyngeal epithelial cells *in vitro. Microbial. Pathogen.*, 4:267–278.

11. Anderson, B., and Svanborg-Eden, C. (1989): Attachment of *Streptococcus pneumoniae* to human pharyngeal epithelial cells. *Respiration*, 55(Suppl. 1):49–52.

12. Ando, M., Sugimoto, M., Nishi, R., et al. (1984): Surface morphology and function of human pulmonary alveolar macrophages from smokers and nonsmokers. *Thorax*, 39:850–856.

13. Angelillo, V.A., Bedi, S., Durfee, D., Dahl, J., Patterson, A.J., and O'Donohue, W.J. (1985): Effects of low and high carbohydrate feedings in ambulatory patients with chronic obstructive pulmonary disease and chronic hypercapnia. *Ann. Intern. Med.*, 103:883–885.

14. Annesi, I., and Kauffmann, F. (1986): Is respiratory mucus hypersecretion really an innocent disorder? *Am. Rev. Respir. Dis.*, 134:688–693.

15. Anthonisen, N.R., (1989): Prognosis in chronic obstructive pulmonary disease: results from multicenter clinical trials. *Am. Rev. Respir. Dis.*, 140:S95–S99.

16. Anthonisen, N.R., Manfreda, J., Warren, C.P.W., Hershfield, E.S., Harding, G.K.M., and Nelson, N.A. (1987): Antibiotic therapy in exacerbations of chronic obstructive pulmonary disease. *Ann. Int. Med.*, 106:196–204.

17. Anthonisen, N.R., Wright, E.C., and Hodgkin, J.E. (1986): IPPB Trial Group. Prognosis in chronic obstructive pulmonary disease. *Am. Rev. Respir. Dis.*, 133:14–20.

18. Anthonisen, N.R., Wright, E.C., and the IPPB trial group. (1986): Bronchodilator response in chronic obstructive pulmonary disease. *Am. Rev. Respir. Dis.*, 133:814–819.

19. Apicella, M.A., Dudas, K.C., Campagnari, A., Rice, P., Mylotte, J.M., and Murphy, T.F. (1985): Antigenic heterogeneity of lipid A of *Hemophilus influenzae. Infect. Immun.*, 50:9–14.

20. Arora, N.S., and Rochester, D.F. (1982): Effect of body weight and muscularity on human diaphragm muscle mass, thickness and area. *J. Appl. Physiol.*, 52(1):64–70.

21. Arora, N.S., and Rochester, D.F. (1982): Respiratory muscle strength and maximal voluntary ventilation in undernourished patients. *Am. Rev. Respir. Dis.*, 126:5–8.

22. Arora, N.S., and Rochester, D.F. (1987): COPD and human diaphragm dimensions. *Chest*, 91:719–724.

23. Asmundsson, T., and Kilburn, K.H. (1969): Survival of acute respiratory failure: a study of 239 episodes. *Ann. Intern. Med.*, 70:471–485.

24. ATS Scientific Assembly on Clinical Problems Take Group (1987): Standards for the diagnosis and care of patients with chronic obstructive pulmonary disease (COPD) and asthma. *Am. Rev. Respir. Dis.*, 136:225–244.

25. Aubier, M., De Troyer, A., Sampson, M., Macklem, P.T., and Roussos, C. (1981): Aminophylline improves diaphragmatic contractility. *N. Engl. J. Med.*, 305:249–252.

26. Aubier, M., Murciano, D., Mal, H., and Pariente, R. (1987): Role de la fatigue des muscles respiratoires dans le sevrage de la ventilation artificielle. In: *Ventilation Artificielle Conventionnelle et Ventilation a Haute Frequence*, edited by F. Clerque and J.J. Rouby, pp. 153–164. Arnette, Paris.

27. Aubier, M., Murciano, D., Milic-Emili, J., et al. (1987): Effects of the administration of O_2 on ventilation and blood gases in patients with chronic obstructive disease during acute respiratory failure. (correspondence) *Am. Rev. Respir. Dis.*, 135:274.

28. Auerbach, O., Hammond, E.C., Kirman, D., Garfinkel, L., and Stout, A.P. (1967): Histologic changes in bronchial tubes of cigarette-smoking dogs. *Cancer*, 20:2055–2066.

29. Austin, T. (1970): The relationship between arterial blood saturation, carbon dioxide tension, and pH and airway resistance during 30% oxygen breathing in chronic bronchitis with airways obstructions. *Am. Rev. Respir. Dis.*, 102:382–387.

30. Bakalitz, L.O., Tallon, B.M., Hoepf, T., DeMaria, T.F., Birck, H.G., and Lim, D.J. (1988): Frequency of fimbriation of nontypable *Hemophilus influenzae* and its ability to adhere to chinchilla and human respiratory epithelium. *Infect. Immun.*, 56:331–335.

31. Barbers, R.G., Gong, H., Jr., Tashkin, D.P., Oishi, J., and Wallace, J.M. (1987): Differential examination of bronchoalveolar lavage cells in tobacco cigarette and marijuana smokers. *Am. Rev. Respir. Dis.*, 135:1271–1275.

32. Barenkamp, S.J., Munson, R.S., Jr., and Granoff, D.M. (1982): Outer membrane protein and biotype analysis of pathogenic nontypable *Haemophilus Influenzae. Infect. Immun.*, 36:535–540.

33. Barnes, P.J. (1989): A new approach to the treatment of asthma. *N. Engl. J. Med.*, 321:1517–1527.

34. Bates, D.V. (1973): The fate of the chronic bronchitic: a report of the ten-year follow-up in the Canadian Department of Veteran's Affairs coordinated study of chronic bronchitis. *Am. Rev. Respir. Dis.*, 108:1043–1065.

35. Bates, J.H. (1982): The role of infection during exacerbations of chronic bronchitis. *Ann. Int. Med.*, 97:130–131.

36. Beachey, E.H. (1981): Bacterial adherence: adhesin-receptor interactions mediating the attachment of bacteria to mucosal surfaces. *J. Infect. Dis.*, 143:325–345.

37. Beachey, E.H., and Courtney, H.S. (1989): Bacterial adherence of group A streptococci to mucosal surfaces. *Respiration, 55*(Suppl. 1):33–40.
38. Beaty, T.H., Menkes, H.A., Cohen, B.H., et al. (1984): Risk factors associated with longitudinal change in pulmonary function. *Am. Rev. Respir. Dis., 129*:660.
39. Becklake, M.R. (1989): Occupational exposures: evidence for a causal association with chronic obstructive pulmonary disease. *Am. Rev. Respir. Dis., 140*:S85–S91.
40. Benhamou, D., Girault, C., Faure, C., Portier, F., and Muir, J.-F. (1992): Nasal mask ventilation in acute respiratory failure. *Chest, 102*:912–917.
41. Bergofsky, E.H. (1983): Tissue oxygen delivery and cor pulmonale in chronic obstructive pulmonary disease. *N. Engl. J. Med., 308*:1092–1094.
42. Bishop, J.M., and Cross, K.W. (1984): Physiological variables and mortality in patients with various categories of chronic respiratory disease: WHO multicenter study. *Bull. Eur. Physiopathol. Respir., 20*:495–500.
43. Bishop, J.M., and Cross, K.W. (1984): Physiological variables and mortality in patients with various categories of chronic respiratory disease: WHO multicenter study. *Bull. Eur. Physiopathol. Respir., 20*:495–500.
44. Blake, G.H., Abell, T.D., and Stanley, W.G. (1988): Cigarette smoking and upper respiratory infection among recruits in basic combat training. *Ann. Intern. Med., 109*:198–202.
45. Bone, R.C. (1980): Treatment of respiratory failure due to advanced chronic obstructive lung disease. *Arch. Intern. Med., 140*:1018–1021.
46. Bone, R.C. (1981): Acute respiratory failure and chronic obstructive lung disease: recent advances. *Med. Clin. No. Amer., 65*:563–578.
47. Bone, R.C. (1993): Acute respiratory failure: definition and overview. In: *Diagnostic Procedures: Pulmonary and Critical Care Medicine*, Vol. 1, edited by R.C. Bone, D.R. Dantzker, R.B. George, R.A. Mathay, and H.Y. Reynolds, pp. 1–7. Mosby Year Book, St. Louis, Mo.
48. Bosken, C.H., Hards, J., Gatter, K., and Hogg, J.C. (1992): Characterization of the inflammatory reaction in the peripheral airways of cigarette smokers using immunocytochemistry. *Am. Rev. Respir. Dis., 145*:911–917.
49. Boucher, R.G., Stutts, M.J., and Gatzky, J.T. (1981): Regional differences in bioelectric properties and ion flow on excised canine airways. *J. Appl. Physiol., 51*:706–714.
50. Boudier, C., Pelletier, A., Gast, A., Tournier, J.M., Pauli, G., and Bieth, J.G. (1987): The elastase inhibitory capacity and the α_1-proteinase inhibitor and bronchial inhibitor content of bronchoalveolar lavage fluids from healthy subjects. *Biol. Chem. Hoppe Seyler, 369*:981–990.
51. Boushey, S.F., Thompson, H.K., North, L.B., Beale, A.R., and Snow, T.R. (1973): Prognosis in COPD. *Am. Rev. Respir. Dis., 108*:1373–1382.
52. Bradley, B.L., Azzawi, M., Jacobson, M., et al. (1991): Eosinophils, T-lymphocytes, mast cells, neutrophils, and macrophages in bronchial biopsy specimens from atopic subjects with asthma: comparison with biopsy specimens from atopic subjects without asthma and normal control subjects and relationship to bronchial hyperresponsiveness. *J. Allergy Clin. Immunol., 88*:661–674.
53. Braun, N.M.T., and Marino, N. (1984): Effect of daily intermittent rest of respiratory muscles in patients with chronic airflow limitation. *Chest, 85*:595.
54. Brent, B.N., Berger, H.J., Matthay, R.A., Mahler, D., Pytlik, L., and Zaret, B.L. (1982): Physiologic correlates of right ventricular ejection fraction in chronic obstructive pulmonary disease: a combined radionuclide and hemodynamic study. *Am. J. Cardiol., 50*:255–262.
55. Brumfitt, W., Willoughby, M.L.N., and Bromley, L.L. (1957): An evaluation of sputum examination in chronic bronchitis. *Lancet, 2*:1306–1309.
56. Burk, R.H., and George, R.B. (1973): Acute respiratory failure in chronic obstructive pulmonary disease in immediate and long-term prognosis. *Arch. Intern. Med., 132*:865–868.
57. Burnett, D., Crocker, J., and Stockley, R.A. (1983): Cathepsin B-like cysteine proteinase activity in sputum and immunohistologic identification of cathepsin B in alveolar macrophages. *Am. Rev. Respir. Dis., 128*:915–919.
58. Burnett, D., and Stockley, R.A. (1980): The electrophoretic mobility of α_1-antitrypsin in sputum and its relationship to protease inhibitory capacity, leucocyte elastase concentrations and acute respiratory infection. *Physiol. Chem. Hoppe Seyler, 361*:781–789.
59. Burnett, D., and Stockley, R.A. (1985): Cathepsin B-like cysteine proteinase activity in sputum and bronchoalveolar lavage samples: relationship to inflammatory cells and effects of corticosteroids on antibiotic treatment. *Clin. Sci., 68*:469–474.
60. Burnett, D., and Stockley, R.A. (1993): Low molecular weight elastase inhibitors in cells and tissues of alveolar regions: seek and ye shall find. *Am. J. Respir. Cell. Mol. Biol., 8*:119–120.
61. Burrows, B. (1984): Possible pathogenetic mechanisms in chronic airflow obstruction. *Chest, 85*(Suppl.):13–15.
62. Burrows, B., Bloom, J.W., Traver, G.A., and Cline, M.G. (1987): The course and prognosis of different forms of chronic airways obstruction in a sample from the general population. *N. Engl. J. Med., 317*:1309–1314.

63. Burrows, F., and Earle, R.H. (1969): Course and prognosis of chronic obstructive lung disease. *N. Engl. J. Med.*, 280:397–404.
64. Burrows, B., Fletcher, C.M., Heard, B.E., et al. (1966): The emphysematous and bronchial types of chronic airways obstruction: a clinicopathological study of patients in London and Chicago. *Lancet*, i:830–835.
65. Burrows, B., Knudson, R.J., Camilli, A.E., Lyle, S.K., and Lebowitz, M.D. (1987): The "horse-racing effect" and predicting decline in forced expiratory volume in one second from screening spirometry. *Am. Rev. Respir. Dis.*, 135:788–793.
66. Burrows, B., Knudson, R.J., Cline, M.G., and Lebowitz, M.D. (1977): Quantitative relationships between cigarette smoking and ventilatory function. *Am. Rev. Respir. Dis.*, 115:195–205.
67. Burrows, B., Knudson, R.J., Cline, M.G., and Lebowitz, M.D. (1988): A reexamination of risk factors for ventilatory impairment. *Am. Rev. Respir. Dis.*, 138:829–836.
68. Burrows, B., Lebowitz, M.D., Barbee, R.A., Knudson, R.J., and Halonen, M. (1983): Interactions of smoking and immunologic factors in relation to airways obstruction. *Chest*, 84:657–661.
69. Buscho, R.O., Saxtan, D., Shultz, P.S., Finch, E., and Mufson, M.A. (1978): Infections with viruses and *Mycoplasma pneumoniae* during exacerbations of chronic bronchitis. *J. Infect. Dis.*, 137:377–383.
70. Buttle, D.J., Burnett, D., and Abrahamson, M. (1990): Levels of neutrophil elastase and cathepsin B activities, and cystatins human sputum: relationship to inflammation. *Scand. J. Clin. Lab. Invest.*, 50:509–516.
71. Calverley, P.M.A., Brezinova, V., Douglas, N.J., et al. (1982): The effect of oxygenation on sleep quality in chronic bronchitis and emphysema. *Am. Rev. Respir. Dis.*, 126:206–210.
72. Camilli, E.A., Burrows, B., Knudson, R.J., Lyle, S.K., and Lebowitz, M.D. (1987): Longitudinal changes in forced expiratory volume in one second in adults. *Am. Rev. Respir. Dis.*, 135:794–799.
73. Camner, P., Philipson, K., and Arvidsson, T. (1973): Withdrawal of cigarette smoking: a study on tracheobronchial clearance. *Arch. Environ. Health*, 26:90–92.
74. Campagnari, A.A., Gupta, M.R., Dudas, K.C., Murphy, T.F., and Apicella, M.A. (1987): Antigenic diversity of lipooligosaccharides of nontypable *Haemophilus influenzae*. *Infect. Immun.*, 55:882–887.
75. Cantin, A., and Woods, D.E. (1993): Protection by antibiotics against myeloperoxidase-dependent cytotoxicity to lung epithelial cells *in vitro*. *J. Clin. Invest.*, 91:38–45.
76. Carilli, A.D., Gohd, R.S., and Gordon, W. (1964): A virologic study of chronic bronchitis. *N. Engl. J. Med.*, 270:123–127.
77. Carilli, A.D., Kotzen, L.M., and Fischer, M.J. (1973): The chest roentgenogram in smoking females. *Am. Rev. Respir. Dis.*, 107:133–136.
78. Carp, H., Miller, F., Hoidal, J.R., and Janoff, A. (1982): Potential mechanism of emphysema: alpha-1-proteinase inhibitor recovered from lungs of cigarette smokers contains oxidized methionine and has decreased elastase inhibitory capacity. *Proc. Natl. Acad. Sci. USA*, 79:2041–2045.
79. Centers for Disease Control (1989): Pneumococcal polysaccharide vaccine. *MMWR*, 38:64–76.
80. Chervinsky, P. (1977): Double-blind study of ipratropium bromide, a new anticholinergic bronchodilator. *J. Allergy Clin. Immunol.*, 59:22–30.
81. Chodosh, S. (1991): Treatment of acute exacerbations of chronic bronchitis: state of the art. *Am. J. Med.*, 91(Suppl. 6A):87S–92S.
82. Chrystyn, H., Mulley, B.A., and Peake, M.D. (1988): Dose response relation to oral theophylline in severe chronic obstructive airways disease. *Br. Med. J.*, 297:1506–1510.
83. Ciba Guest Symposium Report (1959): Terminology, definitions and classification of chronic pulmonary emphysema and related conditions. *Thorax*, 14:286–299.
84. Cohen, A.B., and James, H.L. (1982): Reduction of the elastase in inhibitory capacity of alpha-1-antitrypsin by peroxides in cigarette smoke: an analysis of the brands and the filters. *Am. Rev. Respir. Dis.*, 126:25–30.
85. Cole, P. (1989): Host-microbe relationships in chronic respiratory infection. *Respiration*, 55(Suppl. 1):5–8.
86. Cole, P.J. (1985): Investigation of disordered respiratory defenses. *Clin. Immunol. Allergy*, 5:549–568.
87. Cole, P.J., Roberts, D.E., Higgs, E., and Prior, C. (1985): "Colonising microbial load": a cardinal concept in the pathogenesis and treatment of progressive bronchiectasis due to "vicious circle" host mediated damage [abstract]. *Thorax*, 40:227.
88. Cosio, M., Ghezzo, M.S.C., Hogg, J.C., Corbin, R., Loveland, M., Dosman, J., and Macklem, P.T. (1977): The relations between structural changes in small airways and pulmonary function tests. *N. Engl. J. Med.*, 298:1277–1281.
89. Cosio, M.G., Hale, K.A., and Niewoehner, D.E. (1980): Morphologic and morphometric effects of prolonged cigarette smoking on the small airways. *Am. Rev. Respir. Dis.*, 122:265–271.

90. Costabel, U., and Guzman, J. (1992): Effect of smoking on bronchoalveolar lavage constituents. *Eur. Respir. J.*, 5:776–779.

91. Coultas, D.B. (1991): The physician's role in smoking cessation. *Clin. Chest Med.*, 12:755–768.

92. Craven, D.E., Kunches, L.M., Kilinsky, V., Lichteberg, D.A., Make, B.J., and McCabe, W.R. (1986): Risk factors for pneumonia and fatality in patients receiving continuous mechanical ventilation. *Am. Rev. Respir. Dis.*, 133:792–796.

93. Creeth, J.M., Bhaskar, K.R., Horton, J.R., Das, I., Lopez-Vidriero, M.T., and Reid, L. (1977): The separation and characterization of bronchial glycoproteins by density-gradient methods. *Biochem. J.*, 167:557–569.

94. Cullen, J.H., and Kaemmerlen, J.T. (1968): Acute ventilatory failure in chronic obstructive lung disease. *Am. Rev. Respir. Dis.*, 98:998–1001.

95. Dardes, N., Campo, S., Chiappini, M.G., Re, M.A., Ciccairello, P., and Vulterini, S. (1986): Prognosis of COPD patients after an episode of acute respiratory failure. *Eur. J. Respir. Dis.*, 69(Suppl. 146):377–381.

96. Daughton, D.M., Heatley, S.A., Prendergast, J.J., et al. (1991): Effect of transdermal nicotine delivery as an adjunct to low-intervention smoking cessation therapy. *Arch. Intern. Med.*, 151:749–752.

97. Davis, A.L., Brabow, E.J., Kaminski, T., et al. (1965): Bacterial infection and some effects of chemoprophylaxis in chronic pulmonary emphysema. II. Chemoprophylaxis with daily chloramphenicol. *Am. Rev. Respir. Dis.*, 92:900–913.

98. Derenne, J.-P., Fleury, B., and Pariente, R. (1988): Acute respiratory failure of chronic obstructive pulmonary disease. *Am. Rev. Respir. Dis.*, 138:1006–1323.

99. Djukanovic, R., Roche, W.R., Wilson, J.W., et al. (1990): Mucosal inflammation in asthma. *Am. Rev. Respir. Dis.*, 142:434–457.

100. Doern, G.V., Miller, M.J., and Winn, R.E. (1981): *Branhamella (Neisseria) catarrhalis* systemic disease in humans. *Arch. Intern. Med.*, 141:1690–1692.

101. Dolan, M.C. (1985): Carbon monoxide poisoning. *Can. Med. Assoc. J.*, 133:392–397.

102. Dompeling, E., van Schayck, C.P., van Grunsven, P.M., et al. (1993): Slowing the deterioration of asthma and chronic obstructive pulmonary disease observed during bronchodilator therapy by adding inhaled corticosteroids. *Ann. Int. Med.*, 118:770–778.

103. Driver, A.G., McAlevy, M.T., and Smith, J.L. (1982): Nutritional assessment of patients with chronic obstructive pulmonary disease and acute respiratory failure. *Chest*, 82:568–571.

104. Dunnill, M.S. (1960): The pathology of asthma, with special reference to changes in the bronchial mucosa. *J. Clin. Pathol.*, 13:27.

105. Dunnill, M.S. (1987): Chronic bronchitis. In: *Chronic Bronchitis, Asthma*, 2nd Edition, pp. 41–59. Churchill Livingstone, Edinburgh, Scotland.

106. Dunnill, M.S., Massarella, G.R., and Anderson, J.A. (1969): A comparison of the quantitative anatomy of the bronchi in normal subjects, in status asthmaticus, in chronic bronchitis, and in emphysema. *Thorax*, 24:176–179.

107. Eadie, M.B., Stott, E.J., and Grist, N.R. (1966): Virological studies in chronic bronchitis. *Br. Med. J.*, 2:671.

108. Edson, R.S. (1986): A newly recognized lower-respiratory pathogen. *Diagnosis*, (Nov):53–55.

109. Efthimiou, J., Fleming, J., Gomes, C., and Spiro, S.G. (1988): The effect of supplementary oral nutrition in poorly nourished patients with chronic obstructive pulmonary disease. *Am. Rev. Respir. Dis.*, 137:1075–1082.

110. Eliasson, O., Hoffman, J., Trueb, D., Frederick, D., and McCormick, J.R. (1986): Corticosteroids in COPD: a clinical trial and reassessment of the literature. *Chest*, 89:484–490.

111. Elmes, P.C., Fletcher, C.M., and Dutton, A.A.C. (1957): Prophylactic use of oxytetracycline for exacerbations of chronic bronchitis. *Br. Med. J.*, 2:1272–1275.

112. Elmes, P.C., King, T.K.C., Langlands, J.H.M., Mackay, J.A., Wallace, W.F.M., Wade, O.L., and Wilson, T.S. (1965): Value of ampicillin in the hospital treatment of exacerbations of chronic bronchitis. *Brit. Med. J.*, 2:904–908.

113. Emerman, C.L., Connors, A.F., Lukens, T.W., May, M.E., and Effron, D. (1989): A randomized controlled trial of methylprednisolone in the emergency treatment of acute exacerbations of COPD. *Chest*, 95:563–567.

114. Ericksson, S. (1964): Pulmonary emphysema and alpha-1-antitrypsin deficiency. *Acta Med. Scand.*, 175:197–205.

115. Fahy, J.V., Schuster, A., Ueki, I., Boushey, H.A., and Nadel, J.A. (1992): Mucus hypersecretion in bronchiectasis. *Am. Rev. Respir. Dis.*, 146:1430–1433.

116. Feldhoff, P.A., Bhavanandan, V.P., and Davidson, E.A. (1979): Purification, properties and analysis of human asthmatic bronchial mucin. *Biochemistry*, 18:2430–2436.

117. Fels, A.O.S., and Cohn, Z.A. (1986): The alveolar macrophage. American Physiological Society, 353–369.

118. Ferguson, G.T., and Cherniack, R.M. (1993): Management of chronic obstructive pulmonary disease. *N. Engl. J. Med.*, 328:1017–1022.

119. Filley, G.F., Beckwitt, H.J., Reeves, J.T., and Mitchell, R.S. (1968): Chronic obstructive bronchopulmonary disease: oxygen transport in two clinical types. *Am. J. Med.*, 44:26–38.
120. Finckh, E.S., and Bader, L. (1974): Pulmonary damage from Hong Kong influenza. *Aust. N.Z., J. Med.*, 4:16–22.
121. Finlay, M., Middleton, H.C., Peake, M.D., et al. (1983): Cardiac output, pulmonary hypertension, hypoxaemia and survival in patients with chronic obstructive airways disease. *Eur. J. Respir. Dis.*, 64:252–263.
122. Fiore, M.C., Baker, L.J., and Deeren, S.M. (1993): Cigarette smoking: the leading preventable cause of pulmonary diseases. In: *Diagnostic Procedures: Pulmonary and Critical Care Medicine*, Vol. 1. edited by, Bone, R.C., Dantzker, D.R., George, R.B., Mathay, R.A., and Reynolds, H.Y., pp. 1–19. Mosby Year Book, St. Louis, Mo.
123. Fisher, G.L., McNeill, K.L., Finch, G.L., Wilson, F.D., and Golde, D.W. (1982): Functional evaluation of lung macrophages from cigarette smokers and nonsmokers. *J. Reticuloendoth. Soc.*, 32:311–312.
124. Flenley, D.C., and Warren, P.M. (1980): Abnormalities of gas exchange in chronic bronchitis and emphysema, during acute exacerbations, on exercise, and during sleep. *Rev. Fr. Mal. Respir.*, 115–124.
125. Fletcher, C., and Peto, R. (1977): The natural history of chronic airflow obstruction. *Brit. Med. J.*, 1:1645–1648.
126. Fletcher, C., Peto, R., Tinker, C., and Speizer, F.E. (1976): *The Natural History of Chronic Bronchitis and Emphysema.* Oxford University Press, New York.
127. Fletcher, E.C., Luchett, R.A., Miller, T., et al. (1989): Pulmonary vascular hemodynamics in chronic lung disease patients with and without oxyhemoglobin desaturation during sleep. *Chest*, 95:157–166.
128. Flint, F.J. (1954): Cor pulmonale: incidence and aetiology in an industrial city. *Lancet*, 2:51–58.
129. Fournier, M., Lebargy, F., Leroy Ladurie, F., Lenormand, E., and Pariente, R. (1989): Intraepithelial T-lymphocyte subsets in the airways of normal subjects and/or patients with chronic bronchitis. *Am. Rev. Respir. Dis.*, 140:737–742.
130. Fox, B.F., Bull, T.B., Makey, A.R., and Rawbone, R. (1981): The significance of ultrastructural abnormalities in human cilia. *Chest*, 80(Suppl.):796–804.
131. Foxman, B., Higgins, I.T.T., and Oh, M.S. (1986): The effects of occupation and smoking on respiratory disease mortality. *Am. Rev. Respir. Dis.*, 134:649–652.
132. Frasca, J.M., Auerbach, O., Carter, H.W., and Parks, V.R. (1983): Morphologic alterations induced by short-term cigarette smoking. *Am. J. Pathol.* 111:11–20.
133. Fraser, R.G., Fraser, R.S., Renner, J.W., et al. (1976): The roentgenologic diagnosis of chronic bronchitis. *Radiology*, 120:1–9.
134. Fujita, J., Nelson, N.L., Daughton, D.M., Dobry, C.A., Spurzem, J.R., Irino, S., and Rennard, S.I. (1990): Evaluation of elastase and antielastase balance in patients with bronchitis and pulmonary emphysema. *Am. Rev. Respir. Dis.*, 142:57–62.
135. Gadek, J., Fells, G.A., and Crystal, R.G. (1979): Cigarette smoking induces functional antiprotease deficiency in lower respiratory tract of humans. *Science*, 206:1315–1316.
136. Gaertner, M., Chau, N., Ludwiczak, E., Polu, J.M., and Sadoul, P. (1983): Long-term prognosis of chronic bronchitis following the first episode of acute respiratory decompensation. *Rev. Fr. Mal. Respir.*, 11:739–750.
137. Ghafouri, M.A., Patil, K.D., and Kass, I. (1984): Sputum changes associated with the use of ipratropium bromide. *Chest*, 86:387–393.
138. Gillespie, D.J., Marsh, H.M.M., Diverthie, M.B., and Meadows, J.A., III. (1986): Clinical outcome of respiratory failure in patients requiring prolonged (>24 hours) mechanical ventilation. *Chest*, 90:364–369.
139. Glynn, A.A. (1959): Antibodies to *Hemophilus influenzae* in chronic bronchitis. *Br. Med. J.*, 2:911–914.
140. Glynn, A.A., and Michaels, L. (1960): Bronchial biopsy in chronic bronchitis and asthma. *Thorax*, 15:142–153.
141. Goldstein, N., and Doring, G. (1986): Lysosomal enzymes from polymorphonuclear leukocytes and proteinase inhibitors in patients with cystic fibrosis. *Am. Rev. Respir. Dis.*, 134:49–56.
142. Goldstein, R.S., Ramcharan, V., Bowes, G., et al. (1984): Effect of supplemental nocturnal oxygen on gas exchange in patients with severe obstructive lung disease. *N. Engl. J. Med.*, 310:425–429.
143. Gong, H., Jr., Fligiel, S., Tashkin, D.P., and Barbers, R.G. (1987): Tracheobronchial changes in habitual, heavy smokers of marijuana with and without tobacco. *Am. Rev. Respir. Dis.*, 136:142–149.
144. Goodman, R.M., Yergin, B.M., Landa, J.F., Golinvaux, M.H., and Sackner, M.A. (1978): Relationship of smoking history and pulmonary function tests to tracheal mucous velocity in nonsmokers, young smokers, ex-smokers, and patients with chronic bronchitis. *Am. Rev. Respir. Dis.*, 117:205–214.

145. Gottlieb, L.S., and Balchum, D.J. (1973): Course of chronic obstructive pulmonary disease following first onset of respiratory failure. *Chest,* 63:5–8.
146. Graham, D.E., and Koren, H.S. (1990): Biomarkers of inflammation in ozone-exposed humans. *Am. Rev. Respir. Dis.,* 142:152–156.
147. Green, B.A., Metalf, B.J., Quinn-Dey, T., Kirkley, D.H., Quataert, S.A., and Deich, R.A. (1990): A recombinant non-fatty acylated form of the Hi-PAL (P6) protein of *Hemophilus influenzae* elicits biologically active antibody against both nontypeable and type b *H. influenzae. Infect. Immun.,* 58:3272–3278.
148. Gross, N.J., and Skorodin, M.S. (1984): Anticholinergic, antimuscarinic bronchodilators. *Am. Rev. Respir. Dis.,* 129:856–870.
149. Gross, N.J., and Skorodin, M.S. (1984): Role of the parasympathetic system in airway obstruction due to emphysema. *N. Engl. J. Med.,* 311:421–425.
150. Gump, D.W., Phillips, C.A., Forsyth, B.R., McIntosh, K., Lamborn, K.R., and Stouch, W.H. (1976): Role of infection in chronic bronchitis. *Am. Rev. Respir. Dis.,* 113:465–474.
151. Gurwitz, D., Mindorff, C., and Levison, H. (1981): Increased incidence of bronchial reactivity in children with a history of bronchiolitis. *J. Pediatr.,* 98:551–555.
152. Haas, H., Morris, J.F., Samson, S., Kilbourn, J.P., and Kim, P.J. (1977): Bacterial flora of the respiratory tract in chronic bronchitis: comparison of transtracheal, fiberbronchoscopic, and oropharyngeal sampling methods. *Am. Rev. Respir. Dis.,* 116:41–47.
153. Haase, E.M., Campagnari, A.A., Sarwar, J., Shero, M., Wirth, M., Cumming, C.U., and Murphy, T.F. (1991): Strain-specific and immunodominant surface epitopes of the P2 porin protein of nontypeable *Hemophilus influenzae. Infect. Immun.,* 59:1278–1284.
154. Hager, H., Verghese, A., Alvarez, S., and Berk, S.L. (1987): *Branhamella catarrhalis* respiratory infections. *Rev. Infect. Dis.,* 9:1140–1149.
155. Hanski, E., Horwitz, P.A., and Caparon, M.G. (1992): Expression of protein F, the fibronectin-binding protein of *Streptococcus pyogenes* JRS4, in heterologous streptococcal and enterococcal strains promotes their adherence to respiratory epithelial cells. *Infect. Immun.,* 60:5119–5125.
156. Hasty, D.L., Ofek, I., Courtney, H.S., and Doyle, R.J. (1992): Multiple adhesins of streptococci. *Infect. Immun.,* 60:2147–2152.
157. He, X.-Z., Chen, W., Liu, Z.-Y., et al. (1991): An epidemiological study of lung cancer in Xuau Wei county, China: current progress. Case-control study on lung cancer and cooking fuel. *Environ. Health Perspect.,* 94:9–13.
158. Heino, M., Juntunen-Backman, K., Leijala, M., Rapola, J., Laitinen, L.A. (1990): Bronchial epithelial inflammation in children with chronic cough after early lower respiratory tract illness. *Am. Rev. Respir. Dis.,* 141:428–432.
159. Hendley, J.O., Fishburne, H.B., and Gwaltney, J.M. (1972): Coronavirus infections in working adults. *Am. Rev. Respir. Dis.,* 105:805–811.
160. Higgins, M. (1991): Risk factors associated with chronic obstructive lung disease. *Ann. NY Acad. Sci.,* 624:7–17.
161. Higgins, M., and Keller, J. (1975): Familial occurrence of chronic respiratory disease and familial resemblance in ventilatory capacity. *J. Chron. Dis.,* 28:239.
162. Higgins, M.W., and Keller, J.B. (1989): Trends in COPD morbidity and mortality in Tecumseh, Michigan. *Am. Rev. Respir. Dis.,* 140:542.
163. Higgins, M.W., Keller, J.B., Becker, M., et al. (1982): An index of risk for obstructive airways disease. *Am. Rev. Respir. Dis.,* 125:144.
164. Hill, N.S. (1987): The cardiac exam in lung disease. *Clin. Chest Med.,* 8:273–285.
165. Hill, N.S. (1988): The use of theophylline in "irreversible" chronic obstructive pulmonary disease. *Arch. Intern. Med.,* 148:2579–2584.
166. Hill, N.S., (1993): Noninvasive ventilation. *Am. Rev. Respir. Dis.,* 147:1050–1055.
167. Hill, S.L., Morrison, H.M., Burnett, D., and Stockley, R.A. (1986): Short-term response of patients with bronchiectasis to treatment with amoxycillin given in standard or high doses orally or by inhalation. *Thorax,* 41:559–565.
168. Hirata, T., Matsunobe, S., Matsui, Y., Kado, M., Mikiya, K., and Oshima, S. (1990): Effect of erythromycin on the generation of neutrophil chemiluminescence *in vitro. Nippon-Kyobu-Shikkan-Gakkai-Zasshi,* 28:1066–1071.
169. Hoepelman, A.I.M., and Tuomanen, E.I. (1992): Consequences of microbial attachment: directing host cell functions with adhesins. *Infect. Immun.,* 60:1729–1733.
170. Hogg, J.C., Macklem, P.T., and Thurlbeck, W.M. (1968): Site and nature of airway obstruction in chronic obstructive lung disease. *N. Engl. J. Med.,* 278:1355–1360.
171. Hoogsteden, H.C., van Hal, P.Th.W., Wijkhuijs, J.M., Hop, W., Verkaik, A.P.K., and Hilvering, C. (1991): Expression of the CD11/CD18 cell surface adhesion glycoprotein family on alveolar macrophages in smokers and nonsmokers. *Chest,* 6:1567–1571.
172. Hubbard, R.C., Ogushi, F., Fells, G.A., Cantin, A.M., Jallat, S., Courtney, M., and Crystal, R.G. (1987): Oxidants spontaneously released by alveolar macrophages of cigarette smokers can inactivate the active site of α1-antitrypsin, rendering it ineffective as an inhibitor of neutrophil elastase. *J. Clin. Invest.,* 80:1289–1295.

173. Hudson, L.D. (1987): Acute respiratory failure in patients with chronic obstructive pulmonary disease. In: *Acute Respiratory Failure,* edited by R.C. Bone, R.B. George, and L.D. Hudson, pp. 155–172. Churchill Livingstone, New York.

174. Hudson, L.D., and Monti, C.M. (1990): Rationale and use of corticosteroids in chronic obstructive pulmonary disease. *Med. Clin. No. Amer.,* 74:661–690.

175. Hultgren, S.J., Normark, S., and Abraham, S.N. (1991): Chaperone-assisted assembly and molecular architecture of adhesive pili. *Annu. Rev. Microbiol.,* 45:383–415.

176. Hunninghake, G.W., and Crystal, R.G. (1983): Cigarette smoking and lung destruction. *Am. Rev. Respir. Dis.,* 128:833–838.

177. Hunninghake, G.W., Davidson, J.M., Rennard, S.I., Szapiel, S., Gadek, J.E., and Crystal, R.G. (1981): Elastin fragments attract macrophage precursors to diseased sites in pulmonary emphysema. *Science,* 212:929–937.

178. Hunter, A.M.B., Carey, M.A., and Larsh, H.W. (1981): The nutritional status of patients with chronic obstructive pulmonary disease. *Am. Rev. Respir. Dis.,* 124:376–381.

179. Iravani, J., and Melville, G.N. (1974): Long-term effect of cigarette smoke on mucociliary function in animals. *Respiration,* 31:358–366.

180. Jakab, G.J. (1990): Sequential virus infections, bacterial superinfections, and fibrogenesis. *Am. Rev. Respir. Dis.,* 142:374–379.

181. Janoff, A. (1985): Elastase and emphysema. Current assessment of the protease-antiprotease hypothesis. *Am. Rev. Respir. Dis.,* 132:411–417.

182. Jeffrey, P.K. (1991): Morphology of the airway wall in asthma and in chronic obstructive pulmonary disease. *Am. Rev. Respir. Dis.,* 143:1152–1158.

183. Jeffery, P.K., and Reid, L.M. (1981): The effect of tobacco smoke, with or without phenylmethyloxadiazole (PMO), on rate bronchial epithelium: a light and electron microscopic study. *J. Pathol.,* 133:341–359.

184. Jenkins, S.C., and Moxham, J. (1987): High-dose salbutamol in chronic bronchitis: comparison of 400 μg, 1 mg, 1.6 mg, 2 mg and placebo delivered by Rotahaler. *Br. J. Dis. Chest,* 81:242–247.

185. Johnson, A.P., and Inzana, T.J. (1986): Loss of ciliary activity in organ cultures of rat trachea treated with lipooligosaccharide from *Hemophilus influenzae.* J. Med. Microbiol., 22:265–268.

186. Johnston, R.N., McNeill, R.S., Smith, D.H., Dempster, M.B., Nairn, J.R., Purvis, M.S., Watson, J.M., and Ward, F.G. (1969): Five-year winter chemoprophylaxis for chronic bronchitis. *Br. Med. J.,* 4:265–269.

187. Jones, C.H., Jacob-Dubuisson, F., Dodson, K., Kuehn, D.M., Slonim, L., Striker, R., and Hultgren, S.J. (1992): Adhesion presentation in bacteria requires molecular chaperones and ushers. *Infect. Immun.,* 60:4445–4451.

188. Joseph, M., Tonnel, A.B., Capron, A., and Voison, C. (1980): Enzyme-release and superoxide anion production by human alveolar macrophages stimulated with immunoglobulin E. *Clin. Exp. Immunol.,* 40:416–422.

189. Kanner, R.E., Renzetti, A.D., Klauber, M.R., Smith, C.B., and Golden, C.A. (1979): Variables associated with changes in spirometry in patients with obstructive lung diseases. *Am. J. Med.,* 67:44–50.

190. Kark, J.D., Lebiush, M., and Rannon, L. (1982): Cigarette smoking as a risk factor for epidemic A(H₁N₁) influenza in young men. *N. Engl. J. Med.,* 307:1042–1046.

191. Kattan, M., Keens, T.G., Lapierre, J.-G., Levison, H., Bryan, A.C., and Reilly, B.J. (1977): Pulmonary function abnormalities in symptom-free children after bronchiolitis. *Pediatrics,* 59:683–688.

192. Kauffmann, F., Drouet, D., Lelouch, J., et al. (1982): Occupational exposure and 12-year spirometric changes among Paris area workers. *Brit. J. Industr. Med.,* 39:221–232.

193. Kaufmann, F., Tager, I.B., Munoz, A., et al. (1989): Familial factors related to lung function in children aged 6–10 years: results from the PAARC epidemiologic study. *Am. J. Epidemiol.,* 129:1289.

194. Kerby, G.R., Mayer, L.S., and Pingleton, S.K. (1987): Nocturnal positive pressure ventilation via nasal mask. *Am. Rev. Respir. Dis.,* 135:738–740.

195. Kerstjens, H.A.M., Brand, P.L.P., Hughes, M.D., et al. (1992): A comparison of bronchodilator therapy with or without inhaled corticosteroid therapy for obstructive airways disease. *N. Engl. J. Med.,* 327:1413–1419.

196. Klein, A., Lamblin, G., Lhermitte, M., et al. (1988): Primary structure of neutral oligosaccharides derived from respiratory-mucus glycoproteins of a patient suffering from bronchiectasis, determined by combination of 500-MHz ¹H-NMR spectroscopy and quantitative sugar analysis. 1. Stucture of 16 oligosaccharides having the Galβ(1–3) GalNAc-ol core (type 1) or the Galβ (1–3)[GlcNAcβB1–6]GalNAc-ol core (type 2). *Eur. J. Biochem.,* 171:631–642.

197. Koch-Brandt, C.I. (1991): Glycoprotein synthesis and secretion: translation and targeting. *Am. Rev. Respir. Dis.,* 144:S29–S32.

198. Kollberg, H., Mossberg, B., Afzelius, B.A., Philipson, K., and Camner, P. (1978): Cystic fibrosis compared with the immotile cilia syndrome. *Scand. J. Respir. Dis.,* 59:297–306.

199. Koyama, S., Rennard, S.I., Daughton, D., Shoji, S., and Robbins, R.A. (1991): Bronchoalveolar

lavage fluid obtained from smokers exhibits increased monocyte chemokinetic activity. *J. Appl. Physiol.*, 70(3):1208–1214.

200. Kramps, J.A., Rudolphus, A., Stolk, J., Willems, L.N.A., and Dijkman, J.H. (1991): Role of antileukoprotease in the human lung. *Ann. NY Acad. Sci.*, 624:97–108.

201. Krivan, H.C., Roberts, D.D., and Ginsburg, V. (1988): Many pulmonary pathogenic bacteria bind specifically to the carbohydrate sequence GalNacB1-4Gal found in some glycolipids. *Proc. Natl. Acad. Sci. USA*, 85:6157–6161.

202. Krzyanowski, M., and Jedrychowski, W. (1990): Occupational exposure and incidence of chronic respiratory symptoms among residents of Cracow followed for 13 years. *Int. Arch. Occup. Environ. Health*, 62:311–317.

203. Krzyzanowski, M., and Kauffmann, F. (1988): The relation of respiratory symptoms and ventilatory function to moderate occupational exposure in a general population. *Int. J. Epidemiol.*, 17:397–406.

204. Kuehn, M.J., Heuser, J., Normark, S., and Hultgren, S.J. (1991): P pili in uropathogenic *E. coli* are composite fibres with distinct fibrillar adhesive tips. *Nature*, 356:252–255.

205. Kunkel, S.L., Standiford, T., Kasahara, K., and Strieter, R.M. (1991): Interleukin-8 (IL-8): the major neutrophil chemotactic factor in the lung. *Exp. Lung Res.*, 17:17–23.

206. Kuo, C.-D., Shiao, G.-M., and Lee, J.-D. (1993): The effects of high-fat and high-carbohydrate diet loads on gas exchange and ventilation in COPD patients and normal subjects. *Chest*, 104:189–196.

207. Lamblin, G., Boersma, A., Klein, A., Roussel, P., Van Halbeek, H., and Vliegenthart, J.F.G. (1984): Primary structure determination of five sialylated oligosaccharides derived from bronchial mucus glycoproteins of patients suffering from cystic fibrosis. *J. Biol. Chem.*, 259:9061–9068.

208. Lamblin, G., Lhermitte, M., Boersma, A., Roussel, P., and Reinhold, V. (1980): Oligosaccharides of human bronchial glycoproteins: neutral di- and trisaccharides isolated from a patient suffering from chronic bronchitis. *J. Biol. Chem.*, 255:4595–4598.

209. Lamblin, G., Lhermitte, M., Klein, A., Houdret, N., Scharfman, A., Ramphal, R., and Roussel, P. (1991): The carbohydrate diversity of human respiratory mucins: a protection of the underlying mucosa? *Am. Rev. Respir. Dis.*, 144:S19–S24.

210. Lamy, M.E., Pouthier-Simon, F., and Debacker-Willame, E. (1973): Respiratory viral infections in hospital patients with chronic bronchitis. *Chest*, 63:336–341.

211. Laraya-Cuassay, L.R., DeForest, A., Huff, D., Lischner, H., and Huang, N.N. (1977): Chronic pulmonary complications of early influenza virus infection in children. *Am. Rev. Respir. Dis.*, 116:617–625.

212. Laurell, C.B., and Ericksson, S. (1963): The electrophoretic alpha-1-globulin pattern of serum in alpha-1-antitrypsin deficiency. *Scand. J. Clin. Lab. Invest.*, 15:132–140.

213. Laurenzi, G.A., Potter, R.T., and Kass, E.H. (1961): Bacteriologic flora of the lower respiratory tract. *N. Engl. J. Med.*, 265:1273–1278.

214. Lebowitz, M.D. (1989): 2. Trends from cohort studies. The trends in airway obstructive disease morbidity in the Tucson epidemiological study. *Am. Rev. Respir. Dis.*, 140:S35–41.

215. Lebowitz, M.D., Knudson, R.J., and Burrows, B. (1975): Tucson epidemiologic study of obstructive lung diseases. 1. Methodology and prevalence of disease. *Am. J. Epidemiol.*, 102:137.

216. Lee, T.H. (1987): Interactions between alveolar macrophages, monocytes, and granulocytes. *Am. Rev. Respir. Dis.*, 135:S14–S17.

217. Lees, A.W., and McNaught, W. (1959): Bacteriology of lower-respiratory-tract secretions, sputum, and upper-respiratory-tract secretions in "normals" and chronic bronchitis. *Lancet*, 2:1112–1115.

218. Leffler, H., and Svanborg-Eden, C. (1980): Clinical identification of a glycosphingolipid receptor for *Escherichia coli* attaching to human urinary tract epithelial cells and agglutinating human erythrocytes. *Fems. Microbiol. Lett.*, 8:127–134.

219. Lewis, M.I., Sieck, G.C., and Fournier, M. (1986): Effect of nutritional deprivation on diaphragmatic contractility and muscle size. *J. Appl. Physiol.*, 60:596–603.

220. Lopez-Vidriero, M.T. (1989): Mucus as a natural barrier. *Respiration*, 55(Suppl. 1):28–32.

221. Lourenco, R.V., Loddenkemper, R., and Carton, R.W. (1972): Patterns of distribution and clearance of aerosols in patients with bronchiectasis. *Am. Rev. Respir. Dis.*, 106:857–866.

222. Low, R.B., Davis, G.S., and Giancola, M.S. (1978): Biochemical analyses of bronchoalveolar lavage fluids of healthy human volunteer smokers and nonsmokers. *Am. Rev. Respir. Dis.*, 118:863–887.

223. Lund, B., Lindberg, F., Marklund, B.I., and Normark, S. (1987): The papG protein is the a-D-galactopyranosyl-(1-4)-B-D-galactopyranose-binding adhesin of uropathogenic *Escherichia coli*. *Proc. Natl. Acad. Sci.*, 84:5898–5902.

224. Mahler, D.A., Brent, B.N., Loke, J., Zaret, B.L., and Matthay, R.A. (1984): Right ventricular performance and central haemodynamics during upright bicycle exercise in patients with chronic obstructive pulmonary disease. *Am. Rev. Respir. Dis.*, 130:722–729.

225. Mahler, D.A., Matthay, R.A., Snyder, P.E., Wells, C.K., and Loke, J. (1985): Sustained-release theophylline reduces dyspnea in nonreversible obstructive airway disease. *Am. Rev. Respir. Dis.*, 131:22–25.
226. Malkamaki, M., Honkanen, E., Leinonen, M., et al. (1983): *Branhamella catarrhalis* as a cause of bacteremic pneumonia. *Scan. J. Infect. Dis.*, 15:125.
227. Marlin, G.E., Hartnett, B.J.S., Berend, N., and Hacket, N.B. (1978): Assessment of combined oral theophylline and inhaled b-adrenoceptor agonist bronchodilator therapy. *Br. J. Clin. Pharmacol.*, 5:45–50.
228. Marthan, R., Castaing, Y., Manier, G., and Guenard, H. (1985): Gas exchange alteration in patients with chronic obstructive lung disease. *Chest*, 87:470–475.
229. Martin, T.R., Lewis, S.W., and Albert, R.K. (1982): The prognosis of patients with chronic obstructive pulmonary disease after hospitalization for acute respiratory failure. *Chest*, 82:310–314.
230. Martin, T.R., Raghu, G., Maunder, R.J., and Springmeyer, S.C. (1985): The effects of chronic bronchitis and chronic airflow obstruction on lung cell populations recovered by bronchoalveolar lavage. *Am. Rev. Respir. Dis.*, 132:254–260.
231. Mason, M.J., and Von Epps, D.E. (1989): *In vivo* neutrophil emigration in response to interleukin-1 and tumor necrosis factor-alpha. *J. Leucocyte Biol.*, 45:62.
232. Mathay, R.A., Berger, H.J., Davies, R., et al. (1982): Improvement in cardiac performance by oral long-acting theophylline in chronic obstructive pulmonary disease. *Am. Heart J.*, 104:1022–1026.
233. Mathay, R.A., Berger, H.J., Loke, J., et al. (1978): Effects of theophylline upon right and left ventricular performance in chronic obstructive pulmonary disease. *Am. J. Med.*, 65:903–910.
234. Matthys, H., Muller, M., and Konietzko, N. (1974): Quantitative and selective bronchial clearance studies using ^{99M}Tc-sulfate particles. *Scand. J. Respir. Dis.*, 55(Suppl. 85):33–37.
235. Matthys, H., Vastag, E., Koehler, K., Daikeler, G., and Fisher, J. (1983): Mucociliary clearance in patients with chronic bronchitis and bronchial carcinoma. *Respiration*, 44:329–337.
236. May, J.R. (1953): The bacteriology of chronic bronchitis. *Lancet*, 2:534–537.
237. May, J.R. (1965): Antibodies to *Hemophilus influenzae* in the sera of patients with chronic bronchitis. *J. Pathol. Bacteriol.*, 90:163–174.
238. McDowell, E.M., Barrett, L.A., Harris, C.C., and Trump, B.F. (1976): Abnormal cilia in human bronchial epithelium. *Arch. Pathol. Lab. Med.*, 100:429–436.
239. McLeod, D.T., Ahmad, F., Capewell, S., Croughan, M.J., Calder, M.A., and Seaton, A. (1986): Increase in bronchopulmonary infection due to *Branhemella catarrhalis*. *Br. Med. J.*, 292:1103–1105.
240. McLeod, D.T., Ahmad, F., Power, J.T., Calder, M.A., and Seaton, A. (1983): Bronchopulmonary infection due to *Branhamella catarrhalis*. *Br. Med. J.*, ii:1446–1447.
241. McLeod, R., Mack, D.G., McCleod, E.G., Campbell, E.J., and Estes, R.G. (1985): Alveolar macrophage function and inflammatory stimuli in smokers with and without obstructive lung disease. *Am. Rev. Respir. Dis.*, 131:377–384.
242. McNamara, M.J., Phillips, I.A., and Williams, O.B. (1969): Viral and *Mycoplasma pneumoniae* infections in exacerbations of chronic lung disease. *Am. Rev. Respir. Dis.*, 100:19–24.
243. Mecikalski, M.B., Cutillo, A.G., and Renzetti, A.D., Jr. (1984): Effect of right-to-left shunting on alveolar dead space. *Bull. Eur. Physiopathol. Respir.*, 20:513–519.
244. Medical Research Council Working Party. (1981): Long-term domiciliary oxygen therapy in chronic hypoxic cor pulmonale complicating chronic bronchitis and emphysema. *Lancet*, 1:681–686.
245. Medical Research Council Working Party on Trials of Chemotherapy in Early Chronic Bronchitis. (1966): Value of chemoprophylaxis and chemotherapy in early chronic bronchitis. *Br. Med. J.*, 1:317–322.
246. Meduri, G.U., Abou-Shala, N., Fox, R.C., et al. (1991): Noninvasive face mask mechanical ventilation in patients with acute hypercapnic respiratory failure. *Chest*, 100:445–454.
247. Metcalf, J.P., Thompson, A.B., Gossman, G.L., Nelson, K.J., Koyama, S., Rennard, S.I., and Robbins, R.A. (1991): GcGlobulin functions as a co-chemotaxin in the lower respiratory tract. *Am. Rev. Respir. Dis.*, 143:844–849.
248. Miller, B.G., and Jacobsen, M. (1985): Dust exposure, pneumoconiosis and mortality of coal miners. *Br. J. Ind. Med.*, 42:723–733.
249. Miller, D.L., and Jones, R. (1964): The bacterial flora of the upper respiratory tract and sputum of working men. *J. Pathol. Bacteriol.*, 87:182–186.
250. Minette, A. (1986): Is chronic bronchitis also an industrial disease? *Eur. J. Respir. Dis.*, 69(Suppl. 146):87–98.
251. Miro, A.M., Shivaram, U., and Hertig, I. (1993): Continuous positive airway pressure in COPD patients in acute hypercapnic respiratory failure. *Chest*, 103:266–268.
252. Mitchell, R.S., Stanford, R.E., Johnson, J.M., et al. (1976): The morphologic features of the bronchi, bronchioles and alveoli in chronic airway obstruction. *Am. Rev. Respir. Dis.*, 114:137–145.

253. Miyatake, H., Taki, F., Taniguchi, H., Suzuki, R., Takagi, K., and Satake, T. (1991): Erythromycin reduces the severity of bronchial hyperresponsiveness in asthma. *Chest*, 99:670–673.
254. Monod, H., and Scherrer, J. (1965): The work capacity of a synergic muscular group. *Ergonomics*, 8:329–337.
255. Monto, A.S., and Bryan, E.R. (1978): Susceptibility to rhinovirus infection in chronic bronchitis. *Am. Rev. Respir. Dis.*, 118:1101–1103.
256. Monto, A.S., Higgins, M.W., and Ross, H.W. (1975): The Tecumseh Study of Respiratory Illness. III. Acute infection in chronic respiratory disease and comparison groups. *Am. Rev. Respir. Dis.*, 111:27–36.
257. Monto, A.S., and Ross, H.W. (1978): The Tecumseh Study of Respiratory Illness. X. Relation of acute infections to smoking, lung function and chronic symptoms. *Am. J. Epidemiol.*, 107:57–64.
258. Morgan, W.K.C. (1978): Industrial bronchitis. *Brit. J. Indust. Med.*, 35:285–291.
259. Morrison, D.A., Adcock, K., Collins, C.M., Goldman, S., Caldwell, J.H., and Schwartz, M.I. (1987): Right ventricular dysfunction and the exercise limitation of chronic obstructive pulmonary disease. *J. Am. Coll. Cardiol.*, 9:1219–1229.
260. Morrison, H.M., Kramps, J.A., Afford, S.C., Burnett, D., Dijkman, J.H., and Stockley, R.A. (1987): Elastase inhibitors in sputum from bronchitic patients with and without α_1-proteinase inhibitor deficiency: partial characterization of a hitherto unquantified inhibitor of neutrophil elastase. *Clin. Sci.*, 73:19–28.
261. Morrow, P.E. (1984). Toxicological data on NO_2: an overview. *J. Toxicol. Environ. Health*, 13:205–227.
262. Mossberg, B., Björkander, J., Afzelius, B., and Camner, P. (1982): Mucociliary clearance in patients with immunoglobulin deficiency. *Eur. J. Respir. Dis.*, 63:570–578.
263. Moser, K.M., Shibel, E.M., and Beamon, A. (1973): Acute respiratory failure in obstructive lung disease: long-term survival after treatment in an intensive care unit. *J.A.M.A.*, 225:705–707.
264. Mullen, J.B.M., Wright, J.L., Wiggs, B.R., Pare, P.D., and Hogg, J.C. (1985): Reassessment of inflammation of airways in chronic bronchitis. *Br. Med. J.*, 291:1235–1239.
265. Murciano, D., Aubier, M., Lecocguic, Y., and Pariente, R. (1984): Effects of theophylline on diaphragmatic strength and fatigue in patients with chronic obstructive pulmonary disease. *N. Engl. J. Med.*, 311:349–353.
266. Murciano, D., Auclair, M.-H., Pariente, R., and Aubier, M. (1989): A randomized, controlled trial of theophylline in patients with severe chronic obstructive pulmonary disease. *N. Engl. J. Med.*, 320:1521–1525.
267. Murphy, T.F., and Apicella, M.A. (1987): Nontypable *Hemophilus influenzae:* a review of clinical aspects, surface antigens, and the human immune response to infection. *Rev. Infect. Dis.*, 9:1–15.
268. Murphy, T.F., Bartos, L.C., Campagnari, A.A., Nelson, M.B., and Apicella, M.A. (1986): Antigenic characterization of the P6 protein of nontypable *Hemophilus influenzae. Infect. Immun.*, (Dec):774–779.
269. Murphy, T.F., Dudas, K.C., Mylotte, J.M., and Apicella, M.A. (1983): A subtyping system for nontypeable *Haemophilus influenzae* based on outer-membrane proteins. *J. Infect. Dis.*, 147:838–846.
270. Murphy, T.F., Nelson, M.B., Dudas, K.C., Mylotte, J.M., and Apicella, M.A. (1985): Identification of a specific epitope of *Hemophilus influenzae* on a 16,600-dalton outer membrane protein. *J. Infect. Dis.*, 152:1300–1307.
271. Murphy, T.F., Nelson, M.B., and Apicella, M.A. (1992): The P6 outer membrane of nontypeable *Hemophilus influenzae* as a vaccine antigen. *J. Infect. Dis.*, 165(Suppl. 1):S203–S205.
272. Murphy, T.F., and Sethi, S. (1992): Bacterial infection in chronic obstructive pulmonary disease. *Am. Rev. Respir. Dis.*, 146:1067–1083.
273. Musher, D.M., Kubitschek, K.R., Crennan, J., and Baughn, R.E. (1983): Pneumonia and acute febrile tracheobronchitis due to *Hemophilus influenzae. Ann. Intern. Med.*, 99:444–450.
274. Nagai, A., West, W.W., Paul, J.L., and Thurlbeck, W.M. (1985): The National Institutes of Health intermittent positive-pressure breathing trial: pathology studies. I. Interrelationship between morphologic lesions. *Am. Rev. Respir. Dis.*, 132:937–945.
275. Nagai, A., West, W.W., and Thurlbeck, W.M. (1985): The National Institutes of Health intermittent positive-pressure breathing trial: pathology studies. II. Correlation between morphologic findings, clinical findings, and evidence of expiratory airflow obstruction. *Am. Rev. Respir. Dis.*, 132:946–953.
276. Nakamura, H., Yoshimura, K., Jaffe, H.A., and Crystal, R.G. (1991): Interleukin-8 gene expression in human bronchial epithelial cells. *J. Biol. Chem.*, 266:19611–19617.
277. Nathan, C.F. (1987): Secretory products of macrophages. *J. Clin. Invest.*, 79:319–326.
278. National Center for Health Statistics (1987): Current estimates from the National Health Interview Survey, United States 1986. In: *Vital and Health Statistics*. Series 10, No. 164. DHHS Publication No. (PHS) 87–1592. U.S. Government Printing Office, Washington, D.C.

279. Nelson, M.B., Apicella, M.A., Murphy, T.F., Vankeulen, H., Spotila, L.D., and Rekosh, D. (1988): Cloning and sequencing of *Haemophilus influenzae* outer membrane protein P6. *Infect. Immun.*, 56:128–134.
280. Nelson, M.B., Munson, R.S., Apicella, M.A., Sikkema, D.J., Molleston, J.P., and Murphy, T.F. (1991): Molecular conservation of the P6 outer membrane protein among strains of *Hemophilus influenzae:* analysis of antigenic determinants, gene sequences, and restriction fragment length polymorphisms. *Infect. Immun.*, 59:2658–2663.
281. Nicotra, M.B., Rivera, M., and Awe, R.J. (1982): Antibiotic therapy of acute exacerbations of chronic bronchitis. *Ann. Intern. Med.*, 97:18–21.
282. Nicotra, B., Rivera, M., Luman, J.I., and Wallace, R.J. (1986): *Branhamella catarrhalis* as a lower respiratory tract pathogen in patients with chronic lung disease. *Arch. Intern. Med.*, 146:890–893.
283. Niewoehner, D.E., Kleinerman, J., Rice, D.B., and Div, M. (1974): Pathologic changes in the peripheral airways of young cigarette smokers. *N. Engl. J. Med.*, 291:755–758.
284. Ninane, G., Joly, J., and Kraytman, M. (1978): Bronchopulmonary infection due to *Branhamella catarrhalis:* eleven cases assessed by transtracheal puncture. *Br. Med. J.*, 1:276–278.
285. Nisar, M., Walshaw, M., Earis, J.E., Pearson, M.G., and Calverley, P.M.A. (1990): Assessment of reversibility of airway obstruction in patients with chronic obstructive airways disease. *Thorax*, 45:190–194.
286. Nocturnal Oxygen Therapy Trial Group (1980): Continuous or nocturnal oxygen therapy in hypoxemic chronic obstructive lung disease: a clinical trial. *Ann. Intern. Med.*, 93:391–398.
287. Oliver, R.M., Fleming, J.S., and Waller, D.G. (1993): Right ventricular function at rest and during exercise in chronic obstructive pulmonary disease. *Chest*, 103:74–80.
288. Orie, N.G.M., Sluiter, H.J., deVries, K., Tammeling, G.J., and Witkop, J. (1961): The host factor in bronchitis. In: *Bronchitis,* edited by N.G.M. Orie and H.J. Sluiter, pp. 43–59. Van Gorcum Press, Asen, The Netherlands.
289. Oswald, N.C., Harold, J.T., and Martin, W.J. (1953): Clinical patterns of chronic bronchitis. *Lancet*, 2:639–643.
290. Ozaki, T., Hayashi, H., Tani, K., Ogushi, F., Yasuoka, S., and Ogura, T. (1992): Neutrophil chemotactic factors in the respiratory tract of patients with chronic airway disease or idiopathic pulmonary fibrosis. *Am. Rev. Respir. Dis.*, 145:85–91.
291. Parker, D.R., O'Connor, G.T., Sparrow, D., Segal, M.R., and Weiss, S.T. (1990): The relationship of nonspecific airway responsiveness and atopy to the rate of decline of lung function. *Am. Rev. Respir. Dis.*, 141:589–594.
292. Passamonte, P.M., and Martinez, A.J. (1984): Effect of inhaled atropine or metaproterenol in patients with chronic airway obstruction and therapeutic serum theophylline levels. *Chest*, 85:610–615.
293. Pauwels, R. (1986): The clinical relevance of airway inflammation. *Eur. J. Respir. Dis.*, 69(Suppl. 147):88–92.
294. Pauwels, R.A. (1989): New aspects of the therapeutic potential of theophylline in asthma. *J. Allergy Clin. Immunol.*, 83:548–553.
295. Pavia, D. (1987): Acute respiratory infections and mucociliary clearance. *Eur. J. Respir. Dis.*, 71:219–226.
296. Pearlman, R.A. (1987): Variability in physicians' estimates of survival for acute respiratory failure in chronic obstructive pulmonary disease. *Chest*, 91:515–521.
297. Pedersen, M., and Stafanger, G. (1983): Bronchopulmonary symptoms in primary ciliary dyskinesia. *Eur. J. Respir. Dis.*, 64(Suppl. 127):118–128.
298. Pederson, L.L., and Baskerville, J.C. (1983): Multivariate prediction of smoking cessation following physician advice to quit smoking: a validation study. *Prev. Med.*, 12:430–436.
299. Pennington, J.E., Rossing, T.H., Boerth, L.W., and Lee, T.H. (1985): Isolation and partial characterization of a human alveolar macrophage-derived neutrophil-activating factor. *J. Clin. Invest.*, 75:1230–1237.
300. Pennock, B.E., Crawshaw, L., Kaplan, P.D., Koliner, C., Carlin, B., Shively, J., and Magovern, J.A. (1992): Additional experience with BIPAP/nasal mask in patients with acute respiratory failure. *Am. Rev. Respir. Dis.*, 145:A525.
301. Peto, R., Speizer, F.E., Cochrane, A.L., Moore, F., Fletcher, C.M., Tinker, C.M., Higgins, I.T.T., Gray, R.G., Richards, S.M., Gilliland, J., and Norman-Smith, B. (1983): The relevance in adults of airflow obstruction, but not of mucus hypersecretion, to mortality from chronic lung disease. *Am. Rev. Respir. Dis.*, 128:491–500.
302. Petrof, B.J., Legare, M., Goldberg, P., Milic-Emili, J., and Gottfried, S.B. (1990): Continuous positive airway pressure reduces work of breathing and dyspnea during weaning from mechanical ventilation in severe chronic obstructive pulmonary disease. *Am. Rev. Respir. Dis.*, 141:281–289.
303. Petty, T.L. (1990): Definitions in chronic obstructive pulmonary disease. *Clin. Chest Med.*, 11:363–373.

304. Pines, A. (1967): Controlled trials of a sulphonamide given weekly to prevent exacerbations of chronic bronchitis. *Br. Med. J.*, 3:202–204.
305. Pines, A., Greenfield, J.S.B., Raafat, H., and Siddiqui, G. (1972): Chloramphenicol and ampicillin compared in elderly patients with severe purulent exacerbations of bronchitis. *Brit. J. Dis. Chest*, 66:116–120.
306. Pines, A., Raafat, H., Plucinski, K., Greenfield, J.S.B., and Solari, M. (1968): Antibiotic regimens in severe and acute purulent exacerbations of chronic bronchitis. *Br. Med. J.*, 2:735–738.
307. Pingleton, S.K. (1986): Nutrition in acute respiratory failure. *Lung*, 164:127–137.
308. Porras, O., Svanborg-Eden, C., Lagergard, T., et al. (1985): Method for testing adherence of *Hemophilus influenzae* to human buccal epithelial cells. *Eur. J. Clin. Microbiol.*, 4:310–315.
309. Postlethwaite, A.E., and Kang, A.H. (1976): Collagen and collagen peptide–induced chemotaxis of human blood monocytes. *J. Exp. Med.*, 143:1299–1307.
310. Postma, D.S., DeVries, K., Koëter, G.H., and Sluiter, H.J. (1986): Independent influence of reversibility of airflow obstruction and nonspecific hyperreactivity on the long-term course of lung function in chronic airflow obstruction. *Am. Rev. Respir. Dis.*, 134:276–280.
311. Postma, D.S., Gimeno, F., Van der Weele, L.Th., and Sluiter, H.J. (1985): Assessment of ventilatory variables in survival prediction of patients with chronic airflow obstruction: the importance of reversibility. *Eur. J. Respir. Dis.*, 67:360–368.
312. Postma, D.S., Peters, I., Steenhuis, E.J., and Sluiter, H.J. (1988): Moderately severe chronic airflow obstruction. Can corticosteroids slow down obstruction? *Eur. Respir. J.*, 1:22–26.
313. Postma, D.S., and Sluiter, H.J. (1989): Prognosis of chronic obstructive pulmonary disease: the Dutch experience. *Am. Rev. Respir. Dis.*, 140:S100–105.
314. Postma, D.S., Steenhuis, E.J., van der Weele, L.Th., and Sluiter, H.J. (1985): Severe chronic airflow obstruction: can corticosteroids slow down progression? *Eur. J. Respir. Dis.*, 67:56–64.
315. Pridie, R.B., Datta, N., Massey, D.G., et al. (1960): A trial of continuous winter chemotherapy in chronic bronchitis. *Lancet*, 2:723–727.
316. Ramphal, R., Carnoy, C., Fievre, S., et al. (1991): *Pseudomona aeruginosa* recognizes carbohydrate chains containing type 1 (Galβ1-3GlcNAc) or type 2 (Galβ1-4GlcNAc) disaccharide units. *Infect. Immun.*, 59:700–704.
317. Rankin, J.A. (1989): The contribution of alveolar macrophages to hyperreactive airway disease. *J. Allergy Clin. Immunol.*, 83:722–729.
318. Read, R.C., Wilson, R., Rutman, A., Lund, V., Todd, H.C., Brain, A.P.R., Jeffery, P.K., and Cole, P.J. (1991): Interaction of nontypable *Haemophilus influenzae* with human respiratory mucosa *in vitro*. *J. Infect. Dis.*, 163:549–558.
319. Reid, L., O'Sullivan, D.D., and Bhaskar, K.R. (1987): Pathophysiology of bronchial hypersecretion. *Eur. J. Respir. Dis.*, 71(Suppl. 153):19–25.
320. Rennard, S.I., Daughton, D., Fujita, J., Oehlerking, M.B., Dobson, J.R., Stahl, M.G., Robbins, R.A., and Thompson, A.B. (1990): Short-term smoking reduction in associated with reduction in measures of lower respiratory tract inflammation in heavy smokers. *Eur. Respir. J.*, 3:752–759.
321. Reynolds, H.Y., Fulmer, J.D., Kazmierowski, J.A., Roberts, W.C., Frank, M.M., and Crystal, R.G. (1977): Analysis of cellular and protein content of bronchoalveolar lavage fluid from patients with idiopathic pulmonary fibrosis and chronic hypersensitivity pneumonitis. *J. Clin. Invest.*, 59:165–175.
322. Reynolds, H.Y., and Newball, H.H. (1974): Analysis of proteins and respiratory cells obtained from human lungs by bronchial lavage. *J. Lab. Clin. Med.*, 84:559–573.
323. Richman-Eisenstat, J.B.Y., Jorens, P.G., Herbert, C.A., Ueki, I., and Nadel, J.A. (1993): Interluekin-8: an important chemoattractant in sputum of patients with chronic inflammatory airway diseases. *Am. J. Physiol.*, 264:L413–L418.
324. Robbins, R.A., Gossman, G.L., Nelson, K.J., Koyama, S., Thompson, A.B., and Rennard, S.I. (1990): Inactivation of chemotactic factor inactivator by cigarette smoke. *Am. Rev. Respir. Dis.*, 142:763–768.
325. Rodnick, J.E., and Gude, J.K. (1988): The use of antibiotics in acute bronchitis and acute exacerbations of chronic bronchitis. *West. J. Med.*, 149:347–351.
326. Rolfe, M.W., Kunkel, S.L., Standiford, T.J., et al. (1991): Pulmonary fibroblast expression of interleukin-8: a model for alveolar macrophage-derived cytokine networking. *Am. J. Respir. Cell. Mol. Biol.*, 5:493–501.
327. Ross, C.A., McMichael, S., Eadie, M.B., et al. (1966): Infective agents and chronic bronchitis. *Thorax*, 21:461.
328. Rott, H.-D. (1983): Genetics of Kartagener's syndrome. *Eur. J. Respir. Dis.*, 64(Suppl. 127):1–4.
329. Royal College of Physicians of London (1962): *Smoking and Health*, pp. 27–31. Pitman Medical, London.
330. Roussos, C.S. (1984): Ventilatory muscle fatigue governs breathing frequency. *Bull. Eur. Physiopathol. Respir.*, 20:445–452.

331. Roussos, C.S., and Macklem, P.T. (1977): Diaphragmatic fatigue in man. *J. Appl. Physiol.*, 43:189–197.
332. Rubin, B.K. (1988): Immotile cilia syndrome (primary ciliary dyskinesia) and inflammatory lung disease. *Clin. Chest Med.*, 9:657–668.
333. Russell, M.A.H., Stapleton, J.A., Jackson, P.H., et al. (1987): District programme to reduce smoking: effect of clinic-supported brief intervention by general practitioners. *Br. Med. J.*, 295:1240–1244.
334. Sachs, D.P.L. (1991): Advances in smoking cessation treatment. *Curr. Pulmonol.*, 12:139–198.
335. Saetta, M., Di Stefano A., Maestrelli, P., Ferraresso, A., Drigo, R., Potena, A., Ciaccia, A., and Fabbri, L.M. (1993): Activated T-lymphocytes and macrophages in bronchial mucosa of subjects with chronic bronchitis. *Am. Rev. Respir. Dis.*, 147:301–306.
336. Sahn, S.A. (1978): Corticosteroids in chronic bronchitis and pulmonary emphysema. *Chest*, 73:389–396.
337. Salvato, G. (1968): Some histological changes in chronic bronchitis and asthma. *Thorax*, 23:168–172.
338. Samet, J.M., Marbury, M.C., and Spengler, J.D. (1987): Health effects and sources of indoor air pollution. Part 1. *Am. Rev. Respir. Dis.*, 136:1486–1508.
339. Samet, J.M., Tager, I.B., and Speizer, F.E. (1983): The relationship between respiratory illness in childhood and chronic airflow obstruction in adulthood. *Am. Rev. Respir. Dis.*, 127:508–523.
340. Sanders, J.S., Berman, T.M., Bartlett, M.M., and Kronenberg, R.S. (1980): Increased hypoxic ventilatory drive due to administration of aminophylline in normal men. *Chest*, 78:279–282.
341. Sauret, J.M., Guitart, A.C., Rodriguez-Frojan, G., and Cornudella, R. (1991): Intermittent short-term negative pressure ventilation and increased oxygenation in COPD patients with severe hypercapnic respiratory failure. *Chest*, 100:455–459.
342. Schwartz, J.L. (1991): Methods for smoking cessation. *Clin. Chest Med.*, 12:737–753.
343. Schwartz, D.A., Landas, S.K., Lassise, D.L., Burmeister, L.F., Hunninghake, G.W., and Merchant, J.A. (1992): Airway injury in swine confinement workers. *Ann. Intern. Med.*, 116:630–635.
344. Seriff, N.S., Khan, F., and Lazo, B.J. (1973): Acute respiratory failure: current concepts of pathophysiology and management. *Med. Clin. No. Amer.*, 57:1539–1550.
345. Sexton, K., Spengler, J.D., and Treitman, R.D. (1984): Effects of residential wood combustion on indoor air quality: a case study in Waterbury, Vermont. *Atmos. Environ.*, 18:1371–1383.
346. Seybold, Z.V., Abraham, W.M., Gazeroglu, H., and Wanner, A. (1992): Impairment of airway mucociliary transport by *Pseudomonas aeruginosa* products. *Am. Rev. Respir. Dis.*, 146:1173–1176.
347. Sheehan, J.K., Thornton, D.J., Somerville, M., and Carlstedt, I. (1991): 1. Mucin structure. The structure and heterogeneity of respiratory mucus glycoproteins. *Am. Rev. Respir. Dis.*, 144: S4–S9.
348. Shennib, H., Mulder, D.S., and Chiu, R.C. (1985): Replenishing the starved patient: when do lung immune cells recover? *Chest*, 87:138–139.
349. Sherrill, D.L., Lebowitz, M.D., and Burrows, B. (1990): Epidemiology of chronic obstructive pulmonary disease. *Clin. Chest Med.*, 11:375–387.
350. Shim, C.S., and Williams, M.H. (1984): Effect of bronchodilator therapy administration by canister versus jet nebulizer. *J. Allergy Clin. Immunol.*, 68:387–390.
351. Sibille, Y., and Reynolds, H.Y. (1990): Macrophages and polymorphonuclear neutrophils in lung defense and injury. *Am. Rev. Respir. Dis.*, 141:471–501.
352. Simberkoff, M.S., Cross, A.P., Al-Ibrahim, M., Baltch, A.L., Geiseler, P.J., Nadler, J., et al. (1986): Efficacy of pneumococcal vaccine in high-risk patients. *N. Engl. J. Med.*, 315:1318–1327.
353. Sisson, J.H., Tuma, D.J., and Rennard, S.I. (1991): Acetaldehyde-mediated cilia dysfunction in bovine bronchial epithelial cells. *Am. J. Physiol.*, 260:L29–L36.
354. Sleigh, M.A., Blake, J.R., and Liron, N. (1988): State of the art. The propulsion of mucus by cilia. *Am. Rev. Respir. Dis.*, 137:726–741.
355. Sluiter, H.J., Blokzijl, E.J., Vandijl, W., et al. (1972): Conservative and respirator treatment of acute respiratory insufficiency in patients with chronic obstructive lung disease: a reappraisal. *Am. Rev. Respir. Dis.*, 105:932–943.
356. Smith, J.P., Stone, R.W., and Muschenheim, C. (1968): Acute respiratory failure in chronic lung disease. *Am. Rev. Respir. Dis.*, 97:791–803.
357. Smith, C.B., Golden, C., Kanner, R.E., and Renzetti, A.D. (1976): *Hemophilus influenzae* and *Hemophilus parainfluenzae* in chronic obstructive pulmonary disease. *Lancet*, 1:1253–1255.
358. Smith, C.B., Golden, C.A., Kanner, R.E., and Renzetti, A.D. (1980): Association of viral and *Mycoplasma pneumoniae* infections with acute respiratory illness in patients with chronic obstructive pulmonary diseases. *Am. Rev. Respir. Dis.*, 121:225–232.
359. Smith, C.B., Golden, C., Klauber, M.R., et al. (1976): Interactions between viruses and bacteria in patients with chronic bronchitis. *J. Infect. Dis.*, 134:552–561.

360. Snider, G.I. (1988): Chronic bronchitis and emphysema. In: *Textbook of Respiratory Medicine,* edited by J.F. Murray and J.A. Nadel, pp. 1069–1106. W.B. Saunders, Philadelphia/Harcourt Brace Jovanovich, New York.

361. Snider, G.L. (1989): 1. Changes in COPD occurrence. Chronic obstructive pulmonary disease: a definition and implications of structural determinants of airflow obstruction for epidemiology. *Am. Rev. Respir. Dis.,* 140:S3–8.

362. Snider, G.L., Ciccolella, D.E., Morris, S.M., Stone, P.J., and Lucey, E.C. (1991): Putative role of neutrophil elastase in the pathogenesis of emphysema. *Ann. NY Acad. Sci.,* 624:45–59.

363. Snider, G.L. (1992): Emphysema: the first two centuries—and beyond. *Am. Rev. Respir. Dis.,* 146(Part I):1334–1344.

364. Snider, G.L. (1992): Emphysema: the first two centuries—and beyond. *Am. Rev. Respir. Dis.,* 146:1615–1622.

365. Speizer, F.E., Rosner, B., and Tager, I.B. (1976): Familial aggregation of chronic respiratory disease: use of national health interview survey data for specific hypothesis testing. *Int. J. Epidemiol.,* 5:167.

366. Speizer, F.E., and Tager, I.B. (1979): Epidemiology of chronic mucus hypersecretion and obstructive airways disease. *Epidemiol. Rev.,* 1:124.

367. Speizer, F.E., and Tager, B. (1979): Epidemiology of chronic mucus hypersecretion and obstructive airways disease. *Epidemiol. Rev.,* 1:124–142.

368. Spiteri, M.A., and Rotondetto, S. (1993): Antibiotics in the treatment of bronchitis: effect on mucociliary kinetics. In: *Highlights in Pneumology,* edited by A. Pezza and F. DeBlasio, pp. 9–18. La Bronchite Cronica, Naples, Italy.

369. Srinivasan, G., Raff, M.J., Templeton, W.C., et al. (1981): *Branhamella catarrhalis* pneumonia: report of two cases and review of the literature. *Am. Rev. Respir. Dis.,* 123:553.

370. Standiford, T.J., Kunkel, S.L., Kasahara, K., et al. (1991): Interleukin-8 gene expression from human alveolar macrophages: the role of adherence. *Am. J. Respir. Cell. Mol. Biol.,* 5:579–585.

371. Stanley, P.J., Wilson, R., Greenstone, M.A., Mackay, I.S., and Cole, P.J. (1985): Abnormal nasal mucociliary clearance in patients with rhinitis and its relationship to concomitant chest disease. *Br. J. Dis. Chest,* 79:77–82.

372. Stark, J.E., Heath, R.B., and Curwen, M.P. (1965): Infection with parainfluenza viruses in chronic bronchitis. *Thorax,* 20:124.

373. Stockley, R.A., Hill, S.L., and Burnett, D. (1991): Proteinases in chronic lung infection. *Ann. NY Acad. Sci.,* 624:257–266.

374. Stockley, R.A., and Morrison, H.M. (1990): Elastase inhibitors of the respiratory tract. *Eur. Respir. J.,* 3(Suppl. 9):9S–15S.

375. Stockley, R.A., Morrison, H.M., Kramps, J.A., et al. (1986): Elastase inhibitors of sputum sol phase: variability, relationship to neutrophil elastase inhibition, and effect of corticosteroid treatment. *Thorax,* 41:442–447.

376. Stockley, R.A. (1988): Chronic bronchitis: the antiproteinase/proteinase balance and the effect of infection and corticosteroids. *Clin. Chest Med.,* 9:643–656.

377. Stone, P.J., Calore, J.D., McGowan, S.E., Bernardo, J., et al. (1983): Functional alpha$_1$-protease inhibitor in the lower respiratory tract of cigarette smokers is not decreased. *Science,* 221:1187–1189.

378. Strandling, J.R. (1986): Hypercapnea during oxygen therapy in airway obstruction: a reappraisal. *Thorax,* 41:897–902.

379. Stromberg, N., Marklund, B.I., Lund, B., Liver, D., Hamers, A., Gaastra, W., Karlsson, K.-A., and Normark, S. (1990): Host specificity of uropathogenic *Escherichia coli* depends on differences in binding specificity to Galα(1-4) Gal-containing isoreceptors. *EMBO J.,* 9:2001–2010.

380. Stromberg, N., Nyholm, P.-G., Pascher, I., and Normark, S. (1991): Saccharide orientation at the cell surface affects glycolipid receptor function. *Proc. Natl. Acad. Sci.* 88:9340–9344.

381. Stuart-Harris, C.H., Hanley, T., Clifton, M., Platts, M.M., Hammond, J.D.S., and Whitaker, W. (1957): *Chronic Bronchitis, Emphysema and Cor Pulmonale,* pp. 199–236. John Wright and Sons, Bristol, England.

382. Suhs, R.H., and Feldman, H.A. (1965): Pneumococcal types detected in throat cultures from a population of "normal" families. *Am. J. Med. Sci.,* 250:424–427.

383. Susuki, Y., Nagao, Y., Kato, H., et al. (1986): Human influenza A virus hemagglutinin distinguishes sialyloligosaccharides in membrane-associated gangliosides as its receptor which mediates the adsorption and fusion processes of virus infection. *J. Biol. Chem.,* 261:17057–17061.

384. Tager, I.B., Rosner, B., Tishler, P.V., et al. (1976): Household aggregation of pulmonary function and chronic bronchitis. *Am. Rev. Respir. Dis.,* 114:485.

385. Tager, I.B., Segal, M.R., Speizer, F.E., and Weiss, S.T. (1988): The natural history of forced expiratory volumes. *Am. Rev. Respir. Dis.,* 138:837–849.

386. Tager, I., and Speizer, F.E. (1975): Medical progress: role of infection in chronic bronchitis. *N. Engl. J. Med.,* 292:563–571.

387. Tager, I.B., Tishler, P.V., Rosner, B., et al. (1978): Studies of the familial aggregation of chronic bronchitis and obstructive airways disease. *Int. J. Epidemiol.*, 7:55.

388. Takizawa, T., and Thurlbeck, W.M. (1971). Muscle and mucous gland size in the major bronchi of patients with chronic bronchitis, asthma and asthmatic bronchitis. *Am. Rev. Respir. Dis.*, 104:331–336.

389. Tao, X., Hong, C.J., Yu, S., Chen, B., et al. (1992): Priority among air pollution factors for preventing chronic obstructive pulmonary disease in Shanghai. *Sci. Total Environ.*, 127:57–67.

390. Tashkin, D.P., Ashutosh, A., Bleecker, E.R., et al. (1986): Comparison of the anticholinergic bronchodilator ipratropium bromide with metaproterenol in chronic obstructive pulmonary disease. *Am. J. Med.*, 81(Suppl. 5A):81–89.

391. Tenney, S.M., and Mithoefer, J.C. (1982): The relationship of mixed venous oxygenation to oxygen transport, with special reference to adaptations to high altitude and pulmonary disease. *Am. Rev. Respir. Dis.*, 125:474–479.

392. Terblanche, A.P., Opperman, L., Nel, C.M., et al. (1992): Preliminary results of exposure measurements and health effects of the Vaal Triangle Air Pollution Health Study. *S. Ar. Med. J.*, 81:550–567.

393. Thom, T.J. (1989): International comparisons in COPD mortality. *Am. Rev. Respir. Dis.*, 140:S27–34.

394. Thompson, A.B., Daughton, D., Robbins, R.A., Ghafouri, M.A., Oehlerking, M., and Rennard, S.I. (1989): Intraluminal airway inflammation in chronic bronchitis. *Am. Rev. Respir. Dis.*, 140:1527–1537.

395. Thompson, A.B., Mueller, M.B., Heires, A.J., et al. (1992): Aerosolized beclomethasone in chronic bronchitis. *Am. Rev. Respir. Dis.*, 146:389–395.

396. Thompson, A.B., and Rennard, S.I. (1988): Assessment of airways inflammation utilizing bronchoalveolar lavage. *Clin. Chest Med.*, 9:635–642.

397. Thornton, D.J., Davies, J.R., Kraayenbrink, M., Richardson, P.S., Sheehan, J.K., and Carlstedt, I. (1990): Mucus glycoproteins from "normal" human tracheobronchial secretion. *Biochem. J.*, 265:179–186.

398. Thurlbeck, W.M. (1978): Diaphragm and body weight in emphysema. *Thorax*, 33:483–487.

399. Thurlbeck, W.M., Henderson, J.A., Fraser, R.G., and Bates, D.V. (1970): Chronic obstructive lung disease: a comparison between clinical, roentgenologic, functional and morphologic criteria in chronic bronchitis, emphysema, asthma and bronchiectasis. *Medicine*, 49:81–145.

400. Tiep, B.L. (1990): Long-term home oxygen therapy. *Clin. Chest Med.*, 11:505–521.

401. Toews, G.B., Vial, W.C., Dunn, M.M., et al. (1984): The accessory cell function of alveolar macrophages in specific T-cell proliferation. *J. Immunol.*, 132:181–186.

402. Tonnesen, P., Fryd, V., Hansen, M., et al. (1988): Effect of nicotine chewing gum in combination with group counseling on the cessation of smoking. *N. Engl. J. Med.*, 318:15–18.

403. Tonnesen, P., Norregaard, J., Simoneen, K., et al. (1991): A double-blind trial of a 16-hour transdermal nicotine patch in smoking cessation. *N. Engl. J. Med.*, 325:311–315.

404. U.S. Department of Health and Human Services (1989): *The Health Consequences of Smoking: 25 Years of Progress.* DHHS Publication No. [CDC]89-8411.

405. U.S. Department of Health and Human Services (1990): The health benefits of smoking cessation. *A Report of the Surgeon General* DHHS Publication No. [CDC]90-8416. U.S. Government Printing Office, Rockville, Md.

406. U.S. Public Health Service (1984): The health consequences of smoking: chronic obstructive lung disease. *A Report of the Surgeon General*. DHHS Publication No. (PHS) 84-50205.

407. Valentin-Weigand, P., Grulich-Henn, J., Chhatwal, G.S., Muller-Berghaus, G., Blobel, H., and Preissner, K.T. (1988): Mediation of adherence of streptococci to human endothelial cells by complement S protein (vitronectin). *Infect. Immun.*, 56:2851–2855.

408. van Alphen, L., Geelen-van den Broek, L., and van Ham, M. (1990): In vivo and in vitro expression of outer membrane components of *Hemophilus influenzae. Microb. Pathog.*, 8:279–288.

409. van der Baan, S., Veerman, A.J.P., Weltevreden, E.F., and Feenstra, L. (1983): Kartagener's syndrome: clinical symptoms and laboratory studies. *Eur. J. Respir. Dis.*, 64(Suppl. 127):91–95.

410. Vathenen, A.S., Britton, J.R., Ebden, P., Cookson, J.B., Wharrad, H.J., and Tattersfield, A.E. (1988): High-dose inhaled albuterol in severe chronic airflow limitation. *Am. Rev. Respir. Dis.*, 138:850–855.

411. Velluti, G., Capelli, O., Lusuardi, M., Braghiroli, A., and Azzolini, L. (1984): Bronchoalveolar lavage in the normal lung. II. Cell distribution and cytomorphology. *Respiration*, 46:1–7.

412. Verdugo, P. (1991): Mucin exocytosis. *Am. Rev. Respir. Dis.*, 144:S33–S37.

413. Viegi, G., Paoletti, P., Prediletto, R., et al. (1987): Prevalence of respiratory symptoms in an unpolluted area of northern Italy. *Eur. Respir. J.*, 1:311.

414. Vishwanath, S., and Ramphal, R. (1985): Tracheobronchial mucin receptor for *Pseudomonas aeruginosa:* predominance of aminosugars in binding sites. *Infect. Immun.*, 48:331–335.

415. Von Essen, S. (1993): Bronchitis in agricultural workers. *Seminars in Respir. Med.*, 14:60–72.

416. Von Essen, S.G., Robbins, R.A., Thompson, A.B., et al. (1988): Mechanisms of neutrophil recruitment to the lung by grain dust exposure. *Am. Rev. Respir. Dis.*, 138:921–927.
417. Von Essen, S.G., Thompson, A.B., Robbins, R.A., et al. (1990): Lower respiratory tract inflammation in grain farmers. *Am. J. Ind. Med.*, 17:75–76.
418. Wagner, P.D., Dantzker, D.R., Dueck, R., Clausen, J.L., and West, J.B. (1977): Ventilation-perfusion inequality in chronic obstructive pulmonary disease. *J. Clin. Invest.*, 59:203–216.
419. Wahl, S.M., Hunt, D.A., Wakefield, L.M., McCartney-Francis, N., Wahl, L.M., Robert, A.B., and Sporn, M.B. (1987): Transforming growth factor type β induces monocyte chemotaxis and growth factor production. *Proc. Natl. Acad. Sci.* (USA), 84:5788–5792.
420. Wallace, R.J., Nash, D.R., and Steingrube, V.A. (1990): Antibiotic susceptibilities and drug resistance in *Moraxella (Branhamella) catarrhalis. Am. J. Med.*, 88(Suppl. 5A):46S–50S.
421. Wallace, R.J., Jr., Steingrube, V.A., Nash, D.R., et al. (1989): BRO β-lactamases of *Branhamella catarrhalis* and subgenus *Moraxella,* including evidence for chromosomal β-lactamase transfer by conjugation in *B. catarrhalis, M. nonliquefaciens,* and *M. lacunata. Antimicrob. Agents Chemother.*, 33:1845–1854.
422. Wanner, A. (1990): The role of mucus in chronic obstructive pulmonary disease. *Chest*, 97:11S–15S.
423. Watson, D.A., and Musher, D.M. (1990): Interruption of capsule production in *Streptococcus pneumoniae* serotype 3 by insertion of transposon Tn916. *Infect. Immun.*, 58:3135–3138.
424. Weir, D.C., and Burge, P.S. (1993): Effects of high-dose-inhaled beclomethasone dipropionate, 750 μg and 1500 μg twice daily, and 40 mg per day oral prednisolone on lung function, symptoms, and bronchial hyperresponsiveness in patients with nonasthmatic chronic airflow obstruction. *Thorax*, 48:309–316.
425. Weir, D.C., Gove, R.I., Robertson, A.S., and Burge, P.S. (1990): Corticosteroid trials in nonasthmatic chronic airflow obstruction: a comparison of oral prednisolone and inhaled beclomethasone dipropionate. *Thorax*, 45:112–117.
426. Weir, D.C., Robertson, A.S., Gove, R.I., and Burge, P.S. (1990): Time course of response to oral and inhaled corticosteroids in nonasthmatic chronic airflow obstruction. *Thorax*, 45:118–121.
427. Weitzenblum, E., Sautegeau, A., Ehrhart, M., et al. (1984): Long-term course of pulmonary arterial pressure in chronic obstructive pulmonary disease. *Am. Rev. Respir. Dis.*, 130:993–998.
428. West, J.B. (1971): Causes of carbon dioxide retention in lung disease. *N. Engl. J. Med.*, 284:1232–1236.
429. West, J.B. (1977): Ventilation-perfusion relationship. *Am. Rev. Respir. Dis.*, 116:919–943.
430. Wiedemann, H.P., and Matthay, R.A. (1990): Cor pulmonale in chronic obstructive pulmonary disease. *Clin. Chest Med.*, 11:523–545.
431. Williams, J.H., Jr., and Moser, K.M. (1986): Pneumococcal vaccine and patients with chronic lung disease. *Ann. Intern. Med.*, 104:106–109.
432. Wilson, D.O., Rogers, R.M., and Hoffman R.M. (1985): Nutrition and chronic lung disease. *Am. Rev. Respir. Dis.*, 132:1347–1365.
433. Wilson, D.O., Rogers, R.M., Sanders, M.H., Pennock, B.E., and Reilly, J.J. (1986): Nutritional intervention in malnourished patients with emphysema. *Am. Rev. Respir. Dis.*, 134:672–677.
434. Wilson, D.O., Rogers, R.M., Wright, E.C., and Anthonisen, N.R. (1989): Body weight in chronic obstructive pulmonary disease. *Am. Rev. Respir. Dis.*, 139:1435–1438.
435. Wilson, R., and Cole, P.J. (1988): The effect of bacterial products on ciliary function. *Am. Rev. Respir. Dis.*, 138:S49–S53.
436. Wilson, R., Pitt, T., Taylor, G., et al. (1987): Pyocyanin and 1-hydroxyphenazine produced by *Pseudomonas aeruginosa* inhibit the beating of human respiratory cilia *in vitro. J. Clin. Invest.*, 79:221–229.
437. Wilson, R., Roberts, D., and Cole, P. (1985): Effect of bacterial products on human ciliary function *in vitro. Thorax*, 40:125–131.
438. Wilson, R., Sykes, D., Currie, D.C., and Cole, P.J. (1986): Beat frequency of cilia from sites of purulent infection. *Thorax*, 41:453–458.
439. Woodward, H., Horsey, B., Bhavanandan, V.P., and Davidson, E.A. (1982): Isolation, purification and properties of respiratory mucus glycoproteins. *Biochem.*, 21:694–701.
440. Wright, J.L., Lawson, L.M., Padre, P.D., Wiggs, B.J., Kennedy, S., and Hogg J.C. (1983): Morphology of peripheral airways in current smokers and ex-smokers. *Am. Rev. Respir. Dis.*, 127:1474–1477.
441. Xipung, X.U., Dockery, D.W., Ware, J.H., Speizer, F.E., and Ferris, B.G., Jr. (1992): Effects of cigarette smoking on rate of loss of pulmonary function in adults: a longitudinal assessment. *Am. Rev. Respir. Dis.*, 146:1345–1348.
442. Zakrzewski, J.H., Barnes, N.C., Costello, J.F., and Piper, P.J. (1987): Lipid mediators in cystic fibrosis and chronic obstructive pulmonary disease. *Am. Rev. Respir. Dis.*, 136:779–782.
443. Ziment, I. (1987): Theophylline and mucociliary clearance. *Chest*, 92(Suppl. 1):38S–43S.
444. Ziment, I. (1990): Pharmacologic therapy of obstructive airway disease. *Clin. Chest Med.*, 11:461–486.

Respiratory Infections: Diagnosis and Management, 3d ed.,
edited by James E. Pennington.
Raven Press, Ltd., New York © 1994

10

Community-Acquired Pneumonia and Acute Bronchitis

James E. Pennington

University of California, San Francisco, California 94143

Pneumonia is no longer "Captain of the men of death" (36). In fact, the availability of antimicrobial agents has resulted in a precipitious fall in death rates associated with community-acquired bacterial pneumonia (23). As an example of this remarkable progress, survival among patients with untreated bacteremic pneumococcal pneumonia at Boston City Hospital, between 1929 and 1935, was recorded as 17% (42). Therapy with antisera improved this survival rate to 53%. However, in a more recent clinical series (1952–1962), Austrian and Gold (1) recorded an 85% survival rate for a similar group of patients receiving penicillin treatment for bacteremic pneumococcal pneumonia. The impact of antimicrobial therapy on mortality associated with nonpneumococcal bacterial pneumonia is less well documented. It has, in fact, only been during the antimicrobial era that significant increases in the incidence of community-acquired nonpneumococcal bacterial pneumonias have occurred. However, it is clear that appropriate specific therapy for nonpneumococcal bacterial pneumonias will result in lower mortality (25). Finally, while so-called atypical pneumonias are infrequently life-threatening, the correct approach to management will often result in decreased morbidity (31), and in some cases, mortality (35).

Despite these encouraging observations, there continues to be a small but rather persistent mortality rate associated with community-acquired pneumonia (Table 10-1). It should be noted that these mortality data are recorded for patients hospitalized due to their pneumonia. Undoubtedly, the mortality rate for the large number of pneumonias treated in the ambulatory setting ("walking pneumonia") is much lower (6). In a series of articles by Woodhead and colleagues, the relationship between severity of community-acquired pneumonia, the necessity for hospitalization, and outcome is clear. For those cases requiring hospitalization, the mortality was 11.5%, while for those treated in the ambulatory setting, the mortality was less than 1% (46). In a subset of patients requiring intensive care unit treatment, mortality reached 54% (47). Thus, a sense of clinical urgency accompanies each case of community-acquired pneumonia, since the potential for a fatality is surely present and may be unpredictable during the early phase of illness. For example, a presumptive diagnosis of pneumococcal pneumonia in a patient with Legionnaires' disease may be disastrous, since penicillin has no therapeutic value for *Legionella pneumophila*. Further, penicillin treatment for a patient presumed to have pneumococcal pneu-

TABLE 10–1. *Mortality from community-acquired pneumonia requiring hospitalization*

Series (ref.)	Patient types	Number of cases	Mortality (%)
Austrian, 1964 (1)	Pneumococcal	1130	13
Mufson, 1967 (33)	General	427	10
Sullivan, 1972 (41)	General	292	24
Dorff, 1973 (9)	General	148	17.5
Fraser, 1977 (18)	Legionnaires' disease	182[a]	16
Garb, 1978 (19)	Elderly	35	20
Ebright, 1980 (11)	General	106	13
MacFarlane, 1982 (30)	General	127	15
Woodhead, 1985 (47)	Intensive care	50	54
Multicenter, 1987 (7)	General	453	5.7
Marrie, 1989 (32)	Hospital	719	21
Pachon, 1990 (37)	Hospital	67	20.8
Torres, 1991 (43)	Intensive care	92	22

[a]81% hospitalized.

monia who actually has staphylococcal, Klebsiella, or Hemophilus pneumonia would be a major error. This concern for diagnostic or at least therapeutic accuracy in the early management of community-acquired pneumonia (i.e., the first 24 to 48 hours) is particularly critical in elderly patients where very little temporal margin of error exists.

Since in many cases the exact etiology for community-acquired pneumonia is difficult or impossible to determine, the clinician must have a management strategy for this illness which is not dependent upon precise diagnosis in each case. This requires an understanding of the clinical spectrum of community-acquired pneumonias and an awareness of which antimicrobial agents offer coverage of the necessary pathogens in specific settings. This chapter is designed to first discuss the clinical spectrum of community-acquired pneumonia, including incidence and etiology. Then, a clinical approach is described which takes into account the difficulties in achieving specificity of diagnosis during the initial period of management.

INCIDENCE AND ETIOLOGY

Whereas respiratory infection is a common illness among otherwise normal, healthy individuals, true pneumonia appears to occur in only a fraction of these cases. Dingle and associates (8) prospectively recorded respiratory illness among 292 people in 61 families from 1948 to 1950. A total of 4,428 respiratory infections occurred, but in only 29 patients was primary atypical pneumonia observed (0.7%), and only three cases of pneumococcal pneumonia (0.1%) occurred. These data have been used to provide an estimate that about 250,000 to 400,000 cases of pneumococcal pneumonia occur in the United States per year. More recent surveys suggest that 214 million episodes of respiratory tract infections occur each year in ambulatory patients in the United States, and that among these, 1.5% (3.3 million episodes) are pneumonias (20). In addition, it is estimated that bacterial pneumonias now account for over 500,000 hospital admissions per year in the United States for patients 15 years of age or greater (20).

Since pneumonias are not reportable, however, the true incidence of community-acquired pneumonia is impossible to determine. Further compounding this problem, a large number of patients with pneumonia are treated without hospitalization. In one clinical series, it was observed that only one of every two patients reporting to the emergency room with pneumonia required hospitalization (15). More recent data suggest that 3 of 4 patients with pneumonia are now treated in the ambulatory setting (20). Thus, the possibility of at least deriving incidence and etiologic data for pneumonias from retrospective analyses of hospital discharge records does not exist for a sizable number of pneumonia cases.

A number of factors conspire to make a precise determination of etiologic categories for community-acquired pneumonia impossible. The difficulty of obtaining a good quality sputum specimen for microscopic and bacteriologic examination (34), or for that matter, the difficulty of obtaining any sputum in some patients; the lack of sensitivity of sputum smears (39), or cultures (2); the logistical difficulties of obtaining acute and convalescent viral, Mycoplasma, Chlamydia and Legionella sp serologies, plus the nonavailability of cultures for these agents in many laboratories; and finally the inaccuracy of diagnosis of anaerobic pneumonias without invasive diagnostic techniques (3), are all important reasons why the true incidence of specific etiologies cannot be determined.

However, despite these adverse epidemiologic, microbiologic, and clinical conditions, a large number of clinical studies have been designed to document specific etiologies for community-acquired pneumonias (Table 10-2). It must be emphasized that the rather high ratio of bacterial to viral etiologies in these series reflects the

TABLE 10–2. *Etiologies for community-acquired pneumonias*

Series (ref.)	Number of patients	Etiologies (%)				
		Bacteria	(Pneumo-coccus)[a]	Virus, Mycoplasma, Chlamydia	Legionella	Unknown
Pre-Legionella Series						
Mufson, 1967 (33)	427	47	("Most")	20	—	33
Lepow, 1968 (27)	98	47	("Most")	11	—	42
Fiala, 1969 (16)	192	67	(83)	Uncertain	—	33
Fekety, 1971 (15)	100	66	(94)	5	—	29
Sullivan, 1972 (41)	292	57	(62)	?[b]	—	43
Dorff, 1973 (9)	148	74	(65)	9	—	17
Post-Legionella Series						
MacFarlane, 1982 (30)	127	82	76[c]	16.5	15	3
Klimek, 1983 (26)[d]	204	100	36	—	14	—
Woodhead, 1985 (47)	50	44	32	6	30	18
Berntsson, 1986 (5)[e]	54	21	9	55	0	41
Multicenter, 1987 (7)	453	53	42[c]	34	2	33
Woodhead, 1987 (46)	236	49	(36)	16	0.4	45
Marrie, 1989 (32)[f]	719	—	—	—	2	49
Pachon, 1990 (37)	67	30	(37)	—	10	52
Torres, 1991 (43)	92	28	(50)	—	14	48

[a]Percentage of total bacteria that are pneumococcus.
[b]Serologic evidence for viral infection in about 10% of "Bacteria" and "Unknown" categories.
[c]Sputa tested for pneumococcal antigen by counter-current immunoelectrophoresis.
[d]Series limited to bacterial pneumonias.
[e]Ambulatory pneumonias.
[f]Atypical pneumonias only.

hospitalized status of the patient populations, and in a number of cases, a high incidence of underlying medical illnesses. Bacterial etiologies appear to be much less common in ambulatory pneumonias (5,6). In fact, it is safe to say that presence of underlying illness is often a determining factor for whether a patient with community-acquired pneumonia will require hospitalization. Thus, while these series record a preponderance of bacterial etiologies in hospitalized patients, others estimate that at least half, and probably more, of all cases of community-acquired pneumonias are viral or mycoplasmal (5,6,23).

Bacterial pneumonia and pneumococcal pneumonia have generally been considered to be synonymous. In 1948, for example, Dowling (10) found that among 2,500 cases of bacterial pneumonia, 98.1% were caused by *Diplococcus pneumoniae* (now *Streptococcus pneumoniae*). Table 10-2 illustrates that the clinical series reported during the 1960s emphasized the high incidence of pneumococcal etiologies. As early as 1966, however, a word of warning was sounded (40). It was becoming clear that the frequency of certain high-risk patient groups, particularly the elderly, presenting from the community with nonpneumococcal bacterial pneumonias was increasing. This is shown in Table 10-2 by more recently reported series. Most recent series have continued to document this trend (11,19,26). Fortunately, there is some predictability regarding the likely etiologic agents in specific high-risk patient groups. In alcoholics, for example, bacterial pneumonia is often caused by the pneumococcus, Klebsiella, *Hemophilus influenzae,* or Staphylococcus. In patients with recent viral influenza, the concerns are pneumococcus, Staphylococcus, or *H. influenzae.* Likewise, the elderly and the patient with chronic lung disease have a predictable group of bacterial etiologies. These are reviewed in detail in the section on clinical management, because an understanding of which etiologies occur in which patient groups is crucial in selecting presumptive antibiotic therapy for a new case of pneumonia. The most encouraging observation to date has been the exceedingly low incidence of highly antibiotic resistant gram-negative bacteria (e.g., *Pseudomonas aeruginosa* and *Serratia marcescens*), even among high-risk patient groups developing pneumonia in the community (9,19,41).

The true incidence of anaerobic etiologies of community-acquired pneumonias is uncertain. In some series employing invasive diagnostic methods, anaerobic bacteria have been cultured from lower respiratory specimens in 20 to 30% of cases of community-acquired pneumonia (4). However, other reports suggest that anaerobic pneumonias account for only 3 to 4% of cases (9,26). It is safe to say that clinically apparent anaerobic pneumonias, lung abscess, and empyemas are considerably less common presentations than aerobic bacterial or atypical pneumonias.

Finally, it must be pointed out that in virtually every clinical series recording etiologic agents for community-acquired pneumonia, there is a sizable number of cases in which no specific etiology could be determined (Table 10-2). In their analysis of 100 cases of community-acquired pneumonia requiring hospitalization at Johns Hopkins Hospital, Fekety and associates (15) began their description of the data by stating, "It must be emphasized that this analysis had to be based on clinical diagnoses. Even with all of the laboratory data and clinical observations at hand, it was difficult to be certain of the cause of the pneumonia in most of the patients." Recent advances in serologic techniques have provided more sensitive diagnostic methods. For example, prospective screening for Legionella and Chlamydia obviously increases diagnostic yields (Table 10-2). Also, use of countercurrent immunoelectrophoresis to detect pneumococcal antigen in sputa (30) appears to enhance the diagnosis of pneumococcal infection. However, since pneumococci are often resident respiratory flora, the validity of this technique could be questioned. All in all, when clinicians have access only to noninvestigational, readily available diagnostic methods, the percentage of unknown etiologies for cases of community-acquired pneumonia remains high. The reasons for this frustrating fact were outlined above. Nevertheless, the major issue remains, what is the appropriate management strategy for cases of pneumonia of unknown etiology?

PATHOGENESIS

The pathogenesis for specific etiologic agents causing community-acquired pneumonia is discussed in the relevant chapters. Several issues lend themselves to a general discussion, however. First is the role of colonization of the respiratory tract in predisposing to community-acquired pneumonia. It is hard to postulate that this is the first step in etiology for pneumococcal pneumonia since the carrier rate for pneumococcus in the upper airways is quite high, yet the incidence of actual pneumonia is quite low. Rather, it is likely that host alterations occur which allow the pneumococcus to proceed from upper to lower airway. In contrast, there is evidence that increased rates of upper airway colonization with gram-negative enteric bacilli occur in patient groups at risk for pneumonia with these pathogens, such as alcoholics (31) and the elderly (44). Thus, investigations regarding factors that increase respiratory adherence of gram-negative bacilli among high-risk individuals in the community are warranted.

Next is the controversial issue of whether viral respiratory infection is a frequent and predisposing event among patients who develop bacterial pneumonias. It is clear that for influenza A there is an increased risk of subsequent bacterial pneumonia following viral infection (29). Further, in surveying individuals with bacterial pneumonia, a large number will report on antecedent upper respiratory infection. This was found in one-third of the patients with pneumococcal pneumonia, reported by Fekety et al. (15). However, when viral and mycoplasmal cultures and serologies were carefully studied among patients with bacterial pneumonia, a close association between these infections could not be established in two separate studies (16,27). In contrast, the analysis by Fekety et al. (15) did suggest such a relationship. Thus, this point remains controversial and will probably continue to be so until more complete methods for serologic screening become available.

Finally, the relationship of host to pathogen is a central issue for community-acquired pneumonias as it is for any infectious disease. The exact mechanism by which specific host factors select for specific types of respiratory pathogens is not completely understood. Some of these issues are, in fact, discussed in other chapters in this text. Let it suffice to say that specific host factors do appear to increase the likelihood of developing pneumonia (9,15,41), and that certain factors select for a rather precise list of etiologic agents (see Table 10-2). The most general of statements is that for normal adult hosts, pneumococcus, virus, and mycoplasma comprise the list of common etiologies for community-acquired pneumonia. It is possible that Legionnaires' disease (13) and *Chlamydia pneumoniae* (22) should also be added to this short list. For most complicated patients, there generally is an expansion of nonpneumococcal bacterial etiologies.

CLINICAL APPROACH

The two questions confronting the clinician for community-acquired respiratory infection are (i) is this bronchitis or pneumonia? and (ii) what is the etiology? Physical examination and chest x-ray should resolve the first question. The second question will require a multifactorial analysis. A presumptive answer to this question must be determined on the day of presentation in order to guide management. That, of course, eliminates the use of such potentially helpful items as sputum and blood cultures, as well as acute and convalescent serologies for virus, Mycoplasma, Chlamydia, or Legionella sp. Although microscopic examination of sputum may be useful in some cases, a surprisingly large number of patients produce either no sputum (dehydration, atypical pneumonia) or poor quality sputum specimens. The following is a clinical approach to the early management of patients with community-acquired pneumonia.

The Setting

Where and when was the pneumonia acquired? What are the underlying host risk factors? These are critical questions when constructing a list of likely etiologies. About 90 to 95% of normal adults developing pneumonia in the usual community setting will be infected with either virus, *Mycoplasma pneumoniae,* or *Streptococcus pneumoniae* ("the Big Three"). The endemic incidence of Legionella sp and *Chlamydia pneumoniae* pneumonia in the community is uncertain but best estimates are from 2 to 5%. Certainly these agents are common enough that they should also be kept in mind in approaching the normal adult developing pneumonia in the community. In the altered host, however, a variety of additional nonpneumococcal bacterial etiologies must be considered. Fortunately, these are rather predictable (Table 10-3).

Special attention should be given to pneumonias developing in unusual settings. College dormitories or military barracks are notorious for outbreaks of *Mycoplasma*

TABLE 10–3. *Empiric treatment of suspected bacterial pneumonia in the high-risk patient*

Underlying condition	Usual pathogens	Presumptive therapy
Recent influenza	Pneumococcus; *Staphylococcus aureus; Hemophilus influenzae*	Cephalosporin with *H. flu.* activity (i.e., 2nd or 3rd generation)
Alcoholism	Pneumococcus; Klebsiella; *Staphylococcus aureus; Hemophilus influenzae*	As above
Chronic bronchitis	Pneumococcus; *Hemophilus influenzae; Moraxella catarrhalis*	Ampicillin, or cephalosporin with *H. flu.* activity
Aspiration pneumonia	Mouth anaerobes	Clindamycin or penicillin G
Old age (residence in a nursing home)	Pneumococcus; Klebsiella; *Staphylococcus aureus; Hemophilus influenzae;*	Cephalosporin with *H. flu.* activity
Gay male, IV drug addict, hemophilia	Pneumococcus; *H. influenzae; Pneumocystis carinii*	Ampicillin, or cephalosporin with *H. flu.* activity[a]

[a]Strong suspicion for pneumocystis should prompt aggressive diagnostic approach.

pneumoniae. More recently, *Chlamydia pneumoniae* (TWAR agent) has been implicated in such settings. Nursing homes are associated with increased rates of gram-negative pneumonia (particularly Klebsiella). Seasonal issues are also important. For example, the coincidence of influenza season and a reported outbreak in the community may lower the clinician's threshold for trying amantadine therapy early in a suspected case of viral pneumonia. Further, Legionnaires' disease appears to be more frequent in late summer and early fall. Needless to say, exposure resulting from an unusual occupation or from travel must be considered (e.g., travel to a Q-fever zone, or frequent handling of psittacine birds).

Physical and Laboratory Examinations

It is unlikely that physical examination will offer enough specificity that treatment can be selected on that basis. For example, the relative bradycardia reported in Legionnaires' disease (25) is interesting but hardly pathognomonic. In addition, hematologic and chemistry tests may suggest certain infections but are not specific. An elevated leukocyte count with a shift to the left is actually consistent with any infectious etiology, and a low white cell count does not exclude a bacterial etiology (particularly in the elderly). Needless to say, a leukocyte count of 25,000/mm^3 with 98% polymorphonuclear leukocytes (PMNs) is suggestive of a bacterial etiology. However, a more frequent example is 11,500/mm^3 with 68% PMNs, a totally nonspecific value. Chemistries are even less specific (48), despite such reports as liver function abnormalities and hypophosphatemia associated with Legionnaires' disease.

Chest X-Ray

Pneumonia or no pneumonia, that is the question, and the chest x-ray should assist in the answer. Further, the presence of lung abscess, lobar collapse, and pleural effusion can all be useful in management decisions (e.g., obstruction, aspiration, fluid for diagnostic tap). However, it is unlikely that the pattern of infiltrate will provide an etiology. A long list of pattern-etiology associations has been developed, but there are as many exceptions (perhaps more) as there are examples of conformity to the rules. Although one recent report suggests that alveolar densities, as contrasted to interstitial patterns, are more often associated with bacterial etiologies (28), this unsurprising finding does not exclude a bacterial etiology in association with interstitial patterns.

Serologies and Cultures

Although serologies and cultures are beyond the proposed scope of this discussion since they are not available during the early management period (the first 24 to 48 hours), some comments will be made. Specific serologies for viral, Mycoplasma, Chlamydia, and Legionella sp are available at certain reference laboratories. Unfortunately, they rely upon a host immune response, which generally takes 1 to 5 weeks to occur. More rapid diagnostic methods for Legionnaires' disease are being developed, the most widely available being direct fluorescent antibody stains of sputum or transtracheal aspirates (TTA), and also cultures of blood and TTA onto special media. A nonspecific antibody, "cold agglutinin," may rise during Mycoplasma infections. Unfortunately, this antibody also requires 7 to 14 days of infection before becoming positive and is present in only about 50% of cases. Further, other respiratory infections (e.g., influenza) have been reported to cause an elevation of cold agglutinins. In summary, serologies are more useful for the epidemiologist than for "day-one" clinical management.

The usefulness of sputum and blood cultures for bacteria has been discussed elsewhere. In summary, the sensitivity of sputum cultures for pneumococci appears to be only about 50% (2). Thus, if numerous pneumococci are seen on sputum smear but do not grow in culture, that does not exclude a pneumococcal diagnosis. Blood cultures may be helpful, as they are positive in 10–30% of bacterial pneumonias. Further, they may be positive when sputum is not (2). In addition to the pneumococcus, *Hemophilus* influenzae is also a fastidious organism and may be difficult to cultivate from sputum. Further, Legionella sp may be impossible to isolate from sputum, even if selective media are used, due to overgrowth of oral flora. Finally, certain respiratory bacterial pathogens do grow readily on routine sputum culture, including staphylococci and aerobic gram-negative enteric bacilli (e.g., Klebsiella, *E. coli*). The major limiting factor for sputum culture in community-acquired pneumonia remains the lack of sensitivity for the most common respiratory pathogens. Perhaps these bacteriologic limitations are not of such major clinical consequence after all, as indicated by a recent report showing that clinical outcome was not influenced by the ability to make a bacteriologic diagnosis (28).

Sputum Examination

Sputum may or may not be available for examination. Even if the patient can produce sputum, there appears to be a 75% chance that the specimen will be of poor quality (i.e., contaminated with mouth flora) (34). The ideal specimen has been described elsewhere. In one study, for collection of sputum, patients were coached and observed, and carefully controlled microscopic methods for sputum gram-stain exam were used, yet there was a 38% false-negative rate for proven cases of pneumonococcal pneumonia (39). Despite these discouraging words, it is the obligation of each clinician to attempt to obtain and properly examine a sputum specimen. In some instances, this maneuver will be extremely rewarding. In any event, while sputum is certainly less than the ideal diagnostic specimen, it is usually the only specimen available on day one of pneumonia (i.e., "This is the best of all possible worlds," Pangloss, Voltaire's *Candide*).

When the clinician is confronted with no sputum or with a poor quality sputum specimen, what alternatives exist for making an early diagnosis? Invasive methods, such as transtracheal aspiration, shielded-tip bronchoscopy, or percutaneous, thin-needle lung aspiration, have all been proposed. However, for an uncomplicated case of community-acquired pneumonia, or for an uncooperative patient (e.g., an agitated, hypoxemic elderly patient, or a combative alcoholic), it is unlikely that invasive techniques will be needed (first instance) or feasible (second instance). Rather, the clinician must understand the most likely etiologic agents in that setting and use empiric ("presumptive") treatment.

Empiric Therapy for Community-Acquired Pneumonia

The choice of therapy for patients unable to produce a good quality sputum for microscopic examination takes into consideration the clinical points above. The two most important issues are (i) is the presentation "viral-like" ("atypical pneumonia") or "bacterial-like"?; and (ii) does the host have additional risk factors?

Normal Host

Figure 10-1 depicts the two basic pneumonia syndromes which over the years have been called atypical and typical pneumonia. By and large, the normal host can be presumed to have either virus, Mycoplasma, Chlamydia pneumoniae, pneumococcus, or Legionnaires' disease. The former three etiologies tend to present with a viral-like illness, while the pneumococcus presents as a bacterial illness. Legionnaires' disease is unpredictable, and may present with features of both syndromes (24). The presence or absence of diarrhea has not been reliable in ruling Legionnaires' disease in or out (48). In my experience, the most common presentation for sporadic community-acquired Legionnaires' disease has been first as a prodromal illness, systemic in nature, followed by a consolidating pneumonia with many of the features of pneumococcal infection (pleuritis, leukocytosis). These patients generally are treated with penicillins, cephalosporins, and even aminoglycosides, on the presumption that their impressive lobar pneumonia is bacterial. Lack of sputum production, even after 1 or 2 days of intravenous hydration, should place this diagnosis in doubt, however. While Legionella sp are indeed bacterial agents, they only respond to erythromycin (or perhaps doxycycline or co-trimoxazole). Thus, in such a patient, if the "usual bacterial drugs" aren't working, a trial of intravenous erythromycin (1 g every 6 hours) is next. Responses generally become evident as early as 24–48 hours after starting erythromycin if the patient actually has Legionnaires' disease.

It can be seen from Figure 10-1 that erythromycin is an ideal empiric agent when the diagnosis is uncertain in the normal host. Obviously, this agent will not help the patient with viral pneumonia, but differentiating between viral, Mycoplasma, Chlamydia and Legionnaires' disease is usually impossible during early management. It is clear that for Mycoplasma (38) and Legionnaires' disease (25), erythromycin is quite useful. If the patient receives erythromycin but actually has pneumococcal pneumonia, this antibiotic has also been shown to work well for that pathogen. It has also recently been proposed that the newer, long-acting macrolides, azithromycin and clarithromycin, possess the usual erythromycin spectrum, plus added coverage for *Hemophilus influenzae*. More clinical experience with these new agents in treatment of *H. flu.* pneumonia is needed, however. In selecting the dosage and route for erythromycin therapy, an intravenous route (1 g every 6 hours) is generally used for the initial 72 hours of treatment in patients with advanced pneumonias. Oral erythromycin, 500 mg four times daily, may be used in less ill patients and may be used to follow up intravenous therapy when employed. If Mycoplasma is suspected (or proven), a 10-day course is sufficient. If Legionnaires' disease is suspected (or proven) a 3-week course is recommended. For *Chlamydia pneumoniae,* a 2-week regimen is advised. Since in most cases the etiology will be unknown, it is perhaps wisest to use at least a 2-week regimen for all cases.

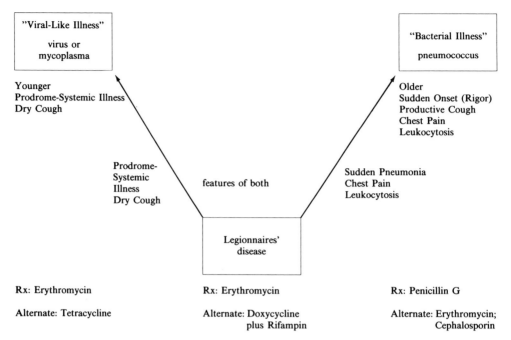

FIG. 10–1. Management of community-acquired pneumonia in the normal host according to presenting clinical syndrome.

Complicated Host

Table 10-3 lists the most frequent underlying medical conditions that alter the etiologic considerations for community-acquired pneumonia, lists the usual etiologies, and offers an appropriate choice for empiric treatment pending further evaluation (e.g., culture results). Several points should be stressed regarding this scheme. (i) This table applies only if the clinician suspects a bacterial etiology. Further, if gram-stained sputum reveals a diagnostic flora (e.g., gram-positive cocci in clusters), this "empiric" approach will not be necessary. (ii) There are alternative antibiotic choices that could be used (although they generally require the use of multiple agents, e.g., ampicillin plus oxacillin instead of 2^d or 3^d generation cephalosporins). (iii) In certain communities, ampicillin-resistant *H. influenzae* has become common among patients with chronic bronchitis (45); thus ampicillin may not be the initial choice for pneumonia in these patients. Also, for patients with chronic bronchitis, suspicion that *Moraxella catarrhalis* rather than *H. influenzae* is involved argues against ampicillin as the initial therapeutic choice. (iv) Some may choose to be even more aggressive and add an aminoglycoside if gram-negative pneumonia is suspected. It should be pointed out that highly resistant gram-negative pathogens (e.g., Pseudomonas) are rarely encountered in this setting, however. It would also be possible to add an aminoglycoside later, if the clinical course so dictated.

Where to Treat the Pneumonia

Whether or not to hospitalize a patient for treatment of community-acquired pneumonia has both clinical as well as economical implications. In an attempt to evaluate proposed guidelines for when to admit such patients for inpatient treatment, Fine and colleagues (17) evaluated 280 patients presenting to a major municipal hospital with community-acquired pneumonia. A published set of criteria, the Appropriateness Evaluation Protocol (21), was used to evaluate the need for admission. These criteria included severe vital sign abnormalities, hypoxemia, mental status change, evidence of suppuration in metastatic location, severe laboratory abnormalities, and acute coexistent medical condition (e.g., myocardial infarction). No weight was given to chronic illness, home conditions, or subjective clinical judgment. Among 280 patients, 110 met these admission criteria and 108 were admitted. However, in 76 additional cases (i.e., 45%), the patient was also admitted, despite not meeting the published criteria. This was usually because the clinician felt uncomfortable about factors not reflected in the guidelines. This conservative clinical approach was justified, as over one-third of the cases not meeting the guidelines for admission progressed to complicated courses of illness. In summary, there is no substitute for clinical judgment in determining when to admit the patient. Particular concern should be present when patients have chronic underlying illness and/or a high-risk bacterial etiologic agent is involved (17).

An even more expensive location for pneumonia management would be the intensive care unit. Predictive factors (respiratory rate ≥ 30, diastolic bp ≤ 60 mm Hg, and BUN ≥ 20 mg/dl) have recently been proposed which might allow for selecting the highest-risk patients for this special care (7,14). However, a prospective evaluation using these selection criteria for ICU admission has not been reported.

ACUTE BRONCHITIS

In many ways, acute bronchitis in the normal host simply represents a less extensive version of community-acquired pneumonia. In fact, acute bronchitis appears to be much more common than frank pneumonia (8,20). In the absence of chronic bronchopulmonary disease (e.g., chronic bronchitis, bronchiectasis, cystic fibrosis), the etiologic agents causing acute bronchitis are virtually identical to those discussed above for community-acquired pneumonia. Specifically, these include viral agents, particularly adenovirus or influenza in adults, and respiratory syncytial or parainfluenza virus in children; *Mycoplasma pneumoniae,* particularly in children and younger adults; and occasionally, the pneumococcus. To date, Legionella sp infections limited to the tracheobronchial tree are not well described. If the patient has chronic bronchopulmonary disease, then additional bacterial etiologies may account for an episode of acute bronchitis (e.g., *Hemophilus influenzae* in chronic bronchitis or bronchiectasis; *Pseudomonas aeruginosa* or *Staphylococcus aureus* in cystic fibrosis). Thus, just as for community-acquired pneumonia, consideration of the host status should provide initial etiologic clues in acute bronchitis.

In evaluating the patient with acute bronchitis, the initial concern generally is whether or not the condition has progressed to pneumonia. A symptomatic patient with a negative physical exam (e.g., afebrile, clear chest) is unlikely to have pneumonia. However, when the chest exam is positive, a chest x-ray may be required to exclude parenchymal infiltration.

Differentiating between viral, mycoplasmal, and bacterial etiologies is also an initial concern. An otherwise normal host, who is not dehydrated, should be able to provide a purulent sputum specimen if bacterial infection is present. In fact, in a relatively healthy patient with an acute cough, and productive of purulent sputum, many would automatically begin oral penicillin or erythromycin, with no further diagnostic workup. If the patient has underlying disease, however, careful microbiological evaluation of the sputum should be carried out. How closely such a patient should be followed, and when or if a chest x-ray should be obtained, must remain individualized clinical decisions. Even more problematic is the relatively well but acutely symptomatic patient without a productive cough. In the absence of physical or radiographic signs of pneumonia, is antibiotic therapy indicated? As with "atypical pneumonia," the question is whether or not a viral or mycoplasmal etiology exists. In children, the empiric use of erythromycin for this syndrome is almost routine; however, in adults, a "waiting period" is generally advocated, followed by a trial of erythromycin if the dry cough persists longer than 5 days.

One of the most frustrating sequelae to acute bronchitis is the so-called postviral bronchial hyperreactivity syndrome (12). The patient need not be atopic or asthmatic to experience this condition, although it occurs more commonly in such patients. Clinically, the patient experiences an acute episode of apparent viral bronchitis, followed by many weeks of dry cough and a tendency to bronchospasm. Throughout this period, airways are hyperreactive to cold, dry air, smoke, or dust. The pathogenesis of this syndrome is somewhat obscure but denuded respiratory mucosa and loss of the normal protective epithelial mucous layer have been demonstrated. Treatment is usually symptomatic, although glucocorticosteroids are occasionally employed. Regular use of inhalant bronchodilators may be particularly useful until the normal homeostasis of the respiratory tract returns. Unfortunately, this often takes from 4 to 6 weeks.

REFERENCES

1. Austrian, R., and Gold., J. (1964): Pneumococcal bacteremia with especial reference to bacteremic pneumococcal pneumonia. *Ann. Int. Med.,* 60:759–776.
2. Barrett-Connor, E. (1971): The nonvalue of sputum culture in the diagnosis of pneumococcal pneumonia. *Am. Rev. Respir. Dis.,* 103:845–848.
3. Bartlett, J. (1979): Anaerobic bacterial pneumonitis. *Am. Rev. Respir. Dis.,* 119:19–23.
4. Bartlett, J.G. (1987): Anaerobic bacterial infections of the lung. *Chest,* 91:901–909.
5. Berntsson, E., Lagergard, T., Strannegard, O., and Trollfors, B. (1986): Etiology of community-acquired pneumonia in out-patients, *Eur. J. Clin. Microbiol.,* 5:446–447.
6. Billie, J., Moser, F., and Francioli, P. (1986): Etiology of community-acquired pneumonia. *Eur. J. Clin. Microbiol.,* 5:389–390.
7. British Thoracic Society and the Public Health Laboratory Service. (1987): Community-acquired pneumonia in adults in British hospitals in 1982–1983: a survey of aetiology, mortality, prognostic factors and outcome. *Quar. J. Med.,* 62:195–220.
8. Dingle, J.H., Badger, G.F., Feller, A.E., Hodges, R.G., Jordan, W.S., Jr., and Rammelkamp, C.H., Jr. (1953): A study of illness in a group of Cleveland families. I. Plan of study and certain general observations. *Am. J. Hyg.,* 58:16–30.
9. Dorff, G.J., Rytel, M.W., Farmer, S.G., and Scanlon, G. (1973): Etiologies and characteristic features of pneumonias in a municipal hospital. *Am. J. Med. Sci.,* 266:349–358.
10. Dowling, H.F. (1948): *The Acute Bacterial Disease,* p. 102. W.B. Saunders, Philadelphia.
11. Ebright, J.R., and Rytel, M.W. (1980): Bacterial pneumonia in the elderly. *J. Am. Ger. Soc.,* 28:220–223.
12. Empey, D.W., Laitinen, L.A., Jacobs, L., Gold, W.M., and Nadel, J.A. (1976): Mechanisms of bronchial hyperreactivity in normal subjects after upper respiratory tract infection. *Am. Rev. Respir. Dis.,* 113:131–139.
13. England, A.C., III, Fraser, D.W., Plikaytis, B.D., Tsai, T.F., Storch, G., and Broome, C.V. (1981): Sporadic legionellosis in the United States: the first thousand cases. *Ann. Int. Med.,* 94:164–170.
14. Farr, B.M., Sloman, A.J., and Fisch, M.J. (1991); Predicting death in patients hospitalized for community-acquired pneumonia. *Ann. Intern. Med.,* 115:428–436.

15. Fekety, F.R., Jr., Caldwell, J., Gump, D., Johnson, J.E., Mᶜxson W., Mulholland, J., and Thoburn, R. (1971): Bacteria, viruses, and mycoplasmas in acute pneumonia in adults. *Am. Rev. Respir. Dis.,* 104:499–507.
16. Fiala, M. (1969): A study of the combined role of viruses, mycoplasmas and bacteria in adult pneumonia. *Am. J. Med. Sci.,* 257:44–51.
17. Fine, M.J., Smith, D.N., and Singer, D.E. (1990): Hospitalization decision in patients with community-acquired pneumonia: a prospective cohort study. *Am. J. Med.,* 89:713–721.
18. Fraser, D.W., Tsai, T.R., Orenstein, W., Parkin, W.E., Beecham, H.J., Sharrar, R.G., Harris, J., Mallison, G.F., Martin, S.M., McDade, J.E., Shepard, C.C., Brachman, P.S., and the field investigation team. (1977): Legionnaires' disease: description of an epidemic of pneumonia. *N. Engl. J. Med.,* 297:1189–1197.
19. Garb, J.L., Brown, R.B., Garb, J.R., and Tuthill, R.W. (1978): Differences in etiology of pneumonias in nursing home and community patients. *J.A.M.A.,* 240:2169–2172.
20. Garibaldi, R.A. (1985): Epidemiology of community-acquired respiratory tract infections in adults. *Am. J. Med.,* (suppl 6B), 78:32–37.
21. Gertman, P., and Restuccia, J. (1981): The appropriateness evaluation protocol: a technique for assessing unnecessary days of hospital care. *Med. Care,* 19:855–871.
22. Grayston, J.T. (1992): Infections caused by *Chlamydia pneumoniae* strain TWAR. *Clin. Infect. Dis.,* 15:757–761.
23. Hall, W.H. (1959): The specific diagnosis and treatment of the pneumonias. *Med. Clin. North Am.,* 43:191–207.
24. Helms, C.M., Viner, J.P., Sturm, R.H., Renner, E.D., and Johnson, W. (1979): Comparative features of pneumococcal, mycoplasmal, and Legionnaires' disease pneumonias. *Ann. Intern. Med.,* 90:543–547.
25. Kirby, B.D., Snyder, K.M., Meyer, R.D., and Finegold, S.M. (1980): Legionnaires' disease: report of sixty-five nosocomially acquired cases and review of the literature. *Medicine,* 59:188–203.
26. Klimek, J.J., Ajemian, E., Fontecchio, S., Gracewski, J., Klemas, B., and Jimenez, L. (1983): Community-acquired bacterial pneumonia requiring admission to hospital. *Am. J. Infect. Control,* 11:79–82.
27. Lepow, M.L., Balassanian, N., Emmerich, J., Roberts, R.B., Rosenthal, M.S., and Wolinsky, E. (1968): Interrelationships of viral, mycoplasmal, and bacterial agents in uncomplicated pneumonia. *Am. Rev. Respir. Dis.,* 97:533–545.
28. Lévy, M., Dromer, F., Brion, N., Leturdu, F., and Carbon, C. (1988): Community-acquired pneumonia, importance of initial noninvasive bacteriologic and radiographic investigations. *Chest,* 92:43–48.
29. Louria, D.B., Blumenfeld, H.L., Ellis, J.T., Kilbourne, E.D., and Rogers, D.E. (1959): Studies on influenza in the pandemic of 1957–58. II. Pulmonary complications of influenza. *J. Clin. Invest.,* 38:213–265.
30. MacFarlane, J.T., Finch, R.G., Ward, M.J., and Macrae, A.D. (1982): Hospital study of adult community-acquired pneumonia. *Lancet,* 2:255–258.
31. Mackowiak, P.A., Martin, R.M., Jones, S.R., and Smith, J.W. (1978): Pharyngeal colonization by gram-negative bacilli in aspiration-prone persons. *Arch. Intern. Med.,* 138:1224–1227.
32. Marrie, T.J., Durant, H., and Yates, L. (1989): Community-acquired pneumonia requiring hospitalization: 5-year prospective study. *Rev. Infect. Dis.,* 11:586–599.
33. Mufson, M.A., Chang, V., Gill, V., Wood, S.C., Romansky, M.J., and Chanock, R.M. (1967): The role of viruses, mycoplasmas and bacteria in acute pneumonia in civilian adults. *Am. J. Epidem.,* 86:526–544.
34. Murray, P.R., and Washington, J.A., II. (1975): Microscopic and bacteriologic analysis of expectorated sputum. *Mayo Clin. Proc.,* 50:339–344.
35. Noriega, E.R., Simberkoff, M.S., Gilroy, F.J., and Rahal, J.J., Jr. (1974): Life-threatening mycoplasma pneumoniae pneumonia. *J.A.M.A.,* 229:1471–1472.
36. Osler, W. (1901): *The Principles and Practice of Medicine,* p. 108, 4th edition. Appleton and Co., New York.
37. Pachon, J., Prados, M.D., Capote, F., Cuello, J.A., Garnacho, J., and Verano, A. (1990): Severe community-acquired pneumonia, etiology, prognosis, and treatment. *Am. Rev. Respir. Dis.,* 142:369–373.
38. Rasch, J.R., and Mogabgab, W.J. (1966): Therapeutic effect of erythromycin on mycoplasma pneumoniae pneumonia. In: *Antimicrobial Agents and Chemotherapy—1965.* pp. 693–699. Amer. Soc. Microbiol., Washington, D.C.
39. Rein, M.F., Gwaltney, J.M., O'Brien, W.M., Jennings, R.H., and Mandell, G.L. (1978): Accuracy of gram's stain in identifying pneumococci in sputum. *J.A.M.A.,* 239:2671–2673.
40. Shulman, J.A., Phillips, L.A., and Petersdorf, R.G. (1966): Errors and hazards in the diagnosis and treatment of bacterial pneumonias. *Ann. Int. Med.,* 62:41–58.
41. Sullivan, R.J., Jr., Dowdle, W.R., Marine, W.M., and Hierholzer, J.C. (1972): Adult pneumonia in a general hospital. *Arch. Intern. Med.,* 129:935–942.

42. Tilghman, R.C., and Finland, M. (1937): Clinical significance of bacteremia in pneumococcal pneumonia. *Arch. Intern. Med.,* 59:602–619.
43. Torres, A., Serra-Batlles, J., Ferrer, A., Jiménez, P., Celis, R., Cobo, E., and Rodriguez-Roisin, R. (1991): Severe community-acquired pneumonia, epidemiology and prognostic factors. *Am. Rev. Respir. Dis.,* 144:312–318.
44. Valenti, W.M., Trudell, R.G., and Bentley, D.W. (1978): Factors predisposing to oropharyngeal colonization with gram-negative bacilli in the aged. *N. Engl. J. Med.,* 298:1108–1112.
45. Wallace, R.J., Jr., Steele, L.C., Brooks, D.L., Forrester, G.D., Garcia, J.G.N., Luman, J.I., Wilson, R.W., Shepherd, S., and McLarty, J. (1988): Ampicillin, tetracycline, and chloramphenicol-resistant *Hemophilus influenzae* in adults with chronic lung disease, relationship of resistance to prior antimicrobial therapy. *Am. Rev. Respir. Dis.,* 137:695–699.
46. Woodhead, M.A., and MacFarlane, J.T. (1987): Prospective study of the aetiology and outcome of pneumonia in the community. *Lancet,* 1:671–674.
47. Woodhead, M.A., Macfarlane, J.T., Rodgers, F.G., Laverick, A., Pilkington, R., and Macrae, A.D. (1985): Aetiology and outcome of severe community-acquired pneumonia. *J. Infect.,* 10:204–210.
48. Yu, V.L., Kroboth, F.J., Shonnard, J., Brown, A., McDearman, S., and Magnussen, M. (1982): Legionnaires' disease: new clinical perspective from a prospective pneumonia study. *Am. J. Med.,* 73:357–361.

Respiratory Infections: Diagnosis and Management, 3d ed.,
edited by James E. Pennington.
Raven Press, Ltd., New York © 1994

11

Hospital-Acquired Pneumonia

James E. Pennington

University of California, San Francisco, California 94143

The lung is now the second most common site of hospital-acquired infection, accounting for approximately 15% of all nosocomial infections in the United States (16,17,32,64,136). In contrast to other frequently involved organs (urinary tract and skin), for which mortalities range from 1 to 4%, mortality rates associated with nosocomial pneumonia range from 20 to 50% (13,50,136,137). In fact, it has been estimated that as many as 15% of all deaths occurring in hospitalized patients are directly related to nosocomial pneumonia (53). Thus, hospital-acquired pneumonia is currently the most common fatal nosocomial infection in this country.

INCIDENCE AND MORTALITY

The National Nosocomial Infections Study (NNIS), reporting for the year 1984, recorded an annual incidence of nosocomial lower respiratory infection of approximately 0.60% (6.0 cases/1000 discharges) (17). The incidence was much lower in nonteaching hospitals (0.42%) and small teaching hospitals (0.54%), when compared to larger teaching hospitals (0.77%). In a separate study, the incidence of bacteremic nosocomial pneumonia was noted to be 10 times greater in a teaching as compared to a nonteaching hospital (13). The incidence of nosocomial pneumonia is particularly common on medical-surgical services (0.5–1.0%) (17). An even higher incidence of nosocomial pneumonia occurs in respiratory intensive care units, 20% (137); postoperative patients, 17.5% (45); and neonatal intensive care units, 7% (61).

The mortality from nosocomial pneumonia correlates with the severity of underlying diseases. In one series, including a large number of nonteaching hospital patients, the overall mortality from nosocomial pneumonia was 20% (136), whereas mortality rates of 50% or greater have been typical for nosocomial pneumonia in teaching hospitals (50,137). Bacteremia occurs in approximately 2 to 6% of nosocomial pneumonias (17,136), and is associated with a threefold increase in mortality when present (136). Of interest has been the relationship between etiologic agent and mortality from nosocomial pneumonia. The mortality associated with gram-negative bacillary pneumonias is generally about 50% (50,137); mortality from gram-positive pneumonias is considerably lower, reported to be 5 to 24% (50,137). Death rates associated with *Pseudomonas aeruginosa* pneumonia are particularly high, with rates of 70 to 80% reported in several series (13,109,137,141). The 25% mortality reported for nosocomial Legionnaires' disease (72) may be somewhat overstated in that a number of fatal cases were diagnosed retrospectively, without a trial of specific therapy. On the other hand, since nosocomial Legionnaires' disease occurs predominantly in compromised hosts, mortality might be expected to be higher than that reported for sporadic community-acquired Legionnaires' disease. Viral nosocomial pneumonias are usually not fatal, but deaths can occur, particularly in children with congenital heart disease (84) or in adults with debilitating diseases (96).

It is of interest that while mortality for nosocomial pneumonia has been reported ranging from 20 to 50%, this is crude, rather than attributable mortality. Recent estimates of attributable mortality indicate that only about one-third of fatalities are caused directly by the pneumonia itself (147). In a recent report from Spain, mortality from nosocomial pneumonia among ventilated patients in an intensive care unit was 42%, whereas mortality among similar patients without pneumonia was 37% (124). It appeared that pneumonia added little to the risk of dying among already critically ill patients. Thus it might be that critical care patients develop pneumonia because they are dying rather than die because they develop pneumonia. Without doubt, the occurrence of pneumonia among hospitalized patients increases morbidity, including time in intensive care units (124); however, the precise relationship between the pneumonia and outcome is often obscured by the complex status of critically ill patients.

ETIOLOGIES

Fifty to 60% of all hospital-acquired pneumonias are caused by aerobic gram-negative bacilli (17,64). Although single pathogenic isolates have usually been identified, in 10 to 20% of cases, polymicrobial gram-negative pneumonias are reported (13,17). The NNIS data for 1984 indicate that six of the seven most common etiologic agents causing nosocomial pneumonia are gram-negative rods (Table 11-1). The predominance of gram-negative bacillary pathogens as etiologic agents for nosocomial pneumonia has been noted for community hospitals (136), as well as teaching centers (137). Among gram-positive bacteria, *Staphylococcus aureus* is by far the most common (17), with *Streptococcus pneumoniae* accounting for less than 3% of nosocomial pneumonias (17).

TABLE 11–1. *Seven most frequent etiologic agents causing hospital-acquired pneumonia in the United States, 1985 to 1988*

Pathogen	Frequency (%)
Pseudomonas aeruginosa	17.2
Staphylococcus aureus	14.6
Enterobacter sp	10.4
Klebsiella sp	7.4
Escherichia coli	6.4
Hemophilus influenzae	6.4
Serratia marcescens	4.5

Adapted from Horan, Culver, and Jarvis (64).

Among less frequent etiologies of nosocomial pneumonia, several may be more common than is generally acknowledged. For example, epidemic viral pneumonia usually caused by respiratory syncytial virus and influenza A has been recognized in the hospital setting (49,55,56,57,63,71,84,88,145,148). However, only with prospective monitoring and careful evaluation of specimens by a diagnostic virology laboratory can the true incidence of endemic viral pneumonias in the hospital setting be determined. In one survey, it was reported that viral agents accounted for 20% of all nosocomial lower respiratory infections during a 17-month surveillance period in a general hospital (145). The majority of nosocomial viral pneumonia cases in that study occurred on pediatric wards. Others have observed that viral etiologies are, in fact, the most common cause of nosocomial respiratory infections on the pediatric ward (55). It appears that nosocomial viral respiratory infections are much less common on adult medical and surgical wards (71).

Legionella sp also account for a certain number of cases of nosocomial pneumonia (12,42,47,72,78,90,154). The diagnosis of pneumonia caused by *Legionella* sp requires special serologic and microbiologic techniques, so its precise frequency is presently unknown. Estimates of frequency range from 3 to 10% (4,35,90). In hospital settings with contamination of potable water by *Legionella* sp, this pathogen may account for up to 30% of all nosocomial pneumonias. However, using prospective monitoring, others have documented extremely low frequencies of *Legionella* nosocomial pneumonias (48). Two more recent reports from Canada have confirmed this finding. One prospective study was conducted at a 1,100-bed tertiary care hospital over a one-year period (81). Respiratory specimens from clinical cases of nosocomial pneumonia were cultured using selective media for Legionella. In addition, acute and convalescent sera were collected for serologic studies, including *Chlamydia,* respiratory viruses, *Mycoplasma,* and *Legionella* sp. Nosocomial pneumonia occurred in 5.7 per 1,000 discharges (135 cases). However, only four *Legionella,* one *Mycoplasma,* one *Chlamydia,* and seven viral cases were identified. In a separate report, a four-year prospective surveillance study was conducted in an 800-bed, tertiary care hospital to determine the incidence of Legionella causing nosocomial pneumonia (86). Among 813 cases of pneumonia, only 3.8 percent were definitely and 2.5 percent were possibly caused by Legionella. Thus, whereas certain medical centers encounter a cluster of nosocomial *Legionella* pneumonias due to environmental factors, it appears that overall, Legionella and other atypical etiologic agents cause a small percentage of nosocomial pneumonias.

Hemophilus influenzae is a relatively frequent respiratory isolate among hospitalized patients with chronic lung diseases (133), but has otherwise rarely been associated with nosocomial pneumonia (17). Recent reports, however, suggest an increasing frequency of this agent (64), most likely related to smoking (34). Also, enterococcal pneumonia has been documented as a superinfection among patients receiving broad-spectrum cephalosporin therapy (8). In addition, certain hospital centers experience sporadic outbreaks of nosocomial pneumonia caused by nonfermentative gram-negative bacilli such as *Acinetobacter* sp (15) and *Pseudomonas* sp. (100). These outbreaks are often associated with local factors, such as contamination of respiratory equipment, or carriage on skin of individual health care personnel. Finally, although aspiration of upper airway secretions clearly predisposes to nosocomial pneumonia (see below), large-volume aspirations leading to anaerobic lung infection appear to be rare in the hospital setting (17).

FACTORS PREDISPOSING TO HOSPITAL-ACQUIRED PNEUMONIA

Endotracheal intubation is the single most important factor predisposing to nosocomial pneumonia. Both short-term intubations for surgery and longer term intubation for respiratory failure are associated with the highest reported frequencies (17 to 21%) for nosocomial pneumonia (29,45,137). In fact, the incidence of nosocomial pneumonia for intubated patients appears to be four times higher than that for nonintubated patients, and tracheostomy further increases the risk (33). In one prospective study, 21% of 233 intubated patients developed nosocomial pneumonia, and associated mortality was 34% (30). The major risk factors associated with pneumonia in the intubated patients were presence of intracranial pressure monitors, fall-winter season, use of cimetidine (see below), and tubing changes every 24 instead of 48 hours (30). A number of other factors likely account for the enhanced risk of pneumonia among intubated patients. Apart from the obvious fact that such patients are often the most critically ill, the presence of an endotracheal tube eliminates the action of the inertial filtration system of the nose and conducting airways, and the mucociliary clearance system of the airways. Also, mechanical irritation and injury of respiratory mucosa could predispose to local colonization of airways with potential bacterial pathogens (121).

It is well known that respiratory equipment can be a source for bacteria-causing nosocomial pneumonia. In past years, the major risk of infection was associated with contaminated mainstream reservoir nebulizers, designed to deliver aerosols of small particle size suspended in the effluent gas (39,112,113,123). The large body of data implicating nebulization equipment with increased risk of gram-negative pneumonia has led to the current trend in respiratory therapy to utilize cascade humidifiers. The cascade humidifiers allow gas to bubble through water prior to delivery, but do not generate microaerosols which can become contaminated (134). Despite these advances in design, respiratory equipment continues to serve as a source of bacterial contamination (29,32). For example, side-arm medication nebulizers can become contaminated with bacteria after a single use (31). Also, condensate in dependent regions of disposable tubing can become contaminated (29). Evidence now suggests that less frequent (48 hour) rather than more frequent (24 hour) tubing changes result in a lower risk of pneumonia, presumably due to less frequent manipulation of tubes and possible reflux of condensate into airways (28,29,30,32). In fact, one recent study from Paris compared a group of 73 mechanically ventilated patients who had circuit tubing changed either every 48 hours (n = 38) or not at all (n = 35) (36). There was no difference in the incidence of pneumonia between the group with changed tubing versus without. The level of bacterial colonization was likewise similar between groups. It thus appears that reduced frequency of circuit tubing changes can be recommended, with obvious cost benefits.

Antibiotic use in the hospital setting has also been associated with increased risk for nosocomial pneumonia (67,82,140). These so-called superinfections presumably occur as a consequence of selection for more resistant bacterial pathogens during treatment of a primary infection. In one report, 149 patients treated in the hospital with penicillin or erythromycin for community-acquired bacterial pneumonia experienced a 16% incidence of pulmonary superinfections (140). Etiologic agents were either gram-negative bacilli or *S. aureus*.

A recent report from Sweden challenges this concept, however (101). Among 245 patients treated in-hospital for community-acquired pneumonia, 93 (38%) developed airway colonization, usually with gram-negative bacteria or *Candida* sp. Only two patients developed lower respiratory superinfection. Of interest was an association between airway colonization and increased mortality. Mortality, however, was not related to increased nosocomial pneumonia.

Nosocomial pneumonias are particularly common in postsurgical patients. One series reported that 50% of all nosocomial pneumonias occurred in postoperative patients (40). Others have reported a 17.5% incidence of nosocomial pneumonia among patients undergoing elective thoracic or abdominal procedures (45). Obesity, advanced age, and severity of underlying disease were all associated with increased risk for nosocomial pneumonia in that study. Considering that intubation and prophylactic antibiotics are commonly used in surgical patients, it is not surprising that nosocomial pneumonias are particularly common on the surgical service. Other conditions associated with an increased risk for nosocomial pneumonias include chronic lung disease (67,133), malnutrition (95), and advanced age (47,58,59,137).

PATHOGENESIS

Although hospital-acquired pneumonias may occur as metastatic infections secondary to bacteremia, the infrequent association of nosocomial pneumonia with bacteremias suggests that primary respiratory infection is by far the most common route. The majority of nosocomial pneumonias appear to result from aspiration of potential pathogens that have colonized the mucosal surfaces of the upper airways (67,125). In one study (67), 213 patients admitted to a medical intensive care unit were monitored with frequent cultures of the posterior oropharynx. Ninety-five patients (45%) became colonized with aerobic gram-negative bacilli by the end of 1 week in the hospital. Of these 95 colonized patients, subsequent nosocomial pneumonia developed in 22 (23%). Pneumonia developed in only 4 of 118 noncolonized patients (3.3%). In that same study, the risk of airway colonization increased as a function of time in the hospital. In separate observations, a direct correlation was made between the degree of illness and the risk of airway colonization with gram-negative bacilli (66). Surveillance cultures of oropharyngeal flora revealed aerobic gram-negative bacilli in 0% of psychiatry patients, 16% of moderately ill patients, and 57% of moribund patients. The carriage rate of aerobic gram-negative rods among normal volunteers was 2%.

It thus appears that colonization of the upper respiratory tract with potentially pathogenic bacteria is the critical first event in the pathogenesis of nosocomial bacterial pneumonia. Consequently, prevention of upper airway colonization with bacterial pathogens represents an important potential method for decreasing the incidence of nosocomial pneumonia. There is considerable interest in identifying the sources of colonizing bacterial flora. A fecal to oral route of bacterial contamination of airways has long been suspected for bedridden patients. This route cannot readily explain the frequency of colonization by organisms such as *P. aeruginosa* or *Acinetobacter*, however, since these organisms are considered unusual inhabitants of the human gastrointestinal tract. In one study, daily cultures were monitored from rectal, hypopharyngeal, and tracheal sites in 21 patients requiring prolonged intubation (131). Enterobacteriaceae were commonly cultured from the hypopharynx and rectum prior to their appearance in tracheal cultures, whereas non-Enterobacteriaceae (e.g., *P. aeruginosa*, *Acinetobacter*) were rarely found in those sites prior to their appearance in the trachea. This suggested that environmental sources existed primarily for non-Enterobacteriaceae, and that colonizing Enterobacteriaceae originated primarily from the patients' endogenous flora. A view at variance with this has been expressed by Olson et al. (100). In their report, a high rate of gastrointestinal colonization with *P. aeruginosa* occurred among patients in the ICU. It was suggested that endogenous sources could frequently account for clinical *P. aeruginosa* infections, and measures aimed at barrier protection and cross-contamination among patients could fail. A more recent report also supports the view that colonization with *P. aeruginosa* upon admission to the hospital is more common than previously believed (92). Finally, it has been suggested that an important vector for transmission of environmental flora could be the hands of health care personnel (85). Although hand washing and other infection control methods can reduce cross-contamination with certain potential pathogens, it appears that the patient's endogenous flora will continue to provide a source for upper airway colonization.

Several reports suggest that the use of gastric alkalinization to prevent stress ulcers and bleeding in hospitalized patients is producing larger numbers of patients with extensive bacterial overgrowth in the upper gastrointestinal tract. This in turn appears to lead to airway colonization secondary to aspiration of gastric microflora (38,114). Indeed, in one report, use of cimetidine was a major risk factor for nosocomial pneumonia in the intensive care unit (30). Furthermore, a recent controlled trial demonstrated a greater frequency of nosocomial pneumonia in patients receiving gastrointestinal bleeding prophylaxis by gastric alkalinization as compared to patients receiving sucralfate, a compound that does not act to raise gastric pH (37). More recently, a study has compared the incidence of pneumonia among 55 patients randomized to receive stress ulcer prophylaxis with H_2 blockers versus 49 patients treated with sucralfate (69). Pneumonia occurred in 46% of those receiving H_2 blockers versus 27% receiving sulcralfate. Finally, it is noteworthy that Cook et al. (25) have utilized meta analysis to combine data from eight separate studies examining this issue. Surprisingly, their findings suggest no increased risk of pneumonia among patients with pharmacologically elevated gastric pH as compared to controls. They did note a 45% decrease in risk of pneumonia, however, if sulcralfate, an agent that does not act by raising gastric pH, was used for ulcer prophylaxis as compared to the pH elevating agents. Their conclusion was that larger prospective trials would be required to allow conclusions regarding these concepts.

Several studies have suggested that the respiratory epithelium in hospitalized patients has increased affinity for the attachment of gram-negative bacilli (65,68,95), and that *in vitro* bacterial adherence assays using buccal cells from various patient groups may predict for subsequent bacterial colonization of airways (65,68). Most studies have utilized buccal cells for *in vitro* adherence assays, but data indicate that tracheal cells may be even more useful for such studies (96). The mechanisms by which aerobic gram-negative bacilli become more adherent to airway mucosa of hospitalized or otherwise debilitated patients have also been studied. Bacterial lectins, such as the pili on cell membranes of *P. aeruginosa,* have been identified as important in adherence to airway mucosa (121,153). Receptors on respiratory epithelial cells could also be important in mediating attachment of gram-negative bacilli. For example, a sialic acid moiety on cell surfaces or in tracheal mucin has been implicated as a receptor for *P. aeruginosa* (120). Also, considerable data have been collected suggesting that the mucosal cell surface glycoprotein, fibronectin, plays an integral part in modulating oropharyngeal bacterial ecology. Under normal conditions, buccal cells are coated with fibronectin, which in turn selects for adherence of gram-positive cocci (1). Fibronectin also appears to prevent adherence of *P. aeruginosa* to buccal cells (151). Of particular interest are studies documenting increased levels of salivary protease in seriously ill hospitalized patients (151). Increased protease content of saliva was associated with loss of fibronectin from buccal cell surfaces and increased adherence (*in vitro*) and colonization (*in vivo*) of airway mucosa with gram-negative bacilli. One study identified polymorphonuclear leukocytes in airway secretions as the source of this protease (97). The implications of the preceding biochemical and biophysical observations are uncertain, but could form the basis for new strategies in prevention or reversal of airway bacterial colonization among patient populations at high risk for nosocomial pneumonia.

DIAGNOSIS

Given the high incidence of airway colonization with potential bacterial pathogens, and the complex clinical status of patients in the intensive care unit, it is not surprising that the diagnosis of nosocomial pneumonia can be difficult. For example, patients in the intensive care unit generally have abnormal chest x-rays, whether or not lung infection is present. Similarly, fever and leukocytosis are common in such patients, irrespective of pneumonia, and cough and sputum production have little relevance in the obtunded and intubated patient. Even when the tracheobronchial secretions are purulent, the differentiation between tracheobronchitis and pneumonia can be difficult.

Nosocomial pneumonia is particularly difficult to diagnose in patients with adult respiratory distress syndrome. In one report (3), histopathologic and clinical diagnoses were correlated for 30 consecutive adult patients who died with adult respiratory distress syndrome. Premortem diagnoses of pneumonia were correlated with histologic findings suggesting lung infection. Overall, nosocomial bacterial pneumonia was misdiagnosed by clinicians in 30% of the patients.

In another study, premortem diagnoses of pneumonia in patients with Adult Respiratory Distress (ARDS) correlated with postmortem evidence of lung infection in 19 of 21 cases (7). However, pneumonia was also found in postmortem examination of lungs in 16 patients in whom no premortem diagnosis was made, suggesting that clinicians most often err by underdiagnosis of this condition. Despite these difficulties, clinical experience, coupled with careful physical and microbiologic observations, should assist the clinician in this difficult setting. Questions useful in evaluating these patients include: Has there been a change in clinical status, unexplained by other events (e.g., myocardial infarction, pulmonary embolism)? Has there been a sudden increase in lung infiltrate, a drop in arterial pO_2, or a change in fever pattern? Most important has there been an increase in quantity and purulence of respiratory secretions? Whereas such criteria for nosocomial pneumonia might lack both sensitivity and specificity, they could be the only available parameters for the clinician.

In addition to the clinical decision of whether or not a nosocomial pneumonia exists is the decision regarding etiology. Sputum, or respiratory secretions (obtained by endotracheal aspiration), should be examined microscopically using a gram stain. Unfortunately, these specimens are often contaminated with upper airway flora. Likewise, cultures of such specimens could or could not reflect the microbiology of infected lung tissues. In one series, the difficulty in reproducing growth of a single, known bacterial pathogen from multiple respiratory specimens in the hospital setting resulted in a 55% incidence of uncertain etiologies for nosocomial pneumonia (50). Isolation of a single organism from blood cultures can help in deciphering between contaminating and infecting bacterial isolates in sputum.

In an attempt to circumvent these diagnostic difficulties, a number of invasive diagnostic methods have been developed by which noncontaminated respiratory specimens can be obtained directly from the site of infection (5,150,129). These methods are probably impractical for widespread use, however; in fact, they have met with some controversy regarding their actual usefulness. Perhaps the most extensively studied invasive diagnostic approach is bronchoscopic quantitative culture of lower respiratory fluids using a plugged tip bronchoscope containing a protected specimen sampling brush (18). It has also been suggested that quantitative cultures with $\geq 10^3$ colony-forming units of bacteria correlate with clinical pneumonia (18,129). Original work with this technique attempted to verify diagnostic accuracy using lung biopsy samples ("gold standard"), taken immediately postmortem (18). However, a false-positive rate of 40% was observed. Other studies using this method have also noted false-negative results in patients receiving antibiotics. For example, in a report by Fagan et al. (43), 147 mechanically ventilated patients with new pulmonary infiltrates and purulent tracheal secretions underwent bronchoscopy with protected brush cultures. In only 45 of these patients did cultures yield $>10^3$ cfu bacteria. In 11 of these 45, a clinical diagnosis of pneumonia was not confirmed. Of even greater interest, however, was that among the 102 patients with negative cultures, antibiotics were employed in 76, which could have accounted for the lack of bacterial growth. Needless to say, the potential for false-negative results in this report is high.

Recently, two studies have addressed another liability of bronchoscopic airway sampling, that of expense and need for expertise. In one report, 28 patients on ventilators who were at high risk of pneumonia underwent bronchial lavage via bronchoscope guidance versus via blind single-lumen plugged-tip No. 14 French catheter wedged into a distal airway (118). Correlation of quantitative cultures between the methods was good. Also, cultural results were correlated with a clinical scoring system to determine accuracy of diagnosing pneumonia. Correlations were again good. It should be noted, however, that using clinical criteria for comparisons with quantitative cultures cannot be considered a "gold standard," as discussed above. Another study has compared bronchoscopic quantitative cultures using a protected specimen brush versus a blindly introduced or bronchoscopically guided, plugged-tip, telescoping catheter (111). Among 55 patients on ventilators, 78 episodes of suspected pneumonia were investigated using each of these methods. The two procedures gave similar results in 58 episodes and were discordant in 20 episodes. False-positives occurred with catheter cultures in 10 of 61 cases considered not to have pneumonia; false-negatives occurred with the brush cultures in 6 of 17 patients thought to have pneumonia. Presence or absence of pneumonia was determined primarily by clinical evaluation, however, further obscuring the ability to draw conclusions from the study.

Even more recently, Rouby et al. (126) employed minibronchoalveolar lavage in 69 mechanically ventilated patients suspected as having pneumonia, and in whom follow-up postmortem lung cultures and histologic exams were made ("gold standard"). When correlations were made between premortem cultures and lung cultures, false-positive and false-negative results were each 30%. Thus, after several years of reports using a variety of invasive methods to diagnosis nosocomial pneumonia in ventilated patients, the literature remains unconvincing that this time-consuming, expensive, and invasive methodology should be widely adopted in the intensive care unit. Traditional clinical evaluation is clearly associated with an intrinsic error rate of about 30% in this setting, but actual clinical accuracy appears to be similar to that obtained using invasive methodologies. Until more appropriate studies using "gold standard" diagnostic end points are described, routine use of invasive diagnostic methodologies for nosocomial pneumonia does not seem clinically necessary or cost effective.

TREATMENT

Conventional treatment of hospital-acquired pneumonia involves the use of intra-venous antibiotics, along with the usual supportive measures (e.g., tracheal suction, oxygen, assisted ventilation). In many cases, the etiology of the infection is unclear and broad-spectrum antibiotic coverage is necessary. Even when specific etiologic agents have been identified, it is common for combination therapy with aminogly-cosides and beta-lactams to be employed (105,129). A number of developments have occurred in recent years, however, that may alter this traditional approach.

If microscopic examination of sputum or tracheal aspirate smears does not provide a presumptive diagnosis, empiric choices for initial antimicrobial therapy must be made for suspected cases of nosocomial pneumonia. In selecting appropriate empiric therapy, clinical considerations include: Has the patient recently received antibiotics that could select for more resistant organisms? Does the patient have underlying chronic bronchitis, which would increase the risk of *Hemophilus influenzae;* or cys-tic fibrosis, which would increase the risk of *Pseudomonas aeruginosa* and *Staph-ylococcus aureus?* Have recent surveillance cultures of the patient's sputum been consistently positive for a particular organism? Also important is the recent experi-ence with nosocomial pathogens in a given hospital or intensive care unit. For ex-ample, has there been a particularly high incidence of pneumonias caused by mul-tiantibiotic-resistant *Acinetobacter* or *Serratia* during recent months? Furthermore, have *Legionella* sp been noted in the patient's hospital? Relevant to pediatric and psychiatric wards are outbreaks of viral or *Mycoplasma* respiratory infections in the community. Also important in making an empiric therapeutic decision is an under-standing of which pathogens are most likely to cause nosocomial pneumonia (see section on Etiologies above).

Empiric treatment of nosocomial pneumonia should include coverage for aerobic gram-negative bacilli, including highly resistant organisms such as *P. aeruginosa, Serratia marcescens,* and *Acinetobacter,* as well as for *S. aureus.* Based upon these considerations, several regimens have been employed for empiric treatment of nos-ocomial pneumonia. In Table 11-2 are selections of empiric therapy of nosocomial pneumonia, both in general and in specialized situations. In each case, combination therapy has been advocated, and an aminoglycoside has been included in each reg-imen.

Although combination antibiotic regimens, generally including an aminoglycoside, are considered standard therapy for nosocomial pneumonia (80,105), considerable interest has developed in the use of single-agent ("monodrug") coverage for life-threatening nosocomial infections (54,99,135). Most clinical studies of broad-spec-

TABLE 11–2. *Choices of antimicrobial agents for empiric treatment of hospital-acquired pneumonia*

Potential pathogens	Therapeutic agents

All patients
  Staphylococcus aureus
  Aerobic gram-negative bacilli (including
    Pseudomonas aeruginosa)
  Mouth flora (anaerobes)
	Nafcillin plus aminoglycoside; or
	  Cephalosporin plus aminoglycoside; or
	  Clindamycin plus aminoglycoside; or
	  Broad-spectrum penicillin[a] plus
	    aminoglycoside

Patients with chronic lung disease
  Add *Hemophilus influenza*
	Cephalosporin with *H. flu.* activity (i.e., second
	  or third generation) plus aminoglycoside

Large aspiration Maximize anaerobe coverage	Clindamycin or cefoxitin plus aminoglycoside
Legionella sp endemic	Include erythromycin

[a]For patients with sputum gram stains clearly indicative of gram-negative pathogens.

trum beta-lactam antibiotics as monodrug coverage for nosocomial sepsis have not been limited to treatment of pneumonia. However, several reports have examined this approach specifically for pulmonary indications (24,51,70,102,128,129,130,143). In general, clinical efficacy of monodrug empiric treatment of nosocomial sepsis has been equivalent to that with combination regimens (54,99,135). However, problems have also been associated with this approach (Table 11-3). These include emergence of antibiotic-resistant bacteria while on therapy (24,115,149), and in some cases serious bacterial superinfections have occurred (24). Another concern about the monodrug approach to empiric therapy is whether or not single agents would be as effective as combination regimens for treatment of *P. aeruginosa* pneumonia (102,129). Because mortalities associated with *P. aeruginosa* pneumonia are substantially higher than mortalities associated with other gram-negative bacillary pneumonias (13,104,137), optimal empiric coverage for this nosocomial pathogen is desirable. Numerous reports have described *in vitro* synergism for beta-lactam/aminoglycoside combinations against isolates of *P. aeruginosa* (41). Likewise, *in vivo* studies using animal models of *P. aeruginosa* pneumonia (110,127) have demonstrated improved

TABLE 11–3. *Limitations of newer antibiotics as single-agent treatment of nosocomial pneumonia*

Cefotaxime Ceftizoxime Ceftriaxone	Weak *P. aeruginosa* activity
Cefoperazone Ceftazidime	Weak *S. aureus* activity
Imipenem	Induced resistance CNS toxicity at high doses
Timentin	Questionable *S. aureus* efficacy
Extended-spectrum penicillins	No *S. aureus* activity
Aztreonam	Limited spectrum (no *Staphylococcus* or anaerobe activity) Resistance, especially *P. aeruginosa*
Quinolones	No anaerobe activity Resistance, especially *P. aeruginosa*

therapeutic efficacy for combination regimens as compared to single beta-lactam agents.

Clinical reports offer mixed messages on this issue. One retrospective series reported no advantage of adding an aminoglycoside to beta-lactams (94); another perspective (but not randomized) study showed a significant advantage of combined therapy in 28 patients with bacteremic *P. aeruginosa* pneumonia (62). Thus, it may be that monodrug therapies of nosocomial pneumonia would best be reserved for infections in which *P. aeruginosa* has been excluded as the etiologic agent.

Further comment regarding the role of aminoglycosides in treating gram-negative pneumonia is warranted. Although some consider this class of agent to be the cornerstone of therapy for serious gram-negative respiratory infections (83,91,142), others question the usefulness of aminoglycosides in treating pneumonia (10,93). It has been proposed, for example, that the narrow therapeutic ratios for aminoglycosides in serum, and the difficulty in penetration of aminoglycosides from blood into the infected respiratory tissues, can result in local drug concentrations insufficient to treat infecting organisms (103). On the other hand, evidence also exists that aminoglycosides are more active than β-lactam antimicrobial agents against certain resistant gram-negative bacilli (such as *P. aeruginosa*) (14,27). Two separate reports have documented the importance of achieving high peak serum levels of aminoglycosides (≥ 6 μg/ml for gentamicin or tobramycin; ≥ 24 μg/ml for amikacin) in order to treat gram-negative pneumonia successfully with these agents (91,98). Several other approaches have been utilized to improve delivery of aminoglycosides into infected lung tissues. These include computer-assisted individualized dosing (19), bolus dosing with unconventionally large doses (87), and direct instillation of aminoglycoside into the respiratory tract via an endotracheal or tracheostomy tube (73,74). In one prospective randomized study (73), groups of patients with nosocomial gram-negative pneumonia were treated with systemic antibiotics along with either 25 mg of sisomicin in saline suspension instilled into the respiratory tract every 8 hours, or saline-placebo instillations. More patients in the group receiving local aminoglycoside treatment experienced improvement, and superinfections with resistant flora were no different between the groups.

A double-blind randomized trial of endobronchial tobramycin versus placebo treatment of gram-negative bacterial pneumonia was reported (11). Patients with endobronchial tubes or tracheostomies in place and documented gram-negative pneumonia were randomized to receive conventional parenteral antibiotics (β-lactam plus aminoglycoside) with intratracheal instillation of 40 mg of tobramycin in solution every 8 hours, versus the same parenteral therapy with intratracheal saline instillations every 8 hours. Of 85 patients enrolled, only 41 were evaluable. Gram-negative pathogens were eradicated from sputum more frequently in the group receiving endobronchial tobramycin (68% vs. 31% in controls). However, clinical improvement was virtually identical between the endobronchial tobramycin group (80%) and the placebo group (81%). Local instillations were well tolerated and superinfections were not a problem. Although the results of this trial were not dramatic, it should be noted that the evaluable group had unusually good responses overall, suggesting that the nonevaluable cases were more complex. Perhaps the nonevaluable group comprised precisely the type of patient who might benefit most from innovative new therapies. Despite this moderately encouraging experience, further investigation of local aminoglycoside therapy for pneumonia will be necessary before the relative risks and benefits can be defined.

In addition to antibiotics, there is growing interest in immunologic methods of treatment of gram-negative pneumonia (106,107,108). A number of passive immune preparations, including the J-5 cross-protective monoclonal antibodies (155) and hyperimmune *Pseudomonas* globulin and monoclonal antibodies (20,22,60,106), are potentially valuable agents for treatment of gram-negative pneumonias. Clinical data are insufficient, however, to establish a definitive therapeutic role for passive immune preparations in nosocomial pneumonia at this time.

PREVENTION

The primary objective in preventing nosocomial pneumonia is to reduce the acquisition of potential bacterial pathogens in upper airways and thus to reduce the potential for aspiration of these organisms into the lower respiratory tract. Three general approaches have been utilized to achieve this objective. These include: (i) attention to environmental factors (e.g., hand washing, specialized isolation procedures, monitoring of respiratory equipment for bacterial contamination); (ii) prophylactic antibiotics; and (iii) immunologic intervention. Great emphasis has been placed upon reducing oropharyngeal bacterial colonization by infection control procedures within the patient's environment. It is clear that careful monitoring, decontamination, and adherence to the usage guidelines of respiratory equipment will decrease the incidence of nosocomial gram-negative pneumonia (113). Nevertheless, a nationwide survey on the impact of infection control measures documented only a 13% reduction in incidence of nosocomial pneumonia when strict measures were instituted in medical intensive care units (119). Although infection control guidelines for the prevention of nosocomial pneumonia have been published (132), a number of these recommendations are empiric rather than based upon controlled observations. For example, the recommendation that breathing circuit tubing be changed every 24 hours appears to be arbitrary. In one report, no significant increase in bacterial contamination of tubing was noted between 24 and 48 hours of use (28). In fact, changes every 48 hours appear to result in a decreased rate of pneumonia (30). It was estimated that $30 million could be saved annually in the United States if tubing changes were carried out every 48 hours instead of every 24 hours as recommended in the published guidelines (28). In another report, the recommendations that side-arm medication nebulizers be changed every 24 hours was shown to be inappropriate; significant contamination of nebulizers occurred after a single use (31). These published guidelines contain many other commonsense recommendations, such as washing hands between patient contacts, wearing sterile gloves for endotracheal suctioning, and avoiding contact between infected hospital personnel and high-risk patients. Remarkably few of the precepts have been carefully studied, however.

A number of groups have utilized endobronchial prophylactic antibiotics in an attempt to reduce the incidence of nosocomial pneumonia. In one study, aerosolized gentamicin was employed in burn patients with inhalation injury (79). Pulmonary and septic complications were not reduced in the gentamicin group, and the use of prophylactic gentamicin aerosol was associated with isolation of antibiotic-resistant *Pseudomonas* and *Klebsiella* from sputum. In a separate study, hospitalized patients with tracheostomies were randomized to receive endotracheal instillations of gentamicin (80 mg every 8 hours, suspended in 10 ml of saline) versus saline alone (76). Prophylactic gentamicin instillations resulted in fewer episodes of purulent sputum, documented chest infiltrates, and positive sputum cultures. However, a slight increase in gentamicin resistance was noted among respiratory isolates from the drug-treated group. In a subsequent study (75), an aminoglycoside-polymyxin B combination was employed in order to reduce resistant flora. Bronchial irritation was noted with that regimen, however. Finally, an extensive analysis of prophylactic polymyxin B aerosol for patients in a respiratory intensive care unit has been described (44,52,77). Early reports were encouraging, with both reduced colonization of airways (52) and reduced incidence of pneumonia (77) observed in patients receiving polymyxin B. In the final phase of this study, however, emergence of antibiotic-resistant respiratory pathogens and increased pneumonia-related mortalities were both observed (44). Based upon these data, routine use of prophylactic endobronchial antibiotics could not be recommended.

Since oropharyngeal or gastrointestinal bacterial flora appear to be a major source of airway colonization in hospitalized patients, several groups in Europe have employed topical prophylactic antibiotics for "decontamination" of the oropharynx and gastrointestinal tract in patients at high risk for nosocomial pneumonia. This methodology has become known as selective decontamination of the digestive tract (SDD) (122). In one study (139), trauma patients requiring assisted ventilation for more than 5 days received daily polymyxin, tobramycin, and amphotericin B, applied to oropharyngeal mucosa, and also instilled via gastric feeding tube. In order to prevent the emergence of resistant bacteria, intravenous cefotaxime was also given. Although this study was not controlled, the incidence of nosocomial pneumonia was less than the incidence during the 2-year period prior to institution of antibiotic prophylaxis. In a separate and controlled study, also conducted in intubated critically ill patients, topical polymyxin, gentamicin, and amphotericin B were applied daily to the oropharynx and nostrils, and polymyxin plus gentamicin were also instilled via gastric feeding tube (144). Systemic antibiotics were not employed in this study. Pneumonia occurred in 1 of 19 (5%) patients receiving the topical prophylaxis, and 9 of 20 (45%) controls. There was no difference in mortality between the groups, however.

More recent reports continue to highlight the controversies and inconsistencies with SDD. A prospective, randomized study from The Netherlands randomized 56 patients on mechanical ventilation to receive SDD using norfloxacin, polymyxin, and amphotericin B, plus 5 days of intravenous cefotaxime, versus no prophylaxis (2). Pneumonia occurred in only 6% of the prophylaxis group versus 70% in the control group. Mortalities among groups were too low for comparison, raising the issue of small sample size. In a separate report from Switzerland, a double-blind, placebo-controlled study was conducted using oropharyngeal decontamination among 52 ventilated patients (117). Polymyxin, neomycin, and vancomycin (or placebo) were applied to the oropharynx 6 times daily. No antibiotic was given via nasogastric tube. Pneumonia occurred in 78% of controls and 16% of prophylaxed patients ($p < 0.0001$). Subsequent need for treatment with parenteral antibiotics was more frequent in controls, as well. Mortality among the groups was identical, however, and the authors speculated that huge sample sizes would be needed to show differences in mortality. In a recent multicenter study from France, 445 mechanically ventilated patients were randomized to receive either tobramycin, colistin, and amphotericin B via nasogastric tube and as oropharyngeal paste versus placebo (46). The primary efficacy criteria were mortality in the intensive care unit and 60-day mortality. SDD did not reduce mortality, nor was the occurrence of pneumonia reduced by SDD. The sample size was large enough to result in enough deaths (75 with SDD and 67 in placebo groups) to make useful comparisons. Of interest in this study was that SDD did result in decreased gram-negative pneumonia (p = 0.01), whereas *Staphylococcus* sp pneumonias occurred at increased frequency in the SDD group (p = 0.06). Although these shifts in microbiological distribution among groups did not affect survival, one wonders if adding vancomycin to the SDD group would have resulted in an overall reduction in pneumonias in that group. Given the infrequent occurrence of fungal pneumonias in ventilated patients, one also wonders if using amphotericin B in SDD regimens is necessary.

In another report (21), 150 patients were admitted to surgical trauma, and medical intensive care units were randomized to prophylactic gentamicin, nystatin, and polymyxin (oral paste and oral liquid) plus cefotaxime intravenous for the first 3 days, versus usual care (controls). Pulmonary infections were reduced in the SDD group (14 controls vs. 4 antibiotics; p = 0.05). However, numbers of days in the ICU and hospital and mortality rates were not affected. Finally, a group from The Netherlands has recently used meta-analysis to assess whether the net impression of published trials of SDD support the claim of reduced nosocomial pneumonia and reduced mortality in the intensive care unit (146). Results from 11 controlled studies, dating from 1984 to 1990, were included. Half of the studies used historical controls and half were prospective. A variety of SDD regimens were employed. Overall, a significant reduction in pneumonia was noted, both in historical as well as prospective controlled studies. However, no significant reduction in mortality could be detected in either group. It was concluded that cost-benefit assessment and morbidity parameters must be evaluated in future studies of SDD. Obviously, this relatively expensive approach to prophylaxis of nosocomial pneumonia will remain controversial for some time to come.

Another approach to prevention of nosocomial pneumonia is immunoprophylaxis (104,107,136). There are several approaches to providing immune enhancement of lung defenses. One is to provide organism-specific immunization for pathogens known to be associated with particularly high mortalities. This approach has been evaluated for *P. aeruginosa* pneumonia, using prophylactic immunization with a lipopolysaccharide (LPS) vaccine (116). Although results from that study suggested that immunization reduced the incidence and mortality of *Pseudomonas* pneumonia, the experience was limited to only 34 vaccinated patients. Other concerns for active vaccination with *P. aeruginosa* vaccines include the side effects associated with LPS vaccine, the fact that *P. aeruginosa* accounts for only 10 to 15% of nosocomial pneumonias, and importantly, the insufficient time to develop a full immune response in acutely hospitalized patients. Recent development of a hyperimmune anti-*Pseudomonas* globulin (22) and monoclonal antibodies (60) offers the potential for rapid immunization using passive administration of type-specific antibodies.

An alternative, and perhaps even more rational, immunologic approach would be to confer protection against the wide range of gram-negative bacillary species which serve as potential pathogens for the human respiratory tract. So-called cross-protective vaccines or antisera, such as the J-5 mutant of *Escherichia coli* 0111, might be candidate immunogens. Recent clinical studies with J-5 monoclonal antibody suggest a therapeutic role for gram-negative septicemia (155). In a separate study, however, the prophylactic administration of J-5 antisera did not protect against nosocomial pneumonia (6). In a recent trial Cometta et al. (23) reported that prophylactic use of a broad-spectrum anti-LPS immunoglobulin preparation was unsuccessful in reducing gram-negative pneumonia in 108 surgical ICU patients, as compared to 112 placebo-treated controls. However, in the same trial, a group of 109 patients who received conventional commercial intravenous immunoglobulin did show reduced rates of nosocomial pneumonia (p < 0.02). The reason for this discrepancy is unclear.

REFERENCES

1. Abraham, S.N., Beachey, E.H., and Simpson, W.A. (1983): Adherence of *Streptococcus pyogenes*, *Escherichia coli*, and *Pseudomonas aeruginosa* to fibronectin-coated and uncoated epithelial cells. *Infect. Immun.*, 41:1261–1268.
2. Aerdts, S.J.A., van Dalen, R., Clasener, A.L., Festen, J., van Lier, H.J.J., and Vollaard, E.J. (1991): Antibiotic prophylaxis of respiratory tract infection in mechanically ventilated patients. *Chest*, 100:783–791.
3. Andrews, C.P., Coalson, J.J., Smith, J.D., and Johanson, W.G., Jr. (1981): Diagnosis of nosocomial bacterial pneumonia in acute, diffuse lung injury. *Chest*, 80:254–258.
4. Balows, A., and Fraser, D.W. (1979): International symposium on Legionnaires' disease. *Ann. Intern. Med.*, 90:481–714.
5. Bartlett, J.G. (1983): Invasive diagnostic techniques in respiratory infections. In: *Respiratory Infections: Diagnosis and Management*, edited by J. E. Pennington, pp. 57–77. Raven Press, New York.
6. Baumgartner, J., McCutchan, J.A., Van Melle, G., Vogt, M., Luethy, R., Glauser, M.P., Ziegler, E.J., Klauber, M.R., Muehlen, E., Chiolero, R. and Geroulanos, S. (1985): Prevention of gram-negative shock and death in surgical patients by antibody to endotoxin core glycolipid. *Lancet*, 2:59–63.
7. Bell, R.C., Coalson, J.J., Smith, J.D., and Johanson, W.G., Jr. (1983): Multiple organ system failure and infection in adult respiratory distress syndrome. *Ann. Intern. Med.*, 99:293–298.
8. Berk, S.L., Verghese, A., Holtsclaw, S.A., and Smith, J.K. (1983): Enterococcal pneumonia. Occurrence in patients receiving broad-spectrum antibiotic regimens and enteral feeding. *Am. J. Med.*, 74:153–154.
9. Blumenfeld, H.L., Kilbourne, E.D., Louria, D.B., and Robers, D.E. (1959): Studies on influenza in the pandemic of 1957–1958. I. An epidemiologic, clinical and serologic investigation of an intra-hospital epidemic, with a note on vaccination efficacy. *J. Clin. Invest.*, 38:199–212.
10. Bodem, C.R., Lampton, L.M., Miller, D.P., Tarka, E.F., and Everett, E.D. (1983): Endobronchial pH: relevance to aminoglycoside activity in gram-negative bacillary pneumonia. *Am. Rev. Respir. Dis.*, 127:39–41.
11. Brown, R.B., Kruse, J.A., Counts, G.W., Russell, J.A., Christou, N.V., Sands, M.L., and the Endotracheal Tobramycin Study Group. (1990): Double-blind study of endotracheal tobramycin in the treatment of gram-negative bacterial pneumonia. *Antimicrob. Agents Chemother.*, 34:269–272.
12. Brown, A., Yu, V.L., Elder, E.M., Magnussen, M.H., and Kroboth, F. (1980): Nosocomial outbreak of Legionnaires' disease at the Pittsburgh Veterans Administration Medical Center. *Trans. Assoc. Am. Physicians*, 93:52–59.
13. Bryan, C.S., and Reynolds, K.L. (1984): Bacteremic nosocomial pneumonia: analysis of 172 episodes from a single metropolitan area. *Am. Rev. Respir. Dis.*, 129:668–671.
14. Bundtzen, R.W., Gerger, A.U., Cohn, D.L., and Craig, W.A. (1981): Postantibiotic suppression of bacterial growth. *Rev. Infect. Dis.*, 3:28–37.
15. Buxton, A.E., Anderson, R.L., Werdegar, D., and Atlas, E. (1978): Nosocomial respiratory tract infection and colonization with *Acinetobacter calcoaceticus*: epidemiologic characteristics. *Am. J. Med.*, 65:507–513.
16. Centers for Disease Control (1985): National Nosocomial Infections Study report, annual summary 1983. *M.M.W.R.*, 33:9SS–21SS.
17. Centers for Disease Control (1986): National Nosocomial Infections Study report, annual summary 1984. *M.M.W.R.*, 35:17S–29S.
18. Chastre, J., Viau, F., Brun, P., Pierre, J., Dauge, M-C., Bouchama, A., Akesbi, A., and Gibert, C. (1984): Prospective evaluation of the protected specimen brush for the diagnosis of pulmonary infections in ventilated patients. *Am. Rev. Respir. Dis.*, 130:924–929.
19. Cipolle, R.J., Seifert, R.D., Zaske, D.E., and Strate, R.G. (1980): Hospital acquired gram-negative pneumonias: response rate and dosage requirements with individualized tobramycin therapy. *Ther. Drug Monitoring*, 2:359–363.
20. Class, I., Junginger, W., and Kloss, T. (1987): *Pseudomonas* immunoglobulin in surgical intensive care patients on mechanical ventilation. *Infection*, 15S:67–70.

21. Cockerill, F.R., III, Muller, S.R., Anhalt, J.P., Marsh, H.M., Farnell, M.B., Mucha, P., Gillespie, D.J., Ilstrup, D.M., Larson-Keller, J.J., and Thompson, R.L. (1992): Prevention of infection in critically ill patients by selective decontamination of the digestive tract. *Ann. Intern. Med.,* 117:545–553.

22. Collins, M.S., and Roby, R.E. (1984): Protective activity of an intravenous immune globulin (human) enriched in antibody against lipopolysaccharide agents of *Pseudomonas aeruginosa.* *Am. J. Med.,* 76:168–174.

23. Cometta, A., Baumgartner, J-D., Lee, M.L., Hanique, G., and Glauser, M.-P. (1992): Prophylactic intravenous administration of standard immune globulin as compared with core-lipopolysaccharide immune globulin in patients at high risk of postsurgical infection. *N. Engl. J. Med.,* 327:234–240.

24. Cone, L.A., Woodard, D.R., Stoltzman, D.S., and Byrd, R.G. (1985): Ceftazidime versus tobramycin-ticarcillin in the treatment of pneumonia and bacteremia. *Antimicrob. Agents Chemother.,* 28:33–36.

25. Cook, D.J., Laine, L.A., Guyatt, G.H., and Raffin, T.A. (1991): Nosocomial pneumonia and the role of gastric pH. *Chest,* 100:7–13.

26. Cordes, I.G., Wiesenthal, A.M., Gorman, G.W., Phair, J.P., Sommers, H.M., Brown, A., Yu, V.L., Magnussen, M.H., Meyer, R.D., Wolf, J.S., Shands, K.N., and Fraser, D.W. (1981): Isolation of *Legionella pneumophila* from hospital shower heads. *Ann. Intern. Med.,* 94:195–197.

27. Corrado, M.L., Landesman, S.H., and Cherubin, C.D. (1980): Influence of inoculum size on activity of cefoperazone, cefotaxime, moxalactam, piperacillin, and *N*-formimidoyl thienamycin (MK 0787) against *Pseudomonas aeruginosa.* *Antimicrob. Agents Chemother.,* 18:893–896.

28. Craven, D.E., Connolly, M.G., Jr., Lichtenberg, D.A., Primeau, P.J., and McCabe, W.R. (1982): Contamination of mechanical ventilators with tubing changes every 24 or 48 hours. *N. Engl. J. Med.,* 306:1505–1509.

29. Craven, D.E., and Driks, M.R. (1987): Nosocomial pneumonia in the intubated patient. *Sem. Resp. Infect.,* 2:20–33.

30. Craven, D.E., Kunches, L.M., Kilinsky, V., Lichtenberg, D.A., Make, B.J., and McCabe, W.R. (1986): Risk factors for pneumonia and fatality in patients receiving continuous mechanical ventilation. *Am. Rev. Respir. Dis.,* 133:792–796.

31. Craven, D.E., Lichtenberg, D.A., Goularte, T.A., Make, B.J., and McCabe, W.R. (1984): Contaminated medication nebulizers in mechanical ventilator circuits: source of bacterial aerosols. *Am. J. Med.,* 77:834–838.

32. Craven, D.E., Steger, K.A., and Barber, T.W. (1991): Preventing nosocomial pneumonia: state of the art and perspectives for the 1990s. *Am. J. Med.,* 91(Suppl. 3B):44S–53S.

33. Cross, A.S., and Roup, B. (1981): Role of respiratory assistance devices in endemic nosocomial pneumonia. *Am. J. Med.,* 70:681–685.

34. Dilworth, J.P., White, R.J., and Brown, E.M. (1991): Oropharyngeal flora and chest infection after upper abdominal surgery. *Thorax,* 46:165–167.

35. Dondero, T.J., Jr., Rendtorff, R.C., Mallison, G.F., Weeks, R.M., Levy, J.S., Wong, E.W., and Schaffner, W. (1980): An outbreak of Legionnaires' disease associated with a contaminated air-conditioning cooling tower. *N. Engl. J. Med.,* 7:365–370.

36. Dreyfuss, D., Djedaini, K., Weber, P., Brun, P., Lanore, J.-J., Rahmani, J., Boussougant, Y., and Coste, F. (1991): Prospective study of nosocomial pneumonia and of patient and circuit colonization during mechanical ventilation with circuit changes every 48 hours versus no change. *Am. Rev. Respir. Dis.,* 143:738–743.

37. Driks, M.R., Craven, D.E., Bartolome, R., Celli, B.R., Manning, M., Burke, R.A., Garvin, G.M., Kunches, L.M., Farber, H.W., Wedel, S.A., and McCabe, W.R. (1987): Nosocomial pneumonia in intubated patients given sucralfate as compared with antacids or histamine type 2 blockers. *N. Engl. J. Med.,* 317:1376–1382.

38. Du Moulin, G.C., Paterson, D.G., Hedley-Whyte, J., and Libson, A. (1982): Aspiration of gastric bacteria in antacid-treated patients: a frequent cause of postoperative colonisation of the airway. *Lancet,* 1:242–245.

39. Edmondson, E.B., Reinarz, J.A., Pierce, A.K., and Sanford, J.P. (1966): Nebulization equipment: a potential source of infection in gram-negative pneumonias. *Am. J. Dis. Child.,* 111:357–360.

40. Eickhoff, J.C. (1980): Pulmonary infections in surgical patients. *Surg. Clin. No. Amer.,* 60:175–183.

41. Eliopoulos, G.M., and Moellering, R.C., Jr. (1982): Antibiotic synergism and antimicrobial combinations in clinical infections. *Rev. Infect. Dis.,* 4:282–293.

42. England, A.C., III, and Fraser, D.W. (1981): Sporadic and epidemic nosocomial legionellosis in the United States. *Am. J. Med.,* 70:707–711.

43. Fagon, J.-Y., Chastre, J., Hance, A.J., Guiguet, M., Trouillet, J.-L., Domart, Y., Pierre, J., and Gibert, C. (1988): Detection of nosocomial lung infection in ventilated patients: use of a pro-

tected specimen brush and quantitative culture techniques. *Am. Rev. Respir. Dis.,* 138:110–116.

44. Feeley, T.W., Du Moulin, G.C., Hedley-Whyte, J. Bushnell, L.S., Gilbert, J.P., and Feingold, D.S. (1975): Aerosol polymyxin and pneumonia in seriously ill patients. *N. Engl. J. Med.,* 293:471–475.

45. Garibaldi, R.A., Britt, M.R., Coleman, M.L., Reading, J.C., and Pace, N.L. (1981): Risk factors for postoperative pneumonia. *Am. J. Med.,* 70:677–680.

46. Gastinne, H., Wolff, M., Delatour, F., Faurisson, F., and Chevret, S. (1992): A controlled trial in intensive care units of selective decontamination of the digestive tract with nonabsorbable antibiotics. *N. Engl. J. Med.,* 326:594–599.

47. Gerber, J.E., Casey, C.E., Martin, P., and Winn, W.C., Jr., (1981): Legionnaires' disease in Vermont, 1972–1976. *Am. J. Clin. Pathol.,* 76:816–818.

48. Girod, J.C., Reichman, R.C., Winn, W.C., Jr., Klaucke, D.N., Vogt, R.L., and Dolin, R. (1982): Pneumonic and nonpneumonic forms of legionellosis. *Arch. Intern. Med.,* 142:545–547.

49. Glezen, W.P. (1983): Viral pneumonia as a cause and result of hospitalization. *J. Infect. Dis.,* 147:765–770.

50. Graybill, J.R., Marshall, L.W., Charache, P., Wallace, C.K., and Melvin, V.B. (1973): Nosocomial pneumonia. *Am. Rev. Respir. Dis.,* 108:1130–1140.

51. Greenberg, R.N., Reilly, P.M., Luppen, K., Ballinger, M., and McMillian, R. (1985): Aztreonam therapy for gram-negative pneumonia. *Am. J. Med.,* 78S:31–33.

52. Greenfield, S., Teres, D., Bushness, L.S., Hedley-Whyte, J., and Feingold, D.S. (1973): Prevention of gram-negative bacillary pneumonia using aerosol polymyxin as prophylaxis. *J. Clin. Invest.,* 52:2934–2940.

53. Gross, P.A., Neu, H.C., Aswapokee, P., Van Antwerpe, C., and Aswapokee, N. (1980): Deaths from nosocomial infections: experience in a university hospital and a community hospital. *Am. J. Med.,* 68:219–223.

54. Guerra, J.G., Casalino, E., Palomino, J.C., Barboza, E., del Castillo, M., del Riego, M.G., Huapaya, V., and de Mayolo, E.A. (1985): Imipenem/cilastatin versus gentamicin/clindamycin for the treatment of moderate to severe infections in hospitalized patients. *Rev. Infect. Dis.,* 7S:463–470.

55. Hall, C.B. (1981): Nosocomial viral respiratory infections: perennial weeds on pediatric wards. *Am. J. Med.,* 70:670–676.

56. Hall, C.B., and Douglas, R.G. Jr. (1975): Nosocomial influenza infection as a cause of intercurrent fevers in infants. *Pediatrics,* 55:673–677.

57. Hall, C.B., Douglas, R.G. Jr., Geiman, J.M., and Messner, M.K. (1975): Nosocomial respiratory syncytial virus infections. *N. Engl. J. Med.,* 293:1343–1346.

58. Hanson, L.C., Weber, D.J., and Rutala, W.A. (1992): Risk factors for nosocomial pneumonia in the elderly. *Am. J. Med.,* 92:161–166.

59. Harkness, G.A., Bentley, D.W., and Roghmann, K.J. (1990): Risk factors for nosocomial pneumonia in the elderly. *Am. J. Med.,* 89:457–464.

60. Hector, R.F., Collins, M.S., and Pennington, J.E. (1989): Treatment of experimental *Pseudomonas aeruginosa* pneumonia with a human IgM monoclonal antibody. *J. Infect. Dis.,* 160:483–489.

61. Hemming, V.G., Overall, J.C., Jr., and Britt, M.R. (1976): Nosocomial infections in a newborn intensive care unit. *N. Engl. J. Med.,* 294:1310–1316.

62. Hilf, M., Yu, V.L., Sharp, J., Zuravleff, J.J., Korvick, J.A., and Muder, R.R. (1989): Antibiotic therapy for *Pseudomonas aeruginosa* bacteremia: outcome correlations in a prospective study of 200 patients. *Am. J. Med.,* 87:540–546.

63. Hoffman, P.C., and Dixon, R.E. (1977): Control of influenza in the hospital. *Ann. Intern. Med.,* 87:725–728.

64. Horan, T., Culver, D., and Jarvis, W. (1988): Pathogens causing nosocomial infections. *Antimicrob. Newslett.,* 5:65–67.

65. Johanson, W.G., Jr., Higuchi, J.G., Chaudhuri, T.R., and Woods, D.E. (1980): Bacterial adherence to epithelial cells in bacillary colonization of the respiratory tract. *Am. Rev. Respir. Dis.,* 121:55–63.

66. Johanson, W.G., Jr., Pierce, A.K., and Sanford, J.P. (1969): Changing pharyngeal bacterial flora of hospitalized patients. *N. Engl. J. Med.,* 281:1137–1140.

67. Johanson, W.G., Jr., Pierce, A.K., Sanford, J.P., and Thomas, G.D. (1972): Nosocomial respiratory infections with gram-negative bacilli. *Ann. Intern. Med.,* 77:701–706.

68. Johanson, W.G., Jr., Woods, D.E., and Chaudhuri, T. (1979): Association of respiratory tract colonization with adherence of gram-negative bacilli to epithelial cells. *J. Infect. Dis.,* 139:667–673.

69. Kappstein, I., Schulgen, G., Friedrich, T., Hellinger, P., Benzing, A., Geiger, K., and Daschner, F.D. (1991): Incidence of pneumonia in mechanically ventilated patients treated with sucralfate

or cimetidine as prophylaxis for stress bleeding: bacterial colonization of the stomach. *Am. J. Med.*, 91(Suppl. 2A):125S–131S.

70. Khan, F.A., and Basir, R. (1989): Sequential intravenous-oral administration of ciprofloxacin vs. ceftazidime in serious bacterial respiratory tract infections. *Chest*, 96:528–537.
71. Kimball, A.M., Foy, H.M., Cooney, M.K., Allan, I.D., Matlock, M., and Plorde, J.J. (1983): Isolation of respiratory syncytial and influenza viruses from the sputum of patients hospitalized with pneumonia. *J. Infect. Dis.*, 147:181–184.
72. Kirby, B.D., Snyder, K.M., Meyer, R.D., and Finegold, S.M. (1980): Legionnaires' disease: report of sixty-five nosocomially acquired cases and review of the literature. *Medicine*, 59:188–205.
73. Klastersky, J., Carpentier-Meunier, F., Kahan-Coppens, L., and Thys, J.P. (1979): Endotracheally administered antibiotics for gram-negative bronchopneumonia. *Chest*, 75:586–591.
74. Klastersky, J., Geuning, C., Mouawad, E., and Daneau, D. (1972): Endotracheal gentamicin in bronchial infections in patients with tracheostomy. *Chest*, 61:117–120.
75. Klastersky, J., Hensgens, C., Noterman, J., Mouawad, E., and Meunier-Carpentier, F. (1975): Endotracheal antibiotics for the prevention of tracheobronchial infections in tracheotomized unconscious patients: a comparative study of gentamicin and aminosidinpolymyxin B combination. *Chest*, 68:302–306.
76. Klastersky, J., Huysmans, E., Weerts, D., Hensgens, C., and Daneau, D. (1974); Endotracheally administered gentamicin for the prevention of infections of the respiratory tract in patients with tracheostomy: a double-blind study. *Chest*, 65:650–654.
77. Klick, J.M., Du Moulin, G.C., Hedley-Whyte, J., Teres, D., Bushnell, L.S., and Feingold, D.S. (1975): Prevention of gram-negative bacillary pneumonia using polymyxin aerosol as prophylaxis. II. Effect on the incidence of pneumonia in seriously ill patients. *J. Clin. Invest.*, 55:514–519.
78. Korvick, J.A., Yu, V.L., and Fang, G. (1987): Legionella species as hospital-acquired respiratory pathogens. *Sem. Resp. Infect.*, 2:34–47.
79. Levine, B.A., Petroff, P.A., Slade, C.L., and Pruitt, B.A. Jr. (1978): Prospective trials of dexamethasone and aerosolized gentamicin in the treatment of inhalation injury in the burned patient. *J. Trauma*, 18:188–193.
80. Levison, M.E., and Kaye, D. (1985): Pneumonia caused by gram-negative bacilli: an overview. *Rev. Infect. Dis.*, 7S:656–665.
81. Louie, M., Dyck, B., Parker, S., Sekla, L., and Nicolle, L.E. (1991): Nosocomial pneumonia in a Canadian tertiary care center: a prospective surveillance study. *Infect. Control Hosp. Epidemiol.*, 12:356–363.
82. Louria, D.B., and Kaminski, T. (1962): The effects of four antimicrobial drug regimens on sputum superinfection in hospitalized patients. *Am. Rev. Respir. Dis.*, 85:649–665.
83. Louria, D.B., Young, L., Armstrong, D., and Smith, J.K. (1969): Gentamicin in the treatment of pulmonary infections. *J. Infect. Dis.*, 119:483–485.
84. MacDonald, N.E., Hall, C.B., Suffin, S.C., Alexson, C., Harris, P.J., and Manning, J.A. (1982): Respiratory syncytial viral infection in infants with congenital heart disease. *N. Engl. J. Med.*, 307:397–400.
85. Maki, D.G., Alvarado, C.J., Hassemer, C.A., and Zilz, M.A. (1982): Relation of the inanimate hospital environment to endemic nosocomial infection. *N. Engl. J. Med.*, 25:1562–1566.
86. Marrie, T.J., MacDonald, S., Clarke, K., and Haldane, D. (1991): Nosocomial Legionnaires' disease: lessons from a four-year prospective study. *Am. J. Infect. Control*, 19:79–85.
87. Martin, A.J., Smalley, C.A., George, R.H., Healing, D.E., and Anderson, C.M. (1980): Gentamicin and tobramycin compared in the treatment of mucoid *Pseudomonas* lung infections in cystic fibrosis. *Arch. Dis. Child.*, 55:604–607.
88. Mathur, U., Bentley, D.W., and Hall, C.B. (1980): Concurrent respiratory syncytial virus and influenza A infections in the institutionalized elderly and chronically ill. *Ann. Intern. Med.*, 93:49–52.
89. Meibalane, R., Sedmak, G.V., Sasidharan, P., Garg, P., and Grausz, J.P. (1977): Outbreak of influenza in a neonatal intensive care unit. *J. Pediatr.*, 91:974–976.
90. Meyer, R.D., and Edelstein, P.H. (1983): *Legionella* pneumonias. In: *Respiratory Infections: Diagnosis and Management*, edited by J.E. Pennington, pp. 283–297. Raven Press, New York.
91. Moore, R.D., Smith, C.R., and Lietman, P.S. (1984): Association of aminoglycoside plasma levels with therapeutic outcome in gram-negative pneumonia. *Am. J. Med.*, 77:657–662.
92. Murthy, S.K., Baltch, A.L., Smith, R.P., Desjardin, E.K., Hammer, M.C., Conroy, J.V., and Michelsen, P.B. (1989): Oropharyngeal and fecal carriage of *Pseudomonas aeruginosa* in hospital patients. *J. Clin. Microbiol.*, 27:35–40.
93. Neu, H.C. (1982): Clinical use of aminoglycosides. In: *The Aminoglycosides, Microbiology, Clinical Use and Toxicology*, edited by A. Whelton and H.C. Neu, pp. 611–628. Marcel Dekker, New York.
94. Nichols, L., and Maki, D.G. (1985): The emergence of resistance to beta-lactam antibiotics dur-

ing treatment of *Pseudmonas aeruginosa* lower respiratory tract infections: Is combination therapy the solution? *Chemoterapia*, 4:102–109.

95. Niederman, M.S., Merrill, W.M., Ferranti, R.D., Pagano, K.M., Palmer, L.B., and Reynolds, H.Y. (1984): Nutritional status and bacterial binding in the lower respiratory tract in patients with chronic tracheostomy. *Ann. Intern. Med.*, 100:795–800.

96. Niederman, M.S., Rafferty, T.D., Sasaki, C.T., Merrill, W.M., Matthay, R.A., and Reynolds, H.Y. (1983): Comparison of bacterial adherence to ciliated and squamous epithelial cells obtained from the human respiratory tract. *Am. Rev. Respir. Dis.*, 127:85–90.

97. Nogare, A.R.D., Toews, G.B., and Pierce, A.K. (1987): Increased salivary elastase precedes gram-negative bacillary colonization in postoperative patients. *Am. Rev. Respir. Dis.*, 135:671–675.

98. Noone, P., Pattison, J.R., and Garfield Danies, D. (1974): The effective use of gentamicin in life-threatening sepsis. *Postgrad. Med. J.*, 50S:9–16.

99. Oblinger, M.J., Bowers, J.T., Sande, M.A., and Mandell, G.L. (1982): Moxalactam therapy versus standard antimicrobial therapy for selected serious infections. *Rev. Infect. Dis.*, 4S:639–649.

100. Olson, B., Weinstein, R.A., Nathan, C., Chamberline, W., and Kabins, S.A. (1984): Epidemiology of endemic *Pseudomonas aeruginosa:* why infection control efforts have failed. *J. Infect. Dis.*, 150:808–816.

101. Örtqvist, A., Hammers-Berggren, S., and Kalin, M. (1990): Respiratory tract colonization and incidence of secondary infection during hospital treatment of community-acquired pneumonia. *Eur. J. Clin. Microbiol. Infect. Dis.*, 9:725–731.

102. Peloquin, C.A., Cumbo, T.J., Nix, D.E., Sands, M.F., and Schentag, J.J. (1989): Evaluation of intravenous ciprofloxacin in patients with nosocomial lower respiratory tract infections. *Arch. Intern. Med.*, 149:2269–2273.

103. Pennington, J.E. (1981): Penetration of antibiotics into respiratory secretions. *Rev. Infect. Dis.*, 3:67–73.

104. Pennington, J.E. (1983): *Pseudomonas aeruginosa* pneumonia: the potential for immune intervention. In: *Seminars in Infectious Diseases*, edited by L. Weinstein and B.N. Fields, pp. 71–80. Thieme-Stratton, New York.

105. Pennington, J.E. (1985): Nosocomial respiratory infection. In: *Principles and Practice of Infectious Diseases*, 2nd Edition, edited by F.L. Mandell, R.G. Douglas, Jr., and J.E. Bennett, pp. 1602–1625. John Wiley and Sons, New York.

106. Pennington, J.E. (1987): New therapeutic approaches to hospital-acquired pneumonia. *Sem. Resp. Infect.*, 2:67–73.

107. Pennington, J.E. (1992): Immunological perspectives in prevention and treatment of nosocomial pneumonia. *Intensive Care Med.*, 18:S35–S38.

108. Pennington, J.E., Pier, G.B., and Small, G.J. (1986): Efficacy of intravenous immune globulin for treatment of experimental *Pseudomonas aeruginosa* pneumonia. *J. Crit. Car.*, 1:4–10.

109. Pennington, J.E., Reynolds, H.Y., and Carbone, P.P. (1973): *Pseudomonas* pneumonia: a retrospective study of 36 cases. *Am. J.Med.*, 55:155–160.

110. Pennington, J.E., Schiff, J.B., and Johnson, C.B. (1984): Therapeutic lessons learned from pneumonia models. In: *Current Aspects of Bacterial and Non-Bacterial Pneumonias*, edited by H. Lode, B. Kemmerich, and J. Klastersky, pp. 61–69. Georg Thieme Verlag, Stuttgart, Germany.

111. Pham, L.H., Brun-Guisson, C., Legrand, P., Rauss, A., Verra, F., Brochard, L., and Lemaire, F. (1991): Diagnosis of nosocomial pneumonia in mechanically ventilated patients. *Am. Rev. Respir. Dis.*, 143:1055–1061.

112. Pierce, A.K., and Sanford, J.P. (1973): Bacterial contamination of aerosols. *Arch. Intern. Med.*, 131:156–159.

113. Pierce, A.K., Sanford, J.P., Thomas, G.D., and Leonard, J.S. (1970): Long-term evaluation of decontamination of inhalation-therapy equipment and the occurrence of necrotizing pneumonia. *N. Engl. J. Med.*, 282:528–531.

114. Pingleton, S.K., Hinthorn, D.R., and Liu, C. (1986): Enteral nutrition in patients receiving mechanical ventilation. *Am. J. Med.*, 80:827–832.

115. Platt, R., Ehrlich, S.L., Afarian, J., O'Brien, T.F., Pennington, J.E., and Kass, E.H. (1981): Moxalactam therapy of infections caused by cephalothin resistant bacteria: influence of serum inhibitory activity on clinical response; acquisition of antibiotic resistance during therapy. *Antimicrob. Agents Chemother.*, 20:351–355.

116. Polk, H.C., Jr., Borden, S., and Aldrett, J.A. (1973): Prevention of *Pseudomonas* respiratory infection in a surgical intensive care unit. *Ann. Surg.*, 177:607–615.

117. Pugin, J., Auckenthaler, R., Lew, D.P., and Suter, P.M. (1991): Oropharyngeal decontamination decreases incidence of ventilator-associated pneumonia. *J.A.M.A.*, 265:2704–2710.

118. Pugin, J., Auckenthaler, R., Mili, N., Janssens, J.-P., Lew, P.D., and Suter, P.M. (1991): Diagnosis of ventilator-associated pneumonia by bacteriologic analysis of bronchoscopic and non-bronchoscopic "blind" bronchoalveolar lavage fluid. *Am. Rev. Respir. Dis.*, 143:1121–1129.

119. Quade, D., Culver, D.H., Haley, R.W., Whaley, F.S., Kalsbeek, W.D., Hardison, C.D., Hohn-

son, R.E., Stanley, R.C., and Shachtman, R.H. (1980): The SENIC sampling process: design for choosing hospitals and patients and results of sample selection. *Am. J. Epidemiol.*, 111:486–502.

120. Ramphal, R., and Pyle, M. (1983): Evidence for mucins and sialic acid as receptors for *Pseudomonas aeruginosa* in the lower respiratory tract. *Infect. Immun.*, 41:339–344.

121. Ramphal, R., Sadoff, J.C., Pyle, M., and Silipigni, J.D. (1984): Role of pili in the adherence of *Pseudomonas aeruginosa* to injured tracheal epithelium. *Infect. Immun.*, 44:38–40.

122. Ramsay, G., and Reidy, J.J. (1990): Selective decontamination in intensive care practice: a review of clinical experience. *Intensive Care Med.*, 16:S217–S223.

123. Reinarz, J.A., Pierce, A.K., Mays, B.B., and Sanford, J.P. (1965): The potential role of inhalation therapy equipment in nosocomial pulmonary infection. *J. Clin. Invest.*, 44:831–839.

124. Rello, J., Quintana, E., Ausina, V., Castella, J., Luquin, M., Net, A., and Prats, G. (1991): Incidence, etiology, and outcome of nosocomial pneumonia on mechanically ventilated patients. *Chest*, 100:439–444.

125. Reynolds, H.Y. (1987): Bacterial adherence to respiratory tract mucosa—a dynamic interaction leading to colonization. *Sem. Resp. Infect.*, 2:8–19.

126. Rouby, J.-J., De Lassale, E.M., Poete, P., Nicolas, M.-H., Bodin, L., Jarlier, V., Le Charpentier, Y., Grosset, J., and Viars, P. (1992): Nosocomial bronchopneumonia in the critically ill: histologic and bacteriologic aspects. *Am. Rev. Respir. Dis.*, 146:1059–1066.

127. Rusnak, M.G., Drake, T.A., Hackbarth, C.J., and Sande, M.A. (1984): Single versus combination antibiotic therapy for pneumonia due to *Pseudomonas aeruginosa* in neutropenic guinea pigs. *J. Infect. Dis.*, 149:980–985.

128. Salata, R.A., Gebhart, R.L., Palmer, D.L., Wade, B.H., Scheld, W.M., Groschel, D.H.M., Wenzel, R.P., Mandell, G.L., and Duma, R.J. (1985): Pneumonia treated with imipenem/cilastatin. *Am. J. Med.*, 78S:104–109.

129. Scheld, W.M., and Mandell, G.L. (1991): Nosocomial pneumonia: pathogenesis and recent advances in diagnosis and therapy. *Rev. Infect. Dis.*, 13:S743–S751.

130. Schentag, J.J., Reitberg, D.P., and Cumbo, T.J. (1984): Cefmenoxime efficacy, safety, and pharmacokinetics in critical care patients with nosocomial pneumonia. *Am. J. Med.*, 77S:34–42.

131. Schwartz, S.N., Dowling, J.N., Benkovic, C., DeQuittner-Buchanan, M., Prostko, T., and Yee, R.B. (1978): Sources of gram-negative bacilli colonizing the tracheae of intubated patients. *J. Infect. Dis.*, 138:227–231.

132. Simmons, B.P., and Wong, E.S. (1982): Guidelines for prevention of nosocomial pneumonia. *Infect. Control*, 3:327–333.

133. Simon, H.B., Southwick, F.S., Moellering, R.C., and Sherman, E. (1980): *Hemophilus influenzae* in hospitalized adults: current perspectives. *Am. J. Med.*, 69:219–226.

134. Shultze, T., Edmondson, E.B., Pierce, A.K., and Sanford, J.P. (1967): Studies of a new humidifying device as a potential source of bacterial aerosols. *Am. Rev. Respir. Dis.*, 96:517–519.

135. Smith, C.R., Ambinder, R., Lipsky, J.J., Petty, B.G., Israel, E., Levitt, R., Mellits, E.D., Rocco, L., Longstreth, J., and Lietman, P.S. (1984): Cefotaxime compared with nafcillin plus tobramycin for serious bacterial infections: a randomized, double-blind trial. *Ann. Intern. Med.*, 101:469–477.

136. Stamm, W.E., Martin, S.M., and Bennett, J.V. (1977): Epidemiology of nosocomial infections due to gram-negative bacilli: aspects relevant to development and use of vaccines. *J. Infect. Dis.*, 136S:151–160.

137. Stevens, R.M., Teres, D., Skillman, J.J., and Feingold, D.S. (1974): Pneumonia in an intensive care unit. *Arch. Intern. Med.*, 134:106–111.

138. Stout, J., Yu, V.L., Vickers, R.M., Zuravleff, J., Best, M., Brown, A., Yee, R.B., and Wadowsky, R. (1982): Ubiquitousness of *Legionella pneumophila* in the water supply of a hospital with epidemic Legionnaires' disease. *N. Engl. J. Med.*, 306:466–468.

139. Stoutenbeek, C.P., van Saene, H.K.F., Miranda, D.R., and Zandstra, D.F. (1984): The effect of selective decontamination of the digestive tract on colonisation and infection rate in multiple trauma patients. *Intensive Care Med.*, 10:185–192.

140. Tillotson, J.R., and Finland, M. (1969): Bacterial colonization and clinical superinfection of the respiratory tract complicating antibiotic treatment of pneumonia. *J. Infect. Dis.*, 119:597–624.

141. Tillotson, J.R., and Lerner, A.M. (1968): Characteristics of non-bacteremic *Pseudomonas* pneumonia. *Ann. Intern. Med.*, 68:295–307.

142. Trenholme, G.M., McKellar, P.P., Rivera, N., and Levin, S. (1977): Amikacin in the treatment of gram-negative pneumonia. *Am. J. Med.*, 62:949–953.

143. Trenholme, G.M., Pottage, J.C., Jr., and Karakusis, P.H. (1985): Use of ceftazidime in the treatment of nosocomial lower respiratory infections. *Am. J. Med.*, 79S:32–36.

144. Unertl, K., Ruckdeschel, G., Selbmann, H.K., Jensen, U., Forst, H., Lenhart, F.P., and Peter, K. (1987): Prevention of colonization and respiratory infections in long-term ventilated patients by local antimicrobial prophylaxis. *Intensive Care Med.*, 13:106–113.

145. Valenti, W.M., Hall, C.B., Douglas, R.G., Jr., Menegus, M.A., and Pincus, P.H. (1979): Nosocomial viral infections. 1. Epidemiology and significance. *Infect. Control*, 1:33–37.

146. Vandenbroucke-Grauls, C.M.J.E., and Vandenbroucke, J.P. (1991): Effect of selective decontamination of the digestive tract on respiratory tract infections and mortality in the intensive care unit. *Lancet*, 338:859–862.

147. Wenzel, R.P. (1989): Hospital-acquired pneumonia: overview of the current state of the art for prevention and control. *Eur. J. Clin. Microbiol. Infect. Dis.*, 8:56–60.

148. Wenzel, R.P., Deal, E.C., and Hendley, J.O. (1977): Hospital-acquired viral respiratory illness on a pediatric ward. *Pediatrics*, 60:367–371.

149. Winston, D.J., McGrattan, M.A., and Busuttil, R.W. (1984): Imipenem therapy of *Pseudomonas aeruginosa* and other serious bacterial infections. *Antimicrob. Agents Chemother.*, 26:673–677.

150. Winterbauer, R.H., and Dreis, D.F. (1987): New diagnostic approaches to the hospitalized patient with pneumonia. *Sem. Resp. Infect.*, 2:57–66.

151. Woods, D.E., Straus, D.C., Johanson, W.G., Jr., and Bass, J.A. (1981): Role of fibronectin in the prevention of adherence of *Pseudomonas aeruginosa* to buccal cells. *J. Infect. Dis.*, 143:784–790.

152. Woods, D.E., Straus, D.C., Johanson, W.G., Jr., and Bass, J.A. (1981); Role of salivary protease activity in adherence of gram-negative bacilli to mammalian buccal epithelial cells *in vivo*. *J. Clin. Invest.*, 68:1435–1440.

153. Woods, D.E., Straus, D.C., Johanson, W.G., Jr., Berry, V.K., and Bass, J.A. (1980): Role of pili in adherence of *Pseudomonas aeruginosa* to mammalian buccal epithelial cells. *Infect. Immun.*, 29:1146–1151.

154. Yu, V.L., Kroboth, F.J., Shonnard, J., Brown, A., McDearman, S., and Magnussen, M. (1982): Legionnaires' disease: new clinical perspective from a prospective pneumonia study. *Am. J. Med.*, 73:357–361.

155. Ziegler, E.J., Fisher, C.J., Sprung, C.L., Straube, R.C., Sadoff, J.C., Foulke, G.E., Wortel, C.H., Fink, M.P., Dellinger, R.P., Teng, N.N.H., Allen, I.E., Berger, H.J., Knatterud, G.L., LoBuglio, A.F., Smith, C.R., and the HA-1A Sepsis Study Group. (1991): Treatment of gram-negative bacteremia and septic shock with HA-1A human monoclonal antibody against endotoxin. *N. Engl. J. Med.*, 324:429–436.

Respiratory Infections: Diagnosis and Management, 3d ed.,
edited by James E. Pennington.
Raven Press, Ltd., New York © 1994

12

Infections of the Lower Respiratory Tract in Infancy and Early Childhood

Hugh E. Evans and Nelson L. Turcios

*Department of Pediatrics, New Jersey Medical School,
Newark, New Jersey 07103-2757*

This chapter summarizes the essential features of lower respiratory tract infections that occur in infants and children. It is a complex subject with a changing pattern of etiologic agents, increasing awareness of pathogenetic mechanisms, and extensive diagnostic and therapeutic innovation. Recent developments include the impact of AIDS which has led to a new entity—lymphocytic interstitial pneumonitis, as well as opportunistic infections including *Pneumocystis carinii* pneumonitis, cytomegalovirus pneumonia, fungal infections, and others.

Lower respiratory infections of infancy and childhood differ fundamentally from those of adulthood (9). Anatomic and immunologic immaturity, a more diverse set of etiologic agents, nonspecificity of clinical signs, avoidance of invasive diagnostic procedures, unavailability of sputum for microbiologic examination, and relative frequency of noninfectious etiology and pathogenesis (aspiration, foreign body, congenital defect) are some of the recognized differences. They intensify the challenge in management of infants and young children with lower respiratory infection.

In infancy and early childhood significant airway obstruction is more likely in an inflammatory process than in later life, due to the following anatomic and physiologic differences (4):

1. Collateral ventilation (such as the pores of Kohn and canals of Lambert) is underdeveloped in infancy, and therefore an obstructed unit is more likely to develop atelectasis.
2. Peripheral airways contribute a greater proportion than do central airways to total pulmonary resistance in the first 5 years of life. Hence, inflammation in the peripheral airways in children under 5 years has a greater effect on total resistance than it does in older children.
3. The cross-sectional area of the airways is smaller in infancy. Resistance is inversely proportional to the fourth power of the radius. Therefore, decreased caliber of the airways among infants, who have narrower lumens to start with, has a particularly severe effect.
4. Airway closure is more likely to occur in the lungs of infants because they have low recoil pressure and low lung volumes.
5. Infants' chest walls are more compliant. A negative intrathoracic pressure is developed during inspiration, and is increased because of the airway obstruc-

tion. This negative pressure exerts a force that draws in the infant's rib cage, and breathing becomes inefficient because the ribs are drawn in to a greater extent than fresh air.

The precise dimensions of immunologic immaturity are not well defined (23). However, the full-term neonate has, at best, 50% of adult concentration of total complement and most of its components. This contributes to a relative inadequacy of PMN chemotaxis. IgM and IgA concentrations in umbilical cord serum are negligible and do not attain adult levels until 2–4 years and 8–10 years, respectively. The normal (adult standards) IgG levels decline in the first year of life, reaching a nadir at 6–9 months of age, a time of "physiologic hypogammaglobulinemia." T-cell function is difficult to assess completely but is also reduced in infancy. This is the only time in life when the individual may be normally "immunodeficient."

Heterogeneity of etiologic agents is important to consider because each of the three age ranges in this group—neonatal, infancy, and childhood—has its own microbial prevalence spectrum. Clinical presentations can be especially misleading. A febrile convulsion, rather than respiratory distress, could be the initial manifestation of lower respiratory tract infection in patients from 6 months to 5 years of age. Conversely, fever, retractions, and tachypnea could be due to salicylate poisoning rather than respiratory infection. Moreover, even if these signs were due to infection, the diagnosis could just as likely be sepsis or meningitis, even in the absence of systemic or neurologic findings. Invasive procedures such as bronchoscopy, bronchoalveolar lavage, or lung biopsy are unusual in pediatrics. Infants do not bring up sputum, and adequate sputum specimens in older children are rarely obtained. Hence, this material is rarely available for stain or culture. Noninfectious etiologies and pathogenesis, including aspiration pneumonia (milk, hydrocarbons), congenital anomalies ("H" shaped T-E fistula, cleft palate, hiatus hernia with gastroesophageal reflex), and foreign bodies (peanuts) can simulate pulmonary disorders due to infectious agents. These are some considerations that contribute to the particular, if not unique, diagnostic and therapeutic problems of lower respiratory tract infection in infants and young children.

Most lower respiratory tract infections, that is, inflammation below the epiglottis, can be grouped anatomically by clinical and radiographic findings into four syndromes: laryngotracheitis, tracheobronchitis, bronchiolitis, and pneumonia. The first two are referred to elsewhere in this book. The latter two will be discussed here.

NEONATAL PNEUMONIA (6,8)

Pneumonia is a common form of neonatal infection and an important cause of perinatal mortality. Such infection, either bacterial or viral, can be acquired before, during, or shortly after birth. Pneumonia can be acquired (1) *transplacentally* as part of a generalized intrauterine infection, which can occur in the TORCH syndrome (toxoplasmosis, rubella, cytomegalovirus, herpes simplex), *Listeria, Treponema pallidum,* and, very rarely, *Mycobacterium tuberculosis*; (2) *intrapartum* by aspiration of infected amniotic fluid or vaginal bacteria during labor or delivery with onset of illness in the first few days of life and most commonly associated with group B streptococcus (GBS) or other bacteria such as *Escherichia coli, Klebsiella, Enterobacter, Listeria, T. pallidum,* and *Chlamydia;* and (3) *postnatally* due to the same pathogens, or *Staphylococcus, Pseudomonas, Serratia,* and *Candida.* Viral pneumonia is noted at or shortly after birth, and outbreaks have been reported to follow introduction of respiratory syncytial virus, adenovirus, coxsackie, parainfluenza, influenza A and B, and ECHO virus into the nursery. A break in hand washing technique; spread of organisms from one infant to another, or from the hands of nursery personnel; and contaminated isolette reservoirs have lead to such outbreaks. *Pneumocystis carinii* pneumonia has been noted in debilitated premature and full-term infants as well as in a small number of healthy full-term babies.

Pulmonary infection due to *Moraxella catarrhalis* has been reported in infants with endotracheal intubation and frequent endotracheal tube suction. It has been recommended that initial antibiotic therapy for severe pneumonia in mechanically ventilated young infants be tailored to cover *M. catarrhalis*—a potential nosocomial pathogen. Sepsis, meningitis, and osteomyelitis are often found with bacterial pneumonia, especially during epidemics.

When pneumonia is acquired perinatally, it is often termed *congenital pneumonia,* and usually results from ascending bacterial infection following prolonged rupture of the membranes in excess of 24 hours, although occasionally they are intact. In some instances, chorioamnionitis occurs first and induces rupture of the membranes. Like other infections, pneumonia can be associated with any obstetric abnormality, including premature rupture of the membranes, prolonged or otherwise difficult labor, maternal infection, premature labor, and fetal distress. Pneumonia can also occur in a healthy term infant delivered after an apparently uneventful pregnancy and labor.

Prolonged exposure to infectious agents is reflected by vasculitis in the umbilical cord, chorioamnionitis, and elevated cord serum IgM immunoglobulin levels at delivery.

Clinical Findings

In neonatal pneumonia, clinical findings are nonspecific, so a high index of suspicion is the key to an early diagnosis. Typical manifestations include apnea, anorexia, lethargy, hypothermia, tachycardia, and bradycardia. The presence of tachypnea, cyanosis, grunt, flaring of alae nasi, and sternal and subcostal retractions can focus attention on the lungs in these infants. Crackles on auscultation and dullness to percussion are occasionally found. Physical findings can be minimal, even with extensive disease shown on x-ray. Mixed metabolic and respiratory acidosis are typical.

Radiologic Signs

Findings on chest films are variable; they include unilateral or bilateral streaky infiltrates, lobar consolidations, or the "ground-glass" appearance of the respiratory distress syndrome (RDS). Indeed, the clinical and radiologic picture of RDS is mimicked by GBS, *E. Coli,* and other infectious pneumonias, so that administration of antibiotics to infants with respiratory distress (RDS) is a widely accepted practice.

Complications recognized on x-ray include pneumatoceles seen with *E. coli, Klebsiella pneumoniae,* and *Staphylococcus aureus,* as well as other agents, and lung abscess with *S. aureus* infection. Rapidly progressive consolidation even in the absence of pneumatoceles or empyema suggests *S. aureus* infection. A miliary distribution of the infiltrates is consistent with *Listeria.* Conversely, bronchopneumonic infiltrates, common among sick neonates, can represent infection with the agents cited or aspiration of sterile or infected fluid, or segmental atelectasis. Air fluid levels found in the lungs on chest film are consistent with necrotizing pneumonia, empyema, bronchopleural fistula, infected lung cyst, or lung abscess. CT scan permits unequivocal identification of a lung abscess in the presence of extensive pulmonary density. Sudden deterioration with tachypnea and cyanosis should raise the suspicion of pneumothorax.

Diagnostic Tests

Generalized neonatal infection is suggested by elevated ratios of immature to total white blood cell counts, leukopenia, elevated C-reactive protein, and erythrosedimentation rate (ESR) levels. These findings, however, have not been evaluated specifically in pneumonia. Blood, cerebrospinal fluid (CSF), and tracheal cultures can reveal the etiologic agent, but organisms isolated from surface areas (skin, external auditory canals), nares, and throat could reflect normal flora and hence do not help to establish the etiology.

Latex agglutination assay of body fluids for group B streptococcal polysaccharide antigen allows for specific diagnosis before results of blood and CSF cultures are available. Serologic studies should be performed if intrauterine infection is suspected, and cord immunoglobulins should be measured, although not all infants with intrauterine pneumonia will have increased IgM levels.

Therapy

Treatment is similar to that of any systemic neonatal infection. Ampicillin and either an aminoglycoside or cefotaxime are appropriate initially, following diagnostic procedures. The initial choices should reflect recent microbiologic experience of the specific neonatal unit. If an etiologic agent is subsequently identified, its sensitivities and the clinical course would guide changes in further management.

The dose of ampicillin varies from 50 to 100 mg/kg/day in two divided doses for those under 1 week to 100–150 mg/kg/day in three divided doses for older neonates. For group B streptococcal disease, penicillin G is given in a dose of 50,000 units/kg/day if the infant is under 7 days; 75–100,000 units/kg/day in divided doses, as for ampicillin, is preferred for older neonates. The precise dose varies with birth weight (over or under 2.5 kg) and age (over or under 1 week). For staphylococcal pneumonia, methicillin in a dose of 100 mg/kg/day divided into two or three doses for those under 2 weeks of age and 200–250 mg/kg/day into four to six doses for older infants is appropriate. Vancomycin (25–50 mg/kg/day) should be given in pneumonia caused by methicillin-resistant *S. aureus* or coagulase-negative staphylococci, whereas *Pseudomonas* infections can be treated with ticarcillin (200–300 mg/kg/day) or ceftazidime (100–150 mg/kg/day) together with an aminoglycoside, tobramycin, or gentamicin (5–7.5 mg/kg/day), which will cover other gram-negative bacteria as well. Acyclovir (250 mg/square meter/day) should be started if herpes simplex virus pneumonia is suspected.

Duration of therapy varies with the organism, extent of disease, and clinical response. A minimum of 10–14 days is needed, and more often 3–4 weeks are required for infection due to gram-negative organisms or *S. aureus*.

Two agents of particular concern are *Chlamydia trachomatis* and *Mycobacterium tuberculosis*.

Chlamydia trachomatis (2,13)

Chlamydia are gram-negative bacteria that, due to certain metabolic deficiencies, are obligate intracellular parasites. Three species are presently recognized within the genus: *C. trachomatis, C. psittaci,* and *C. pneumoniae* (formerly termed the TWAR strain). *C. psittaci* strains are only occasional, accidental causes of an acute febrile respiratory tract infection with systemic symptoms, and *C. pneumoniae,* whose peak age of initial infection is between 5 and 20 years, will not be discussed here.

C. trachomatis exists mainly in a genital reservoir. Infants acquire infection from infected mothers during their passage through the birth canal. Either the conjunctiva or the respiratory tract or both can serve as a portal of entry. Acquisition occurs in about 50% of infants born vaginally of infected mothers and in some infants born by cesarean section with intact membranes. The risk of conjunctivitis is 25 to 50% and the risk of pneumonia is 5 to 20%. The nasopharynx is the most commonly infected anatomic site.

Neonatal inclusion conjunctivitis is a well-known entity. It usually becomes evident at 3–5 days or as late as 14 days. When present, it provides the earliest clinical evidence of natally acquired infection, and it requires a complete course of both oral and topical treatment.

The chlamydial respiratory tract involvement ranges from asymptomatic infection to a syndrome of afebrile pneumonia. Chlamydial pneumonia is an afebrile illness of the first 3 months of life. A paroxysmal, staccato cough and tachypnea with respiratory rates ranging from 40 to 80 breaths/minute are characteristic but not always present. Inspiratory crackles can be present; wheezing is rare. Radiographic findings can include symmetrical hyperinflation, bilateral interstitial infiltrates, scattered atelectatic patches, and narrowed upper mediastinal silhouette.

Arterial blood gases often show PaO_2 in the range of 50–60 mm/Hg but $PaCO_2$ levels within normal limits. A peripheral blood eosinophilia (>300 cells/mm^3) is often found. Serum immunoglobulin abnormalities are the rule. IgM levels are always elevated (>110 mg/dL); IgG levels are high in most cases (>500 mg/dL). IgA is sometimes elevated.

The diagnosis of chlamydial pneumonia requires evidence that the infant is infected with *C. trachomatis* and that the infection is etiologically, rather than coincidentally, related to the illness. Tissue culture with irradiated McCoy cells offers the most sensitive and specific method for identification of infection, except in infants recently or currently treated with antimicrobials that inhibit *C. trachomatis.* Direct fluorescent staining for elementary bodies using monoclonal antibody is a practical alternative to culture for the detection of *C. trachomatis* in the nasopharyngeal and conjunctival secretions. Serologic methods for confirmation of *C. trachomatis* include indirect microimmunofluorescence or enzyme-linked immunoassay and requires demonstration of a significant rise in *C. trachomatis* antibody titer or the demonstration of *C. trachomatis*–specific IgA or IgM antibody. Serum IgM levels, both total and *Chlamydia*-specific, can be helpful in differentiating chlamydial infections that are only coincidentally related to respiratory illness and those that are actually responsible for the respiratory illness.

During the first 3 months of life, pneumonia, as well as otitis media, laryngitis, and nasopharyngitis, can follow in half of the cases with conjunctivitis. Hence, oral erythromycin estolate (30–50 mg/kg/day) as well as erythromycin eye ointment should be used for 14 days. Clinical improvement usually begins between the third and fifth days of treatment, and complete resolution is the case by the 14th day. However, in follow-up studies of children 7 to 8 years of age, after treatment for chlamydial pneumonia, mild pulmonary function abnormalities, including limitations in expiratory flow parameters and by history, were reported in a third of these children.

Congenital Tuberculosis (26)

Congenital tuberculosis could become an important concern as immigrant groups enter urban areas in the United States from Southeast Asia and the Caribbean Islands. Transplacental transmission leads to widespread dissemination, predominantly to the liver or lungs. The extent of involvement can be determined by blood oxygen levels. These are low in the fetus, and hence tubercle growth could be inhibited. Conversely, higher oxygen levels following delivery can favor its multiplication.

Congenital tuberculosis is rare; just over 300 cases have been reported. Although this number represents a small fraction of childhood tuberculosis, the incidence of congenital tuberculosis is expected to rise during the next few years as more childbearing women infected with the human immunodeficiency virus acquire tuberculosis as an opportunistic infection.

There are several ways in which tuberculosis in the fetus and newborn can be acquired: transplacental spread via the umbilical vein; aspiration or inhalation *in utero* or during birth of infected amniotic fluid; and acquisition of organisms from the mother or attendant by inhalation, ingestion, or contamination of traumatized skin or mucous membranes.

Affected infants are frequently born prematurely, but signs of disease usually do not appear for several days and are nonspecific. The most common manifestations are fever, cough, anorexia, poor weight gain, tachypnea, lymphadenopathy, and hepatosplenomegaly. Most of these infants have abnormalities on their chest roentgenograms; in about half of them a miliary pattern is present.

The tuberculin skin test is usually negative. Positive smear and/or culture results can often be obtained from tracheal aspirates, gastric washings, urine, liver, or lung biopsy specimens. The spinal fluid should be examined, even if the infant is asymptomatic, to evaluate the presence of central nervous system disease. The course may be fulminant with a mortality rate of about 50%, almost entirely due to the failure to establish the diagnosis antemortem. Complications include airway obstruction due to massive mediastinal lymphadenopathy, extensive pneumonia, or meningitis.

Neonatal antituberculous therapy is not standardized; however, when the mother is known to have active pulmonary tuberculosis, it is recommended that the newborn be separated from her immediately after delivery until maternal infectivity is no longer present and until the infant has been evaluated for the presence of tuberculous infection or disease and either started on chemotherapy or vaccinated with Bacillus Calmette-Guerin (BCG). The newborn infant should have a chest film and tuberculin test. If both are negative, some centers (including our own) treat prophylactically with isoniazid-INH-(10 mg/kg/day) because the infant could have already acquired tuberculous infection. The drug is given for at least 3 months, at which time the skin test and chest x-ray are repeated. If they remain negative and the infant is asymptomatic, INH could be discontinued.

The infant with a positive tuberculin test and negative chest film should be given INH for 1 year. If the chest film is also positive, rifampin (RIF) (15 mg/kg/day) and pyrazinamide (PZA) (20 mg/kg/day) should be added after cultures are obtained, including cerebrospinal fluid.

If noncompliance in administration of INH is of particular concern, BCG vaccine following a normal chest x-ray and negative tuberculin test can be administered. A tuberculin test should be carried out 6 weeks later to be sure it has become positive, as a result of the BCG vaccination. Uncertainties in management are compounded by the inconsistent efficacy of BCG as well as insufficient knowledge of pharmacokinetics and the efficacy of INH, RIF, and PZA in the newborn.

PNEUMONIA IN INFANCY AND EARLY CHILDHOOD (10,7,21)

It has been estimated that more than 1 million cases of pneumonia occur every year among children in the United States, and that more than 75% of the pneumonias occur in children under the age of 5 years.

Poverty, crowding, urban environment, premature birth, and exposure to tobacco smoke all predispose to infection. Other predisposing elements include the use of immunosuppressant therapy, ventilatory support in intensive care units, and several medico-surgical conditions known to increase the colonization and infection with a variety of respiratory pathogens. Other recognized factors include: anatomic defects, congenital or acquired; immunodeficiencies, congenital or acquired; congestive heart failure; and cystic fibrosis.

THE VIRAL PNEUMONIAS (11)

The pathogens causing pneumonia vary with the age of the patient, the immunologic status of the host, and environmental conditions. However, respiratory viruses are responsible for most lower respiratory tract infections in children. It is estimated that about 85% of pneumonias in children are due to viruses through a direct invasion of the lower respiratory tract or an indirect facilitation of entrance by bacterial pathogens.

There are epidemiologic and experimental data, suggesting that viral inoculation takes place by direct contact, droplet nuclei, or aerosol. The small airways and alveoli seem to be the primary target of viral invasion.

Both epidemiologic and virologic studies have revealed that most lower respiratory tract disease occurs during epidemics with the major respiratory viruses: respiratory syncytial virus, parainfluenza, and influenza. Adenoviruses and picornaviruses have also been associated with lower respiratory infections during nonepidemic periods. Among bacteria, *S. pneumoniae* is the leading organism, and *H. influenzae* type b and *S. aureus* should also be considered. Under certain conditions, *Moraxella catarrhalis* and group A streptococci are occasional pathogens in infants and young children.

TABLE 12–1. *Relative frequency of agents causing community-acquired pneumonia in otherwise healthy children*

Age group	Most common	Frequency	
		Occasional	Rare
Neonate (<1 mo.)	Group B streptococci *Escherichia coli* Respiratory viruses Enteroviruses	*H. influenzae* (nontypeable) *S. pneumoniae,* *Klebsiella,* and other gram- negative enteric bacilli Group A streptococci *Staphylococcus* *aureus* Varicella Cytomegalovirus Herpes simplex	Mycobacteria
Young infants (1–3 mo.) Febrile	Respiratory viruses Enteroviruses	Group B streptococci *H. influenzae* type b *S. pneumoniae* *S. aureus* Group A streptococci *Bordetella pertussis*	Varicella Cytomegalovirus Mycobacteria Gram-negative enteric bacilli
Afebrile	*Chlamydia*	Cytomegalovirus Ureaplasma *Pneumocystis carinii*	
Infants and young children	Respiratory viruses *S. pneumoniae* *H. influenzae* type b	*B. pertussis* *S. aureus* Group A streptococci *M. catarrhalis*	Mycobacteria
Older children (>5 yrs.) and adolescent	*Mycoplasma* *S. pneumoniae* Respiratory viruses	*S. aureus* Group A streptococci Mycobacteria	

From J.R. Gilsdorf, 1987, Community-acquired pneumonia in children. *Semin. Respir. Infect.,* 2:146–151; with permission.

It appears that the earliest histopathologic lesion associated with viral pneumonia is probably destruction of ciliated epithelium associated with mononuclear cells infiltration into the submucosa and surrounding perivascular areas. The sloughing of cellular debris into the lumen, accompanied by mucus and inflammatory cells, produces either partial or complete airway obstruction. Partial obstruction can cause air trapping, as airways are apt to collapse during expiration. Complete obstruction can result in atelectasis. The mononuclear cells' inflammatory response will also be accompanied by edema of the submucosa, which can extend into the alveoli and interstitial space. The interstitial infiltration rarely progresses to fibrosis. In general, the host immune response, including interferon, cytotoxic cells, and specific antibody, limits the progression of the infection and helps promote recovery.

Other etiologic associations that are potentially important during infancy and childhood include some of the viral exanthems, such as varicella, measles, and rubella. Infectious mononucleosis (due to Epstein-Barr virus) can cause pneumonia in school-aged children and adolescents. Pneumonia is a rare complication of salmonellosis, and it is more often found in the elderly than in children.

Respiratory Syncytial Virus (19,20)

Respiratory syncytial virus (RSV) is the most important cause of acute lower respiratory infection in infants. Although bronchiolitis is its best-recognized clinical form, most have radiographic evidence of pneumonitis. However, there is no clear clinical distinction between bronchiolitis and pneumonia. Upper respiratory infection is the most common form of involvement with the first infection.

The RSV envelope contains two antigenic subtypes, which determine its infectivity: (i) The F (fusion) protein, antigenically constant, fuses cell membranes of contiguous cells in culture, producing large syncytia. (ii) The G (large) glycoprotein has different epitopes for the two subtypes A and B. The age of the patient is the major determinant of the response to the F glycoprotein. RSV rarely causes disease in infants younger than 1 month; this is probably due to the protective effect of specific neutralizing antibody that is passively transferred from mother to infant. All term newborns have antibody levels similar to those of their mothers. This protective effect can be surmounted, however, by a large inoculating dose of RSV. Thus, the level of antibody may be important. This would explain why serious RSV infections do not usually occur in the first month of life but occur later when maternal antibody is present, but in lower levels. Preexisting antibody titer determines the response to G glycoprotein.

The detection in respiratory secretions of children with severe lower respiratory tract infections of high IgE antibody specific for RSV, accompanied by detectable histamine release, raises the possibility that the inflammatory response to infection could be enhanced by the release of chemical mediators of atopy. This would result in edema, mucus production, and bronchospasm, which could contribute to the development of pneumonia.

Two major subtypes of respiratory syncytial virus have been identified: A and B. Several clinical observations have suggested that A-subtype infections are more severe. The finding that A-subtype infections were more severe might have important implications for vaccine development, studies of the virulence of RSV, clinical management (i.e., selection for antiviral therapy), and long-term prognosis.

RSV is the only respiratory virus that occurs in consistent annual epidemics each year, usually from November to March with predictable intervals, as the sole or nearly sole cause of severe lower respiratory infection of infancy requiring hospitalization. An infant under the age of 1 year has about a 50% chance of being infected, and by 2 years of age virtually 100% of children have had at least one infection. During the epidemic period, except when it is interrupted by epidemic influenza, RSV accounts for 90% of the lower respiratory tract disease in preschool children. It causes 5 to 40% of pneumonias in infants, 60 to 90% of cases of bronchiolitis, and is rarely recovered from those without respiratory disease.

Its severity is greater in male infants, especially those of 2–5 months. Infants in day care centers could have increased prevalence of initial infection. Infection, which can be mild, especially in middle-class families and those living in rural or suburban areas, leads to antibody development in 25 to 50% of infants at 1 year of age, 95% at 5 years, and 100% in adults. Reinfection is common in older children and adults. Immunity induced by a single infection has no effect on the severity of illness associated with reinfection 1 year later. In fact, a significant reduction in the severity of RSV illness has been shown to occur only after the third infection.

Spread is intrafamilial with an older child (2 to 14 years) as the index case and both infants and adults secondarily infected. Nosocomial spread to other infants and hospital staff may be extensive. During infection, RSV is shed in nasal secretions in large quantities and for prolonged periods. Viral excretion is common until at least the sixth day of infection, and in 50% of infections shedding persists for at least 10 days. The ability of respiratory syncytial virus to spread widely is difficult to understand because the agent is unstable at temperature and humidity extremes. RSV spread is not likely by small-particle aerosol (as with influenza) but through direct contact with large droplets of respiratory secretions or by self-inoculation after touching contaminated surfaces. Large droplets of secretions remain infectious on countertops for over 6 hours and on cloth and paper tissue for 30 minutes. Hence efforts to control the nosocomial spread of RSV should concentrate on good hand washing rather than such respiratory precautions as masks or gowns.

Parainfluenza Viruses

After RSV, parainfluenza viruses are the next most common cause of acute lower respiratory infection in children. As a group they account for almost as many hospitalizations each year as RSV. Their seasonal patterns differ markedly. RSV produces annual midwinter epidemics. Parainfluenza virus types 1 and 2 occur biannually in autumn, and parainfluenza type 3 is endemic. Like RSV, parainfluenza virus type 3 can cause serious lower respiratory infection in infants. Although infections with RSV and parainfluenza type 3 virus occur with almost the same frequency in the first year of life, infection with parainfluenza type 3 is much less likely to produce lower respiratory tract involvement. Parainfluenza types 1 and 2 do not produce serious infections before 6 months of life. Croup is the most prominent illness for these viruses, but pneumonia is a common manifestation.

Influenza Viruses

Influenza viruses rank just behind RSV and parainfluenza viruses as an important cause of lower respiratory infection in infants and preschool children. There are three influenza virus types distinct in their nucleoprotein and matrix antigens: A, B, and C. Influenza A and B are the most prevalent. Change in antigenic composition occurs from time to time primarily among A serotypes but also among the B serotypes. New variants emerge for which immunity acquired from previous infection or vaccination may not be protective.

Spread is often by aerosol, so that laryngotracheitis is a common manifestation particularly in infants. Influenza virus infection destroys the ciliated respiratory epithelium. Destruction of the respiratory epithelium can also predispose to secondary bacterial pneumonia; infections with staphylococci, pneumococci, and *H. influenzae* are frequent complications of influenza virus infection.

Amantadine shortens the course of uncomplicated influenza A infections in otherwise healthy children and young adults if administered within the first 48 hours. Amantadine is not effective for influenza B. Rimantadine, an analogue of amantadine, is as effective without having the side effects of amantadine. Ribavirin by aerosol appears to shorten the course of both influenza A and B in adolescents. It is possible that the combination of amantadine or rimantadine and ribavirin will be the treatment of choice for children with severe influenza A pneumonias.

Adenoviruses

Adenoviruses are present throughout the year. The serotypes that infect children most commonly (types 1, 2, 5, and 6) usually involve the upper respiratory tract, and they are responsible for the most cases of exudative pharyngitis in children under 2 years of age. These viruses frequently cause otitis media.

Adenovirus types 3 and 7 are a common cause of pharyngoconjunctival fever in adolescents and young adults. These viruses, along with types 11 and 21, can cause a severe necrotizing pneumonia in infants with a high mortality rate and pathologic findings consistent with bronchiolitis obliterans.

THE BACTERIAL PNEUMONIAS (1,22)

The frequency with which the common pyogenic bacterias such as *S. pneumoniae* and *H. influenzae* cause pneumonia in otherwise healthy infants and children is difficult to assess, because invasive diagnostic procedures are not justified in those conditions. Recent studies have revealed that bacteria may account for as many as 30% of cases in out-patients. In immunologically intact children between 1 and 5 years, most cases of bacterial pneumonia are caused by *S. pneumoniae* or *H. influenzae*. However, there has been a marked decrease in *H. influenzae* pneumonia since the advent of the conjugate vaccine. In older children and adolescents, bacterial pneumonia is usually caused by *M. pneumoniae* or *S. pneumoniae*. Antibodies to *C. pneumoniae* strain TWAR, which has emerged as an important pathogen in the last 5 to 6 years, are seen in 15 to 40% of children under 15 years of age. The pathogen is associated with bronchitis and pharyngitis, as well as pneumonia that clinically resembles *M. pneumoniae*. Staphylococcal pneumonia has been rare in recent years; however, its potentially high morbidity and mortality requires prompt recognition.

Group B Streptococci

Group B streptococci are associated with infections at any age, but are more common in infants under 3 months. Acquisition by neonates is usually vertical, from the maternal genital tract *in utero,* or during passage through the birth canal.

Group B streptococci are subdivided into five serotypes (Ia, Ib, Ic, II, and III) based on specific polysaccharide antigens. Serotypes I and II are usually associated with lung disease, and type III with meningitis.

Although the mortality of group B streptococcal pneumonia has been high (up to 60%), recent studies suggest improvement with prompt therapy. Some infants experience a second episode of infection a few days after antibiotic therapy has been completed. This recurrence could be the result of exogenous recolonization or reinvasion of the streptococci, which persist in mucous membranes after penicillin therapy.

Streptococcus pneumoniae

Pneumococci are a major cause of pneumonia in infants and children. The incidence is highest in infants younger than 2 years of age, with a peak between 3 and 5 months. Black children are affected more frequently. Socioeconomic factors, sickle cell anemia, and nephrosis can be predisposing factors.

Pneumococci are subdivided into some 84 serotypes. In children, types 1, 3, 6A, 14, 18C, and 23F are responsible for 60 to 70% of pneumococcal infection.

Pneumococcal disease correlates with the seasonal variations of other respiratory tract infections, with the highest incidence in winter and spring. Patients with asplenia or functional hyposplenia, as well as those with Hodgkin's disease or those receiving immunosuppressive therapy, are at special increased risk of developing pneumococcal disease, including pneumonia.

Penicillin is the treatment of choice in pneumococcal pneumonia. However, penicillin-relatively-resistant pneumococci has been reported in some areas of the country.

Hemophilus influenzae Type b

H. influenzae is a major cause of invasive diseases, including bacteremia, meningitis, and pneumonia. Other manifestations are otitis media, epiglottitis, cellulitis, arthritis, and osteomyelitis. The incidence of pneumonia is higher in children younger than 5 years of age, with a peak between 4 and 7 months of age.

These gram-negative rods occur in encapsulated and nonencapsulated forms. Based on their polysaccharide, the encapsulated forms are divided into six capsular types (A to F). Almost 95% of invasive disease, including pneumonia, is caused by serotype B. The noncapsular forms are normal colonizers of the nasopharynx, and, although a major cause of otitis media and sinusitis, rarely cause bacteremic disease or pneumonia in children.

Once the diagnosis of *H. influenzae* pneumonia is made, based on a positive culture, identification of beta-lactamase-positive strains and susceptibility testing must be done, as a few strains are beta-lactamase-negative but still ampicillin-resistant. In a hospitalized patient, a cephalosporin (cefuroxime, ceftriaxone, or cefotaxime) is effective.

Staphylococcal Pneumonia

Staphylococcal pneumonia is most common in the first year of life, especially the first 3 months. It is more frequent in boys and occurs more often in the winter months. Previous use of antibiotics, or a viral infection (adenovirus, influenza), are typical background features. The organism has a special predilection for children with leukemia and for infants and children with cystic fibrosis.

Staphylococci are frequently found on the skin and on nasal and other mucous membranes. Three major species are recognized: *S. aureus, S. epidermidis,* and *S. saprophyticus.* Coagulase formation characterizes most of the *S. aureus* strains.

A person colonized in the nose and throat or perineal region is the major source of the organism. *S. aureus* is carried in the anterior nares in up to 70% of normal individuals. Transmission of *S. aureus* usually occurs by direct contact or by spread of heavy particles. Wounds, skin disease, intravenous drug abuse, use of steroids, wide-spectrum antibiotic administration, and diabetes mellitus increase the likelihood of infection.

Systemic and respiratory signs are comparable with other types of pneumonia. Rapid progression, even over a few hours, of both clinical and radiologic findings is typical of staphylococcal pneumonia. Early in the illness, consolidation is the most common radiologic finding, often associated with pleural effusions in 60% of cases. Empyema or multiple lung abscesses are also characteristic. Pneumothorax has been reported in 40% of cases. It is associated with sudden severe decompensation and can be due to localized bronchial wall necrosis. Pneumatoceles usually appear during the convalescent phase. They can persist for months to years in asymptomatic children without clinical significance and can be due to the passage of air into interstitial spaces in areas of alveolar or bronchial necrosis. They are usually multiple, thin-walled, cyst-like, airfilled cavities, and are typical of staphylococcal pneumonia (Fig. 12.1).

The organism is usually penicillin-resistant; therefore the initial therapeutic approach should include a drug resistant to inactivation by penicillinase. Antibiotic therapy for neonates was described earlier. Methicillin-resistant *S. aureus* (MRSA) accounts for more than 10% of the cultures. Vancomycin should be given when these organisms are isolated.

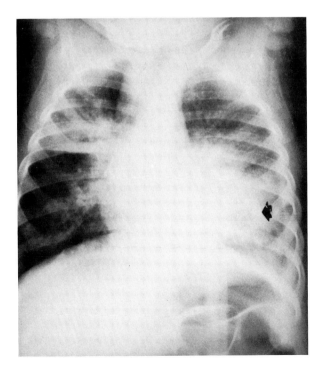

FIG. 12–1. Staphylococcal pneumonia. Massive bilateral infiltrates. Pleural fluid on left. Probable necrotizing pneumonia on left lingular area (age 10 months).

PERTUSSIS

Pertussis, commonly referred to as "whooping cough," is caused by *Bordetella pertussis*. It is very contagious, especially for children under 5 years of age and those not adequately immunized. An identical illness can be caused by adenoviruses, influenza viruses, and other agents.

Pertussis classically begins with mild upper respiratory tract symptoms with cough (catarrhal stage) that can progress to severe paroxysmal coughing episodes (paroxysmal stage), often with a characteristic inspiratory whoop, followed by vomiting. Fever is absent or minimal. Symptoms subsequently fade gradually (convalescent phase). Adolescents and adults may present with persistent cough and no inspiratory whoop. In infants younger than 6 months, apnea is a common manifestation and whoop can be absent. Duration of the illness in uncomplicated cases is 6 to 10 weeks. Mortality is highest in the first year of life.

Erythromycin estolate is effective in eradicating the organism from the nasopharynx, but not in shortening the paroxysmal stage of the disease.

CLINICAL MANIFESTATIONS OF PNEUMONIA

The onset of pneumonia can include anorexia, lethargy, irritability, tachypnea, cough, intercostal retractions, flaring of alae nasi, nasal discharge, conjunctivitis, and otitis media; often there is no fever. Physical findings vary with the severity of the illness. Cyanosis can be apparent in the nail beds or lips. Rapid pulse, increased respiratory rate, and crackles are typical. If bronchiolitis is present, expiratory and inspiratory wheezing are characteristic.

RADIOLOGIC FINDINGS IN PNEUMONIA (3)

Diagnosis requires radiographic evidence of pulmonary inflammation. Although symptoms and auscultatory findings can be highly suggestive, radiographic examination is necessary, not only for confirmation but also for evaluation of the extent of pulmonary involvement and possible complications such as pleural effusion and atelectasis. A chest x-ray should be obtained in children with fever in conjunction with one or more of the following pulmonary findings: tachypnea; respiratory distress defined as nasal flaring, grunting or intercostal retractions; crackles or decreased breath sounds.

Patterns of radiographic abnormalities in pneumonia are not accurate in differentiating between bacterial and nonbacterial etiology in most cases. However, chest x-ray findings reported in viral infections include poorly defined multilobar infiltrates with a perihilar predilection. Atelectasis involving the right upper or middle lobes is considered to be associated with viral pneumonia. Bacterial pneumonias are reported to produce well-defined infiltrates usually involving one lobe and located in the mid or peripheral areas. The presence of fluid in the pleural space and abscess, pneumatocele, or bullae are considered due to bacterial infection. Occasionally a mass is simulated (Fig. 12.2). The association of lobar infiltration only with bacterial infection, and of a diffuse or disseminated pattern only with a viral etiology, has not been validated in the literature. Further compounding the problem is the occurrence of viral infection in 25 to 75% of patients with bacterial pneumonia.

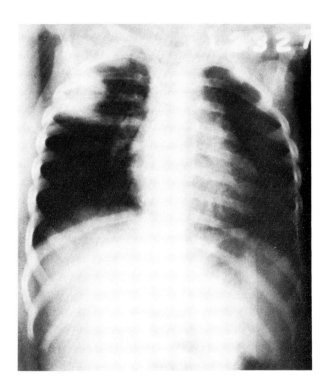

FIG. 12–2. Right upper lobe pneumonia, simulating a mass. Etiology: pneumococcus (age 9 months).

ETIOLOGIC DIAGNOSTIC TESTS

Etiologic diagnoses are difficult for a number of reasons. Sputum samples are hard to obtain from children under 4 years, and antibody tests and cultures are often misleading for some of the most common pathogens, including *C. pneumoniae, Staphylococcus,* pneumococcus, and *Hemophilus.* Diagnosis of pneumonia is often difficult and in many cases cannot be made despite multiple diagnostic tests. Invasive diagnostic procedures are justified only in severely ill, usually compromised children. Other tests are often helpful, but all have limitations.

The most critical question in the treatment is to differentiate viral from the diverse bacterial causes. Clinical findings are nonspecific as are the radiographic abnormalities. Leukocytosis of 15,000/mm³ or higher or an increased sedimentation rate are not sufficiently specific to identify children with bacterial pneumonia and provide a basis for antimicrobial therapy.

Positive bacterial cultures of blood and pleural fluid provide definitive evidence of bacterial pneumonia, but respiratory tract cultures are less helpful. However, blood cultures are positive in less than 10% of outpatient children with pneumonia, and in only about 20% of children with pneumococcal pneumonia. Gram stain and culture of sputum expectorated or aspirated by deep tracheal suction can be helpful in adults, but adequate sputum samples in children are seldom obtained. Nasopharyngeal and throat cultures are of no value, because results of cultures of the upper respiratory tract correlate poorly with those of lung aspirates, and pharyngeal carriage of pulmonary pathogens among healthy children is common.

Bacterial antigen detection tests on nasopharyngeal secretions, serum and urine from children with pneumonia, using the counterimmunoelectrophoresis (CIE) and latex agglutination (LA) methods, have shown an apparent higher sensitivity of antigen detection tests than blood cultures, but presently only LA tests on concentrated urine appear to be clinically useful. These tests have several limitations and should be considered to provide only presumptive evidence of bacterial pneumonia. Furthermore, bacterial antigen detection tests of urine and sera, utilizing LA, are much less sensitive in the diagnosis of bacteremic pneumococcal pneumonia than in the case of *H. influenzae*. At present, bacterial antigen tests on urine or other body fluids, although occasionally valuable in the early diagnosis of bacterial pneumonia, are not routinely recommended for nonhospitalized children with pneumonia.

Isolation of viruses in tissue culture is the standard method of virus diagnosis. Several methods for the rapid detection of viral antigen have been found to be useful. These include immune electron microscopy, fluorescent antibody (FA), enzyme-linked immunosorbent assay (ELISA), enzyme-linked fluorescent assay, and tissue culture amplification (TCA). The tests that have found practical application for respiratory viruses are FA, ELISA, and TCA. FA has the broadest application. ELISA kits are available for identification of several viruses. Rapid diagnostic tests for the identification of RSV and *C. trachomatis* in nasopharyngeal secretions, based on their immunofluorescence or enzyme-linked immunosorbent assays, are important in the diagnosis of pneumonia caused by these now treatable infections.

In the usual clinical practice, serologic tests are less helpful but can be important under certain circumstances. For most respiratory virus infections, antibodies in serum and secretions do not develop until the patient is recovering. Cytomegalovirus (CMV) is an important exception, among those organisms that may cause pneumonia in the neonatal period; measurement of specific IgM antibodies to CMV can be diagnostic in such cases. Testing of paired serum specimens to measure a rise in antibodies to respiratory viruses can be important for severe infections that produce complications, such as bronchiolitis obliterans, myocarditis, or encephalitis.

Complement fixation (CF) tests are available for most of the respiratory viruses, especially for adenoviral and influenza infection.

A new, promising diagnostic method includes the use of genetic probes, such as random chromosomal fragments and ribosomal RNA or DNA probes. They produce simple fingerprinting patterns that will distinguish virtually any infectious agent.

It is more practical to design treatment around the most likely pathogens for the age group. In the first 3 months of life, *C. trachomatis* (vertically transmitted), respiratory syncytial virus (RSV), and parainfluenza are most frequent. From 4 months to 2 years, RSV, parainfluenza, influenza, and adenoviruses are most common, along with pneumococcus and *Hemophilus;* from 2 to 5 years, respiratory viruses and pneumococcus are the chief pathogens.

Ambulatory infants with lower respiratory tract disease of uncertain pathology will probably do well on amoxicillin, to cover pneumococcus and *Hemophilus* species. Hospitalized children without RSV should be given cefuroxime, which is effective against *S. aureus, Hemophilus,* and pneumococcus.

BRONCHIOLITIS (5,16,25,27,28)

Bronchiolitis is one of the most common disorders of the lower respiratory tract among infants. It is nearly always of viral etiology, peaks at 6 months of age or earlier, often occurs in epidemic form, and can lead to nosocomial spread. It is rarely fatal but has potential long-term implications for development of abnormal lung function, subsequent illness in childhood, and chronic respiratory impairment in adults. Host response to the major pathogen, the respiratory syncytial virus, is unusual in that antibodies (maternal or vaccine acquired) not only fail to confer protection, but can be associated with more severe illness. Infection is more severe in neonates, especially premature, or those infants with underlying pulmonary disease, immunodeficiency, or congenital heart disease. Respiratory syncytial virus is the most common etiology, but other viral agents, including adenovirus (types 3, 7, 21), parainfluenza virus (types 1 and 3), influenza, and enterovirus have been identified, as well as *Mycoplasma pneumoniae*.

Clinical Features

Bronchiolitis, because it begins in conjunctival or nasal mucosa, typically starts out as an upper respiratory infection. Nasal discharge, cough, and sometimes a low-grade fever precede the onset of tachypnea, chest retractions, and wheezing by 1 to 3 days. Apnea with cyanosis and/or bradycardia occurs in 20% of cases in infants under 6 months of age. Physical findings usually include increased respiratory rate, commonly to rates above 50 breaths/min, chest retractions, and wheezes throughout the lungs. Signs of dehydration secondary to reduced fluid intake produced by the respiratory distress can be present. Abnormalities in gas exchange—mismatching of ventilation and perfusion—produce hypoxemia. Despite severe alterations in gas exchange, cyanosis is detectable in only a small number of infants. Increased respiratory rate is a more reliable indicator of altered gas exchange. The faster the respiratory rate, the more severe the hypoxemia. Carbon dioxide retention reflects severe illness, especially in infants less than 3 months of age.

Radiographic Findings

The radiographic manifestations of bronchiolitis are nonspecific and include hyperinflation with low, flat diaphragms, increased antero-posterior thoracic diameter, and prominent retrosternal space. Most also show interstitial infiltrates and patchy atelectasis.

Pathophysiology

A variety of histopathologic changes start on the 5th day (range 4–6) of the incubation period. Inflammatory changes occur in small peripheral airways associated with peribronchiolar infiltration with lymphocytes. Further changes include edema of the walls, submucosa and adventitia, necrosis of epithelium of the bronchioles, and plugging of the lumen of the airways. Hyperaeration is due to partial obstruction of airways and a ball valve mechanism permitting air to flow initially during inspiration but obstructing it during expiration. Atelectasis can occur secondary to complete airway obstruction. Lung mechanisms are adversely affected, with an increase in total lung capacity, residual volume, and functional residual capacity. Airway resistance is increased and compliance is decreased. There is also increased work of breathing. Regeneration of respiratory epithelium occurs after a few days, but cilia do not regenerate until late. Destruction of small airways by the inflammatory process may predispose to future hyperreactivity of the airways.

Diagnostic Tests

The standard for diagnosis of RSV infection is viral culture. However, the role of viral isolation in management is limited because it could take 2 to 3 weeks for a positive result.

Enzyme immunoassay offers a more rapid and highly reliable diagnosis for RSV. Abbott ELISA is the most sensitive, specific, rapid, and easy-to-perform test. This method, which takes only a few hours, can identify viral antigen in nasopharyngeal secretions by using enzyme-tagged antibodies that bind to infected cells and can be identified by a photometric assay. Direct fluorescent antibody technique is the more reliable method for RSV detection in the community hospital laboratory.

Management

Exposure of infants with cardiopulmonary disease to RSV should be kept to a minimum; therefore, if possible, they should not be admitted to the hospital during the season of peak RSV activity. Infants with moderate-to-severe respiratory distress should be hospitalized. In-hospital therapy has four components: supportive care, detection and treatment of complications, protecting others, and the use of specific antiviral agents.

The mainstay of supportive care is the use of supplemental, humidified oxygen because nearly all hospitalized children are hypoxemic. Fluids to correct dehydration should be given, keeping in mind that excessive fluid administration could produce worsening of airway obstruction. In an attempt to reduce oxygen consumption, nursing should be provided in a neutral environment. Careful monitoring to detect complications such as hypoxemia, apnea, and respiratory failure must be implemented. Recent studies have reported some improvement in the bronchial obstruction with the use of albuterol by aerosol. Strict hand washing and avoidance of infant-to-infant contact must be enforced.

Most investigators agree that ribavirin—a synthetic nucleoside that resembles guanosine and inosine and has broad-spectrum antiviral activity against RNA and DNA viruses—is indicated in infants with underlying lung disease such as bronchopulmonary dysplasia, chronic lung infection, cystic fibrosis, immunodeficiencies, and congenital heart disease, and in infants who are severely ill as shown by hypoxemia with increasing levels of carbon dioxide. The drug is administered by a small-particle aerosol generator (SPAG) at a concentration of 20 mg/ml in oxygen tent, hood, mask, or through ventilator tubing for 12 to 18 hours for 3 to 5 days. Clinical trials have shown that aerosolized ribavirin improves arterial oxygenation saturation, attenuates the severity of the disease, and diminishes viral shedding.

Prognosis

In general, most infants with bronchiolitis, receiving appropriate supportive care, improve within 3 to 5 days. The respiratory rate becomes normal and radiographic abnormalities clear by the second week. Children who as infants were hospitalized with bronchiolitis continue to have small but significant pulmonary function abnormalities, increased bronchial hyperreactivity, and recurrent obstructive lower airway disease.

There is a strong association between confirmed RSV bronchiolitis and the subsequent development of asthma with a reported frequency as high as 30 to 50%. Increased levels of histamine and arachidonic acid metabolites in secretions of infants with bronchiolitis and in serum of children with asthma further support a common pathogenesis between bronchiolitis and asthma.

BRONCHIOLITIS OBLITERANS (12)

One possible outcome, especially in cases following adenoviruses types 7 and 21 infection, is bronchiolitis obliterans, a chronic form of bronchiolitis characterized by destruction of the mucosa lining small bronchi and bronchioles which become filled with fibrous tissue. There is obliteration of the lumen of terminal bronchioles with dilatation of the distal respiratory bronchioles. Vessels are narrowed and areas of overdistention, atelectasis, and fibrosis occur within the alveolar region of the lung. Destruction of terminal bronchioles contributes to the "pruning" effect seen on bronchography. Pulmonary angiography shows decreased vascularity in the involved lung. The eventual outcome may be unilateral hyperlucent lung, characterized by poor perfusion and ventilation, airflow obstruction, and reduced vital capacity. Clinically, the course is often marked by recurrent wheezing, chronic cough, and recurrent chest infection.

Treatment is nonspecific. Lobar collapse can be persistent, or there can be reexpansion, even after several years. Remarkably, some patients are asymptomatic and the disease is diagnosed in a routine chest x-ray examination. Surgical intervention is controversial in cases of unilateral hyperlucent lung, and, as in bronchiolitis obliterans, therapy is conservative. The sequence of bronchiolitis obliterans leading to unilateral hyperlucent lung is the result of not only adenovirus bronchiolitis but also influenza A, measles, pertussis, *Mycoplasma,* foreign body, inhalation of nitric acid or hydrochloric acid, hydrocarbon ingestion, and radiation therapy. There is no clear association of bronchiolitis obliterans with RSV infections.

MEASLES PNEUMONIA

Measles pneumonia, caused by the measles virus alone, usually occurs early in the disease. More commonly, pneumonia occurs later, after the rash fades, in association with secondary bacterial or viral invaders. Among the bacterial pathogens, the most common are staphylococci, pneumococci, *H. influenzae,* and hemolytic streptococci. Respiratory viruses, especially adenoviruses and herpesviruses, have also been reported as secondary invaders.

An acute inflammatory process involving the epithelial lining of the entire respiratory tract from the nasal mucosa to the bronchioles is characteristic of measles. Laryngotracheitis is a prominent component of this disease, expressed as a croupy, barking cough. Bronchiolar obstruction can occur causing hyperaeration. There is also an interstitial pneumonia with peribronchial infiltration by mononuclear cells. Desquamated cells that line the alveolar wall can simulate a hyaline membrane.

The frequency of lower respiratory tract complications is greatly influenced by the widespread use of the vaccine and varies from epidemic to epidemic and from country to country. Despite the availability of measles vaccine for immunization, measles are still the most common cause of bronchopneumonia in developing countries where a high mortality rate is closely associated with severe malnutrition.

A related entity, giant cell interstitial pneumonia, has been described in histologic examination of lung tissue in some patients with preceding measles. In the absence of clinical evidence of measles, the disease has been termed *Hecht's pneumonia*. Giant cell pneumonia is known to affect children with underlying conditions involving the reticuloendothelial or hematopoietic system, children treated with antimetabolites, those with altered immune states, and children with acquired immunodeficiency syndrome. Clinically, this disease cannot be distinguished from other pneumonias.

Atypical measles pneumonia can occur many years later in children immunized with killed measles vaccine, no longer available today. In contrast to typical measles, the rash appears first on the palms and soles and spreads to the trunk, often sparing the face. Later, respiratory symptoms and signs develop that suggest pneumonia, which can be confirmed by chest x-ray.

VARICELLA PNEUMONIA

Primary varicella pneumonia appears to be a manifestation of a progressive varicella syndrome. It occurs in the absence of underlying disease and more commonly in adults than in children with chickenpox. The onset of pneumonia is usually 2 to 5 days after the appearance of the rash, but it can occur before the rash.

Primary varicella pneumonia can also occur as part of a fatal progressive varicella syndrome in infants born to mothers who have chickenpox within 4 days before or 1 day after delivery. It can also occur in two clinical forms of dissemination in immunocompromised children: severe multisystem involvement or a mild clinical syndrome.

The chest x-ray is typical with diffuse infiltrates in nummular, or "coin-shaped," form, sometimes known as a "snowball" appearance. In some cases, its appearance must be distinguished from a metastatic malignancy.

There are no well-controlled trials of antiviral therapy for varicella pneumonia. Treatment with either acyclovir or vidarabine does not alter the natural course. To possibly be effective, antiviral therapy should be given early in the course of the disease. Its administration in the immunocompetent patient is a matter of clinical judgment in those under 13 years of age. However, treatment is recommended for all patients older than 13 years.

HIV-infected children can acquire varicella and develop severe disease characterized by pneumonia, encephalitis, hepatitis, pancreatitis, and a protracted course. Therefore, these children, as well as other immunocompromised patients, should be treated aggressively. Intravenous acyclovir is effective against varicella and should be started in HIV-infected children as soon as there is evidence of disease.

PNEUMONIAS IN IMMUNOCOMPROMISED INFANTS AND CHILDREN

In the immunosuppressed child, pneumonia is a frequent, often severe complication, due mostly to agents that would be unusual in the immunologically intact patient. They include opportunistic agents such as *Pneumocystis carinii*, cytomegalovirus, *Mycobacterium avium-intracellulare*, fungi, bacteria such as *S. pneumonia*, *H. influenzae* type b, *S. aureus*, *Pseudomonas* and other gram-negative bacilli, and *M. tuberculosis*, and viruses such as measles, RSV, parainfluenza, and adenovirus.

Children with AIDS commonly develop pulmonary infections. The usual presentation is recurrent interstitial pneumonitis. Due to the complexity of the disease and, in particular, the involvement of the patient's immune system, the clinical and radiographic findings are often atypical. The differential diagnosis of interstitial pneumonitis in pediatric AIDS includes lymphocytic interstitial pneumonitis, infectious agents (*Pneumocystis carinii*, cytomegalovirus, measles virus), and oxygen toxicity and/or mechanical ventilation (barotrauma), as well as chronic aspiration, which could be due to the encephalopathy often present in AIDS patients.

Lymphocytic Interstitial Pneumonitis (14)

The etiology of lymphocytic interstitial pneumonitis (LIP), in general and in HIV-infected children, is unknown. It could be related directly to HIV infection or to a coinfection. The detection by *in situ* hybridization of HIV-RNA, the isolation of HIV from bronchial alveolar fluid, and the higher levels of HIV-specific antibodies (anti-p24 and anti-gp41) in lung fluid of patients with HIV infection and LIP supports a causative role for HIV infection in the development of LIP. Some evidence supports a role for coinfection, specifically Epstein-Barr virus (EBV), in the pathogenesis of LIP. EBV genome has been detected by *in situ* hybridization in the lungs of HIV-infected children. LIP could be a response to polyclonal B-cell activation by EBV.

The spectrum of pulmonary lymphoid lesions in HIV-infected children ranges from the classic diffuse infiltrates of LIP to nodular infiltrates of pulmonary lymphoid hyperplasia (PLH). In LIP, there are diffuse interstitial and peribronchial infiltrates that consist of lymphocytes, plasma cells, plasmacytoid lymphocytes, and immunoblasts. PLH is characterized by peribronchial lymphoid nodules of 0.5 to 2.0 mm in diameter. The presence of overlapping features of LIP and PLH in lung biopsies of children with AIDS could represent a continuum of pulmonary lesions in HIV-infected children.

Initially, LIP produces few signs and symptoms. There could be a slight cough or the absence of respiratory signs. The presence of LIP is often first suggested by characteristic findings on chest radiograph of bilateral diffuse reticulo-nodular infiltrates. The mild clinical findings do not parallel the severity of the radiographic changes. LIP is usually associated with the presence of generalized lymphadenopathy, hepatosplenomegaly, enlarged parotid glands, and increased immunoglobulin levels. As LIP progresses, the presence of chronic lung disease could be evident by chronic cough, digital clubbing, tachypnea, and cyanosis.

In some children, the natural course of LIP seems to be static; in others it seems to slowly progress over months or years. Early in the course of LIP, chest radiographs show nodules approximately 1 mm in diameter. In later stages, the nodules can be 2 to 3 mm in diameter, and upper mediastinal adenopathy can be present.

Children with LIP frequently develop superimposed pneumonia. Fever, tachypnea, crackles, and hypoxia dominate the clinical picture. There can be leukocytosis, increased C-reactive protein, and a positive blood culture. Coalescence of the nodules can be seen on chest x-rays. The most commonly isolated organisms include *H. influenzae type b* and *S. pneumoniae*.

A presumptive diagnosis of LIP can be made on the basis of lung infiltrates that persist for at least 2 months, with no causative organism isolated and no response to therapy. A definitive diagnosis of LIP is made by lung biopsy that shows the typical lymphocytic infiltrates. No laboratory findings are specific for LIP.

In a child with radiographic evidence of reticulo-nodular infiltrates and significant manifestations of respiratory involvement, LIP alone must be differentiated from LIP complicated with a superimposed pneumonia, *Pneumocystis carinii* pneumonitis, miliary tuberculosis, or other primary pneumonia.

Early LIP requires no specific therapy. As LIP progresses, children can develop repeated bouts of hypoxia and hypercarbia. These incidents are usually discrete, and frequently associated with an intercurrent respiratory tract infection. With the progression of the lung disease, children can become chronically hypoxemic. At this point corticosteroids should be started and continued until there is clinical improvement. Severe cardiopulmonary complications such as bronchiectasis and cor pulmonale then ensue. These children need continuous supplemental oxygen, bronchodilators, diuretics, and, in some cases, inotropic agents. Children with LIP usually have longer survival than children with other HIV infection–associated diseases.

Pneumocystis carinii Pneumonitis (24)

Pneumocystis carinii pneumonitis (PCP) is a unique infection of the immunocompromised host. Unlike in other opportunistic infections, the process and the causative agent remain confined to the lungs in most cases, even in fatal ones.

PCP infection has been described in patients with a variety of immunologic disorders, but cellular immune defect has been generally accepted as more apt to predispose to PCP infection than defects in humoral immunity. Patient populations predisposed to infection with this organism include children with immunodeficiencies, children receiving immunosuppressive drugs, particularly corticosteroids, malnourished children, and debilitated, premature infants.

In premature infants, the onset is slow, with nonspecific manifestations such as poor feeding, tachypnea, and perioral cyanosis. Fever is usually absent, and crackles are often heard. The respiratory distress becomes severe in 1 to 2 weeks, with marked nasal flaring, tachypnea, chest retractions, and cyanosis. If untreated, the mortality is as high as 50%.

In immunocompromised children and adults, the onset is abrupt and fever is usually present. The absence of crackles is a usual feature. The disease follows a rapidly progressive course ending fatally in almost all cases.

In children with AIDS, the course of infection can follow either of the clinical types described above or have an intermediate course. Infants with perinatally acquired HIV infection can develop PCP during the first year of life, frequently as an early manifestation of HIV infection with or without other abnormalities. Early in the disease the chest x-ray can be normal. The disease can have a rapid progression manifested by increased respiratory distress and hypoxia. The white blood cells (WBC) count is usually normal, but LDH levels are frequently elevated to more than three times normal values. As the disease progresses, the chest x-ray reveals bilateral diffuse alveolar infiltrates radiating from the hilum, which are difficult to distinguish from pneumonias from other causes.

P. carinii pneumonitis is the most common and serious opportunistic infection in HIV-infected children. Even with the effective anti-*Pneumocystis* therapy now available, mortality from PCP in infants and children is high. Therefore, prevention is of critical importance.

At the present time, it is impossible to predict with certainty which children will or will not acquire PCP. It appears, however, that children who have significant involvement of their immune systems, as reflected by decreased age-adjusted CD4 + levels, are at increased risk of developing PCP, just as are adults. With the progression of HIV infection, CD4 + lymphocyte counts fall. *P. carinii* pneumonitis should be suspected in any infant at risk for HIV infection or known to be infected if respiratory symptoms develop. Therefore, prophylactic antibiotics should be started in the HIV-positive infant depending on the age and CD4 + counts. Definitive diagnosis relies on the histopathologic demonstration of organisms in the lung. Examination of specimens obtained by deep endotracheal suctioning often demonstrates the organism. Bronchoalveolar lavage is another useful alternative. Open lung biopsy and percutaneous lung puncture are the most reliable methods of diagnosis. The specimen should be stained using the methenamine-silver nitrate method of Gomori.

Clinical features are not enough to distinguish PCP from other opportunistic infections. In addition, PCP has been found in association with CMV infection, as well as other viral, bacterial, and fungal infections. An LDH determination, CD4 + lymphocyte counts, and arterial blood gases can help determine the therapeutic plan to follow. Trimethoprin-sulfamethoxazole (TMP-SMX) should be included as part of the initial antibiotic regimen if PCP is suspected. If the patient shows deterioration over the first 5 days of therapy or no improvement, pentamidine isethionate should be considered.

PREVENTION OF LOWER RESPIRATORY INFECTIONS (15,17,18)

Worldwide, acute respiratory infections are a leading cause of death in infants and young children. The attack rates of respiratory infections in children in both the developed and developing nations are similar, therefore variations in morbidity and mortality among countries are related largely to differences in availability of health care and nutrition.

Several host factors contribute to the morbidity and mortality of respiratory infections, malnutrition perhaps more than any other. Malnourished children are at increased risk of developing severe pneumonia with significant morbidity and mortality. Malnutrition is less common in breast-fed than in bottle-fed infants. Breast-fed infants have reduced risk of developing bronchiolitis from RSV and parainfluenza virus.

Minor changes in the environment, immunopreventive measures, and chemopro-phylaxis can prevent the development of serious illness involving the upper and lower respiratory tract.

There is sufficient evidence to support the association of passive smoking with an increased incidence of respiratory infections, particularly bronchitis and pneumonia, during the first year of life. Maternal smoking shows a much stronger effect than paternal smoking, especially in infants. Parents should be advised to stop smoking, or to at least avoid smoking in the house or in the immediate proximity of their children whenever possible.

Viral Infections

Respiratory Syncytial Virus

As infection is acquired by direct inoculation of large-particle secretions from con-taminated surfaces through finger-to-nose or -eye contact, careful hand washing can reduce spread in the hospital and in the home as well.

Influenza

Inactivated split virus vaccine is recommended for children with impaired cardiac, pulmonary, immune, renal, or metabolic function. Medical personnel should also receive the vaccine to reduce the introduction of infection to high-risk patients under their care. Amantadine offers short-term protection and can be used in high-risk children who require protection until vaccine-induced immunity develops and in those who have eggs allergy or other contraindication.

Adenovirus

A live attenuated oral vaccine (types 4, 7, and 21) has been used successfully to prevent acute respiratory infections in military personnel. As infection with this agent is sometimes acquired by self-inoculation, hand washing is helpful in reducing the spread of illness due to adenovirus.

Measles

Live attenuated measles vaccine is highly effective in preventing measles. Ex-posed susceptible children should receive a preventive dose of human immune glob-ulin, followed by immunization 3 months later.

Varicella

Varicella-zoster immune globulin can provide protection for exposed, susceptible, high-risk newborns, infants, and children. A live attenuated vaccine is presently un-der investigation in the United States and is in use in Japan and other nations.

Bacterial Infections

Group B Streptococci

Parenteral administration of ampicillin to high-risk, colonized, pregnant women (i.e., those with premature onset of labor, premature rupture of membranes, or fever) throughout labor has been demonstrated to decrease transmission of Group B streptococci to the infant and rates of disease in infants. Intrapartum treatment with ampicillin for a woman with a previously infected infant to prevent a subsequent neonatal infection is recommended. Treatment of the twin of an index case is indicated because of the high frequency of coinfection in both infants.

Chlamydia trachomatis

The identification and treatment of women with *C. trachomatis* genital tract infection during pregnancy can prevent disease in the infant. Pregnant women at high risk for *C. trachomatis* infection should be screened. Some experts advocate general testing of pregnant women.

Streptococcus pneumoniae

The 23-valent pneumococcal vaccine is indicated in children 2 years and older with increased risk of acquiring pneumococcal pneumonia and bacteremia. Included in this high-risk category are children with sickle cell disease, functional or anatomic asplenia, nephrotic syndrome or chronic renal failure, conditions associated with immunosuppression (e.g., organ transplant), and HIV infection.

Hemophilus influenzae Type b

All children should be immunized with an *H. influenzae* type b conjugate vaccine initially at approximately 2 months of age or as soon as possible thereafter with repeat administration at 4 and 6 months. Rifampin prophylaxis is indicated in all children exposed to a person with invasive *H. influenzae* type b disease regardless of their immunization status.

Pertussis

Pertussis vaccine is effective in reducing susceptibility to whooping cough but is toxigenic and probably the least immunogenic of the routinely used vaccines. Erythromycin given in the catarrhal stage can ameliorate the disease. After paroxysms are established, however, erythromycin is recommended primarily to limit the spread of the organisms to others. Household and other close contacts should receive prophylactic erythromycin for 10 days and a DPT booster if they are under 7 years old and have not received a booster within the past 6 months. There is an acellular vaccine recommended now for booster use only.

M. tuberculosis

Protection against exposure by closely monitoring children who come in contact with infected persons is an ideal form of prevention.

Pneumocystis carinii

Prophylactic administration of TMP-SMX or other agents to immunodeficient children is recommended in the following situations: prior PCP, fewer than 1,500 CD4+ cells in the first year with progressive decrease, and infants with established HIV infection.

REFERENCES

1. Arguedas, A.G., Stutman, H.R., and Marks, M.I. (1990): Bacterial pneumonia. In: *Kendig's Disorders of the Respiratory Tract in Children,* 5th Edition, edited by V. Chernick, W.B. Saunders, Philadelphia; 371–380.
2. Beem, M., and Saxon, E. (1982): *Chlamydia trachomatis* infections of infants. In: *Chlamydial Infections,* edited by P.A. Mardh, K.K. Holmes, J.D. Oriel, et al. Elsevier Biomedical Press, New York.
3. Bettenay, F., DeCampo, J, and McCrossin, D. (1988): Differentiating bacterial from viral pneumonia in children. *Pediatr. Radiol.,* 18:453–454.
4. Bryan, A.C., and Wohl, M.E.B. (1986): Respiratory mechanics in children. In: *The Respiratory System: Handbook of Physiology,* Sec. 3, Vol. 3, edited by A.P. Fishman, Williams and Wilkins, Baltimore.
5. Christensen, M., and Flanders, R. (1988): Comparison of the Abbott and Ortho enzyme immunoassays and cell culture for the detection of respiratory syncytial virus in nasopharyngeal specimens. *Diagn. Microbiol. Infect. Dis.,* 9:245.
6. Cowles, T., and Gonik, B. (1992): Perinatal infections. In: *Neonatal-Perinatal Medicine,* 5th Edition, edited by A. Fanaroff and R. Martin, Mosby Year Book, St Louis, MO.
7. Denny, F.W. (1987): Acute respiratory infections in children: etiology and epidemiology. *Ped. in Rev.,* 9(5):135–146.
8. Dyson, C., Poonyth, H.D., Watkinson, M., and Rose, S.J. (1990): Life-threatening *B. catarrhalis* pneumonia in young infants. *J. Infect.,* 21(3):305–307.
9. Eichenwald, H.D. (1978): Acute infections of respiratory tract. II. Lower airway: larynx, trachea, bronchi, lungs and pleura. *J. Cont. Edu. Pediatr.,* 20:14–28.
10. Gilsdorf, J.R. (1987): Community-acquired pneumonia in children. *Sem. Resp. Infect.,* 2:146–151.
11. Glezen, W.P. (1991): Viral respiratory infections. *Pediatr. Ann.,* 20(8):413–418.
12. Graham, P.S., and Hall, C.B. (1989): Nosocomial viral respiratory infections. *Sem. Resp. Infect.,* 4(4):253–260.
13. Hammerschlag, M.R. (1992): Is that pulmonary infection due to *C. pneumoniae? J. Respir. Dis.,* 13(10):1385–1397.
14. Hardy, K.A., Schidlow, D.V., and Zaeri, N. (1988): Obliterative bronchiolitis in children. *Chest,* 93:460.
15. Hoppenbrouwers, T. (1990): Airways and air pollution in childhood: state of the art. *Lung,* 168(Suppl.):335–346.
16. Issacs, D., Moxon, E., Harvey, D., Kovar, I., Madeley, C., Richardson, R., Levin, M., Whitelaw, A., and Modi, N. (1988): Ribavirin in respiratory syncytial virus infection. *Arch. Dis. Child.,* 63:986–990.
17. Karzon, D.T. (1991): Control of acute lower respiratory illness in the developing world: an assessment of vaccine intervention. *Rev. Infect. Dis.* 13(Suppl. 6):S571–S577.
18. Marcy, S.M. (1985): Prevention of respiratory infections. *Pediatr. Infect. Dis.,* 4(4):442–446.
19. McConnochie, K.M., Hall, C.B., Walsh, E.E., and Roghman, K.J. (1990): Variation in severity of respiratory syncytial virus infections with subtype. *J. Pediatr.,* 117(1):52–62.
20. McIntosh, K., and Chanock, R.M. (1990): Respiratory syncytial virus. In: *Virology,* 2nd Edition, edited by B.N. Fields, D.M. Knipe, R.M. Chanock et al. Raven Press, New York.
21. Peter, G. (1988): The child with pneumonia: diagnostic and therapeutic considerations. *Pediatr. Infect. Dis. J.,* 7:453–456.

22. Red Book (1991): *Report of the Committee on Infectious Diseases,* 22nd Edition. American Academy of Pediatrics, Elk Grove, Ill.
23. Reynolds, H.Y., and Merrill, W.W. (1981): Pulmonary immunology: humoral and cellular immune responsiveness of the respiratory tract. In: *Current Pulmonology,* Vol. 3, edited by D.H. Simmons. John Wiley and Sons, New York.
24. Scott, G.B., and Mastrucci, M.T. (1992): Pulmonary complications of HIV-1 infection in children. In: *HIV Infections in Infants and Children,* edited by R. Rogev and E. Connor. C.V. Mosby, St. Louis, Mo.
25. Tompkins, L.S. (1992): Current concepts: the use of molecular methods in infectious diseases. *N. Engl. J. Med.,* 327(18):1290–1297.
26. Turcios, N.L., and Evans, H.E. (1989): Establishing the diagnosis of tuberculosis in children. *J. Respir. Dis.,* 10(5):15–31.
27. Volovitz, B., Welliver, R., De Castro, G., Krystofik, D., and Ogra, P. (1988): The release of leukotrienes in the respiratory tract during infection with respiratory syncytial virus: role in obstructive airway disease. *Pediatr. Res.,* 24:504–507.
28. Wohl, M.E.B. (1990): Bronchiolitis. In: *Kendig's Disorders of the Respiratory Tract in Children,* 5th edition, edited by V. Chernick. W.B. Saunders, Philadelphia; 360–370.

Respiratory Infections: Diagnosis and Management, 3d ed., edited by James E. Pennington.
Raven Press, Ltd., New York © 1994

13

Pneumonia in the Elderly

Anthony L. Esposito

Division of Infectious Diseases, St. Vincent's Hospital, 25 Winthrop Street, Worcester, Massachusetts 01604

For decades, physicians have been intrigued by the unique manifestations of pneumonia in the elderly. In the early 19th century, Hourman and Dechambre (48–50) published a landmark series of articles in which they detailed the subtle features of the disease. Moreover, employing autopsy data, they identified age-related changes in the mechanics of respiration as important factors in the pathogenesis of the infection, which produced many of the "sudden deaths of old age" at their institution. Half a century later, in his textbook of medicine, Sir William Osler provided generations of physicians with insights into the clinical manifestations of the infection which remain unexcelled. Indeed, Osler's characterization of pneumonia as "the captain of the men of death" (79) continues to convey the gravity of the illness.

Pneumonia in the aged represents a clinical problem of enormous magnitude. For example, attack rates for pneumococcal pneumonia among persons 65 years of age and older have been estimated to be 12–14/1,000, a figure three- to fivefold greater than that reported in younger adults (14,31,57,64,73,107). Hospitalization is necessary in 90% of geriatric patients with pneumonia, and the average length of stay for aged individuals is almost twice that for younger adults (27,90). Seventy percent of deaths due to pneumococcal pneumonia occur in the elderly (90), and infection of the lower respiratory tract represents the leading infectious cause of death in persons 65 years of age and older (59). Moreover, demographic changes will likely result in a substantial increase in the extent of the problem over the next four decades. In 1980, 11% of the population in the United States, or 22 million, were 65 years of age or older; by the year 2030, 17%, or 48 million Americans, will be elderly (12).

Although many of the clinical aspects of pneumonia in the aged have been well described, information on the pathogenesis of the infection remains scant. In fact, the effects of normal aging on lung host defenses are largely unknown. The reluctance of physicians to perform elective bronchoscopy on otherwise healthy elderly persons and the absence, until recently, of animal models of aging are two important factors that have impeded research. The indifference of physicians toward old age could also have contributed to a lack of investigative interest. Indeed, ambivalence toward the problem was expressed by Sir William Osler: in 1892 he characterized pneumonia as "the special enemy of old age" (74); 6 years later he wrote, "Pneumonia may well be called the friend of the aged. Taken off by it in an acute, short, often painless illness, the old man escapes those 'cold gradations of decay' so distressing to himself and his family" (78).

In this chapter, the impact of normal aging on host defenses will be detailed, and the importance of concomitant pulmonary or systemic diseases in predisposing the elderly to infection of the lower respiratory tract will be assessed; because bacteria represent the pathogens most frequently isolated from aged patients with pneumonia, host defenses against that group of microbes will be emphasized. The salient clinical features and the microbiology of pneumonia in the geriatric patient will be reviewed. Finally, the management and prophylaxis of the infection will be discussed.

PATHOGENESIS

The protection of the lungs from infectious agents results from a complex interaction between anatomic barriers and cleansing actions present in upper airways and cellular and humoral responses operant in the terminal airspaces. Detailed reviews of pulmonary defense mechanisms are provided in other chapters of this book. In general, colonization of the oropharynx with potential pathogens represents the critical first step in the evolution of most bacterial pneumonias. The effects of the normal aging process on the factors that impede colonization with virulent organisms, such as the glycoprotein content of saliva, have not been fully characterized. Salivary immunoglobulin A (IgA) levels appear to remain unaltered. In fact, Finkelstein et al. (30) noted that the salivary IgA concentrations of 21 randomly selected aged persons were significantly greater than those of 17 younger controls.

The prevalence of oropharyngeal colonization with *Streptococcus pneumoniae* does not appear to increase with age, although definitive data from subjects greater than 65 years of age are not available (21,31,91). However, the oropharyngeal carriage rate of *Staphylococcus aureus* and aerobic gram-negative bacilli tends to be greater in the aged. In a throat culture survey of subjects who had received no antibiotics within 4 weeks, Valenti et al. (108) isolated aerobic gram-negative bacilli from 8% of a younger control group and from 19% of persons 65 years or older who lived independently, 23% of aged nursing home residents, 42% of chronically hospitalized patients, and 60% of geriatric patients on an acute care ward of a chronic disease hospital. The authors noted that the risk of colonization increased in elderly individuals who were unable to ambulate without assistance, who had difficulty performing activities of daily living, and who had bladder incontinence, chronic cardiac or respiratory disease, or a deteriorating clinical status. Phair et al. (85) demonstrated that among relatively fit persons admitted to the hospital, oropharyngeal colonization with *Staphylococcus aureus* and gram-negative bacilli occurred almost exclusively in individuals 60 years of age or older. Seven percent of the aged patients, all of whom were colonized, developed pneumonia; in contrast, none of the younger persons became infected. The authors were not able to correlate deficiencies of immune function or defects in the inflammatory response with the occurrence of either colonization or pneumonia. Irwin et al. (53) have illustrated the transient nature of upper airway colonization among the elderly. In a prospective, weekly prevalence survey of aged residents of a skilled nursing facility, the authors noted that colonization with aerobic gram-negative bacilli rarely lasted more than 3 consecutive weeks in the individual patient. Almost 50% of the patients were never colonized, and the noncolonized individuals were clinically indistinguishable from those who harbored gram-negative bacilli. Pneumonia did not occur in any patient during the survey. Similarly, Sveinbjornsdottir et al. (102) found that the oropharyngeal carriage of gram-negative bacilli among hospitalized elderly subjects was transient and associated with prior antibiotic use; of note, the rates of colonization were greatest upon admission but declined during the hospital stay.

Most bacterial pneumonias result from the clinically inapparent aspiration of oropharyngeal contents. The effects of normal aging on the mechanical factors that prevent aspiration, such as epiglottic function and deglutination, remain to be assessed. Esophageal dysfunction has been presumed to result from aging and to contribute to the occurrence of aspiration. Soergel et al. (97) found a high prevalence of aperistalsis after swallowing, frequent nonperistaltic contractions, and defective relaxation of the lower esophageal sphincter in nonagenarians with senile dementia, diabetes mellitus, or peripheral neuropathy. However, esophageal manometric studies performed by Hollis and Castell (47) in healthy 70- to 80-year-old subjects and in younger controls failed to detect differences in the prevalence of aperistalsis, spontaneous contractions, or defective lower esophageal sphincter function. Amplitudes of esophageal contractions were significantly decreased in the octagenarians, but the propagation of peristaltic waves was similar in all groups. Thus, a role for "presbyesophagus" in predisposing to aspiration remains to be established.

Age-related alterations in the mechanics and patterns of respiration suggest that the elderly are at greater risk for nocturnal aspiration. Senescence is associated with a loss of elastic tissue surrounding alveoli and alveolar ducts, an increase in the anteroposterior diameter of the chest due to rib and vertebral calcification, and a weakening of the muscles of respiration (72). These changes likely impair cough effectiveness. Disturbances in the patterns of respiration during sleep have been noted in greater than one-third of normal old people (13). Periods of apnea or hypopnea lasting 10 seconds and longer are commonly observed, and these usually result in the interruption of sleep. Although it is not known if apneic spells are directly associated with aspiration, the insomnia that aged individuals with disordered sleep patterns experience does lead to sedative use, which can predispose to aspiration.

Geriatric patients with altered states of consciousness due to medications or central nervous system disease are clearly at risk to aspirate. Employing a radioactive tracer technique, Huxley et al. (51) detected aspiration in two-thirds of elderly patients with stupor or coma. Because only a single test was administered and because a number of the patients had equivocal results, it is likely that with repeat evaluations aspiration would have been detected in all of the subjects. Dysphagia and mechanical devices increase the likelihood of aspiration; the dysphagia can be due to carcinoma of the oropharynx or esophagus, stricture of the esophagus, or central nervous system disease, such as bulbar or pseudobulbar palsy. By mechanically disrupting anatomic barriers, nasogastric or tracheostomy tubes also predispose to aspiration. The importance of nasogastric tubes as risk factors for pneumonia has been emphasized by recent studies which have indicated that 31–58% of patients with those devices will develop the infection (15,16,45,83,99). The risk of pneumonia in patients with nasogastric tubes appears to be independent of the underlying disease for which the device was placed; for example, in a study of late-stage demented patients by Peck et al. (83), aspiration pneumonia occurred in 58% of the subjects with nasogastric tubes and in 19% of controls.

Under normal circumstances, inhaled or aspirated microbes contained in large particles (2–3 microns) undergo inertial deposition on the mucosal surfaces of the upper respiratory tract because of flow turbulence and directional changes. Within a few hours these particles are mechanically removed by mucociliary transport or coughing. Employing different techniques, Goodman et al. (36) and Puchelle et al. (88) have demonstrated that nonsmoking, healthy aged persons have a significantly slower mucociliary clearance rate than do younger adults. Moreover, the tracheal mucous velocity of elderly smokers with chronic bronchitis is less than that of age-matched nonsmokers. Whether the decline in mucociliary transport present in normal aged individuals results from morphological or functional abnormalities of the ciliated epithelial cells lining the tracheobronchial tree or from alterations in the quantity or rheologic properties of the secretions coating the airways remains unknown. In any case, in the otherwise healthy aged person, abnormalities in mucociliary transport likely enhance the risk that aspirated particles will reach the terminal airspaces; in the senescent individual with chronic bronchitis and an abnormality of the cough, gag, or swallow reflex, the deposition of oropharyngeal secretions into the lower respiratory tract must be a frequent event.

Immunocompetent T- and B-cells reside within lymphoid tissue along the upper respiratory tract and within the bronchoalveolar spaces. T-lymphocytes secrete lymphokines which modulate the activities of the resident macrophage. For example, by enhancing the microbicidal potential of lung macrophages, the sensitized T-lymphocyte appears essential in controlling facultative intracellular pathogens, such as *Mycobacterium tuberculosis*. The normal aging process is associated with qualitative changes in the T-lymphocytes circulating in the peripheral blood (39,113,114). *In vitro*, T-cells from the aged exhibit attenuated responses to a variety of mitogens. *In vivo*, delayed cutaneous hypersensitivity reactions to both common and foreign test antigens tend to be blunted. The depression in T-lymphocyte function in healthy aged individuals is accentuated in the presence of chronic disease states, such as uremia and protein-calorie malnutrition. Gillis et al. (34) have documented that lymphokine production by T-cells from the aged is attenuated. Unfortunately, the influence of aging on the pulmonary T-lymphocyte populations remains unknown. Finally, immunoglobulins present in respiratory secretions are synthesized locally by B-lymphocytes or derived by transport from the intravascular pool. Specific IgG antibodies promote the lysis of gram-negative bacilli in the presence of complement, and opsonizing antibodies facilitate the phagocytosis of encapsulated organisms by bronchoalveolar macrophages and polymorphonuclear leukocytes. Because of age-related changes in helper T-lymphocyte function, the elderly exhibit a depressed antibody response to many new antigens (87). However, antibody responses to previously encountered antigens appear to remain intact. In any case, the impact of senescence on B-cell number and function within the lower respiratory tract has not been elucidated.

Information concerning the effects of aging on immunoglobulins within the lungs remains very limited; in a recent study of normal, nonsmoking subjects, Thompson et al. (104) found that the concentration of IgG in bronchoalveolar lavage fluid was significantly higher in the aged subjects versus the young and middle-aged controls. In contrast, substantial data are available concerning extrapulmonary immunoglobulin levels. The total concentration of serum IgG remains stable throughout life (11,85). However, the levels of antibodies against some bacterial pathogens appear to decline over time. In 1932, Sutliff and Finland (101) demonstrated that whole blood from persons 64 years of age and older was less frequently bactericidal against pneumococcal serotypes I, II, and III than was that obtained from younger subjects. Ammann et al. (1) detected a wide range of antibody concentrations to types 3 and 8 *S. pneumoniae* among relatively fit aged individuals; of note, the mean levels were significantly lower in the aged subjects versus the younger controls. In some populations, such as geriatric patients with chronic obstructive lung disease, antibody levels in excess of those considered protective are routinely detected (60). Norden (71) found that the prevalence of naturally occurring serum bactericidal antibodies to type b *Hemophilus influenzae* was 29% in persons 20 to 29 years of age and 8% in octagenarians. However, because these reports represent cross-sectional surveys, it remains unknown whether aged individuals who lack immunoglobulins to *S. pneumoniae* or *H. influenzae* ever possessed such antibodies. Clearly, longitudinal studies will be necessary in order to determine the effect of aging on the levels of serum antibodies against common bacterial pathogens.

The relative importance of locally produced IgA in protecting the lungs against bacterial pathogens remains uncertain. This class of immunoglobulins opsonizes bacteria poorly and does not fix complement in the classical manner. However, because IgA antibodies do agglutinate bacteria, perhaps resulting in more efficient removal by mucociliary transport, and because they inhibit the adherence of bacteria to respiratory epithelial cells, impeding colonization, these immunoglobulins do play a role in lung host defense. Limited data are available concerning the effect of age on the production of IgA within the tracheobronchial tree. Thompson et al. (104) observed that the amount of IgA present in the bronchoalveolar lavage fluid of elderly subjects was similar to that found in younger controls. Serum and salivary levels of IgA remain constant or increase in later life (11,89).

The critical importance of the bronchoalveolar macrophage in maintaining the sterility of the lower respiratory tract has become firmly established. The influence of advanced age on the resident macrophage population has yet to be determined. Information does exist concerning the peripheral blood monocyte. Munan and Kelly (68) surveyed over 2,000 healthy persons 10 to 96 years of age and determined that the total number of monocytes in the peripheral circulation remains stable through life. Gardner et al. (33) evaluated monocyte function in relatively fit, hospitalized, aged and younger patients and in nonhospitalized young controls. Significant differences could not be detected in the ability of monocytes from any of these groups to respond to chemotactic factors or to ingest and kill *Candida albicans*. It is tempting to extrapolate these data to the bronchoalveolar macrophage; however, although the peripheral blood monocyte and the pulmonary macrophage share a common origin, these cells possess substantial metabolic and functional differences. Preliminary observations indicate that the number of macrophages lining the tracheobronchial tree is not reduced in the elderly (104).

Although the effects of normal aging on the antimicrobial activities of the bronchoalveolar macrophage remain to be elucidated, it is likely that many elderly people harbor functionally inadequate cells. This assumption is based on the fact that the prevalence of diseases that are known to adversely affect the lung macrophage is high in the elderly. These disorders include systemic problems such as uremia, diabetes mellitus, and malnutrition, as well as pulmonary disorders such as hypoxemia, retained pulmonary secretions, cigarette smoking, and viral infection.

Antecedent infection with influenza A substantially predisposes the elderly individual to bacterial infection of the lower respiratory tract. Epidemiologic data obtained from pandemic and epidemic outbreaks have invariably shown that the highest fatality rates occur in persons 65 years of age or older, even though attack rates are greater in children and young adults (4,35). Aged patients with underlying cardiac or pulmonary disease are at greatest risk for complications of influenza. The specific aberrations in lung host defenses produced by the influenza A virus include a disruption of mucociliary transport, a predisposition to oropharyngeal colonization with pathogenic bacteria, and an attenuation in the bactericidal capacities of the bronchoalveolar macrophage and circulating neutrophil. Infection with influenza B, rhinoviruses, and other respiratory viruses probably results in less disruption of pulmonary defenses in that pneumonia appears to be a relatively uncommon complication, even in debilitated individuals (40,66,109).

Complement and polymorphonuclear leukocytes represent two components of the acute inflammatory response critical to the control of bacterial infection within the lower respiratory tract. Phair et al. (85) and others (70,80) have concluded that aging is not associated with changes in the opsonic capacity of serum or in the function of the classical or alternate complement pathways. An elevation in the concentration of C3 in the sera of apparently well, senescent subjects has been noted; the significance of this observation is unknown. The number of polymorphonuclear leukocytes in the peripheral blood remains unaltered throughout life (55,86). However, neutrophil reserves can be diminished in the aged. Timaffy (105) observed a blunted leukocyte response in aged subjects challenged intravenously with a lipopolysaccharide extract from *Shigella*. In younger persons, the mean increase above baseline was 109%; in the aged, the mean rise was 30%. Because the number of immature neutrophils increased markedly in the younger patients after challenge, Timaffy concluded that the attenuated response observed in the elderly was due to inadequate bone marrow reserves. On the other hand, the chemotactic responsiveness, oxidative metabolism, and phagocytic and bactericidal capacities of circulating neutrophils appear to remain unaltered in fit elderly individuals (18).

During the past two decades, a number of animal models of aging have been developed. These models have been used extensively in immunogerontological studies, and much of the data initially obtained from these systems have been confirmed in studies in humans (103). In addition to investigations of systemic immune function, studies of aging and lung host defense have been performed in animal models (25). Of note, in experiments in which C57BL/6 mice were screened for the presence of protective antibodies and underlying diseases, age-related differences in survival rates following infection with type 3 *S. pneumoniae, Klebsiella pneumoniae,* and *Staphylococcus aureus* have not been observed (25).

Although the studies performed in C57BL/6 mice have not revealed age-associated changes in survival rates, they have demonstrated substantial differences in the mechanisms through which the senescent animals respond to bacteria in the lower respiratory tract (25). Whether or not similar changes in local host defenses are present in humans remains to be determined. Nevertheless, the observations in the C57BL/6 mouse suggest that whereas advanced age could be associated with differences in pulmonary antimicrobial systems, those differences do not necessarily lead to an enhanced risk of infection of the lower respiratory tract or to an increased likelihood of a fatal outcome. In addition, the data from the animal models support the concept that factors beyond advanced age play important roles in determining infection risk and outcome; these factors include the existence of underlying disease, the use of immunosuppressive drugs, and the presence or absence of immunity against potential respiratory tract pathogens.

The majority of geriatric patients who experience community-acquired pneumonia have a substantial number of underlying medical conditions, including chronic obstructive pulmonary disease, ischemic heart disease, diabetes mellitus, malignancy, neurological impairment, and protein-calorie malnutrition (23,63,67,107,111,116). These conditions substantially enhance the susceptibility of the aged individual to infection of the lower respiratory tract by altering local or systemic host defenses; the mechanisms by which these conditions predispose to infection are summarized elsewhere (25). In most reports, geriatric patients hospitalized with community-acquired pneumonia have more associated medical conditions than do younger patients; for example, Marrie (63) found that in patients 30 years of age or younger the number of comorbid diseases was less than one; among patients 71 to 80 years of age, the number was almost three. It has also been noted that aged patients with pneumonia are characteristically receiving a variety of pharmacologic agents prior to the onset of their infection; for example, in one study of bacteremic pneumococcal pneumonia, 50% of the geriatric patients were taking nonsteroidal antiinflammatory agents, 44% were prescribed digitalis preparations, 33% were receiving sedatives or hypnotics, and 33% were being administered two or more of these drugs (23). Because a variety of pharmacologic agents can disrupt one or more components of host defense (24), the clinical observations raise the possibility that common drugs also contribute to predisposing the aged host to infection of the lungs.

Recent investigations have focused on risk factors for hospital-acquired (i.e., nosocomial) pneumonia in the elderly. Harkness et al. (43) identified neurological disease, renal dysfunction, an altered level of consciousness, a deteriorating clinical status, disorientation, difficulties in activities of daily living, aspiration, difficulty with oropharyngeal secretions, and the presence of a nasogastric tube as significant risk factors; through a logistic regression analysis, the best predictors were difficulty with oropharyngeal secretions and the presence of a nasogastric tube. Hanson et al. (41) found that the risk of nosocomial pneumonia was increased among geriatric patients with poor nutrition, neuromuscular disease, aspiration, a depressed level of alertness, intubation, admission to an intensive care unit, and nasogastric tube use; logistic regression analysis revealed a low serum albumin, a diagnosis of neuromuscular disease, and the presence of an endotracheal tube to be strong independent risk factors for the infection. These studies again emphasize the importance of debilitating underlying disease in the pathogenesis of pneumonia in the elderly.

CLINICAL FEATURES

A few contemporary publications detailing the clinical features of pneumonia in the aged have appeared in the medical literature (23,27,44); however, these reports have largely confirmed the accuracy of prior descriptions. Indeed, many physicians acknowledge that Sir William Osler's observations remain as insightful today as they were a century ago. Emphasizing the subtle manifestations of the infection, he writes: "In the old and debilitated, a knowledge that the onset of pneumonia is insidious and that the symptoms are ill-defined and latent should place the practitioner on his guard and make him very careful in the examination of the lungs in doubtful cases" (75). According to Osler, "At the extremes of life, pneumonia presents with certain well-marked features. . . . In old age, pneumonia may be latent, coming on without a chill; the cough and expectoration are slight. . . . The amount (of sputum produced) is very variable and in old people there may be none" (76). Osler noted, "In children and healthy adults the fever is usually higher than in old persons. . . . In healthy individuals and children, the pulse (at presentation) is full and bounding. . . . In the old and feeble, the pulse may be small and rapid from the onset" (77). He cautions the physician that in the elderly the examination can be misleading as "the physical signs (are typically) ill-defined and changeable" (77). Finally, Osler recognized the frequency with which aged patients with pneumonia experience changes in mental status: "These cases of cerebral pneumonia (in adults) are commonly associated with a very high fever. In senile and alcoholic patients, however, the temperature may be low but the brain symptoms pronounced" (76).

The most characteristic laboratory finding in the aged patient with pneumonia is a normal or mildly elevated total leukocyte count, although a frank leukocytosis can be present. Immature polymorphonuclear neutrophils and "toxic granulations" are often prominent. A frank neutropenia has long been recognized as an ominous prognostic sign. Multiple metabolic derangements are common; these include uremia, hyperglycemia, hyponatremia, hypernatremia, and hypophosphatemia. Arterial blood gases can reveal a profound hypoxemia produced by the acute infection, as well as by concomitant congestive heart failure or underlying obstructive pulmonary disease or both. The chest radiograph usually reveals an infiltrate at the time of presentation. However, the pneumonia could be obscured in the presence of pulmonary edema or by a technically inadequate film. Occasionally, a pulmonary infiltrate will not appear until 24 to 48 hours after admission; the negative initial study is often attributed to "dehydration."

Unlike younger patients, the aged are often incapable of expectorating lower respiratory tract secretions that might aid in establishing an etiologic diagnosis. Moreover, the specimens that are produced are frequently intermingled with oral secretions and debris. Transtracheal aspiration, a procedure that eliminates upper respiratory tract contamination, remains a research technique. Even when available, transtracheal aspiration is contraindicated in the elderly patient who has a disorder of hemostasis or who is not cooperative. Nevertheless, Berk et al. (9) performed the procedure on 32 acutely ill and hypoxemic aged patients without morbidity or mortality; the authors found that the bacteriologic information obtained by the transtracheal aspiration was very useful in the management of their patients. Tracheal suctioning ("snaking") usually represents the only practical means of obtaining lower respiratory tract secretions. Although the culture of sputum obtained by tracheal suction will be contaminated by oropharyngeal flora, the gram stain can provide insight into the etiology of the pneumonia. Tracheal suction is not without risk in the elderly patient, and arrhythmias and cardiac arrest have occurred as a result of the procedure. Because of the problem of obtaining an adequate sputum specimen and because of the inherent difficulties in interpreting the results of sputum gram stains and cultures, blood cultures are essential in the geriatric patient with pneumonia. The isolation of a pathogen from the blood could represent the only means of establishing an etiologic diagnosis and thus of ensuring focused antimicrobial therapy.

ETIOLOGIES

In the preantibiotic era, pneumonia in the aged was invariably attributed to *S. pneumoniae*. Contemporary studies have emphasized the growing importance of other pathogens (111). The pneumococcus remains the bacterium most frequently isolated from geriatric patients, and overall, it is responsible for about 50% of the infections. Garb et al. (32) and others (20,22) have shown that 40–45% of geriatric patients hospitalized with community-acquired pneumonia have nonpneumococcal disease. *H. influenzae, Klebsiella pneumoniae, Staphylococcus aureus, Escherichia coli,* and *Enterobacter* sp are the organisms most frequently isolated. The emergence of these pathogens as frequent causes of community-acquired bacterial pneumonia cannot be explained by prior antibiotic exposure or by improvements in bacteriologic techniques. Oropharyngeal anaerobes and *Mycoplasma pneumoniae* appear to be less-common causes of community-acquired pneumonia in this population.

The prevalence of *Legionella* among geriatric patients with pneumonia is not well established; however, the bacterium can produce both community-acquired and nosocomial infection, and legionellosis should be suspected in the patient who has a pneumonia that is progressive, that has prominent extrapulmonary manifestations, and that fails to respond to beta-lactam antibiotics (penicillins, cephalosporins). Similarly, although *Chlamydia pneumoniae* can cause community-acquired infection in the elderly (65), its importance as a pathogen remains to be defined. Finally, aged individuals immunosuppressed by corticosteroids, malignancies, or infection with the human immunodeficiency virus (HIV) can present with *Pneumocystis carinii* pneumonia (PCP) (42). The possibility of PCP should be considered in the geriatric patient with an atypical pneumonia syndrome characterized by a scantly productive cough, diffuse pulmonary infiltrates, and marked hypoxemia. Influenza A and other viruses represent additional causes of atypical pneumonia in the aged patient. Of note, respiratory syncytial virus (RSV) has been identified as a cause of fatal nursing home and community-acquired pneumonia; patients who survive typically require a prolonged period of convalescence, often lasting 6–8 weeks (62,98).

Fifty percent of geriatric patients hospitalized with nursing home–acquired pneumonia have nonpneumococcal infection; that figure increases to greater than 90% in nursing home patients administered antibiotics prior to admission (32). *H. influenzae, Klebsiella pneumoniae, Staphylococcus aureus, Escherichia coli, Enterobacter* sp, and *Proteus mirabilis* represent the most common isolates in these patients. The spectrum of pathogens producing hospital-acquired pneumonia appears to be similar to that observed in nursing home–acquired disease. Berk et al. (8) have shown that *S. pneumoniae* could be recovered by transtracheal aspiration from only 20% of geriatric patients with hospital-acquired pneumonia. Moreover, in a number of these patients, the aspirate revealed aerobic gram-negative bacilli, including *Klebsiella* sp, *Pseudomonas* sp, and *Serratia* sp, in addition to the pneumococcus. Yamamoto et al. (117) have also emphasized the fact that polymicrobial infection is prevalent in both nursing home–acquired and nosocomial pneumonia and that *S. aureus* and aerobic gram-negative bacilli represent common copathogens in geriatric patients with hospital-associated disease. Of note, Venkatesan et al. (110) have not found a high prevalence of infection due to *S. aureus* or gram-negative bacilli among aged patients with community- or nursing home–acquired pneumonia in the United Kingdom.

Moraxella (Branhamella) catarrhalis is recognized as a bacterium capable of producing community-acquired or nosocomial lower respiratory tract infection in debilitated aged patients (93,95), and group B *Streptococcus* has been identified as a cause of a highly lethal pneumonia in the elderly (112). The aged represent the main reservoir for tuberculosis in the United States, so infection with M. *tuberculosis* should be suspected in the geriatric patient with a subacute pneumonic illness or an apparent acute bacterial pneumonia that only partially responds to antibiotics. Nursing home patients present with either primary or reactivation tuberculosis.

The mortality of aged patients with pneumonia who are treated in-hospital varies with the offending pathogen. Approximately 20% of patients infected with *S. pneumoniae* will expire and up to 70% of those with disease due to *Klebsiella pneumoniae* or another aerobic gram-negative bacillus will succumb. The fatality rates of infection due to *H. influenzae* or *Staphylococcus aureus* appear to be in the range of 30 to 40%. Because 90% of aged patients hospitalized with pneumonia have other debilitating illnesses, the relative contribution to mortality made by underlying disorders appears to be substantial. Indeed, in their classic study of bacteremic pneumococcal pneumonia, Austrian and Gold (2) make the following observation: "Comparable in importance to age in its influence on prognosis was the presence or absence of complicating pre-existing illness." Contemporary studies have identified apyrexia, hypoalbuminemia, bed-ridden status, admission from a nursing home, and other factors that reflect advanced degrees of debilitation as significant predictors of mortality (52,64,110).

TREATMENT

Details concerning antimicrobial therapies and adjunctive interventions are presented in other chapters of this book. Nevertheless, a few aspects of the management of the aged patient with pneumonia merit emphasis. First, not all geriatric patients with pneumonia require hospitalization. Although relatively few studies have attempted to define the criteria necessary for ambulatory treatment, some information has become available. In general, ambulatory management is feasible if the elderly patient has no problem that requires stabilization (i.e., hypotension, hypoxemia), no factor indicating a poor prognostic outcome (i.e., neutropenia, multiple lobe involvement), and no functional or social impairment to care outside of the hospital (29). In a study of ambulatory patients of all ages with pneumonia, Black et al. (10) concluded that serious comorbid conditions and preexisting lung disease were among the most important factors supporting the need for hospitalization; of note, advanced age alone was not identified in the multivariate analysis as a factor that significantly impacted on the decision concerning hospitalization versus outpatient management.

Because of the high prevalence of nonpneumococcal infection, penicillin alone should not be employed as the initial therapy in the aged patient who cannot produce a quality sputum specimen. Pending the analysis of subsequent sputum gram stains and the results of cultures of blood and lower respiratory tract secretions, patients with community-acquired pneumonia should receive a second-generation cephalosporin (cefuroxime) or trimethoprim-sulfamethoxazole. Patients with nursing home–acquired infection can be given a second-generation (cefuroxime) or third-generation (ceftriaxone) cephalosporin; trimethoprim-sulfamethoxazole can be utilized in the patient intolerant to beta-lactam drugs. The management of geriatric patients with nosocomial pneumonia will be guided by a consideration of the area of the hospital in which the infection evolves (ward versus intensive care unit) and by a knowledge of the antimicrobial susceptibility patterns of pathogens prevalent within the specific institution; in general, a third-generation cephalosporin (ceftriaxone or ceftazidime) plus clindamycin would usually be appropriate. Critically ill patients with either community-acquired or nosocomial infections should also be considered candidates for erythromycin, the antibiotic of choice for Legionnaires' disease. Aminoglycosides should be reserved for use in seriously ill patients with infection due to *Klebsiella pneumonia, Pseudomonas aeruginosa,* or another aerobic gram-negative bacillus; in general, aminoglycosides should be used in combination with a beta-lactam drug, such as a third-generation cephalosporin, and they should be continued only until the patient demonstrates clinical improvement.

Untoward reactions to antimicrobials occur more frequently in the aged (26). The most common and serious antibiotic-related adverse reactions are usually a consequence of toxic serum levels which are caused by age-related changes in renal function. The normal aging process is associated with a decline in the glomerular filtration rate which is not reflected in the serum creatinine. Thus, dosing of drugs, especially aminoglycosides, should be guided by a measured creatinine clearance or by an estimated creatinine clearance that is derived from a formula that takes into account the patient's age and body weight. In any case, blood urea nitrogen, creatinine, and antibiotic levels must be monitored closely in patients administered aminoglycoside antibiotics. In addition, the aged are at greater risk than younger adults for other complications of antibiotic therapy, especially disease due to *Clostridium difficile.*

The management of the aged patient includes vigorous supportive measures in addition to judicious antimicrobial treatment. Hypoxemia, hyperglycemia, azotemia, hypophosphatemia, and other metabolic derangements should be quickly identified and corrected. Circulatory disorders, such as congestive heart failure, must also be addressed promptly. Antipyretics should be used with caution, and patients with extreme pyremia should have their temperatures lowered by gentle mechanical maneuvers, such as alcohol sponging. Caloric intake can be supplemented by parenteral feeding to avoid a state of negative nitrogen balance. Frequent turning in bed will prevent decubiti, and passive range of motion exercises will delay the development of contractures. Chest physiotherapy and intermittent positive pressure breathing treatments have not been proved to accelerate the rate of resolution of pneumonia but can be of value in selected patients.

PREVENTION

Efforts to reduce pneumonia attack and mortality rates have focused on the immunoprophylaxis of infection due to influenza A and *S. pneumoniae.* The administration of the influenza vaccine to adults of all ages during epidemics provides an overall protection rate of 80 to 90%. Moreover, the vaccine is effective in preventing infection in the elderly. In a study of relatively fit members of a retirement community, Stuart et al. (100) observed that among 3,338 recipients of monovalent influenza

A vaccine, 73% demonstrated a fourfold or greater rise in antibody titer. The highest postvaccination mean titers occurred in persons also immunized the previous year. Compared to unvaccinated residents of the community, immunized subjects experienced fewer febrile illnesses and hospitalizations during the 1965–66 influenza A epidemic. Barker and Mullooly (5) retrospectively analyzed influenza-related hospitalizations and deaths among elderly members of a prepaid health plan. These authors found that during the 1972–73 epidemic, vaccination reduced hospitalizations by an estimated 70% and deaths by 87%. In a study of geriatric home residents, Ferry et al. (28) noted a reduction in the severity of influenzal illnesses in vaccinated subjects, although the attack and death rates were similar in the immunized and control groups; in contrast, in a study of similar patients, Gross et al. (38) found that vaccination reduced the number of episodes of respiratory tract infection and prevented deaths.

Among nursing home residents, influenza vaccination programs have been associated with reductions in attack, complication, and mortality rates (82); nevertheless, because of poor vaccine acceptance among staff members and antigenic drift in the prevalent strains, outbreaks of disease do occur among well-immunized nursing home populations (17). Moreover, because senescence and concomitant disease can produce immunologic deficiencies, some aged individuals will not benefit from the influenza vaccine. Bandriss et al. (3) have demonstrated that although 72% of their ambulatory, institutionalized subjects had a fourfold or greater rise in antibody titer and 92% had postvaccination titers of 1:40 or greater, some patients failed to develop protective levels, even upon repeat vaccination. To enhance the generation of an immune response to the influenza vaccine, alternate methods of immunization are being explored. In a randomized, double-blind study, Treanor et al. (106) administered an inactivated trivalent influenza vaccine parenterally along with either a placebo or a live attenuated influenza A vaccine intranasally to elderly nursing home residents; the investigators found that the recipients of the intranasal vaccine experienced significantly fewer episodes of laboratory-confirmed influenza A infections.

In the setting of an epidemic of influenza A, the administration of amantidine hydrochloride should be considered for high-risk, nonimmunized patients pending vaccination or during the first two weeks after vaccination. The maximum dose of amantidine should be 100 mg daily. To reduce the likelihood of central nervous system toxicity, especially seizures, the specific dose should be based on the patient's measured or calculated creatinine clearance.

Because *S. pneumoniae* has long been recognized as the most prevalent pathogen in aged patients with bacterial pneumonia, attempts have been made throughout this century to control the infection with vaccines. In Kaufman's preantibiotic era study of over 10,000 chronically ill patients, approximately two-thirds of whom were elderly, vaccination with capsular polysaccharides from pneumococcal types I, II, and III resulted in reductions in attack, complication, and mortality rates (57). With the introduction of penicillin in the 1940s, interest in vaccination quickly waned. Penicillin dramatically enhanced the outcome for patients of all ages with serious pneumococcal infections. However, the impact on fatality rates was most striking in the youngest age groups. Thus, when compared to therapy with pneumococcal antiserum, penicillin reduced the death rate from bacteremic pneumococcal pneumonia in patients under 50 years of age from 40 to 8%; in older individuals, it fell from 64 to 28% (2).

A resurgence of interest in the immunization of the aged against infection with *S. pneumoniae* has resulted, in part, from the observation that in spite of the availability of potent antibiotics and sophisticated life-support facilities, deaths from pneumococcal pneumonia remain common. Indeed, among geriatric patients with bacteremic pneumococcal pneumonia, the case-fatality rates do not appear to have changed substantially since the advent of penicillin almost 50 years ago, and mortality rates approaching 50% continue to be reported (2,67,116). The persistently high fatality rates have been attributed to irreversible physiologic derangements that occur consequent to inadequacies in host defense and that supervene prior to medical intervention.

The contemporary pneumococcal vaccines (14- and 23-valent) contain capsular polysaccharide antigens from the serotypes associated with 70 to 80% of infections in the aged (6,7,107). In healthy, ambulatory elderly subjects, the polysaccharide vaccine is immunogenic (1,7). The percentage of fit individuals responding to immunization with a significant increase in antibody titers appears comparable to that observed in younger adults, and the postimmunization antibody levels are equal to those usually associated with protection. In addition, vaccination does increase antibody levels in many high-risk aged populations, such as patients with chronic obstructive pulmonary disease (19,60) and nursing home residents (6,92). However, in studies of elderly patients with chronic bronchitis, Musher et al. (69) have shown that the correlation between the presence of type-specific anticapsular antibodies and efficient opsonophagocytosis may be poor; thus, these studies suggest that although a vaccine may be immunogenic, it may not be protective.

Although a series of epidemiological evaluations have demonstrated that the pneumococcal vaccine is 60–70% effective in protecting elderly patients, practitioners have remained skeptical, in part because of the failure of clinical trials to confirm a benefit. In a randomized, prospective investigation of older, debilitated patients, Simberkoff et al. (95) administered the 14-valent vaccine or placebo to 2,295 male subjects with one or more underlying diseases; differences in attack rates for pneumococcal pneumonia or bronchitis between the vaccine and placebo recipients were not detected. Similar observations have been made by Leech et al. (61) in a smaller study of patients with chronic obstructive lung disease.

The definitive answer concerning the efficacy of the pneumococcal vaccine and the explanation for the disappointing outcomes of the clinical trials has likely been provided in a hospital-based, case-control study by Shapiro et al. (94). That investigation involved 1,054 patients infected with *S. pneumoniae* and a similar number of controls. Shapiro and colleagues found that the overall protective efficacy was 56%; among "immunocompetent" vaccine recipients, the calculated efficacy was 61%, but among "immunosuppressed" recipients, the vaccine was not protective. An analysis of the data for the "immunocompetent" patients also showed that the protective benefit of the vaccine was inversely related to age and that the benefit waned over time for recipients of all ages. Thus, based upon the data of Shapiro et al. (94) and the results of prior clinical and epidemiological investigations, the following conclusions seem reasonable: first, geriatric patients who have no immunosuppressive conditions will generate an immune response to the pneumococcal vaccine and will be protected from infection with *S. pneumoniae;* second, because immunity following vaccination fades, aged patients who are at high risk but relatively immunocompetent should be considered candidates for revaccination every

5–7 years; and finally, elderly individuals "immunosuppressed" by conditions such as disseminated cancer, lymphoma, splenectomy, multiple myeloma, monoclonal gammopathy, leukemia, and myelodysplasia do not respond to the polysaccharide vaccine and are not protected.

Because nasogastric tubes present a substantial risk for pneumonia, the benefit of alternate methods of enteral feeding are being explored. Strong et al. (99) found that nasogastric and nasoduodenal tubes produced similar rates of aspiration pneumonia among neurologically impaired patients of all ages. In a small, randomized, prospective study, Park et al. (81) did not detect significant differences in the frequency of aspiration pneumonia in patients with nasogastric tubes versus those given a feeding gastrostomy; other studies have also suggested that feeding gastrostomies do not reduce the incidence of pneumonia (15,16,45,54). In contrast, data from studies by Kaplan et al. (56) and Weltz et al. (115) indicate that surgically or endoscopically placed jejunostomy tubes can significantly reduce incidence of aspiration pneumonia; unfortunately, postoperative deaths, late surgical complications, and mechanical problems with the tubes are common.

SUMMARY

The assumption that biologic aging results in alterations in the capacity of the host to respond to potential pulmonary pathogens appears reasonable. However, the effects of normal aging on lung defense mechanisms remain largely unknown, and the relative roles that aging and concomitant disease play in enhancing the susceptibility of the senescent host to infection of the lower respiratory tract have yet to be determined. Research is necessary to not only advance our understanding of pathogenic mechanisms but to also improve our ability to prevent the infection. To clinicians, the problem of pneumonia in the elderly continues to present challenges in diagnosis and management.

REFERENCES

1. Ammann, A.J., Schiffman, G., and Austrian, R. (1980): The antibody responses to pneumococcal capsular polysaccharides in aged individuals. *Proc. Soc. Exp. Biol. Med.*, 164:312–316.
2. Austrian, R., and Gold, J. (1964): Pneumococcal bacteremia with special reference to bacteremic pneumococcal pneumonia. *Ann. Intern. Med.*, 60:759–778.
3. Bandriss, M.W., Betts, R.F., Mathur, U., and Douglas, R.G. (1981): Responses of elderly subjects to monovalent A/USSR/77 (H1N1) and trivalent A/USSR/77 (H1N1)-A/Texas/77(H3N2)-B/Hong Kong/72 vaccines. *Am. Rev. Respir. Dis.*, 124:681–684.
4. Barker, W.H., and Mullooly, J.P. (1980): Impact of epidemic type A influenza in a defined adult population. *Am. J. Epidemiol.*, 112:798–813.
5. Barker, W.H., and Mullooly, J.P. (1980): Influenza vaccination of elderly persons: reduction in pneumonia and influenza hospitalizations and deaths. *J.A.M.A.*, 244:2547–2549.
6. Bentley, D.W. (1981): Pneumococcal vaccine in the institutionalized elderly: review of past and recent studies. *Rev. Infect. Dis.*, 3(Suppl.):61–70.
7. Bentley, D.W., Simon, S.E., Douglas, R.G., and Robertson, R.G. (1974): Responses to pneumococcal vaccine in healthy elderly volunteers. *Clin. Res.*, 22:435 (abstract).
8. Berk, S.L., Gallemore, G.M., and Smith, J.K. (1981): Nosocomial pneumococcal pneumonia in the elderly. *J. Am. Geriatr. Soc.*, 29:319–321.
9. Berk, S.L., Holtsclaw, S.A., Kahn, A., and Smith, J.K. (1981): Transtracheal aspiration in severely ill elderly patients with bacterial pneumonia. *J. Am. Geriatr. Soc.*, 29:228–231.
10. Black, E.R., Mushlin, A.I., Griner, P.F., Suchman, A.L., James, R.L., and Schoch, D.R. (1991): Predicting the need for hospitalization of ambulatory patients with pneumonia. *J. Gen. Intern. Med.*, 6:394–400.

11. Buckley, C.S., III, Buckley, E.G., and Dorsey, F.C. (1974): Longitudinal changes in serum immunoglobulin levels in older humans. *Fed. Proc.*, 33:2036–2039.
12. Butler, R.N. (1981): Introduction to the second conference on the epidemiology of aging. In: *Epidemiology of Aging*, edited by S.G. Haynes and M. Feinleib, pp. 1–4. DHEW Publication No. (PGS) 80-969.
13. Carskadon, M.A., and Dement, W.C. (1981): Respiration during sleep in the aged human. *J. Gerontol.*, 4:420–423.
14. Centers for Disease Control (1984): Update: pneumococcal polysaccharide virus usage. *Morbid. Mortal. Week. Rep.*, 33:273–281.
15. Ciocon, J.O., Silverstone, F.A., Graver, L.M., and Foley, C.J. (1988): Tube feedings in elderly patients: indications, benefits, and complications. *Arch. Intern. Med.*, 148:429–433.
16. Cogen, R., and Weinryb, J. (1989): Aspiration pneumonia in nursing home patients fed via gastrostomy tubes. *Am. J. Gastroenterol.*, 84:1509–1512.
17. Coles, F.B., Balzano, G.J., and Morse, D.L. (1992): An outbreak of influenza A (H3N2) in a well immunized nursing home population. *J. Am. Geriatr. Soc.*, 40:589–592.
18. Corberand, J., Laharraque, P., and Fillola, G. (1986): Neutrophils of healthy aged humans are normal. *Mech. Aging Dev.*, 36:57–63.
19. Davis, A.L., Aranda, C., Christianson, L., and Schiffman, G. (1981): Pneumococcal antibodies in patients with chronic obstructive pulmonary disease and their response to pneumococcal capsular polysaccharides. *Rev. Infect. Dis.*, 3(Suppl.):183.
20. Dorff, G.J., Rytell, M.W., Farmen, S.G., and Scanlong, G. (1973): Etiologies and characteristic features of pneumonias in a municipal hospital. *Am. J. Med. Sci.*, 266:349–358.
21. Dowling, J.N., Sheehe, P.R., and Feldman, H.A. (1971): Pharyngeal pneumococcal acquisitions in "normal" families: a longitudinal study. *J. Infect. Dis.*, 124:9–17.
22. Ebright, J.R., and Rytel, M.W. (1980): Bacterial pneumonia in the elderly. *J. Am. Geriatr. Soc.*, 28:220–223.
23. Esposito, A.L. (1984): Community-acquired bacteremic pneumococcal pneumonia: effect of age on manifestations and outcome. *Arch. Intern. Med.*, 149:945–948.
24. Esposito, A.L. (1988): The effect of common pharmacologic agents on pulmonary antibacterial defenses: implications for the geriatric patient. *Clin. Chest Med.*, 8:373–380.
25. Esposito, A.L. (1991): Pulmonary host defenses. In: *Respiratory Infections in the Elderly*, edited by M.S. Neiderman, pp. 25–45. Raven Press, New York.
26. Esposito, A.L., and Gleckman, R.A. (1980): Antibiotic-related adverse reactions of special significance in the elderly. *Geriatrics*, 35:26–37.
27. Fedullo, A.J., and Swinburn, A.J. (1985): Relationship of patient age to clinical features and outcome for in-hospital treatment of pneumonia. *J. Gerontol.*, 40:29–33.
28. Ferry, B.J., Evered, M.G., and Morrison, E.I. (1979): Different protection rates in various groups of volunteers given subunit influenza virus in 1976. *J. Infect. Dis.*, 139:237–241.
29. Fine, M.J. (1990): Pneumonia in the elderly: the hospital admission and discharge decisions. *Sem. Resp. Dis.*, 5:303–313.
30. Finkelstein, M.S., Tanner, M., Shenkman, L., Gottlieb, D., and Freedman, M.L. (1980): Salivary and serum IgA levels in a geriatric outpatient population. *Gerontologist*, 20(Suppl. 2):104.
31. Foy, H.J., Wentworth, B., Kenny, G.E., Kloeck, J.M., and Grayston, J.T. (1975): Pneumococcal isolations from patients with pneumonia and control subjects in a prepaid medical group. *Am. Rev. Respir. Dis.*, 111:595–601.
32. Garb, J.L., Brown, R.B., Garb, J.R., and Tuthill, R.W. (1975): Differences in etiology of pneumonia in nursing home and community patients. *J.A.M.A.*, 240:2169–2172.
33. Gardner, I.D., Lim, S.T., and Lawton, J.W. (1981): Monocyte function in aging humans. *Mech. Aging. Dev.*, 16:233–239.
34. Gillis, S., Kozas, R., Durante, M., and Weksler, M.E. (1981): Immunological studies of aging: decreased production of and response to T-cell growth factor by lymphocytes from aged humans. *J. Clin. Invest.*, 67:937–942.
35. Glezen, W.P., and Couch, R.B. (1978): Interpandemic influenza in the Houston area, 1974–76. *N. Engl. J. Med.*, 298:587–592.
36. Goodman, R.M., Yergin, B.M., Landa, J.F., Golinvaux, M.H., and Sacker, M.A. (1978): Relationship of smoking history and pulmonary function tests to tracheal mucous velocity in nonsmokers, young smokers, ex-smokers and patients with chronic bronchitis. *Am. Rev. Respir. Dis.*, 117:205–214.
37. Green, G.M., Jakab, G.J., Low, R.B., and Davis, G.S. (1977): Defense mechanisms of the respiratory membrane. *Am. Rev. Respir. Dis.*, 115:479–514.
38. Gross, P.A., Quinnan, G.V., Rodstein, M., et al. (1988): Association of influenza immunization with reduction in mortality in an elderly population. *Arch. Intern. Med.*, 148:562–565.
39. Grossman, J., Baum, J., Gluckman, J., Fusner, J., and Condemi, J.J. (1975): The effect of aging and acute illness on delayed hypersensitivity. *J. Allergy Clin. Immunol.*, 55:268–275.
40. Hall, W.N., Goodman, R.A., Noble, G.R., Kendal, A.P., and Steece, R.S. (1981): An outbreak of influenza B in an elderly population. *J. Infect. Dis.*, 144:297–302.

41. Hanson, L.C., Weber, D.J., and Rutala, W.A. (1992): Risk factors for nosocomial pneumonia in the elderly. *Am. J. Med.*, 92:161–166.
42. Hargreaves, M.R., Fuller, G.N., and Gazzard, B.G. (1988): Occult AIDS: *Pneumocystis carinii* pneumonia in elderly people. *Br. Med. J.*, 297:721–722.
43. Harkness, G.A., Bentley, D.W., and Roghmann, K.J. (1990): Risk factors for nosocomial pneumonia in the elderly. *Am. J. Med.*, 89:457–463.
44. Harper, C., and Newton, P. (1989): Clinical aspects of pneumonia in the elderly veteran. *J. Am. Geriatr. Soc.*, 37:867–872.
45. Hassett, J.M., Sunby, C., and Flint, L.M. (1988): No elimination of aspiration pneumonia in neurologically disabled patients with feeding gastrostomy. *Surg. Gynecol. Obstet.*, 167:383–388.
46. Hayashi, M., and Huber, G.L. (1980): Airway defenses. *Sem. Resp. Med.*, 1:233–239.
47. Hollis, J.B., and Castell, D.O. (1974): Esophageal function in elderly men. *Ann. Intern. Med.*, 80:371–374.
48. Hourman and Dechambre (1835): Recherches pour servir a l'histoire des vieillards faites à la Salpetriere. Maladies des organes de la respiration. *Arch. Gen. Med.* (Paris), 8:405–435.
49. Hourman and Dechambre (1836): Pneumonie chez les vieillards: characteres anatomiques. *Arch. Gen. Med.* (Paris), 10:269–296.
50. Hourman and Dechambre (1836): Pneumonie des vieillards: Etiologie et symptomatologie. *Arch. Gen. Med.* (Paris), 12:164–182.
51. Huxley, E.J., Viroslav, J., Gray, W.R., and Pierce, A.K. (1978): Pharyngeal aspiration in normal adults and patients with depressed consciousness. *Am. J. Med.*, 64:564–568.
52. Ichikawa, Y., Tokunaga, N., Kakizoe, Y., et al. (1992): Host factors which influence the outcome of pneumonia in the elderly. *Jap. J. Thoracic Dis.*, 30:209–215.
53. Irwin, R.S., Whitaker, S., Pratter, M.R., Milland, C.E., Tarpey, J.T., and Corwin, R.W. (1982): The transiency of oropharyngeal colonization with gram-negative bacilli in residents of a skilled nursing facility. *Chest*, 81:31–35.
54. Jarnagin, W.R., Duh, Q.Y., Mulvihill, S.J., et al. (1992): The efficacy and limitations of percutaneous endoscopic gastrostomy. *Arch. Surg.*, 127:261–264.
55. Jernigan, J.A., Gudat, J.C., Blake, J.L., Bowen, L., and Lezotte, D.C. (1980): Reference values for blood findings in relatively fit elderly persons. *J. Am. Geriatr. Soc.*, 28:308–314.
56. Kaplan, D.S., Murthy, U.K., and Linscheer, W.G. (1989): Percutaneous endoscopic jejunostomy: long-term follow-up of 23 patients. *Gastrointest. Endoscopy*, 35:403–406.
57. Kauffman, P. (1974): Pneumonia in old age: active immunization against pneumonia with pneumococcus polysaccharide: results of a six-year study. *Arch. Intern. Med.*, 79:518–531.
58. Kazmierowski, J.A., Aduan, R.P., and Reynolds, H.Y. (1977): Pulmonary host defense: coordinated interaction of mechanical, cellular and humoral immune systems of the lung. *Bull. Eur. Physiopath. Resp.*, 13:103–116.
59. Kovar, M.D. (1977): Health of the elderly and use of health services. *Public Health Rep.*, 92:9–19.
60. Landsman, S.H., Smith, P.M., and Schiffman, G. (1983): Pneumococcal vaccine in elderly patients with COPD. *Chest*, 48:433–435.
61. Leech, J.A., Gervis, A., and Ruben, F.L. (1987): Efficacy of pneumococcal vaccine in severe obstructive pulmonary disease. *Can. Med. Assoc. J.*, 136:361–365.
62. Levenson, R.M., and Kantor, O.S. (1987): Fatal pneumonia in an adult due to respiratory syncytial virus. *Arch. Intern. Med.*, 147:791–792.
63. Marrie, T.J. (1990): Epidemiology of community-acquired pneumonia in the elderly. *Sem. Resp. Dis.*, 5:260–268.
64. Marrie, T.J., Durant, H., and Yates, L. (1989): Community-acquired pneumonia requiring hospitalization: 5-year prospective study. *Rev. Infect. Dis.*, 11:586–599.
65. Marrie, T.J., Grayston, J.T., Wang, S.P., and Kuo, C.C. (1987): Pneumonia associated with the TWAR strain of *Chlamydia*. *Ann. Intern. Med.*, 106:507–511.
66. Mathur, U., Bentley, D.W., and Hall, C.B. (1980): Concurrent respiratory syncytial virus and influenza A infections in the institutionalized elderly and chronically ill. *Ann. Intern. Med.*, 93:49–52.
67. Mufson, M.A., Kruss, D.M., Wasil, R.E., and Metzger, W.I. (1974): Capsular types and outcome of bacteremic pneumococcal disease in the antibiotic era. *Arch. Intern. Med.*, 134:505–510.
68. Munan, L., and Kelly, A. (1979): Age-dependent changes in blood monocyte populations in man. *Clin. Exp. Immunol.*, 35:1961–1962.
69. Musher, D.M., Chapman, A.J., Goree, A., Jonsson, S., Briles, D., and Baughn, R.E. (1986): Natural and vaccine-related immunity to *Streptococcus pneumoniae*. *J. Infect. Dis.*, 154:245–255.
70. Nagaaki, K., Hiramatsu, S., Inai, S., and Sasaki, A. (1980): The effect of aging on complement activity (CH50) and complement protein levels. *J. Clin. Lab. Immunol.*, 3:45–50.
71. Norden, C.W. (1974): Prevalence of bactericidal antibodies to *Hemophilus influenzae*, type b. *J. Infect. Dis.*, 130:489–494.

72. Ohar, S., Shasti, S.R., and Lenora, R.A. (1976): Aging and the respiratory system. *Med. Clin. No. Amer.*, 50:1121–1139.
73. Oseasohn, R., Skipper, S.E., and Tempest, B. (1978): Pneumonia in a Navajo community: a two-year experience. *Am. Rev. Respir. Dis.*, 117:1003–1009.
74. Osler, W. (Editor) (1892): *The Principles and Practice of Medicine*, 1st Edition, p. 511. D. Appleton, New York.
75. Ibid., p. 529.
76. Ibid., p. 520.
77. Ibid., pp. 525–526.
78. Osler, W. (Editor) (1898): *The Principles and Practice of Medicine*, 3rd Edition, p. 109. D. Appleton, New York.
79. Osler, W. (Editor) (1901): *The Principles and Practice of Medicine*, 4th Edition, p. 108. D. Appleton, New York.
80. Palmblad, J., and Haak, A. (1978): Aging does not change blood granulocyte bactericidal capacity and levels of complement factors 3 and 4. *Gerontology*, 24:381–385.
81. Park, R.H., Allison, M.C., Lang, J., et al. (1992): Randomised comparison of percutaneous endoscopic gastrostomy and nasogastric tube feeding in patients with persisting neurological dysphagia. *Br. Med. J.*, 304:1406–1409.
82. Patriarca, P.A., Arden, N.H., Koplan, J.P., and Goodman, R.A. (1987): Prevention and control of type A influenza infections in nursing homes. *Ann. Intern. Med.*, 107:732–740.
83. Peck, A., Cohen, C.E., and Mulvihill, M.N. (1990): Long-term enteral feeding of aged demented nursing home patients. *J. Am. Geriatr. Soc.*, 38:1195–1198.
84. Phair, J.P., Kauffman, C.A., and Bjornson, A. (1977): Investigation of host defense mechanisms in the aged as determinants of nosocomial colonization and pneumonia. *J. Reticuloendothel. Soc.*, 23:397–405.
85. Phair, J.P., Kauffman, C.A., Bjornson, A., Gallagher, J., Adams, L., and Hess, E.V. (1978): Host defenses in the aged: evaluation of components of the inflammatory and immune responses. *J. Infect. Dis.*, 138:67–73.
86. Polednak, A.P. (1978): Age changes in differential leukocyte count among female adults. *Human Biol.*, 50:301–311.
87. Price, G.B., and Makinodan, T. (1972): Immunologic deficiencies in senescence. I. Characterization of intrinsic deficiencies. *J. Immunol.*, 108:403–412.
88. Puchelle, E., Zahm, J.M., and Bertrand, A. (1979): Influence of age on mucociliary transport. *Scand. J. Respir. Dis.*, 60:307–313.
89. Radl, J., Sepers, J.M., Skvaril, F., Morell, A., and Hijmons, W. (1975): Immunoglobulin patterns in humans over 95 years of age. *Clin. Exp. Immunol.*, 22:84–90.
90. Roden, D.R., and Platt, W.G. (Editors) (1978): *A Study to Estimate the Prevalence and Costs of Pneumonia*, pp. 14–24. Pracon, Washington, D.C.
91. Rosenau, M.J., Felton, L.D., and Atwater, R.M. (1926): An epidemiologic study of pneumonia and its spread. *Am. J. Hygiene*, 6:463–483.
92. Ruben, F.L., and Uhrin, M. (1985): Specific immunoglobulin-class antibody responses in the elderly before and after 14-valent pneumococcal vaccine. *J. Infect. Dis.*, 151:845–849.
93. Scrinivasan, E.B., Raff, M.J., Templeton, W.C., Givens, S.J., Graves, C., and Melo, J.C. (1981): *Branhamella catarrhalis* pneumonia: report of two cases and review of the literature. *Am. Rev. Respir. Dis.*, 123:553–555.
94. Shapiro, E.D., Berg, A.T., Austrian, R., et al. (1991): The protective efficacy of polyvalent pneumococcal vaccine. *N. Engl. J. Med.*, 325:1453–1460.
95. Simberkoff, M., Cross, A.P., Al-Ibrahim, M., et al. (1986): Efficacy of pneumococcal vaccine in high-risk patients: results of a Veterans Administration Cooperative Study. *N. Eng. J. Med.*, 315:1318–1327.
96. Slevin, J.S., Aitken, J., and Thornley, P.E. (1984): Clinical and microbiologic features of *Branhamella catarhallis* bronchopulmonary infections. *Lancet*, 1:7812–7813.
97. Soergel, K.H., Zboralske, F.F., and Amberg, J.R. (1964): Prebyesophagus: esophageal motility in nonagenarians. *J. Clin. Invest.*, 43:1472–1479.
98. Sorvillo, F.J., Huie, S.F., Strassburg, M.A., Butsumyo, A., Shandera, W.X., and Fannin, S.L. (1984): An outbreak of respiratory syncytial virus pneumonia in a nursing home for the elderly. *J. Infect.*, 9:252–256.
99. Strong, R.M., Condon, S.C., Solinger, M.R., Namihas, B.N., Ito-Wong, L.A., and Leuty, J.E. (1992): Equal aspiration rates from postpylorus and intragastric-placed small-bore nosogastric feeding tubes: a randomized, prospective study. *J. Parenteral Enteral Nutrition*, 16:59–63.
100. Stuart, W.H., Dull, H.B., Newton, L.H., Mcqueen, J.L., and Schiff, E.R. (1969): Evaluation of monovalent influenza vaccine in a retirement community during the epidemic of 1965–1966. *J.A.M.A.*, 309:232–238.
101. Sutliff, W.D., and Finland, M. (1932): Antipneumococcic immunity reactions in individuals of different ages. *J. Exp. Med.*, 55:837–852.

102. Sveinbjornsdottir, S., Gudmundsson, S., and Briem, H. (1991): Oropharyngeal colonization in the elderly. *Eur. J. Clin. Micro. Infect. Dis.,* 10:959–963.
103. Thoman, M.L., and Weigle, W.O. (1989): The cellular and subcellular basis of immunosenescence. *Adv. Immunol.,* 46:221–261.
104. Thompson, A.B., Scholer, S.G., Daughton, D.M., Potter, J.F., and Rennard, S.I. (1992): Altered epithelial lining fluid parameters in old normal individuals. *J. Gerontol.,* 47:M171–M176.
105. Timaffy, M. (1962): A comparative study of bone marrow function in young and old individuals. *Gerontol. Clin.,* 4:13–18.
106. Treanor, J.J., Mattison, H.R., Dumyati, G., et al. (1992): Protective efficacy of combined live intranasal and inactivated influenza A vaccines in the elderly. *Ann. Intern. Med.,* 117:625–633.
107. Valenti, W.N., Jenzer, M., and Bentley, D.W. (1978): Type-specific pneumococcal respiratory disease in the elderly and chronically ill. *Am. Rev. Respir. Dis.,* 177:233–238.
108. Valenti, W.M., Randall, R.G., and Bentley, D.W. (1978): Factors predisposing to oropharyngeal colonization with gram-negative bacilli in the aged. *N. Engl. J. Med.,* 298:1108–1111.
109. Van Voris, L.P., Belshe, R.B., and Shaffer, J.L. (1982): Nosocomial influenza B virus infection in the elderly. *Ann. Intern. Med.,* 96:153–158.
110. Venkatesan, P., Gladman, J., MacFarlane, J.T., et al. (1990): A hospital study of community-acquired pneumonia in the elderly. *Thorax,* 45:254–258.
111. Verghese, A., and Berk, S.L. (1983): Bacterial pneumonia in the elderly. *Medicine,* 62:271–285.
112. Verghese, A., Berk, S.L., Boelen, L.J., and Smith, J.K. (1982): Group B streptococcal pneumonia in the elderly. *Arch. Intern. Med.,* 142:1642–1645.
113. Waldorf, D.S., Wilkens, R.F., and Decker, J.L. (1968): Impaired delayed hypersensitivity in an aging population. *J.A.M.A.,* 203:831–834.
114. Weksler, M.E., and Hutteroth, T.H. (1974): Impaired lymphocyte function in aged humans. *J. Clin. Invest.,* 53:99–103.
115. Weltz, C.R., Morris, J.B., and Mullen, J.L. (1992): Surgical jejunostomy in aspiration risk patients. *Ann. Surg.,* 215:140–145.
116. Woodhead, M.A., MacFarlane, J.T., Rodgers, F.G., Laverick, A., Pilkington, R., and MacRea, A.D. (1985): Aetology and outcome of severe community-acquired pneumonia. *J. Infect.,* 10:204–210.
117. Yamamoto, K., Yamada, Y., Hayashi, Y., et al. (1990): Studies of polymicrobial infection in pneumonia by transtracheal aspiration in the elderly. *J. Jap. A. Infect. Dis.,* 64:1433–1438.

Respiratory Infections: Diagnosis and Management, 3d ed.,
edited by James E. Pennington.
Raven Press, Ltd., New York © 1994

14

Pneumonia in the Immunocompromised Host

Christopher H. Fanta and James E. Pennington

*Departments of Medicine of the Brigham and Women's Hospital and Harvard Medical
School, Boston Massachusetts 02115; and University of California,
San Francisco, California 94143*

The student of medicine usually acquires knowledge by the detailed examination of individual disease entities: their epidemiology, pathophysiology, clinical presentation, diagnosis, and treatment. The physician practicing medicine, on the other hand, more often is faced with a clinical condition lacking an etiologic label, a constellation of symptoms and signs for which the cause still remains to be discovered. This chapter addresses the clinical problem of pulmonary infiltrates in the immunocompromised host from the point of view of the approach to the undiagnosed patient. We will discuss what diagnostic clues can be learned from history and physical examination, review which laboratory tests are of value and which are not, and examine the yield of various invasive diagnostic procedures. Given the myriad of specific causes for this syndrome, some infectious and others not, the temptation when faced with such a patient is to throw up one's hands in dismay and automatically conclude that open lung biopsy or multiple drug empiric antibiotic therapy are one's only options. Our contention is that a systematic approach to the immunocompromised host with pulmonary infiltrates can narrow the differential diagnosis and in many cases lead to more rational selection of diagnostic tests and therapeutic interventions.

Despite the advances of modern immunology, immunosuppression is still defined by the susceptibility to infection of certain populations rather than by specific laboratory tests of white blood cell or antibody function. For the purposes of this discussion, we will focus on patients immunocompromised by virtue of (i) lymphoma or leukemia; (ii) other malignancies and the chemotherapeutic drugs given for these neoplasias; (iii) organ transplantation and attendant immunosuppressive therapy; (iv) neutropenia (fewer than 500 circulating neutrophils per mm³, from any cause); or (v) immunosuppressive drugs, including high-dose corticosteroids, given for any indication. Other immunocompromised patient populations, such as those with hypogammaglobulinemia, complement deficiencies, asplenia, collagen-vascular disorders, and acquired immune deficiency syndrome, will not be specifically considered here.

The magnitude of the problem of pulmonary infections in these patient groups is immense. In patients with lymphoma who are receiving intensive chemotherapy, the lung is the most common site of serious infections, and deaths from infection are most often associated with pneumonia (8). Patients with acute leukemia in relapse suffer an episode of pneumonia once every 60 days of patient risk (54). Interstitial pneumonias occur in as many as 55% of bone marrow transplant recipients who survive 30 days posttransplantation, with an associated mortality of approximately 66% (12,64). In a review of renal allograft recipients over a 12-year period at one institution, pulmonary diseases (of which two-thirds were infectious) complicated 20% of all transplants and were associated with 50% of the fatalities (47). Progress in the duration of survival in many of these conditions awaits our ability to prevent, or to diagnose and effectively treat, these common and devastating pulmonary complications (53).

A partial listing of the spectrum of pulmonary diseases to which the immunocompromised host is susceptible appears in Table 14-1, divided into infectious, noninfectious, and unknown etiologies. It is important to emphasize that two or more processes can coexist in the lungs at one time. For instance, we have seen in a renal transplant patient diffuse pulmonary infiltrates due to coexistent pneumocystis, cytomegalovirus, and cryptococcus. Figure 14-1 is the chest radiograph of a woman with breast cancer and three distinct pulmonary processes: lymphangitic spread of her breast cancer, radiation fibrosis, and a nocardial abscess.

HISTORICAL DATA

Cough and dyspnea are the most common complaints in patients symptomatic from their pulmonary infiltrates. Most patients with pulmonary infections, even in the presence of neutropenia, manifest a fever; but fever is by no means a reliable sign of infection. Many noninfectious processes elicit fever as part of the inflammatory response, including radiation pneumonitis, cytotoxic drug-induced lung dis-

TABLE 14–1. *Pulmonary infiltrates in the immunocompromised host:*
a partial listing of causes

Infectious	Noninfectious	Unknown cause
Bacterial	Pulmonary edema	Nonspecific interstitial
S. aureus	Cytotoxic drug-induced lung	pneumonia (or organizing
Gram-negative bacilli	injury	pneumonia)
Legionella sp	Radiation pneumonitis/fibrosis	
Nocardia	Leukostasis	
Viral	Leukoagglutinin reaction	
Cytomegalovirus	Spread of underlying neoplasm	
Herpes simplex	Leukemic cell lysis	
Adenovirus	Pulmonary hemorrhage	
Varicella-zoster		
Parainfluenza virus		
Human herpes virus 6		
Fungal		
Cryptococcus		
Aspergillus		
Mucormycosis		
Candida		
Mycobacterial		
M. tuberculosis		
Parasitic		
Pneumocystis		
Strongyloides		
Toxoplasma		

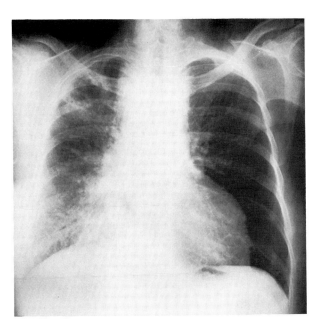

FIG. 14–1. Forty-six-year-old woman following mastectomy for breast cancer with (i) radiation fibrosis, (ii) lymphangitic spread of cancer, and (iii) nocardial abscess in right upper lobe.

ease, and nonspecific interstitial pneumonitis. Furthermore, fever may be caused by the underlying neoplasm (particularly, Hodgkin's disease and some non-Hodgkin's lymphomas) or by occult infection unrelated to the pulmonary process. The absence of fever, however, argues against an infectious pneumonia.

One's differential diagnosis of pulmonary pathogens in a particular case will be influenced in part by the nature of the underlying immunocompromising condition. Patients with cell-mediated immune deficiency, such as occurs in lymphomas, organ transplantation, and high-dose steroid therapy, are prone to infection with herpes-group viral agents (especially cytomegalovirus), *Pneumocystis,* cryptococcus, *Nocardia,* and *Legionella.* On the other hand, patients immunocompromised by virtue of granulocytopenia are predisposed to infection with gram-negative bacilli, staphylococcus, and the fungi *Apsergillus,* mucor, and *Candida.* As an example, a patient with lymphoma having corticosteroid therapy withdrawn, who then develops diffuse bilateral pulmonary infiltrates, is suspect for having *Pneumocystis.* On the other hand, the neutropenic patient with leukemia, receiving a course of empiric broad-spectrum antibiotics for fever of unknown cause, who then develops a new pulmonary infiltrate, has a history suggestive of fungal (e.g., *Aspergillus*) pneumonia.

The time of onset as well as the tempo of the illness also may focus the differential diagnosis. Cytomegalovirus pneumonia occurs 1 to 6 months following renal transplantation, but is uncommon before or after this period (18,52). This relatively limited time frame could reflect the pathogenic observation that in most cases, the source of cytomegalovirus is the donor kidney transplanted into a seronegative recipient (28). Among the noninfectious pulmonary diseases, certain entities also have a predictable time for their radiographic appearance. Radiation pneumonitis typically develops approximately 8 weeks following completion of a course of radiation therapy, and roughly 1 week earlier for every 1,000 rads above a total dose of 4,000 rads (25). Radiation pneumonitis is generally not seen within the first month post-irradiation, except in reirradiated lung (25). Also, an occasional cause of diffuse interstitial infiltrates, called "leukemic cell lysis pneumopathy," develops characteristically within 4 days of the nadir of the white blood cell count in treated myeloblastic leukemia (60). Lysis of interstitial and alveolar blast cells, with release of their toxic intracellular constituents, is postulated as the mechanism for the observed interstitial inflammation and diffuse alveolar damage. Although bleomycin-induced interstitial pneumonitis is in large part dose related, with appearance of life-threatening lung damage only after cumulative doses, greater than 150 mg (56), toxic reactions to the drug have been observed at lower doses, especially when the drug is used as part of combination chemotherapy programs (5); thus, no minimum dose excludes the diagnosis of bleomycin lung injury with complete assurance (48). Leukoagglutinin reaction is a sudden diffuse vascular endothelial injury that appears to result from the interaction of antibodies in transfused blood products with the recipient's white blood cells; a pattern of pulmonary edema develops within minutes to hours of transfusion (61).

In this context, one should be alert to the potentiation of pulmonary toxicity from the interactions of certain therapeutic agents. In particular, high inspired oxygen concentrations may precipitate interstitial inflammation in patients receiving bleomycin therapy (23), and amphotericin B appears to interact with white blood cell transfusions to cause leukoagglutinin reactions (65).

Disease tempo is another important historical observation. Pulmonary infections in compromised patients can be differentiated according to their rate of progression (52). In Table 14-2 the course of untreated disease is categorized as rapid, subacute, or insidious. The acute, often fulminant onset of *Pneumocystis* pneumonia is notorious: disease may progress from mild breathlessness, fever, nonproductive cough, and a minimally abnormal chest radiograph to overwhelming dyspnea, hypoxemia, and diffuse pulmonary infiltrates within a matter of a few days. The indolent form of *Pneumocystis* pneumonia, with symptoms extending over many days to weeks, appears to be unique to patients with the acquired immunodeficiency syndrome. Bacterial infections (including *Legionella*), particularly in the neutropenic host, can also spread to multilobe involvement within days. Although cytomegalovirus pneumonia may also have an explosive onset, it more often evolves over a period of 1 to 2 weeks, a tempo similar to that for *Aspergillus* or mucormycosis. Nonspecific interstitial pneumonitis is similar to cytomegalovirus pneumonia in this regard. Nocardiosis, tuberculosis, and the slower growing fungal infections (e.g., cryptococcosis) usually follow a more insidious course. Their development over weeks to months may mimic other noninfectious pulmonary processes such as growth of metastatic malignancy, drug-induced lung injury, or the appearance of radiation fibrosis.

Increasingly, prophylactic measures are being employed to prevent pulmonary infections in immunocompromised patients, especially among patients receiving organ and bone marrow transplants. For instance, low doses of trimethoprim-sulfameth-

TABLE 14–2. *Tempo of pulmonary infections in compromised patients*

Rapid	Subacute	Insidious
Pneumocystis	Cytomegalovirus	*Nocardia*
Bacterial (especially gram-negative, S. aureus, Legionella)	*Aspergillus*/mucor	Cryptococcus
Cytomegalovirus	Cryptococcus	Tuberculosis
Aspergillus		

oxazole are now commonly administered for several months following transplantation, with a consequent marked reduction in the incidence of *Pneumocystis* and nocardial infections. As a result, the differential diagnosis of new pulmonary infiltrates will be strongly influenced by a history of the use of antibiotic prophylaxis.

Finally, two points in the clinical history referable to noninfectious etiologies for pulmonary infiltrates are worthy of emphasis. The first is that in patients with underlying cancer or lymphoma, disease activity should be assessed in other potential metastatic sites besides the lungs. The patient with breast cancer whose bibasilar interstitial infiltrates appear in concert with new hepatic and bony lesions may be suspected of having lymphangitic carcinomatosis, whereas the appearance of the same pulmonary infiltrates in a woman whose breast cancer is responding to treatment, with no evident disease outside of her lungs, is likely to have a different etiology for her new lung infiltrates. The second point is that a careful review of fluid balance is always appropriate in the immunocompromised patient with diffuse pulmonary infiltrates. Large-volume loads are often given in conjunction with certain chemotherapeutic agents or for resuscitation of the hypotensive, septic patient. Impaired renal function, atherosclerotic heart disease, adriamycin cardiotoxicity, or other poorly defined factors can impair the normal ability to compensate for large infusions of fluids, with the resultant development of pulmonary edema. Early interstitial phase pulmonary edema can resemble interstitial inflammatory processes such as mycoplasma or viral pneumonia, cytotoxic drug-induced lung disease, or nonspecific interstitial pneumonitis (see Fig. 14-2). The late alveolar-filling phase of pulmonary edema can be difficult to differentiate radiographically from *Pneumocystis* or cytomegalovirus pneumonia.

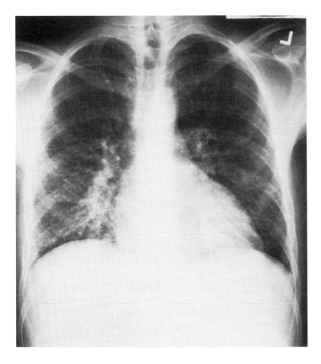

FIG. 14–2. Eighteen-year-old man with acute myelogenous leukemia and adriamycin cardiotoxicity, whose chest x-ray shows interstitial pulmonary edema.

PHYSICAL EXAMINATION

Physical examination of the immunocompromised patient with pneumonia may be frustratingly unrevealing. Even in the face of life-threatening dyspnea and hypoxemia, with widespread infiltrates on chest radiograph, auscultation of the lungs may be normal or reveal only minimal end-inspiratory rales (31). Particularly in neutropenic patients, with their impaired inflammatory response to infection, the usual physical findings in chest infection can be lacking. However, to conclude from this that physical examination is worthless in this setting would be a great error. Clues to diagnosis or guides to the optimal diagnostic procedures may be derived from pulmonary and extrapulmonic findings in such patients.

What information can chest examination add to that obtainable from the readily available chest x-ray film? First, rales could become audible even before infiltrates appear radiographically and could be the first clue to an infiltrative lung process. Similarly, when the chest x-ray film shows an early unilateral infiltrate, examination can reveal the presence of bilateral disease, altering diagnostic considerations. Second, the presence of localized, monophonic wheezing would suggest a partially obstructed bronchus, which might be radiographically inapparent. In the absence of voluminous tracheobronchial secretions, this finding usually indicates neoplastic involvement of an airway and would guide one toward bronchoscopy for tissue confirmation. Third, a pleural friction rub may be the only sign of active pleural inflammation. Its presence in the setting of a rapidly progressing pulmonary infiltrate suggests a virulent bacterial or fungal (usually aspergillus) infection. Further, a pleural friction rub is strong evidence against pneumocystis as the sole etiology. Finally, and perhaps most importantly, physical examination is often superior to chest x-ray in suggesting the overall severity of the illness. Respiratory rate alone may provide critical information about the extent of physiologic derangement, thereby directing the rapidity and course of the diagnostic evaluation.

When pulmonary infection spreads outside of the thorax, the extrapulmonic manifestation may be the best clue to the etiology of the pulmonary disease. The scope of this chapter permits only a superficial description of some of the extrapulmonic signs of disseminated infection. For instance, an indurated, ulcerated, painless round skin lesion with a central black eschar and surrounding erythema—ecthyma gangrenosum—suggests gram-negative septicemia, particularly due to pseudomonas infection, but must be distinguished by examination of biopsy or aspirate material from invasive fungal infection, such as aspergillus. Disseminated cryptococcus or nocardia may cause cutaneous papules or nodules with surrounding erythema, which may give an appearance similar to neoplastic involvement. Appropriate stains and cultures of skin biopsies may give the first clue to the nature of the concurrent pulmonary process (66).

In the eye, yellow-white retinal patches, perhaps with surrounding hemorrhage, may be the earliest manifestation of disseminated cytomegalovirus infection (36). Discrete choroidal lesions, yellowish-white and with indistinct margins, may be found on fundoscopic exam in some patients with disseminated candidiasis or aspergillosis (39). Necrotizing nasal lesions, sometimes with frank septal perforation, may be caused not only by mucormycosis but also by aspergillus and invasive gram-negative bacilli. Identification of such a physical finding and sampling of material from the nose may eliminate the need for a more morbid lung biopsy procedure (2).

Neurologic examination may detect signs of meningitis (consider cryptococcus, tuberculosis, or neoplasia), a space-occupying brain lesion (nocardia, mucormycosis, or neoplasia), or encephalitis (herpes simplex or toxoplasmosis). The necessity for cerebrospinal fluid sampling may be suggested on the basis of the physical examination, and may lead to the diagnosis of a perplexing pulmonary infiltrate.

Finally, in the patient with diffuse, bilateral pulmonary infiltrates, physical examination may be the best test for the presence of congestive heart failure. Detection of a laterally displaced cardiac impulse, jugular venous distention, and an early diastolic gallop has spared more than one patient an unnecessary lung biopsy for pulmonary edema.

THE CHEST RADIOGRAPH

Occasionally, the radiographic pattern of pulmonary infiltrates is so characteristic that the etiology is apparent simply by inspection of the x-ray film. In most cases, however, the x-ray film allows one to limit the list of differential diagnoses by assigning the process to one of several broad categories (Table 14-3). At the least, one can use the chest film to distinguish focal from diffuse disease, and thus direct the choice of biopsy techniques, if lung sampling is indicated.

Radiation pneumonitis and fibrosis generally have a radiographic appearance that is pathognomonic. Nothing else causes infiltrates with linear margins that defy anatomic boundaries but obey precisely the radiation field. Fibrosis uniformly follows acute radiation pneumonitis, and with fibrosis comes contracture and volume loss ("cicatrization atelectasis"). Review of the ports used during delivery of radiation to the thorax often suffices to establish the diagnosis in the immunocompromised patient who has received radiation therapy. Although diffuse, bilateral infiltrates have been attributed in at least one series of patients to unilateral pulmonary irradiation (6), this unexplained phenomenon is exceedingly rare and does not gainsay the general rule.

The air crescent sign is a radiographic finding highly suggestive, though not pathognomonic, for invasive aspergillosis (13), particularly in the more advanced stages. Fungal invasion of blood vessels leads to necrosis of lung tissue and the creation of a sequestrum of devitalized tissue. The appearance of a crescentic rim of air peripherally located within a preexisting nodule or infiltrate, as seen in Figure 14-3, should suggest the diagnosis of invasive aspergillosis (and must not be confused with sap-

TABLE 14–3. *Radiographic patterns of pulmonary infiltrates in immunocompromised patients*

Diffuse	Nodular or cavitary	Focal
Common		
Pneumocystis	Cryptococcus	Bacteria, including *Nocardia*
Cytomegalovirus	*Nocardia*	Cryptococcus
Pulmonary edema	Bacterial lung abscess	*Aspergillus*
NIP	Neoplastic	Mucor
Drug-induced	*Aspergillus*	NIP
Lymphangitic carcinomatosis		
Uncommon		
Cryptococcus	*Legionella*	TB
Aspergillus	Septic emboli	Viral
Candida		*Legionella*
Hemorrhage		
Leukemic involvement		

NIP, nonspecific interstitial pneumonitis.

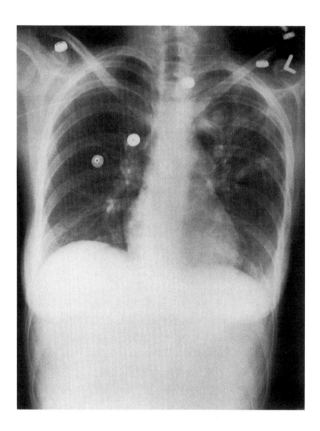

FIG. 14–3. Nineteen-year-old woman with acute myelogenous leukemia, neutropenia, fever despite broad-spectrum antibiotics, and invasive aspergillosis causing a left upper lobe cavity and fungus ball.

rophytic colonization of a preexisting cavity, as in aspergilloma). Other, less common causes of this finding in the compromised host include a cavitating carcinoma, tuberculosis, and bacterial lung abscess (22). Unfortunately, the majority of cases of invasive aspergillosis are associated with more nonspecific radiographic patterns.

In a group of patients dying with leukemia and found at autopsy to have pulmonary infection, the most common antemortem misdiagnosis was congestive heart failure (9). In our experience, the converse situation is also common; namely, that pulmonary edema is frequently mistaken for an opportunistic infection in immunocompromised patients with fever. For this reason, it is worth emphasizing the radiographic features that, if present, favor the diagnosis of congestive heart failure. These include cardiomegaly, engorgement of the pulmonary arteries and blurring of vascular markings, redistribution of blood flow to upper lung zone vessels, horizontal lines of septal edema (Kerley B lines), and pleural effusions, including fluid in the fissures (see Fig. 14-2).

Although a large number of different types of infection can cause bilateral, multilobar infiltrates, relatively few give a diffuse, relatively uniform, bilateral pattern of involvement mimicking pulmonary edema. Pneumocystis and viral (most commonly, cytomegalovirus) pneumonias (and occasionally, pneumonia due to mycoplasma) may take this form. Although atypical presentations have been described, in general pneumocystis pneumonia manifests as bibasilar and perihilar air space (alveolar) infiltrates without pleural effusion or hilar lymphadenopathy. In its earliest stages, patchy involvement may give a reticulonodular appearance; as the disease advances, frank consolidation develops (15). On the other hand, cytomegalovirus may elicit predominantly interstitial inflammation, causing a fine reticular or reticulonodular pattern similar to that of interstitial pulmonary edema. With the formation of intraalveolar hyaline membranes and the accumulation of inflammatory cells in the alveolar spaces, alveolar infiltrates (acinar shadows and air bronchograms) may be added to the interstitial pattern (1). Other noninfectious causes of diffuse pulmonary infiltrates in immunosuppressed patients include cytotoxic drug-induced pulmonary injury, leukemic and neoplastic infiltrates, leukoagglutinin reaction, leukemic cell lysis pneumopathy, and pulmonary hemorrhage. Fungal or bacterial infections are uncommon causes of this diffuse pattern (55). In a number of series, the most common pathologic finding in patients with diffuse pulmonary infiltrates was the entity of nonspecific interstitial pneumonitis (3,38,41).

The radiographic finding of solitary or multiple nodules, or nodular-appearing infiltrates, narrows the differential diagnosis considerably. *Nocardia* and cryptococcus infections commonly present in this manner, and on occasion may be associated with pleural effusions and hilar lymphadenopathy. Metastatic spread of cancer or lymphoma, septic emboli, bacterial lung abscesses, and rarely, *Legionella* infections may give a similar radiographic pattern. Cavitation may complicate any of these nodule-forming processes or may appear as part of necrotizing infiltrative bacterial, fungal, or mycobacterial disease.

A localized patchy infiltrate or bronchopneumonia provides the least informative x-ray pattern. Bacterial, viral, fungal, mycobacterial, neoplastic, and nonspecific etiologies can all present in this way, and the presence or absence of airspace consolidation generally adds little useful information. Statistically, gram-negative bacilli (e.g., *E. coli, Klebsiella, Enterobacter, Pseudomonas*) account for most localized pneumonias in immunocompromised hosts, but the radiographic appearance rarely, if ever, excludes the multiple other potential etiologies.

Hilar and/or mediastinal adenopathy would be a distinctly unusual finding in viral, pneumocystis, and most bacterial pneumonias. Exceptions include the rare "atypical pneumonias": pneumonic tularemia and psittacosis. Mycobacterial infection and the endemic fungal pneumonias, histoplasmosis and coccidioidomycosis, commonly cause adenopathy; nocardia and cryptococcal pneumonias infrequently do. In some cases one must also consider the possibility of neoplastic lymphadenopathy due to spread of the primary malignancy, especially cancers and lymphomas.

LABORATORY DIAGNOSIS

In the immunologically normal person with pneumonia, sputum smear and culture, blood culture, and sometimes acute and convalscent antibody titers are the standard tools for etiologic diagnosis. In the immunocompromised host at risk for opportunistic infection, the problem is more complex. Sputum is often not available for examination, especially in neutropenic patients. The spectrum of potential infectious agents is broader, while at the same time techniques for culture or serologic diagnosis may be lacking for some entities. To compound the problem, appropriate therapy often must be chosen immediately, because the tenuous clinical condition of the patient will not tolerate delay; yet at the same time the patient may be too ill for definitive biopsy procedures to be performed safely because of severe hypoxemia or thrombocytopenia.

Given this compelling need for accurate, noninvasive diagnostic techniques, it is not surprising that a great deal of research is ongoing in this area. New techniques are constantly being developed and tested, so that what follows, while reflecting the present state of our knowledge, will undoubtedly need to be updated in future years. Details about the means of diagnosis for individual infections can be found elsewhere in this book in chapters devoted to specific diseases. In this section we ask the more general question of what tests are available to those of us facing the undiagnosed immunocompromised patient with pneumonia.

Skin Tests

In brief, skin testing is of little or no value in the diagnosis of acute infections in the compromised host. This includes skin tests that under other circumstances may provide valuable information about the presence of disease, such as the *Aspergillus* skin test in allergic bronchopulmonary aspergillosis. Even patients with active tuberculosis are generally nonreactive to standardized PPD antigen when undergoing immunosuppressive chemotherapy.

Serology

Analysis of blood samples for circulating antigens or specific antibodies may prove of value in certain limited clinical situations. In renal, bone marrow, or cardiac transplant recipients, in whom diffuse interstitial pulmonary infiltrates develop, an immunofluorescent antibody titer against cytomegalovirus of $\geq 1 : 16$ or a fourfold rise in complement fixation antibody titers over pretransplant levels would suggest a diagnosis of cytomegalovirus pneumonia (38). The test is not sensitive (7), however, and cytomegalovirus pneumonia may occur in the absence of seroconversion, a situation with a particularly poor prognosis (38). Circulating cryptococcal antigen, detectable in serum by a latex agglutination test, has been reported in some cases of diffuse cryptococcal pneumonia (21). Although highly specific (in the absence of latex-fixation positive rheumatoid arthritis), its sensitivity is low. When pulmonary infiltrates are accompanied by signs and symptoms of meningeal irritation, cryptococcal antigen should be sought in cerebrospinal fluid samples. A titer of $\geq 1 : 8$ is generally diagnostic of cryptococcal meningitis and would suggest that cryptococcus is the cause of the pulmonary disease as well.

Indirect fluorescent antibody tests are available for diagnosis of legionella infection, but they require acute and convalescent blood samples and testing for antibodies against multiple serotypes. Radioimmunoassay and enzyme-linked immunosorbent assay (ELISA) techniques are being developed for detection of legionella antigens in urine (33). Research continues on serologic tests to distinguish invasive from noninvasive fungal infections. Immunodiffusion and counterimmunoelectrophoresis techniques have been applied in aspergillus infection (34) and gas-liquid chromatography and other techniques used to detect invasive candidiasis (32). As yet, none of these serologies appears entirely reliable, nor are these tests widely available.

Staining Techniques

Sputum, transtracheal aspirate, or bronchial washings may contain pathogenic material that, when properly stained, gives immediate diagnostic information (see Table 14-4). Besides the routine gram and acid-fast (Ziehl-Neelsen or rapid Kinyoun)

TABLE 14-4. *Staining and cultivation techniques for selected opportunistic organisms*

| Organism | Staining techniques | | Culture techniques | |
	Fresh material	Fixed tissue	Medium	Period of incubation (time to preliminary identification)
Legionella sp	Direct immunofluorescent antibody	Dieterle, acid-fast	Charcoal yeast extract	3–5 days, sometimes up to 10 days
Nocardia	Modified acid-fast, gram	Modified acid-fast, gram	Sabouraud	Minimum of 5 days, up to 4 weeks
Cryptococcus	India ink	H&E, PAS, MSS, mucicarmine	Sabouraud	4–7 days; some strains 4–6 weeks
Aspergillus	Potassium hydroxide	H&E, PAS, MSS	Blood agar, Sabouraud	1–2 weeks
Mucor (Phycomyces)	Potassium hydroxide	H&E, MSS	Sabouraud	1–2 weeks
Candida	Wet mount	H&E, PAS, MSS	Blood agar, Sabouraud	1–14 days
Mycobacterium tuberculosis	Acid-fast (Ziehl-Neelson, Kinyoun)	Acid-fast stains	Lowenstein-Jensen	Up to 4–6 weeks[a]
Pneumocystis	MSS	MSS	—	—
Cytomegalovirus	Tzanck preparation, Wright-Giemsa	H&E	Cell culture (fibroblasts)	2–10 days when inoculum high, up to 6 weeks[b]

H&E, hemotoxylin and eosin; MSS, methenamine silver stain; PAS, periodic acid-Schiff.
[a]Nucleic acid hybridization techniques for rapid identification in culture are becoming available (see ref. 49).
[b]Rapid identification by means of centrifugation culture and monoclonal antibody detection of early antigens is newly possible (see ref. 11).

stains, special preparations can be applied in certain selected clinical settings. India ink staining of a wet preparation may reveal the encapsulated budding yeast forms of cryptococcus. Methenamine silver nitrate or toluidine blue O stains of air-dried smears reveal the cyst walls of pneumocystis, which may be found in sputum, especially specimens of sputum that have been induced with the inhalation of hypertonic saline by ultrasonic nebulization. Direct fluorescent antibody staining techniques provide a sensitive means of identifying legionella, but the organisms are not often expectorated into the sputum and the special antibodies to all serotypes are not widely available. If metastatic cancer is suspected, it is worthwhile submitting sputum for cytologic examination with Papanicolaou staining. A variety of additional stains are available for demonstration of organisms in tissue section, often providing definitive diagnosis, but these are not relevant to the present discussion of noninvasive techniques.

Cultures

Bacterial cultures of sputum and blood should routinely be performed in all patients. In addition, special culture media are available for growth of certain opportunistic bacteria, viruses, and fungi. Unfortunately, sputum is often not produced, or when available, frequently does not contain any pathogenic organisms. Furthermore, whereas growth of an organism from tissue samples is usually diagnostic, cultivation from sputum only raises the suspicion of etiologic association. For some organisms, such as staphylococcus, gram-negative bacilli, and candida, colonization is common; other organisms, such as aspergillus, cryptococcus, and nocardia, which may be saprophytes in normal hosts, are almost always pathogenic in immunocompromised patients with pneumonia.

For practical decision-making in the case of immunosuppressed patients with pulmonary infiltrates, it is important to know what length of time is needed to identify specific organisms by culture techniques. This information is depicted in Table 14-4 and can be summarized as follows: rapid growth rate: most bacteria, some candida species; intermediate growth rate: legionella, nocardia, cryptococcus, aspergillus, and cytomegalovirus; slow growth rate: mycobacteria. New techniques for the rapid identification of cytomegalovirus (11) and mycobacteria (49) in culture are becoming available. Pneumocystis has not yet been reproducibly grown *in vitro*.

BIOPSY TECHNIQUES

Historical information, physical examination, chest radiography, and diagnostic laboratory studies often serve to limit the differential diagnostic possibilities, and in some cases will lead to a specific etiologic diagnosis. Most often, however, one cannot definitively establish the exact nature of the pulmonary infiltrate on the basis of these criteria alone. In one prospectively studied group of 80 immunocompromised patients with diffuse pulmonary infiltrates, a specific etiologic diagnosis was made by blood and sputum cultures in only four patients, and by serologies in another four (total of 10%) (55).

In those cases in which establishing a specific diagnosis is mandated by the potential implications for the patient's management, lung biopsy becomes the diagnostic procedure of choice. Thoracotomy with open lung biopsy is the traditional means of obtaining lung tissue for histologic examination, special stains, and cultures. The surgeon can provide the pathology and microbiology laboratories with an ample piece of lung tissue and assure a diagnostic accuracy of at least 90%, with specific etiologic diagnoses established in approximately 60–70% of cases (24). Despite the grave medical condition of many of the operated patients, overall surgical mortality from open lung biopsy is less than 5% in the experience of some surgeons (51,59). And at least in one series, the results of open biopsy led to a change in therapy in as many as one-half of the patients (51).

The major drawbacks of the open biopsy procedure are the requirement for general anesthesia, the pain of the operative incision, and occasional surgical complications, particularly delayed pneumothorax and prolonged need for assisted ventilation. These considerations have led to a search for simpler, less "invasive" means of sampling lung tissue. A number of techniques have evolved, including percutaneous needle aspiration and biopsy (4), fluoroscopically guided bronchial brushing (20), thorascopic lung biopsy (14), and transbronchial lung biopsy and bronchoalveolar lavage via the fiberoptic bronchoscope (19,58).

Percutaneous needle aspiration and bronchoscopic lung sampling are the two most widely used of these techniques. The safety of the former procedure has been enhanced by the recent trend toward use of thinner needles, for example, 22-gauge spinal needles, thereby decreasing the incidence of pneumothoraces. Although sometimes a small core of lung tissue is obtained, in general the result is a fluid aspirate for cytologic examination, special stains, and cultures. Because material is not reliably obtained for histologic evaluation, diagnosis cannot be established in conditions in which histopathology is needed, such as radiation pneumonitis or pulmonary hemorrhage. Considerable success with percutaneous needle aspiration and biopsy has been reported in pediatric cases (30) and in recipients of heart transplants (51). In our experience, the technique is particularly valuable for diagnosis of peripheral nodular or cavitary infiltrates.

On the other hand, transbronchial lung biopsy, together with the bronchial washings and brushings and bronchoalveolar lavage obtained at the same fiberoptic bronchoscopic procedure, has its highest yield in diffuse pulmonary infiltrates (26). With transbronchial forceps biopsy, one or more small pieces (approximately 1.0 to 3.0 mm in diameter) of lung tissue can be reliably obtained. When pathologic changes are widespread throughout the lungs, even such minute fragments often contain diagnostic information. For instance, an interstitial pneumonitis with intranuclear and intracytoplasmic inclusion bodies in the alveolar lining cells establishes a diagnosis of cytomegalovirus pneumonia even in the absence of viral isolation, and tissue invasion by fungal hyphae distinguishes colonization from invasive fungal disease. A specific etiologic diagnosis can be made using the transbronchial lung biopsy in about 40 to 50% of cases, and more often when the prevalence of infection as the cause of the infiltrates is high (17).

There is a major difficulty, however, in interpretation of transbronchial lung biopsy results when the findings are a nonspecific interstitial pneumonitis or organizing pneumonia. In 20 to 40% of immunocompromised patients with pulmonary infiltrates, such nonspecific pathologic changes are the only abnormality present in the lungs, even on open biopsy or postmortem examination. However, a number of specific infectious and neoplastic diseases also can elicit nonspecific inflammatory reactions in areas adjacent to the primary disease processes. Thus, because of the vagaries of tissue sampling, a transbronchial lung biopsy containing nonspecific interstitial inflammation or organizing pneumonia may or may not reflect the nature of the disease in the remainder of the lungs. Recent studies of this particular problem have found that an alternative, specific diagnosis can be made in as many as 30% of patients with a nonspecific transbronchial lung biopsy (40,44). Given this unacceptably high "false-negative" rate, whenever possible a nonspecific transbronchial biopsy should be followed by open lung biopsy (59).

The major advantage of the transbronchial lung biopsy over an open procedure is its relative lack of morbidity. Complications are infrequent: significant bleeding and pneumothorax requiring chest tube placement each occur in less than 5% of cases. Fiberoptic bronchoscopy with brushings and biopsy is contraindicated by severe hypoxemia (arterial oxygen tension < 60 mm Hg despite supplemental inspired oxygen) and by bleeding disorders (platelet count < 50,000/mm^3 after platelet transfusion), blood urea nitrogen > 50 mg/dl with prolonged bleeding time, or uncorrectable prothrombin time).

The introduction of a relatively simple diagnostic technique, bronchoalveolar lavage performed through the fiberoptic bronchoscope, has had a major impact on the evaluation of infiltrates in immunocompromised hosts. The procedure involves wedging the tip of the bronchoscope into a subsegmental bronchial lumen, and then instilling approximately 100–150 ml of normal saline into the lung in 20–50 ml aliquots, aspirating the lavage fluid after each aliquot. Usually, approximately half of the instilled volume is retrieved. The fluid bathes distal bronchioles and alveoli; the predominance of pulmonary alveolar macrophages in the cellular differential of the lavage fluid testifies to alveolar sampling. It is estimated that as many as 1 million alveoli are sampled by this method (as opposed to the 25–50 alveoli included in a successful transbronchial forceps biopsy of the lung). The procedure can be completed easily within 10–15 minutes, and it can safely be performed in patients who are intubated and receiving positive pressure ventilation without risk of pneumothorax and bronchopleural fistula. Likewise, the risk of hemorrhage is far less than for biopsy techniques.

Extensive experience with bronchoalveolar lavage has been obtained in patients with the acquired immune deficiency syndrome, where the sensitivity of the technique for diagnosing pneumocystis pneumonia exceeds 90%. Fewer reports have been published describing the results of bronchoalveolar lavage in the diagnosis of pulmonary infiltrates in patients with other immunocompromising illnesses. Stover and colleagues reported making a specific diagnosis by analysis of bronchoalveolar lavage fluid alone in 66% of 97 patients with diffuse pulmonary infiltrates and a variety of causes for immunosuppression (58). Thirty-eight of 46 opportunistic infections (83%) were correctly diagnosed by examination and culture of the lavage fluid. Other studies have documented the utility of bronchoalveolar lavage among recipients of bone marrow (10,57) and kidney (29) transplants. Another recent report (42) describes results of 150 diagnostic bronchoalveolar lavage procedures in a variety of immunocompromised patients (only 4% AIDS). The diagnostic yield was only 39%; however, in 46 of the 150 patients no subsequent diagnosis was ever made by clinical, autopsy, or other means. The sensitivity of this technique may be enhanced by new methods for rapid identification of pathogens in the lavage fluid. These include nucleic acid probes for *in situ* hybridization, used to detect cytomegalovirus and legionella (16,37) and monoclonal antibodies to early antigens expressed by cytomegalovirus in cell culture (11). Complications of the procedure are few; the most common one is arterial oxygen desaturation, which can be effectively monitored by means of oximetry. Because of the sensitivity and safety of the procedure, fiberoptic bronchoscopy with bronchoalveolar lavage is probably the initial procedure of choice in patients with diffuse infiltrates who are thought to have infection or hemorrhage as likely etiologic possibilities.

LUNG SAMPLING VS. EMPIRIC THERAPY

It has recently been commented that no prospective trial has ever demonstrated improved survival in immunocompromised patients who undergo lung biopsy as opposed to those who receive empiric therapy based on clinical presentation and laboratory data collected noninvasively (50). One prospective randomized trial compared immediate lung biopsy with empiric trimethoprim-sulfamethoxazole and erythromycin therapy followed by delayed open lung biopsy if no clinical improvement had occurred after 4 days of therapy (45). Most of the 22 nonneutropenic patients entered into the study had an underlying lymphoma. Nineteen of the 22 entered the study with diffuse pulmonary infiltrates; the remaining 3 patients had hypoxemia of unknown etiology. There were 3 deaths directly attributable to complications of the lung biopsy, and there was no significant difference in survival rates for the two groups. It should be noted that the only infectious etiology identified in this study was *Pneumocystis carinii,* found in 9 of the 14 biopsy specimens obtained. Thus, in this select population, the prevalence of pneumocystis pneumonia was very high, accounting for the success of empiric therapy with trimethoprim-sulfamethoxazole and erythromycin (8 of 10 patients improved without need of delayed open lung biopsy). A variety of other, retrospective studies have analyzed the impact of lung biopsy by comparing the outcome of patients who had a specific diagnosis established by lung biopsy with the outcome of patients who had a nonspecific result (27,46,62). In general, patients with a specific diagnosis following lung biopsy had no better chance of survival than patients with nonspecific findings. Note that this is not the same as saying that survival is not improved by making a specific diagnosis.

We agree that prospective studies are needed to assess the effect of lung sampling versus empiric therapy on survival in immunocompromised patients with pulmonary infiltrates. In the meantime, however, physicians faced with an ill patient with an undiagnosed pulmonary infiltrate may be unable to design a rational therapeutic regimen without additional diagnostic information: should the renal transplant recipient with diffuse pulmonary infiltrates unresponsive to trimethoprim-sulfamethoxazole therapy receive pentamidine for presumed pneumocystis pneumonia, an experimental antiviral therapy (and adjustment of immunosuppressive medications) for possible cytomegalovirus infection, or possibly an intensified regimen of immunosuppressive therapy for pulmonary vasculitis (e.g., in a patient who had end-stage renal failure secondary to Wegener's granulomatosis)? Furthermore, in such a clinical setting, empiric therapy would probably be inadequate for the occasional patient with disseminated herpes simplex pneumonia or miliary tuberculosis, whereas a specific diagnosis might lead to curative treatment. In other circumstances, the differential diagnosis may include not only opportunistic infection but also neoplasia or cytotoxic drug-induced lung disease. The treatment would differ in each case and be for the most part mutually exclusive; an empiric regimen covering all possibilities could not rationally be designed. Thus, we would argue that lung sampling procedures are indicated whenever there is a reasonable possibility of establishing a treatable diagnosis for which empiric therapy cannot safely be given. The risks of multidrug empiric, and potentially inappropriate, therapy must be weighed against the morbidity and mortality of the lung sampling procedure. The latter is fortunately quite small for bronchoalveolar lavage with or without transbronchial lung biopsy.

GENERAL APPROACH

Given the variety of infectious and noninfectious causes of pulmonary infiltrates in immunocompromised hosts, the diversity of the underlying disease processes causing immunosuppression, and the spectrum of clinical severities, no one algorithm is likely to summarize a suitable approach to all patients. In some, making no intervention at all may be appropriate. In others, when history, examination, and initial laboratory studies do not yield an answer, an aggressive diagnostic evaluation in search of a specific diagnosis may be warranted. In still others, where the clinical condition makes the risk of invasive biopsy procedures unacceptably high, empiric therapy is often justified. Empiric therapy is also warranted if the likelihood of identifying a *treatable* cause of the pulmonary infiltrates is considered remote. The following discussion depicts, in broad outline form, one general strategy for management of patients with this pulmonary problem.

When clinical information does not exclude bacterial infection as the cause of the pulmonary infiltrates, empiric antibiotics should be started promptly. Especially in the neutropenic host, at risk for bacteremia and septic shock from a pulmonary site of infection, broad-spectrum antibiotic coverage within a few hours of presentation is mandated. Combination antibiotic regimens to cover staphylococcus and resistant gram-negative bacilli, including pseudomonas, are usually required. For instance, one might use a third-generation cephalosporin (e.g., ceftazidime) and an aminoglycoside, or the combination of a broad-spectrum penicillin (e.g., ticarcillin or piperacillin) and an aminoglycoside, with oxacillin or vancomycin added for better staphylococcal coverage, as indicated.

When pneumocystis pneumonia is suggested by the clinical setting and diffuse bilateral pulmonary infiltrates, we favor immediate institution of therapy with trimethoprim-sulfamethoxazole, followed by lung sampling within 24 to 48 hr. In the patient able to tolerate an invasive procedure, we consider definitive confirmation of a diagnosis of pneumocystis preferable to a full course of empiric therapy for suspected disease: (i) alternative or additional treatable infections may be found on biopsy; (ii) treatment failures (35) can be managed correctly if the diagnosis has been established; and (iii) patients with noninfectious causes for their infiltrates can be spared 2 weeks of unnecessary antibiotic therapy. An alternative approach would be to perform an invasive diagnostic procedure only in those patients who fail to improve after approximately 4 days of empiric treatment (45). This option may result in the eventual inability to perform a procedure due to clinical deterioration, however.

In patients with diffuse infiltrates in whom diagnostic material is sought with an invasive procedure, choice is usually made between open lung biopsy versus fiberoptic bronchoscopy with bronchoalveolar lavage and transbronchial lung biopsy. Local practices at different medical centers vary widely in this regard. In most instances, we favor fiberoptic bronchoscopy as the initial procedure, because of its generally good yield and low morbidity. If a nonspecific result is obtained (as many as 50% of cases), we would then proceed to open lung biopsy if the chance of obtaining a treatable diagnosis that could not be readily managed with empiric therapy outweighed the risks of the procedure. Thoracotomy with lung biopsy is recommended as the initial procedure under three major conditions. First, patients who are hypoxemic despite supplemental oxygen or unable to cooperate with fiberoptic bronchoscopy are best referred for thoracotomy. Second, when a disease with nonspecific pathologic findings is strongly suspected, such as cytotoxic drug-induced pneumonitis, open biopsy is preferred, to avoid possible sampling error as a cause of nonspecific interstitial pneumonitis on transbronchial lung biopsy. Third, when the course of the disease is so rapid that the first biopsy procedure must be definitive, the sequential approach is abandoned and open biopsy done first.

Localized infiltrates are more often bacterial in origin and therefore are more likely to respond to empiric antibacterial antibiotic therapy, although clinical and radiographic improvement may be delayed in immunocompromised patients. When noninvasive studies suggest a nonbacterial cause or do not yield a specific etiology, especially in the face of disease progression, lung sampling is again indicated. If infection is strongly suspected, fiberoptic bronchoscopy can be used not only for the purposes of lavage and biopsy, but also to obtain uncontaminated bacteriologic samples from the lower respiratory tract using special double-sheathed microbiologic sampling brushes (63). Percutaneous needle aspiration is preferable for discrete nodules or cavities. Again, as for diffuse pulmonary infiltrates, open lung biopsy gives the highest yield, but also the greatest morbidity.

Some patients with localized infiltrates will be unable to tolerate any invasive diagnostic procedures, necessitating continued empiric choices. Depending on the clinical setting, this may mean initiating intravenous erythromycin for possible Legionnaire's disease (e.g., progressive consolidated pneumonia), or adding amphotericin B for possible fungal infection (e.g., focal infiltrates, neutropenia, antecedent antibiotic therapy, and recent chemotherapy and/or corticosteroids) (43). A schema illustrating these diagnostic and therapeutic options appears in Figure 14-4.

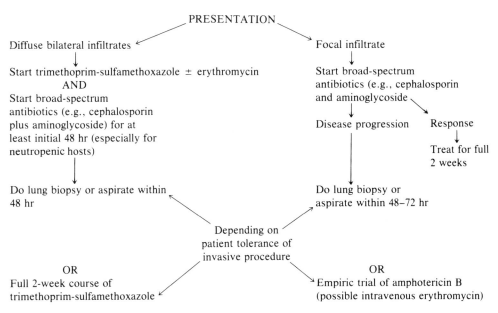

FIG. 14–4. Management schema for fever and pulmonary infiltrates in the compromised host. (Modified from Fanta and Pennington [17].)

In the future, new developments in this field are likely to decrease reliance on empiric forms of therapy. On the one hand, sophisticated radioimmunoassay, immunodiffusion, and ELISA techniques will allow diagnosis of more infections to be made simply by analyzing blood or urine specimens. On the other hand, newer therapies, particularly for fungal and viral infections, will broaden the potential therapeutic options available to the clinician, necessitating more accurate matching of specific drugs to specific diseases. Finally, one can predict advances in disease prevention, replacing empiric therapy with effective means of prophylaxis.

REFERENCES

1. Abdallah, P.S., Mark, J.S.B., and Merigan, T.C. (1976): Diagnosis of cytomegalovirus pneumonia in compromised hosts. *Am. J. Med.,* 61:326–332.
2. Aisner, J., Murillo, J., Schimpff, S.C., and Steere, A.C. (1979): Invasive aspergillosis in acute leukemia: correlation with nose cultures and antibiotic use. *Ann. Intern. Med.,* 40:4–9.
3. Armstrong, D. (1976): Interstitial pneumonia in the immunosuppressed patient. *Transplant. Proc.,* 8:657–661.
4. Bandt, P.D., Blank, N., and Castellino, R.A. (1972): Needle diagnosis of pneumonitis: value in high-risk patients. *J.A.M.A.,* 220:1578–1580.
5. Bauer, K.A., Skarin, A.T., Balikian, J.P., Garnick, M.B., Rosenthal, D.S., and Canellos, G.P. (1983): Pulmonary complications associated with combination chemotherapy programs containing bleomycin. *Am. J. Med.,* 74:557–563.
6. Bennett, D.E., Million, R.R., and Ackerman, L.V. (1969): Bilateral radiation pneumonitis: a complication of the radiotherapy of bronchogenic carcinoma. *Cancer,* 23:1001–1018.
7. Betts, R.F., and Hanshaw, J.B. (1977): Cytomegalovirus (CMV) in the compromised host(s). *Ann. Rev. Med.,* 28:103–110.
8. Bishop, J.F., Schimpff, S.C., Diggs, C.H., and Wiernik, P.H. (1981): Infections during intensive chemotherapy for non-Hodgkin's lymphoma. *Ann. Intern. Med.,* 95:549–555.
9. Bodey, G.P., Powell, R.D., Jr., Hersh, E.M., Yeterian, A., and Freireich, E.J. (1966): Pulmonary complications of acute leukemia. *Cancer,* 19:781–793.
10. Cordonnier, C., Bernaudin, J.-F., Fleury, J., Feuilhade, M., Haioun, C., Payen, D., Huet, Y., Atassi, K., and Vernant, J.-P. (1985): Diagnostic yield of bronchoalveolar lavage in pneumonitis occurring after allogeneic bone marrow transplantation. *Am. Rev. Respir. Dis.,* 132:1118–1123.
11. Crawford, S.W., Bowden, R.A., Hackman, R.C., Gleaves, C.A., Meyers, J.D., and Clark, J.G. (1988): Rapid detection of cytomegalovirus pulmonary infection by bronchoalveolar lavage and centrifugation culture. *Ann. Intern. Med.,* 108:180–185.
12. Crawford, S.W., and Hackman, R.C. (1993): Clinical course of idiopathic pneumonia after bone marrow transplantation. *Am. Rev. Respir. Dis.,* 147:1393–1400.
13. Curtis, A. McB., Smith, G.J.W., and Ravin, C.E. (1979): Air crescent sign of invasive aspergillosis. *Radiology,* 133:17–21.
14. Dijkman, J.H., van der Meer, J.W.M., Bakker, W., Wever, A.M.J., and van der Broek, P.J. (1982): Transpleural lung biopsy by the thorascopic route in patients with diffuse interstitial pulmonary disease. *Chest,* 82:76–83.
15. Doppman, J.L., and Geelhoed, G.W. (1976): Atypical radiographic features in *Pneumocystis carinii* pneumonia. *Natl. Cancer Inst. Monogr.,* 43:89–95.
16. Edelstein, P.H., Bryan, R.N., Enns, R.K., Kohne, D.E., and Kacian, D.L. (1987): Retrospective study of Gen-Probe rapid diagnostic system for detection of legionellae in frozen clinical respiratory tract samples. *J. Clin. Microbiol.,* 25:1022–1026.
17. Fanta, C.H., and Pennington, J.E. (1981): Fever and new lung infiltrates in immunocompromised hosts. *Clin. Chest Med.,* 2:19–39.
18. Fanta, C.H., and Pennington, J.E. (1985): Pulmonary infections in the transplant patient. In: *Progress in Transplantation,* vol. 2, edited by P.J. Morris and N.L. Tilney, pp. 207–230. Churchill Livingstone, New York.
19. Feldman, N.T., Pennington, J.E., and Ehrie, M.G. (1977): Transbronchial lung biopsy in the compromised host. *J.A.M.A.* 238:1377–1379.
20. Finley, R., Kieff, E., Thomsen, S., Fennessy, J., Beem, M., Lerner, S., and Morello, J. (1974): Bronchial brushing in the diagnosis of pulmonary disease in patients at risk for opportunistic infection. *Am. Rev. Respir. Dis.,* 109:379–387.
21. Fisher, B.D., and Armstrong, D. (1977): Cryptococcal interstitial pneumonia: value of antigen determination. *N. Engl. J. Med.,* 297:1440–1441.

22. Gold, W., Vellend, H., and Brunton, J. (1992): The air crescent sign caused by *Staphylococcus aureus* lung infection in a neutropenic patient with leukemia. *Ann. Intern. Med.*, 116:910–911.
23. Goldiner, P.L., Carlon, G.C., Cvitkovic, E., Schweizer, O., and Howland, W.S. (1978): Factors influencing postoperative morbidity and mortality in patients treated with bleomycin. *Br. Med. J.*, 1:1664–1667.
24. Greenman, R.L., Goodall, P.T., and King, D. (1975): Lung biopsy in immunocompromised hosts. *Am. J. Med.*, 59:488–496.
25. Gross, N.J. (1977): Pulmonary effects of radiation therapy. *Ann. Intern. Med.*, 86:81–92.
26. Haponik, E.F., Summer, W.R., Terry, P.B., and Wang, K.P. (1982): Clinical decision making with transbronchial lung biopsies: the value of nonspecific histologic examination. *Am. Rev. Respir. Dis.*, 125:524–529.
27. Haverkos, H.W., Dowling, J.N., Pasculle, A.W., Myerowitz, R.L., Lerberg, D.B., and Hakala, T.R. (1983): Diagnosis of pneumonitis in immunocompromised patients by open lung biopsy. *Cancer*, 52:1093–1097.
28. Ho, M., Suwansirikul, S., Dowling, J.N., Youngblood, L.A., and Armstrong, J.A. (1975): The transplanted kidney as a source of cytomegalovirus infection. *N. Engl. J. Med.*, 293:1109–1112.
29. Hopkin, J.M., Turney, J.H., Young, J.A., Adu, D., and Michael, J. (1983): Rapid diagnosis of obscure pneumonia in immunosuppressed renal patients by cytology of alveolar lavage fluid. *Lancet*, 2:299–301.
30. Hughes, W.T., Feldman, S., Chaudhary, S.C., Ossi, M.J., Cox, F. and Sanyal, S.K. (1978): Comparison of pentamidine isethionate and trimethoprim sulfamethoxazole in the treatment of *Pneumocystis carinii* pneumonia. *J. Pediatr.*, 92:285–291.
31. Hughes, W.T., Sanyal, S.K., and Price, R.A. (1976): Signs, symptoms, and pathophysiology of *Pneumocystis carinii* pneumonitis. *Natl. Cancer Inst. Monogr.*, 43:77–84.
32. Kiehn, T.E., Bernard, E.M., Gold, J.W.M., and Armstrong, D. (1979): Candidiasis: detection by gas-liquid chromatography of *d*-arabinitol, a fungal metabolite, in human serum, *Science*, 206:577–580.
33. Kohler, R.B., Zimmerman, S.E., Wilson, E., Allen, S.D., Edelstein, P.H., Wheat, J., and White, A. (1981): Rapid radioimmunoassay diagnosis of Legionnaires' disease: detection and partial characterization of urinary antigen. *Ann. Intern. Med.*, 94:601–605.
34. Ma, P. (1980): The microbiology laboratory in diagnosis and therapy. In: *Infections in the Abnormal Host*, edited by M.H. Grieco, pp. 797–847. Yorke Medical Books, New York.
35. Mitsuyasu, R.T., Corwin, H.L., Harris, A.A., Trenholme, G.M., Levin, S., and Karakusis, P.H. (1982): Failure of trimethoprim-sulfamethoxazole in the therapy of recurrent *Pneumocystis carinii* pneumonia. *Am. Rev. Respir. Dis.*, 125:762–765.
36. Murray, H.W., Knox, D.L., Green, W.R., and Susel, R.M. (1977): Cytomegalovirus retinitis in adults: a manifestation of disseminated viral infection. *Am. J. Med.*, 63:574–584.
37. Myerson, D., Hackman, R.C., and Meyers, J.D. (1984): Diagnosis of cytomegaloviral pneumonia by in situ hybridization. *J. Infect. Dis.*, 150:272–277.
38. Neiman, P.E., Reeves, W., Ray, G., Flournoy, N., Lerner, K.G., Sale, G.E., and Thomas, E.D. (1977): A prospective analysis of interstitial pneumonia and opportunistic viral infection among recipients of allogeneic bone marrow grafts. *J. Infect. Dis.*, 136:754–767.
39. Newton, J.C. (1980): Intraocular manifestations of systemic infections. In: *Infections in the Abnormal Host*, edited by M.H. Grieco, pp. 746–755. Yorke Medical Books, New York.
40. Nishio, J.N., and Lynch, J.P., III (1980): Fiberoptic bronchoscopy in the immunocompromised host: the significance of a "non-specific" transbronchial biopsy. *Am. Rev. Respir. Dis.*, 121:307–312.
41. Pennington, J.E., and Feldman, N.T. (1977): Pulmonary infiltrates and fever in patients with hematologic malignancy: assessment of transbronchial biopsy. *Am. J. Med.*, 62:581–587.
42. Pisani, R.J., and Wright, A.J. (1992): Clinical utility of bronchoalveolar lavage in immunocompromised hosts. *Mayo Clin. Proc.*, 67:221–227.
43. Pizzo, P.A., Robichaud, K.J., Gill, F.A., and Witebsky, F.G. (1982): Empiric antibiotic and antifungal therapy for cancer patients with prolonged fever and granulocytopenia. *Am. J. Med.*, 72:101–111.
44. Poe, R.H., Utell, M.J., Israel, R.H., Hall, W.J., and Eshleman, J.D. (1979): Sensitivity and specificity of the nonspecific transbronchial lung biopsy. *Am. Rev. Respir. Dis.*, 119:25–31.
45. Potter, D., Pass, H.I., Brower, S., Macher, A., Browne, M., Thaler, M., Cotton, D., Hathorn, J., Wesley, R., Longo, D., Pizzo, P., and Roth, J.A. (1985): Prospective randomized study of open lung biopsy versus empirical antibiotic therapy for acute pneumonitis in nonneutropenic cancer patients. *Ann. Thorac. Surg.*, 40:422–427.
46. Puksa, S., Hutcheon, M.A., and Hyland, R.H. (1983): Usefulness of transbronchial biopsy in immunosuppressed patients with pulmonary infiltrates. *Thorax*, 38:146–150.
47. Ramsey, P.G., Rubin, R.H., Tolkoff-Rubin, N.E., Cosimi, A.B., Russell, P.S., and Greene, R. (1980): The renal transplant patient with fever and pulmonary infiltrates: etiology, clinical manifestations, and management. *Medicine*, 59:206–222.

48. Richman, S.D., Levenson, S.M., Bunn, P.A., Flinn, G.S., Johnston, G.S., and DeVita, V.T. (1975): ^{67}Ga accumulation in pulmonary lesions associated with bleomycin toxicity. *Cancer*, 36:1966–1972.
49. Roberts, M.C., McMillan, C., and Coyle, M.B. (1987): Whole chromosomal DNA probes for rapid identification of Mycobacterium tuberculosis and Mycobacterium avium complex. *J. Clin. Microbiol.*, 25:1239–1243.
50. Robin, E.D., and Burke, C.M. (1986): Lung biopsy in immunosuppressed patients. *Chest*, 89:276–278.
51. Rossiter, S.J., Miller, D.C., Churg, A.M., Carrington, C.B., and Mark, J.B.D. (1979): Open lung biopsy in the immunosuppressed patient: Is it really beneficial? *J. Thorac. Cardiovasc. Surg.*, 77:338–343.
52. Rubin, R.J., Wolfson, J.S., Cosimi, A.B., and Tolkoff-Rubin, N.E. (1981): Infection in the renal transplant recipient. *Am. J. Med.*, 70:405–411.
53. Shelhamer, J.H., Toews, G.B., Masur, H., Suffredini, A.F., Pizzo, P.A., Walsh, T.J., and Henderson, D.K. (1992): Respiratory disease in the immunosuppressed patient. *Ann. Intern. Med.*, 117:415–431.
54. Sickles, E.A., Young, V.M., Greene, W.H., and Wiernik, P.H. (1973): Pneumonia in acute leukemia. *Ann. Intern. Med.*, 79:528–534.
55. Singer, C., Armstrong, D., Rosen, P.P., Walzer, P.D., and Yu, B. (1979): Diffuse pulmonary infiltrates in immunosuppressed patients: prospective study of 80 cases. *Am. J. Med.*, 66:110–120.
56. Sostman, H.D., Matthay, R.A., and Putman, C.E. (1977): Cytotoxic drug-induced lung disease. *Am. J. Med.*, 62:608–615.
57. Springmeyer, S.C., Hackman, R.C., Holle, R., Greenberg, G.M., Weems, C.E., Myerson, D., Meyers, J.D., and Thomas, E.D. (1986): Use of bronchoalveolar lavage to diagnose acute diffuse pneumonia in the immunocompromised host. *J. Infect. Dis.*, 154:604–610.
58. Stover, D.E., Zaman, M.B., Hajdu, S.I., Lange, M., Gold, J., and Armstrong, D. (1984): Bronchoalveolar lavage in the diagnosis of diffuse pulmonary infiltrates in the immunosuppressed host. *Ann. Intern. Med.*, 101:1–7.
59. Toledo-Pereyna, L.H., DeMeester, T.R., Kinealey, A., MacMahon, H., Churg, A., and Golomb H. (1980): The benefits of open lung biopsy in patients with previous non-diagnostic transbronchial lung biopsy: guide to appropriate therapy. *Chest*, 77:647–650.
60. Tryka, A.F., Godleski, J.J., and Fanta, C.H. (1982): Leukemic cell lysis pneumopathy: a complication of treated myeloblastic leukemia. *Cancer*, 50:2763–2770.
61. Ward, H.N. (1970): Pulmonary infiltrates associated with leukoagglutinin transfusion reaction. *Ann. Intern. Med.*, 73:689–694.
62. Williams, D., Yungbluth, M., Adams, G., and Glassroth, J. (1985): The role of fiberoptic bronchoscopy in the evaluation of immunocompromised hosts with diffuse pulmonary infiltrates. *Am. Rev. Respir. Des.*, 131:880–885.
63. Wimberley, N., Faling, L.J., and Bartlett, J.G. (1979): A fiberoptic bronchoscopy technique to obtain uncontaminated lower airway secretions for bacterial culture. *Am. Rev. Respir. Dis.*, 119:337–343.
64. Winston, D.J., Gale, R.P., Meyer, D.V., and Young, L.S. (1979): UCLA bone marrow transplantation group: infectious complications of human bone marrow transplantation. *Medicine*, 58:1–31.
65. Wright, D.G., Robichaud, K.J., Pizzo, P.A., and Deisseroth, A.B. (1981): Lethal pulmonary reactions associated with the combined use of amphotericin B and leukocyte transfusions. *N. Engl. J. Med.*, 304:1185–1189.
66. Utz, J.P., and Shadomy, H.J. (1979): Deep fungous infections. In: *Dermatology in General Medicine*, 2nd Edition, edited by T.B. Fitzpatrick, A.Z. Eisen, K. Wolff, I.M. Freedberg, and K.F. Austen, pp. 1533–1563. McGraw-Hill, New York.

Respiratory Infections: Diagnosis and Management, 3d ed.,
edited by James E. Pennington.
Published by Raven Press, Ltd., New York, 1994

15

Diagnosis and Therapy of Pulmonary Disease in Patients Infected with Human Immunodeficiency Virus

Jeffrey R. Dichter, Anthony F. Suffredini, and Henry Masur

*Critical Care Medicine Department, National Institutes of Health,
9000 Rockville Pike, Bethesda, Maryland 20892*

Pulmonary disease is one of the most common complications of HIV infection. Pneumonia due to opportunistic pathogens such as *Pneumocystis carinii* (PCP), cytomegalovirus (CMV), *Cryptococcus neoformans,* and *Histoplasma capsulatum* have been well recognized. There is now increasing recognition that common community-acquired pathogens such as *Streptococcus pneumoniae, Hemophilus influenzae, Mycoplasma pneumoniae, Chlamydia pneumoniae* (TWAR), influenza, respiratory syncytial virus (RSV), and *Legionella* species also cause disease in patients with HIV infection (50). Thus, there is an impressive spectrum of microbial processes that can cause pneumonia in this patient population.

Infection is not the only process that can cause pulmonary disease in patients with HIV infection. When a patient presents with pulmonary dysfunction, clinicians must consider congestive heart failure due to HIV or drug-related cardiomyopathy, pulmonary hemorrhage due to thrombocytopenia or Kaposi's sarcoma, neoplasia (e.g., lymphoma or Kaposi's sarcoma), or pulmonary emboli due to catheter-related thrombosis or thrombophlebitis. The differential diagnosis for pulmonary dysfunction is thus extensive (Table 15-1).

Over the past 5 years there has been substantial progress in the management of pulmonary complications of HIV, probably more progress than in most other areas of management for this patient population. Knowledge of natural history, diagnosis, therapy, and prevention has made rapid advances. These advances have allowed many pneumonias to be prevented. When pneumonia does occur, it can be diagnosed earlier and treated more effectively, often on an out-patient basis. These advances have decreased the adverse impact pneumonia has on the quality and duration of survival and on the cost of patient care.

It is also important to recognize that the causes of pulmonary dysfunction in the HIV-infected population are changing as demographics, prophylaxis, and life expectancy change. The differential diagnosis of patients in North America is not identical to that of patients in South America, Africa, or Asia. Even in North America, the differential diagnoses in Los Angeles and New York are not identical to the differential diagnoses in the Ohio River Valley or in Phoenix, Arizona. Intravenous drug

TABLE 15–1. *Pulmonary diseases in HIV-infected patients as a function of the total CD4 lymphocyte count*

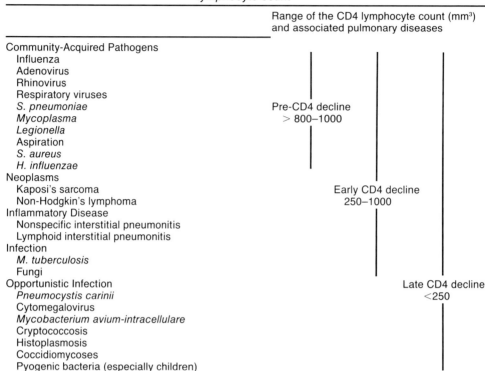

	Range of the CD4 lymphocyte count (mm³) and associated pulmonary diseases
Community-Acquired Pathogens	
Influenza	
Adenovirus	
Rhinovirus	
Respiratory viruses	
S. pneumoniae	Pre-CD4 decline
Mycoplasma	> 800–1000
Legionella	
Aspiration	
S. aureus	
H. influenzae	
Neoplasms	
Kaposi's sarcoma	Early CD4 decline
Non-Hodgkin's lymphoma	250–1000
Inflammatory Disease	
Nonspecific interstitial pneumonitis	
Lymphoid interstitial pneumonitis	
Infection	
M. tuberculosis	
Fungi	
Opportunistic Infection	Late CD4 decline
Pneumocystis carinii	<250
Cytomegalovirus	
Mycobacterium avium-intracellulare	
Cryptococcosis	
Histoplasmosis	
Coccidiomycoses	
Pyogenic bacteria (especially children)	

users, prisoners, and hospitalized patients are likely to develop processes different from that of suburban homosexual men. Prophylaxis against PCP, and longer survival with low CD4 and T-lymphocyte counts, is also changing the spectrum of pathogens that are being seen.

This chapter reviews a clinical approach to pneumonia in patients with HIV infection and focuses on the infectious causes of pulmonary dysfunction in these patients. Clinicians need to consider the entire spectrum of potential causative processes, however, rather than assume that pulmonary dysfunction is necessarily infectious in etiology. Until antiretroviral therapy or immunomodulation is successful at reversing the immunologic decline that is the hallmark of HIV infection, effective management of the infectious complications will be an essential element for this patient population.

DIFFERENTIAL DIAGNOSIS

In Table 15-1 are the infectious processes that can cause pneumonia in patients with HIV infection. The clinical manifestations of these pneumonias overlap considerably. The tempo of disease progression, the presence of rigors, the radiologic pattern, and the white blood count help narrow the differential diagnosis to some extent. However, each infectious process has the potential to present atypically. Moreover, some processes are occasionally caused by a mixed infection of two or more organisms, or they can reflect infection superimposed on another process such as tumor. Thus, an important principle of management is to establish the specific etiology by a specific microbiologic test. A substantial number of cases that might appear to be community-acquired viral processes are, in fact, Pneumocystis carinii pneumonia. Similarly, many cases that appear clinically to be PCP are, in fact, caused by *Histoplasma capsulatum, M. tuberculosis,* or nonspecific interstitial pneumonitis (9,30,68,69). Thus, a specific diagnosis should be established for an HIV-infected patient presenting with pulmonary symptoms or signs.

Some nonspecific tests have been advocated as useful for screening patients with pulmonary symptoms prior to establishing a specific diagnostic test. Gallium scans, white blood cell scans, pulmonary function tests, and serum lactic dehydrogenase (LDH) levels have some utility; however, none provides specific information (20,44,46,73,75,77,88,89). It is probably unwise to rely on any of these techniques to make a specific diagnosis, or to exclude infection as the cause of pulmonary dysfunction. Whether the information derived from such tests merits the time and expense they require is a subject of debate. Likewise, screening of asymptomatic patients for declining pulmonary diffusing capacity as an early indicator of lung infection has not been a useful strategy (39).

Circulating CD4 and T-lymphocyte counts are useful for predicting what types of infection should be considered (Table 15-1) (46,58). Some infectious agents need to be considered at any CD4+ T-lymphocyte count. These include the common community-acquired pathogens such as influenza, respiratory syncytial virus (RSV), *Streptococcus pneumoniae, Hemophilus influenza, Mycoplasma pneumoniae,* and *Legionella* species (63,87). Some opportunistic processes, such as PCP and CMV, need not be considered at high CD4+ T-lymphocyte counts: at such counts their occurrence is extremely unusual. Only when the counts fall below 200–300/mm^3 do these pathogens need to be considered (46,58). Thus, the CD4+ T-lymphocyte count is a crucial determinant of how the diagnostic evaluation should be directed and as to what empiric antibiotics should be chosen pending the results from a final diagnostic procedure.

Prophylactic antibiotics also have a profound influence on the cause of pneumonia. Patients receiving trimethoprim-sulfamethoxazole (TMP-SMX) prophylaxis for PCP are extremely unlikely to develop PCP if they are actually taking the drug as prescribed (13,45). These patients are probably less likely to develop pneumonia due to *S. pneumoniae* and *H. influenzae* (and *Toxoplasma gondii*). In contrast, breakthrough episodes of PCP are fairly common in patients receiving aerosol pentamidine or dapsone prophylaxis (13,45). Thus, knowledge of what prophylactic regimen the patient is receiving is an important determinant of management.

HIV risk factors are another determinant of the differential diagnoses. Kaposi's sarcoma occurs in homosexual men but almost never in any other risk group (67).

Lastly, geography is an important issue in predisposing patients from endemic areas to specific infectious agents. In Indianapolis, for example, pulmonary histoplasmosis is almost as common as PCP and presents identically (30,84). In France, pulmonary toxoplasma is often described (57,64). In Korea, *Penicillium marneffe* is being described with increasing frequency. In New York and Haiti tuberculosis can occur in as many as 50% of AIDS patients (24,60). Physicians caring for HIV-infected patients must be cognizant of the patterns of disease in the geographic area where they practice and in areas where the patient has resided and traveled.

Epidemiologic data are also important for determining appropriate empiric anti-biotic therapy. Although trimethoprim-sulfamethoxazole (or other PCP drug) should be included for most, if not all, patients with respiratory symptoms, bacterial patho-gens are a significant consideration in other risk categories. For instance, among IV drug users anti-staphylococcus therapy (nafcillin and a cephalosporin, or vancomycin and possibly an aminoglycoside) is appropriate; for patients with nosocomial pneu-monias coverage for hospital-acquired pathogens (aminoglycoside, semisynthetic penicillin, and possibly vancomycin) is usually required; and for community-ac-quired infections antibiotics for atypical pneumonitides (erythromycin) might be in-dicated.

It is important to point out that attention must be paid to protecting other patients and visitors to a hospital as well as health care employees from communicable in-fectious processes (12). In those communities where the frequency of *M. tubercu-losis* is considered significant, tuberculosis must be considered in every patient with pulmonary dysfunction, and appropriate respiratory isolation should be instituted until it is excluded as a diagnosis.

DIAGNOSTIC TECHNIQUES

A major goal of management in the HIV-infected patient should be to establish a specific cause of pulmonary dysfunction. A prompt pulmonary evaluation is appro-priate even if symptoms or signs are minimal, and even if the chest radiograph is normal in a symptomatic patient. A key to improving prognosis is the prompt insti-tution of the appropriate therapy (4,20,32). There are considerable data to support an observation that is intuitively obvious: the less pulmonary dysfunction that is present when therapy is initiated, the better the patient's prognosis (3,4,20,32).

As with any patient population, HIV-infected patients with pulmonary dysfunc-tion should have a chest radiograph and a sputum gram stain. If pleural fluid is pres-ent, it should be sampled and examined for infection and tumor. If the diagnosis is not unequivocal from this initial workup, then blood culture and serum cryptococcal antigen should be obtained. Sputum stain and culture for mycobacteria should also be routine in most regions.

If the sputum gram stain is not diagnostic, a workup for PCP should be instituted in patients with CD4+ T-lymphocyte counts below 200–300/μL. Most patients should be able to produce an adequate induced sputum sample, and the diagnostic sensitivity and specificity should be very high using published methods (see Table 15-2) (38). More than a dozen hospitals, including community and university facili-ties, report a sensitivity over 75%, but such results require coordination among res-piratory therapy and clinical pathology and adherence to well-formulated protocols (23). In patients receiving aerosol pentamidine for PCP prophylaxis, the yield of induced sputum and bronchoscopy for pneumocystis may be reduced substantially in some laboratories (31,42). Rarely, other opportunistic pathogens such as histo-plasmae, cryptococci, or coccidiomycosis can be recognized morphologically on sputum smears (7,30,65).

If the induced sputum does not reveal pneumocystis, tuberculosis, or a convincing bacterial process, further workup is indicated (Fig. 15-1). Flexible fiberoptic bron-choscopy is performed when a patient cannot produce sputum, the sputum analysis is negative, or the patient deteriorates while receiving therapy based on a sputum analysis. The sensitivity for pneumocystis using bronchoalveolar lavage is 87–89%,

TABLE 15–2. *Microbiologic evaluation of induced sputum and bronchoalveolar lavage*

	Stains	Pathogen identified
Induced sputum[a]	methenamine silver	*Pneumocystis carinii*
	Giemsa	
	Diff-Quick	
	toluidine blue-O	
	immunofluorescence	
	acid-fast	Mycobacteria
	gram stain	Bacteria
Bronchoalveolar lavage pellet	gram stain	Bacteria
	wet mount	Fungus
	methenamine silver	
	Giemsa	
	toluidine blue-O	*Pneumocystis carinii*
	immunofluorescence	
	acid-fast	Mycobacteria
	Legionella direct fluorescent antibody	*Legionella* sp
	cytologic evaluation	Tumor
		Virus cytopathic effect
		Pneumocystis carinii

[a]Induced sputum obtained by inhalation of 3% saline via ultrasonic nebulizer; specimen liquified by reducing agent and then concentrated by cytocentrifugation, and stained.

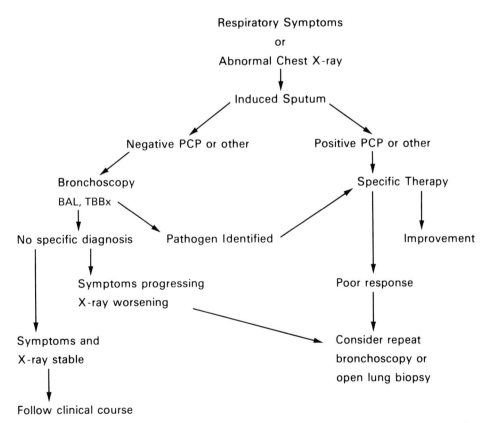

FIG. 15–1. Pulmonary dysfunction in patients infected with human immunodeficiency virus. (PCP, *P. carinii* pneumonia; BAL, bronchoalveolar lavage; TBBₓ, transbronchial biopsy)

and, when combined with transbronchial biopsies, the diagnostic sensitivity increases to 94–100% (5,55). This technique should rarely, if ever, fail to diagnose PCP, even if the patient has received several days of empiric therapy or aerosolized pentamidine. A transbronchial biopsy should be done initially if CMV is to be a major diagnostic consideration, because this process must be established by histology (36,74).

We routinely stain the pellet obtained from bronchoalveolar lavage for gram-positive and gram-negative bacteria, acid-fast bacilli, fungal organisms, and pneumocystis. Cultures of the pellet should be obtained for routine bacteria, fungal species, and mycobacterial species. If clinically indicated, we will obtain viral cultures for respiratory pathogens (e.g., respiratory syncytial virus, influenza, parainfluenza, adenovirus). Cultures of lavage for cytomegalovirus have no diagnostic importance in the absence of histologic evidence of cytomegalovirus pneumonia (2,29,48,74).

Contraindications to fiberoptic bronchoscopy include severe hypoxemia ($PaO_2 <$ 100 mmHg while breathing FiO_2 of 1.0), high levels of positive end expiratory pressure (PEEP) if the patient is being mechanically ventilated, and a bleeding diathesis (thrombocytopenia or elevated prothrombin or partial thromboplastin times) if transbronchial biopsies are contemplated.

Reassessment of the patient should occur if the bronchoalveolar lavage and transbronchial biopsies are unrevealing for a specific pulmonary process. If stable, the patient can be followed, and if deterioration occurs clinically or radiographically a repeat bronchoscopy or open lung biopsy should be performed.

The yield of open lung biopsy for opportunistic infections following an adequate evaluation with bronchoalveolar lavage and transbronchial biopsies will be low (18). Open lung biopsy is often necessary, however, to establish a diagnosis of lymphoma, Kaposi's sarcoma, cytomegalovirus, or fungus (especially *Aspergillus*). Kaposi's sarcoma is evident on endobronchial inspection, implying (but not assuring) that parenchymal disease could be due to this tumor (22,62). However, transbronchial biopsy produces too much crush artifact to permit accurate diagnosis of Kaposi's sarcoma in most situations. Computer-assisted tomographic (CAT) scans are helpful in that they can demonstrate a suggestive (but not diagnostic) nodular pattern. Most centers perform very few open lung biopsies per year because the diagnostic sensitivity of bronchoalveolar lavage is so high.

SPECIFIC PATHOGENS: DIAGNOSIS, THERAPY, AND PREVENTION

Pneumocystis carinii Pneumonia (PCP)

PCP usually presents as a diffuse pulmonary infiltrate associated with fever, chest tightness, cough, and dyspnea. Extrapulmonary manifestations occur but are unusual.

PCP is most readily diagnosed by induced sputum examination. The yield in many laboratories is 70–95%, although the sensitivity is reduced by 20% if patients have received aerosolized pentamidine (42). Essentially, all cases of PCP can be diagnosed by BAL: transbronchial or open lung biopsy should rarely be necessary. *Pneumocystis* must be recognized histologically: Giemsa, toluidine blue–O, methenamine silver, gram stain, and immunofluorescent monoclonal antibody techniques are all very sensitive and very specific in experienced laboratories (Table 15-2). The immunofluorescent stain is the most sensitive and the most specific in some laboratories (23,38). Human *Pneumocystis* cannot be cultured and serologies are not useful diagnostically.

TMP-SMX is the therapy of choice for PCP of any severity in patients who can tolerate it (Table 15-3). TMP-SMX is at least as effective as any other regimen, but many patients (20–40%) cannot tolerate it due to rash, fever, leukopenia, transaminase elevation, renal dysfunction, nausea, or vomiting (45). The hematologic, renal, and perhaps the hepatic abnormalities appear to be dose-related (70). Using a regimen of TMP 5 mg/kg q 8h with sulfamethoxazole 25 mg/kg q 8h can result in less toxicity than the same doses given q 6h. Peak sulfa levels should be maintained in the 100–150 µg/ml level, but need only be checked if patients are doing poorly in terms of inefficacy or toxicity. Clinicians are less hesitant now compared to 5–10 years ago about treating through mild or moderate toxicity, and achieving at least 10–14 days of TMP-SMX therapy. Prognosis is directly related to the room air partial pressure of oxygen PaO_2 at the time therapy is initiated. For patients who initiated therapy when their initial PO_2 is greater than 70 mmHg, mortality should occur in less than 5% of cases (27,52).

There is an expanding list of useful alternative therapies for patients unable to tolerate TMP-SMX. Intravenous pentamidine has been the major alternative for two decades, but this drug is well recognized to be toxic as well as inconvenient and expensive, the latter because it must be given intravenously. Intravenous pentamidine is also less desirable in an era when other pancreatic toxic antiviral drugs, such as dideoxycytidine and dideoxyinosine, are being used. It remains, however, the alternative of choice for patients with severe PCP because it can be given parenterally and is very effective. Aerosolized pentamidine should not be used for therapy except in a research protocol because its efficacy is low (76).

For patients with mild PCP (initial room air PaO_2 greater than 70 torr), two oral regimens are reasonable alternatives for TMP-SMX–intolerant patients. Atovaquone is not as effective as TMP-SMX, but it is extremely well tolerated (27). Clindamycin-primaquine is effective but is associated with considerable diarrhea, rash, and hepatic toxicity (53,66,79). TMP-dapsone is used as first-line therapy at some centers in preference to TMP-SMX because it is very effective and better tolerated than TMP-SMX. How often patients will tolerate TMP-dapsone if they are intolerant of TMP-SMX is not clear.

Trimetrexate is approved for therapy of moderate-to-severe PCP. It has the advantage of being well tolerated, and it is administered parenterally, which is desirable for patients with severe disease. Overall, it is not as effective, however, as TMP-SMX, and is indicated only for patients who are failing or intolerant of both TMP-SMX and parenteral pentamidine (71).

The most important advance in the therapy of PCP is the recognition that adjunctive corticosteroids improve the survival of patients who present with an initial room air PaO_2 less than 70 mmHg. Corticosteroid therapy is now standard practice for the patient population, regardless of what specific anti-pneumocystis agent is administered. Serious adverse effects are rare, although metabolic disturbances, oral candidiasis, and reactivation of mucocutaneous HSV does occur. The initial recommended dose of corticosteroids is 40 mg of prednisone q 12h po for 5 days, then 40 mg/d for 5 days, and then 20 mg/d for 11 days (52).

TABLE 15–3. *Therapy of specific pulmonary pathogens in patients with HIV infection*

Pulmonary process	Therapy	Prophylaxis
Infectious		
Pneumocystis carinii pneumonia	Trimethoprim-sulfamethoxazole (iv, po) Pentamidine (iv) Trimetrexate ($\pm$ sulfa) (iv) with leucovorin Dapsone-trimethoprim (po) Pyrimethamine-sulfadiazine Clindamycin and primaquine (po)	Trimethoprim-sulfamethoxazole (po) Pentamidine (inhaled) Sulfadoxine-pyrimethamine (po) Dapsone (po) Dapsone-pyrimethamine (po)
	Adjunctive therapy: Corticosteroids therapy (iv, po)	
Cytomegalovirus	Ganciclovir (iv) Foscarnet (iv)	
	Adjunctive therapy: Hyperimmune globulin (iv)	
Herpes simplex Measles Influenza	Acyclovir (po, iv)	Passive postexposure immunoglobulin Influenza vaccine Amantadine
Respiratory syncytial virus	Ribavirin (aerosol)	
Mycobacterium tuberculosis	Isoniazid, rifampin, pyrazinamide, and ethambutol (po)	Isoniazid for sensitive strains Rifampin and pyrazinamide for resistant strains (investigational)
Mycobacterium avium-intracellulare	Ethambutol (po), clofazamine (po), ciprofloxacin (po), and clarithromycin (po)	Rifabutin

Condition	Treatment	
Nocardiosis	Trimethoprim-sulfamethoxazole (po, iv)	
Fungal disease		
Cryptococcus neoformans	Amphotericin (iv) ± flucytosine (po)	Itraconazole
	Fluconazole (po)	
Histoplasma capsulatum	Amphotericin (iv) ± flucytosine (po)	Itraconazole
Coccidioides immitis	Amphotericin (iv) ± flucytosine (po)	Itraconazole
Candidiasis	Amphotericin (iv) ± flucytosine (po)	Fluconazole
Neoplasms		
Kaposi's sarcoma	Single or combination chemotherapy	Anti-*Pneumocystis* prophylaxis
	Radiation therapy for symptomatic airway or parenchymal lesions	
Lymphoma		
non-Hodgkin's	Multidrug chemotherapy	
Inflammatory Pulmonary Disease		
Lymphoid interstitial pneumonitis	Corticosteroids (iv, po)	
Nonspecific interstitial pneumonitis	No therapy indicated	
Diffuse alveolar damage	Corticosteroids (iv) ?	
Congestive Heart Failure		
Cardiomyopathy	Diuretics	
	Digoxin, inotropic agents	
	Afterload reduction	

PCP prophylaxis is indicated for anyone with a CD4+ T-lymphocyte count below 200/μL, in the presence of oropharyngeal candidiasis or persistent fever, or with a previous episode of PCP (13). TMP-SMX is preferred because it is more effective than other regimens, and because it has useful activity against toxoplasmosis, routine bacterial pathogens, and perhaps other pathogens such as isospora or cyclospora. A dose of TMP 160 mg/SMX 800 mg given once daily 2, 3, or 7 days per week is acceptable: the latter is usually recommended. Aerosol pentamidine is an alternative for the 20–40% of patients who cannot tolerate TMP-SMX. Pyrimethamine (75 mg) plus dapsone (200 mg) once weekly is equally effective against PCP but more effective against toxoplasmosis. What fraction of TMP-SMX–intolerant patients can tolerate pyrimethamine-dapsone is unknown (13).

Tuberculosis

M. Tuberculosis occurs in 50% of HIV-infected patients in Haiti and is quite prevalent in several large cities in North America, especially among populations traditionally at high risk for TB (9,10,15,24,61,72,78). *M. tuberculosis* can be present as classic, upper lobe reactivated disease. However, many cases of tuberculosis in patients with HIV infection are primary, and secondary cases frequently have presentations that are not classic (11,16). Patients with HIV and tuberculosis can have CD4+ T-lymphocyte counts that are either high or low. Preliminary reports suggest that reactivated disease is said to be characteristic of the population with more than 200–300 cells/μL, and primary disease is said to be more common in patients with CD4+ T-lymphocyte counts below 110/μL (16,58).

About half of cases of pulmonary *M. tuberculosis* in patients with HIV infection can be diagnosed by sputum smear. When a pulmonary secretion is smear-positive for acid-fast bacilli, the organism is much more likely to be *M. tuberculosis* than *M. avium* complex. For culture results, the opposite is true (51). A distressing number of cases of pulmonary tuberculosis are culture-positive but smear-negative, even when multiple smears are performed. Thus, appropriate isolation procedures should be maintained until a final diagnosis is established because of the risk of nosocomial spread of tuberculosis. Initial therapy for tuberculosis consists of a four-drug regimen: Isoniazid, rifampin, ethambutol, and pyrizinamide for 6 months (14). An initial three-drug regimen without pyrizinamide is recommended only in areas where almost no resistance occurs, or when the isolate's susceptibility is known. The response to therapy is, in general, favorable, and maintenance therapy is not required (14).

All PPD-positive patients with HIV infection (defined as PPD induration greater than 5 mm) should receive 1 year of isoniazid. If the strain causing the conversion is known or likely to be INH-resistant, regimens including two drugs (e.g., pyrizinamide and rifampin or ethambutol) are often used. More data are needed about the efficacy of prophylaxis on this patient group (11).

Mycobacterium avium complex (MAC) is frequently cultured from respiratory secretions or tissue. MAC almost never, however, causes pulmonary dysfunction in this patient population (25,26,54,59,83). Mediastinal adenopathy can occasionally be present, but well-documented cases of inflammatory lung disease due to MAC in AIDS patients are rare.

CMV

The frequency of CMV inclusion bodies in the lungs has been reported to be as high as 40–50%, yet CMV pneumonia is seldom documented antemortem. This may be because clinicians are reluctant to obtain lung biopsies, and it would appear that CMV pneumonia does not occur very frequently until patients have extremely advanced HIV disease (28,82,86).

CMV pneumonia presents as diffuse infiltrates. There is no highly suggestive clinical or radiologic feature, although CMV pneumonia is almost never seen in patients with CD4+ T-lymphocyte counts over 100 cells/μL. CMV pneumonia must be documented histologically. Cultures of blood, bronchoalveolar lavage, or lung tissue are nonspecific, and these cultures are often positive in patients with CD4+ T-lymphocyte counts below 100 cells/μL and no pulmonary dysfunction (2,29,48,49). CMV pneumonia is a patchy disease, and a transbronchial biopsy can miss areas of lung with typical inclusion bodies (28,74,82). Conversely, a few inclusion bodies can be seen in patients with no important CMV pneumonia; patients with PCP treated only for PCP have equal likelihood of survival regardless of the presence of CMV inclusion bodies (2,29). Thus, diagnosis is not precise. It must be based on seeing many inclusion bodies in lung tissue in the absence of other likely pathogens.

Reports of successful therapy with either parenteral ganciclovir or parenteral foscarnet are increasing. Many clinicians also administer intravenous immunoglobulin based on reports from bone marrow transplant recipients. Prognosis most likely depends on how extensive the pneumonia is (i.e., how hypoxemic patients are) when therapy is initiated.

Streptococcus pneumoniae and *Hemophilus influenzae*

There is increasing appreciation for the morbidity that *S. pneumoniae, H. influenzae,* and other common pathogens cause in the upper and lower respiratory systems of HIV-infected patients. Sinusitis, otitis, bronchitis, and pneumonia occur with substantial frequency in patients with HIV infection (8,43,92).

Fungal Infections

Pneumonitis due to fungal disease is an uncommon complication of HIV infection, and the clinical presentations are usually nonspecific. Serum immunological titers (i.e., cryptococcal and histoplasma antigens, coccioidomycosis antibody titer) are helpful when positive, although definitive diagnosis requires isolation of the fungal organism from tissue or fluid.

Cryptococcus neoformans is probably the most common HIV-related fungal infection involving the lungs. Pneumonitis usually presents after involvement of other organs and is only rarely (4–6%) a primary manifestation of cryptococcal disease (7,37,91). When pulmonary involvement is the initial manifestation, a complete evaluation for involvement at other sites should be performed, especially the bone marrow and meninges (7,37,91).

Histoplasma capsulatum is endemic in the areas of the Ohio and Mississippi river valleys, and nearly always presents as disseminated disease in HIV infection. Infection results from both reactivation of latent disease and primary pulmonary infection, although which mechanism is most significant is controversial (30,69,84). *Coccidioides immitis* is found only in the southwestern United States and should be considered as a potential pathogen given the appropriate geographic history (6).

Other fungal pathogens, such as *Candida* and *Aspergillus,* are only rarely encountered as primary pulmonary pathogens. *Aspergillus,* however, has been reported as a late cause of pulmonary disease, usually in patients receiving corticosteroids or broad-spectrum antibiotics, and in those who are neutropenic (17,35).

Neoplastic Diseases

Kaposi's sarcoma (KS) is seen almost exclusively in homosexual men and can be encountered at any stage of HIV infection. Approximately one-third of patients with cutaneous KS or other organ involvement will develop pulmonary involvement; only rarely will the lungs be affected exclusively. Radiographic findings of nodular infiltrates with pleural effusion is highly suggestive of KS (19,34,47,56,62,81,85).

Non-Hodgkin's lymphoma is the second most common HIV-related malignant neoplasm and affects all groups of patients. It is occurring with increased frequency as patients live longer with low CD4 lymphocyte counts. It is usually an aggressive, high-grade B-cell variety, and the sites commonly involved include the central nervous system, GI tract, and liver; thoracic involvement is unusual (1,21,33,40,41,85,90).

Non-Neoplastic Diseases

Interstitial pneumonitis in association with HIV infection is predominantly of two types: nonspecific interstitial pneumonitis (NIP) and lymphoid interstitial pneumonitis (LIP). NIP can account for up to 32% of episodes of pneumonitis in adults, and can be present in nearly half of asymptomatic patients (68). NIP is usually a mild illness, which stabilizes or resolves without therapy.

LIP is encountered primarily in children with HIV infection. Respiratory symptoms are usually more severe, and extrathoracic involvement, including adenopathy and lymphocytic infiltrations of the kidney, liver, bone marrow, and GI tract, is common. Significant respiratory compromise can occur; corticosteroid therapy is beneficial in some patients (80,85).

Both NIP and LIP can mimic other conditions. Their diagnosis requires a tissue specimen that is pathologically consistent with these conditions, and the absence of other causative pathogens (80,85).

CONCLUSION

Over the past decade, substantial progress has been made in the diagnosis, therapy, and prevention of pulmonary disease in patients with HIV infection. Early diagnosis, corticosteroid therapy for severe disease, and aggressive prophylaxis have, for example, substantially decreased the toll PCP has taken on this population. For the remainder of the 1990s, the challenges will include providing access to these advances for all patients with HIV infection, and continuing progress in treating other pulmonary pathogens such as tuberculosis and CMV. The goal in the 1990s should be to continue to extend the duration and quality of survival for patients infected with HIV.

REFERENCES

1. Bermudez, M.A., Grant, K.M., Rodvien, R., and Mendes, F. (1989): Non-Hodgkin's lymphoma in a population with or at risk for acquired immunodeficiency syndrome: indications for intesive chemotherapy. *Am. J. Med.*, 86:71–76.
2. Bozzette, S.A., Arcia, J., Bartok, A.E., et al. (1992): Impact of *Pneumocystis carinii* and cytomegalovirus on the course and outcome of atypical pneumonia in advanced human immunodeficiency virus disease. *J. Infect. Dis.*, 165:93–98.
3. Bozzette, S.A., Sattler, F.R., Chiu, J., et al. (1990): A controlled trial of early adjunctive treatment with corticosteroids for *Pneumocystis carinii* pneumonia in the acquired immunodeficiency syndrome. *N. Engl. J. Med.*, 323:1451–1457.
4. Brenner, M., Ognibene, F.P., Lack, E.E., et al. (1987): Prognostic factors and life expectancy of patients with acquired immunodeficiency syndrome and *Pneumocystis carinii* pneumonia. *Am. Rev. Respir. Dis.*, 136:1199–1206.
5. Broaddus, C., Dake, M.D., Stulbarg, M.S., et al. (1985): Bronchoalveolar lavage and transbronchial biopsy for the diagnosis of pulmonary infections in the acquired immunodeficiency syndrome. *Ann. Intern. Med.*, 102:747–752.
6. Bronimann, D.A., Adam, R.D., Galgiani, J.N., et al. (1987): Coccidioidomycosis in the acquired immunodeficiency syndrome. *Ann. Intern. Med.*, 106:372–379.
7. Cameron, M.L., Bartlett, J.A., Gallis, H.A., and Waskin, H.A. (1991): Manifestations of pulmonary cryptococcosis in patients with acquired immunodeficiency syndrome. *Rev. Infect. Dis.*, 13:64–67.
8. Casadevall, A., Dobroszycki, J., Small, C., and Pirofski, L.-A. (1992): *Hemophilus influenzae* type b bacteremia in adults with AIDS and at risk for AIDS. *Am. J. Med.*, 92:587–590.
9. Centers for Disease Control. (1988): Tuberculosis and human immunodeficiency virus infection: recommendations of the Advisory Committee for the elimination of tuberculosis. *M.M.W.R.*, 38:236–250.
10. Centers for Disease Control. (1989): Prevention and control of tuberculosis in correctional institutions: recommendations of the Advisory Committee for the elimination of tuberculosis. *M.M.W.R*, 38:313–320.
11. Centers for Disease Control. (1989): Tuberculosis and human immunodeficiency virus infection: Recommendations of the Advisory Council for the Elimination of Tuberculosis. *M.M.W.R.*, 38:236–250.
12. Centers for Disease Control. (1991): Nosocomial transmission of multi-drug resistant tuberculosis among HIV-infected persons: Florida and New York, 1988–1991. *M.M.W.R.*, 70:585–591.
13. Centers for Disease Control. (1992): Recommendations for prophylaxis against *Pneumocystis carinii* pneumonia for adults and adolescents infected with human immunodeficiency virus. *M.M.W.R.*, 41(RR-4):1–11.
14. Centers for Disease Control. (1993): Initial therapy for tuberculosis in the era of multidrug resistance. Recommendations of the Advisory Council for the Elimination of Tuberculosis. *M.M.W.R.*, 42(RR-7):1–8.
15. Chaisson, R.E., Schecter, G.F., Theuer, C.P., Rutherford, G.W., Echenberg, D.F., and Hopewell, P.C. (1987): Tuberculosis in patients with the acquired immunodeficiency syndrome: clinical features response to therapy and survival. *Am. Rev. Respir. Dis.*, 136:570–574.
16. Chaisson, R.E., and Slutkin, G. (1989): Tuberculosis and human immunodeficiency virus infection. *J. Infect. Dis.*, 159:96–100.
17. Denning, D.W., Follansbee, S.E., Scolaro, M., Edelstein, H., and Stevens, D.A. (1991): Pulmonary aspergillosis in the acquired immunodeficiency syndrome. *N. Engl. J. Med.*, 324:654–662.
18. Fitzgerald, W., Bevelaqua, F.A., Garay, S.M., and Aranda, C.P. (1987): The role of open lung biopsy in patients with the acquired immunodeficiency syndrome. *Chest*, 91:659–661.
19. Garay, S.M., Belenko, M., Fazzini, E., and Schinella, R. (1987): Pulmonary manifestations of Kaposi's sarcoma. *Chest*, 91:39–43.
20. Garay, S.M., and Greene, J. (1989): Prognostic indicators in the initial presentation of *Pneumocystis carinii* pneumonia. *Chest*, 95:769–772.
21. Gill, P.S. (1991): Pathogenesis of HIV-related malignancies. *Curr. Opin. Oncol.*, 3:867–871.
22. Gill, P.S., Akil, B., Colletti, P., et al. (1989): Pulmonary Kaposi's sarcoma: clinical findings and results of therapy. *Am. J. Med.*, 87:57–61.
23. Glenny, R.W., and Pierson, D.J. (1992): Cost reduction in diagnosing *Pneumocystis carinii* pneumonia. *Am. Rev. Respir. Dis.*, 145:1425–1428.

24. Handwerger, S., Mildvan, D., Senie, R., and McKinley, F.W. (1987): Tuberculosis and the acquired immunodeficiency syndrome at a New York city hospital: 1978–1985. *Chest*, 91:176–180.
25. Horsburgh, C.R. (1991): *Mycobacterium avium* complex infection in the acquired immunodeficiency syndrome. *N. Engl. J. Med.*, 324:1332–1338.
26. Horsburgh, C.R., and Selik, R.M. (1989): The epidemiology of disseminated nontuberculous mycobacterial infection in the acquired immunodeficiency syndrome (AIDS). *Am. Rev. Respir. Dis.*, 139:4–7.
27. Hughes, W., Leoung, G., Kramer, F., et al. (1993): Comparison of Atovaquone (566C80) with trimethoprim-sulfamethoxazole to treat *Pneumocystis carinii* pneumonia in patients with AIDS. *N. Engl. J. Med.*, 328:1521–1527.
28. Jacobson, M.A., and Mills, J. (1988): Serious cytomegalovirus disease in the acquired immunodeficiency syndrome (AIDS). *Ann. Intern. Med.*, 108:585–594.
29. Jacobson, M.A., Mills, J., Rush, J., et al. (1991): Morbidity and mortality of patients with AIDS and first-episode *Pneumocystis carinii* pneumonia unaffected by concomitant pulmonary cytomegalovirus infection. *Am. Rev. Respir. Dis.*, 144:6–9.
30. Johnson, P.C., Khardori, N., Najjar, A.F., Butt, F., Mansell, P.W., and Sarosi, G.A. (1988): Progressive disseminated histoplasmosis in patients with acquired immunodeficiency syndrome. *Am. J. Med.*, 85:152–158.
31. Jules-Elysee, K., Stover, D.E., Zaman, M.B., Bernard, E.M., and White, D.A. (1990): Aerosolized pentamidine: effect on the diagnosis and presentation of *Pneumocystis carinii* pneumonia. *Ann. Intern. Med.*, 112:750–757.
32. Kales, C.P., Murren, J.R., Torres, R.A., and Crocco, J.A. (1987): Early predictors of in-hospital mortality for *Pneumocystis carinii* pneumonia in the acquired immunodeficiency syndrome. *Arch. Intern. Med.*, 147:1413–1417.
33. Kaplan, L.D., Abrams, D.I., Feigal, E., et al. (1989): AIDS-associated non-Hodgkin's lymphoma in San Francisco. *J.A.M.A.*, 261:719–724.
34. Kaplan, L.D., Hopewell, P.C., Jeffe, H., Goodman, P.C., Bottles, K., and Volberding, P. (1988): Kaposi's sarcoma involving the lung in patients with acquired immunodeficiency syndrome. *J. AIDS*, 1:23–30.
35. Klapholz, A., Salomon, N., Perlamn, D.C., and Talavera, W. (1991): Aspergillosis in the acquired immunodeficiency syndrome. *Chest*, 100:1614–1618.
36. Klatt, E.C., and Shibata, D. (1988): Cytomegalovirus infection in the acquired immunodeficiency syndrome: clinical and autopsy findings. *Arch. Pathol. Lab. Med.*, 112:540–544.
37. Kovacs, J.A., Kovacs, A.A., Polis, M., et al. (1985): Cryptococcosis in the acquired immunodeficiency syndrome. *Ann. Intern. Med.*, 103:533–538.
38. Kovacs, J.A., Ng, V., Masur, H., et al. (1988): Diagnosis of *Pneumocystis carinii* pneumonia: improved detection in sputum using monoclonal antibodies. *N. Engl. J. Med.*, 318:589–593.
39. Krale, P.A., Rosen, M.J., Hopewell, P.C., Markowitz, N., et al. (1993): A decline in the pulmonary diffusing capacity does not indicate opportunistic lung disease in asymptomatic persons infected with human immunodeficiency virus. *Am. Rev. Respir. Dis.*, 148:390–395.
40. Levine, A.M., Gill, P.S., Meyer, P.R., et al. (1985): Retrovirus and malignant lymphoma in homosexual men. *J.A.M.A.*, 254:1921–1925.
41. Levine, A.M., Meyer, P.R., Begandy, M.K., et al. (1984): Development of B-cell lymphoma in homosexual men: clinical and immunologic findings. *Ann. Intern. Med.*, 100:7–13.
42. Levine, S.J., Masur, H., Gill, V.J., et al. (1991): Effect of aerosolized pentamidine prophylaxis on the diagnosis of *Pneumocystis carinii* pneumonia by induced sputum examination in patients infected with the human immunodeficiency virus. *Ann. Rev. Respir. Dis.*, 144:760–776.
43. Magnenat, J.-L., Nicod, L.P., Auckenthaler, R., and Junod, A.F. (1991): Mode of presentation and diagnosis of bacterial pneumonia in human immunodeficiency virus–infected patients. *Am. Rev. Respir. Dis.*, 144:917–922.
44. Mason, G.R., Duane, B.B., Mena, I., and Effros, R.M. (1987): Accelerated solute clearance in *Pneumocystis carinii* pneumonia. *Am. Rev. Respir. Dis.*, 135:864–868.
45. Masur, H. (1992): Prevention and treatment of Pneumocystis pneumonia. *N. Engl. J. Med.*, 327:1853–1860.
46. Masur, H., Ognibene, F.P., Yarchoan, R., et al. (1989): CD4 counts as predictors of opportunistic pneumonias in human immunodeficiency virus infected individuals. *Ann. Intern. Med.*, 111:223–231.
47. Meduri, G.U., Stover, D.E., Lee, M., Myskowski, P.L., Caravelli, J.F., and Zaman, M.B. (1986): Pulmonary Kaposi's sarcoma in the acquired immune deficiency syndrome: clinical radiographic and pathologic manifestations. *Am. J. Med.*, 81:11–18.
48. Miles, P.R., Baughman, R.P., and Linnemann, C.C. (1990): Cytomegalovirus in the bronchoalveolar lavage fluid of patients with AIDS. *Chest*, 97:1072–1076.
49. Millar, A.B., Patou, G., Miller, R.F., et al. (1990): Cytomegalovirus in the lungs of patients with AIDS: respiratory pathogen or passenger? *Am. Rev. Respir. Dis.*, 141:1474–1477.

50. Murray, J.F., and Mills, J. (1990): Pulmonary infectious complications of human immunodeficiency virus infection. *Am. Rev. Respir. Dis.*, 141:1356–1372, 1582–1598.
51. Nassos, P.S., Yajko, D.M., Sanders, C.A., and Hadley, W.K. (1991): Prevalence of *Mycobacterium avium* complex in respiratory specimens from AIDS and non-AIDS patients in a San Francisco hospital. *Am. Rev. Respir. Dis.*, 143:66–68.
52. The National Institutes of Health–University of California Expert Panel for Corticosteroids as Adjunctive Therapy for Pneumocystis Pneumonia. (1990): Consensus statement on the use of corticosteroids as adjunctive therapy for Pneumocystis pneumonia in the acquired immunodeficiency syndrome. *N. Engl. J. Med.*, 323:1500–1504.
53. Noskin, G.A., Murphy, R.L., Black, J.R., and Phair, J.P. (1992): Salvage therapy with clindamycin/primaquine for Pneumocystis pneumonia. *Clin. Infect. Dis.*, 14:183–188.
54. O'Brien, R.J., Miller, B., Pitchenik, A., et al. (1987): Topics in pulmonary medicine symposium: mycobacterial diseases in AIDS. *Am. Rev. Respir. Dis.*, 136:1027–1030.
55. Ognibene, F.P., Shelhamer, J., Gill, V., et al. (1982): The diagnosis of *Pneumocystis carinii* pneumonia in patients with the acquired immunodeficiency syndrome using subsegmental bronchoalveolar lavage. *Am. Rev. Respir. Dis.*, 129:929–932.
56. Ognibene, F.P., Steis, R.G., Macher, A.M., et al. (1985): Kaposi's sarcoma causing pulmonary infiltrates and respiratory failure in the acquired immunodeficiency syndrome. *Ann. Intern. Med.*, 102:471–475.
57. Oksenhendler, E., Cadranel, J., Sarfati, C., et al. (1990): *Toxoplasma gondii* pneumonia in patients with the acquired immunodeficiency syndrome. *Am. J. Med.*, 88:5-18N–5-21N.
58. Phair, J., Muñoz, A., Detels, R., et al. (1990): The risk of *Pneumocystis carinii* pneumonia among men infected with human immunodeficiency virus type 1. *N. Engl. J. Med.*, 322:161–165.
59. Pitchenik, A. (1988): The treatment and prevention of mycobacterial disease in patients with HIV infection. *AIDS*, 2(Suppl. 1):S177–S182.
60. Pitchenik, A., Burr, J., Suarez, M., Fertel, D., Gonzalez, G., and Moas, C. (1987): Human T-cell lymphotrophic virus-III (HTLV-III) seropositivity and related disease among 71 consecutive patients in whom tuberculosis was diagnosed. *Am. Rev. Respir. Dis.*, 135:875–879.
61. Pitchenik, A.E., Cole, C., Russell, B.W., Fischl, M.A., Spira, T.J., and Snider, D.E. (1984): Tuberculosis atypical mycobacteriosis and the acquired immunodeficiency syndrome among Haitian and non-Haitian patients in South Florida. *Ann. Inter. Med.*, 101:641–645.
62. Pitchenik, A.E., Fischl, M.A., and Saldana, M.J. (1985): Kaposi's sarcoma of the tracheobronchial tree: clinical bronchoscopic and pathologic features. *Chest*, 87:122–124.
63. Polsky, B., Gold, J.W., Whimbey, E., et al. (1986): Bacterial infections in patients with the acquired immunodeficiency syndrome. *Ann. Intern. Med.*, 104:38–41.
64. Pomeroy, C., and Filice, G.A. (1992): Pulmonary toxoplasmosis: a review. *Clin. Infect Dis.*, 14:863–870.
65. Roberts, G.D. (1975): Detection of fungi in clinical specimens by phase-contrast microscopy. *J. Clin. Microbiol.*, 2:261–265.
66. Ruf, B., and Pohle, H.D. (1989): Clindamycin/primaquine for *Pneumocystis carinii* pneumonia. *Lancet*, 2:626–627.
67. Rutherford, G.W., Schwarcz, S.K., Lemp, G.F., et al. (1989): The epidemiology of AIDS-related Kaposi's sarcoma in San Francisco. *J. Infect. Dis.*, 159:569–572.
68. Suffredini, A.F., Ognibene, F.P., Lack, E.E., et al. (1987): Nonspecific interstitial pneumonitis: a common cause of pulmonary disease in the acquired immunodeficiency syndrome. *Ann. Intern. Med.*, 107:7–13.
69. Salzman, S.H., Smith, R.L., and Aranda, C.P. (1988): Histoplasmosis in patients at risk for the acquired immunodeficiency syndrome in a nonendemic setting. *Chest*, 93:916–921.
70. Sattler, F.R., Cowan, R., Nielson, D.M., and Ruskin, J. (1988): Trimethoprim-sulfamethoxazole compared with pentamidine for treatment of *Pneumocystis carinii* pneumonia in the acquired immunodeficiency syndrome: a prospective noncrossover study. *Ann. Intern. Med.*, 109:280–287.
71. Sattler, F.R., Frame, P., Davis, R., et al. (n.d.): Comparison of trimetrexate with leucovorin versus trimethoprim-sulfamethoxazole for moderate-to-severe episodes of *Pneumocystis carinii* pneumonia in patients with AIDS. (Submitted.)
72. Selwyn, P.A., Hartel, D., Lewis, V.A., et al. (1989): A prospective study of the risk of tuberculosis among intravenous drug users with human immunodeficiency virus infection. *N. Engl. J. Med.*, 320:545–550.
73. Shaw, R.J., Roussak, C., Forster, S.M., Harris, J.R., Pinching, A.J., and Mitchell, D.M. (1988): Lung function abnormalities in patients infected with the human immunodeficiency virus, with and without overt pneumonitis. *Thorax*, 43:436–440.
74. Smith, C.B. (1989): Cytomegalovirus pneumonia: state of the art. *Chest*, 95:(Suppl.):182S–187S.
75. Smith, D.E., McLuckie, A., Wyatt, J., and Gazzard, D. (1988): Severe exercise hypoxemia with normal or near normal x-rays: a feature of *Pneumocystis carinii* infection. *Lancet*, 1:1049–1051.

76. Soo Hoo, G.W., Mohsenifar, Z., and Meyer, R.D. (1990): Inhaled or intravenous pentamidine therapy for *Pneumocystis carinii* pneumonia in AIDS: a randomized trial. *Ann. Intern. Med.*, 113:195–202.
77. Stover, D.E., and Meduri, G.U. (1988): Pulmonary function tests. *Clin. Chest Med.*, 9:473–479.
78. Sunderan, G., McDonald, R.J., Maniatis, T., Oleske, J., Kapila, R., and Reichman, L.B. (1986): Tuberculosis as a manifestation of the acquired immunodeficiency syndrome (AIDS). *J.A.M.A.*, 256:362–366.
79. Toma, E., Fournier, S., Dumont, M., Bolduc, P., and Deschamps, H. (1994): Clindamycin/primaquine versus trimethoprim-sulfamethoxazole as primary therapy for *pneumocystis carinii* pneumonia in AIDS: a randomized, double blind pilot trial. *Clinic. Infect. Dis.*, 17:178–184.
80. Travis, W.D., Fox, C.H., Devaney, K.O., et al. (1992): Lymphoid pneumonitis in 50 adult patients infected with the human immunodeficiency virus: lymphocytic interstitial pneumonitis versus nonspecific interstitial pneumonitis. *Human Pathol.*, 23:529–541.
81. Travis, W.D., Lack, E.E., Ognibene, F.P., Suffredini, A.F., and Shelhamer, J. (1989): Lung biopsy interpretation in the acquired immunodeficiency syndrome: experience at the National Institutes of Health with literature review. *Prog. AIDS Pathol.*, 1:51–84.
82. Wallace, J.M., and Hannah, J. (1987): Cytomegalovirus pneumonitis in patients with AIDS: findings in an autopsy series. *Chest*, 92:198–203.
83. Wallace, J.M., and Hannah, J.B. (1988): *Mycobacterium avium* complex infection in patients with acquired immunodeficiency syndrome: a clinicopathologic study. *Chest*, 93:926–932.
84. Wheat, L.J., Slama, T.G., and Zeckel, M.L. (1985): Histoplasmosis in the acquired immunodeficiency syndrome. *Am. J. Med.*, 78:203–210.
85. White, D.A., and Matthay, R.A. (1989): Noninfectious pulmonary complications of infection with the human immunodeficiency virus. *Am. Rev. Respir. Dis.*, 140:1763–1787.
86. Wilkes, M.S., Fortin, A.H., Felix, J.C., Godwin, T.A., and Thompson, W.G. (1988): Value of necropsy in acquired immunodeficiency syndrome. *Lancet*, 2:85–88.
87. Witt, D.J., Craven, D.E., and McCabe, W.R. (1987): Bacterial infections in adults with the acquired immune deficiency syndrome (AIDS) and AIDS-related complex. *Am. J. Med.*, 82:900–906.
88. Woolfenden, J.M., Carrasquillo, J.A., Larson, S.M., et al. (1987): Acquired immunodeficiency syndrome: Ga-67 citrate imaging. *Radiology*, 162:383–387.
89. Zaman, M.K., and White D.A. (1988): Serum lactate dehydrogenase levels and *Pneumocystis carinii* pneumonia: diagnostic and prognostic significance. *Am. Rev. Respir. Dis.*, 137:796–800.
90. Ziegler, J.L., Beckstead, J.A., Volberding, P.A., et al. (1984): Non-Hodgkin's lymphoma in 90 homosexual men: relation to generalized lymphadenopathy and the acquired immunodeficiency syndrome. *N. Engl. J. Med.*, 311:565–570.
91. Zuger, A., Louie, E., Holzman, R.S., Simberkoff, M.S., and Rahal, J.J. (1986): Cryptococcal disease in patients with the acquired immunodeficiency syndrome: diagnostic features and outcome of treatment. *Ann. Intern. Med.*, 104:234–240.
92. Zurlo, J.J., Feuerstein, I.M., Lebovics, R., and Lane, H.C. (1992): Sinusitis in HIV-1 infection. *Am. J. Med.*, 93:157–162.

Respiratory Infections: Diagnosis and Management, 3d ed.,
edited by James E. Pennington.
Raven Press, Ltd., New York © 1994

16

Aspiration Pneumonia, Lung Abscess, and Empyema

Sydney M. Finegold

*Departments of Medicine and Microbiology and Immunology, UCLA School of
Medicine, Los Angeles, California 90073*

The use of the term *aspiration pneumonia* has led to a great deal of confusion. It is important to keep in mind that there are four major clinical pictures associated with aspiration (2,15). One is airway obstruction related to aspiration of particulate matter, foreign bodies, or large volumes of inert fluids. The second syndrome is a chemical pneumonitis. The major cause of this is aspiration of liquid gastric contents, but other causes are inhalation of exogenous chemicals, lipoid pneumonitis, and smoke inhalation (9,15,17,24,25). The third category is infectious pneumonitis. Infectious problems can follow aspiration of particulate matter or chemical pneumonitis, or relate to inhalation of oropharyngeal secretions containing bacteria. The fourth category is drowning.

BACKGROUND FACTORS

The common denominator for all these problems is a breakdown of the normal protective mechanisms. Specific predisposing conditions include reduced levels of consciousness, dysphagia, and mechanical interference with the cardiac sphincter caused by nasogastric tubes.

In individuals with pulmonary complications of aspiration, the major predisposing conditions are alcoholism, seizure disorders, general anesthesia, cerebrovascular accidents, esophageal disease, nasogastric tube feeding, and drug addiction (1–3, 9,15,24,25). Periodontal disease and gingivitis are other important background factors (1,3).

Aspiration of even small quantities of oropharyngeal secretions can present a very large bacterial inoculum to the lung. Such secretions will contain 10^7 anaerobes and 10^6 aerobes and facultatives in as little as 0.1 ml (11,12,17). In contrast, inhalation of air containing 15 organisms/m^3 for 1 hr introduces only 10 bacteria into the lungs (17).

About 50% of normal subjects and 70% of subjects with impaired consciousness aspirate during sleep. Furthermore, for reasons still not entirely clear, the defense mechanisms of the lung are not as efficient in handling aspirated bacteria as they are for inhaled (aerosolized) organisms. The efficiency of the antibacterial mechanisms under normal circumstances accounts for the normal sterility of the distal airways and the lung parenchyma.

As indicated, the normal oral flora consists of 10^8 anaerobes/ml (chiefly various species of *Bacteroides, Prevotella, Porphyromonas, Fusobacterium,* and anaerobic cocci) and 10^7 aerobes/ml (chiefly streptococci). Under certain circumstances, there can be significant modification of the indigenous flora (11). Counts of anaerobes are lower than usual in edentulous subjects and higher in patients with gingivitis and periodontal disease, for example. Alcoholics and patients who are acutely or chronically ill (whether or not they are hospitalized or in a nursing home) often demonstrate oropharyngeal colonization with gram-negative bacilli, particularly if they undergo endotracheal intubation and especially if they also receive histamine type 2 blockers or antacids (1,3,10,17,26).

PATHOPHYSIOLOGY

The various types of pleuropulmonary infection relating to aspiration—pneumonitis, necrotizing pneumonia (multiple excavations 1 cm in diameter or less), lung abscess (one or more cavities >1 cm in diameter communicating with a bronchus), and empyema—should be considered as one process with a continuum of changes (1). The initial stage, pneumonitis, consists of alveolar filling with edema and inflammatory cells. The distribution of the lesion is very distinctive in two respects (1,7). First, the disease has a definite predilection for dependent segments, particularly the superior segments of the lower lobes and the posterior segments of the upper lobes. Second, the process, based on the pleural surface, can lead to pyramidal-shaped lesions with the apex toward the hilum (accounting for the confusing term *bronchial embolus*). Small-volume aspirations are usually not as strongly oriented toward dependent segments and peripheral location, at least at the outset.

The most common site of aspiration pneumonia is the posterior segment of the right upper lobe, with the same segment on the left less commonly affected (7). Next in frequency of involvement are the apical segments of both lower lobes. The inhaled material—saliva; nasal, oral, or nasopharyngeal secretions; blood; vomitus—is distributed according to gravity and the posture of the subject. Such inhalation occurs in many situations, for example, during sleep, deep narcosis, and anesthesia, and after oral surgery. Normally, the inhaled matter is handled effectively by ciliary action, cough, and alveolar macrophages. If the protective mechanisms are not effective, infection can result. Endotracheal tubes impair coughing, impede pulmonary clearance mechanisms, and allow leakage of oropharyngeal secretions into the tracheobronchial tree. Thick or particulate matter and foreign bodies are not easily removed and can produce bronchial obstruction and atelectasis. In pneumonia following aspiration of gastric contents, gastric acid and enzymes are the primary offending agents (9,15,17,25).

Generally, there is no significant vascular involvement in either necrotizing pneumonia or lung abscess. However, pulmonary embolus (septic or bland) can be the initial event. Once underway, the infection itself can give rise to pulmonary arteritis, as in infection caused by *Pseudomonas* sp.

Other important mechanisms leading to necrotizing pulmonary infection include the following: seeding as a result of bacteremia, with or without endocarditis; extension of infection by way of lymphatics and through the diaphragm (or defects in it); infection within or distal to a neoplastic obstruction of airways; and infection secondary to trauma to the chest (1,11).

With delay in treatment, or with inadequate therapy, the process goes on to necrotizing pneumonia or lung abscess, the latter usually bounded by fibrosing inflammatory response, which minimizes extension of the process. Peripheral extension of anaerobic pneumonias to the pleural surface leads to pleural thickening and fibrosis or empyema. With the anaerobes, at least, the specific organisms involved do not determine the nature, extent, or severity of the pleuropulmonary infectious process except for *Fusobacterium necrophorum,* which is especially virulent (1,11). Both the size of the bacterial inoculum and the role of associated organisms and host defenses are uncertain, but likely important. Strain differences in virulence, probably related primarily to toxin or enzyme production, can be important; this applies to nonanaerobes as well. Organisms such as *Staphylococcus aureus* and *Klebsiella pneumoniae,* which produce potent extracellular enzymes, are more likely to lead to pulmonary parenchymal necrosis and empyema than organisms such as *Streptococcus pneumoniae* which do not produce such products.

ETIOLOGY

Anaerobes

Ninety percent of cases of aspiration pneumonia and lung abscess involve anaerobic bacteria (3). In spontaneously occurring empyema (not related to prior surgery or trauma), anaerobes are found in 75% of cases (5). In these conditions, anaerobic bacteria are found to the exclusion of other kinds of bacteria in one-third of cases. So-called nonspecific lung abscess is virtually always caused by anaerobes (4).

The anaerobic bacteria that are most important as causes of pulmonary infections are listed in Table 16-1. Of these, the anaerobes most often involved are the pigmented *Prevotella* and *Porphyromonas, Prevotella oris* and *P. buccae, Fusobacter-*

TABLE 16–1. *Major anaerobes encountered in pleuropulmonary infection*

Gram-negative bacilli
  Pigmented *Prevotella* and *Porphyromonas*
  Prevotella oris, P. buccae
  Prevotella oralis group
  Bacteroides ureolyticus group (especially *B. gracilis*)
  Bacteroides fragilis group
  Fusobacterium nucleatum
  F. necrophorum, F. naviforme, F. gonidiaformans
Gram-positive cocci
  Peptostreptococcus (especially *P. magnus, P. asaccharolyticus, P. prevotii, P. anaerobius, P. micros*)
  Microaerophilic streptococci (*S. intermedius* and others)
Gram-positive nonsporing bacilli
  Actinomyces sp
  Propionibacterium propionicus
  Bifidobacterium dentium
Gram-positive spore-forming bacilli
  Clostridium (especially *C. perfringens, C. ramosum*)

ium nucleatum, and various anaerobic streptococci (*Peptostreptococcus,* anaerobic strains of *Streptococcus,* and microaerophilic streptococci) (1,3–5,11,12,20,23). *Bacteroides fragilis* group strains are found in 5% of cases (23), and other β-lactamase-producing (penicillin-resistant) *Bacteroides, Prevotella,* and *Porphyromonas* sp are found in 30–35% of cases (11,14,20,23). *Fusobacterium necrophorum,* found frequently in the pre-antimicrobic era, is no longer encountered commonly. Spirochetes (*Treponema* sp) are common and are often associated with *F. nucleatum* (so-called fusospirochetal disease), but their significance is doubtful. On the basis of experimental work, the pigmented gram-negative anaerobic rods may be key pathogens in this kind of mixed infection. The microaerophilic cocci are identical with species classified as aerobic (facultative) and officially belong in the genus *Streptococcus;* however, anaerobic techniques are often required for their isolation and characterization (11).

Occasionally, subphrenic abscess or other intraabdominal infection will extend directly or indirectly to involve the lung. In this situation and with intestinal obstruction, *Bacteroides fragilis* is much more common than in the usual type of aspiration pneumonia (3).

Aerobes

The major aerobic and facultative causes of aspiration pneumonia and/or empyema are *Staphylococcus aureus, Streptococcus pyogenes,* other *Streptococcus* species, and various gram-negative bacilli, including *Klebsiella pneumoniae, Enterobacter, Serratia,* and *Pseudomonas aeruginosa* (3,13,22,27). Occasionally, other gram-negative bacilli, such as *Escherichia coli* and *Proteus* sp, may be implicated. Uncommon but important causes of cavitating pneumonia are *Nocardia* sp, *Legionella* sp, and *P. pseudomallei.*

Tuberculosis should always be considered in necrotizing pneumonia, and fungal infection (particularly histoplasmosis, coccidioidomycosis, and aspergillosis) can also produce this type of pathology. Bronchogenic cysts commonly contain fluid that can constitute a good culture medium for various organisms. Factors that favor aspiration of oropharyngeal flora or that interfere with drainage can lead to infection of lung cysts. The bacteriology of these infected lung cysts is not unlike that of lung abscess.

Lung abscess is the primary manifestation of pleuropulmonary amebiasis, but pleural complications can occur as well.

CLINICAL PICTURE

The initial lesion in bacterial infection following aspiration is pneumonitis without distinctive features except for predisposition to aspiration, a relatively insidious onset in some patients, and involvement of dependent segments of lung (1,3). After 1 or 2 weeks, tissue necrosis leading to abscess formation or empyema occurs in many of the patients. Excavation may lead to solitary lung abscess or multiple small areas of necrosis of the lung, with or without air-fluid levels (necrotizing pneumonia). Following cavitation, putrid sputum is often noted in 50% or more of patients. Hemoptysis is often seen as well.

The usual picture is that of an acute pneumonic process, with fever, malaise, dry cough, and, frequently, pleuritic pain, but the onset is sometimes much more insidious. Weeks to months of malaise, low-grade fever, and cough, with significant weight loss and anemia, can precede consolidation. Neoplasia is a serious diagnostic consideration in such patients.

The physical findings are those of a local pneumonia, with or without pleurisy; later, amphoric or cavernous breath sounds are often noted. Radiography occasionally reveals mediastinal lymphadenopathy in addition to the usual findings, making the differential diagnosis more difficult. Clubbing of the fingers occurs occasionally. There can also be other findings related to the pathogenetic factors: diseased gums, presence of an endotracheal tube, absence of the gag reflex, and evidence of alcoholism (1,3). Leukocytosis and anemia are often present.

The severity of the illness varies considerably among patients. Those with acute necrotizing pneumonia, however, are often quite ill.

DIAGNOSIS

The following are important clues to the diagnosis: observed aspiration or predisposition to aspiration; disease in a dependent segment; cavitation or abscess formation, with or without empyema; foul-smelling sputum or empyema fluid; periodontal disease or gingivitis; and distinctive microscopic morphology of organisms from empyema fluid, transtracheal aspirate, or other source free of normal flora (11). On gram stain, pigmented *Prevotella* and *Porphyromonas* appear as small, pale-staining, gram-negative coccobacillary forms. *F. nucleatum* is seen as long, thin, tapering pale-staining gram-negative cells arranged end-to-end in pairs sometimes containing irregular gram-positive granules. Anaerobic and microaerophilic streptococci appear as very small gram-positive cocci in chains. Discharges with foul odor are definitive evidence of involvement of anaerobes in the infective process. However, the absence of such odor does not exclude this possibility because the odor appears only after cavitation or abscess formation has taken place, and certain organisms, particularly microaerophilic and some anaerobic cocci, often do not produce the metabolic end products responsible for foul or putrid odor.

Expectorated sputum cannot be used for anaerobic culture because of the presence of large numbers of anaerobes from the indigenous flora of the upper respiratory tract that contaminate such specimens. When empyema is present, empyema fluid constitutes an excellent source for specific diagnosis. Positive blood cultures can also provide the diagnosis; bacteremia is not common, however, in aspiration pneumonia. Furthermore, not all of the organisms involved in the pulmonary process will necessarily be recovered on blood culture. Transtracheal aspiration bypasses the normal flora of the upper respiratory tract, when properly done, and provides a reliable specimen for anaerobic and aerobic culture (6,18). Aside from its importance in terms of cultivation of the anaerobic flora, transtracheal aspiration can be extremely useful in distinguishing between colonization of the upper respiratory tract with aerobic and facultative potential pathogens and true involvement of these organisms in a pulmonary infection. Unfortunately, the procedure is seldom done now and therefore may be done improperly, and contamination with indigenous flora can be a problem (23). The procedure should not be used in individuals with a significant bleeding tendency or in those in whom it is difficult to provide adequate oxygenation. Percutaneous transthoracic aspiration is associated with a risk of pneumothorax and provides a very small specimen that is difficult to protect from exposure to air. A suitable alternative for patients in whom transtracheal aspiration isn't feasible (unable to cooperate, bleeding tendency, intubated, or tracheotomized) is sampling with a bronchial brush protected within a telescoping plugged double catheter via a fiberoptic bronchoscope (8,21,28,29). It is absolutely essential that the techniques as outlined in detail by Broughton et al. (8) be used exactly as described and that cultures be done quantitatively. Growth at a 10^{-3} dilution is considered significant. The amount of the secretions collected by the brush is 0.001 ml to 0.01 ml, so the 10^{-3} dilution represents 10^5 to 10^6 organisms/ml of lower respiratory tract secretions. The small volume of material obtained and the difficulty one would encounter in arranging for anaerobic transport are a concern; nevertheless, good results appear to have been obtained in a small number of cases of anaerobic pulmonary infection (28). Use of a plugged telescoping catheter without a bronchial brush has also been advocated and offers some advantages. Quantitative culture of fluid obtained by bronchoalveolar lavage (during or without bronchoscopy) also provides reliable results in bacterial pneumonias (19). Little information is available on recovery of anaerobes from such specimens, but the limited studies done so far are promising (16).

It is important to keep in mind that specimens for anaerobic culture must be placed under anaerobic conditions in an appropriate transport tube immediately after being obtained from the patient. Without this precaution, a significant number of anaerobes could die en route to the laboratory. It is usually desirable to aspirate the material to be cultured into a syringe, to expel all bubbles of air or gas from the syringe and needle, and then to transfer the specimen to a tube which has been gassed out with oxygen-free gas for transport to the laboratory (11). Small vials nearly filled with anaerobic semi-solid transport medium are useful for bronchial brush specimens.

For aerobic bacteria such as *S. aureus* and various gram-negative bacilli, expectorated sputum is still a problem because of the frequent oropharyngeal colonization with such organisms mentioned in the introduction; distinction between organisms that are merely colonizers and those involved in an infectious process often is impossible. Use of the Mayo Clinic criteria for a satisfactory sputum specimen (>25 polymorphonuclear leukocytes and/or <10 squamous epithelial cells per 100× microscopic field) may be helpful; pure growth or nearly pure growth of one organism from such a specimen is likely to be significant. More important, absence of *S. aureus* and/or gram-negative bacilli from expectorated sputum in a particular patient can be taken to mean that these organisms are not involved in aspiration pneumonia or lung abscess.

The coexistence of carcinoma and lung abscess can take several forms and be a difficult diagnostic problem. There can be secondary infection within a necrotic tumor, infection distal to an obstructing carcinoma, or a spillover abscess in the same lobe as the tumor, in another lobe, or even in the other lung (7). Lung abscess in an edentulous person very often indicates bronchogenic carcinoma (1).

Diagnosis of empyema is based on the demonstration of purulent pleural fluid. Ultrasound and computerized tomographic scanning can be most useful for detection and localization of empyemas. The following characteristics of the pleural fluid should always be noted: (i) volume; (ii) color, consistency, and odor; (iii) specific gravity; (iv) pH; (v) total protein content; (vi) red and white blood cell count and differential; (vii) gram stain and acid-fast stain; (viii) wet mount for fungi; (ix) culture for aerobic and anaerobic bacteria; (x) culture for tubercle bacilli and fungi; and (xi) cytology. The fluid can vary from moderately cloudy material with fibrinous webs to actual pus. Pus associated with infection caused by group A streptococci is typically thin and turbid and can be blood-tinged. Leukocyte counts of empyema fluid are variable early in the illness; cells are almost exclusively polymorphonuclear leukocytes. The presence of significant numbers of mononuclear cells indicates either sterile effusion or granulomatous infection. When the specific gravity is 1.018 or higher, the protein concentration above 3 g/100 ml, and the lactic dehydrogenase level above 550 units, the effusion is inflammatory in origin. With infectious empyemas, the pH is less than 7.20 and usually <7.0. Both infections and malignant neoplasms can give rise to inflammatory exudates. Leukocyte counts >25,000/mm³, glucose concentration <40 mg/dL, and pleural fluid lactate level >45 mg/dL, along with a low pH, indicate the likelihood of empyema. The microbiologic examination of empyema fluid is of the greatest significance and must always include microscopic examination of a gram-stained smear. Clues to specific causes are quickly obtained by this simple examination. Counter-immunoelectrophoresis, coagglutination, or latex-particle agglutination can be useful in detecting soluble polysaccharide of pneumococci or *Hemophilus* sp. Thick, purulent exudates that are sterile on culture sometimes relate to previous antimicrobial therapy. Much more commonly, however, such empyema fluids yield anaerobic or other microorganisms with special growth requirements.

TREATMENT

Antimicrobial therapy is the keystone of treatment. Prolonged therapy is important to prevent relapse; the actual duration of treatment must be individualized, but periods of 1 to 3 or more months are often required. Drainage is crucial in the case of empyema.

Drugs effective against various anaerobes are listed in Table 16-2. Chloramphenicol is uniformly active. Tetracycline is not effective because many anaerobes are now resistant. Penicillin G is more active than most of the other penicillins and the cephalosporins; penicillin and ampicillin are roughly comparable. However, these compounds are not suitable often because of beta-lactamase production by anaerobes and other organisms. Because very high concentrations can be safely attained in the blood, ticarcillin, piperacillin, and mezlocillin originally were active against 95% of strains of the *B. fragilis* group. These agents are also active against most other anaerobes and against a number of gram-negative bacilli including a variable percent of strains of *P. aeruginosa*. They are not active against *S. aureus*. Cefoxitin, a β-lactamase-resistant cephamycin, is active against 70 to 75% of the *B. fragilis* group strains and against most other anaerobes except for one-third of clostridia of species other than *C. perfringens*. Cefoxitin is also active against *S. aureus* (except for the methicillin-resistant variety which requires vancomycin therapy) and some of gram-negative bacilli (but not *Enterobacter* or *Pseudomonas*).

Clindamycin and metronidazole are usually very effective, but some anaerobic cocci are resistant to both drugs, and *Actinomyces* and *Propionibacterium* are usually resistant to metronidazole. Unfortunately, 15–30% of strains of the *Bacteroides fragilis* group have now been found to be resistant to the broad-spectrum penicillins

TABLE 16–2. *In vitro susceptibility of anaerobes to antimicrobial agents*

Bacteria	Penicillin G	Broad-spectrum penicillins[b]	Cefoxitin	Beta-lactam plus β-lactamase inhibitor[c]	Imipenem	Clindamycin	Metronidazole	Chloramphenicol
Microaerophilic and anaerobic streptococci	+++ - +++++	+++	+++	+++	+++	++ - +++	++	+++
Bacteroides fragilis group	+	++ - +++	++ - +++	+++	+++	++ - +++	+++	+++
Other Bacteroides, Prevotella, and Porphyromonas	++	++ - +++	+++	+++	+++	+++[a]	+++	+++
Fusobacterium sp	+++	++ - +++	+++	+++	+++	++ - +++	+++	+++
Actinomyces, Propionibacterium	++++	+++	+++	+++	+++	+++[a]	+	+++

+ Poor or inconsistent activity; ++ Moderate activity; +++ Good activity; ++++ Good activity, good pharmacologic characteristics, low toxicity, low cost, drug of choice.

[a]A few strains are resistant.

[b]Piperacillin, ticarcillin, mezlocillin.

[c]Ampicillin/sulbactam, amoxicillin/clavulanate, ticarcillin/clavulanate, piperacillin/tazobactam.

such as piperacillin, and to clindamycin and cefoxitin in a number of hospitals in the United States.

Imipenem, a new, broad-spectrum beta-lactam agent, and the combination of ticarcillin and clavulanic acid (a beta-lactamase inhibitor) and of piperacillin and tazobactam are active against essentially all anaerobes and most of the nonanaerobes important in hospital-acquired aspiration pneumonia. Ampicillin/sulbactam is very active against anaerobes but has less activity against nonanaerobic gram-negative rods.

Patients with necrotizing pneumonia or other pleuropulmonary infection that may be caused by anaerobes should be treated with either clindamycin plus penicillin, metronidazole plus penicillin, a beta lactam/beta-lactamase inhibitor combination, imipenem, or chloramphenicol.

The usual adult patient with anaerobic lung abscess is not critically ill and generally responds quite satisfactorily to therapy. There have been reports of treatment failures related to β-lactamase–producing anaerobes. Preferred alternatives to penicillin G are indicated in the preceding paragraph.

Vancomycin is generally reserved for the treatment of methicillin-resistant (MRSA) staphylococcal infections, but it is sometimes useful in gram-positive anaerobic infections. For non-MRSA staphylococcal infections a penicillinase-resistant penicillin is preferable, but one of the parenteral cephalosporins or vancomycin can be used in the event of allergy. For infections involving *Klebsiella pneumoniae, Pseudomonas aeruginosa,* or other facultative or aerobic gram-negative bacilli, options include aminoglycosides such as amikacin, a carboxy or ureido penicillin, ticarcillin plus clavulanic acid, piperacillin plus tazobactam, imipenem, ceftazidime, ciprofloxacin, and other agents.

Postural drainage is an important component of therapy for lung abscess. Bronchoscopy is occasionally helpful in effecting good drainage, permitting removal of foreign bodies, and enabling biopsy diagnosis of tumors. Tracheostomy and frequent suctioning are often required in selected patients.

Surgical resection of lung abscess is rarely required unless there is a coexisting malignancy. There is a hazard of uncontrollable spread before medical control can be achieved. Surgical drainage of a lung abscess through the chest wall is almost never indicated.

The principles of treatment of empyema include the use of appropriate antimicrobials, the provision of adequate drainage, and the obliteration of dead space. Therapy should be prolonged, often for months.

In the early exudative phase of empyema, intermittent, closed drainage by repeated thoracenteses can provide adequate drainage. However, if the patient remains toxic or if fluid reaccumulates rapidly, continuous closed drainage by intercostal catheter, is required. Open drainage at this stage could result in collapse of the lung. Most patients with pleural fluid pH less than 7.0 will require tube drainage and most with a pH higher than 7.3 will not require drainage at all. During the fibrinopurulent phase, thoracenteses are unsatisfactory, and delay in instituting adequate drainage only allows further coagulation and loculation. Closed intercostal drainage with suction can be effective, but open drainage with rib resection may be required. Drainage tubes should not be removed until the cavity is totally obliterated and any bronchopleural fistula is well sealed. Enzymatic debridement has been disappointing.

Decortication (removal of the entire empyema sac) allows free expansion of the lung to obliterate dead space; this procedure is sometimes required. More extreme procedures are rarely necessary; these include a modified thoracoplasty with resection of most of the extrapleural contents, or the creation of an Eloesser flap. At times, a muscle flap is required to close a bronchopleural fistula.

PROGNOSIS

The prognosis depends on the type of underlying or predisposing pathologic processes, if any, and, in the case of acute, severe necrotizing pneumonias, the speed with which appropriate therapy is instituted. Anaerobic lung abscess carries an overall mortality rate of 15% or less (4). The case fatality rate is significantly higher in acute pneumonias caused by *Staphylococcus aureus, Klebsiella* sp, *Pseudomonas* sp, and in anaerobic necrotizing pneumonias (1).

The most common complication is empyema, with or without bronchopleural fistula. Mortality rates for empyema are usually 5–20%. Generalized infection occurs occasionally. The spillover of pus sometimes leads to the spread of infection and even, rarely, to asphyxiation. Other complications are now rare; these include brain or other distal abscesses, severe hemorrhage, and secondary amyloidosis. Superinfections caused by other bacteria or by fungi can occur in relation to antimicrobial therapy. In chronic lung abscess, there can be local bronchiectasis with subsequent recurrences of acute pneumonitis in the involved area. Loss of a variable amount of lung volume sometimes occurs.

Carcinoma is diagnosed relatively easily in patients with infection distal to the tumor. On the other hand, abscesses excavated in neoplasms present a serious paradox in that there will often be subjective and objective evidence of response to antibacterial therapy. It is sometimes impossible to detect the neoplasm without thoracotomy. Such abscesses can achieve stability and even apparent cure with "residual fibrosis," only to reappear as inoperable carcinoma as long as 2 to 3 years later. Factors increasing the likelihood of a primary malignancy include the edentulous state, a history of cigarette smoking in the older age groups, the absence of precipitating causes for abscess (particularly aspiration), the location of an abscess in a nondependent bronchopulmonary segment, and the presence of hemoptysis or localized wheeze.

Most forms of empyema respond well to therapy, although the course of illness is frequently prolonged. The major complications of empyema are metastatic infection and chronic empyema. Rarely, there can be perforation through the chest wall or into the lung itself. Failure to obliterate the pleural space during the course of management of acute empyema can lead to chronic empyema.

PREVENTION

Precautions should be taken to minimize the possibility of aspiration. Care should be observed in feeding feeble or confused patients and patients with swallowing difficulties. The head of the bed should be elevated for a time after feeding by gastric tube. In the case of gross aspiration, immediate clearing of the airway by postural drainage and suctioning, preferably by bronchoscopy, is important.

Histamine type 2 blockers or antacids have commonly been used to prevent upper gastrointestinal bleeding due to stress ulcers in critically ill patients. This leads to elevated gastric pH and gastric and pharyngeal (by the retrograde route) colonization with gram-negative bacilli (10).

Proper treatment of periodontal disease and gingivitis minimizes pulmonary complications. Acute pneumonias and bacteremias should be treated promptly with appropriate drugs. This is particularly important in necrotizing pneumonias because of the frequency of empyema in this condition. Good surgical technique and careful asepsis in the operating room and elsewhere in the hospital minimize postoperative empyema.

REFERENCES

1. Bartlett, J.G., and Finegold, S.M. (1974): Anaerobic infections of the lung and pleural space. *Am. Rev. Respir. Dis.*, 110:56–77.
2. Bartlett, J.G., and Gorbach, S.L. (1975): The triple threat of aspiration pneumonia. *Chest*, 68:560–566.
3. Bartlett, J.G., Gorbach, S.L., and Finegold, S.M. (1974): The bacteriology of aspiration pneumonia. *Am. J. Med.*, 56:202–207.
4. Bartlett, J.G., Gorbach, S.L., Tally, F.P., and Finegold, S.M. (1974): Bacteriology and treatment of primary lung abscess. *Am. Rev. Respir. Dis.*, 109:510–518.
5. Bartlett, J.G., Gorbach, S.L., Thadepalli, H., and Finegold, S.M. (1974): Bacteriology of empyema. *Lancet*, 1:338–340.
6. Bartlett, J.G., Rosenblatt, J.E., and Finegold, S.M. (1973): Percutaneous transtracheal aspiration in the diagnosis of anaerobic pulmonary infection. *Ann. Intern. Med.*, 79:535–540.
7. Brock, R.C. (1952): *Lung Abscess.* Charles C. Thomas. Springfield, Ill.
8. Broughton, W.A., Bass, J.B., and Kirkpatrick, M.B. (1987): The technique of protected brush catheter bronchoscopy. *J. Critical Illness*, 2:63–70.
9. Bynum, L.J., and Pierce, A.K. (1976): Pulmonary aspiration of gastric contents. *Am. Rev. Respir. Dis.*, 114:1129–1136.
10. Driks, M.R., Craven, D.E., Celli, B.R., Manning, M., Burke, R.A., Garvin, G.M., Kunches, L.M., Farber, H.W., Wedel, S.A., and McCabe, W.R. (1987): Nosocomial pneumonia in intubated patients given sucralfate as compared with antacids or histamine type 2 blockers. *N. Engl. J. Med.*, 317:1376–1382.
11. Finegold, S.M. (1977): *Anaerobic Bacteria in Human Disease.* 710 pp. Academic Press, New York.
12. Finegold, S.M., and George, W.L. (Editors) (1989): *Anaerobic Infections in Humans.* Academic Press, San Diego, Calif.
13. Finland, M., and Barnes, M.W. (1978): Changing ecology of acute bacterial empyema: occurrence and mortality at Boston City Hospital during 12 selected years from 1935 to 1972. *J. Infect. Dis.*, 137:274–291.
14. George, W.L., Kirby, B.D., Sutter, V.L., Citron, D.M., and Finegold, S.M. (1981): Gram-negative anaerobic bacilli: their role in infection and patterns of susceptibility to antimicrobial agents. II. Little-known *Fusobacterium* species and miscellaneous genera. *Rev. Infect. Dis.*, 3:599–626.
15. Hamelberg, W., and Bosomworth, P.P. (1968): *Aspiration Pneumonitis.* Charles C. Thomas, Springfield, Ill.
16. Henriquez, A.H., Mendoza, J., and Gonzalez, P.C. (1991): Quantitative culture of bronchoalveolar lavage from patients with anaerobic lung abscesses. *J. Infect. Dis.*, 164:414–417.
17. Johanson, W.G., Jr., and Harris, G.D. (1980): Aspiration pneumonia, anaerobic infections, and lung abscess. *Med. Clin. No. Amer.*, 64:385–394.
18. Jordan, G.W., Wong, G.A., and Hoeprich, P.D. (1976): Bacteriology of the lower respiratory tract as determined by fiberoptic bronchoscopy and transtracheal aspiration. *J. Infect. Dis.*, 134:428–435.
19. Kahn, F.W., and Jones, J.M. (1987): Diagnosing bacterial respiratory infection by bronchoalveolar lavage. *J. Infect. Dis.*, 155:862–869.
20. Kirby, B.D., George, W.L., Sutter, V.L., Citron, D.M., and Finegold, S.M. (1980): Gram-negative anaerobic bacilli: their role in infection and patterns of susceptibility to antimicrobial agents. I. Little-known *Bacteroides* species. *Rev. Infect. Dis.*, 2:914–951.
21. Lorch, D.G., Jr., John, J.F., Jr., Tomlinson, J.R., Miller, K.S., and Sahn, S.A. (1987): Protected transbronchial needle aspiration and protected specimen brush in the diagnosis of pneumonia. *Am. Rev. Respir. Dis.*, 135:565–569.
22. Lutz, A., Grooten, O., and Berger, M.A. (1963): Considérations à propos des germes isolés dans 638 cas de pleuresies purulentes. *Strasbourg Med.*, 2:119–128.
23. Marina, M., Strong, C.A., Civen, R., Molitoris, E., and Finegold, S.M. (1993): Bacteriology of anaerobic pleuropulmonary infection: preliminary report. *Clin. Infect. Dis.* 16:Suppl. 4: S256–262.

24. Ribaudo, C.A., and Grace, W.J. (1971): Pulmonary aspiration. *Am. J. Med.,* 50:510–520.
25. Ruggera, G., and Taylor, G. (1976): Pulmonary aspiration in anesthesia. *West. J. Med.,* 125:411–414.
26. Tryba, M. (1987): Risk of acute stress bleeding and nosocomial pneumonia in ventilated intensive care unit patients: sucralfate versus antacids. *Am. J. Med.,* 83:Suppl. 3 B:117–124.
27. Weese, W.C., Shindler, E.R., Smith, I.M., and Rabinovich, J. (1973): Empyema of the thorax then and now. *Arch. Intern. Med.,* 131:516–520.
28. Wimberley, N.W., Bass, J.B., Jr., Boyd, B.W., Kirkpatrick, M.B., Serio, R.A., and Pollock, H.M. (1982): Use of a bronchoscopic protected catheter brush for the diagnosis of pulmonary infections. *Chest,* 81:556–562.
29. Wimberley, N., Faling, L.J., and Bartlett, J.G. (1979): Fiberoptic bronchoscopy technique to obtain uncontaminated lower airway secretions for bacterial culture. *Am. Rev. Respir. Dis.,* 119:337–343.

Respiratory Infections: Diagnosis and Management, 3d ed.,
edited by James E. Pennington.
Raven Press, Ltd., New York © 1994

17

Pulmonary Infections in Cystic Fibrosis: Pathogenesis and Therapy

Stephen A. Chartrand and Melvin I. Marks

*Department of Pediatrics, Creighton University School of Medicine, 601 North 30th
Street, Omaha, Nebraska 68131; and Memorial Miller Children's Hospital,
2801 Atlantic Avenue, Long Beach, California 90801-1428*

Cystic fibrosis (CF) is the most common lethal genetic disorder among Caucasian children, affecting an estimated 30,000 persons in the United States (27). The autosomal recessive trait for CF is carried by 3.3% of the white population of the United States with an observed disease incidence of 1 : 3,500; the disease is less common in U.S. black children (1 : 14,000), Hispanics (1 : 11,500), and American Indians (1 : 10,500). In the United States, 95% of patients are white, with a slightly higher proportion of men (52–54%) (27).

Gene linkage experiments have now mapped the CF gene locus to the long arm of human chromosome 7, within band q 31. The most common mutation at this site is a 3-base pair deletion which results in the loss of a phenyalanine residue at position 508, referred to as ΔF508 (48). The defective protein coded by this mutation is known as the cystic fibrosis transmembrane regulator (CFTR). This abnormal regulatory protein produces a chloride ion (Cl^-) conductance (permeability) defect that significantly decreases the electrochemical gradient for sodium ion (Na^+) movement into the CF duct cell and may explain the elevated Na^+/Cl^- concentrations found in the sweat of CF patients. The ΔF508 mutation makes up 70–80% of CF genes, but over 120 different gene mutations have now been identified around this locus. These different mutations somewhat determine the major phenotypic differences in CF patients who bear the different genotypes (49). For example, 99% of CF patients homozygous for the ΔF508 allele suffer pancreatic insufficiency compared to one-third of those with other mutations. Detection of CF carriers (i.e., heterozygotes) is now possible, but is generally restricted to relatives of CF patients. Nevertheless, there is still no unifying concept to adequately explain the pathogenesis of CF. Serous exocrine secretions, such as sweat, are abnormally concentrated but have normal water content. On the other hand, sodium absorption in airway epithelium, but not in sweat glands, is abnormally elevated. Mucous airway secretions, then, contain decreased water and electrolyte concentrations with twice the usual ratio of macromolecules (mucins) to electrolytes. These glycoprotein mucins form thick gels that alter the rheologic properties of the mucus. In the tracheobronchial tree, thick, tenacious sputum obstructs the airways and apparently contributes to progressive suppurative pneumonia. Yet respiratory tract histology in CF patients is normal at birth (78), suggesting that some of these changes may be the result, rather than the cause, of infection. Other factors such as defective mucociliary transport and aberrant local immunity can also be important (see below).

Seventy percent of CF cases are diagnosed during the first year of life (median age, 7 months). These infants with CF can present with a wide range of symptoms largely referable to gastrointestinal or respiratory manifestations. These include meconium ileus at birth (16% of patients), recurrent diarrhea and malabsorption, failure to thrive, and progressive cough. Therapy is primarily directed at improving nutrition by exocrine pancreatic enzyme replacement and management of pulmonary infections. The leading causes of morbidity in CF patients are protein-calorie malnutrition, cardiac failure, and progressive pulmonary insufficiency caused by chronic necrotizing bronchopneumonia. Early diagnosis of CF by neonatal screening and early therapy can reduce morbidity (130). Neonatal screening is possible with a blood test for immunoreactive trypsinogen which identifies almost 100% of CF patients (20,79). False-positives, however, are common and should always be confirmed with sweat testing and DNA analysis.

Life expectancy for CF patients in 1950 was only 5 years. By 1900 this had increased to 28.5 years, and one-third of all CF patients are now over 18 years of age; more than 7% of patients are 31 years of age or older. Cardiorespiratory complications secondary to infection are the cause of death in 80% of patients (27).

PULMONARY INFECTION

Clinical Features

Many of the features of pulmonary infection in CF are nonspecific. The young infant could develop a persistent, dry cough after a seemingly benign respiratory infection. In a few patients the cough is associated with choking, gagging, and subsequent vomiting of swallowed purulent sputum. Occasionally sudden airway embarrassment resulting from mucous plugging will occur. Persistence of cough, an increased quantity of lower respiratory secretions, and repeated lower respiratory infections can herald the presence of CF. Increased sleeping respiratory rate, weight loss, and wheezing are often noted. At an early age, bronchiolar constriction is reversible and can be confused with asthma. Moreover, the auscultatory findings between episodes are often normal at this stage. Some infants with CF present with recurrent pneumonia, particularly of the right upper lobe, or an acute episode of staphylococcal pneumonia with pneumothorax and/or empyema.

As the pulmonary disease progresses, fever, productive cough, and chest pain often predominate. Long-standing infection is usually associated with purulent sputum, intercostal retractions, digital clubbing, increased antero-posterior diameter of the chest, and exercise intolerance. Rales and rhonchi are consistent findings at this stage, and wheezing is often present. Both hyperresonance caused by air trapping and dullness resulting from consolidation are seen. Acute exacerbations of pulmonary infection are characterized by fever, weight loss, increased dyspnea and sputum production, and worsening cyanosis. Accumulating lung damage first produces reactive pulmonary hypertension, then fixed pulmonary vascular obstruction and an exuberant proliferation of collateral bronchial vessels. Inexorably, right ventricular hypertrophy and congestive heart failure ensue, often complicated by cor pulmonale and hemoptysis.

Chronic pansinusitis resulting from mucous gland obstruction and infection is universal in children with CF, and nasal polyposis is common (106).

Pulmonary Function

Pulmonary function studies are the most accurate and objective measure of changing obstructive airway disease. Forced vital capacity (FVC) and forced expiratory volume at one second (FEV_1) are the most useful because performance variability is minimal and can be measured with an office-based spirometer (18). Prior to that time, blood gas analysis is the only consistently reliable tool for routine clinical use.

The initial pulmonary dysfunction in cystic fibrosis is obstruction of the small airways resulting in widespread ventilation–perfusion inequalities. Often these early changes are not detectable clinically, roentgenographically, or by routine pulmonary airflow studies. Even with normal pulmonary airflow rates and lung volume, however, there is an early decrease in arterial oxygen tension, a significant alveolar–arterial oxygen difference, and increased residual volume/total lung capacity ratio (57). This is likely due to nonuniform distribution of small airway obstruction with mucus.

With the inevitable but often erratic progression of pulmonary disease, increased airway resistance can be detected by other pulmonary function tests such as helium flow volume curves and forced expiratory flow during the middle half of ventilation (FEF 25–75%). Gurwitz et al. (35) demonstrated an average exponential decline of 8% per year for this test, but there is great variability between patients in this regard. Arterial hypoxemia due to nonuniform distribution of ventilation is progressive in CF patients and correlates well with clinical pulmonary status. Significant CO_2 retention, on the other hand, is usually absent until the preterminal stage of pulmonary involvement.

Radiographic Features

Early radiographic changes in CF include increased bronchovascular markings with bronchial thickening ("tram-tracks") and localized obstructive emphysema reflecting the increased residual volume (36). Patches of atelectasis and infiltration are common at this stage, especially in the upper lobes and on the right. Diffuse peripheral rounded lesions of bronchiectasis often come and go at first, but eventually become permanent. Hilar adenopathy, hyperinflation, and segmental or lobar atelectasis are seen as the disease progresses. Ultimately, extensive bronchiectasis with cyst formation and diffuse infiltrates are seen. With abscess formation throughout the periphery of the lung, the radiograph can show a "snowflake" or "honeycomb" appearance. (See Fig. 17-1.) Asymptomatic subpleural emphysema, pneumothorax, or even pneumomediastinum can be present. The roentgenographic findings are included in numerous clinical scoring systems widely used for following the progression of pulmonary disease in CF patients. The Brasfield score, for example, grades five different categories: air-trapping, linear markings, cystic-nodular lesions, large lesions, and general severity. The Shwachman-Kulczycki clinical score is the system most widely employed for assessing the patient's overall condition. Equal weight is given to each of four categories (activity level, pulmonary physical findings and cough, growth and nutrition, radiographic changes), with 100 points representing a

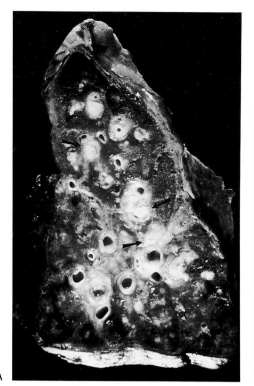 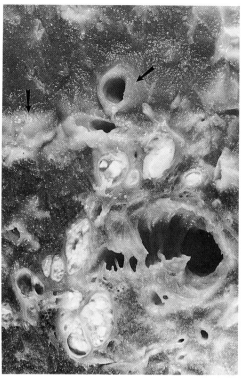

FIG. 17–1. (A) Lung specimen from a patient with cystic fibrosis. Note bronchiectasis with mucopurulent airway plugging (*arrows*), peribronchial infiltrates, and multiple peripheral abscesses. **(B)** Close-up view of same specimen. Note dense peribronchial infiltrates (*arrows*). (Courtesy of T. Pysher.)

perfect score. Both of these systems correlate well with pulmonary function tests and arterial oxygen tension.

In some patients, radiographic changes are reversible during the first year of treatment. Patients whose x-rays return to near normal in the first year after diagnosis have a significantly improved long-term survival rate compared to those without similar improvement.

Pulmonary Histopathology

Lung tissue obtained from neonates who die of meconium ileus is histologically normal. However, pulmonary histopathology can develop by 1 to 2 weeks, as shown by Bedrossian (11). Bronchial changes predominated, especially in younger infants, and included the following: epithelial metaplasia with loss of cilia, predominance of mucous versus serous acini in hyperplastic bronchial glands, goblet cell hyperplasia, acute and chronic inflammatory infiltrates, bronchiectasis, and mucopurulent plugging of the airways. Mucosal and submucosal inflammatory infiltrates were prominent and mucopurulent airway plugging was present in two-thirds of the patients at 4 months of age. (See Fig. 17-2.) Bronchiectasis increased in severity with age, affecting 75% of 2-year-old patients and 100% of older children. Parenchymal changes

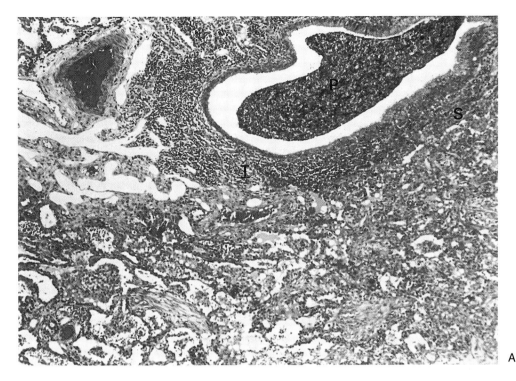

A

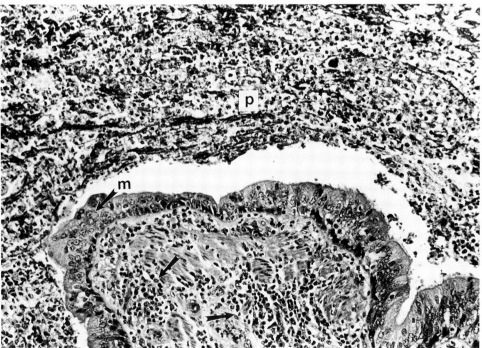

B

FIG. 17–2. (A) Pulmonary histopathology in cystic fibrosis. Section shows characteristic in-spissated mucopurulent airway plug (P) with intense peribronchial infiltrate (I). Alveoli show pulmonary edema and acute and chronic inflammation. × 40, H & E. **(B)** Advanced pulmonary lesion with squamous epithelial metaplasia (m) and mucopurulent airway plugging (p). Also note extensive submucosal plasma cell infiltrate (*arrows*). × 100, H & E.

other than pneumonia (emphysema, hemorrhage) were less common. Chronic organized alveolar inflammatory exudate was present in the lungs of all patients examined after the first 2 years of age. Air trapping was common but emphysema with destruction of the alveolar septae was infrequent and absent in children under 2 years old. When present, emphysema never involved more than 10% of the lung. Apical bullae, commonly seen in the lungs of older CF patients, can spontaneously rupture, leading to recurrent pneumothorax. Twenty percent of the patients had significant pulmonary hemorrhages associated with bronchiectasis and hyperplasia of the bronchial arteries. Surprisingly, the incidence of this finding did not increase with age, although hemoptysis is usually seen only in those patients with advanced disease. The Reid index (ratio of bronchial mucous gland layer to total bronchial wall diameter) was significantly increased, consistent with mucous gland and goblet cell hyperplasia.

Sputum Characteristics

Early in the course of pulmonary disease in CF patients, tracheobronchial secretions are usually yellow or green-tinged with frequent mucous plugs. With disease progression, they become more discolored and blood-tinged. During respiratory exacerbations, the sputum can be grossly purulent. CF sputum is thick and mucoid in appearance, and, at postmortem, it is sometimes possible to stretch tracheobronchial secretions great distances because of their elastic, gelatinous character.

CF sputum is a complex mixture of leukocytes, red blood cells, water, electrolytes, proteins, DNA, organic acids, bacteria, and extracellular bacterial products. Unfortunately, the constituents of CF pulmonary secretions have rarely been examined from patients free of pulmonary infection. Patients old enough to produce adequate sputum specimens reliably are generally those with established infection, and their sputum reflects chronic inflammatory processes.

The sodium and water content of tracheobronchial secretions is decreased in CF patients, primarily due to increased sodium reabsorption across respiratory epithelial surfaces, the opposite of the situation in sweat glands (113). This abnormality is specific for CF homozygotes and has been shown *in vitro* by measurement of bioelectrical potential differences across respiratory epithelia, and *in vivo* in infants as young as 3 months of age (52). Studies with cultured CF epithelial cells indicate that the quality and quantity of secreted mucins do not differ from normal controls. This again suggests a regulatory defect, perhaps involving free water resorption. The total sputum protein content is markedly elevated in CF patients, primarily as the consequence of bacterial-induced tissue injury.

With progressive lung injury, large numbers of red and white blood cells and their breakdown products (e.g., lysosyme) and increased DNA concentrations are present in the sputum. Bacteria are present in densities up to 10^8 colony-forming units per milliliter of sputum. These components, along with the extracellular mucopolysaccharide of *Pseudomonas aeruginosa,* contribute to the viscosity of the respiratory secretions and the resultant airway obstruction.

Microbial Flora

Sputum cultures from expectorating patients accurately reflect bacteria isolated from the lower airway but are most useful when plated quantitatively on selective media (122,124). Oropharyngeal cultures are less sensitive but fairly specific when *P. aeruginosa* is isolated (87). *Staphylococcus aureus* is still the initial pulmonary bacterial pathogen in most CF patients (2,27). *Staphylococcus aureus* is ubiquitous in the environment and is commonly found in the nasopharynx of normal children during viral respiratory infections, or following antibiotic therapy. In normal individuals, the bacterium is readily cleared from the respiratory tract, although persistent nasal carriage is described. In CF patients, *S. aureus* sputum colonization can be intermittent and is not associated with a particular phage type. The reason for initial *S. aureus* colonization is unclear, but its persistence could be due to toxin-mediated airway injury and ineffective ciliary clearance due to the abnormal CF mucus. Three decades ago, *S. aureus* was the most common bacterial isolate from sputum in CF patients. Today it is grown from 28% of patients and is the predominant pathogen only in children less than 1 year of age (2,27).

Pseudomonas aeruginosa is occasionally isolated early in the course of CF pulmonary disease. However, it will not adhere to normal airway epithelium in the absence of damage, malnutrition, prior infection, or co-infection with a virus or other bacterium. It is thought that early staphylococcal-induced airway injury predisposes to subsequent pseudomonal colonization (2,17,68). This can be enhanced by antimicrobial therapy directed at *S. aureus* (8). Initially, rough (nonmucoid) *Pseudomonas* colonial forms predominate, possibly because of their increased adherence (compared with mucoid forms) to the upper respiratory tract of CF patients. This adherence can be the result of decreased epithelial surface fibronectin caused by the increased concentration of salivary proteases seen in CF patients (131). In any event, it appears that initial attachment of *P. aeruginosa* to respiratory epithelial cells is more dependent on bacterial fimbriae acting as cell surface adhesions than to alginic acid (mucoid exopolysaccharide) (80). There is no evidence that bacterial exoproducts (elastase, toxin A, etc.) are important for initial respiratory tract colonization. *Pseudomonas* strains initially colonizing CF patients are similar morphologically and biochemically to those in the gastrointestinal tract of many well subjects; however, they are in an abnormal location and have some other distinct characteristics. The phenotypic heterogeneity of the bacterial populations in the sputum of CF patients is impressive. For example, a single sputum specimen from a patient with moderate-to-severe illness can contain several different serotypes of *P. aeruginosa,* each with a specific antimicrobial susceptibility pattern (101). DNA probe studies, however, indicate that these isolates frequently derive from a single parent strain (2,77). With time, the majority of *Pseudomonas* isolates appear as mucoid or gelatinous colonies on agar, as first reported by Doggett et al. in 1964 (22). Extracellular alginate produced by mucoid strains enhances colonization of the bronchopulmonary tree, possibly through interactions with ciliary receptors (64). Such colonial forms can be found in 70–90% of CF patients with moderate to severe pulmonary disease. The majority of *Pseudomonas* strains from CF patients are serum sensitive, which perhaps, in part, explains why bacteremia is so rare in these patients.

Hemophilus influenzae is most frequently isolated after age one year, often in association with *S. aureus* or *P. aeruginosa* (2,7,27,68). In one study, *Hemophilus* was the predominant or even sole bacterial isolate recovered in 29% of infants (2). Unless selective media are employed (9,127), the presence of *Hemophilus* will not be appreciated because of their fastidious nutritional requirements and the relatively rapid growth of *S. aureus* and *P. aeruginosa*. These isolates of *H. influenzae* are generally nontypeable. The fact that they do not invade may be referable to their lack of capsule, and the component host defenses present in CF patients. Occasionally, encapsulated strains (type B) are isolated; these should be considered potentially pathogenic.

Pseudomonas cepacia, which is only distantly related to *P. aeruginosa,* is nonpathogenic in normal, healthy individuals. A dramatic increase in the incidence of pulmonary *P. cepacia* colonization was first noted in the early 1980s in certain CF populations with advanced lung disease (33,43). It is rarely, if ever, found in patients under 10 years of age (2,27). For example, the overall prevalence of *P. cepacia* in CF patients at the Cleveland Clinic increased from 5.1% to 20.0% from 1979 to 1983 (122). Surveillance in more than 100 United States CF centers has shown that, since 1986, when centers started routinely using *P. cepacia* selective media for sputum cultures, the annual incidence and prevalence of *P. cepacia* infection have plateaued at 1% and 3.5%, respectively (120). This discrepancy could be partially explained by the use of selective laboratory media for isolation (128) and possibly nosocomial transmission. Evidence for the latter also comes from the Cleveland Clinic, where *P. cepacia* colonization was correlated with recent or concurrent hospitalization. When strict separation of colonized and noncolonized patients was instituted, the incidence fell from 8.2% to 1.7% in 1 year (122). A recent study using molecular techniques documented person-to-person transmission of *P. cepacia* (59). Moreover, the significance of *P. cepacia* in CF sputum is unclear. Although initially *P. cepacia* was thought to be a harbinger of rapid clinical demise, some colonized patients survive for long periods with no change in status (30). This suggests a less pathogenic role, a concept supported by animal studies of pseudomonal pneumonia (33). Conversely, several CF patients have developed sepsis and bacteremia due to *P. cepacia* (16,90)—an event rarely seen with *P. aeruginosa.* These strains are highly resistant to multiple antibiotics, so selective pressure can favor their growth in patients who have received prolonged antimicrobial therapy.

Other gram-negative nonfermentative bacilli are frequently and sometimes persistently isolated from sputum in CF patients (51). These include *Pseudomonas maltophilia, Pseudomonas fluorescens/putida, Pseudomonas alcaligenes, Pseudomonas stutzeri, Achromobacter xylosidans, Flavobacterium* sp, and CDC groups IVe and Ve. Of these, only *P. maltophilia* is present in significant numbers (10^6–10^8 cfu/ml in ~7% of CF patients) and elicits a host immune response similar to *S. aureus* and *P. aeruginosa* (7).

The significance of Enterobacteriaceae in CF sputum is unclear. Sixty-eight percent of patients in one study harbored these bacteria at some point, most commonly *Escherichia coli, Klebsiella* sp, and *Enterobacter* sp, in that order (102). Interestingly, mucoid *E. coli* strains are occasionally seen. The mucoid material differs antigenically and biochemically from *Pseudomonas* (colanic acid in *E. coli,* mannuronic and guluronic acids in *P. aeruginosa*), and likely represents an expression of mucoid-governing genes that are regulated by the environment in which the bacteria grow (63).

Other organisms such as *Candida albicans, Aspergillus* sp, and mycobacteria can also be found in CF sputum, although their pathogenicity is not always certain. In one study, *Aspergillus* was isolated from 57% of CF patients (75). Some of these patients with advanced lung disease also had an increased incidence of *Aspergillus* serum precipitins along with other evidence of sensitization to *Aspergillus* antigens. Allergic bronchopulmonary aspergillosis has been reported in atopic CF patients, even in the absence of severe lung damage, and can respond to steroid treatment (17). Pulmonary candidiasis is rare and usually secondary to prolonged antibiotic and/or steroid therapy. Although anaerobic bacteria have been isolated from CF sputum, their pathogenic role has not been explored.

PATHOGENESIS OF PULMONARY INJURY IN CF

Staphylococcus

Although much remains to be learned about the pathogenesis of respiratory infections in patients with CF, bacteria play a major role in the resultant pulmonary injury. Having colonized the sputum, *S. aureus* can injure pulmonary tissue by several mechanisms, including the elaboration of extracellular toxins. The necrotic and leukotoxic properties of alpha and delta toxins produce bronchial wall injury and abscess formation, eventually leading to bronchiectasis. Serum antibody titers against alpha toxin and the cell wall teichoic acid are significantly elevated in CF patients chronically infected with *S. aureus;* these titers fall with effective antibiotic treatment, analogous to the serologic response to various *P. aeruginosa* exoproducts (see below). Coagulase action on fibrin leads to walling off of abscesses and contributes to both the gelatinous character of the sputum and resistance to clearance by mechanical and immunological host defenses. The host response to *Staphylococcus* can also be injurious secondary to the release of lysosomal enzymes from phagocytes and inflammatory edema. Immunopathic injury due to immune complexes is also postulated.

Pseudomonas

Pseudomonas aeruginosa elaborates numerous extracellular products that directly or indirectly induce pulmonary injury in CF patients (126). The mucoid exopolysaccharide originating from certain "smooth" strains is a polyanionic alginic acid-like matrix comprised primarily of D-mannuronic and L-guluronic acids (24). This alginate layer lends the organism a mucoid or gelatinous appearance on primary isolation agar. It is likely that most *Pseudomonas* isolates possess the genetic coding for mucopolysaccharide production when grown in an appropriate environment. The increased isolation rate of these strains in advanced disease can reflect either local adaptation by strains previously in the lung or *de novo* acquisition and decreased clearance of the mucoid forms. Small amounts of slime polysaccharide interfere with antibody coating and can inhibit phagocytosis and killing of *P. aeruginosa in vitro* (6,99). (See Fig. 17-3.) A rise in antibody titers against the mucopolysaccharide is associated with bacterial clearance in animal models of *P. aeruginosa* pneumonia. Similarly, high serum titers of mucoid-exopolysaccharide-specific killing antibody is associated with a lack of detectable *P. aeruginosa* colonization in older, relatively healthy CF patients (85). Unfortunately, alginic acid antigen excess in the CF lung can lead to immune complex deposition and inflammatory lung damage (132) (see below). Mucoid capsular material can also inactivate complement, a feature that could partially explain its antiphagocytic activity (114). Both mucoid and nonmucoid *Pseudomonas* can form extensive fiber-enclosed microcolonies in the bronchi of CF patients that could interfere with normal pulmonary defense mechanisms (phagocytosis, opsonization, surfactant, ciliary clearance) (13,56). (See Fig. 17-4.) The diffusion of positively charged antibiotics, such as aminoglycosides, through

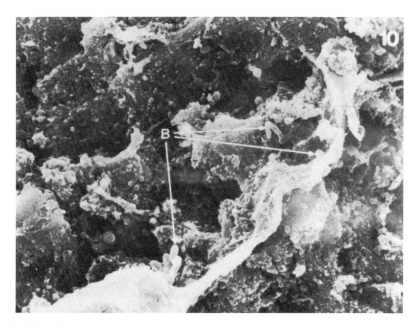

FIG. 17–3. Scanning electron micrograph of *Pseudomonas*-infected rat lung tissue showing rod-shaped bacterial cells (B) embedded in amorphous slime and exudate. (Reproduced with permission from Lam et al., ref. 56.)

the negatively charged exopolysaccharide can be retarded, leading to decreased susceptibility of these strains to antimicrobials *in vivo* (107). Seale et al. (101), however, found no *in vitro* differences in antibiotic susceptibility of isogenic mucoid versus nonmucoid isolates.

Exotoxin A is a heat-labile, single-chain polypeptide "proenzyme" that, like diphtheria toxin, catalyzes the adenine diphosphate (ADP)-ribosylation of elongation factor 2. The effect on the ribosome is to halt protein synthesis, leading to cell death and necrosis. Exotoxin A is produced by about 90% of *P. aeruginosa* strains and probably plays a major role in the pathogenesis of tissue injury in CF patients. The highest titers of serum antibodies to toxin A in CF patients are present in patients with severe pulmonary disease (50).

Eighty-six percent of *Pseudomonas* isolates from CF patients produce proteases, usually elastase, collagenase, and fibrinolysin. As noted under "Immunopathic Factors" below, recent studies have incriminated elastase as a major factor in the immunopathogenesis of chronic lung infection. The antibody response to these enzymes in CF patients also correlates positively with severity of the pulmonary disease (50).

The endotoxin activity of *Pseudomonas* lipopolysaccharide is low, and it probably contributes little to the pathogenesis of lung injury but could stimulate local inflammation.

Other Bacteria

The mechanism of pulmonary injury caused by other bacteria such as *H. influenzae, P. cepacia, P. maltophilia,* or mucoid *E. coli* has not been critically evaluated.

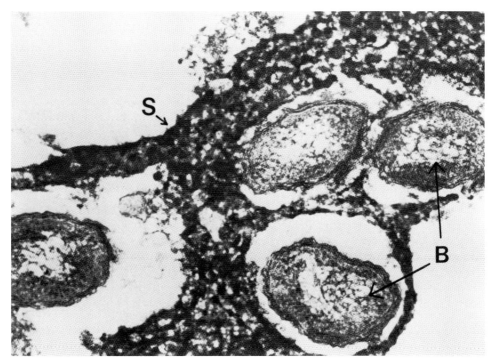

FIG. 17–4. Electron micrograph of alveolar material obtained at post mortem from *P. aeruginosa*-infected CF patient. Note the thick mass of fibrous exopolysaccharide (S) material surrounding the gram-negative bacteria (B). (Reproduced with permission from ref. 56, Lam et al.)

Nonbacterial Infections

Nonbacterial respiratory infections in CF patients have received little attention. Epidemiologic factors to consider in such studies include season, age, epidemics, and definition of infection. These studies indicate that at least 20% of respiratory exacerbations are secondary to respiratory viruses, *Mycoplasma pneumoniae, Chlamydia,* and so forth (68,84). Abman et al. (1) reported that respiratory syncytial virus (RSV) was a frequent cause of early hospitalization in young CF patients, and was often associated with significant morbidity, including prolonged hospitalization, the need for mechanical ventilation, and persistent oxygen requirement at discharge. Compared to a control group of CF patients, chronic respiratory symptoms and low chest x-ray scores were more common in the RSV-infected group at follow-up. In a study of older CF patients, multiple nonbacterial respiratory infections were documented during a single 8-month period, although two-thirds of these were also associated with bacterial infections (84). Respiratory syncytial virus was the most common nonbacterial pathogen isolated (9% of all infections), and such infections were frequently associated with a rise in antipseudomonal antibodies. These two studies suggest a synergistic role for viruses, especially RSV, in the pathogenesis of pulmonary injury. In a study by Mearns (68), 18% of nonbacterial infections in CF patients were caused by mycoplasma. Airway dysfunction with either viral or mycoplasma infection can be critical for CF patients, and the direct cytotoxicity and inflammation caused by these organisms contributes to progressive tissue destruction. Depression of serum complement during viral lower respiratory infections in CF can reflect consumption by immune complexes with resultant pulmonary injury, an attractive hypothesis to explain viral-bacterial synergistic pulmonary injury (117).

Immunopathic Factors

It is generally agreed that early pulmonary pathology in CF is mediated by bacteria and their extracellular products. The pathogenesis of the chronic pulmonary damage is less well understood (65), but accumulating data now suggest a major role for local immune dysfunction due to both opsonophagocytic (immunoglobulin and complement) and cellular factors.

Chronically infected CF patients produce markedly elevated titers of local and systemic antipseudomonal antibodies directed against lipopolysaccharide (LPS) (the major opsonic immunodeterminant), mucoid expolysaccharide, and bacterial exoproducts (elastase, exotoxin-A, exotoxin-S, etc.). Several investigators, however, have shown that such antibodies possess deficient opsonophagocytic activity, particularly for *P. aeruginosa* LPS. In a series of elegant experiments, Fick et al. (25,26) have shown that extracellular proteases (primarily elastase) from mucoid and nonmucoid *P. aeruginosa* are able to cleave off the Fab and F_c fragments of immunoglobulins, rendering these antibodies incapable of interacting with receptor sites on pulmonary macrophages or polymorphonuclear (PMN) cells. Immunoglobulins from CF patients were no more sensitive to cleavage than controls. In CF patients, the predominant immunoglobulin subclass response to LPS is IgG3 and IgG4 (71), the latter being somewhat less sensitive to this proteolytic cleavage. This may not be beneficial, however, because Moss et al. (73) have shown that anti-LPS IgG4 acts as a blocking antibody that also inhibits opsonophagocytosis in CF patients. In addition, elastase levels in CF sputum are so markedly elevated that even the more resistant IgG2 is efficiently cleaved. This "self-defense" mechanism by *P. aeruginosa* can limit the effectiveness of antipseudomonal vaccines unless they can be administered prior to the onset of *Pseudomonas*-associated endobronchial inflammation.

In the absence of opsonically functional immunoglobulin, phagocytosis by pulmonary PMNs is critically dependent on complement-phagocyte interaction. However, excessive pseudomonal elastase activity in the lungs of CF patients can directly damage important cell surface receptors on PMNs, rendering them functionally impotent. *In vitro, Pseudomonas* elastase reduces PMN C3b receptors by as much as 90%, dramatically reducing phagocytosis of both mucoid and nonmucoid *P. aeruginosa* (12). In addition, elastase damages the remaining iC3b ligand on the bacterium, making it unrecognizable by the complementary PMN receptor. According to Berger (12), such an "opsonin-receptor mismatch could result in severe impairments in phagocytosis."

Because pulmonary macrophages depend on the same types of complement receptors as PMNs, Berger postulates that they, too, could be damaged by pseudomonal proteases with similar deleterious effects on phagocytosis. Macrophage-lymphokine interactions can also be subject to suppression by lymphokine inhibitory factors (see below). These factors, along with IgG4 nonopsonic antibody, could partially explain the pulmonary macrophage hyporesponsiveness seen in CF patients (121,123). Due to the failure of pulmonary macrophages to clear the infection, excessive infiltration of the lung by PMNs can cause additional injury. Elastase from PMNs directly damages lung tissue (118), whereas cellular breakdown products—especially DNA—increase sputum viscosity and decrease local pH.

Sorensen et al. (111) have noted lymphocyte hyporesponsiveness in CF patients persistently infected with *P. aeruginosa*. This defect is generalized to several gram-negative bacteria and involves all *Pseudomonas* strains tested. In contrast, lymphocyte responses to *S. aureus, H. influenzae, Streptococcus pyogenes,* phytohemagglutinin, and concanavalin A remain normal. Although lymphokine destruction probably occurs in CF sputum, elaboration of phenazine pigments (pyocyanin) by *P. aeruginosa* can act as another line of bacterial self-defense (76). Pyocyanin inhibits lymphocyte proliferation by decreasing T-cell IL-2 production and preventing expression of IL-2 receptors in T-lymphocytes. T-cells are the major source of macrophage-activating factors, which could augment the macrophage hyporesponsiveness noted earlier. Many of the host–parasite relationships in CF pulmonary infection are characterized by chronicity of infection, immune hyporesponsiveness locally and systemically, and subsequent "turning off" or "paralysis" of the immune response. This tolerance-like effect for cellular immunity could be an attempt by the host to prevent progressive and continuing immune-mediated lung injury. Consistent with this theory is the observation that the number of circulating T-lymphocytes correlates with severity of disease, suggesting that cell-mediated tissue injury also contributes to progressive lung damage in CF (41).

The association of high antipseudomonal precipitin titers (39) and elevated acute phase reactants (haptoglobin, ceruloplasmin, hemopexin) with advanced lung infection indicates that such antibodies do not prevent ongoing tissue damage and, in fact, could reflect a type III hypersensitivity reaction (40). Formation of local and circulating immune complexes is associated with chronic lung infection among CF patients. CF patients chronically infected with mucoid *P. aeruginosa* have a higher frequency of soluble immune complexes in their sputum than those without *Pseudomonas* colonization (95). British workers have found extensive immune complex deposition in the lungs and other organs of patients dying with CF (67). Some of these complexes involved human tissue antigens, a finding supported by the presence of isoantibodies in CF serum (115). Moss et al. (72) have demonstrated antipseudomonal and antistaphylococcal specificity in immune complexes isolated from CF patients and a concordance between immune complex titers and deteriorating pulmonary function. Complement consumption is increased in the serum of patients with *P. aeruginosa* precipitins (96), and activated complement appears in the sputum, where it is associated with an increased inflammatory response (97).

Local immunopathology in CF patients can also manifest as respiratory allergy and bronchial hyperreactivity. Twenty-four percent of CF patients in one study had clinical and laboratory evidence of respiratory allergies, including a marked degree of reversible airway obstruction (86). Reversible airway disease is often demonstrated in up to one-half of CF patients, even without allergic manifestations. This usually correlates with poor pulmonary function and exaggerated respiratory distress. Immunoglobulin E antibodies to *P. aeruginosa* and *Aspergillus* sp have also been demonstrated in the sera of CF patients.

MANAGEMENT

The management of bronchopulmonary infections in cystic fibrosis is complex and controversial. We shall attempt to outline only the most commonly used and newer treatment modalities.

Supplemental oxygen administration is standard for all acute infections, but mist tent therapy has been largely abandoned. Studies fail to show a benefit of mist therapy and suggest the additional risk of superinfection (55,74). Aggressive chest physiotherapy has been shown to significantly slow the rate of decline in pulmonary function in patients with mild to moderate CF (88). Regular exercise (23) and nutritional therapy are also important in enhancing host resistance and recovery from infection.

Antimicrobial Therapy

Prophylaxis

Should prophylactic antibiotic treatment be administered to all patients from the time of diagnosis? Although this question has not been answered, particularly in relation to the first critical infectious episode, continuous antistaphylococcal therapy is prescribed by many in hope of preventing early airway damage. A nationwide collaborative study is currently under way to address this important issue.

Sputum Colonization

CF patients with established bronchopulmonary disease and colonization by one or more of the three major bacterial respiratory pathogens have intermittent respiratory exacerbations and relatively stable periods in between. In the absence of signs of acute infection, the use of antibiotics directed at one or more of these pathogens is controversial. Many practitioners administer oral antibiotics active against *S. aureus* or *H. influenzae,* or both, on a chronic intermittent basis. Support for this comes from a controlled trial of cephalexin in patients with mild to moderate disease (60). Treatment decreased the frequency of respiratory infections and the need for hospitalization for those patients initially colonized with *S. aureus* and/or *H. influenzae*. Unfortunately, patients colonized with *P. aeruginosa* at the beginning of the study showed increased colonization by this organism and clinical deterioration. Some physicians prescribe oral chloramphenicol, trimethoprim/sulfamethoxazole, or amoxicillin/clavulanate to control *H. influenzae* colonization and note clinical improvement (106), but controlled evaluations of this approach are lacking. Chloramphenicol treatment risks hematopoietic toxicity and trimethoprim is inactivated by the elevated thymidine content of CF sputum. Clavulanate could hasten the development of bacterial resistance by derepression of chromosomal beta lactamase in *P. aeruginosa*.

Danish investigators prospectively studied the value of early antipseudomonal therapy in preventing chronic colonization with *P. aeruginosa* in CF patients (125). Whenever *P. aeruginosa* was isolated from sputum cultures, patients were treated with either placebo or oral ciprofloxacin along with aerosolized colistin for 3 weeks.

During 27 months of follow-up, significantly fewer treated patients became acutely or chronically colonized by *P. aeruginosa*.

Acute Exacerbations

Another strategy is to treat only acute exacerbations of pulmonary infection in CF patients. Acute respiratory exacerbations are characterized by malaise, anorexia, weight loss, increased cough, dyspnea (increased rate and work of breathing), increased quantity and purulence of sputum, and, usually, a deterioration in arterial pO_2. Fever and leukocytosis could or could not be present.

The benefit of therapy targeted against *P. aeruginosa*–associated exacerbations is supported by several studies (42) but challenged by others (31). With increasing severity of lung damage, even temporary pulmonary eradication of *Pseudomonas* becomes impossible. During acute pulmonary exacerbations, quantitative cultures reveal $\geq 10^8$ bacteria per milliliter of sputum; with therapy this falls by 1 to 2 logs, but the decrease is short lived, and, in fact, sometimes there is no change in bacterial density even with clinical improvement (10,66,69,129). This has led some to question whether anti-*Pseudomonas* therapy is even necessary for CF patients with advanced lung disease (10). Most clinicians, however, believe empirical anti-*Pseudomonas* therapy to be beneficial. Part of the difficulty lies in differentiating patients who have acute infections with viruses or other respiratory pathogens and in whom *P. aeruginosa* temporarily proliferates and increases its noxious effects on the pulmonary tissue, from those who have intercurrent infection in which the *Pseudomonas* plays little role in the acute symptomatology. Until methods are developed to distinguish between the two, empiric recommendations include treatment of *P. aeruginosa* (and usually *S. aureus* and *H. influenzae*, if they are also present) during acute pulmonary exacerbations in these patients.

Treatment of acute pulmonary exacerbations usually requires combined antibiotic therapy with a beta-lactam plus an aminoglycoside. The availability of new antipseudomonal cephalosporins (ceftazidime), penems (imipenem), monobactams (aztreonam), and beta-lactamase inhibitors (ticarcillin/clavulanic acid) has raised the possibility of single-drug therapy, especially for outpatient administration. Short-term comparative studies suggest that monotherapy is equivalent to conventional combinations, but the emergence of bacterial resistance can severely limit such long-term strategies. For example, Giwercman et al. (29) have demonstrated high levels of chromosomal (Class I) beta-lactamase activity in the sputum of CF patients who were treated with various β-lactam antibiotics for 2 weeks. This may be due to both *in vivo* selection of derepressed mutants and reversible induction with antibiotic exposure. Ceftazidime, for example, is a potent inducer of the normally repressed Class I enzyme, and widespread use of ceftazidime can result in the spread of multiresistant *P. aeruginosa* in CF centers (81). Although imipenem is less likely to induce the chromosomal enzyme, imipenem resistance due to alterations in membrane permeability can rapidly appear (19,82). Aztreonam is four-fold less active than ceftazidime or imipenem against *P. aeruginosa* and also induces the chromosomal enzyme, to which it is susceptible (45). Ticarcillin plus clavulanate is unlikely to be effective because clavulanate does not inhibit chromosomal beta-lactamase and actually induces derepression of this enzyme. Tazobactam is a more potent inhibitor of the Class I enzyme than either clavulanate or sulbactam and has recently been combined with piperacillin. This combination was more active than piperacillin alone against β-lactamase-producing *P. aeruginosa,* but achievable sputum levels and clinical efficacy of piperacillin/tazobactam in CF patients remain unknown (28). It should be noted that both beta-lactam and aminoglycoside antibiotics have increased renal clearance in CF patients (46,47). Accordingly, higher doses than usual may be required (Table 17-1).

Oral Quinolone Therapy

Until recently, antibiotic therapy of CF patients required hospitalization and intravenous treatment (or home intravenous treatment) because there was no orally available drug active against *P. aeruginosa.* The quinolones, however, represent a new class of antimicrobials with the following general characteristics: broad *in vitro* activity versus gram-positive and gram-negative bacteria, including *P. aeruginosa;* bactericidal activity unaffected by pH changes such as occur in CF sputum; good oral

TABLE 17–1. *Suggested dosages for various antimicrobials used in treating pulmonary infections in cystic fibrosis*

Antibiotic	Antimicrobial spectrum for CF patients	Dose (mg/kg/day)	Dose interval (hr)	Route
Dicloxacillin	S. aureus	100	6	p.o.
Cephalexin	S. aureus, some H. influenzae	100	6	p.o.
Amoxicillin	H. influenzae	100	8	p.o.
Chloramphenicol	H. influenzae	75	6	p.o.
Ticarcillin	Pseudomonas	400–500	6	i.v.
Piperacillin	Pseudomonas	400–500	6	i.v.
Azlocillin	Pseudomonas H. influenzae Enterobacteriaceae	400–500	6	i.v.
Ceftazidime	Pseudomonas H. influenzae Enterobacteriaceae	150	8	i.v.
Cefsulodin	Pseudomonas	150	6–8	i.v.
Imipenem	S. aureus Pseudomonas H. influenzae Enterobacteriaceae	90–100	6	i.v.
Aztreonam	Pseudomonas Enterobacteriaceae H. influenzae	150	6–8	i.v.
Ciprofloxacin	S. aureus Pseudomonas H. influenzae Enterobacteriaceae	(1500–2000 mg/day)	12	p.o. (i.v.)[a]
Gentamicin	Pseudomonas	7.5–10.0	6–8	i.v.
Tobramycin	Pseudomonas	10.0–12.0	6–8	i.v.
Amikacin	Pseudomonas	22.0–30.0	6–8	i.v.
Methicillin	S. aureus	200	6	i.v.
Nafcillin	S. aureus	200	6	i.v.
Ketoconazole	C. albicans	5.0–10.0	24	p.o.
Amantadine	Influenza A	5.0–10.0	12	p.o.

[a]Investigational.

absorption (60–80%) with a large volume of distribution, including lung; no cross-resistance with other classes of antibiotics; absence of significant oto- or nephrotoxicity; no significant synergistic or antagonistic interactions with other classes of antibiotics. To date, quinolones have not been approved for use in children due to weight-bearing cartilage dysplasia seen in immature experimental animals. However, Schaad et al. (92) found no evidence of knee joint arthropathy by magnetic resonance imaging in 13 CF patients who received ciprofloxacin for 3 months at 30 mg/kg/day. Monotherapy with oral ciprofloxacin, pefloxacin, and ofloxacin for acute respiratory exacerbations in CF patients is as effective as traditional intravenous treatment with β-lactamase plus aminoglycosides. Peak serum concentrations of quinolones are higher and the volume of distribution somewhat lower in CF patients. Similar to conventional therapy, *Pseudomonas* is not eradicated from CF sputum and emergence of resistant strains occurs regularly. *In vitro* susceptibility usually returns, however, when quinolones are withheld for a few months. Overall, tolerance to the quinolones has been satisfactory (15,32,34,37,45,91,100,104). A few patients experienced continued clinical improvement after stopping ciprofloxacin, but most returned to "baseline" within a short time. Optimal strategies for timing, dose, and duration of quinolone therapy in CF patients are yet to be determined.

Aerosol Antibiotics

As discussed earlier, the site of pulmonary infection in CF patients is the bronchial lumen, not the parenchyma. Most antibiotics penetrate poorly into CF sputum where the relatively low pH and high ionic concentration are particularly inhibitory to the positively charged aminoglycosides. Many physicians, therefore, advocate the use of aerosolized antibiotics, particularly aminoglycosides. There are few prospective studies to evaluate this approach, however, and results are conflicting (61). A 6-month, double-blind, randomized, crossover study of young adult CF patients chronically infected with *P. aeruginosa* favored the use of aerosolized carbenicillin and gentamicin (38). Shaad et al. (94) studied the efficacy of adding aerosolized amikacin to intravenous amikacin plus ceftazidime during acute pulmonary exacerbations. Significantly more of the patients receiving aerosol drug had complete eradication of *P. aeruginosa* at the end of therapy (70% vs. 42%, $p < 0.02$). However, both regimens resulted in similar improvements in clinical, radiologic, laboratory, and pulmonary function outcomes, and within 4–6 weeks most patients were recolonized with *P. aeruginosa*. The authors concluded that the addition of aerosolized aminoglycoside was of no clinical benefit. Conversely, in a multicenter trial sponsored by the CF Foundation, aerosolized tobramycin 3 times/day for 30 days was associated with a significant improvement in pulmonary function tests when compared to saline placebo (18). By 12 weeks of treatment, however, pulmonary function had returned to enrollment values (110). Sputum density of *P. aeruginosa* decreased by 3 log cfu/gram, coincident with a reduction in cough frequency and sputum production; weight gain was also observed. Almost three-fourths of patients in the treatment group became colonized by tobramycin-resistant *P. aeruginosa*, but one year later all sputum isolates were again susceptible. Other investigators have confirmed the bacteriologic and clinical benefits to aerosolized tobramycin therapy but also found transient bacterial resistance to be a problem (62).

Specific Recommendations

Specific antibiotics, dosages, and their antimicrobial activity are listed in Table 17-1. Of note, a recent study documented the safety of aztreonam in CF patients who had previously had severe hypersensitivity reactions to the β-lactam antibiotics, including anaphylactic shock (44). Two investigational "fourth-generation" cephalosporins, cefepime and cefpirome, have moderate antipseudomonal activity *in vitro*, but more importantly appear resistant to the Class I enzyme (14). Clinical studies with these drugs in CF are now in progress (4). In selecting an appropriate combination of antibiotics, both the relative bioactivity and sputum penetration of the candidate drugs must be considered. Unfortunately, the number of well-controlled studies on sputum antibiotic penetration in CF is limited. Of those few published studies, the experimental designs differ significantly, making comparisons difficult (108,112).

Long-Term Intensive Chemotherapy

Following in-patient treatment of an acute pulmonary exacerbation, there is a high incidence of clinical relapse or recrudescence in the ensuing weeks to months. Because each flare-up can cause cumulative irreversible lung damage, prevention of such episodes can ultimately prolong survival. Studies are planned to assess the value of prolonged antibiotic treatment following acute exacerbations.

Hospitalization for Lung Clean-Up

Some physicians recommend elective "lung clean-up" hospitalization for their CF patients. During a 3–7 day period patients undergo a vigorous program of intensive chest physiotherapy combined with antimicrobials directed at *Pseudomonas*. Only one study (119) has shown a long-term benefit of this approach, and sputum bacterial densities often return to pretreatment levels in a short time. A less costly and more convenient regimen is to administer chest physiotherapy and intravenous antimicrobials at home, via Hickman, Broviac, or totally implantable central venous catheters. Such out-of-hospital therapy has been shown safe and effective for most CF patients who overwhelmingly prefer this mode of treatment (70,116).

Steroid Therapy

As noted earlier, there is a clear association between chronic inflammation and severity of pulmonary disease in advanced CF. To investigate the possible role of immunosuppression on slowing the progression of lung injury, Auerbach et al. (5) administered alternate-day prednisone to 45 CF patients aged 1–12 years in a randomized double-blind placebo-controlled trial. After 4 years, the prednisone-treated group had significantly better outcomes for height, weight, pulmonary function tests, erythrocyte sedimentation rate, and serum IgG levels. The United States Cystic Fibrosis Foundation has now sponsored a multicenter, double-blind, placebo-controlled study of alternate-day prednisone in CF patients with mild to moderate pulmonary disease (89). Initial results confirmed the beneficial effects of both high-dose (2 mg/kg) and low-dose (1 mg/kg) treatment. However, an interim analysis has shown an increased frequency of cataracts, growth retardation, and glucose abnormalities in the high-dose group, leading to premature termination of that arm of the study. Final results of the low-dose regimen are pending.

Investigational Therapy

As noted earlier, excessive sodium reabsorption in CF respiratory epithelium contributes to the thickened, viscous endobronchial secretions in CF patients. Amiloride is a sodium channel blocker that inhibits excessive reabsorption of sodium *in vitro* and *in vivo* when applied to the luminal surface of the airway epithelium of CF patients. Knowles et al. (53) demonstrated that daily aerosol treatments with amiloride decreased sputum viscosity in CF patients and significantly slowed the deterioration in vital capacity while improving mucociliary and cough clearance. These results have now been confirmed by other investigators (3). Similarly, local application of the nucleotide secretagogues adenine triphosphate (ATP) and uridine triphosphate (UTP) stimulate increased chloride secretion across the epithelial luminal surface of respiratory epithelial cells. Knowles et al. (54) subsequently demonstrated that a combination of ameloride and ATP or UTP leads to enhanced *in vitro* liquefaction of airway secretions in CF patients.

Research into the use of recombinant DNase to help liquefy CF sputum is also an exciting area of current investigation. As noted earlier, high levels of leukocyte-derived DNA are a major component of the viscous endobronchial secretions that plug the airways in CF patients. Aerosolized human recombinant DNase has been shown to greatly reduce the viscosity of purulent CF sputum, transforming it within minutes from a nonflowing viscous jell to flowing liquid (103). A single 10-day course of aerosolized DNase was safe and resulted in significant improvement in pulmonary function in one large-scale study (109).

Lung Transplantation

As discussed earlier, progressive endobronchial infection and inflammation culminate in premature cardiorespiratory death for 80% of CF patients. Clinical deterioration is often hastened by the onset of right heart failure or cor pulmonale secondary to combined hypoxemia and high pulmonary vascular resistance. Until the advent of lung transplantation, only palliative treatment was available for such patients. Combined heart-lung transplants were first attempted for CF patients 10 years ago and today have a 70% one-year actuarial survival rate (21). More recently, double-lung, sequential single-lung, and now isolated lobar transplants have all been attempted with generally similar results (105). The transplanted lung retains the physiologic characteristics of the donor, and rejection and *Pseudomonas* infections are no more common in CF versus non-CF patients after transplant.

Vaccines

Children with CF should receive routine childhood vaccinations at the usual times and doses. The use of pneumococcal vaccination in these patients is debatable; however, it seems reasonable to prevent even the few episodes of pneumococcal pneumonia expected by use of this vaccine in children over 2 years of age. Currently available *Pseudomonas* vaccines have not been shown beneficial in the treatment of established CF pulmonary infections (58,83). Schaad et al. (93) administered a *Pseudomonas* polysaccharide-toxin A conjugate vaccine prophylactically to CF patients not yet colonized with *P. aeruginosa*. Immunization produced opsonic and toxin-neutralizing antibodies, but there was no significant change in clinical status after one year. Yearly influenza boosters should be given to ensure immunity against the ever-changing antigenic composition of influenza strains anticipated each winter. Future strategies could include vaccines against viruses and mycoplasma as well as antitoxic or antiinflammatory therapies or immunomodulation.

ACKNOWLEDGMENT

The authors wish to thank Elaine Neppl for typing the manuscript.

REFERENCES

1. Abman, S.H., Ogle, J.W., Butler-Simon, N., et al. (1988): Role of respiratory syncytial virus in early hospitalizations for respiratory distress of young infants with cystic fibrosis. *J. Pediatr.*, 113:826–830.
2. Abman, S.H., Ogle, J.W., Harbeck, R.J., et al. (1991): Early bacteriologic, immunologic, and clinical courses of young infants with cystic fibrosis identified by neonatal screening. *J. Pediatr.*, 119:211–217.
3. App, E.M., King, M., Helfesrieder, R., et al. (1990): Acute and long-term amiloride inhalation in cystic fibrosis lung disease: A rational approach to cystic fibrosis therapy. *Am. Rev. Respir. Dis.*, 141:605–612.
4. Arguedas, A.G., Stutman, H.R., Zaleska, M., et al. (1992): Cefepime: pharmacokinetics and clinical response in patients with cystic fibrosis. *Am. J. Dis. Child.*, 146:797–802.
5. Auerbach, H.S., Kirkpatrick, J.A., Williams, M., et al. (1985): Alternate-day prednisone reduces morbidity and improves pulmonary function in cystic fibrosis. *Lancet*, ii:686–688.
6. Baltimore, R.S., and Mitchell, M. (1980): Immunologic investigations of mucoid strains of *Pseudomonas aeruginosa:* comparison of susceptibility to opsonic antibody in mucoid and nonmucoid strains. *J. Infect. Dis.*, 141:238–247.
7. Bauernfiend, A., Bertele, R.M., Harms, K., et al. (1987): Qualitative and quantitative microbiological analysis of sputa of 102 patients with cystic fibrosis. *Infection*, 15:270–277.
8. Bauernfiend, A., Emminger, G., Horl, G., et al. (1987): Selective pressure of antistaphylococcal chemotherapeutics in favor of *Pseudomonas aeruginosa* in cystic fibrosis. *Infection*, 15(6):469–470.
9. Bauernfiend, A., Rotter, K., and Weisslen-Pfister, C. (1987): Selective procedure to isolate *Hemophilus influenzae* from sputa with large quantities of *Pseudomonas aeruginosa*. *Infection*, 15:278–280.
10. Beaudry, P.H., Marks, M.I., McDougall, D., Desmond, K., and Rangle, R. (1980): Is anti-*Pseudomonas* therapy warranted in acute respiratory exacerbations in children with cystic fibrosis? *J. Pediatr.*, 97:144–147.
11. Bedrossian, C.W.M., Greenberg, S.D., Singer, D.B., Hansen, J.J., and Rosenberg, H.S. (1976): The lung in cystic fibrosis: quantitative study of pathologic findings among different age groups. *Human Pathol.*, 7:195–204.
12. Berger, M., Tosi, M.F., Nutman, J., et al. (1987): Phagocytic defects in the lung in cystic fibrosis. *Pediatr. Pulmonol.*, 3(Suppl. 1):98–100.
13. Blackwood, L.L., and Pennington, J.E. (1981): Influence of mucoid coating on clearance of *Pseudomonas aeruginosa* from lungs. *Infect. Immun.*, 32:443–448.
14. Bosso, J.A., Saxon, B.A., and Matsen, J.M. (1991): Comparative activity of cefepime, alone and in combination, against clinical isolates of *Pseudomonas aeruginosa* and *Pseudomonas cepacia* from cystic fibrosis patients. *Antimicrob. Agents Chemother.*, 35:783–784.
15. Bosso, J.A., Black, P.G., and Matsen, J.M. (1986): Ciprofloxacin versus tobramycin plus azlocillin in pulmonary exacerbations in adult patients with cystic fibrosis. *Am. J. Med.*, 82(4A):180–184.
16. Boxerbaum, B., and Klinger, J.D. (1984): *Pseudomonas cepacia* bacteremia in cystic fibrosis. *Pediatr. Res.*, 18:269A.
17. Brueton, M.J., Ormerod, L.P., Shah, K.J., and Anderson, C.M. (1980): Allergic bronchopulmonary aspergillosis complicating cystic fibrosis in childhood. *Arch. Dis. Child.*, 55:348–353.

18. Burns, J.L., Ramsey, B.W., and Smith, A.L. (1993): Clinical manifestations and treatment of pulmonary infections in cystic fibrosis. *Adv. Pediatr. Infect. Dis.*, 8:53–66.
19. Buscher, K.H., Cullman, W., Dick, W., et al. (1987): Imipenem resistance in *Pseudomonas aeruginosa* resulting from diminished expression of an outer membrane protein. *Antimicrob. Agents Chemother.*, 31:703–708.
20. Davidson, A.G.F., Wong, L.T.K., Kirby, L.T., et al. (1987): Screening for cystic fibrosis: the Vancouver experience. *Pediatr. Pulmonol.*, 3(Suppl. 1):79–80.
21. deLeval, M.R., Smyth, R., Whitehead, B., et al. (1991): Heart and lung transplantation for terminal cystic fibrosis. *J. Thorac. Cardiovasc. Surg.*, 101:633–642.
22. Doggett, R.G., Harrison, G.M., and Wallis, E.S. (1964): Comparison of some properties of *Pseudomonas aeruginosa* isolated from infections of persons with and without cystic fibrosis. *J. Bacteriol.*, 87:427–431.
23. Edlund, L.D., French, R.W., Herbst, J.J., et al. (1986): Effects of a swimming program in children with cystic fibrosis. *Am. J. Dis. Child.*, 140:80–83.
24. Evans, L.R., and Linker, A. (1973): Production and characterization of the slime polysaccharide of *Pseudomonas aeruginosa. J. Bacteriol.*, 116:915–924.
25. Flick, R.B., Naegel, G.P., Matthay, R.A., and Reynolds, H.Y. (1981): Cystic fibrosis *Pseudomonas* opsonins: inhibitory nature in an *in vitro* phagocytic assay. *J. Clin. Invest.*, 68:899–914.
26. Fick, R.B., Baltimore, R.S., Squier, S.U., et al. (1985): IgG proteolytic activity of *Pseudomonas aeruginosa* in cystic fibrosis. *J. Infect. Dis.*, 151:589–598.
27. FitzSimmons, S.C. (1993): The changing epidemiology of cystic fibrosis. *J. Pediatr.*, 122:1–9.
28. Giwercman, B., Lambert, P.A., Rosdahl, V.T., et al. (1990): Rapid emergence of resistance in *Pseudomonas aeruginosa* in cystic fibrosis patients due to *in vivo* selection of stable partially derepressed β-lactamase producing strains. *J. Antimicrob. Chemother.*, 26:247–259.
29. Giwercman, B., Meyer, C., Lambert, P.A., et al. (1992): High-level β-lactamase activity in sputum samples from cystic fibrosis patients during antipseudomonal treatment. *Antimicrob. Agents Chemother.*, 36:71–76.
30. Gladman, G., Connor, P.J., Williams, R.F., et al. (1992): Controlled study of *Pseudomonas cepacia* and *Pseudomonas maltophilia* in cystic fibrosis. *Arch. Dis. Child*, 67:192–195.
31. Gold , R., Carpenter, S., Heurter, H., et al. (1987): Randomized trial of ceftazidime versus placebo in the management of acute respiratory exacerbations in patients with cystic fibrosis. *J. Pediatr.* 111:907–913.
32. Goldfarb, J., Stern, R.C., Reed, M.D., et al. (1986): Ciprofloxacin monotherapy for acute pulmonary exacerbations in cystic fibrosis. *Am. J. Med.*, 82(4A):174–179.
33. Goldman, D.A., and Kinger, J.D. (1986): *Pseudomonas cepacia:* biology, mechanisms of virulence, epidemiology. *J. Pediatr.*, 108(2):806–812.
34. Grenier, B. (1989): Use of the new quinolones in cystic fibrosis. *Rev. Infect. Dis.*, 11:S1245–S1252.
35. Gurwitz, D., Corey, M., Francis, P.W.J., Crozier, D., and Levison, H. (1979): Perspectives in cystic fibrosis. *Pediatr. Clin. No. Amer.*, 26:603–615.
36. Hodson, C.J., and France, N.E. (1962): Pulmonary changes in cystic fibrosis of the pancreas: a radiopathologic study. *Clin. Radiol.*, 13:54–61.
37. Hodson, M.E., Butland, R.J.E., Roberts, C.M., et al. (1987): Oral ciprofloxacin compared with conventional intravenous treatment for *Pseudomonas aeruginosa* infection in adults with cystic fibrosis. *Lancet*, i:235–237.
38. Hodson, M.E., Penketh, A.R.L., and Balten, J.C. (1981): Aerosol carbenicillin and gentamicin treatment of *Pseudomonas aeruginosa* infection in patients with cystic fibrosis. *Lancet* 2:1137–1139.
39. Hoiby, N., and Hertz, J.B. (1979): Precipitating antibodies against *Escherichia coli, Bacteroides fragilis ss., thetaiotaomicron* and *Pseudomonas aeruginosa* in serum from normal persons and cystic fibrosis patients: determined by means of crossed immunoelectrophoresis. *Acta. Pediatr. Scand.*, 68:495–500.
40. Hoiby, N., Jacobsen, L., Jørgensen, B.A., Lykkegaard, E., and Weeke, B. (1974): *Pseudomonas aeruginosa* infection in cystic fibrosis: Occurrence of precipitating antibodies against *Pseudomonas aeruginosa* in relation to the concentration of sixteen serum proteins and the clinical and radiographical status of the lungs. *Acta. Pediatr. Scand.*, 63:843–848.
41. Hoiby, N., and Mathiesen, L. (1974): *Pseudomonas aeruginosa* infection in cystic fibrosis: Distribution of B and T lymphocytes in relation to the humoral immune response. *Acta. Pathol. Microbiol. Scand.* (B), 82:556–559.
42. Hyatt, A.C., Chipps, B.E., Kumor, K.M., Mellits, E.D., Lietman, P.S., and Rosenstein, B.J. (1981): A double-blind controlled trial of anti-*Pseudomonas* chemotherapy of acute respiratory exacerbations in patients with cystic fibrosis. *J. Pediatr.*, 99:307–311.
43. Isles, A., Levison, H., Newth, C., Corey, M., and Flemming, P. (1984): *Pseudomonas cepacia* infection in cystic fibrosis: an emerging problem. *J. Pediatr.*, 104:206–210.
44. Jensen, T., Pedersen, S.S., Hoiby, N., et al. (1991): Safety of aztreonam in patients with cystic fibrosis and allergy to β-lactam antibiotics. *Rev. Infect. Dis.*, 13:S594–S597.

45. Jensen, T., Pedersen, S.S., Nielsen, C.H., et al. (1987): The efficacy and safety of ciprofloxacin and ofloxacin in chronic *Pseudomonas aeruginosa* infection in cystic fibrosis. *J. Antimicrob. Chemother.*, 20:585–594.

46. Kearns, G.L., Hilman, B.C., and Wilson, J.T. (1982): Dosing implications of altered gentamicin disposition in patients with cystic fibrosis. *J. Pediatr.*, 100:312–318.

47. Kearns, G.L., and Trang, J.M. (1986): Introduction to pharmacokinetics: aminoglycosides in cystic fibrosis as a prototype. *J. Pediatr.*, 108(2):847–853.

48. Kerem, B., Rommens, J.M., and Buchanan, J.A. (1989): Identification of the cystic fibrosis gene: genetic analysis. *Science*, 245:1073–1080.

49. Kerem, E., Corey, M., Kerem, B.S., et al. (1990): The relationship between genotype and phenotype in cystic fibrosis: analysis of the most common mutation (ΔF508). *N. Engl. J. Med.*, 323:1517–1522.

50. Klinger, J.D., Strauss, D.C., Hilton, C.B., and Bass, J.A. (1978): Antibodies to proteases and exotoxin A of *Pseudomonas aeruginosa* in patients with cystic fibrosis: demonstration by radioimmunoassay. *J. Infect. Dis.*, 138:49–58.

51. Klinger, J.D., and Thomassen, M.J. (1985): Occurrence and antimicrobial susceptibility of gram-negative nonfermentative bacilli in cystic fibrosis patients. *Diagnost. Microbiol. Infect. Dis.*, 3:149–158.

52. Knowles, M., Gatzy, J., and Boucher, R. (1981): Increased bioelectric potential difference across respiratory epithelia in cystic fibrosis. *N. Engl. J. Med.*, 305:1489–1495.

53. Knowles, M.R., Church, N.L., Waltner, W.E., et al. (1990): A pilot study of aerosolized amiloride for the treatment of lung disease in cystic fibrosis. *N. Engl. J. Med.*, 322:1189–1194.

54. Knowles, M.R., Clark, L.L., and Boucher, R.C. (1991): Activation of extracellular nucleotides of chloride secretion in the airway epithelia of patients with cystic fibrosis. *N. Engl. J. Med.*, 325:533–538.

55. Kuhn, R.J., Lubin, A.H., Jones, P.R., and Nahata, M.C. (1982): Bacterial contamination of aerosol solutions used to treat cystic fibrosis. *Am. J. Hosp. Pharm.*, 38:308–309.

56. Lam, J., Chan, R., Lam, K., and Costerton, J.W. (1980): Production of mucoid microcolonies by *Pseudomonas aeruginosa* within infected lungs in cystic fibrosis. *Infect. Immun.*, 28:546–556.

57. Lamarre, A., Reilly, B.J., Bryan, A.C., and Levison, H. (1972): Early detection of pulmonary function abnormalities in cystic fibrosis. *Pediatrics*, 50:291–298.

58. Langford, D.T., and Hiller, J. (1984): Prospective, controlled study of a polyvalent pseudomonas vaccine in cystic fibrosis: three-year results. *Arch. Dis. Child.*, 59:1131–1134.

59. LiPuma, J.J., Dasen, S.E., Nielson, D.W., et al. (1990): Person-to-person transmission of *Pseudomonas cepacia* between patients with cystic fibrosis. *Lancet*, 336:1094–1096.

60. Loening-Baucke, V.A., Mischler, E., and Myers, M.G. (1979): A placebo-controlled trial of cephalexin therapy in the ambulatory management of patients with cystic fibrosis. *J. Pediatr.*, 95:630–637.

61. MacLusky, I., Levison, H., Gold, R., et al. (1986): Inhaled antibiotics in cystic fibrosis: is there a therapeutic effect? *J. Pediatr.*, 108(2):861–865.

62. MacLusky, I.B., Gold, R., Corey, M., et al. (1989): Long-term effects of inhaled tobramycin in patients with cystic fibrosis colonized with *Pseudomonas aeruginosa*. *Pediatr. Pulmonol.*, 7:42–48.

63. Macone, A.B., Pier, G.B., Pennington, J.E., Matthews, W.J., and Goldman, D.A. (1981): Mucoid *Escherichia coli* in cystic fibrosis. *N. Engl. J. Med.*, 304:1445–1449.

64. Marcus, H., and Baker, N.R. (1985): Quantitation of adherence of mucoid and non-mucoid *Pseudomonas aeruginosa* to hamster tracheal epithelium. *Infect. Immun.*, 47:723–729.

65. Marks, M.I. (1981): The pathogenesis and treatment of pulmonary infections in patients with cystic fibrosis. *J. Pediatr.*, 98:173–179.

66. Martin, A.J., Smalley, C.A., George, R.H., Healing, D.E., and Anderson, C.M. (1980): Gentamicin and tobramycin compared in the treatment of mucoid *Pseudomonas* lung infections in cystic fibrosis. *Arch. Dis. Child.*, 55:604–607.

67. McFarlane, H., Holzel, A., Brenchley, P., Allan, J.D., Wallwork, J.C., Singer, B.E., and Worsley, B. (1975): Immune complexes in cystic fibrosis. *Br. Med. J.*, 1:423–428.

68. Mearns, M.B. (1980): Natural history of pulmonary infection in cystic fibrosis: In: Perspectives in Cystic Fibrosis. *Proceedings of the 8th International Cystic Fibrosis Conference*, edited by J. Sturgess, pp. 325–334.

69. Michalsen, J., and Bergan, T. (1981): Azlocillin with and without an aminoglycoside against respiratory tract infections in children with cystic fibrosis. *Scand. J. Infect. Dis.*, 29:92–97.

70. Morris, J.B., Occhionero, M.E., Gauderer, M.W.L., et al. (1990): Totally implantable vascular access devices in cystic fibrosis: a four-year experience with fifty-eight patients. *J. Pediatr.*, 117:82–85.

71. Moss, R.B. (1986): IgG subclasses in respiratory disorders: cystic fibrosis. *Monogr. Allergy*, 19:202–209.

72. Moss, R.B., Hus, Y.P., and Lewiston, N.J. (1981): I-Clq-binding and specific antibodies as indicators of pulmonary disease activity in cystic fibrosis. *J. Pediatr.*, 99:215–222.

73. Moss, R.B., Hsu, Y.P., Lewiston, N.J., et al. (1986): Altered antibody isotype in cystic fibrosis: possible role in opsonic deficiency. *Pediatr. Res.*, 20:453–459.

74. Motoyama, E.K., Gibson, L.E., and Zigas, C.J. (1972): Evaluation of mist tent therapy in cystic fibrosis using maximum expiratory flow volume curve. *Pediatrics*, 50:299–306.

75. Nelson, L.A., Collerame, M.L., and Schwartz, R.H. (1979): Aspergillosis and atopy in cystic fibrosis. *Am. Rev. Respir. Dis.*, 120:863–873.

76. Nutman, J., Berger, M., Chase, P.A., et al. (1987): Studies on the mechanism of T cell inhibition by the *Pseudomonas aeruginosa* phenazine pigment pyocyanine. *J. Immunol.*, 138:3481–3487.

77. Ogle, J.W., Janda, J.M., and Woods, D.E. (1987): Characterization and use of a DNA probe as an epidemiological marker for *Pseudomonas aeruginosa*. *J. Infect. Dis.*, 155:119–126.

78. Oppenheimer, E.H. (1981): Similarity of the tracheobronchial mucous glands and epithelium in infants with and without cystic fibrosis. *Human Pathol.*, 12:36–48.

79. Orenstein, D.M. (1993): Cystic fibrosis. *Curr. Prob. Pediatr.*, 23:4–15.

80. Paranchych, W., Sastry, P.A., Volpel, K., et al. (1986): Fimbriae (pili): molecular basis of *Pseudomonas aeruginosa* adherence. *Clin. Invest. Med.*, 9:113–118.

81. Pedersen, S.S., Koch, C., Hoiby, N., et al. (1986): An epidemic spread of multiresistant *Pseudomonas aeruginosa* in a cystic fibrosis center. *J. Antimicrob. Chemother.*, 17:505–516.

82. Pedersen, S.S., Pressler, T., Jensen, T., et al. (1987): Combined imipenem/cilastatin and tobramycin therapy of multiresistant *Pseudomonas aeruginosa* in cystic fibrosis. *J. Antimicrob. Chemother.*, 19:101–107.

83. Pennington, J.E., Reynolds, H.Y., Wood, R.E., Robinson, R.A., and Levine, A.S. (1975): Use of a *Pseudomonas aeruginosa* vaccine on patients with acute leukemia and cystic fibrosis. *Am. J. Med.*, 58:629–636.

84. Peterson, N.T., Hoiby, N., Mordhort, C.H., Lind, K., Flensborg, E.W., and Bruun, B. (1981): Respiratory infections in cystic fibrosis patients caused by virus, chlamydia and mycoplasma: possible synergism with *Pseudomonas aeruginosa*. *Acta. Paediatr. Scand.*, 70:623–628.

85. Pier, G.B., Saunders, J.M., Ames, P., et al. (1987): Opsonophagocytic killing antibody to *Pseudomonas aeruginosa* mucoid exopolysaccharide in older noncolonized patients with cystic fibrosis. *N. Engl. J. Med.*, 317:793–798.

86. Rachelefsky, G.S., Osher, A., Dooley, R.E., Ank, B., and Stiehm, R. (1974): Coexistent respiratory allergy and cystic fibrosis. *Am. J. Dis. Child.*, 128:355–359.

87. Ramsey, B.W., et al. (1991): Predictive value of oropharyngeal cultures for identifying lower airway bacteria in cystic fibrosis patients. *Am. Rev. Respir. Dis.*, 144:331–337.

88. Reisman, J.J., et al. (1988): Role of conventional physiotherapy in cystic fibrosis. *J. Pediatr.*, 113:632–636.

89. Rosenstein, B.J., and Eigen, H. (1991): Risks of alternate-day prednisone in patients with cystic fibrosis. *Pediatrics*, 87:245–246.

90. Rosenstein, B.J., and Hall, D.E. (1980): Pneumonia and septicemia due to *Pseudomonas cepacia* in a patient with cystic fibrosis. *Johns Hopkins Med. J.*, 147:188–189.

91. Rubio, T.T. (1986): Ciprofloxacin: comparative data in cystic fibrosis. *Am. J. Med.*, 82(4A):185–188.

92. Schaad, V.B., Stoupis, C., Wedgewood, J., et al. (1991): Clinical, radiologic and magnetic resonance monitoring for skeletal toxicity in pediatric patients with cystic fibrosis receiving a three-month course of ciprofloxacin. *Pediatr. Infect. Dis. J.*, 10:723–729.

93. Schaad, V.B., Wedgewood, J., Que, J.V., et al. (1991): Safety and immunogenicity of *Pseudomonas aeruginosa* conjugate A vaccine in cystic fibrosis. *Lancet*, 338:1236–1237.

94. Schaad, V.B., Wedgewood-Krucko, J., Suter, S., et al. (1987): Efficacy of inhaled amikacin as adjunct to intravenous combination therapy (ceftazidime and amikacin) in cystic fibrosis. *J. Pediatr.*, 111:599–605.

95. Shiotz, P.O., Hoiby, N., Juhl, F., Permin, H., Nielsen, H., and Svehag, S.E. (1977): Immune complexes in cystic fibrosis. *Acta. Pathol. Microbiol. Scand.* [C], 85:57–64.

96. Shiotz, P.O., Nielsen, H., Hoiby, N., Glikmann, G., and Svehag, S.E. (1978): Immune complexes in the sputum of patients with cystic fibrosis suffering from chronic *Pseudomonas aeruginosa* lung infection. *Acta. Pathol. Microbiol. Scand.* [C], 86:37–40.

97. Schiotz, P.O., Sorensen, H., and Hoiby, N. (1979): Activated complement in the sputum from patients with cystic fibrosis. *Acta. Pathol. Microbiol. Scand.* [C], 87:1–5.

98. Schoumaker, R.A., Shoemaker, R.L., Holm, D.R., et al. (1987): Activation of chloride channels in airway cells by the catalytic subunit of A-kinase and membrane depolarization. *Pediatr. Pulmonol.*, 3(Suppl. 1):116(Abstract no. 33).

99. Schwarzmann, S., and Boring, J.R. (1971): Antiphagocytic effect of slime from a mucoid strain of *Pseudomonas aeruginosa*. *Infect. Immun.*, 3:762–767.

100. Scully, B.E., Nakatomi, M., Ores, C., et al. (1986): Ciprofloxacin therapy in cystic fibrosis. *Am. J. Med.*, 82(4A):196–201.

101. Seale, T.W., Thirkill, H., Tarpay, M., Flux, M., and Rennert, O.M. (1979): Serotypes and antibiotic susceptibilities of *Pseudomonas aeruginosa* isolates from single sputa of cystic fibrosis patients. *J. Clin. Microbiol.*, 9:72–78.

102. Seidmon, E.J., Mosovich, L.L., and Neter, E. (1975): Colonization of *Enterobacteriaceae* of the respiratory tract of children with cystic fibrosis of the pancreas and their antibody response. *J. Pediatr.*, 85;528–533.

103. Shak, S., Capon, D.J., Hellmiss, R., et al. (1990): Recombinant human DNase I reduces the viscosity of cystic fibrosis sputum. *Proc. Natl. Acad. Sci.*, 87:9188–9192.

104. Shalit, I., Stutman, H.R., Marks, M.I., et al. (1986): Randomized study of two dosage regimens of ciprofloxacin for treating chronic bronchopulmonary infection in patients with cystic fibrosis. *Am. J. Med.*, 82(4A):189–195.

105. Shennib, H., Noirclerc, M., Ernst, P., et al. (1992): Double-lung transplantation for cystic fibrosis. *Ann. Thorac. Surg.*, 54:27–32.

106. Schwachman, H. (1978): Cystic fibrosis. *Curr. Prob. Pediatr.*, 8:1–71.

107. Slack, M.P.E., and Nichols, W.N. (1981): The penetration of antibiotics through sodium alginate and through the exopolysaccharide of a mucoid strain of *Pseudomonas aeruginosa*. *Lancet*, 2:502–503.

108. Smith, A.L. (1986): Antibiotic therapy in cystic fibrosis: evaluation of clinical trials. *J. Pediatr.*, 108(2):866–870.

109. Smith, A.L., and DNase Research Consortium. (1992): Efficacy and safety of aerosolized recombinant human DNase in patients with cystic fibrosis. *Clin. Res.*, 40:318A.

110. Smith, A.L., Ramsey, B.W., Hedges, D.L., et al. (1989): Safety of aerosol tobramycin administration for 3 months to patients with cystic fibrosis. *Pediatr. Pulmonol.*, 7:265–271.

111. Sorensen, R.V., Stern, R.C., and Polmar, S.H. (1978): Lymphocyte responsiveness to *Pseudomonas aeruginosa* in cystic fibrosis: relationship to status of pulmonary disease in sibling pairs. *J. Pediatr.*, 93:201–205.

112. Sorgel, F., Stephan, V., Weisemann, H.G., et al. (1987): High-dose treatment with antibiotics in cystic fibrosis: a reappraisal with special reference to the pharmacokinetics of beta-lactams and new fluoroquinolones in adult CF patients. *Infection*, 15:385–396.

113. Sorscher, E.J., and Breslow, J.L. (1982): Cystic fibrosis: a disorder of calcium-mediated secretion and transepithelial sodium transport? *Lancet*, 1:368–370.

114. Spent, D.P., and Kim, Y. (1981): Inactivation of complement of *Pseudomonas aeruginosa* mucoid polysaccharide. *CF Club Abstracts*, p. 47.

115. Stein, A.A., Manlapas, F.C., Soike, K.F., and Patterson, P.R. (1964): Specific isoantibodies in cystic fibrosis: a study of serum and bronchial mucus. *J. Pediatr.*, 65:495–500.

116. Strandvik, B., Hjelte, L., Malmborg, A.S., et al. (1992): Home intravenous antibiotic treatment of patients with cystic fibrosis. *Acta. Pediatr.*, 81:340–344.

117. Strunk, R.C., Sieber, O.F., Taussig, L.M., and Gall, E.P. (1977): Serum complement depression during viral lower respiratory tract illness in cystic fibrosis. *Arch. Dis. Child.*, 52:687–690.

118. Suter, S., Schaad, U.B., and Tegner, H. (1986): Levels of free granulocyte elastase in bronchial secretions from patients with cystic fibrosis: effect of antimicrobial treatment against *Pseudomonas aeruginosa*. *J. Infect. Dis.*, 153:902–909.

119. Szaff, M., Hoiby, N., and Flensborg, E.W. (1983): Frequent antibiotic therapy improves survival of cystic fibrosis patients with chronic *Pseudomonas aeruginosa* infection. *Acta. Pediatr. Scand.*, 72:651–657.

120. Tablan, O.C. (1993): Nosocomially acquired *Pseudomonas cepacia* infection in patients with cystic fibrosis. *Infect. Cont. Hosp. Epidemiol.*, 14:124–126.

121. Thomassen, M.J., Boxerbaum, B., Demko, C.A., Kochenbrod, P.J., Dearborn, D.G., and Wood, R.E. (1979): Inhibitory effect of cystic fibrosis serum on *Pseudomonas* phagocytosis by rabbit and human aelvolar macrophages. *Pediatr. Res.*, 13:1085–1088.

122. Thomassen, M.J., Demko, C.A., Stern, R.C., et al. (1986): *Pseudomonas cepacia:* decrease in colonization in cystic fibrosis patients. *Am. Rev. Respir. Dis.*, 134:669–671.

123. Thomassen, M.J., Demko, C.A., Wood, R.E., et al. (1980): Ultrastructure and function of alveolar macrophages in cystic fibrosis patients. *Pediatr. Res.*, 14:715–721.

124. Thomassen, M.J., Klinger, J.D., and Badger, S.J., et al. (1984): Cultures of thoracotomy specimens confirm usefulness of sputum cultures in cystic fibrosis. *J. Pediatr.*, 104:352–356.

125. Valerius, N.H., Koch, C., and Hoiby, N. (1991): Prevention of chronic *Pseudomonas aeruginosa* colonisation in cystic fibrosis by early treatment. *Lancet*, 338:725–726.

126. Vasil, M.L. (1986): *Pseudomonas aeruginosa:* biology, mechanisms of virulence, epidemiology. *J. Pediatr.*, 108(2):800–805.

127. Welch, D.F. (1984): Clinical microbiology of cystic fibrosis. *Clin. Microbiol. Newsl.*, 6:39–42.

128. Welch, D.F., Muszynski, M.J., Pai, C.H., et al. (1987): Selective and differential medium for recovery of *Pseudomonas cepacia* from the respiratory tracts of patients with cystic fibrosis. *J. Clin. Microbiol.*, 25:1730–1734.

129. Wientzen, R., Prestidge, C.B., Kramer, R.I., McCracken, G.H., and Nelson, J.D. (1980): Acute

pulmonary exacerbations in cystic fibrosis. A double-blind trial of tobramycin and placebo therapy. *Am. J. Dis. Child.*, 134:1134–1138.

130. Wilcken, B., and Chalmers, G. (1985): Reduced morbidity in patients with cystic fibrosis detected by neonatal screening. *Lancet,* ii:1319–1321.

131. Woods, D.E., Bass, J.A., Johanson, W.G., and Strauss, D.C. (1980): Role of adherence in the pathogenesis of *Pseudomonas aeruginosa* lung infection in cystic fibrosis patients. *Infect. Immun.*, 30:694–699.

132. Woods, D.E., and Bryan, L.E. (1985): Studies on the ability of alginate to act as a protective immunogen against infection with *Pseudomonas aeruginosa* in animals. *J. Infect. Dis.*, 151:581–588.

Respiratory Infections: Diagnosis and Management, 3d ed.,
edited by James E. Pennington.
Raven Press, Ltd., New York © 1994

18

Gram-Positive Pneumonia

Barry M. Farr and Gerald L. Mandell

*Department of Internal Medicine, University of Virginia Health Sciences Center,
Charlottesville, Virginia 22908*

Once feared as a rapidly fatal disease of unknown cause, pneumonia was personified by Osler as "the captain of the men of death." The microbial etiology of pneumonia was established a century ago by Klebs, Koch, Fraenkel, and Friedlander. The predominance of gram-positive cocci among causative microbes was demonstrated by Gram in 1884 in a postmortem study of 20 pneumonia patients; this work first described Gram's stain (44). During the following decade Osler meticulously recorded his clinical observations of this disease which at that time caused death in about 30% of patients.

Although no longer regarded as "the captain of the men of death" in the antibiotic era, pneumonia still produces significant morbidity and ranks sixth among the leading causes of mortality in the United States (109). As in the preantibiotic era, gram-positive cocci continue to be responsible for a majority of cases.

ETIOLOGY

Relatively few species of gram-positive cocci are associated with human pneumonia. *Streptococcus pneumoniae* is the documented etiology for approximately one-third of all cases of acute community-acquired pneumonia resulting in hospital admission in developed countries (Table 18-1) and a large proportion of cases in developing countries as well (58,100,111). Patients with pneumonia of undetermined etiology (30–50% of patients in prospective studies employing blood and sputum cultures and serologic tests on all patients) have closely resembled patients with pneumococcal pneumonia in age and sex distribution, mean leukocyte count, and proportion with chest pain, but have been more likely to have received prior antibiotic therapy (30); these data suggest that many of the cases of undetermined etiology may, in fact, be due to *S. pneumoniae*. *Staphylococcus aureus* is also a significant cause of pneumonia, although with a much lower incidence than the pneumococcus.

S. pyogenes and other streptococci have been demonstrated to cause pneumonia rarely; the other streptococci include nonpneumococcal α-hemolytic streptococci (streptococci of the viridans group) (107) and β-hemolytic streptococci in group C (79,99,102,104,117) and group G (123,125). The group B streptococcus is an important etiologic agent of pneumonia in the neonate and has caused rare cases in adults

TABLE 18–1. *Etiologic agents identified in prospective studies in patients with community-acquired pneumonia admitted to hospital (27,29,42,45,57–59,65,100,104)*

	No. studies	No. tested	No. positive	Relative frequency (95% CI)	Range
Bacterial Agents					
S. pneumoniae	10	2,203	584	27% (24.7–28.4%)	8.6–76%
M. pneumoniae	8	1,805	140	8% (6.5–9.0%)	0–18%
H. influenzae	9	1,934	118	6% (5.0–7.2%)	0–12%
Aerobic gram-negative bacilli	10	2,203	126	6% (4.7–6.7%)	0.8–21%
Chlamydia pneumoniae (TWAR)	2	660	40	6% (4.2–7.9%)	6.0–6.1%
L. pneumophila	6	1,530	67	4% (3.4–5.4%)	1–15%
S. aureus	10	2,203	82	4% (2.9–4.5%)	1–9%
C. psittaci	6	1,056	25	2% (1.5–3.3%)	0–6%
C. burnetti	7	1,357	11	1% (0.3–1.3%)	0.8–3%
Viral Agents					
Influenza A	8	1,532	130	8% (7.1–9.9%)	5–15%
Parainfluenza	7	1,405	32	2% (1.5–3.1%)	0–12%
Influenza B	6	1,061	11	1% (0.4–1.6%)	0.8–4%
Respiratory synctial virus	6	1,366	15	1% (0.5–1.7%)	0.6–2%
Adenovirus	7	1,231	9	0.7% (0.3–1.2%)	0.2–3%

(27,124). *Corynebacterium* Group JK, better known for its association with cases of device-associated bacteremia, endocarditis, meningitis, and osteomyelitis, has also been reported to cause rare cases of pneumonia (127). Another diphtheroid-like organism recognized as a rare cause of pneumonia is *Rhodococcus equi* (69).

Gram-positive pneumonia caused by such organisms as *Bacillus anthracis, Mycobacterium tuberculosis, Actinomyces israelli,* and *Nocardia asteroides* will be discussed elsewhere. Gram-positive anaerobic cocci such as peptococcus and peptostreptococcus are frequently seen in the mixed anaerobic infection of aspiration pneumonia and also will be discussed elsewhere.

EPIDEMIOLOGY

The true incidence of the various gram-positive pneumonias is unknown. However, epidemiologic studies have suggested an annual incidence of pneumococcal pneumonia of up to two cases per 1,000 in the general population of the United States. Reasonable estimates indicate as many as 200,000 to 500,000 cases per year of pneumococcal pneumonia comprising 30 to 50% of all community-acquired bacterial pneumonia (Table 18-1). In the past the pneumococcus has caused less than

3% of all nosocomial pneumonias (56,58,131). During the past decade two studies have suggested a higher rate of nosocomial pneumococcal pneumonia in veterans' hospitals (12,22), however; and nosocomial rates have risen in other hospitals as well in the past 5 years, accounting for 6.5% of nosocomial pneumonias in the National Nosocomial Infection Surveillance Program between 1986 and 1990 (59). Penicillin-resistant nosocomial pneumococcal pneumonia has occurred and may be an increasing problem.

Certain occupational groups exhibit higher annual rates; these include military recruits (25 cases/1,000), painters (42 cases/1,000), and welders (12 cases/1,000) (82). The highest reported occupationally related incidence has been among neophyte gold miners in South Africa, where 90 cases/1,000 have been recorded (5). Increased annual attack rates have also been described in the elderly (14 cases/1,000), in recipients of renal or bone marrow transplants (72,129), and in patients with AIDS (98). The exact incidence of pneumonia due to *S. aureus* and *S. pyogenes* is unknown, but staphylococcal pneumonia seems to account for about 2 to 5% of cases occurring in outpatients and up to 16% of nosocomial pneumonias (56,59,68). *S. pyogenes*, which reportedly caused 5% of pneumonia cases in the preantibiotic era, now accounts for less than 1% of all cases, and pneumonia caused by other streptococci is rare (40). Mixed infections due to aerobic pathogens account for less than 10% of cases (20,21,51).

CARRIAGE RATES

Each of the gram-positive cocci associated with pneumonia can be carried in the upper respiratory tract in asymptomatic individuals. The rates and sites of carriage vary among the different organisms.

Pneumococci are carried in the pharynx of over 60% of infants, 25% of children, and in about 5% of childless adults (46,49,53). The rates are increased in crowded conditions and closed populations, such as in military barracks and the gold mining camps of South Africa. There is evidence that carriage rates are higher in winter than in summer months (118), corresponding to the observed higher rates of pneumococcal pneumonia in winter. The organism spreads from person to person but the exact method of transmission is unknown. Large-particle aerosol inhalation or hand contact may be important. Pneumococcal pneumonia occurs 50% more often in men than in women, but whether or not this difference relates to a difference in carriage rates is not known because information on carriage rates by sex is not available (49,53).

S. aureus is most often carried in the nasal vestibule. As in pneumococci, infants have the highest carriage rate (40 to 90%), with a decline after 6 months of age to levels approaching those in adults (48). About 15 to 30% of adults are persistently colonized, whereas the remainder of the population have intermittent, transient colonizations. Transfer of nasal secretions from the hands of a staphylococcal carrier to the hands of uncolonized individuals with subsequent autoinoculation of the nose is believed to be the principal mode of transmission (48). The unwashed hands of health care workers appear to be the vector of *S. aureus* from patient to patient in the hospital (41).

S. pyogenes is carried in the pharynx of about 20% of children (14). Carriage rates in adults are about one-sixth of that in children (25). The exact method of transmission is unknown but presumed to relate to large-particle aerosol inhalation or hand contact (8). Approximately 9% of family members exposed to an index carrier will acquire the organism and develop pharyngeal carriage (25). Carriage rates are increased under crowded conditions such as in military barracks, but epidemics of β-hemolytic streptococcal pneumonia are extremely rare (14,40).

Group C streptococcus is carried in the pharynx of about 3 to 11% of the population, but some infections may be acquired from sick animals (79,117,122). Group G streptococcus is also isolated in approximately 2% of all pharyngeal cultures (123). Viridans streptococci are part of the normal human oral flora.

The gram-positive coccal pneumonias occur more frequently during the winter and the early spring, related either to increased carriage rates of these cocci in the upper respiratory tract as a result of crowding indoors during inclement weather or to the increased incidence of viral respiratory infection during this season. About one-third of patients with pneumococcal pneumonia have a history of a prior upper respiratory infection (34,51,119). Influenza season usually runs from December through February. Coronavirus infections peak in mid-winter, followed by increased rhinovirus activity in the early spring.

Bacterial pulmonary superinfection complicating viral influenza deserves special mention. These cases occur in patients younger and with less underlying disease than pneumonia patients without prior influenza. The pneumococcus remains the most frequent pathogen, accounting for about 46% of cases in two studies, but staphylococcal pneumonia is significantly increased in incidence, being found in up to 20% of these patients (15,110). *S. pyogenes,* although still a relatively rare cause of pneumonia in these patients, can occur in younger adult patients following influenza or measles (40,80). Group C streptococcal pneumonia has also been reported following episodes of bronchitis (117).

The incidence of staphylococcal pneumonia has been reported to be higher in patients institutionalized in mental health care facilities and nursing homes (36,86,97). There is also an increased incidence among hospitalized patients, especially intubated neurosurgical patients (32,66). Group B streptococcal pneumonia usually occurs in patients with predisposing conditions such as diabetes mellitus, central nervous system (CNS) disorders, and chronic obstructive pulmonary disease (27). Group G streptococcal pneumonia has usually been reported in patients with malignancy or alcoholism (123).

The diphtheroid *Rhodococcus equi* causes pneumonia in immunosuppressed patients with AIDS, cancer chemotherapy, or organ transplants (69). Corynebacterium JK has also primarily involved immunosuppressed patients, especially those with hematologic malignancy or bone marrow transplants (127).

PATHOGENESIS

The majority of cases of pneumonia caused by gram-positive cocci appear to follow aspiration of these microorganisms from the upper respiratory tract to the lungs. A small percentage of cases results from hematogenous embolization to the lungs from primary extrapulmonary infections. This is most often seen with staphylococcal infections, especailly endocarditis or septic thrombophlebitis (85,87).

Inhalation of airborne gram-positive cocci will not usually result in pneumonia, presumably because of effective host defenses including filtration, the cough reflex, the mucociliary mechanism, alveolar macrophages, neutrophils, antibody, and complement. Particles smaller than 10 μm may escape upper airway filtration but are usually trapped in mucus lining the lower respiratory tract and swept back into the pharynx on the mucus blanket at a rate of 2 cm/hr.

Aspiration of upper respiratory tract secretions containing colonizing pathogens is prevented in the normal host by intact epiglottic and cough reflexes. These reflexes are impaired by alteration of consciousness, as demonstrated by the fact that small amounts of secretions may be aspirated during sleep in 45% of normal individuals (57). Aspiration of large volumes of oral or nasopharyngeal secretions can result in pneumonia; this often occurs with alcohol abuse, anesthesia, narcotic intoxication, hypothermia, tracheal intubation, tracheostomy, nasogastric suction, protracted emesis, cerebral infarction, seizures, and other disorders of the central nervous system. Acute bacterial pneumonia starts most commonly in the most dependent pulmonary segments, into which aspirated fluid drains; these include the basilar segments of both lower lobes, the right middle lobe, and the posterior segments of the upper lobes (11).

Prior or concomitant viral infection can potentiate the pneumonitic process in several ways. It has been demonstrated that mucin-containing fluids, which are similar to upper respiratory secretions produced during viral coryza, provide the most efficient vehicle for producing experimental pneumonia via bronchial instillation of the bacterial pathogen. These secretions also provide a medium suitable for replication to higher titer in the upper airway prior to aspiration. Influenza virus may further potentiate this process by denuding the respiratory epithelium and thereby interrupting the mucociliary cleansing mechanism and preventing removal of aspirated secretions. The mucociliary cleansing apparatus can also be impaired in smokers and in patients with such congenital conditions as cystic fibrosis or the immotile cilia syndrome.

Dry, air-filled alveoli constitute an unfavorable environment for bacterial replication. It has been shown experimentally that filling these terminal airspaces with fluid greatly enhances the tendency to pneumonia (50); this occurs with aspiration of fluid, congestive heart failure, and noncardiogenic pulmonary edema, including that caused by viral infections such as influenza. With bacterial replication, further exudation of fluid takes place, allowing for spread of the infection through the pores of Kohn and terminal bronchioles.

If preexisting antibodies are present or if the microbe activates the alternative complement pathway, the microbes are opsonized, promoting efficient phagocytosis and limiting spread of the infection. With the pneumococcus, specific antibodies usually develop within 5 to 10 days and patients become essentially immune to reinfection with the particular serotype of pneumococcus. Patients with hypogammaglobulinemia or with multiple myeloma can have recurrent infections with the same type of pneumococcus because of lack of appropriate antibody formation. Patients with complement defects such as those with inherited deficiencies of C3 suffer from recurrent pneumococcal infections (24,47). Also, the defect in the alternative pathway of complement activation seen in sickle-cell disease is associated with recurrent pneumonia.

Polymorphonuclear neutrophils adhere to pulmonary venular endothelium, then migrate into the incipient alveolar exudate, trapping bacteria against the alveolar walls to permit surface phagocytosis (130). This vast outpouring of neutrophils into the exudate imparts the characteristic yellowish-green color to purulent sputum. The early phase of exudate formation is accompanied by a significant amount of erythrocytic diapedesis as well, especially in pneumococcal pneumonia, giving the sputum a blood-tinged or rust color and correlating with the gross pathologic state of "red hepatization." Polymorphonuclear leukocytic and monocytic bactericidal activity can be significantly depressed by influenza virus (1).

The alveolar macrophages ingest alveolar debris and then ascend the mucociliary escalator, which transports them to the pharynx. During this stage the consolidated lung, filled with macrophages and degenerating neutrophils, gives the gross appearance known as "gray hepatization."

When host defenses fail to contain replicating bacteria, there is spread via the thoracic duct to the bloodstream. Bacteremia is detected on presentation in about 25% of cases of pneumococcal pneumonia, about 7% of group A streptococcal pneumonia, and 25% of exogenous staphylococcal pneumonia (6,40). Staphylococcal pneumonia caused by hematogenous spread from another site is associated with bacteremia in 90% of cases if the site is right-sided endocarditis, and in 20 to 50% of cases if the site is septic thrombophlebitis or an infected vascular prosthesis (13).

Bacteria can also spread via lymphatic channels to the pleural space. Pneumococcal pneumonia is complicated by empyema in about 1% of cases, although sterile pleural effusions can occur in up to 25% (82). Parapneumonic effusions are found in about half of patients with staphylococcal pneumonia, and empyema with 10% to 25% (64). Thirty to 40% of group A streptococcal pneumonias are complicated by empyema (40,126).

The pneumococcus produces several toxins of uncertain significance in the pathogenesis of pneumonia; these include neuraminidase, the hemolytic toxin pneumolysin, and a "purpura producing principle." Capsule thickness does correlate with virulence, probably by protecting against phagocytosis.

Despite the toxins elaborated by *S. pneumoniae* and the intense inflammatory response, pneumococcal pneumonia almost never proceeds to necrosis of alveolar architecture or abscess formation (132). By contrast, staphylococcal pneumonia can be associated with such necrosis and abscesses in 15 to 25% of cases (64,126). Abscesses have also been reported with group A streptococcal pneumonia (40). Pulmonary necrosis can thus relate to the many proteolytic toxins elaborated by *S. aureus* and *S. pyogenes* (14,126).

CLINICAL MANIFESTATIONS

History

Pneumococcal pneumonia classically involves a middle-aged or elderly patient, but *S. pneumoniae* is also the most frequent etiologic agent of bacterial pneumonia in infants, children, and young adults (65). A sudden dramatic rigor is often the first symptom followed by sustained high fever and localized pleuritic chest pain, which can be severe (10). Recurrent shaking chills are occasionally noted, but can also be produced by antipyretic administration. Cough develops in up to 90% of patients, usually becoming productive of rust-colored, purulent sputum (52). Dyspnea, weakness, malaise, and myalgias are often present. Many patients complain of anorexia, one-third have nausea and vomiting, and 14% complain of diarrhea (51,52). Febrile, hypoxic elderly patients occasionally develop organic brain syndrome and can be referred by a relative who has observed disorientation.

Physical Examination

The patient can be agitated, cyanotic, and in acute respiratory distress with inter-costal retractions and flaring alae nasi. Most patients are tachypneic, tachycardiac, and febrile (mean temperature = 38°C ± 0.8, S.D.), and the pulse pressure is often exaggerated. Shock can be manifested by profound hypotension. The skin is often flushed, warm, and diaphoretic and, rarely, jaundiced; the mucosae can be cyanotic, depending on the degree of pulmonary vascular shunting. Herpes labialis is present in about 10% of all patients with pneumonia regardless of the microbial etiology (51). Jugular vein distension and dependent edema are often present as signs of congestive cardiac failure, which has been described as both a predisposing factor and a com-plication of bacterial pneumonia. Tracheal deviation can be noted as a result of a large empyema or tension pneumothorax.

Chest wall movement can be asymmetric because of splinting of the involved side, which can also exhibit local tenderness to percussion. Early cases can exhibit only localized fine inspiratory crackles (rales), but there is usually progression to include some if not all of the following abnormalities: dullness to percussion, increased tac-tile fremitus, palpable or audible pleural friction rub, whispered pectoriloquy, bron-chophony or egophony, and bronchial breath sounds. Pleural effusion or empyema is often evidenced by dullness to percussion, decreased tactile fremitus, and dimin-ished breath sounds at the base of the lung.

Cardiac examination often reveals a soft (grade I to II/VI) systolic ejection murmur over the left lower sternal border as a result of increased cardiac output. A holosys-tolic murmur radiating to the axilla or a diastolic blowing murmur along the left sternal border could indicate complicating endocarditis. A ventricular gallop is sometimes present with congestive failure, and a pericardial knock or 3-component friction rub can be heard with pericarditis. Abdominal examination could reveal acute gastric dilation and ileus. Referred pain in the epigastrium occasionally sug-gests an intraabdominal process. Rebound tenderness and abdominal rigidity could be present if peritonitis is a complication.

Joint swelling, erythema, and tenderness could suggest complicating infectious arthritis or crystal-induced arthropathies, which occur more commonly with dehy-dration which can accompany pneumonia. Nuchal rigidity and Kernig's sign can be present with meningitis, and focal neurologic abnormalities with a brain abscess.

It is usually impossible to distinguish pneumonia due to *S. pneumoniae* from that due to *S. aureus, S. pyogenes,* and the other streptococci on the basis of history and physical examination (30,68). Knowledge of the epidemiologic correlates discussed above, however, should arouse clinical suspicion in the appropriate setting (40,86). Staphylococcal skin lesions can be a clue to the presence of staphylococcal pneu-monia in up to 40% of cases (usually with the embolic type of pneumonitis) (126).

Laboratory

Leukocytosis (mean WBC = 15,000 cells/mm^3 ± 8,000 S.D.), with neutrophilia and an increased percentage of immature granulocytes, is seen in most patients, although leukopenia with a left shift can occur in patients with fulminant disease. Serum bilirubin is occasionally elevated as a result of intrahepatic cholestasis or secondary to hemolysis caused by glucose-6-phosphate dehydrogenase deficiency.

Posteroanterior and lateral chest radiographs (see Figs. 18-1, 18-2, and 18-3) usually demonstrate a patchy bronchopneumonia and less often a "classic" segmental or lobar consolidation (39,89). Thus, most pneumococcal pneumonia is not lobar, but most lobar pneumonia is still pneumococcal. It is not usually possible at the time of initial radiography to differentiate the pneumonias caused by the various gram-positive cocci; in fact, it may be difficult to differentiate bacterial from nonbacterial pneumonia (23,67,121). Although cavitating pneumonia is extremely rare with *S. pneumoniae,* this radiologic appearance ("pseudocavitation") can be simulated in older patients with prior emphysema (115,132,133). Abscess formation develops in 15 to 25% of cases of staphylococcal pneumonia (64,126) and has also been reported with *S. pyogenes* pneumonia (40).

Pleural effusions are usually reported to be present in about 25% of cases of pneumococcal pneumonia, but repetitive radiography with decubitus views can find small effusions in up to 57% (120). Effusions are reported in 25 to 50% of staphylococcal pneumonias (64,126).

Staphylococcal pneumonia secondary to septic embolization from right-sided endocarditis, an infected arteriovenous fistula, or septic thrombophlebitis yields a characteristic radiographic appearance with multiple nummular lesions that expand and cavitate within days. Thin-walled pneumatoceles may form with either bronchopneumonia or lobar pneumonia (88,90).

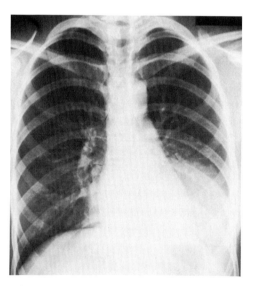
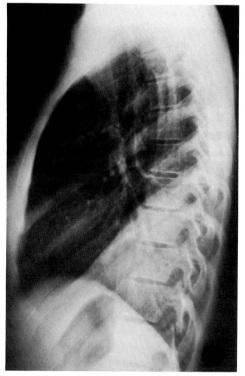

FIG. 18–1. These posteroanterior and lateral radiographs demonstrate a lobar ("typical") pneumococcal pneumonia involving the left lower lobe. Lobar consolidation was the most frequent pattern of pneumococcal pneumonia in the preantibiotic era. (Courtesy of Dr. T.L. Pope, Department of Radiology, University of Virginia.)

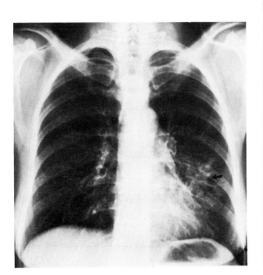
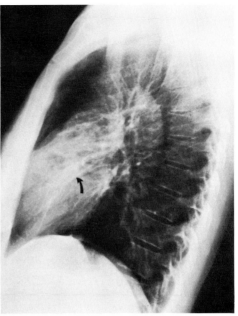

FIG. 18–2. These posteroanterior and lateral radiographs show a patchy ("atypical") pneumococcal bronchopneumonia in the lingula; this is the pattern seen in a majority of pneumococcal pneumonias in the antibiotic era. (Courtesy of Dr. T.L. Pope, Department of Radiology, University of Virginia.)

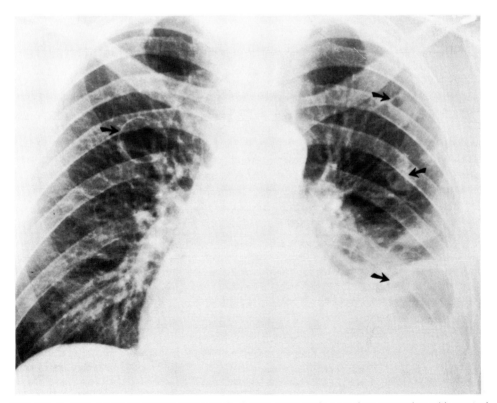

FIG. 18–3. This posteroanterior radiograph shows metastatic round pneumonias with central cavitation in a patient with endocarditis due to *Staphylococcus aureus*. (Courtesy of Dr. T.L. Pope, Department of Radiology, University of Virginia.)

ETIOLOGIC DIAGNOSIS

Examination of the sputum is one of the most important steps in the determination of the causative agent (16,37,38,62). Patients with a dry cough are often able to produce sputum after sitting forward, after chest percussion, or after ultrasonic hypertonic saline nebulation. Approximately 80% of patients hospitalized for pneumonia will produce sputum (51). The quantity and quality of sputum production should be noted. Saliva is not acceptable for analysis. Gram stain of purulent sputum will reveal many granulocytes (pink if appropriately decolorized) and very few oral squamous epithelial cells. The findings of >25 granulocytes and <10 squamous epithelial cells per low power (100×) field has yielded cultural results for expectorated sputum similar to those obtained using culture of transtracheal aspirates (37). If a preponderance of lancet-shaped gram-positive cocci (i.e., pneumococci) is seen with more than 10 cocci per oil immersion field, then the sensitivity for detecting pneumococci in the sputum is about 62% and the specificity about 85% (101). If gram-positive, lancet-shaped diplococci are seen, quellung reaction with Omniserum (which contains rabbit antibodies to 82 pneumococcal serotypes) may be confirmatory (77). Type 3 pneumococci can exhibit chaining, but diplococcal morphology is usually preserved within the chains. Staphylococci can be identified by the presence of grape-like clusters of cocci. *S. pyogenes* or other streptococci may be present in pairs or chains. A mixed flora can be seen with mixed anaerobic infections in aspiration pneumonia. Occasionally, mixed aerobic-anaerobic infections are seen in these patients. Mixed oral flora can also be present in specimens with salivary contamination.

Sputum culture was once considered the definitive diagnostic procedure in bacterial pneumonia, but studies have shown that sputum culture is only positive for pneumococci in about one-half of patients with pneumonia and pneumococcal bacteremia (9). Similarly, expectorated sputum culture is positive in only about one-half of patients with pneumonia diagnosed as pneumococcal by transtracheal aspiration (10). Higher sensitivity of sputum culture for pneumococci has been reported with anaerobic incubation (26).

Transtracheal aspiration, although potentially useful in occasional cases, is rarely performed because of an unacceptable complication rate. It carries risks of hemorrhage, hypoxemia, arrhythmias, pneumothorax, and asphyxiation, and has resulted in death. This procedure is contraindicated in patients with coagulopathies, thrombocytopenia, thrombocytopathy (as occurs in uremia), severe hypoxemia, and severe cough. Actively uncooperative patients should not undergo this procedure because of possible injury (116).

A variety of rapid diagnostic tests have been used to identify pneumococcal polysaccharide in sputum, blood, or urine. Counterimmunoelectrophoresis (CIE), for example, can be performed in 2 to 3 hours and is positive in about one-half of the patients with nonbacteremic pneumococcal pneumonia when performed on both urine and serum, and in half of bacteremic patients when performed only on serum. Sputum CIE is positive in about three-fourths of pneumonia patients with a positive pneumococcal culture, but unlike the culture can remain positive after antibiotic therapy (51,78,106). The overall sensitivity in urine is about 50% and in serum about 10%, but these values would be higher in the subset with bacteremia. The CIE can give positive results with sputum from patients with chronic bronchitis but does not give positive results on respiratory secretions of patients with colds and pharyngeal pneumococcal carriage. In one large study the rate of positive-sputum CIE results for pneumococcal antigen was not higher in patients with a history of chronic bronchitis than it was in patients who did not have chronic bronchitis (51). Latex agglutination, coagglutination, and enzyme-linked immunoassay (ELISA) tests have also been studied and appear to be more sensitive and as specific as the CIE in diagnosing the microbial etiology of pneumonia. From these data it appears that antigen detection by one of these methods could be a useful adjunctive test, especially when sputum is unavailable, as in the pediatric patient, or when antibiotics have already been started which can quickly render cultures negative (78,82).

Serologic studies can also be useful in diagnosing pneumonia due to *S. pyogenes* in which antistreptolysin O or anti-DNase B titers are elevated. A simple slide hemagglutination test (Streptozyme) appears to have equal sensitivity to the usual battery of antistreptococcal antibody tests (14). Teichoic acid antibodies are usually present in significant titers with staphylococcal pneumonia occurring as a complication of staphylococcal endocarditis (63), but the diagnosis is usually clear from culture results.

COMPLICATIONS

Patients with pneumonia caused by the gram-positive cocci could develop any of a number of complications. Respiratory complications include empyema, adult respiratory distress syndrome, and respiratory failure. Meningitis, endocarditis, arthritis, peritonitis, cellulitis, and brain abscess have all been reported (75). Rarely, patients with pneumococcal pneumonia present with simultaneous endocarditis and meningitis (Austrian's syndrome). A fulminant pneumococcal septicemia with rapid demise occurs in asplenic individuals and sickle-cell anemia patients. Disseminated intravascular coagulation can also occur in such patients.

DIAGNOSIS

Fever, leukocytosis with an increase of immature granulocytes, and purulent sputum with neutrophils and gram-positive bacteria on gram stain in a patient with a new pulmonary infiltrate strongly indicate acute pneumonia caused by gram-positive organisms. An accurate gram stain is of paramount importance in differentiating gram-positive cocci from other etiologic agents that can cause the same syndrome, such as *Hemophilus influenzae*.

A detailed discussion of techniques for making an etiologic diagnosis is presented elsewhere. Multiple diseases can occasionally mimic acute bacterial pneumonia. These include acute febrile bronchitis, pulmonary infarction, collagen-vascular disease, drug-induced pneumonitis, toxic pneumonitis, hypersensitivity pneumonitis, lung cancer, eosinophilic pneumonia, and radiation pneumonitis.

TREATMENT

Pneumococcal pneumonia should usually be treated in the hospital setting with parenteral therapy. Penicillin G is the drug of choice given as procaine penicillin, 600,000 units intramuscularly twice/day for 7 to 10 days or as aqueous penicillin G

1 million units intravenously every 4 hours (61,93). Broad-spectrum therapy can pre-dispose to pulmonary superinfection. In patients in shock or with empyema, men-ingitis, arthritis, or endocarditis, intravenous therapy with 20 million units per day of aqueous penicillin G should be administered. Young, reliable adult patients with relatively mild disease can be treated with phenoxymethyl penicillin 500 mg orally every 6 hours. Penicillin-allergic patients can be treated with erythromycin intrave-nously or orally, but susceptibility must be checked because of the increasing prev-alence of *S. pneumoniae* resistant to erythromycin (71). Cephalosporins are also used but with special caution, as about 10% of penicillin-allergic patients can expe-rience allergic reactions to cephalosporins. All cephalosporins have inhibitory activ-ity against the pneumococcus *in vitro* but the activity of cefoxitin, moxalactam, and ceftazadime is much less than that of penicillin, and these antibiotics should not be used to treat known pneumococcal infections. Recent reports of pneumococci with multiple antibiotic resistance have originated from South Africa, Australia, Canada, and the United States (84). These organisms are uniformly susceptible to vancomy-cin. One recent study from France demonstrated that their strains of penicillin-resis-tant pneumococci remained susceptible to cefotaxime (42). The newer macrolides such as clarithromycin and azithromycin are usually active against the gram-positive cocci that cause pneumonia, but they have not been shown to have a significant therapeutic advantage when compared in randomized trials with older, less expen-sive oral antibiotics. Pneumococci resistant to erythromycin are usually also resis-tant to these newer macrolides (71).

Significant pleural effusions should be submitted to diagnostic thoracentesis. This is helpful to establish an etiologic diagnosis, and if empyema is found, intercostal drainage should be considered. Some have suggested that pleural fluid pH below 7.20 suggests the need for surgical drainage (70).

Infections known or presumed to be caused by staphylococci should be treated with a penicillinase-resistant penicillin pending susceptibility data (e.g., nafcillin 1.5g intravenously every 4 hours in adults) except in settings with a high prevalence of methicillin-resistant *S. aureus* (MRSA), which would require vancomycin therapy (1g intravenously q 12 in adults with normal renal function). *S. pyogenes* and other streptococci can be effectively treated with 20 million units per day of penicillin G. For penicillin-allergic patients erythromycin has been used as an alternative, but the clinician should be aware of an increasing prevalence of resistance to erythromycin by *S. pyogenes* isolates (103).

Initial antibiotic therapy of pneumonia due to diphtheroids should be with vanco-mycin; for cases due to *Corynebacterium* vancomycin is the drug of choice; for *Rhodococcus,* which causes infection more frequently in horses than humans, eryth-romycin plus rifampin has been the choice for treatment of equine infections with very low mortality rates as compared with other possible regimens (45). Vancomycin can be used for patients who cannot tolerate erythromycin.

Ancillary therapy of the pneumonia patient includes careful monitoring of arterial blood gases and administration of supplemental oxygen when needed. Acute respi-ratory failure requires intubation and mechanical ventilation. Severe pleuritic pain might require meperidine or codeine analgesia, or even an intercostal block with a long-acting local anesthetic such as bupivacaine to relieve pain and improve the pa-tient's cough efficacy. Antipyretics should usually be avoided, as temperature is a good index of response to therapy. Dehydration should be treated with intravenous fluids. Congestive failure could be present, requiring vasodilator and inotropic ther-

apy. Shock necessitates pulmonary artery catheterization for adequate hemodynamic monitoring and therapy. Gastrectasia and ileus would require bowel rest and
nasogastric suction.

Although dramatic response to therapy is often seen, the median duration of fever
is 3 days for pneumococcal pneumonia; up to a week could be required for complete
defervescence (32,51). Longer periods of fever could suggest a mistaken diagnosis,
loculated fluid, an extrapulmonary focus of infection, or a resistant organism. Recurrence of fever after an initial response could be caused by drug fever or superinfection. Complete resolution of radiographic infiltrates could require longer than
6 weeks even in uncomplicated cases of pneumococcal pneumonia (51,60). Resolution of radiographic infiltrate is age dependent; 80% of patients under 35 years
of age resolve their infiltrate in 6 weeks as compared with 40% of those above 65
years of age.

Respiratory isolation is generally regarded as unnecessary for pneumococcal infection, but several outbreaks have been reported in institutional settings such as
jails, boarding houses, and military barracks in recent years (19). Contact isolation
is required for staphylococcal and other streptococcal pneumonias. This involves
wearing a mask when close to the patient (i.e., within 5 feet), wearing a gown if
soiling is likely, and wearing gloves, for touching infective secretions. Care should
be exercised by care-givers to avoid self-contamination in handling respiratory secretions.

PROGNOSIS

The case fatality rate of pneumococcal pneumonia in the preantibiotic era was
about 30%. With antibiotic treatment this rate has fallen to 5 to 10% (51). With pneumococcal bacteremia the case fatality rate has ranged from 10 (51,60) to 30%
(6,43,55,83). The case fatality rate for staphylococcal pneumonia was 50 to 90% in
the preantibiotic era and has remained as high as 20% with therapy (64).

PREVENTION

Because of the continued morbidity and mortality resulting from pneumococcal
pneumonia despite the easy availability of effective antibiotics, interest has rekindled
in the pneumococcal vaccine (2,4,94,96). The vaccine now licensed in the United
States contains antigens from 23 serotypes of pneumococci: 1, 2, 3, 4, 5, 6B, 7F, 8,
9N, 9V, 10A, I IA, 12F, 14, 15B, 17F, 18C, 19A, 19F, 20, 22F, 23F, and 33F. These
types account for about 85% of cases of bacteremic pneumococcal infection in the
United States. The vaccine has been shown to produce antibody responses in about
85% of those vaccinated. The response to vaccination is poorer in those with impaired immune systems. The vaccine has been proven to be effective in eliciting
antibodies in normal volunteers and will produce antibody rises (although dim-
inshed) in splenectomized patients. It is not effective in children under 2 years of
age. It has therefore been recommended for persons over 2 years of age without a
spleen or with splenic dysfunction (as in sickle-cell anemia) or with certain other
chronic diseases: diabetes mellitus, chronic cardiopulmonary disease, renal failure,
nephrotic syndrome, and liver disease. It is also recommended for patients over 50
years of age without chronic disease.

Pneumococcal vaccine has been shown to be an effective prophylaxis against pneumococcal pneumonia due to vaccine-type strains in randomized, controlled trials in South African gold miners, and in natives in Papua, New Guinea. These groups differ greatly from the civilian patients at high risk of pneumococcal disease in the United States. Three randomized, controlled trials have been conducted in middle-aged to elderly adults in the U.S. encompassing 44,042 person-years and 874 cases of pneumonia without demonstrating either a reduction in the number of cases of pneumonia or of pneumonia mortality (18,114). Two retrospective studies have suggested an efficacy of about 65% in prevention of pneumococcal bacteremia (17,113). A third retrospective study showed no benefit (35). The largest case control study to date showed 56% efficacy in preventing bacteremic pneumococcal infection (85% of cases were associated with pneumonia); efficacy in immunocompetent patients (61%) was higher than in immunosuppressed patients (21%) (112). It seems prudent to administer the vaccine to those at higher risk of pneumococcal infections.

Pneumococcal vaccine is injected intramuscularly or subcutaneously at a dose of 0.5 ml. Most patients experience local reactions such as soreness and induration. Occasionally fever is noted. Rarely, serious anaphylactoid reactions have been described. Revaccination appears to be safer than originally believed and is now recommended for those without a spleen or with other conditions associated with a rapid fall in pneumococcal antibodies (e.g., after 3 to 5 years in children under 10 years of age with nephrotic syndrome, asplenia, or sickle-cell anemia; and after 6 years in adults with nephrotic syndrome, renal failure, or an organ transplant) (19,95).

Annual influenza vaccine is indicated for much the same patient group described as candidates for the pneumococcal vaccine. Such prophylaxis of influenza can reduce the rates of pneumococcal, staphylococcal, and streptococcal pneumonias. Retrospective data suggest that influenza vaccination prevents hospitalization and deaths (7,92,93). Splenectomized children often require prophylactic penicillin in addition to the above immunizations because of their unique susceptibility to pneumococcal bacteremia; this risk appears to be lower in the splenectomized adult.

REFERENCES

1. Abramson, J.S., Mills, E.L., and Giebink, G.S. (1982): Depression of monocyte and polymorphonuclear leukocyte oxidative metabolism and bactericidal capacity by influenza A virus. *Infect. Immun.*, 35:350–355.
2. Austrian, R. (1981): Pneumococcus: the first one hundred years. *Rev. Infect. Dis.*, 3:183–188.
3. Austrian, R. (1981): Pneumonia in the later years. *J. Am. Geriatr. Soc.*, 29:481–489.
4. Austrian, R. (1981): Some observations on the pneumococcus and on the current status of pneumococcal disease and its prevention. *Rev. Infect. Dis.*, 3(Suppl.):S1–S17.
5. Austrian, R., Douglas, R.M., Schiffman, G., Coetzee, A.M., Koornhof, H.J., Hayden-Smith, S., and Reid, R.D. (1976): Prevention of pneumococcal pneumonia by vaccination. *Trans. Assoc. Am. Physicians*, 89:184–194.
6. Austrian, R., and Gold, J. (1964): Pneumococcal bacteremia with especial reference to bacteremic pneumococcal pneumonia. *Ann. Intern. Med.*, 60:759–776.
7. Barker, W.M., and Mullooly J.P. (1980): Influenza vaccination of elderly persons: reduction in pneumonia and influenza hospitalization and deaths. *J.A.M.A.*, 244:2547–2549.
8. Barnham, M., and Kerby, J. (1981): Streptococcus pyogenes pneumonia in residential homes: probable spread of infection from the staff. *J. Hosp. Infect.*, 2:255–257.
9. Barrett-Conner, E. (1971): The nonvalue of sputum culture in the diagnosis of pneumococcal pneumonia. *Am. Rev. Respir. Dis.*, 103:845–848.
10. Bartlett, J.G. (1979): Anaerobic bacterial pneumonitis. *Am. Rev. Respir. Dis.*, 119:19–23.

11. Bartlett, J.G., and Finegold, S.M. (1974): Anaerobic infections in the lung and pleural space. *Am. Rev. Respir. Dis.*, 110:56–77.

12. Bartlett, J.G., O'Keefe, P., Tally, F.P., Louie, T.J., Gorbach, S.L., et al. (1986): Bacteriology of hospital-acquired pneumonia. *Arch. Intern. Med.*, 146:868–871.

13. Bayer, A.S., and Guze, L.B. (1979): *Staphylococcus aureus* bacteremic syndromes: diagnostic and therapeutic update. *D.M.*, 25:1–42.

14. Bisno, A.L. (1990): *Streptococcus pyogenes.* In: *Principles and Practice of Infectious Diseases,* 3rd Edition, edited by G. L. Mandell, R. G. Douglas, and J. E. Bennett, pp. 1519–1528. John Wiley and Sons, New York.

15. Bisno, A.L., Griffin, J.P., Van Epps, K.A., Niell, H.B., and Rytel, M.W. (1971): Pneumonia and Hong Kong influenza: a prospective study of the 1968–1969 epidemic. *Am. J. Med. Sci.*, 261:251–263.

16. Boerner, D.F., and Zwadyk, P. (1982): The value of the sputum gram's stain in community-acquired pneumonia. *J.A.M.A.*, 247:642–645.

17. Bolan, G., Broome, C.V., Facklam, R.R., Plikaytis, B.D., Fraser, D.W., and Schlech, W.F. (1986): Pneumococcal vaccine efficacy in selected populations in the United States. *Ann. Intern. Med.*, 104:1–6.

18. Broome, C.V. (1981): Efficacy of pneumococcal polysaccharide vaccines. *Rev. Infect. Dis.*, 3:S82–S96.

19. Broome, C.V., and Breiman, R.F. (1991): Pneumococcal vaccine—past, present, and future. *N. Engl. J. Med.*, 325:1506–1508.

20. Brown, R.B., Sands, M., and Morris, A.B. (1993): Community-acquired pneumonia caused by mixed aerobic pathogens. *Infect. Dis. Clin. Prac.*, 2:32–39.

21. Brown, R.B., Sands, M., and Ryczak, M. (1986): Community-acquired pneumonia caused by mixed aerobic bacteria. *Chest*, 90:810–814.

22. Schleupner, C.J., and Cobb, D.K. (1992). A study of the etiologies and treatment of nosocomial pneumonia in a community-based teaching hospital. *Infect. Control. Hosp. Epidemiol.* 13;9: 515–525.

23. Courtoy, I., Lande, A.E., and Turner, R.B. (1989): Accuracy of radiographic differentiation of bacterial from nonbacterial pneumonia. *Clin. Peds.*, 28:261–264.

24. Densen, P. (1990): Complement. In: *Principles and Practice of Infectious Diseases,* 3rd Edition, edited by G. L. Mandell, R. G. Douglas, and J. E. Bennett, pp. 62–81. John Wiley and Sons, New York.

25. Dingle, J.H., Badger, G.G., and Jordan, W.S., Jr. (1964): *Illness in the Home: A Study of 25,000 Illnesses in a Group of Cleveland Families.* The Press of Western Reserve University, Cleveland, Ohio.

26. Drew, W.L. (1977): Value of sputum culture in diagnosis of pneumococcal pneumonia. *J. Clin. Microbiol.*, 6:52–55.

27. Dworzack, D.L., Hodges, G.R., Barnes, W.G., and Rosett, W. (1979): Group B streptococcal infections in adult males. *Am. J. Med. Sci.*, 277:67–73.

28. Espersen, F., and Gabrielsen, J. (1981): Pneumonia due to *Staphylococcus aureus* during mechanical ventilation. *J. Infect. Dis.*, 144:19–23.

29. Fang, G.D., Fine, M., Orloff, J., Arisumi, D., Yu, V., Kapoor, W., Grayston, J.T., Wang, S.P., Kohler, R., Muder, R.R., Yee, U.C., Rihs, J.D., and Vickers, R.M. (1990): New and emerging etiologies for community-acquired pneumonia with implications for therapy. *Medicine*, 69:307–316.

30. Farr, B.M., Kaiser, D.L., Harrison, B.D.W., and Connolly, C.K. (1989): Prediction of microbial aetiology at admission to hospital for pneumonia from the presenting clinical features. *Thorax*, 44:1031–1035.

31. Farr, B.M., Sloman, A.J., and Fisch, M.J. (1991): Predicting death in patients hospitalized for community-acquired pneumonia. *Ann. Int. Med.*, 115:428–436.

32. Fekety, F.R., Caldwell, J., Gump, D., Johnson, J.E., Maxson, W., Mulholland, J., et al. (1971): Bacteria, viruses and mycoplasmas in acute pneumonia in adults. *Am. Rev. Respir. Dis.*, 104:499.

33. Fekety, F.R., Jr., and McDaniel, E. (1968): The fever index in evaluation of the course of infectious diseases with special reference to pneumococcal pneumonia. *Yale J. Biol. Med.*, 41:282–288.

34. Fiala, M. (1969): A study of the combined role of viruses, mycoplasmas, and bacteria in adult pneumonia. *Am. J. Med. Sci.*, 257:44–51.

35. Forrester, H.L., Jahnigen, D.W., and LaForce, F.M. (1987): Inefficacy of pneumococcal vaccine in a high-risk population. *Am. J. Med.*, 83:425–430.

36. Garb, J.L., Brown, R.B., Garb, J.R., and Tuthill, R.W. (1978): Differences in etiology of pneumonias in nursing home and community patients. *J.A.M.A.*, 240:2169–2172.

37. Geckler, R.W., Gremillion, D.H., McAllister, C.K., and Ellenbogen, C. (1977): Microscopic and bacteriological comparison of paired sputa and transtracheal aspirates. *J. Clin. Microbiol.*, 6:396–399.

38. Geckler, R.W., McAllister, C.K., Gremillion, D.H., and Ellenbogen, C. (1985): Clinical value of paired sputum and transtracheal aspirates in the initial management of pneumonia. *Chest,* 87:631–635.

39. Geerber, G.J., Farmer, W.C., and Fulkerson, L.L. (1978): Beta-hemolytic streptococcal pneumonia following influenza. *J.A.M.A.,* 240:242–243.

40. Genereux, G.P.M., and Stilwell, G.A. (1980): The acute bacterial pneumonias. *Semin. Roentgenol.,* 15:9–16.

41. Godfrey, M.E., and Smith, I.M. (1958): Hospital hazards of staphylococcal sepsis. *J.A.M.A.,* 166:1197.

42. Goldstein, F.W., Emirian, M.F., and Guerrier, J.F. (1992): Comparative activity of Amoxicillin and Cefotaxime against 392 penicillin-resistant and -susceptible *Streptococcus pneumoniae.* Presented at the 32nd Interscience Conference for Antimicrobial Agents and Chemotherapy, Anaheim, Calif., October 1992 (abstract 1025).

43. Gram, C. (1884): Ueber die isolierte Farbung der Schizomyceten in Schinittund Trockenpraparaten. *Forsch. Med.,* 2:185–189.

44. Gransden, W.R., Eykyn, S.J., and Phillips, I. (1985): Pneumococcal bacteraemia: 325 episodes diagnosed at St. Thomas's Hospital. *Br. Med. J.,* 290:505–508.

45. Gray, B.M. (1992): Case Report: *Rhodococcus Equi* pneumonia in a patient infected by the human immunodeficiency virus. *Am. J. Med. Sci.,* 303:180–183.

46. Gray, B.M., Converse, G.M., III, and Dillon, H.C. (1980): Epidemiologic studies of *Streptococcus pneumoniae* in infants: acquisition, carriage, and infection during the first 24 months of life. *J. Infect. Dis.,* 142:923–933.

47. Guckian, J.C., Christiansen, G.D., and Fine, D.P. (1980): The role of opsonins in recovery from experimental pneumococcal pneumonia. *J. Infect. Dis.,* 142:175–190.

48. Gwaltney, J.M., Jr., and Hayden, F.G. (1982): The nose and infection. In: *The Nose, Upper Airway Physiology and the Atmospheric Environment,* edited by D.F. Proctor and I.M. Andercon, pp. 401–424. Elsevier/North Holland, Amsterdam.

49. Gwaltney, J.M., Jr., Sande, M.A., Austrian, R., et al. (1975): Spread of *Streptococcus pneumoniae* in families. II. Relation of transfer of *S. pneumoniae* to incidence of colds and serum antibody. *J. Infect. Dis.,* 132:62–68.

50. Harford, C.G., and Hara, M. (1950): Pulmonary edema in influenzal pneumonia in the mouse and the relation of fluid in the lung to the inception of pneumococcal pneumonia. *J. Exp. Med.,* 91:245.

51. Harrison, B.D., Farr, B.M., Pugh, S., Selkon, J.B., Prescott, R.J., and Connolly, C.K. (1987): Community-acquired pneumonia in adults in British hospitals in 1982–1983: A BTS/PHLS survey of aetiology, mortality, prognostic factors and outcome. *Q. J. Med.* (New Series), 62:195–220.

52. Helms, C.M., Viner, J.P., Sturm, R.H., Renner, E.D., and Johnson, W. (1979): Comparative features of pneumococcal, mycoplasmal, and Legionnaire's disease pneumonias. *Ann. Intern. Med.,* 90:543–547.

53. Hendley, J.O., Sande, M.A., Stewart, P.M., et al. (1975): Spread of *Streptococcus pneumoniae* in families. I. Carriage rates and distribution of types. *J. Infect. Dis.,* 132:55–61.

54. Holland, W.W., Tanner, E.I., Pereira, M.S., and Taylor, C.E.D. (1960): A study of the aetiology of respiratory disease in a general hospital. *Br. Med. J.,* 1:1917–1922.

55. Hook, E.W., Horton, C.A., and Schaberg, D.R. (1983): Failure of intensive care unit support to influence mortality from pneumococcal bacteremia. *J.A.M.A.,* 249:1055–1057.

56. Horan, T.C., White, J.W., Jarvis, W.R., Emori, T.G., Culver, D.H., Munn, V.P., Thornsberry, C., Olson, D.R., and Hughes, J.M. (1986): Nosocomial infection surveillance, 1984. *M.M.W.R.,* 35:17SS–29SS.

57. Huxley, E.J., Viroslav, J., Gray, W.R., and Pierce, A.K. (1978): Pharyngeal aspiration in normal adults and patients with depressed consciousness. *Am. J. Med.,* 64:564–568.

58. Ikeogu, M.O. (1988): Acute pneumonia in Zimbabwe: bacterial isolates by lung aspiration. *Arch. Dis. Child.,* 63:1266–1267.

59. Jarvis, W.R., and Martone, W.J. (1992): Predominant pathogens in hospital infections. *J. Antimicro. Chem.,* 29(Suppl. A):19–24.

60. Jay, S.J., Johanson, W.G., and Pierce, A.K. (1975): The radiographic resolution of *Streptococcus pneumoniae* pneumonia. *N. Engl. J. Med.,* 293:798–801.

61. Jenkinson, S.G., George, R.B., Light, R.W., and Girard, W.M. (1979): Cefazolin vs. penicillin: treatment of uncomplicated pneumococcal pneumonia. *J.A.M.A.,* 241:2815–2817.

62. Kalin, M., and Lindberg, A.A. (1983): Diagnosis of pneumococcal pneumonia: a comparison between microscopic examination of expectorate, antigen detection and cultural procedures. *Scand. J. Infect. Dis.,* 247–255.

63. Kaplan, M.H., and Tenenbaum, M.J. (1982): *Staphylococcus aureus:* cellular biology and clinical application. *Am. J. Med.,* 72:248–258.

64. Kaye, M.G., Fox, M.J., Bartlett, J.G., Braman, S.S., and Glassroth, J. (1990): The clinical spectrum of *Staphylococcus aureus* pulmonary infection. *Chest,* 97:788–792.

65. Klein, J.O. (1981): The epidemiology of pneumococcal disease in infants and children. *Rev. Infect. Dis.*, 3:246–253.
66. Klimek, J.J., Ajemian, E., Fontecchio, S., Gracewski, J., Klemas, B., and Jiminez, L. (1983): Community-acquired bacterial pneumonia requiring admission to hospital. *Am. J. Infect. Control.*, 11:79–82.
67. Kramer, M.S., Roberts-Bräuer, M.A., and Williams, R.L. (1992): Bias and "Overcall" in interpreting chest radiographs in young febrile children. *Peds.*, 90:11–13.
68. LaForce, F.M. (1981): Hospital-acquired gram-negative rod pneumonias: an overview. *Am. J. Med.*, 70:664.
69. Laskey, J.A., Pulkingham, N., Powers, M.A., and Durack, D.T. (1991): *Rhodococcus equi* causing human pulmonary infection: review of 29 cases. *So. Med. J.*, 84:1217–1220.
70. Light, R.W. (1977): Pleural effusions. *Med. Clin. No. Amer.*, 61:1339–1352.
71. Liñares, J., Mariscal, D., Gomez-Lus, S., Alonso, T., Perez, J.L., Martin, R., and Gomez-Lus, R. (1992): Increase of erythromycin resistance (ER) among clinical isolates of *Streptococcus pneumoniae* (SP). Presented at the 32nd Interscience Conference for Antimicrobial Agents and Chemotherapy, Anaheim, Calif., October 1992 (Abstract 1027).
72. Linnemann, C.C., and First, M.R. (1979): Risk of pneumococcal infection in renal transplant patients. *J.A.M.A.*, 241:2619–2621.
73. Macfarlane, J.T., Finch, R.G., Ward, M.J., and Macrae, A.D. (1982): Hospital study of adult community-acquired pneumonia. *Lancet*, 2:255.
74. Marrie, T.J., Grayston, J.T., Wang, S.-P., and Kuo, C.-C. (1987): Pneumonia associated with the TWAR strain of chlamydia. *Ann. Intern. Med.*, 106:507–511.
75. McGavin, C.R., and Clancy, L.J. (1987): Cellulitis in complicated pneumococcal pneumonia. *Br. J. Dis. Chest*, 71:213–214.
76. McNabb, W.R., Shanson, D.C., Williams, T.D.M., and Lant, A.F. (1984): Adult community-acquired pneumonia in central London. *J. R. Soc. Med.*, 77:550–555.
77. Merrill, C.W., Gwaltney, J.M., Jr., Hendley, J.W., and Sande, M.A. (1973): Rapid identification of pneumococci: gram stain vs. the quellung reaction. *N. Engl. J. Med.*, 288:510–512.
78. Miller, J., Sande, M.A., Gwaltney, J.M., Jr., and Hendley, J.O. (1978): Diagnosis of pneumococcal pneumonia by antigen detection in sputum. *J. Clin. Microbiol.*, 7:459–462.
79. Mohr, D.N., Feist, D.J., Washington, J.A., and Hermans, P.F. (1979): Infections due to group C streptococci in man. *Am. J. Med.*, 66:450–456.
80. Molteni, R.A. (1977): Group A beta-hemolytic streptococcal pneumonia: clinical course and complications of management. *Am. J. Dis. Child.*, 131:1366–1371.
81. Moore, M.A., Merson, M.H., Charache, P., and Shepard, R.H. (1977): The characteristics and mortality of outpatient-acquired pneumonia. *Johns Hopkins M. J.*, 140:9–14.
82. Mufson, M.A. (1990): Streptococcus pneumoniae. In: *Principles and Practice of Infectious Diseases*, 3rd Edition, edited by G.L. Mandell, R.G. Douglas, and J.E. Bennett, pp. 1539–1550. John Wiley and Sons, New York.
83. Mufson, M.A., Oley, G., and Hughes, D. (1982): Pneumococcal disease in a medium-sized community in the United States. *J.A.M.A.*, 248:1486–1489.
84. (1977): Multiple antibiotic resistance of pneumococci—South Africa. *M.M.W.R.*, 26:285–286.
85. Musher, D.M., and Franco, M. (1981): Staphylococcal pneumonia, a new perspective. *Chest*, 79:172–173.
86. Musher, D.M., and McKenzie, S.O. (1977): Infections due to *Staphylococcus aureus*. *Medicine*, 56:383–409.
87. Naraqi, S., and McDonnell, G. (1981): Hematogeneous staphylococcal pneumonia secondary to soft tissue infection. *Chest*, 79:173–175.
88. Olutola, P.S., Komolafe, F., and Onile, B.A. (1984): Multiple staphylococcal pneumatoceles in an adult. *Diag. Imag. Clin. Med.*, 53:306–309.
89. Ort, S., Ryan, J.L., Barden, G., and D'Esopo, N. (1983): Pneumococcal pneumonia in hospital patients: clinical and radiological presentations. *J.A.M.A.*, 249:214–218.
90. Oviawe, O., and Ogundipe, O. (1985): Pneumatoceles associated with pneumonia incidence and clinical course in Nigerian children. *Trop. Geogr. Med.*, 37:264–269.
91. Patriarca, P.A., Weber, J.A., Parker, R.A., Hall, W.N., Kendal, A.P., Bregman, D.J., and Schonberger, L.B. (1985): Efficacy of influenza vaccine in nursing homes. *J.A.M.A.*, 253:1136–1139.
92. Patriarca, P.A., Weber, J.A., Parker, R.A., Orenstein, W.A., Hall, W.N., Kendal, A.P., and Schonberger, L.B. (1986): Risk factors for outbreaks of influenza in nursing homes. *Am. J. Epidemiol.*, 124:114–119.
93. Plaut, M.E., and Perlino, C.A. (1978): Cefamandole vs. procaine penicillin for treatment of pneumonia due to *Streptococcus pneumoniae:* a randomized trial. *J. Infect. Dis.*, 137:S133–S138.
94. (1981): Pneumococcal polysaccharide vaccine. *M.M.W.R.*, 30:410–412.
95. (1989): Pneumococcal polysaccharide vaccine. *M.M.W.R.*, 38:64–76.
96. (1978): Pneumococcal vaccine. *The Medical Letter*, 20:13–14.

97. Polednak, A.P. (1977): Postmortem bacteriology and pneumonia in a mentally retarded population. *Am. J. Clin. Path.*, 67:190–195.
98. Polsky, B., Gold, J.W.M., Whimbey, E., Dry Janski, J., Brown, A.E., Schiffmann, G., and Armstrong, D. (1986): Bacterial pneumonia in patients with the acquired immunodeficiency syndrome. *Ann. Intern. Med.*, 104:38–41.
99. Pratter, M.R., and Irwin, R.S. (1980): Viridans streptococcal pulmonary parenchymal infections. *J.A.M.A.*, 243:2515–2517.
100. Prout, S., Potgieter, P.D., Forder, A.A., Moodie, J.W., and Matthews, J. (1983): Acute community-acquired pneumonias. *S. Afr. Med. J.*, 64:443–446.
101. Rein, M.F., Gwaltney, J.M., Jr., O'Brien, W.M., Jennings, R.H., and Mandell, G.L. (1978): Accuracy of gram's stain in identifying pneumococci in sputum. *J.A.M.A.*, 239:2671–2673.
102. Rizkallah, M.F., Hoffler, E., and Ayoub, E.M. (1988): Serological confirmation of group C streptococcal pneumonia. *J. Inf. Dis.*, 158:1092–1094.
103. Rodriguez-Creixems, M., Pelase, T., Diza, M.D., Muñoz, P., Bernaldo De Quiros, J.C.L., Cercenado, E., and Miralles, P. (1992): Increase isolation and resistance to erythromycin in group A streptococci. Presented at the 32nd Interscience Conference for Antimicrobial Agents and Chemotherapy, Anaheim, Calif., October 1992 (abstract 1029).
104. Rose, H.E., Allen, J.R., and Witte, G. (1980): *Streptococcus zooepidemicus* (group C) pneumonia in a human. *J. Clin. Microbiol.*, 11:76–78.
105. Rudin, J.E., and Wing, E.J. (1986): Prospective study of pneumonia: unexpected incidence of Legionellosis. *So. Med. J.*, 79:417–419.
106. Rytel, M.W., and Preheim, L.C. (1986): Antigen detection in the diagnosis and in the prognostic assessment of bacteria pneumonias. *Diag. Microbiol. Infect. Dis.*, 4:35S–46S.
107. Sarkar, T.K., Murarka, R.S., and Gilardi, G.L. (1989): Primary *streptococcus viridans* pneumonia. *Chest*, 96:831–834.
108. Schwartz, J.S. (1982): Pneumococcal vaccine: clinical efficacy and effectiveness. *Ann. Intern. Med.*, 96:208–220.
109. Schwartz, J.S. (1986): Pneumococcal vaccine. *Ann. Intern. Med.*, 104:118–220.
110. Schwarzmann, S.W., Adler, J.L., Sullivan, R.J., and Marine, W.M. (1971): Bacterial pneumonia during the Hong Kong influenza epidemic of 1968–1969. *Arch. Intern. Med.*, 127:1037–1041.
111. Shann, F., Gratten, M., Germer, S., Linnemann, V., Hazlett, D., and Payne, R. (1984): Aetiology of pneumonia in children in Goroka Hospital, Papua, New Guinea. *Lancet*, Sept. 8:537–541.
112. Shapiro, E.D., Berg, A.T., Austrian, R., Schroeder, D., Parcells, V., Margolis, A., Adair, R.K., and Clemens, J.D. (1991): The protective efficacy of polyvalent pneumococcal polysaccharide vaccine. *N. Engl. J. Med.*, 325:1453–1460.
113. Shapiro, E.D., and Clemens, J.D. (1984): A controlled evaluation of the protective efficacy of pneumococcal vaccine for patients at high risk of serious pneumococcal infections. *Ann. Intern. Med.*, 101:325–330.
114. Simberkoff, M.S., Cross, A.P., Al-Ibrahim, M., Baltch, A.L., Geiseler, J., Nadler, J., Richmond, A.S., Smith, R.P., Schiffman, G., Shepard, D.S., and Van Eeckhout, J.P. (1986): Efficacy of pneumococcal vaccine in high-risk patients. *N. Engl. J. Med.*, 315:1318–1327.
115. Sinclair, V. (1980): Pneumococcal pneumonia complicated by lung abscess. *Physiotherapy*, 66:184–185.
116. Spencer, C.D., and Beaty, H.N. (1972): Complications of transtracheal aspiration. *N. Engl. J. Med.*, 286:304.
117. Stamm, A.M., and Cobbs, C.G. (1980): Group C streptococcal pneumonia: report of a fatal case and review of the literature. *Rev. Infect. Dis.*, 2:889–898.
118. Straker, E., Bradford, A., and Lovell, R. (1939): A study of the nasopharyngeal bacterial flora of different groups of persons observed in London and South-East England during the years 1930–1937. In: *Reports on Public Health and Medical Subjects*, 90:3–51. Ministry of Health, London.
119. Sullivan, R.J., Jr., Dowdle, W.R., Marine, W.M., and Hierholzer, J.C. (1972): Adult pneumonia in a general hospital: etiology and host risk factors. *Arch. Intern. Med.*, 129:935–942.
120. Taryle, D.A., Potts, D.E., and Sahn, S.A. (1978): The incidence and clinical correlates of parapneumonic effusions. *Chest*, 74:170–173.
121. Tew, J., Calenoff, L., and Berlin, B.S. (1977): Bacterial or nonbacterial pneumonia: accuracy of radiologic diagnosis. *Radiology*, 124:607–612.
122. Turner, J.C., Hayden, G.F., Kiselica, D., Lohr, J., Fisburne, C.F., and Murren, D. (1990): Association of group C β-hemolytic streptococci with endemic pharyngitis among college students. *J.A.M.A.*, 264:2644–2647.
123. Vartian, C., Lerner, P.I., Shlaes, D.M., and Gopalakrishna, K.V. (1985): Infections due to Lancefield group G streptococci. *Medicine*, 64:75–88.
124. Verghese, A., Berk, S.L., Boelen, L.J., and Smith, J.K. (1982): Group B streptococcal pneumonia in the elderly. *Arch. Intern. Med.*, 142:1642–1645.

125. Vracin, W., Gage, K., Ortega, G., and Berk, S.L. (1982): Bacteremic group G streptococcal pneumonia. *So. Med. J.,* 75:1427.
126. Waldvogel, F.A. (1990): *Staphylococcus aureus* (including toxic shock syndrome). In: *Principles and Practice of Infectious Diseases,* 3rd Edition, edited by G.L. Mandell, R.G. Douglas, and J.E. Bennett, pp. 1489–1510. John Wiley and Sons, New York.
127. Waters, B.L. (1988): Pathology of culture-proven JK corynebacterium pneumonia. *A.J.C.P.,* 91:616–619.
128. White, R.J., Blainey, A.D., Harrison, K.J., and Clarke, S.K.R. (1981): Causes of pneumonia presenting to a distinct general hospital. *Thorax,* 36:566–570.
129. Winston, D.J., Schiffman, G., Wang, D.C., et al. (1979): Pneumococcal infections after human bone marrow transplantation. *Ann. Intern. Med.,* 91:835–841.
130. Wood, W.B. (1951–1952): Studies of the cellular immunology of acute bacterial infections. *Haney Lect.* (Series 47):72–98.
131. Woodhead, M.A., Macfarlane, J.T., McCracken, J.S., Rose, D.H., and Finch, R.G. (1987): Prospective study of the aetiology and outcome of pneumonia in the community. *Lancet,* March 21:671–674.
132. Yangco, B.G., and Deresinki, S.C. (1980): Necrotizing or cavitating pneumonia due to *Streptococcus pneumoniae:* report of four cases and review of the literature. *Medicine,* 59:449–457.
133. Zishind, M.M., Schwarz, M.I., George, R.B., Weill, H., Shames, J.M., Herbert, S.J., and Ichinose, H. (1970): Incomplete consolidation in pneumococcal lobar pneumonia complicating pulmonary emphysema. *Ann. Intern. Med.,* 72:835–859.

Respiratory Infections: Diagnosis and Management, 3d ed.,
edited by James E. Pennington.
Raven Press, Ltd., New York © 1994

19

Gram-Negative Bacillary Pneumonias

Janice Eisenstadt and Lawrence R. Crane

*Department of Clinical Pathology, The Cleveland Clinic Foundation,
9500 Euclid Avenue, Cleveland, Ohio 44195; and Department of Internal Medicine,
Division of Infectious Diseases, Wayne State University School of Medicine,
4160 John R, Detroit, Michigan 48201*

Gram-negative bacilli (GNB) were first implicated as a pneumonia pathogen in 1880 (6) when the organism was found at autopsies by Friedlander. However, clinicians generally ignored observations that GNBs could be the microbiologic cause of pneumonia. During the preantibiotic era, aerobic GNBs were estimated to be the cause of fewer then 5% of pneumonia cases (113). Clinicians regarded aerobic GNB pneumonias (GNBPs) as medical curiosities until the early 1960s. Since then, GNBPs have been recognized as significant medical problems, especially among hospitalized, chronically ill, elderly, and many immunocompromised patients.

Aerobic GNBPs have become major challenges for modern medicine and are now major causes of community- and hospital-acquired lower respiratory tract infections. Recent studies have shown GNB to make up 58.7% of the pathogens associated with nosocomial pneumonia (25) and as much as 80% of ventilator-associated pneumonias (35). Microbiological trends in nosocomial pneumonia reveal an increasing incidence of pneumonias caused by resistant organisms; *Pseudomonas aeruginosa* and *Enterobacter* and *Acinetobacter* sp are prominent examples (129). The relative incidence of community-acquired gram-negative pneumonias is difficult to determine, but estimates gleaned from community-acquired pneumonias requiring hospital or ICU admission range from 6 to 20% (36,116).

The increasing incidence and the high mortality associated with GNBP have attracted considerable interest by researchers during the past 25 years. As a result, there has been a considerable increase of understanding regarding these disorders. Investigators have delineated several differences between the clinical and epidemiologic features of community-acquired and nosocomial GNBP. Among recent gains have been the identification of risk factors, methods for early determination of microbial cause, and prompt, specific aggressive antimicrobial therapies.

Overview

Pathogenesis

Pneumonia caused by GNB is the result of one of three mechanisms: (i) remotely, because of nebulization with contaminated fluids (called exogenous aspiration); (ii) hematogenous dissemination to the lung; or (iii) resulting from aspiration of colonizing oropharyngeal microorganisms.

Now, exogenous aspiration is more of historical interest than a practical concern. Previously, inadequate sterilization of nebulization reservoirs allowed inhalation of contaminated materials leading to the occurrence of pulmonary infection (117). Pneumonia caused by hematogenous dissemination occurs in burn patients and in patients with infection at a remote site. Hematogenous seeding of the lung can also occur with septic thrombophlebitis and with right-sided endocarditis. Hematogenous GNBPs are most often caused by *Escherichia coli* and *P. aeruginosa* (82). Infection of the lower respiratory tract by facultative gram-negative organisms usually precede colonization of the oropharynx, tracheobronchial tree, or stomach (59,109,135). Alteration in oropharyngeal epithelial surfaces allows for the adherence of gram-negative organisms. The presence of bacterial surface structures (called adhesions) promotes attachment to the epithelial cell surfaces and allows for colonization (83,101). The mechanisms of bacterial adherence are reviewed in detail elsewhere in this text and by Niederman (101).

Colonization of the oropharynx with gram-negative rods in healthy individuals is unusual. Various investigators report colonization rates ranging between 2 and 11.5% (65,80,81,154); in one report the rate was 18% (123). *Klebsiella pneumoniae,* the most common cause for community-acquired gram-negative pneumonia, is found in 1–6% of healthy individuals (95). Colonization with GNB in the normal host is of little clinical significance. In hospital personnel, colonization is transient (65) and not related to direct contact with patients (113). Chronic colonization occurs frequently in persons with chronic bronchitis and in alcoholics (70,87,113,123). Among alcoholics, the incidence of colonization is as high as 29% (87). The colonization rates among hospitalized patients are higher. For example, the incidence increases with ICU admission. It correlates with length of ICU stay and illness severity (66). Colonization usually occurs within 72 hours of admission. Colonization is especially rapid among intubated patients; 25% are colonized within 24 hours, and by one week, the figure is 63–87% (134). *Pseudomonas* species primarily colonize the tracheobronchial tree, in contrast to other GNB that are found in the oropharynx before isolation in the trachea (135). Colonization rates increase among those elderly persons living in chronic care facilities. One study found 9% of older persons who lived independently were colonized with GNB, compared to 60% of older persons who lived in skilled nursing care environments (154). In 1972, Johanson and colleagues (66) described the significance of oropharyngeal colonization and the subsequent development of GNBP. Their study reported that nosocomial pneumonia developed in 12.2% of 213 patients admitted to a medical ICU. Eighty-five percent of patients developing pneumonia were previously colonized before the appearance of infection. Among patients not colonized, only 3.3% went on to develop pneumonia.

Risk Factors

Table 19-1 lists risk factors associated with colonization and infection of the respiratory tract by facultative gram-negative rods. In a recent study of community-acquired pneumonias, 88.2% of those diagnosed with GNBP had one or more of these associated risk factors (36).

The classic clinical manifestations of pneumonia—cough, sputum production, fever, shortness of breath, chills, and pleuritic chest pain—are not useful for defining the etiologic agent. In certain circumstances for which the incidence of GNBP is increased, the signs and symptoms of pneumonia can be mitigated or absent. This can be the case in hematogenously spread pneumonias, pneumonias occurring in the elderly, and in immunosuppressed individuals. Under these circumstances, physical findings are often trivial and sputum scant or nonpurulent. The elderly can present with extrapulmonary symptoms including mental status changes or deterioration of a known chronic illness (102). Physical signs of gram-negative pneumonia in neutropenic patients occurred in fewer than half of autopsy-confirmed cases in one study (166).

Most GNBPs are not associated with bacteremia. Most large series report positive blood cultures in 33–50% of the cases (46). Karnad and colleagues (71) reported an incidence of 14.2% positive blood cultures; others (12,131) have reported as few as 10% of patients with nosocomial pneumonia who had either positive blood or pleural fluid cultures. The incidence of associated bacteremia varies with bacterial etiology. It has been noted that *Pseudomonas aeruginosa* is most commonly associated with bacteremia (71,106).

Most cases of GNBP begin as patchy infiltrates in the lower lobes. Cavitation and empyema are common. Although chest x-rays are unreliable for microbiological diagnosis, they are suggestive in certain instances. Besides *Streptococcus pneumoniae,* lobar pneumonias are often associated with *K. pneumoniae* and *Proteus* sp. The presence of a bulging fissure on x-ray (although an infrequently seen finding) suggests *K. pneumoniae* as the etiologic agent. Infiltrates are more extensive and more likely to be bilateral in patients with bacteremic pneumonia (71). Early necrosis and abscess formation could suggest a GNBP, although this can also be seen in pneumonias caused by pneumococci, staphylococci, *Legionella,* and, rarely, *Mycoplasma.*

The presence of radiographic abnormalities can correlate with the neutrophil count (10,166). Radiographic evidence of pneumonia can be absent in neutropenic patients (especially initially), and pneumonia may go clinically undetected (166). When noninfectious etiologies cause pulmonary infiltrates (as in congestive heart failure, ARDS, malignancy, or pulmonary infarction), it can be exceedingly difficult to distinguish colonization from infection with GNB.

Histologically, GNBP is associated with an increase in both type 2 and interstitial pulmonary cells. There is a concurrent decrease in type 1 and endothelial cells (21). These changes are seen with hypoxia, but gram-negative bacterial infection appears to impart a synergistic effect. Gram-negative bacteria increase the surface tension of rabbit surfactant *in vitro,* whereas gram-positive bacteria do not (122). Lipopolysaccharide itself can cause this effect (29). This effect occurs either through direct effects on surfactant or by effects on type 2 epithelial cells. The change in surfactant decreases total lung capacity, static compliance, and diffusion capacity, and increases pulmonary arterial pressure. Diminished concentrations of surfactant or abnormal surfactant can produce pulmonary edema, hemorrhage, and atelectasis (11). Lipopolysaccharide alone induces inflammation of the lung parenchyma (118).

Gram-negative bacilli are a noteworthy cause of pneumonia because of their high mortality rates. Crude mortality of nosocomial GNBP ranges from 50 to 80% (160). Higher mortality rates are associated with bacteremic pneumonia (12,37,72,106). Increased mortality is also associated with pneumonias caused by *P. aeruginosa* (12,146) and *Acinetobacter baumannii* (35). Gram-negative bacteria are the cause for

TABLE 19–1. *Pathogenesis and pathology of community- and hospital-acquired gram-negative bacillary pneumonias (GNBPs)*

Pathogen	Usual route of infection		Predisposing condition(s)		Hospital epidemiology	
	Community	Hospital	Community	Hospital	Reservoir(s)	Mode(s) of transmission
Klebsiella pneumoniae	Endogenous aspiration	Endogenous aspiration Exogenous aspiration	Alcoholism Diabetes mellitus Cardiopulmonary or renal diseases Malignancy Residents of nursing homes	Cardiac arrest Malignancy Assisted ventilation. Residents of Intensive Care Units, Postoperative state Prior antibiotics Neutropenia Corticosteroids Cytotoxic drugs	Patients: bowel, pharynx, urine Aerosol medication Respiratory equipment	Hands of personnel Aerosol treatment
Enterobacter sp.	Endogenous aspiration Hematogenous	Hematogenous Endogenous aspiration	Drug addiction Alcoholism Malignancy Residents of nursing homes	Burns Malignancy Cardiac arrest	Burns Hydrotherapy ?Urine, bowel	Hands of personnel Hydrotherapy
Serratia marcescens	Endogenous aspiration	Endogenous aspiration Exogenous aspiration		Malignancy Pulmonary disease Drug addiction Postoperative state Assisted ventilation Residents of Intensive Care Units. Prior aminoglycosides (aminoglycoside-resistant *Serratia*) Corticosteroids	Patients: urine, bowel, Disinfectants, Urometers Respiratory equipment	Hands of personnel Bronchoscopes Aerosol treatment, Disinfectants

Organism						
Escherichia coli	Hematogenous	Hematogenous Endogenous aspiration	Diabetes Alcoholism Cardiopulmonary or renal diseases	Cerebrovascular disease. Acute abdominal infections Malignancy Thoracoabdominal surgery	Patients: urine, stool, pharyngeal, secretions	Hands of personnel
Proteus, Morganella, Providencia	Endogenous aspiration	Endogenous aspiration	Alcoholism and chronic lung disease		Patients: urine	Hands of personnel
Acinetobacter calcoaceticus	Endogenous aspiration with secondary bacteremia Airborne	Endogenous aspiration Exogenous aspiration	Alcoholism Pneumoconiosis	Tracheostomy Postoperative state Antibiotic treatment	Aerosol medications Personnel	Aerosol treatment. Hands of personnel
Pseudomonas aeruginosa	Endogenous aspiration Hematogenous (rare)	Endogenous aspiration Hematogenous Exogenous aspiration	Chronic lung disease Malignancy Neutropenia Acquired immunodeficiency syndrome	Burns Residents of intensive care Postoperative state Malignancy Neutropenia	Patients: bowel, urine, pharynx Aerosol treatment Sinks	Hands of personnel Aerosol treatment

two-thirds of all deaths due to pneumonia (108). In the United States, GNBPs cause approximately 45,000 deaths each year.

This chapter outlines GNBP caused by the Enterobacteriaceae, the Pseudomonaceae, and some of the glucose-nonfermenting gram-negative bacteria. Incidence, mortality, and clinical and laboratory characteristics are discussed, and treatment, as we approach it today, is also addressed.

SPECIFIC ETIOLOGIC AGENTS

Enterobacteriaceae and *Klebsiella* sp

Incidence and Mortality (Table 19-2)

The genus *Klebsiella* includes seven species: *pneumoniae, oxytoca, ornithinolytica, planticola, tearigena, rhinoscleromatis,* and *ozaenae. Klebsiella pneumoniae* is the species most commonly associated with pneumonia; *K. oxytoca* rarely causes pneumonia; the rest of the species are not pulmonary pathogens.

Friedlander's bacillus *(K. pneumoniae)* has been known as a virulent pulmonary pathogen since 1882. Today it is recognized as the preeminent microbe causing community-acquired GNBP in the United States. It is now the third leading cause of nosocomial GNBP. The precise incidence of community-acquired GNBPs, including *K. pneumoniae,* is not known. Although studies have both prospectively and retrospectively estimated the incidence, etiology, and risk factors in patients with GNBPs admitted to hospitals, the populations surveyed have been, to date, limited to large city hospitals serving mostly the indigent of their respective communities (4,30,39,43,46,67,71,144,146). In these studies, Friedlander's pneumonia accounted for 1 to 8% of all pneumonia admissions, and 18 to 64% of all community-acquired GNBPs. The incidence of community-acquired *Klebsiella* pneumonia has remained unchanged at Parkland Memorial Hospital for over 20 years, which is the general experience for most city hospitals (14). The incidence of nosocomial *Klebsiella* pneumonias are more precisely known. It accounts for about 20% of all nosocomial GNBPs, representing 7 to 11% of all nosocomial pneumonias (62). Rates range from 6.6 to 8.0 cases/10,000 admissions or discharges (17,18,141,157). Data from the National Nosocomial Infections Surveillance System (NNIS) report a frequency of 6% hospital-wide, and 8% in intensive care units.

Microbiology

Klebsiella pneumoniae are gram-negative, encapsulated, nonmotile rods that form mucoid colonies. It ferments lactose, but does not produce indole or H_2S. The polysaccharide capsule of *K. pneumoniae* is often seen on gram stains of expectorated sputa or transtracheal aspirates as a clear space displacing the background material. Many strains of *Klebsiella* are large, thick rods, four to five times as long as they are wide. Unfortunately, other species of gram-negative bacilli often have a similar appearance on gram stain. It can be serotyped using the Quellung reaction. More than 75 capsular types have been identified. The cost of reagents and technical difficulties limits the utility of direct serotyping of sputum for rapid diagnosis. Serotypes 1–6 cause most pneumonias, although higher numbered serotypes can also

TABLE 19–2. Incidence and mortality of community- and hospital-acquired gram-negative bacillary pneumonias (GNBPs)

Organism	Community-acquired GNBPs (1966–1985)[a]		Nosocomial GNBPs (1977–1988)[b]		
	Total cases (%)	Mortality (%)	Admissions or discharges (rate/10,000)	Total cases (%)	Mortality (%)
Enterobacteriaceae (tribe Klebsiellae)					
Klebsiella pneumoniae	18–64	20–54	6.6–8.0	7.4–21.0	18–30
Enterobacter sp	0–21	14	4.0–5.3	10.4–17.0	13–45
Serratia marcescens	Rare	High	2.4–3.3	4.0–10.0	44–57
Escherichia coli	12–43	29–60	4.1–9.0	6.4–15.0	24–89
Proteus sp. (Morganella sp)	0–10	18	2.4–7.0	3.4–14.0	21
Providencia sp	Rare	—	Rare case reports (140)	—	25
Other Enterobacteriaceae (Shigella, Salmonella-Arizona-Citrobacter, Edwarsiella, Hafnia, Erwinia, unclassified)	Case series of Citrobacter (88); 11% of cases of typhoid fever (143)	—	Rare case reports of Citrobacter (153), Erwina (94), and Hafnia (155) pneumonias	1.0–2.5	—
Acinetobacter baumannii	Case series (2,23,50,124)	33–64	2.0	1.0–3.0	44
Pseudomonas aeruginosa	0–11	72	3.0–9.6	17.2–30.0	24–90

[a]Based on published series from major metropolitan hospitals (30,71,144,146).
[b]Based on reports of the National Nosocomial Infections Studies (17,18,25) and the University of Virginia consortium (157).

cause nosocomial pneumonias. Serotypes 1 to 6 can also cause nonrespiratory infections (146). There is little evidence that certain types are more virulent than others.

Pathogenesis and Pathology (Table 19-1)

Most cases of both community- and hospital-acquired Friedlander's pneumonia occur after endogenous aspiration of oropharyngeal secretions. Patients are the most common reservoirs during nosocomial outbreaks of *Klebsiella* pneumonias. The bowel, the infected urinary tract, the colonized pharynx, and tracheobronchial secretions are the usual sources (95). Hands of hospital personnel (after patient contact) are the usual mode of transmission. Mertz and coinvestigators (93) incriminated contaminated nebulizer aerosols in an outbreak of *Klebsiella* pneumonia at Bellevue Hospital in New York City. However, the natural spread of *Klebsiella* infections by an airborne route with resultant pneumonia has never been convincingly documented.

Classic Friedlander's pneumonia in humans is a lobar consolidation involving the upper lobes of the lung (82,93,147). Bronchopneumonias are not as frequent (82). Diffuse bilateral patchy bronchopneumonias are found in neutropenic patients with Friedlander's pneumonia (166). At postmortem examination, lungs are reddish-gray and consolidated. A characteristic sticky exudate exudes from cut surfaces. There may be multiple abscesses. Alveolar wall necrosis causes alveolar collapse and loss of lung volume. Major pulmonary vessels can thrombose, leading to localized pulmonary gangrene and the formation of a pulmonary sequestrum (28). Enlarged, matted hilar nodes, bronchiectasis, friable blood vessels, and empyema can also be observed.

At histologic section, outpouring of edema fluid, mononuclear cells, and bacteria is seen in early disease. Later, there is alveolar wall destruction, polymorphonuclear leukocytic infiltration, and fibrosis. Intrapulmonary bleeding, pyopneumothorax, and pericarditis are other intrathoracic complications in infected lungs, but sinusitis, mastoiditis, meningitis, splenitis, cystitis, prostatitis, and cholecystitis can also be found at autopsy (82).

Host/Virulence Factors

Klebsiella pneumoniae pneumonia is a disease of the debilitated. Alcoholism, diabetes mellitus, and chronic heart, kidney, lung, and neoplastic diseases are predisposing conditions (82). In various studies the prevalence of *Klebsiella* carriage in throats of normal, nonhospitalized patients ranges between 1 and 6% (95). Carriage rates are much higher, up to 29%, in persons recovering from viral illnesses and in ambulatory alcoholics (42,114). Once established, *Klebsiella* carriage in the throat or nasopharynx can last for as long as 4 months (95). In hospitalized patients an increased colonization rate is associated with tracheal intubation, acidosis, azotemia, extremes in white cell counts, shock, coma, and use of antibiotics (66,146).

In critically ill colonized patients, binding sites for *Klebsiella* are present on the surfaces of oropharyngeal epithelial cells, but not in noncolonized control patients who matched for disease severity. Binding site adherence of *Klebsiella* is inhibited by concanavalin A, but not by bovine serum albumin or phytohemagglutinin (67). Investigators postulate similar high-affinity binding for *Klebsiella* on the oropharyngeal epithelial cells of ambulatory alcoholics (42). Fimbriae or pili, which are present on cell surfaces of most gram-negative bacilli, play a role in attachment to epithelial cells. Fimbriae can also be important in phagocytic attachment. Of interest are observations that the more pathogenic strains of *Klebsiella* lack fimbriae (95). Fimbriated strains are often inhibited from attachment by mannose and thus more easily engulfed by polymorphonuclear leukocytes or monocytes. In animal modes of Friedlander's pneumonia, neutrophils are the primary means of cellular defense.

Rehm et al. (115) studied the relative roles of resident pulmonary alveolar macrophages and neutrophilic granulocytes in the clearance of aerosolized *Klebsiella* from murine lungs. Neutropenic mice readily cleared the lung of *S. aureus* but were unable to clear *K. pneumoniae* or *P. aeruginosa. Staphylococcus aureus* were cleared by alveolar macrophages, but circulating granulocytes play a major role in early clearance of the studied GNB. *In vitro* studies also emphasize the importance of polymorphonuclear neutrophils relative to alveolar macrophages in cellular defense mechanisms against *K. pneumoniae* (41). The polysaccharide capsule on *K. pneumoniae* enhances virulence. Capsular K antigens of *Klebsiella* cross-react with polysaccharide capsules of virulent *S. pneumoniae* and *Hemophilus influenzae* (95). A minor capsular component of *Klebsiella* retards migration of phagocytic cells into foci of infection (73). Heavily encapsulated strains are more virulent in animal models of Friedlander's pneumonia (7). Resistance to phagocytosis by encapsulated strains of *Klebsiella* correlates with increased virulence in animals (55). In turn, phagocytosis of encapsulated strains is enhanced by opsonic antibody, complement, and other heat-labile components (7). Levels of C1 and C3 are low in bronchoalveolar lavage fluid of rat models of Friedlander's pneumonia and are inadequate for opsonization (22). *Klebsiella* capsular polysaccharide suppresses maturation of macrophages, exhibits a strong adjuvant effect, induces interferons, and is pyrogenic in rabbits and lethal to mice (103,162). The relevance of these properties to human disease is not clear.

Clinical and Laboratory Features (59)

The typical patient with community-acquired Friedlander's pneumonia is a chronic alcoholic middle-aged man with chronic pulmonary disease who suddenly becomes acutely ill. An abrupt onset is recorded three-quarters of the time. In the preantibiotic era, an exposure to cold in winter was common; contemporary series do not emphasize this seasonal predilection. Fever, malaise, rigors, dyspnea, cough, sputum, and hemoptysis are usual. The classical sputum is bloody and mucoid with a currant-jelly appearance. Sputum production is prodigious with an average of 120 ml daily. At admission to the hospital, about 20% of patients are jaundiced, reflecting their underlying alcoholic liver disease. If the patient survives, liver functions improve. Physical findings are those of lobar consolidation, with or without an abscess. Alveolar wall necrosis and loss of lung volume can progress to cause a shift of the trachea ipsilaterally, lead to narrowing of intercostal spaces, cause an elevation of the hemidiaphragm, and decrease respiratory movement of the affected hemithorax.

Sputa or transtracheal aspirates reveal polymorphonuclear leukocytes and myriads of encapsulated gram-negative bacilli. In 20 to 66% of patients blood cultures are positive, an ominous finding. Two-thirds of the cases have leukocytosis. Associated neutropenia is a poor prognostic sign. Liver function tests can also be abnormal. On chest x-ray, lobar consolidation is typical, often affecting the right upper lobe.

Bronchopneumonias with diffuse patchy infiltrates are seen in immunosuppressed patients with cancer. In about one-half of community-acquired cases, multiple lobes are involved, and 16 to 50% have abscesses. Pulmonary gangrene, resulting from vascular compromise, is an exceedingly rare complication. Bulging interlobar fissures are a distinctive sign of Friedlander's pneumonia, but are occasionally seen in cases of type 3 pneumococcal pneumonia as well. The bulging fissure is a result of voluminous inflammatory exudate accumulation with an increase in lobar volume. Downward expansion of the upper lobe will indent the minor fissure. The bulging fissure sign is rarely encountered (75). The edges of the infiltrate are classically described as having sharp margins. Metapneumonic empyemas appear with varying frequency. With recovery, reduced lung volumes, fibrosis, and thickened pleura remain. A post-pneumonic empyema infrequently occurs. At times, a chronic thick-walled cavity of noncavitary infiltrate can persist, suggesting tuberculosis (Fig. 19-1A). However, chronic pulmonary infection following acute *Klebsiella* infections with persistent abscess formation and noncavitary infiltrates have not been convincingly distinguished from anaerobic co-infection. Chronic infection can result in pneumopyopericardium or myopericardial involvement (127). Radiologic findings in nosocomial cases are similar to community-acquired pneumonia.

Enterobacter Species

Incidence and Mortality (Table 19-2)

The genus *Enterobacter* includes twelve species, eight of which have been recovered in humans: *cloacae, aerogenes, agglomerans, gergoviae, taylorae, amnigevus, asburiae,* and *sakazakii.* Although all of these species have been isolated from pulmonary specimens, the most common species grown in the clinical microbiology laboratory are *E. cloacae* and *aerogenes* (4,68).

Community-acquired cases of *Enterobacter* pneumonia are rare (30,46,82,144, 146,147). Notably, community-acquired *Enterobacter* pneumonias occur more often in nursing home patients (14.3%) than in age-matched patients living at home (8.6%) (43). The incidence of nosocomial *Enterobacter* pneumonias is on the rise, particularly in critical care units. NNIS reported a rate of 4.1 *Enterobacter* species pneumonias per 10,000 discharges in 1979; the rate had increased to 5.3/10,000 discharges by 1984 (17,18). *Enterobacter* caused 15% of GNBPs in hospitals participating in the CHIP survey, and 5.0% of GNBPs in a cancer hospital (141,153). A cumulative incidence of 10.4% was reported during the 1985–1988 NNIS surveys (25), second only to *P. aeruginosa* as leading causes of nosocomial pneumonia. During the 1980–1986 NNIS surveys, *Enterobacter* sp were reported at an incidence of 9.4%, equal to that of *K. pneumoniae.* It is noteworthy that 74.6% of nosocomial *Enterobacter* pneumonias have occurred in intensive care units (62).

Microbiology

Members of the genus *Enterobacter* are motile, gram-negative bacilli that are often nonencapsulated. Gram stain of sputum from cases of pneumonia show some strains as large, thick, gram-negative bacilli resembling *Klebsiella,* but most are thinner rods.

Pathogenesis and Pathology (Table 19-1)

Fifty percent of nosocomial *Enterobacter* pneumonias usually appear within the first week of hospitalization (141). Infections have become prevalent in burn units (68). Mayhall et al. (89) reported an outbreak of silver sulfadiazine–resistant *E. cloacae* in a burn unit in which four patients had bacteremic pneumonias. Contagion from patient to patient occurred through water used for hydrotherapy or the hands of personnel.

Clinical and Laboratory Features (72,82)

Four community and three nosocomial cases of *Enterobacter* pneumonias were described from Detroit Receiving Hospital (82). Species included *E. aerogenes* (3 times), *E. cloacae* (twice), and unspeciated strains (twice). There were five men 27 to 58 (mean 52) years old. Cases of community-acquired pneumonias included a 27-year-old man who was addicted to heroin, 56- and 61-year-old men with bronchogenic carcinoma, and a final 44-year-old man who suffered from chronic alcoholism. Patients reported fever, dyspnea, and a cough productive of yellow sputum. At x-ray bronchopneumonias, sometimes bilateral and affecting two or more lobes, were seen. No patient had either a lung abscess or empyema, but occasionally these complications have been reported. Ten of eleven *Enterobacter* pneumonias reported by Karnad were nosocomial; four were bacteremic (72). All had serious underlying diseases with a mean age of 65 ± 12 years. Species included *E. aerogenes* (7 times), *E. colacae* (3 times), and *E. agglomerans* (once). Mortality was 45.4% in contrast to only 14.3% in the Detroit series.

Serratia marcescens

Incidence and Mortality (Table 19-2)

For discussions of incidence and mortality, see refs. 4,17,18,25,43,62,141,153, and 157.

Microbiology

Serratia marcescens is an aerobic, motile gram-negative bacillus belonging to the tribe Klebsiellae. About 3 to 5% of strains of *S. marcescens* produce prodigiosin, a pink-to-dark pigment. In patients with pneumonia, these pigmented strains have caused pseudohemoptysis (164). This GNB flourishes in the moist environment often found in hospitals leading to nosocomial outbreaks. During such outbreaks serotyping will distinguish epidemic from commensal strains.

Pathogenesis and Pathology (Table 19-1)

In most major metropolitan hospitals in the United States today, *Serratia* infections of the lungs, genitourinary tract, wounds, and bloodstream are endemic (164). Epidemic spread has occurred both within and between hospitals in the same geographic region (128). The usual means of transmission is by the hands of personnel.

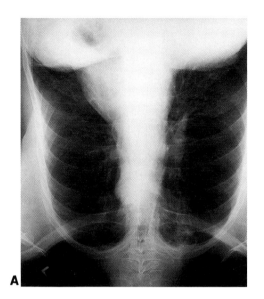

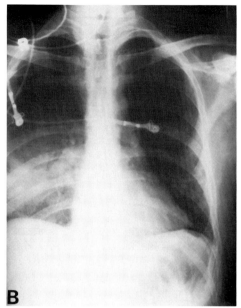

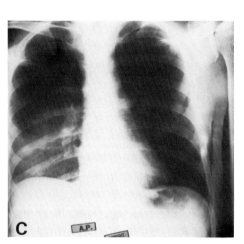

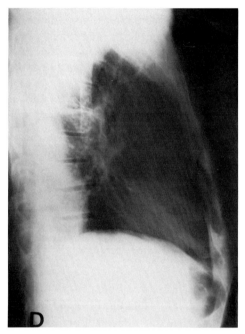

FIG. 19–1. Some x-rays of gram-negative bacillary pneumonias acquired in the hospital or in immunocompromised patients (104). **A:** 74-year-old nursing home resident admitted with fever, cough, purulent sputum. Admitting chest x-ray showed right upper lobe cavitary infiltrate consistent with tuberculosis. Sputum and blood cultures grew *Klebsiella pneumoniae.* Cultures were negative for *M. tuberculosis.* The patient responded to appropriate antimicrobial therapy. **B–D:** *E. coli* nosocomial pneumonia in a patient with an aplastic bone marrow. A 40-year-old man was admitted with mental confusion, diffuse polyneuropathy, and pancytopenia. A diagnosis of arsenic poisoning was made. During the third hospital week, fever, rigors, cough, and rales in the right upper lobe appeared. Chest x-ray **(B)** showed a right lower lobe bronchopneumonia. *E. coli* was grown from urine, sputum, and blood cultures before treatment was begun. On the seventh day of gentamicin therapy, a metapneumonic empyema appeared **(C, D).** Culture of the pleural fluid yielded *E. coli.* The patient responded well to drainage by chest tube after thoracostomy and cefamandole. Unlike some other gram-negative bacillary pneumonias, the clinical and roentgenographic features of nosocomial and community-acquired *E. coli* pneumonia appear to be similar (94).

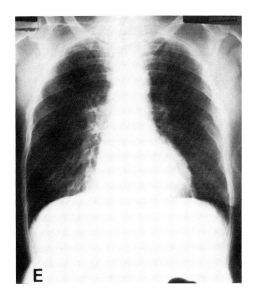
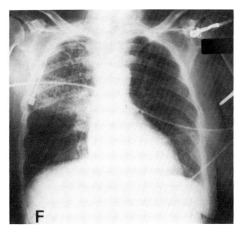

FIG. 19–1 (continued). E, F: Community-acquired *P. aeruginosa* pneumonia in an immuno-compromised patient. Radiographic patterns of gram-negative bacillary pneumonias generally exhibit considerable variability in immunosuppressed patients. A 62-year-old woman with met-astatic carcinoma of the breast was admitted with fevers to 40°C of 1 days' duration. She had been receiving chemotherapy as an outpatient. Aside from fever, chills, and an absent right breast, her physical examination was not remarkable. Her neutrophil count was 475/mm³, and chest x-ray **(E)** showed only pulmonary congestion (31). After cultures, cefazolin, tobramycin, and ticarcillin treatments were begun. The following day, a right upper lobe pneumonia with multiple abscesses was seen **(F)**. At cultures, *P. aeruginosa* grew from blood and sputum. Cefazolin was discontinued. Her neutrophil count increased and she was discharged, much improved, on the 21st hospital day.

Pharyngeal colonization followed by endogenous aspiration leads to pneumonia. The use of contaminated nebulizer reservoirs and fiberoptic bronchoscopes has caused outbreaks of *Serratia* pneumonias (164). Patients at highest risk have often been hospitalized for long periods of time, and the prior use of gentamicin has favored emergence of gentamicin/tobramycin-resistant strains (164).

At autopsy, *S. marcescens* pneumonia is a focal or diffuse bronchopneumonia (49,92). Diffuse pneumonias are common in neutropenic patients (166). Macroscopic abscesses are rare, but 2 to 3 mm abscesses are occasionally found. Peribronchial infiltrates with small areas of central necrosis and hemorrhage are present. Poly-morphonuclear leukocytes are abundant in the outer advancing inflammatory zone (92). In about 75% of cases, vasculitis in scattered veins and arteries are seen, but unlike *P. aeruginosa* vasculitis, intramural GNB are not found (49). After prolonged pneumonias, extensive fibrosis and "honeycombing" are seen. In neutropenic pa-tients without effective inflammatory cellular responses, diffuse hemorrhage and al-veolar necrosis are seen (49).

Host/Virulence Factors

Simberkoff et al. (138,139) studied clinical isolates of *S. marcescens*. All blood culture isolates were resistant to the bactericidal activity of normal serum, and 21%

of isolates from sputa were serum-resistant. Infection with serum-resistant strains also correlated with a poor prognosis. Complement-dependent opsonization by strain-specific IgM antibody to serum-resistant strains resulted in phagocytosis and intracellular killing by neutrophils (139). Opsonic and protective IgG antibodies were complement-independent and directed against somatic (O) antigens of *Serratia* (138).

Clinical and Laboratory Features (92)

Most of the reported cases of *Serratia* pneumonia occurred in hospitalized men over 50 with underlying cardiovascular disease, but anemia, chronic lung disease, malignancy, and drug abuse have also been associated conditions. Often patients have been immediately postoperative in a surgical intensive care unit receiving assisted ventilation. Most cases have occurred after the second week of hospitalization (141). Fever, rigor, and sputum production heralded the onset of pneumonia. Hemoptysis or pseudohemoptysis can be observed. Leukocytosis with shifts to the left is seen. Chest x-ray showed focal patchy bronchopneumonias with a fine nodular pattern without abscesses. Metapneumonic pleural effusions have sometimes followed. Abscess and lobar consolidation are rare. In neutropenic patients, diffuse bilateral mixed alveolar/interstitial pneumonias with a "butterfly" appearance have been seen (166).

Escherichia coli

Incidence and Mortality (Table 19-2)

Escherichia coli infection ranks after *K. pneumonia* as the second most common cause of community-acquired GNBP, representing 2.0 to 3.3% of all pneumonia admissions to city hospitals, and 12 to 45% of community-acquired GNBPs (31,46,53,144,146,147). When first described by Tillotson and Lerner in 1967 (148), the mortality rate of community-acquired *E. coli* pneumonia was 60%. A 1982 report records a death rate of 29% (5), and more recent mortality figures are even lower. During the 1970s and early 1980s, nosocomial case rates were 4.2 to 9.0 per 10,000 admissions or discharges, representing 9 to 15% of nosocomial GNBPs (17,18,141, 153,157). The most recent NNIS reports an incidence of 6.4% (25). Twenty-four to 31% of patients acquiring *E. coli* pneumonia in hospitals die (24,141,153). Mortality is up to 90% in bacteremic cases (69,77).

Microbiology

The "colon bacillus" was isolated in 1885 by Escherich. This gram-negative bacillus can be motile or nonmotile. Somatic (O), flagellar (H), and capsular (K or B) antigens form the basis of typing and, in some instances, have been recognized as virulence factors.

Pathogenesis and Pathology (Table 19-1)

In contrast with other GNBPs, with the exception of *P. aeruginosa,* patients acquire both community and nosocomial *E. coli* pneumonia after bacteremias originating from the genitourinary or gastrointestinal tract (5,90,148). Endogenous aspiration of *E. coli* from a colonized pharyngeal oral flora also causes pneumonia. In busy hospitals multiple antibiotic-resistant Escherichiae have been isolated from hands of working personnel, presumably originating from urine, stool, and pharyngeal secretions of patients. These strains, of course, increase the possible severity of the therapeutic challenge with *E. coli* pneumonia.

At autopsy, diffuse lower lobe, often bilateral, bronchopneumonias are found. Abscesses occasionally are seen (90). In patients surviving for longer than 6 days after onset, empyema with pleural effusion is typical. Intra-alveolar hemorrhage can be seen, but pulmonary arteries and veins are patent. The tracheobronchial mucosa is uninvolved, perhaps because most cases are of hematogenous origin. *Escherichia coli* cholecystitis, diverticulitis, cystitis, pyelonephritis, and meningitis can be present (24).

At histologic section, alveoli are filled with serum and moderate numbers of mononuclear cells. In patients dying after brief courses, red blood cells are also seen, but hemosiderin-laden macrophages are present in cases with prolonged courses. Alveolar cells show cuboidal metaplasia, and the septae are thickened with edema and mononuclear infiltrates. Occasionally, areas of alveolar wall necrosis with predominantly polymorphonuclear leukocytic infiltrate are seen in these zones.

Host/Virulence Factors

Patients with community-acquired *E. coli* pneumonia are usually middle-aged to elderly with underlying diseases including diabetes mellitus, urinary tract infections, cardiac or chronic lung disease, or cirrhosis (5,24,90,148). Strains containing capsular polysaccharide K1 antigen are particularly virulent for newborns and represent the common strain causing neonatal meningitis (126). Similarly, K1 antigen containing strains of *E. coli* more often cause acute pyelonephritis, whereas K1 negative strains are more often associated with acute cystitis or asymptomatic bacteriuria (8). Opsonization of *E. coli* is critical to phagocytosis. Strains from patients with asymptomatic bacteriuria usually are serum-sensitive and activate the alternate complement pathway, whereas isolates from pyelonephritis do not (8). There does not appear to be a relationship between the presence of K antigen, serum sensitivity, or somatic (O) antigen(s) and resultant mortality in adult *E. coli* bacteremia (90). Berk et al. (5) evaluated the role of K1 capsular antigen in *E. coli* pneumonia. Community-acquired cases were caused by K1-positive strains that were of urinary origin. K1-negative strains, too, caused pneumonias, but they were nosocomial infections usually derived directly from the gastrointestinal tract. However, mortality rates were similar in both K1-antigen positive and negative pneumonias (5). To be determined are the roles of the presence of several O antigens; serum resistance; activation of complement; the properdin system; and enterotoxin production in strains of *E. coli* causing pneumonia.

Clinical and Laboratory Features (5,69,148)

Lethargy, chills, fever, cough, purulent sputum, and pleurisy ensue 1 to 3 days before admission. Some have also complained of nonspecific abdominal pain. Others, on drinking sprees, have ignored fever and respiratory symptoms for several days more and presented to emergency rooms with pneumonia and meningitis (24).

Initial temperatures are generally low (100.9 to 101°F), but tachycardia is out of proportion to fevers. In survivors, fevers end by lysis. Physical examinations reveal basilar rales without evidence of consolidation.

White blood cell counts are high with more immature granulocytes in the circulation as well. Patchy lower lobe bronchopneumonias are seen at x-ray. Occasionally, lobar consolidation ($\pm$ abscess) is seen (152). The total lung volume is not decreased. Metapneumonic pleural effusions are usual (see Fig. 19-1, B–D). Similar roentgenographic findings have been reported in neutropenic patients (166). *Escherichia coli* is recovered readily from multiple sites including urine, blood, sputum, and pleural fluid.

Proteus, Providencia, and *Morganella*

Incidence and Mortality (Table 19-2)

For discussions of incidence and mortality, see references 4,17,18,30,39,62,141, 144,146,147, and 157.

Microbiology

Proteus are highly motile gram-negative bacilli that characteristically swarm on agar. There are three species: *mirabilis* and *penneri*, both indole-negative organisms, and *vulgaris,* which is indole-positive. Based on DNA content, two other species, formerly designated *P. morganii* and *P. rettgeri,* have been assigned to other genera, *Providencia rettgeri* and *Morganella morganii. Proteus* sp, *M. morganii*, and *P. rettgeri* are all lactose nonfermenters, and they all produce a powerful urease.

Pathogenesis and Pathology (149) (Table 19-1)

Patients acquire *Proteus* pneumonias after endogenous aspiration of pharyngeal secretions. At autopsy, a dense consolidation with multiple abscesses is found in the affected lung. The pleural space is free of effusion. Alveoli are filled with red blood cells and a mixed exudate consisting of both mononuclear and polymorphonuclear leukocytes. In areas of alveolar necrosis, neutrophils predominate.

Host/Virulence Factors

Proteus pneumonias occurred at Detroit Receiving Hospital in elderly alcoholic men with chronic lung disease (149). Although the most common site of *Proteus* infections is the urinary tract, none of the original Detroit patients had infections at this site. Endogenous aspiration from a colonized oropharynx resulted in these *Proteus* pneumonias. Harrow et al. (57) challenged mice with intravenous *P. mirabilis.* They repeated the experiment with *S. aureus. Proteus* was rapidly cleared from the lungs, but only 2.0% recovery of *S. aureus* was possible at the 4-hr sacrifice. *Proteus* bacilli were engulfed by polymorphonuclear leukocytes, but alveolar macrophages were incapable of phagocytosis of these organisms. On the other hand, Green and Kass (53), using aerosol challenges in mice, found alveolar macrophages the preeminent means of cellular defense. Staphylococci were more rapidly cleared by alveolar macrophages than was *Proteus*.

Clinical and Laboratory Features

In 1968 Tillotson and Lerner (149) described six patients admitted to Detroit Receiving Hospital with pneumonias caused by *P. vulgaris, P. mirabilis,* or *Morganella (Proteus) morganii*. Chronic disease of the lungs (bronchitis, bronchiectasis, emphysema, recurrent pneumonia) was evident in every patient. Bronchitic symptoms worsened 1 to 8 weeks before admission, but 1 to 5 days before admission, rigors, chest pain, fever, dyspnea, and a cough productive of tenacious yellow sputum heralded the onset of pneumonia. Five were chronic alcoholics, and three of them presented in frank delirium tremens. They noted signs of an upper lobe pulmonary consolidation with an ipsilateral shift of the trachea in four patients. Five patients had enlarged livers, which was attributed to alcohol abuse. Leukocytosis with left shifts was present.

Species of *Proteus* (or *Morganella*) were cultured from sputum as the predominant organism and persisted despite suitable antimicrobials for long periods. Throat cultures also revealed *Proteus,* but urine and blood tests were negative. At autopsy of the single fatality, *Proteus vulgaris* was isolated in pure growth from the lung.

Chest x-ray films showed dense infiltrates in the posterior segments of the right upper lobes and superior segments of the right lower lobe. Pneumonias involved a single lobe, and abscesses were evident in five or six cases. Pleural effusions did not occur, and healing left a contracted fibrotic lobe. Similar x-ray findings have been reported by others in both community-acquired and nosocomial infections (152,166).

Four nosocomial cases of *Providencia* pneumonias were reported by Solberg and Matsen (140). Patients were postoperative from thoracoabdominal surgery or had underlying malignancies. Upper lobe consolidations were found in two patients; the others had bronchopneumonias. One of these patients died. A rare case of pulmonary pneumatoceles complicating the course of *Proteus mirabilis* pneumonia was also described (86).

Miscellaneous Enterobacteriaceae

Other genera of the family Enterobacteriaceae include *Shigella;* the *Salmonella-Arizona-Citrobacter* division; *Edwardsiella; Hafnia; Yersinia; Erwinia;* and, in addition, still unclassified organisms. *Yersinia* pneumonias are discussed in a separate chapter of this volume. To date, there are no convincing case reports of GNBPs caused by *Edwardsiella, Shigella,* or other unclassified organisms. Meyers et al. (94) reported a single case of *Erwinia* pneumonia with an associated empyema. This occurred in a patient with a malignant lymphoma during a hospital outbreak. In a review of clinical isolates of *Hafnia* from the Mayo Clinic, the authors reported two fatal secondary pneumonias, one with an associated abscess. One of these patients had underlying chronic renal disease, and the other had a malignant melanoma (155).

Several reports of community-acquired or nosocomial primary *Citrobacter* pneumonias have appeared, generally occurring in patients with malignancies. Acquisition of *Citrobacter* was usually by endogenous aspiration, but bacteremic seeding of lungs has occurred. Chest roentgenograms showed small lower lobe infiltrates with large pleural effusions (88,153). Zornoza et al. (166) described a predominately mixed interstitial and alveolar pattern in neutropenic patients.

A cough can be present in patients with typhoid fever. Occasionally respiratory symptoms can even predominate on presentation, delaying accurate diagnosis (1). As many as 11% of patients with *Salmonella typhi* have pneumonia; many of these pneumonias represent suprainfection (143). Pleuropulmonary disease in nontyphoid *Salmonella* is unusual. Pulmonary disease can occur independently or in association with gastroenteritis. Saphra and Winter (125) reviewed 7,779 cases of salmonellosis and found 85 patients with pneumonias or empyema. Most were elderly with diabetes mellitus or cancers. Lobar and bronchopneumonias were seen. Bacteremic origins were suspected. Fatality rates were high. Occasionally, intrapulmonary abscesses attributable to *Salmonella* pneumonia have been reported in immunocompromised patients (13). Recent reports emphasize the association of Salmonella infection with lymphoma or leukemia (1,13).

Acinetobacter baumannii

Incidence and Mortality (Table 19-2)

For a discussion of incidence and mortality, see references 2,23,47,124,146, and 157. The incidence of pneumonia caused by *Acinetobacter* sp is rising. In the 1984 NNIS survey *Acinetobacter* sp were not ranked as a major cause of nosocomial infection; in the 1989 survey they caused 3% of nosocomial pneumonias (6% in the ICU) (25).

Microbiology

Gram stain of expectorated sputum or transtracheal aspirate reveal *Acinetobacter* as gram-negative nonmotile coccobacilli. Such smears may be misinterpreted as over-decolorized pneumococci, *Neisseria, Hemophilus,* or *Branhamella* (50) (Fig. 19-2). Such a misinterpretation often leads to ineffectual antibiotic treatment. At times, long filamentous bacilli are seen. Some cells retain crystal violet and appear to be gram-positive rods.

The organism has kept taxonomists busy. *Acinetobacter baumannii* was most recently referred to as *Acinetobacter calcoaceticus var. anitratus;* previous designations include *Bacterium anitratum, Herellea vaginicola,* and *Achromobacter anitratus.* Almost all reported cases of *Acinetobacter* pulmonary infections are caused by the specie *baumannii.*

Pathogenesis and Pathology (Table 19-1)

Most *Acinetobacter* cultured from sputum represent transient oropharyngeal colonization or oral contamination. Up to 7% of normal persons carry this GNB in their oropharynx (64); it is not considered part of the normal intestinal flora. It is also a frequent commensal of the skin, found predominately in moist skin areas and conjunctiva. Community-acquired *Acinetobacter* pneumonia is rare, but it is being reported with increasing frequency, especially in tropical developing countries (2). The first case of *Acinetobacter* pneumonia was reported in 1959 (48). *Acinetobacter* pneumonias are seen in elderly persons, often with chronic diseases, particularly

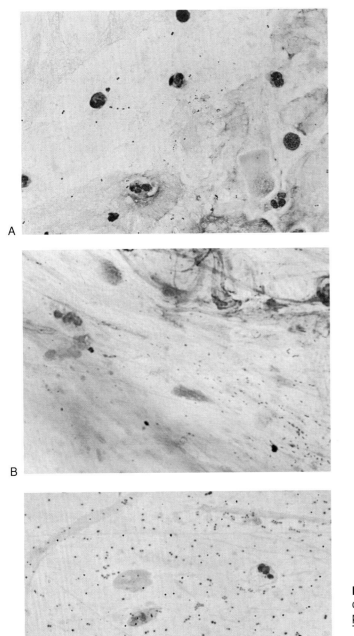

FIG. 19–2. Gram stains of expectorated sputa of patients with pneumonia. The gram stain of patients with *Acinetobacter* pneumonia **(A)** may be misinterpreted as *Hemophillus influenzae* **(B)** or *Moraxella* (Branhamella) pneumonia **(C).**

alcoholism (50,124). In one study of community-acquired disease, three healthy men working in a steel casting foundry acquired *Acinetobacter* pneumonias by an airborne route. Intense exposure to silica and metallic particles in the air can lead to increased susceptibility to infection (23). In the hospital it occurs mainly in intensive care units. Critical care patients at risk typically have tracheotomies or endotracheal tubes. Previous antimicrobial therapy is usual. Environmental isolates in burns units have been well described in nonsterile water supplies and on damp surfaces (165). *Acinetobacter* is the most common gram-negative colonizer of hospital employees' hands (79). Outbreaks of respiratory disease and colonization have previously been associated with contaminated, reusable ventilator equipment (58).

At autopsy, bronchopneumonia with abscesses are found. Abscesses erode into the large bronchi or invaded arteries. Lobar consolidations are occasionally seen. Empyemas occur in half of the cases. Alveoli are filled with erythrocytes, polymorphonuclear leukocytes, and bacteria. Hemosiderin-laden macrophages are seen. In those patients dying during the foundry outbreak, pneumoconiosis was evident (23).

Clinical and Laboratory Features (23,50,124)

Patients with community-acquired *Acinetobacter* pneumonias have usually been middle-aged to elderly men (rarely, women) with antecedent chronic alcoholism, chronic pulmonary disease, and heavy use of cigarettes. Occupational exposure to agents such as silica or metallic particles is an additional risk factor. Before admission to the hospital, patients had been ill for 1 to 7 days with cough, bloody sputum, pleuritic chest pain, and fever. Often a preceding upper respiratory tract infection was noted. Patients were tachypneic, cyanotic, often sitting "bolt upright" with severe respiratory distress. Half the patients were in shock at admission. Lower lobe consolidations, often with pleural effusions, were frequent. Most were leukopenic, and a few had absolute granulocytopenias. Arterial blood gases showed profound hypoxemia. Blood, sputa, and empyema tests frequently yielded *Acinetobacter.*

Lower lobe bronchopneumonias with abscess(es) and prepneumonic empyemas were seen at chest x-ray. Pneumonias progressed rapidly, despite antibiotic therapy, to involve both lungs. Particularly in patients with granulocytopenia or empyema, death occurred within 72 hours. The fatality rate of community-acquired disease is 52% (51).

Outbreaks of multiple-drug-resistant *Acinetobacter baumannii* have been reported in surgical and medical intensive care units since 1978 (16). It is a bacterium of increasing nosocomial importance. Unlike other gram-negative rods causing infection in cancer patients, *Acinetobacter* septicemia is not associated with neutropenia; instead, it occurs in cancer patients with central venous catheters (121). The multidrug-resistant nature of this bacterium, its increasing incidence of nosocomial disease, initial confusion with other, more-common causes of community-acquired pneumonias, and its fulminant course make it a formidable cause of pneumonia.

Pseudomonas aeruginosa

Incidence and Mortality (Table 19-2)

Detroit General and Grady Memorial Hospitals reported that community-acquired *Pseudomonas aeruginosa* pneumonias caused 11% and 6% of GNBPs, respectively

(144,147). The incidence of primary *Pseudomonas* pneumonia among patients transferred to hospitals from nursing homes was 5.7% (43). Mortality in community-acquired cases is 72%.

Pseudomonas causes 17.2% of all nosocomial pneumonias. It outnumbers all other nosocomial GNBPs, including *Klebsiella* (62). *Pseudomonas* sp caused 25% of nosocomial pneumonias in NNIS-participating ICUs during 1989. From 3.0 to 9.6 cases/10,000 admissions or discharges have been reported (17,18,157). Of all nosocomial *P. aeruginosa* pneumonias, most, that is, 75%, originate in intensive care units (62). In a 1974 study, crude mortality of *Pseudomonas* pneumonia in a surgical intensive care unit was 70%, twice the concurrent death rate for other GNBPs (93). Mortality in two recent series of nosocomial *Pseudomonas* pneumonias was 24 and 36% (141,153). In contrast, at the National Cancer Institute (National Institutes of Health), from 1956 to 1970, the mortality was 81% of 36 cases (142). A possible factor in the recent putative difference in mortality between community-acquired and nosocomial *Pseudomonas* pneumonias is earlier use of more-effective antipseudomonal antimicrobial therapy. Nevertheless, mortality rates in bacteremic *P. aeruginosa* pneumonias remain high, ranging from 31 to 90% in recent series (12,71,77,106).

Microbiology

P. aeruginosa is an obligate aerobic, motile, gram-negative bacillus with a single polar flagellum. It is the most frequently isolated organism of the 160 species belonging to the family Pseudomonadacae. It is widely prevalent in the hospital environment, requiring no growth factors, using carbon dioxide as its sole carbon source and ammonium for nitrogen. Some strains produce the soluble blue-green pigment, pyocyanin (aerugiosin). It can also produce fluorescent pigments.

The structure of *P. aeruginosa* resembles that of other gram-negative bacilli. In sputum, they are thin gram-negative rods, but strains from patients with cystic fibrosis have large capsules. Epidemiologists have used various typing systems based on bacteriocin (pyocin) production, seroagglutination to cell wall lipopolysaccharides, or bacteriophages. None of these systems has revealed a special relationship to virulence.

Pathogenesis and Pathology

Pseudomonas aeruginosa pneumonias are acquired in the community after endogenous aspiration from a colonized oropharynx (46,150). Rarely, bacteremic pneumonias have occurred in a community setting (71). Likewise, endogenous aspiration is the usual mode of infection within hospitals. *Pseudomonas* are sometimes present in the pharynx at time of admission to the hospital; more often it is acquired later.

About 5% of healthy adults have a normal oral flora that includes *P. aeruginosa* (123), but 18 to 25% of patients with underlying malignancies are *Pseudomonas* carriers. After 4 weeks' residence in the hospital, 50% of cancer patients are *Pseudomonas* carriers (133). As with *Klebsiella,* critically ill patients develop specific surface-binding sites on their oral epithelial cells for *Pseudomonas* (67). Patients in intensive care or burn units can also acquire these binding sites. The hands of personnel, other patients, or, rarely, sinks serve as reservoirs or vectors (85). Exogenous inhalation from contaminated aerosol medication has caused outbreaks of *P. aeruginosa* pneumonia. In patients with neutropenias or severe burns, hematogenous seeding of the lungs has occurred (63,95,153). In a landmark publication, Pierce et al. (107) described the pathology of fatal cases of nosocomial *P. aeruginosa* pneumonia. Their patients acquired pneumonia during a large outbreak in the Dallas area during the late 1960s. Pneumonias resulted from inhalation of contaminated aerosols (107). Necrotizing pneumonia was characterized by alveolar septal necrosis with necrosis of arterial walls and secondary thrombosis. The alveolar exudate was predominantly mononuclear with some polymorphonuclear leukocytes. Gram-negative bacilli could be seen within alveolar spaces, but microabscesses were not seen (107).

At about the same time, Tillotson and Lerner (150) described a different anatomic pathology in fatal cases of *Pseudomonas* pneumonia acquired in the community by endogenous aspiration of endogenous flora. Infiltrates were diffuse, often bilateral, and occupying the lower lobes. Small pleural effusions were usual. On cut-section, multiple small abscesses were grossly present, and at microscopic examination, marked alveolar cell wall necrosis and microabscesses were characteristic. Areas of focal hemorrhage were seen. There was no arterial wall necrosis, perivascular infiltrate, or thrombosis. When alveolar septa were intact, macrophages, mononuclear cells, and polymorphonuclear leukocytes were found within alveoli. In the patients apparently unrelated to preexisting disease, scattered focal areas of polymorphonuclear leukocytes with recent fibroplasia were found in the spleen, kidneys, heart, and liver.

A different lung pathology occurs in bacteremic *Pseudomonas* pneumonias (38). Pneumonias are usually diffuse and bilateral with small pleural effusions. Gross lesions on cut-section are either (i) nodular, hemorrhagic areas with small central necrotic foci; or (ii) firm, yellow-tan, umbilicated nodules surrounded by dark hemorrhage. Microscopically, hemorrhagic areas are intra-alveolar hemorrhage with patchy alveolar septal necrosis. Inflammatory cells are absent, but myriads of GNB are present. The yellow nodules are microabscesses with mononuclear cells predominating, or they are areas of arterial necrosis and thrombosis. GNB infiltrates the necrotic arterial walls. These patients usually have underlying hematologic malignancies. Ecthyma gangrenosum can occur, and petechial hemorrhages can be seen in viscera.

Host/Virulence Factors

Excluding children with cystic fibrosis, patients with community-acquired *P. aeruginosa* pneumonias are usually middle-aged to elderly men with severe chronic cardiopulmonary disease (150). Outpatient delivery of aggressive cytotoxic cancer chemotherapy has increased the number of admissions of patients with *Pseudomonas* pneumonias (Fig. 19-1, E, F). Recent conference reports suggest that persons with AIDS are at risk of developing community and nosocomial *Pseudomonas* pneumonia. The neonatal unit, burn unit, surgical intensive care unit, oncology unit, HIV/AIDS unit, and postoperative suite are areas of the hospital likely to have patients with *Pseudomonas* pneumonias (19).

Neutropenic patients are especially susceptible to *Pseudomonas* pneumonia (62,105). In leukopenic dogs with experimental *Pseudomonas* pneumonia, granulocyte transfusions plus gentamicin is significantly more effective than gentamicin alone (27). About 85% of all human isolates of *P. aeruginosa* are resistant to lysis by fresh serum; the bacilli are promptly killed. Opsonizing antibody is the principal protective antibody against *Pseudomonas*. These antibodies are type-specific and are directed toward its lipopolysaccharide. Low or absent opsonizing antibody titers in patient's blood are associated with high mortalities. The bulk of the opsonizing *Pseudomonas* antibody is complement-dependent IgM immunoglobulin. IgG opsonizing antibody is also protective and is complement-independent (163).

After parenteral immunization of rabbits with *Pseudomonas* antigens, agglutinating IgG antibody derived by passive diffusion from serum appears in bronchial secretions. Following intranasal vaccination, secretory IgA and IgG are found, suggesting local antibody synthesis (120). The opsonic activity of IgG antibody to *Pseudomonas* is superior to secretory IgA in promoting phagocytosis by either rabbit or human alveolar macrophages (119). Once ingested, intracellular killing is rapid.

Microbial virulence factors of *P. aeruginosa* include the slime layer, lipopolysaccharide, and released proteolytic enzymes and toxins such as exotoxin A, enterotoxin, hemolysins, and leucocidin (59). The slime (capsular) layer inhibits phagocytosis by alveolar macrophages, enhancing adherence to epithelial cells in patients with cystic fibrosis. Pili projecting from the slime also enhance adherence to epithelial cells. It can also induce leukopenia (137). The lipopolysaccharide layer is an endotoxin, but it is not as biologically active as similar substances of Enterobacteriaceae. The pathogenic role of this endotoxin in human pseudomonal infection is unclear. Within the periplasmic space of *Pseudomonas'* cell wall, various proteolytic enzymes, including elastase, caseinase, fibrinolysin, and collagenase are found. Up to 85% of the isolates contain elastase that, although not as lethal to mice as exotoxin A, is also an important virulence factor in *Pseudomonas* pneumonias. Investigators have detected elastase antibodies in patients with *Pseudomonas* pneumonia (161). Intratracheal administration of elastase to experimental animals produces intra-alveolar hemorrhage, necrosis of alveolar septae, and mononuclear cell infiltration, which are also seen in human infection (52,161). Elastase also mediates the necrosis of arterial walls seen in bacteremic *Pseudomonas* pneumonia.

Exotoxin A is the most potent *Pseudomonas* toxin. Sublethal doses to mice cause necrosis of liver cells and elevations in liver enzymes, reminiscent of the liver function abnormalities observed by Tillotson and Lerner (106,150) in patients with *P. aeruginosa* pneumonia. In humans, low levels of serum antibody to exotoxin A correlate with fatal *Pseudomonas* infections, whereas higher antibody titers have been found in patients who recover (111). Phospholipase, a hemolytic toxin, inactivates pulmonary surfactant leading to alveolar collapse (84). The role of *Pseudomonas* enterotoxin is not clear.

Finally, the aftermath of an episode of *Pseudomonas* pneumonia is more severe than one caused by gram-positive bacteria, for example, pneumococcus. The lung usually repairs itself after such an infection, but with *Pseudomonas,* the architecture is disturbed and fibrosis with persistent scarring is a common occurrence.

Clinical and Laboratory Features (63,105,150)

On admission to the hospital, patients with community-acquired *Pseudomonas* are toxic, apprehensive, and confused, and exhibit chills, fever, and coughs that produce yellow or green sputum. Many clinicians have observed relative bradycardia and reversal of the usual diurnal temperature curves. White blood cell counts are elevated with a predominance of immature forms. Even without antecedent hepatic or renal disease, azotemia and abnormal liver function tests are found. At thoracentesis, hemorrhagic pleural effusions can be found.

At chest x-ray bronchopneumonias are diffuse, bilateral, and usually seen in the lower lobe. Infiltrates are nodular with contained radiolucencies that can coalesce with progressive disease. Metapneumonic pleural effusions are frequent.

In neutropenic patients the onset of bacteremic *P. aeruginosa* pneumonia is heralded by the sudden onset of fever, confusion, and dyspnea. Sputum is scanty and a few basilar crackles can be the only physical findings in the lungs. Ecthyma gangrenosum is sometimes seen. At first, chest x-rays show only pulmonary vascular congestion, but central venous pressures are normal (63). Later, patchy, diffuse bilateral pneumonias and abscesses are seen (Fig. 19-1, E, F).

Non-aeruginosa Pseudomonads (excluding *P. mallei* and *P. pseudomallei*)

Pseudomonas cepacia

Reported infections caused by *Pseudomonas cepacia* include pneumonia (156). Children with cystic fibrosis or chronic granulomatous disease are especially at risk. Colonization with *P. cepacia* is frequent in cystic fibrosis patients, and a necrotizing pneumonia associated with bacteremia occurs occasionally. Previously, *P. cepacia* pneumonia was associated with inadequate sterilization of respiratory therapy equipment.

Pseudomonas stutzeri

Pseudomonas stutzeri is rarely associated with clinical disease. To date, three cases of community-acquired pneumonia have been reported (15). All three were seen in severely debilitated patients with either alcoholism or malignancy.

Xanthomonas maltophilia

Formerly designated *Pseudomonas maltophilia*, *Xanthomonas maltophilia* is frequently isolated from respiratory specimens (61). It is a motile, free-living gram-negative nonfermentive bacillus. It possesses polar multitrichous flagella. *Xanthomonas maltophilia* is generally indophenol oxidase-negative. It does oxidize maltose and, usually, dextrose and xylose. It produces a number of enzymes, among them catalases, lipases, esterases, DNase, RNase, hyaluronidase, and mucinase. Production of proteases, hemolysin, and elastases is unusual. These and other genetic, physiologic, and biochemical differences led to the reclassification of *X. maltophilia* from genus *Pseudomonas* (145).

This organism can be isolated from numerous environmental, human, and animal sources. In the past, sources of nosocomial outbreaks of bacterurias and bacteremias included contaminated hospital disinfectants (159) and central venous monitoring devices (40). It is almost always nosocomial in origin; Gardner (44) reported that 97% of the isolates in his study were hospital acquired. In that setting, it often can be isolated in the absence of clinical infection. However, *X. maltophilia* is an opportunistic pathogen that may cause life-threatening illness. Elting and Bodey (34) noted that *Xanthomonas* are not ordinarily found in the GI tract, nor are they generally a colonizer of the skin. Isolation of *X. maltophilia* is especially common in patients with malignancies (34). In one report, patients with acute leukemia were more likely to be infected (41%) than to be colonized (11%), as were neutropenic patients (41% vs. 5%) (74).

A serologic typing system based on somatic O antigens has enabled about 94% of isolates to be typed. Serotype 3 is the most frequent (20.7%) isolate (130).

Previous antimicrobial therapy is strongly correlated to presence of either colonization or infection (74). Other risk factors include presence of central venous catheters (34,58), prolonged hospitalization (74), neutropenia, and leukemia.

Xanthomonas maltophilia pneumonia is generally a diffuse, bilateral process with multilobar involvement (34). In Elting's (34) study 34% of those with *X. maltophilia* septicemia had pulmonary infection. Bacteremic leukemia patients can develop ecthyma gangrenosum (34).

Morrison et al. (97) reported a crude mortality rate of 43% in 99 patients with nosocomial *X. maltophilia* infection. Risk factors for death included a pneumonia (74,97), intensive care, and age greater than 40 years. Mortality for patients with pneumonia was 59%. In response to therapy, bacteremic *Xanthomonas* pneumonia is lower (29%) than *Xanthomonas* bacteremias originating elsewhere (77%) (34). *Xanthomonas maltophilia* is often found in mixed culture (34,97). Higher mortality occurs when the organism grows in mixed cultures (61).

ANTIMICROBIAL THERAPY

Initial Antimicrobial Treatment

Gram-negative bacillary pneumonias are serious infections with significant mortality. Physicians should maintain a high index of suspicion in their diagnosis, especially among hospitalized patients and persons admitted from chronic care facilities. The selection of appropriate treatment is ultimately guided by identification of the responsible microbial pathogen. Carefully collected specimens of sputum, pleural fluids, and blood should be obtained. Consideration should be given to performing bronchoalveolar lavage with protected brush biopsy specimens before therapy, when these procedures are most likely to be diagnostic. This chapter has emphasized that certain clinical, radiographic, and laboratory features can suggest a bacteriologic diagnosis of GNBP before culture results are available. Unfortunately, deviations from "classic" patterns of disease are common, particularly in immunosuppressed hosts (108,166). Initial therapy will then by necessity be empiric.

Empirical therapy should not be withheld pending identification of a definitive causative organism. Concerning nosocomial disease, awareness of the incidence of offending organisms within a specific hospital locale is often crucial in selecting initial therapy. Careful study of antibiograms focused on the changing trends in a hospital's microbial resistance patterns can yield life-saving results. The results of susceptibility testing will vary among institutions and hospital sites based upon patterns of antimicrobial use, the characteristics of the patient population, and the nature of endemic bacterial strains.

When a pathogen has been isolated, antibiotic selection is generally based on *in vitro* susceptibility testing such as minimum inhibitory concentrations (MICs). However, neither MICs nor minimum bacteriocidal concentrations (MBCs) reflect all factors necessary to predict a successful treatment outcome (60). The ability of an antimicrobial to inhibit bacterial growth for a time after drug levels have dipped below the MIC (the postantibiotic effect) (56) illustrates this point. MICs do not reflect the immunocompetence of the host or drug pharmacokinetics like tissue distribution (104). Variable dosing regimens with altered serum levels and the development of antimicrobial resistance are also not reflected in MICs. Antibiotic concentrations in the lung parenchyma approach serum levels, but those in bronchial secretions are considerably lower. Because purulent tracheobronchitis often accompanies GNBPs, high antibiotic doses could be required to achieve therapeutic levels in bronchial secretions. Each of these factors must be considered in association with the MIC in selection of appropriate antimicrobial therapy.

Initial Empiric Therapy: Considerations

Monotherapy

Empiric monotherapy for GNBP has several disadvantages, including (i) limited antimicrobial spectrum; (ii) increased incidence of development of resistance while on single-drug therapy, especially in organisms with inducible mechanisms of resistance; (iii) absence of synergy; (iv) increased incidence of the development of suprainfection when a patient receives single-drug therapy; and (v) the lack of large, controlled clinical trials. For these reasons, we cannot support the use of monotherapy for initial, empirical therapy of GNBP.

Combination Therapy

Beta-Lactam /Aminoglycoside Combination

Combination therapy with a beta-lactam/aminoglycoside offers the theoretical advantages of broad-spectrum, rapidly bacteriocidal therapy with better clinical outcomes associated with synergistic bacteriocidal effects (33). For example, Hilf and co-workers (60) have reported improved survival when bacteremic *P. aeruginosa* pneumonia is treated with a beta-lactam/aminoglycoside combination therapy. Combination therapy has also been seen to limit the development of resistance in the course of receiving therapy (3). Because of these advantages, combination antibiotic therapy with a beta-lactam and an aminoglycoside has become a standard empirical regimen for GNBP.

Aminoglycosides penetrate poorly into bronchial secretions (104), and they are inactivated in the acidic intrabronchial milieu (9). As a result, they are not suitable for monotherapy of gram-negative pneumonias (3,104). They exhibit synergy with beta-lactam antibiotics (32). Aminoglycosides exhibit concentration-dependent killing which achieves rapid bacteriocidal effects when adequate peak serum levels are obtained. Peak levels of 7 µg/ml or greater for gentamicin and tobramycin, or 28 µg/ml or greater for amikacin, have been shown to be important for successful treatment outcome of pneumonia (96). Drug toxicity has occurred when trough levels exceed therapeutic ranges by twofold or greater for gentamicin/tobramycin and >10 µg/ml for amikacin.

The significant toxicities of aminoglycosides have led to alternative dosing and delivery regimens. The postantibiotic effect (56) and adaptive resistance (26) of aminoglycosides permit once-daily drug-dosing regimens. Once-daily dosing can be effective in limiting the nephro- and ototoxicity potentially associated with aminoglycoside use. Single daily dosing has been found to be effective even for *Pseudomonas* pneumonia in non-neutropenic patients (112). The local use of aminoglycoside (either through aerosolized or endotracheal administration) has also had promise (64) for diminishing organ-specific toxicity. Although many studies have been conducted with aerosolized and endotracheally administered aminoglycosides, there has not been convincing evidence for their benefit (64). In contrast to the aminoglycosides, beta-lactam antibiotics do not exhibit a postantibiotic effect. For that reason, pharmacodynamic models suggest that long half-life, frequent dosing, or continuous-infusion beta-lactams might be optimal in the management of gram-negative infections.

There are several choices of beta-lactams. Of the cephalosporins, first- and second-generation cephalosporins lack sufficient gram-negative activity to be appropriate empirical antimicrobials for treatment of GNBP. An antipseudomonal cephalosporin such as cefoperazone or ceftazidime would be a reasonable empirical choice. Cefepime is a fourth-generation cephalosporin not yet released in the United States (56). This drug has an extended spectrum of activity against gram-negative bacilli including *P. aeruginosa* (56,76), and it is stable to chromosomal and plasmid beta-lactamases produced by many gram-negative bacteria.

The antipseudomonal penicillins consist of the carboxypenicillins and ureidopenicillins. *In vitro* studies of *P. aeruginosa* demonstrate that piperacillin has twice the activity of azlocillin, 4 times that of mezlocillin and ticarcillin, and 8 times the activity of carbenicillin. Ticarcillin is often used in conjunction with clavulanate. However, physicians need to be aware that clavulanate does not bind the type I beta-lactamases produced by *P. aeruginosa,* and by certain strains of *Serratia, Enterobacter,* and *Citrobacter* (78). One trial of ticarcillin/clavulanate in treating ICU patients with suspected pneumonia resulted in a clinical success rate of 96%. In the latter study, microbiologic failures occurred in patients with *P. aeruginosa* pneumonia (136). This militates against the use of ticarcillin/clavulanate for empirical therapy of GNBP.

Imipenem/cilastin has a very broad spectrum, including activity against *P. aeruginosa. Pseudomonas aeruginosa* resistance to imipenem, however, is increasing (45). Clinical trials in febrile neutropenic patients have suggested that imipenem-cilastin monotherapy is as effective as beta-lactam/aminoglycoside combination therapy for gram-negative infections, unless the patient has a *P. aeruginosa* infection (158). For that reason, imipenem/cilastin cannot be recommended for empirical monotherapy.

Double Beta-Lactam Combinations

Double beta-lactam combinations in the treatment of gram-negative infections are attractive in that they can be less toxic than aminoglycoside/beta-lactam combination therapy (54). Certain combinations of 2 beta-lactams can be synergistic when they act at different penicillin-binding proteins, or when one of them inhibits beta-lactamase. On the other hand, there could be problems using these combinations against organisms with inducible chromosomal cephalosporinases. If one drug induces beta-lactamase production resulting in inactivation of the other drug by beta-lactamase activity, then the net effect will be drug antagonism. Bacteria with inducible beta-lactams include *Enterobacter, Serratia, Citrobacter, Proteus, Aeromonas,* and *Pseudomonas* species (54).

The major disadvantages of using double beta-lactam therapy include selection of resistant organisms, possible lack of drug synergy, and the possibility of drug antagonism. There are limited data supporting the clinical utility of double beta-lactam therapy compared to standard therapy. An *in vitro* model has shown higher bactericidal activities for amikacin/beta-lactam combinations versus combinations of double beta-lactams (91).

Alternative Agents

New categories of antimicrobials have gained widespread use in the treatment of gram-negative infections during the past 5 years. Their role in empirical therapy of GNBP remains to be defined in well-designed clinical trials. They include the monobactams and the fluoroquinolones.

Aztreonam, the only available monobactam, has been used as monotherapy for GNBP. Its appeal is in its aminoglycoside-like spectrum without oto- or nephrotoxicity. It is well tolerated. However, as opposed to other beta-lactam antibiotics that bind to multiple penicillin-binding proteins (PBPs), aztreonam specifically binds to only PBP 3, which can account for its slower onset of bactericidal activity (91). In addition, it is not synergistic with beta-lactam antibiotics and is occasionally antagonistic. It does not exhibit a postantibiotic effect. Its pharmacodynamic characteristics are drawbacks in combination therapy compared to the aminoglycosides. Aztreonam is a good alternative for therapy of patients with a history of severe penicillin allergy.

The fluoroquinolones have excellent activity against most Enterobacteriaceae and *P. aeruginosa*. Ciprofloxacin is the most active fluoroquinolone against *P. aeruginosa* to date. There is no apparent synergy or antagonism between fluoroquinolones and the aminoglycosides or with beta-lactams against the Enterobacteriaceae. These drugs do exhibit synergistic activity for 20–50% of *P. aeruginosa in vitro* when combined with imipenem or with anti-*Pseudomonas* penicillins. Similar to the aminoglycosides, the fluoroquinolones exhibit concentration-dependent killing and a postantibiotic effect. Unlike aminoglycosides, the lung tissue concentration of the fluoroquinolones tends to be in excess of serum concentrations achieved (132). Concerns regarding the use of fluoroquinolones include (i) the occasionally rapid development of resistance (99); (ii) primary fluoroquinolone resistance; (iii) suprainfection; and (iv) the lack of large clinical trials in the treatment of seriously ill patients with gram-negative pneumonias. Such trials are under way.

The fluoroquinolones are a promising alternative therapy for GNBPs, including *P. aeruginosa* pneumonia. Their lack of serious toxicities makes them attractive alternatives to aminoglycosides in combination with an antipseudomonal penicillin or cephalosporin for initial empirical therapy of GNBPs.

Definitive Antimicrobial Therapy

When a patient is found to be at risk for gram-negative pneumonia and empirical therapy is started, it is anticipated that a specific pathogen will be isolated from available specimens. With definitive identification of the pathogen, therapy can be modified on the basis of antimicrobial susceptibility. Empirical therapy usually can make the transition to definitive therapy within 48 to 72 hours after the start of treatment. A specific microbiologic diagnosis is not always possible. In such circumstances, it becomes necessary to continue with the initial empirical therapy. Regardless of the setting (community-acquired or nosocomial), our policy is generally to continue dual antimicrobial therapy. In bacteremic GNBP, it is best to continue combination therapy until care is achieved. In nonbacteremic GNBP occurring in nonneutropenic hosts (and when *P. aeruginosa, Serratia, Enterobacter,* or *Citrobacter* species have been eliminated as causative organisms), treatment can be modified. After clinical response is attained, an aminoglycoside initially used can be discontinued, and a single agent (usually a beta-lactam) can be maintained. Treatment should be continued for a minimum of 2 weeks. However, in complicated cases (i.e., when atelectasis, abscess, or empyema is present) treatment needs to be extended further. Defervescence, normalization of elevated white blood cell counts, clearing of infiltrates on chest x-ray, collapse of abscesses, or decreasing pleural or empyema fluids are all indications of responses to therapy.

Klebsiella pneumoniae

Klebsiella sp are generally very responsive to third-generation cephalosporins, although these organisms can be susceptible to even first-generation cephalosporins. Monotherapy is ill-advised; treatment of this infection generally requires a cephalosporin in combination with an aminoglycoside. The uriedopenicillins mezlocillin and piperacillin, as well as ticarcillin/clavulanate, are active against *Klebsiella,* and could be used in the place of cephalosporins. Alternative treatments include trimethoprim-sulfamethoxazole, imipenem, and ciprofloxacin.

Enterobacter species

Most strains of *Enterobacter* are resistant to first-generation cephalosporins. Although the organism demonstrates *in vitro* susceptibility to second- and third-generation cephalosporins, resistance rapidly emerges during treatment, and clinical failure has been reported (20). The mechanism for resistance is the induction of beta-lactamase by the prescribed beta-lactam antibiotic. Chow and colleagues (20) found that 29% of initial blood isolates of this organism were resistant to multiple antibiotics. Patients at risk for multiple-antibiotic-resistant *Enterobacter* received antibiotics (especially cephalosporins) within a 2-week period before isolation of the resistant organism. For that reason, most experienced clinicians now prefer to treat *Enterobacter* pneumonia with tobramycin combined with trimethoprim-sulfamethoxazole. In the laboratory, tobramycin is usually somewhat more active than gentamicin and amikacin against clinical isolates of *Enterobacter.* Trimethoprim-sulfamethoxazole-intolerant patients can receive combination tobramycin and an extended-spectrum penicillin; however, the risk of resistance emerging to either of these drugs during the course of therapy is high (20). Experience in imipenem-cilastin or fluoroquinolone therapy of *Enterobacter* pneumonia is limited.

Serratia marcescens

Gentamicin is usually more active than tobramycin against *S. marcescens.* However, resistance to gentamicin and tobramycin is being encountered with increasing frequency. Amikacin is now the aminoglycoside of choice for *Serratia* pneumonias. The extended spectrum penicillins, ticarcillin/clavulanate, the third-generation cephalosporins, aztreonan, imipenem/cilistatin, and fluoroquinolones are all active *in vitro*. *In vitro* synergy is found with most isolates (110). Since *S. marcescens* produces inducible cephalosporinases, monotherapy is not to be recommended. It has been found that combination of beta-lactam antibiotics with low concentrations of amikacin produced marked synergistic postantibiotic effects on *S. marcescens* (56). No assessments can be drawn regarding the efficacy of these agents in combination, but the therapeutic approach should involve an aminoglycoside other than tobramycin plus a beta-lactam.

Escherichia coli

In earlier studies, antipseudomonal penicillins or cephalosporins in combination with an aminoglycoside were used for *E. coli* pneumonias, but mortality rates were as high as 60% (70,97). Berk and colleagues (6) reported a 29% mortality in patients treated with cefamandole plus amikacin (either alone or together). Their patient population was, however, small, and assignment of therapy was not randomized (6). Our recommendations are for using a third-generation cephalosporin plus gentamicin, as the MICs to *E. coli* are generally lowest with this aminocyclitol. Resistance to ampicillin has been increasing. Previously, high-dose ampicillin (6–12 g/day) had been successfully used in the treatment of *E. coli* pneumonia (98). Ampicillin can no longer be recommended.

Proteus/Morganella/Providencia

Most reported patients with *Proteus/Morganella/Providencia* bacillary pneumonias were cured with the use of a single agent (149). For susceptible strains of *P. mirabilis,* we recommend ampicillin. Most patients other than *P. mirabilis* are predictably sensitive only to aminoglycosides and the third-generation cephalosporins.

Acinetobacter baumannii

As the number of cases of nosocomial *A. baumannii* pneumonia has increased, its susceptibility to standard chemotherapeutic agents has declined. In 1989, Traub and colleagues (151) found sensitivity of nosocomial isolates to trimethoprim-sulfamethoxazole, polymyxin B, sulbactam, doxycycline, and imipenem. Today, *Acinetobacter* strains are encountered that are resistant to all antimicrobial agents except amikacin, imipenem, and ampicillin/sulbactam. Resistance to these antimicrobials has also been reported (151). Antimicrobial selection must be based on susceptibility testing; a combination is preferable.

Pseudomonas aeruginosa

We recommend combination antimicrobial treatment with an antipseudomonal cephalosporin or else an extended-spectrum penicillin plus an aminoglycoside. Imipenem should be used when there is a resistant isolate. Alternative forms of combination therapy, such as double beta-lactam combinations or fluoroquinolone/beta-lactams, should be used with caution, pending the results of clinical trials.

Xanthomonas maltophilia

Xanthomonas maltophilia is resistant to many available antimicrobials. Neither beta-lactam antibiotics nor aminoglycosides are consistently active (100). Trimethoprim-sulfamethoxazole is the only dependendable agent against this bacteria. Other antimicrobials, quinolones, antipseudomonal penicillins, and minocycline are not reliable treatments; alternative therapies generally depend on results of susceptibility testing. This high level of resistance of beta-lactams is the result of constitutive and inducible production of beta-lactamases and the low penetrance of the drugs through the outer membrane of this organism.

SUMMARY

The incidence of community-acquired GNBPs has risen since the preantibiotic era and is likely to increase more with the increasing age of our population and the more common use of chemotherapy in the out-patient setting. GNBP is now the etiology for more than 60% of nosocomial pneumonia. The microbiologic trends in nosocomial disease are toward increasingly more resistant pathogens. There has been a decrease in *E. coli* and *K. pneumoniae,* and an increase in *P. aeruginosa, Enterobacter,* and *Acinetobacter* infections. Definitive information regarding the choice between combination drug treatment and monotherapy is not available. We recommend combination therapy for empirical therapy of GNBP and for definitive therapy of *P. aeruginosa, Enterobacter* sp, and *S. marcesens* infections (3). Optimal dosages, frequencies, and durations of antimicrobial therapy are not known. However, we recommend that treatment continue for 14–21 days. Treatment should be prolonged when pneumonia is complicated or associated with abscess formation. Additional studies could support switching from parenteral to oral therapy once there has been clinical response, thereby minimizing hospital stay.

One sign of progress in the control of GNBP has been a decline in death rates. The arrival of new, highly active antimicrobial therapies is not the only reason for this trend. Other important developments include earlier recognition of infections, improved diagnostic techniques, and newer technologies available for supportive care along with improved strategies for prompt and effective management. The future for improving control of these infections depends on further advances in prevention, diagnosis, and therapy. Of critical need is the ability to reliably distinguish colonization from disease. It will be necessary to control the development of further resistant isolates while advances are made in understanding mechanisms of antimicrobial resistance.

A better understanding of immune mechanisms in respiratory disease and how the immune system might be modulated to improve treatment and survival is of interest. Adjunctive therapies being evaluated in the treatment of patients with GNBPs include the use of type-specific polyvalent, cross-protective vaccines, and hyperimmune sera. Of great importance is the need to develop better strategies for prevention of GNBP. Further study aimed at preventing this type of infection by eliminating the risk factors facing the hospitalized patient is needed.

REFERENCES

1. Aguado, J.M., Obese, G., Cabanillas, J.J., Fernandez-Guerrero, M., and Ales, J. (1990): Pleuropulmonary infections due to nontyphoid strains of *Salmonella. Arch. Intern. Med.,* 150:54–56.
2. Ansley, N.M., Currie, B.J., and Withnall, K.M. (1992): Community-acquired *Acinetobacter* pneumonia in the northern territory of Australia. *Clin. Infect. Dis.,* 14:83–91.
3. Aouon, M., and Klastersky, J. (1991): Drug treatment of pneumonia in the hospital. *Drugs,* 42:962–973.
4. Bartlett, J.G., O'Keefe, P., Tally, F.P., Louie, T.J., and Gorbach, S.L. (1986): Bacteriology of hospital-acquired pneumonia. *Arch. Intern. Med.,* 146:868–887.
5. Berk, S.L., Neumann, P., Holtsclaw, S., et al. (1982): *Escherichia coli* pneumonia in the elderly with reference to the role of *E. coli* K1 capsular polysaccharide antigen. *Am. J. Med.,* 72:899–902.
6. Berk, S.L., and Verghese, A. (1989): Emerging pathogens in nosocomial pneumonia. *Eur. J. Clin. Microbiol. Infect. Dis.,* 8:11–14.
7. Berndt, R.F., Long, G.G., Abeles, F.B., et al (1977): Pathogenesis of respiratory *Klebsiella pneumoniae* infection in rats: bacteriological and histological findings and metabolic alterations. *Infect. Immun.,* 15:586–593.
8. Bjorksten, B., and Kaijser, B. (1978): Interaction of human serum and neutrophils with *Escherichia coli* strains: difference between strains isolated from urine of patients with pyelonephritis or asymptomatic bacteremia. *Infect. Immun.,* 22:308–311.
9. Bodem, C.R., Lampton, L.M., Miller, D.P., Tarka, E.F., and Everett, E.D. (1983): Endobronchial pH: relevance to aminoglycoside activity in gram-negative bacillary pneumonia. *Am. Rev. Respir. Dis.,* 127:39–41.
10. Bodey, G.P., Powell, R.D., Jr., Hersh, E.M., Yeterian, A., and Freireich, J. (1966): Pulmonary complications of acute leukemia. *Cancer,* 19:781–792.
11. Brogen, K.A. (1991): Changes in pulmonary surfactant during bacterial pneumonia. *Antonie van Leeuwenhoek,* 59:215–223.
12. Bryan, C.S., and Reynolds, K.L. (1984): Bacteremic nosocomial pneumonia: analysis of 172 episodes from a single metropolitan area. *Am. Rev. Respir. Dis.,* 129:668–671.
13. Canney, P.A., Larsson, S.N., Hay, J.M., and Yussuf, M.A. (1985): Case report: *Salmonella* pneumonia associated with chemotherapy for non-Hodgkin's lymphoma. *Clin. Rad.,* 36:459–460.
14. Carpenter, J.L. (1990): *Klebsiella* pulmonary infections: occurrence at one medical center and review. *Rev. Infect. Dis.,* 12:672–682.
15. Carratala, J., Salazar, A., Mascaro, J., and Santin, M. (1992): Community-acquired pneumonia due to *Pseudomonas stutzeri. Clin. Infect. Dis.,* 14:792.
16. Castle, M., Tenney, J.H., Weinsteim, M.P., and Eickhof, T.C. (1978): Outbreak of a multiply resistant *Acinetobacter* in a surgical intensive care unit: epidemiology and control. *Heart Lung,* 7:641–644.
17. Centers for Disease Control (March 1982): National Nosocomial Infections Study Report, Annual Summary, 1979. *M.M.W.R.*
18. Centers for Disease Control (March 1986): National Nosocomial Infections Surveillence, Annual Summary, 1984. *M.M.W.R.* 35(1SS):17SS–29SS.
19. Chase, R.A., and Trenholme, G.M. (1986): Overwhelming pneumonia. *Med. Clin. No. Amer.,* 70(4):945–960.
20. Chow, J.W., Fine, M.J., Shlaes, D.M., Quinn, J.P., Hooper, D.C., Johnsons, M.P., Ramphal, R., Wagener, M.M., Miyashiro, M.S., and Yu, V.L. (1991): *Enterobacter* bacteremia: clinical features and emergence of antimicrobial resistance during therapy. *Ann. Intern. Med.,* 115:585–590.
21. Coalson, J.J., King, R.J., Winter, V.T., Prihodda, T.J., Anzueto, A.R., Peters, J.I., and Johansson, W.G., Jr. (1989): O_2- and pneumonia-induced lung injury. I. Pathological and morphometric studies. *J. Appl. Physiol.,* 67:346–356.
22. Coonrod, J.D. (1981): Pulmonary opsonins in *Klebsiella pneumoniae* pneumonia in rats. *Infect. Immun.,* 33:533–539.
23. Cordes, L.G., Brink, E.W., Checko, P.J., et al. (1981): A cluster of *Acinetobacter* pneumonia in foundry workers. *Ann. Intern. Med.,* 95:688–693.
24. Crane, L.R., and Lerner, A.M. (1978): Non-traumatic gram-negative bacillary meningitis in the Detroit Medical Center, 1964–1974 (with special mention of cases due to *Escherichia coli). Medicine* (Baltimore), 57:197–209.

25. Craven, D.E., Steger, K.A., and Barbar, T.W. (1991): Preventing nosocomial pneumonias: state of the art and perspectives for the 1990s. Proceedings of the Third Decennial International Conference on Nosocomial Infections. *Am. J. Med.,* 91(Suppl. 3B):44S–53S.
26. Daikos, G.L., Lolans, V.T., and Jackson, G.G. (1991): First-exposure adaptive resistance to aminoglycoside antibiotics *in vivo* with meaning for optimal clinical use. *Antimicrob. Agents Chemother.,* 35(1):117–123.
27. Dale, D.C., Reynolds, H.Y., Pennington, J.E., et al. (1974): Experimental pneumonia due to *Pseudomonas* in dogs: controlled trial of granulocyte transfusion therapy. *J. Infect. Dis.,* 130:S143–S144.
28. Danner, P.K., McFarland, D.R., and Felson, B. (1968): Massive pulmonary gangrene. *Am. J. Roentgenol.,* 103:548–554.
29. DeLucca, A.J., II, Brogden, K.A., and Engen, R. (1988): *Enterobacter agglomerans* lipopolysaccharide–induced changes in pulmonary surfactant as a factor in the pathogenesis of byssinosis. *J. Clin. Microbiol.,* 26:778–780.
30. Dorff, G.J., Rytel, M.W., Farmer, S.G., et al. (1973): Etiologies and characteristic features of pneumonias in a municipal hospital. *Am. J. Med. Sci.,* 266:349–358.
31. Ebright, J.R., and Rytel, M.W. (1980): Bacterial pneumonia in the elderly. *J. Am. Ger. Soc.,* 28(5):220–223.
32. Edson, R.S., and Terrell, C.L. (1991): The aminoglycosides. *Mayo Clin. Proc.,* 35:873–878.
33. Eliopoulos, G.M., and Moellering, R.C., Jr. (1982): Antibiotic synergism and antimicrobial combinations in clinical infections. *Rev. Infect. Dis.,* 4:282–293.
34. Elting, L.S., and Bodey, G.P. (1990): Septicemia due to *Xanthomonas* species and non-aeruginosa *Pseudomonas* species: increasing incidence of catheter-related infections. *Medicine,* 69:5, 296–306.
35. Fagon, J.-Y., Chastre, J., Domart, Y., Trouillet, J.L., Pierre, J., Darne, C., and Gibert, C. (1989): Nosocomial pneumonia in patients receiving continuous mechanical ventilation. Prospective analysis of 52 episodes with use of protected specimen brush and quantitative culture techniques. *Am. Rev. Respir. Dis.,* 139:877–884.
36. Fang, G.D., Fine, M., Orloff, J. Arisumi, D., Yu, V.L., Kapoor, W., Grayston, J.T., Wang, S.P., Kohler, R., Muder, R.R., Yee, Y.Y., Rihs, J.D., and Vickers, R.M. (1990): New and emerging etiologies for community-acquired pneumonia with implications for therapy. *Medicine,* 69:307–316.
37. Feldman, C., Kallenbach, J.M., Levy, H., Reinach, S.G., Hurwiitz, M.D., Thorburn, J.R., and Koornhof, H.J. (1989): Community-acquired pneumonia of diverse aetiology: prognostic features in patients admitted to an intensive care unit and a "severity of illness" score. *Intensive Care Med.,* 15:302–307.
38. Fetzer, A.F., Werner, A.S., and Hagstrom, J.W.C. (1967): Pathologic features of pseudomonal pneumonia. *Am. Rev. Respir. Dis.,* 96:1121–1130.
39. Fiala, M. (1969): A study of the combined role of viruses, mycoplasmas and bacteria in adult pneumonia. *Am. J. Med. Sci.,* 257:44–51.
40. Fisher, M.C., Long, S.S., Roberts, E.M., Dunn, J.M., and Balsaara, R.K. (1981): *Pseudomonas maltophilia* bacteremia in children undergoing open heart surgery. *J.A.M.A.,* 246:1571–1574.
41. Fukutome, T., Misuyuama, M., Takeya, K., et al. (1980): Importance of antiserum and phagocytic cells in the protection of mice against infection by *Klebsiella pneumoniae. J. Gen. Microbiol.,* 119:225–229.
42. Fuxench-Lopez, Z., and Ramirez-Ronda, C.H. (1978): Pharyngeal flora in ambulatory alcoholic patients. Prevalence of gram-negative bacilli. *Arch. Intern. Med.,* 138:1815–1816.
43. Garb, J.L., Brown, R.B., et al. (1978): Difference in etiology of pneumonias in nursing homes and community patients. *J.A.M.A.,* 240:2169–2172.
44. Gardner, P., Griffin, W.B., Swartz, M.N., and Kunz, L.J. (1970): Non-fermentative gram-negative bacilli of nosocomial interest. *Am. J. Med.,* 48:735–749.
45. Gaynes, R.P., and Culver, D.H. (1992): Resistance to imipenem among selected gram-negative bacilli in the United States. *Infect. Control Hosp. Epidemiol.,* 13:10–14.
46. Gleckman, R.A., and Roth, R.M. (1984): Community-acquired bacterial pneumonia in the elderly. *Pharmacol. Ther.,* 4:81–88.
47. Glew, R.H., Moellering, R.C., and Kunz, L.J. (1977): Infections with *Acinetobacter calcoaceticus (Horella vaginicola):* clinical and laboratory studies. *Medicine* (Baltimore), 56:79–97.
48. Glick, L.M., Moran, G.P., Coleman, J.M., and O'Brien, G.F. (1959): Lobar pneumonia with bacteremia caused by *Bacterium anitratus. Amer. J. Med.,* 27:183–186.
49. Goldstein, J.D., Godleski, J.J., Balikian, J.P., et al. (1982): Pathologic patterns of *Serratia marcescens* pneumonia. *Human Pathol.,* 13:479–484.
50. Goodhart, G.L., Abrutyn, E., Watson, K., et al. (1977): Community-acquired *Acinetobacter calcoaceticus var. anitratus* pneumonia. *J.A.M.A.,* 238:1516–1518.
51. Gottliev, T., and Barnes, D.J. (1989): Community-acquired *Acinetobacter* pneumonia. *Aust. N.Z. J. Med.,* 19:259–260.

52. Gray, L., and Kreger, A. (1979): Microscopic characterization of rabbit lung damage produced by *Pseudomonas aeruginosa* proteases. *Infect. Immun.*, 23:150–159.
53. Green, G.M., and Kass, E.H. (1965): The influence of bacterial species on pulmonary resistance to infection in mice subjected to hypoxia, cold stress, and ethanolic intoxication. *Br. J. Exp. Pathol.*, 46:360–366.
54. Gutmann, L., Williamson, R., Kitzis, M.D., and Acar, J.F. (1986): Synergism and antagonism in double beta-lactam antibiotic combinations. *Am. J. Med.*, 80(Suppl. 5C):21–29.
55. Hall, H.E., and Humphries, J.D. (1958): The relationship between insusceptibility to phagocytosis and virulence of certain *Klebsiella pneumoniae* strains. *J. Infect. Dis.*, 103:157–162.
56. Hanberger, H. (1992): Pharmacodynamic effects of antibiotics. *Scand. J. Infect. Dis.* (Suppl 81):13.
57. Harrow, E.M., Jakab, G.J., Brody, A.R., et al. (1975): The pulmonary response to a bacteremic challenge. *Am. Rev. Respir. Dis.*, 112:7–16.
58. Hartstein, A.I., Reashad, A., Liebler, J.M., Actis, L.A., Freeman, J., Rourke, J.W., Stiboilt, T.B., Tolmaskey, M.E., Ellis, G.R., and Crosa, J.H. (1988): Multiple intensive care unit outbreak of *Acinetobacter calcoaceticus* subspecies *anitratus* respiratory infection and colonization associated with contaminated, reusable ventilator circuits and resuscitation bags. *Am. J. Med.*, 85:624–631.
59. Heyland, D., and Mandell, L.A. (1992): Gastric colonization by gram-negative bacilli and nosocomial pneumonia in the intensive care unit patient. *Chest*, 101(1):187–193.
60. Hilf, M., Yu, V.L., Sharp, J.A., Zuraavleff, J.J., Korvick, J.A., and Muder, R.R. (1989): Antibiotic therapy for *Pseudomonas areuginosa* bacteremia: outcome correlations in a prospective study of 200 patients. *Am. J. Med.*, 887: 540–546.
61. Holmes, R., Lapape, S.P., and Easterling, B.G. (1979): Distribution in clinical material and identification of *Pseudomonas maltophilia*. *J. Clin. Pathol.*, 32:66–72.
62. Hughes, J.M. (1988): Epidemiology and prevention of nosocomial pneumonia. In: *Current Clinical Topics in Infectious Diseases*, Vol. 9, edited by J.S. Remington and M.N. Swartz, pp. 241–259. McGraw-Hill, New York.
63. Iannini, P.B., Claffey, T., and Quintiliani, R. (1974): Bacteremic *Pseudomonas* pneumonia. *J.A.M.A.*, 230:558–561.
64. Ilowite, J.S., Niederman, M.S., and Fein, A.M. (1991): Delivery of topical antibiotics: pharmacokinetics and clinical problems. *Sem. Respir. Infect.* 6(3):158–167.
65. Johanson, W.G., Pierce, A.K., and Sanford, J.P. (1969): Changing pharyngeal flora of hospitalized patients: emergence of gram-negative bacilli. *N. Engl. J. Med.*, 281:1137–1140.
66. Johanson, W.G., Pierce, A.K., Sanford, J.P., et al. (1972): Nosocomial respiratory infection with gram-negative bacilli: the significance of colonization of the respiratory tract. *Ann. Intern. Med.*, 77:701–706.
67. Johanson, W.G., Woods, D.E., and Chaudhuri, T. (1979): Association of respiratory tract colonization with adherence of gram-negative bacilli to epithelial cells. *J. Infect. Dis.*, 139:667–673.
68. John, J.F., Sharbaugh, R.J., and Bannister, E.R. (1982): *Enterobacter cloacae:* bacteremia, epidemiology, and antibiotic resistance. *Rev. Infect. Dis.*, 4:13–28.
69. Jonas, M., and Cunha, B.A. (1982): Bacteremic *Escherichia coli* pneumonia. *Arch. Intern. Med.*, 142:2157–2159.
70. Jordan, G.W., Wong, G.A., and Hoeprich, P.D. (1976): Bacteriology of the lower respiratory tract as determined by fiber-optic bronchoscopy and transtracheal aspiration. *J. Infect. Dis.*, 134:428–435.
71. Karnad, A., Alvarez, S., and Berk, S.L. (1985): Pneumonia caused by gram-negative bacilli. *Am. J. Med.*, 79(Suppl. 1A):61–67.
72. Karnad, A., Alvarez, S., and Berk, S.L. (1987): *Enterobacter* pneumonia. *So. Med. J.*, 80(5): 601–604.
73. Kato, N., Kato, O., and Nakashima, I. (1976): Effect of capsular polysaccharide of *Klebsiella pneumoniae* on host resistance to bacterial infections. II. Effects on peritoneal leukocytes of normal mice and mice infected with virulent *Salmonella enteritidus*. *Jap. J. Microbiol.*, 20:415–423.
74. Khardori, N., Elting, L., Wong, E., Schable, B., and Bodey, G.P. (1990): Nosocomial infections due to *Xanthomonas maltophilia (Pseudomonas maltophilia)* in patients with cancer. *Rev. Infect. Dis.*, 12:6, 997–1003.
75. Korvick, J.A., Hackett, A.K., Yu, V.L., and Muder, R.R. (1991): *Klebsiella* pneumonia in the modern era: clinicoradiographic correlations. *So. Med. J.*, 84:200–204.
76. Kovarik, J., Rosenberg-Arska, M., Visser, M., and Verhoef, J. (1991): Pharmacodynamics of cefepime. *Scand. J. Infect. Dis.*, 74:(Suppl.):270–273.
77. Kreger, B.E., Craven, D.E., Carling, P.C., and McCabe, W.R. (1980): Gram-negative bacteremia. III. Reassessment of etiology, epidemiology and ecology in 612 patients. *Am. J. Med.*, 68:332–343.

78. LaForce, F.M. (1989): Systemic antimicrobial therapy of nosocomial pneumonia: monotherapy versus combination therapy. *Eur. J. Clin. Microbiol. Infect. Dis.*, 8(1):61–68.

79. Larson, E.L. (1981): Persistent carriage of gram-negative bacteria on hands. *Am. J. Infect. Control*, 9:112–119.

80. Laurenzi, G.A., Potter, R.T., and Kass, E.H. (1961): Bacteriologic flora of the lower respiratory tract. *N. Engl. J. Med.*, 265:1273–1278.

81. Lees, A.W., and McNaught, W. (1959): Bacteriology of lower respiratory tract secretions, sputum and upper respiratory tract secretions in "normals" and chronic bronchitis. *Lancet*, 2:1112–1115.

82. Lerner, A.M. (1980): The gram-negative bacillary pneumonias. *Dis. Month*, 27:1–56.

83. Levison, M.E., and Kaye, D. (1985): Pneumonia caused by gram-negative bacilli: an overview. *Rev. Infect. Dis.*, 7(Suppl. 4):S656–S665.

84. Liu, P.V. (1974): Extracellular toxins of *Pseudomonas aeruginosa*. *J. Infect. Dis.*, 130:S94–S102.

85. Lowbery, E.J.L., Thom, B.T., Lilly, A., et al. (1970): Sources of infection with *Pseudomonas aeruginosa* in patients with tracheostomy. *J. Med. Microbiol.*, 3:39–56.

86. Lysy, J., Werczberger, A., Globus, M., and Chowers, I. (1985): Pneumatocele formation in a patient with *Proteus mirabilis* pneumonia. *Postgrad. Med. J.*, 61;255–257.

87. Machowiak, P.A., Martin, R.M., Jones, S.R., and Smith, J.W. (1978): Pharyngeal colonization by gram-negative bacilli in aspiration-prone persons. *Arch. Intern. Med.*, 138:1224–1227.

88. Madrazo, A., Geiger, J., and Lauter, C.B. (1975): *Citrobacter diversus* at Grace Hospital, Detroit, Michigan. *Am. J. Med. Sci.*, 270:497–501.

89. Mayhall, C.G., Lamb, V.A., Gayle, W.E., et al. (1979): *Enterobacter cloacae* septicemia in a burn center: epidemiology and control of an outbreak. *J. Infect. Dis.*, 139:166–171.

90. McCabe, W.R., Kaijser, B., Olling, S., et al. (1978): *Escherichia coli* in bacteremia: K and O antigens and serum sensitivity of strains from adult and neonates. *J. Infect. Dis.*, 138:33–41.

91. McGrath, B.J., Bailey, E.M., Lamp, K.C., and Rybak, M.J. (1992): Pharmacodynamics of once-daily amikacin in various combinations with ceprime, aztreonam, and ceftazidime against *Pseudomonas aeruginosa* in an *in vitro* infection model. *Antimicrob. Agents Chemother.*, 36:2741–2746.

92. Meltz, D.J., and Grieco, M.H. (1973): Characteristics of *Serratia marcescens* pneumonia. *Arch. Intern. Med.*, 132:359–364.

93. Mertz, J.J., Scharer, L., and McClement, J.H. (1967): A hospital outbreak of *Klebsiella* pneumonia from inhalation therapy with contaminated aerosol solutions. *Am. Rev. Respir. Dis.*, 95:454–460.

94. Meyers, B.R., Bottone, E., Hirschman, S.Z., et al. (1972): Infections caused by microorganisms of the genus *Erwinia*. *Ann. Intern. Med.*, 76:9–14.

95. Montgomerie, J.Z. (1979): Epidemiology of *Klebsiella* and hospital-associated infections. *Rev. Infect. Dis.*, 1:736–752.

96. Moore, R.D., Smith, C.R., and Lietman, P.S. (1984): Association of aminoglycoside plasma levels with therapeutic outcome in gram-negative pneumonia. *Am. J. Med.*, 77:657–662.

97. Morrison, A.J., Hoffman, K.K., and Wenzel, R.P. (1986): Associated mortality and clinical characteristics of nosocomial *Pseudomonas maltophilia* in a university hospital. *J. Clin. Microbiol.*, 24:52–55.

98. Neu, H.C. (1980): Optimal antibiotic therapy in bronchopulmonary infections. *Infection*, 8:S62–S69.

99. Neu, H.C. (1992): Quinolone antimicrobial agents. *Ann. Rev. Med.*, 43:465–486.

100. Neu, H.C., Saha, G., and Chin, N.-X. (1989): Resistance of *Xanthomonas maltophilia* to antibiotics and the effect of beta-lactamase inhibitors. *Diag. Microbiol. Infect. Dis.*, 12(3):283–285.

101. Niederman, M.S. (1990): Gram-negative colonization of the respiratory tract: pathogenesis and clinical consequences. *Sem. Respir. Infect.*, 5(3):173–184.

102. Niederman, M.S. (1993): Pneumonia in the elderly. In: *Lung Biopsy in Health and Disease. Vol. 63. Pulmonary Disease in the Elderly Patient*, edited by D.A. Mahler, pp. 279–322. Marcel Dekker, New York.

103. Ohta, M., Mori, M., Nakashima, I., et al. (1979): Adjuvant action of capsular polysaccharide of *Klebsiella pneumoniae* on antibody response. VII. Further purification of the active substance. *Microbiol. Immunol.*, 23:805–813.

104. Pennington, J.E. (1981): Penetration of antibiotics into respiratory secretions. *Rev. Infect. Dis.*, 3:67–73.

105. Pennington, J.E., Reynolds, H.Y., and Carbone, P.P. (1973): *Pseudomonas* pneumonia: a retrospective study of 36 cases. *Am. J. Med.*, 55:155–160.

106. Phair, J.P., Bassaris, H.P., Williams, J.E., and Metzger, E. (1983): Bacteremic pneumonia due to gram-negative bacilli. *Arch. Intern. Med.*, 143:2147–2149.

107. Pierce, A.K., Edmonson, E.B., McGee, G., et al. (1966): An analysis of factors predisposing to gram-negative bacillary necrotizing pneumonia. *Am. Rev. Respir. Dis.*, 94:309–315.

108. Pierce, A.K., and Sanford, J.P. (1974): Aerobic gram-negative bacillary pneumonias. *Am. Rev. Respir. Dis.*, 110:647–658.

109. Pingleton, S.K., Hinthorn, D.R., and Liu, C. (1986): Enteral nutrition in patients receiving mechanical ventilation: multiple sources of tracheal colonization include the stomach. *Am. J. Med.*, 80:827–832.

110. Pogwizd, S.M., and Lerner, S.A. (1976): *In vitro* activity of gentamicin, amikacin, and netilmicin alone and in combination with carbenicillin against *Serratia marcescens*. *Antimicrob. Agents Chemother.*, 10:878–884.

111. Pollack, M., Callahan, L.T., III, and Taylor, N.S. (1976): Neutralizing antibody to *Pseudomonas aeruginosa* exotoxin in human sera: evidence for *in vitro* toxin production during infections. *Infect. Immun.*, 14:942–947.

112. Prins, J.M., Bueller, H.R., Kuijper, E.J., Tange, R.A., and Speelman, P. (1993): Once versus thrice daily gentamicin in patients with serious infection. *Lancet*, 341:335–339.

113. Rahal, J.J., Jr., Meade, R.H., III, Bump, C.M., and Reinauer, A.J. (1970): Upper respiratory tract carriage of gram-negative enteric bacilli by hospital personnel. *J.A.M.A.*, 214:754–756.

114. Ramirez-Ronda, C.H., Ruxench-Lopez, A., and Nevarez, M. (1981): Increased pharyngeal bacterial colonization during viral illness. *Arch. Intern. Med.*, 141:1599–1603.

115. Rehm, S.R., Gross, G.N., and Pierce, A.K. (1980): Early bacterial clearance from murine lungs: species-dependent phagocyte response. *J. Clin. Invest.*, 66:194–199.

116. Rello, J., Quintana, E., Ausina, V., Net, A., and Prata, G. (1993): A three-year study of severe community-acquired pneumonia with emphasis on outcome. *Chest*, 103:232–235.

117. Reubarz, J.A., Pierce, A.K., Mays, B.B., and Sandford, J.P. (1965): The potential role of inhalation therapy equipment in nosocomial pulmonary infection. *J. Clin. Invest.*, 44:831–839.

118. Reynolds, H.Y. (1983): Lung inflammation: role of endogenous chemotactic factors in attracting polymorphonuclear granulocytes. *Am. Rev. Respir. Dis.*, 127:S16–S25.

119. Reynolds, H.Y., Kazmierowski, J.A., and Newball, H.H. (1975): Specificity of opsonic antibodies to enhance phagocytosis of *Pseudomonas aeruginosa* by human alveolar macrophages. *J. Clin. Invest.*, 56:376–388.

120. Reynolds, H.Y., and Thompson, R.E. (1973): Pulmonary host defenses. I. Analysis of protein and lipids in bronchial secretions and antibody responses after vaccination with *Pseudomonas aeruginosa*. *J. Immunol.*, 111:358–368.

121. Rolston, K., Guan, Z., and Bodey, G.P. (1985): *Acinetobacter calcoaceticus* septicemia in patients with cancer. *So. Med. J.*, 78:6, 647–651.

122. Rose, M., and Lindberg, D.A.B. (1968): Effect of pulmonary pathogens on surfactant. *Dis. Chest*, 53:541–544.

123. Rosenthal, S., and Tager, I.B. (1975): Prevalence of gram-negative rods in the normal pharyngeal flora. *Ann. Intern. Med.*, 83:355–357.

124. Rudin, M.L., Michael, J.R., and Huxley, E.J. (1979): Community-acquired *Acinetobacter* pneumonia. *Am. J. Med.*, 67:39–43.

125. Saphra, I., and Winter, J.W. (1957): Clinical manifestations of Salmonellosis in men: an evaluation of 7,779 human infections identified at the New York Salmonella Center. *N. Engl. J. Med.*, 256:1128–1134.

126. Sarff, L.D., McCracken, G.H., Schiffer, M.S., et al. (1975): Epidemiology of *Escherichia coli* K1 in healthy and diseased newborns. *Lancet*, 1:1099–1104.

127. Sastry, C.V., and Scrimgeour, E.M. (1991): Pneumopyopericardium in a Zimbabwean man with *Klebsiella pneumoniae*. *Respir. Med.*, 85:427–429.

128. Schaberg, D.R., Alford, R.H., Anderson R., et al. (1976): An outbreak of nosocomial infection due to multiple resistant *Serratia marcescens:* evidence of interhospital spread. *J. Infect. Dis.*, 134:181–188.

129. Schaberg, D.R., Culver, D.H., and Gaynes, R.P. (1991): Major trends in the microbial etiology of nosocomial infection. *Am. J. Med.*, 91(Suppl.3B):S72–S75.

130. Schable, B., Rhoden, D.L., Hugh, R., Weaver, R.E., Khardor, N., Smith, P.B., Bodey, G.P., and Anderson, R.L. (1989): Serological classification of *Xanthomonas maltophilia (Pseudomonas maltophilia)* based on heat-stable O antigens. *J. Clin. Microbiol.*, 27:1011–1013.

131. Scheckler, W.E., Schiebel, W., and Kresge, D. (1991): Temporal trends in a community hospital. *Am. J. Med.*, 91 (Suppl. 3B):90S–94S.

132. Schentag, J.J. (1992): The antimicrobial efficacy of intravenous ciprofloxacin in severe infection. *Inf. Med.*, 9(Suppl. B):41–57.

133. Schimpff, S.C., Young, V.M., Greene, W.H., et al. (1972): Origin of infection in acute nonlymphocytic leukemia: significance of hospital acquisition of potential pathogens. *Ann. Intern. Med.*, 77:707–714.

134. Schwarz, D.B., Olson, D.E., and Kauffman, C.A. (1984): Tracheal colonization during respiratory failure. *Clin. Res.*, 32:253A.

135. Schwartz, S.N., Dowling, J.N., Benkivic, C., DeQuittner-Buchanan, M. Prostko, T., and Yee,

R. (1978): Sources of gram-negative bacilli colonizing the trachea of intubated patients. *J. Infect. Dis.*, 138:227–231.

136. Schwigon, C.D., Hulla, F.W., Schulze, B., and Maslak, A. (1986): Timinetin in the treatment of nosocomial bronchopulmonary infections in intensive care units. *J. Antimicrob. Chemother.*, 17(Suppl. C):115–122.

137. Sensakovic, J.W., and Bartel, P.F. (1974): The slime of *Pseudomonas aeruginosa:* biological characterization and possible role in experimental infection. *J. Infect. Dis.*, 129:101–109.

138. Simberkoff, M.S., Moldover, M.H., and Rahal, J.J. (1976): Specific and nonspecific immunity to *Serratia marcescens* infection. *J. Infect. Dis.*, 134:348–353.

139. Simberkoff, M.S., Ricupero, I., and Rahal, J.J. (1976): Host resistance to *Serratia marcescens* infection: serum bactericidal activity and phagocytosis by normal blood leukocytes. *J. Lab. Clin. Med.*, 87:206–217.

140. Solberg, C., and Matsen, J.M. (1971): Infections with *Providencia* bacilli: a clinical bacteriologic study. *Am. J. Med.*, 50:241–246.

141. Stamm, W.E., Martin, S.M., and Bennett, J.V. (1977): Epidemiology of nosocomial infections due to gram-negative bacilli: aspects relevant to development and use of vaccines. *J. Infect. Dis.*, 136:5151–5160.

142. Stevens, R.M., Teres, D., Skillman, J.J., et al. (1974): Pneumonia in an intensive care unit. *Arch. Intern. Med.*, 134:106–111.

143. Stuart, B.M., and Pullen, R.L. (1946): Typhoid: clinical analysis of three hundred and sixty cases. *Arch. Intern. Med.*, 78:629–661.

144. Sullivan, R.J., Dowdle, W.R., Marine, W.M., et al. (1972): Adult pneumonia in a general hospital: etiology and host risk factors. *Arch. Intern. Med.*, 129:935–942.

145. Swings, J., DeVos, M., Den Mooter, M., and DeLey, J. (1983): Transfer of *Pseudomonas maltophilia* to the genus *Xanthomonas* as *Xanthomonas maltophilia. Int. J. Syst. Bacteriol.*, 33:4099–4413.

146. Tillotson, J.R., and Finland, M. (1969): Bacterial colonization and clinical superinfection of the respiratory tract complicating antibiotic treatment of pneumonia. *J. Infect. Dis.*, 119:598–623.

147. Tillotson, J.R., and Lerner, A.M. (1966): Pneumonias caused by gram-negative bacilli. *Medicine* (Baltimore), 45:65–76.

148. Tillotson, J.R., and Lerner, A.M. (1967): Characteristics of pneumonias caused by *Escherichia coli. N. Engl. J. Med.*, 227:115–122.

149. Tillotson, J.R., and Lerner, A.M. (1968): Characteristics of pneumonias caused by *Bacillus proteus. Ann. Intern. Med.*, 68:287–294.

150. Tillotson, J.R., and Lerner, A.M. (1968): Characteristics of nonbacteremic *Pseudomonas* pneumonia. *Ann. Intern. Med.*, 68:295–307.

151. Traub, W.M., and Spohr, M. (1989): Antimicrobial drug susceptibility of clinical isolates of *Acinetobacter* species (*A. baumanni, A. haemolyticus* Genospecies 3 and Genospecies 6). *Antimicrob. Agents Chemother.*, 33:1617–1619.

152. Unger, J.D., Rose, H.D., and Unger, G.F. (1973): Gram-negative pneumonia. *Diag. Radiol.*, 107:283–291.

153. Valdivieso, M., Gil-Extemera, B., Zornoza, J., et al. (1977): Gram-negative bacillary pneumonia in the compromised host. *Medicine* (Baltimore), 56:241–254.

154. Valenti, M.W., Trudell, R.G., and Bentley, D.W. (1978): Factors predisposing to oropharyngeal colonization with gram-negative bacilli in the aged. *N. Engl. J. Med.*, 298:1108–1111.

155. Washington, J.A., II, Birk, R.J., and Ritts, R.E. (1971): Bacteriologic and epidemiologic characteristics of *Enterobacter hafniae* and *Enterobacter liquefaciens. J. Infect. Dis.*, 125:379–386.

156. Weinstein, A.J., Moellering, R.C., Jr., Hopkins, C.C., and Goldblatt, A. (1973): *Pseudomonas cepacia* pneumonia. *Am. J. Med. Sci.*, 265:491.

157. Wenzel, R.P. (1981): Surveillance and reporting of hospital acquired infections. In: *CRC Handbook of Hospital Acquired Infections,* edited by R. P. Wenzel, pp. 35–72. CRC Press, Boca Raton, Fla.

158. Winston, D.J., Ho, W.G., Bruchner, D.A., et al. (1991): Beta-lactam antibiotic therapy in febrile granulocytopenic patients: a randomized trial comparing cefoperazone plus piperacillin, ceftazidime plus piperacillin, and imipenem alone. *Ann. Intern. Med.*, 115:849–859.

159. Wishart, M.M., and Riley, T.V. (1976): Infection with *Pseudomonas maltophilia:* hospital outbreak due to contaminated disinfectant. *Med. J. Aust.*, 2:710–712.

160. Wollschlager, C.M., Conrad, A.R., and Khan, F.A. (1988): Common complications in critically ill patients. *Dis. Month*, 34:221–293.

161. Wretlind, B., and Pavlovskis, O.R. (1981): The role of proteases and exotoxin A in the pathogenicity of *Pseudomonas aeruginosa* infections. *Scand. J. Infect. Dis.*, 29:S13–S19.

162. Yokochi, T., Nakashima, I., and Kato, N. (1979): Further studies on generation of macrophages in *in vitro* cultures of mouse spleen cells and its inhibition of the capsular polysaccharide of *Klebsiella pneumoniae. Microbiol. Immunol.*, 23:487–499.

163. Young, L.S. (1974): Role of antibody in infections due to *Pseudomonas aeruginosa*. *J. Infect. Dis.*, 130:S111–S118.
164. Yu, V.L. (1979): *Serratia marcescens*. Hospital prospective and clinical review. *N. Engl. J. Med.*, 300:887–893.
165. Zaer, F., and Deodhar, L. (1989): Nosocomial infections due to *Acinetobacter calcoaceticus*. *J. Postgrad. Med.*, 35:1, 14–16.
166. Zornoza, J., Goldman, A.M., Wallace, S., et al. (1976): Radiologic features of gram-negative pneumonias in the neutropenic patient. *Am. J. Roentgenol.*, 127:989–996.

Respiratory Infections: Diagnosis and Management, 3d ed.,
edited by James E. Pennington.
Raven Press, Ltd., New York © 1994

20

Atypical Pneumonias

Carmelita U. Tuazon and Henry W. Murray

*Department of Medicine, George Washington University, 2150 Pennsylvania Avenue,
N.W., Washington, D.C. 20037; and Department of Medicine, Cornell Medical
College, The New York Hospital, New York, New York 10021*

MYCOPLASMA PNEUMONIAE

Mycoplasma pneumoniae is traditionally regarded as a respiratory tract pathogen of children and young adults. More recent experience, however, indicates that this organism is also an important cause of pneumonia and febrile upper respiratory tract infections in adults of all age groups. In addition, it now appears clear that *M. pneumoniae* infection can also be associated with a wide spectrum of both pulmonary and extrapulmonary syndromes that can be benign and self-limited, moderately troublesome, or sometimes life-threatening (12,62,71,91). Moreover, on occasion, extrapulmonary manifestations actually overshadow or occur in the absence of symptomatic respiratory tract involvement (87).

The Organism

M. pneumoniae is a procaryote that more closely resembles a bacterium than a virus. However, it lacks a cell wall and, not surprisingly, is resistant to cell-wall-active antibiotics. *M. pneumoniae* is bound by a single, triple-layer membrane, stains gram-negative, grows on artificial media supplemented with yeast extract and serum, exhibits hemadsorption, and produces a peroxide hemolysin. The organism is 10×200 nm in size, appears filamentous, and on the end displays a neuramic acid receptor site for attachment to host cell membranes (20).

Epidemiology

Although *M. pneumoniae* infections tend to increase during the fall and early winter (37), there is little hard evidence to indicate seasonality. Children and young adults (under the age of 20 years) are the individuals most often clinically ill with *M. pneumoniae* infections; thus, it is not surprising that simultaneous cases within single households are common. Adulthood, however, offers no barrier to infection. *M. pneumoniae* has been implicated in 11 to 17% of pneumonias in patients older than 40 years (87). Those in enclosed populations (e.g., college students, prisoners, military recruits) appear to be particularly prone to *M. pneumoniae* infections (71), and an epidemic among hospital workers was recently reported.

Pathogenesis

Infection appears to be acquired via inhalation of infected material after exposure to an acutely ill coughing individual (71). The incubation period is approximately 14 days. Intense exposure is probably necessary for infection to result. Nasopharyngeal carriers of *M. pneumoniae* (whose clinical illness has resolved) do not appear to transmit the organism readily.

Because fatal cases of *M. pneumoniae* pneumonia are rare, there is little pathologic data from which to draw pathogenic inferences. Histologic findings from human cases have included tracheal and bronchial mucosa hyperemia, alveolar exudates comprised principally of mononuclear inflammatory cells, plasma cell interstitial space infiltration, and accumulation of monocytes and macrophages in the bronchial epithelial submucosa. Studies using an experimental animal model have demonstrated that *M. pneumoniae* colonies bind via neuramic acid receptors to respiratory tract epithelial cells and initiate local tissue injury. The latter can be mediated by hydrogen peroxide elaborated by the organism itself. *M. pneumoniae* can also penetrate the bronchial mucosa. Polymorphonuclear leukocytes are attracted to deciliated cells, and leukocyte products probably contribute to or perpetuate the superficial inflammatory process. Simultaneously, monocytes, macrophages, and lymphocytes infiltrate submucosal areas as well.

Although an IgM followed by an IgG antibody response typically occurs in *M. pneumoniae* infection, serum antibody does not necessarily confer life-long immunity, and reinfection can occur (38). This lack of protection or partial immunity, despite circulating specific antibody, appears to be particularly evident in individuals who are seropositive from prior upper respiratory illnesses but who have not developed pneumonia. In contrast, prior pneumonia due to *M. pneumoniae* seems to confer substantial protection against serologically recognized reinfection (32). It is pertinent to note, however, that locally secreted nasopharyngeal IgA appears to be effective in inhibiting *M. pneumoniae* binding to the respiratory tract epithelium, suggesting a role for a local immune response.

There is a growing body of evidence to suggest that immune mechanisms, rather than actual direct infection, play a role in the development of clinically apparent *M. pneumoniae* pneumonia as well as some of the extrapulmonary complications. Thus, despite the potential to cause disease in practically any organ, bodily fluid, or mucosal or serosal surface, *M. pneumoniae* is seldom isolated from clinical material except from sputum or nasopharyngeal secretions. Moreover, *M. pneumoniae* or its antigen has seldom been demonstrated in the lungs of patients with fatal pulmonary infection (87). Evidence has recently been reported, however, to support the notion that repeated subclinical *M. pneumoniae* infections with consequent sensitization of T-lymphocytes (32) and probably other components of the immune system (e.g., autoantibodies) might be necessary before manifestations such as pneumonitis develop (71). For instance, circulating *M. pneumoniae* immune complexes, which in one study were detected in 41% of infected patients (5), can contribute to target organ injury in the lung, brain, synovium, or elsewhere. Levels of IgG immune complex have been reported to be elevated during the acute phase of illness and can be associated with the degree of pulmonary involvement, whereas IgM rheumatoid factor could play a role in the recovery from *M. pneumoniae* pneumonia (84). Moreover, antithymocyte globulin abrogates or diminishes the severity of experimental *M. pneumoniae* infection in animals (73), and corticosteroids have been used with some beneficial clinical effects in patients with severe *M. pneumoniae* pneumonia (60,91). In our experience, *M. pneumoniae* has also been an infrequent respiratory pathogen in cancer patients receiving immunosuppressive therapy. Furthermore, pneumonia failed to develop in a group of children with immunodeficiency syndromes who had acquired severe *M. pneumoniae* respiratory tract infections (39). These observations suggest, then, that previous sensitization and the vigor of the host immune response could explain in part why some patients with *M. pneumoniae* infection develop pneumonitis rather than bronchitis alone, and why some experience extrapulmonary complications.

Pulmonary Manifestations

Uncomplicated Pneumonia

Clinically apparent pneumonia occurs in less than 10% of patients infected with *M. pneumoniae,* whereas most ill patients develop only pharyngitis or bronchitis (35). Fever, chills, cough, headache, and malaise are common in patients with pneumonia (Table 20-1). Cough is typically nonproductive, but, if obtained, sputum can appear purulent in up to one-third of cases. Although hemoptysis and pleuritic chest pain are rare, *M. pneumoniae* pneumonia occasionally mimics pulmonary embolism with infarction. Substernal (nonpleuritic) chest pain can result from bronchial involvement. Rales and rhonchi are common (Table 20-1), but signs of airspace consolidation are infrequent. In 25 to 50% of pneumonia patients, upper respiratory tract

TABLE 20–1. *Symptoms and signs in patients with* M. pneumoniae

Source: No. of patients:	Biberfield (6) 109	George (42) 90	Grayston (46) 200	Mufson (86) 175	Feizi (31) 40
Symptoms			% of patients		
Fever (>38.9°C)	100	50	74	72	
Chills	73	65	58	78	
Headache	72	40	64	85	25
Cough	100	95	100	93	75
Purulent sputum		20	49		18
Hemoptysis		5			2
Chest pain		30	2	42	
Sore throat	41	25	53	53	25
Rhinorrhea	17	25	25	49	40
Earache		2	35		15
Malaise		40	89	74	60
Anorexia				36	25
Nausea/vomiting	44		29		15
Diarrhea			16		12
Myalgias/arthralgias		20		45	15
Sign					
Rales	82	60		84	
Pharyngitis	57			12	
Lymphadenopathy	28	40		18	19
Myringitis					12
Rash			16		28

From Murray et al. (87).

signs and symptoms occur and include sore throat, rhinorrhea, and earache. Although up to one-third of patients have the latter complaint, bullous or hemorrhagic myringitis is unusual in naturally acquired infection, in contrast with the 27% incidence reported in earlier volunteer studies (100). Musculoskeletal and gastrointestinal symptoms are common but minor complaints. Additional, but less often encountered, findings in patients with *M. pneumoniae* pneumonia include pharyngitis, tonsillar exudates, cervical lymphadenopathy, conjunctivitis, rashes, and pulse-temperature dissociation (87). Generalized lymphadenopathy and splenomegaly are rare. *M. pneumoniae* infection can also precipitate acute clinical exacerbations in patients with chronic obstructive lung disease and bronchospastic episodes in asthmatics.

Within 3 to 10 days in untreated cases, fever, headache, and malaise resolve. Cough and rales abate more slowly, paralleling the clearing of the chest film. Antimicrobial agents such as tetracycline and erythromycin reduce the duration of symptoms and hasten roentgenographic resolution (64,99,119,121,134), but they are not effective in actually eradicating the organism from the respiratory tract (46). Despite appropriate therapy, clinical relapses with reappearance of symptoms and infiltrates can occur 7 to 10 days after an initial response. Moreover, progression of pulmonary infiltrates to involve new parenchymal areas can also occur during therapy (87).

Complicated Pneumonia

Although usually benign and self-limited, the course of *M. pneumoniae* pneumonia is sometimes complicated by severe respiratory syndromes. Patients with sickle-cell anemia can have prolonged and high fever, marked leukocytosis (white blood cell count greater than 30,000/mm^3), multilobe infiltrates, pleuritic pain, and prominent pleural effusions (122). Recently, catastrophic respiratory failure along with the severe hypoxemia seen in the adult respiratory distress syndrome has been reported in five patients with *M. pneumoniae* pneumonia (62). One of the five died. Mixed infections with respiratory viruses including influenza and adenovirus have also been documented, and, infrequently, bacterial pathogens can co-infect or cause subsequent secondary pulmonary infection. One case with simultaneous Legionnaires' disease has also been recorded.

Pleural Effusions

Pleural effusions occur in up to 20% of patients with *M. pneumoniae* pneumonia (33); thus, this manifestation can no longer be considered rare. Effusions have typically been small, unilateral, and transient, and decubitus views are usually required to demonstrate the fluid. Bilateral or massive effusions, although unusual, do occur and often take 3 to 4 weeks to resolve (87). Pleural fluid in *M. pneumoniae* pneumonia usually shows exudative characteristics, a normal glucose level, and variable numbers (up to 10,000 mm^3) of both polymorphonuclear leukocytes and mononuclear cells. In two patients, pleural biopsies have showed no remarkable abnormalities (87). To date, *M. pneumoniae* has been isolated from pleural fluid only once (90).

Miscellaneous

Three cases of lung abscess in patients with laboratory-confirmed *M. pneumoniae* infection have been reported (87), and all three responded slowly to treatment. Other pulmonary complications or findings have included CO_2 retention, residual pleural scarring, the hyperlucent lung syndrome, pneumatoceles, hilar adenopathy, and lobar collapse (87). In a recent study, *M. pneumoniae* has been implicated as a frequent cause of exacerbation of bronchial asthma in adults (118).

Extrapulmonary Manifestations

There are a host of potentially serious nonrespiratory complications that patients with *M. pneumoniae* infection can develop. As can be seen in Table 20-2, virtually any organ system is likely to be involved (87).

Hematologic

Probably best recognized among the extrapulmonary manifestations of *M. pneumoniae* infection is a cold agglutinin, autoimmune hemolytic anemia (30). Although not common, hemolysis can be severe enough to warrant transfusion (warmed packed cells) or systemic corticosteroid therapy. Not infrequent, however, are positive Coombs' tests and mild reticulocytosis, suggesting that subclinical hemolysis in *M. pneumoniae* infection is probably common (87). Overt hemolysis characteristically occurs 2 to 3 weeks after the onset of illness, is transient, and coincides with both recovery from pneumonia and high cold agglutinin titers. On rare occasion, the cold agglutinin response is associated with Raynaud's phenomenon, acrocyanosis, hemoglobinuria, renal failure, chronic cold agglutinin disease, and even death from widespread thrombotic lesions. Disseminated intravascular coagulation can also occur (26).

TABLE 20–2. *Extrapulmonary manifestations of* M. pneumoniae *infections*

Hematologic:	Autoimmune hemolytic anemia, thrombocytopenia, disseminated intravascular coagulation
Gastrointestinal:	Gastroenteritis, anicteric hepatitis, pancreatitis
Musculoskeletal:	Arthralgias, myalgias, polyarthritis
Dermatologic:	Various rashes, erythema nodosum and multiforme, Stevens-Johnson syndrome
Cardiac:	Pericarditis, myocarditis, pericardial effusion, conduction defects
Neurologic:	Meningitis, meningoencephalitis, transverse myelitis, peripheral and cranial neuropathy, cerebellar ataxia
Miscellaneous:	General lymphadenopathy, splenomegaly, interstitial nephritis, glomerulonephritis

From Murray et al. (87,88).

Gastrointestinal

Anorexia can persist for several weeks, but most other gastrointestinal symptoms (see Table 20-1) resolve promptly. Anicteric hepatitis and acute pancreatitis have been reported to develop during the course of *M. pneumoniae* infection (87).

Musculoskeletal

Nonspecific myalgias and arthralgias occur in up to 40% of patients with *M. pneumoniae* pneumonia. A prominent rheumatic syndrome, however, with acute arthritis or severe arthralgias, can also develop during the first 2 weeks of respiratory illness (45). Involvement can be migratory and polyarticular, and the large joints are most often affected. Synovial effusions and morning stiffness can both be troublesome, and resolution of joint complaints can take a year or longer but is usually complete.

Dermatologic

Any one of a variety of mucocutaneous lesions can complicate *M. pneumoniae* infection. In up to 25% of patients, skin lesions occur during the first or second week of respiratory symptoms, and most often these patients are men under the age of 30 years (71). The lesions, which include various rashes, urticaria, erythema nodosum, and erythema multiform, are usually transient and typically not of much clinical significance (87). On occasion, however, extensive vesicular skin eruptions, ulcerative stomatitis and conjunctivitis (the Stevens-Johnson syndrome) can develop and necessitate systemic corticosteroids. *M. pneumoniae* has been isolated from fluid from both bullous and vesicular skin lesions that may be accompanied by urethritis (87).

Cardiac

Approximately 25 cases of pericarditis or myocarditis have been reported in patients with serologically proven *M. pneumoniae* infection (108). One-third of these individuals had no pulmonary infiltrates. Although in most instances cardiac involvement was either asymptomatic or mild, up to 30% of patients had been critically ill with congestive heart failure, pericardial effusion, or heart block; at least three deaths resulted. In one case, *M. pneumoniae* was isolated at autopsy from blood and pericardial fluid (89).

Neurologic

Central and peripheral nervous system disease associated with *M. pneumoniae* infection confirmed by isolation or serology has been well documented (58,70). Aseptic meningitis (modest pleocytosis but occasionally with up to 90 to 100% polymorphonuclear leukocytes), meningoencephalitis, peripheral and cranial neuropathies, transverse myelitis, cerebellar ataxia (children), and acute psychosis have all been reported. Encephalitis can be associated with hemiplegia and coma, and peripheral neuropathy can progress to a disabling Guillain-Barré syndrome. Rarely, patients can present with a stroke syndrome on the basis of cerebral infarction. Cerebrospinal fluid protein values are increased in most cases with neurologic findings, and with the exception of one case of meningoencephalitis with transverse myelitis, cerebrospinal fluid glucose levels have been normal. Complement-fixing antibody can be found in the spinal fluid. Recently, magnetic resonance imaging demonstrated clinically silent lesions of cervical myelitis in two patients with CNS manifestations of *M. pneumoniae* (40).

In 20% of cases of *M. pneumoniae* infection with neurologic manifestations, pulmonary involvement is absent. No correlation has been found between the severity and type of *M. pneumoniae* infection or between the height of the cold agglutinin titer and the subsequent development or extent of neurologic manifestations. *M. pneumoniae* infection has been isolated from the spinal fluid of patients including those presenting with encephalitis (1,34), but in no instance has *M. pneumoniae* been isolated from the brain or other neural tissue. In addition, brain biopsies and autopsy studies have yielded no firm pathogenetic clues. Thus, the pathogenesis of the neurologic complications of *M. pneumoniae* infection remains obscure. Speculative mechanisms include intracerebral intravascular coagulation, direct invasion, neurotoxin elaboration, and immune complex deposition.

Miscellaneous

Additional nonpulmonary manifestations of *M. pneumoniae* infection include cases of inappropriate antidiuretic hormone secretion, congenital central nervous system lesions, a tuboovarian abscess, and immune complex–mediated interstitial nephritis and glomerulonephritis.

Although it is clear that multisystem involvement occurs with *M. pneumoniae* infection in a protean fashion (87), significant morbidity or mortality remain unusual. Since *M. pneumoniae* is seldom isolated from sites distant from the respiratory tract, the pathogenesis of most of these extrapulmonary manifestations remains to be clarified. It is important to note that appropriate antimicrobial therapy does not appear to influence either the development or the course of the systemic complications.

Laboratory Findings and Diagnostic Methods

The white blood cell count is greater than $10,000/mm^3$ in approximately 25% of patients with *M. pneumoniae* pneumonia. Counts as high as 25,000 to $56,000/mm^3$ have been recorded in unusually severe cases. Neutrophilia, lymphocytosis, and monocytosis can all occur, whereas leukopenia is rare. With the exception of occasional rises in hepatic transaminases, routine blood studies are typically normal. False-positive VDRL tests and transient tuberculin anergy can develop. Electrocardiographic changes suggestive of pericarditis or myocarditis can also be noted.

Chest x-ray abnormalities in *M. pneumoniae* pneumonia are highly variable, and have been reviewed in detail elsewhere (8). Infiltrates characteristically are unilateral patchy areas of bronchopneumonia and involve the lower lobes in 75 to 90% of cases. Punctate mottling and centrally dense infiltrates can be helpful diagnostic signs. Lobar consolidation with upper lobe involvement and multilobe infiltrates are unusual. Roentgenographic abnormalities typically resolve within 10 to 20 days, but complete resolution could require 4 to 6 weeks. Residual chest x-ray abnormalities are rare.

The laboratory diagnosis of *M. pneumoniae* infection can be made either by isolation of the organism from an acutely ill individual or by demonstration of an appropriate rise in specific antibody titer. Both techniques require several weeks for positive results, so diagnosis must be based initially on the characteristic history and appropriate clinical findings. Sputum gram stains show a moderate number of leukocytes (either mononuclear or polymorphonuclear cells), but no predominant bacterial pathogen. Routine sputum cultures grow only normal throat flora.

M. pneumoniae is readily isolated from throat washings, sputum, or throat swabs (87). Seven to ten days after isolation in broth media, typical colonies can be observed by means of a binocular microscope. A presumptive identification of *M. pneumoniae* can be made if colonies show hemadsorption of red blood cells. A new cultivation medium has been reported to enhance recovery of *M. pneumoniae* from respiratory secretions (130). Although results are seldom positive, attempts to isolate the organism from bodily fluids, skin lesions, clinically involved tissues, and abscess materials should nonetheless be pursued. *M. pneumoniae* has occasionally been recovered from middle ear and skin vesicle fluid (87), and only once each from blood, pericardial fluid (89), pleural fluid (90), spinal fluid (34), and a tuboovarian abscess (126).

For paired serum samples obtained during the acute and convalescent periods, a fourfold increase in complement fixation titer is considered diagnostic of recent *M. pneumoniae* infection. A high degree of suspicion can be placed on titers greater than or equal to 1 : 64 if only a convalescent serum is available (87). IgM antibody first appears 7 to 9 days after infection, peaks at 4 to 6 weeks, and does not start to decline until 4 to 6 months later. After 2 to 3 years, titers usually fall to levels less than or equal to 1 : 16 (87). Titers, however, remain elevated for a considerably longer period (up to 5 to 9 years) in patients who develop clinically apparent *M. pneumoniae,* as opposed to those who experience only upper respiratory tract infections (36).

One-third to three-fourths of patients with *M. pneumoniae* pneumonia develop high (greater than 1 : 64) or fourfold or greater increases in titers of cold hemaglutinins. These IgM antibodies fix complement and are directed at the erythrocyte I antigens. Elevated cold agglutinin titers are not diagnostic of *M. pneumoniae* infection and can be associated with a variety of other infections as well as connective tissue and neoplastic disorders. In these latter diseases, however, cold agglutinins are usually anti-i. *M. pneumoniae* antigen has been demonstrated by immunoelectrophoretic techniques in the sputum of a small proportion of culture-positive, clinically ill patients (135). Detection of *M. pneumoniae* in respiratory specimens using DNA probe is very sensitive and specific compared to culture (66,128). Direct detection of *M. pneumoniae* antigen in throat swab and sputum specimens from patients with pharyngitis and pneumonia using monoclonal antibody immunoblot assay is sensitive and specific and can be completed within 5 hours (76).

Treatment

The resolution of fever, cough, and the clinical signs of pneumonia, as well as the clearing of roentgenographic abnormalities, are all hastened by tetracycline or erythromycin treatment (2 g per day). Therapy is usually given for 10 to 14 days. Like tetracycline and erythromycin, other agents, including chloramphenicol, clindamycin, and the aminoglycosides, are mycoplasmastatic *in vitro* (71). However, clinical experience with these agents either has been very limited or has shown them to be ineffective (e.g., clindamycin). Penicillin and the cephalosporins are clearly ineffective. Clinical resistance to tetracycline has been observed in two patients with *M. pneumoniae* pneumonia despite *in vitro* sensitivity of the organisms. Both patients responded to erythromycin. As noted, *M. pneumoniae* pneumonia often persists in respiratory tract secretions despite both appropriate drug therapy and a prompt clinical response. In one study, approximately 50% of those originally culture-positive remained so 6 to 13 weeks after treatment (46). Newer macrolides (e.g., clarithromycin) have been shown to be equally effective *in vitro* against *M. pneumoniae* (13). In limited clinical studies azithromycin is equally efficacious in the treatment of *M. pneumoniae* (117).

Efforts have also been directed at production of an effective vaccine. To date, however, killed or inactivated vaccines have not been particularly successful in producing clinically effective serum or local respiratory tract immune responses (71). Current work is directed at the production of an attenuated vaccine and exploration of the possibilities of intranasal inoculation. Recent efforts have been directed in investigating development of vaccine with use of systemic peptides. A P_1-7 gene domain containing epitope has been shown to mediate *M. pneumoniae* cyto adherence (23). The identification of specific T-cell and B-cell epitopes of the P_1 protein which functions as an adhesin and as a major antigen for *M. pneumoniae* has been of interest in the design of systemic vaccines (61).

CHLAMYDIAL PNEUMONIA

Chlamydiae are important causes of both human and veterinary infections. Organ systems involved include respiratory, genital, and ocular. Recently, most research and clinical interests have centered on genital tract infections (110). Within the genus *Chlamydia* there are three species: *Chlamydia psittaci, C. trachomatis*, and *C. pneumoniae. C. psittaci* includes the organisms responsible for human psittacosis and for the avian infections, which may ultimately cause human disease (114). *C. pneumoniae* (also known as TWAR) has been described as a cause of acute respiratory disease with no avian transmission. *C. trachomatis* includes the organisms responsible for trachoma, inclusion conjunctivitis, genital tract infections, and lymphogranuloma venereum (110). The latter organism also has been recovered from nasotracheal and tracheobronchial aspirates of infants with distinctive pneumonia syndrome.

The Organism

The chlamydiae are obligatory intracellular parasites, a feature shared with the viruses. They are also bacteria-like with a discrete cell wall and are susceptible to antimicrobial agents. All members of the genus share a common antigen, but species can be differentiated on the basis of inclusion type: *C. trachomatis* inclusions stain with iodine whereas those of *C. psittaci* and *C. pneumoniae* do not. Another distinguishing feature is the sensitivity of *C. trachomatis* and *C. pneumoniae* to sulfonamides; *C. psittaci* is resistant. Although these organisms possess certain intrinsic synthetic functions, they depend primarily for growth on energy generated by the host cell (85).

CHLAMYDIA PSITTACI

Psittacosis is an uncommon respiratory infection caused by *C. psittaci*. Infection is contracted through exposure to discharges of infected avian species. The human infection can be either a respiratory or a systemic disease. Although many cases are traced to exposure to exotic avian species, psittacosis is also recognized as a serious occupational hazard to people in the poultry business, particularly those in processing plants (114).

Epidemiology

Psittacosis occurs either sporadically or in small outbreaks in all parts of the world. The worldwide distribution of psittacosis has been documented in over 90 species of birds. Both psittacine and nonpsittacine birds can act as hosts, so it has been suggested that *ornithosis* is a more appropriate term (82). Psittacosis persists in this country as an occupational hazard as demonstrated by outbreaks in Texas, Nebraska, and Missouri (29). The turkey serves as a major reservoir for these outbreaks in the United States; in Eastern Europe the duck has been identified as the major source.

C. psittaci is present in the blood, tissues, feathers, and discharges of infected birds (often nestlings). It is a hardy organism and can withstand drying. Diseased birds frequently show only minimal evidence of illness such as ruffled feathers, lethargy, and failure to eat. Whereas many of these young birds die promptly, survivors often become healthy carriers, discharging chlamydia in their feces. Overcrowding, poor sanitation, improper feeding, and insufficient cage or pen conditions contribute to the development of the disease in parakeets in pet shops or during transport. In general, human infections acquired from psittacine birds are more severe than those acquired from pigeons, ducks, chickens, or pheasants. The attack rate and severity of disease are related to the size of the inoculum.

Pathogenesis

Although human infection usually follows inhalation of dried bird excreta, it can also be contracted by handling contaminated plumage or tissues or, rarely, from bites. Person-to-person transmission is rare; however, well-documented cases occurred in a Louisiana epidemic during which 8 of 18 infected patients died (92). The incubation period varies from 7 to 15 days.

After inhalation, the organism disseminates widely and eventually reaches the reticuloendothelial cells of the liver and spleen. After replication in local mononuclear phagocytes, *C. psittaci* spreads hematogenously to the lungs and other organs. The pulmonary lesion usually starts in the hilum, extends peripherally, and tends to be more prominent in the dependent lobes and segments. The initial events are characterized by an outpouring of fluid from capillary vessels filling alveoli and distending interstitial spaces. Polymorphonuclear leukocytes predominate in the early stages, but they soon disappear and are replaced by mononuclear cells. The affected areas become consolidated with a rubbery, gelatinous consistency, and minor hemorrhage can occur, accounting for the occasional occurrence of hemoptysis seen clinically.

Other pathologic changes include nonspecific splenic inflammation and reactive hepatitis (138), fatty degeneration and lymphocytic infiltration of the myocardium, and subendocardial hemorrhage especially in the region of the mitral and aortic valves. In the kidney, hyaline glomerular capillary occlusions can occur. In the central nervous system, fibrinous or gelatinous arachnoiditis about the central sylvian fissures has been described.

Clinical Features

Pulmonary Manifestations

The clinical features of psittacosis are highly variable; however, pulmonary involvement is most common. Illness can vary from a mild and transient viral-like syndrome to an acute disorder with high fever, severe headache, and nonproductive cough that, in rare instances, can progress to hypoxemia, delirium, and death. Acute respiratory insufficiency has been reported in a patient with psittacosis (4). The onset of illness can be insidious but more often starts abruptly with chills and fever up to 39 to 40°C. Malaise, anorexia, arthralgias, and severe myalgias, particularly in the neck and back, are common. Cough is usually prominent and is usually productive of small amounts of mucoid sputum with occasional blood streaking.

The clinical sign is that of an acutely ill, febrile patient with tachypnea and relative bradycardia. High fever can persist for a week or more. A macular rash (Horden's spots) resembling that seen in typhoid has been described. Psittacosis can sometimes mimic bacterial pneumonia with pleuritic chest pain, productive cough, hemoptysis, and physical findings including consolidation and pleural friction rubs (116). However, rales without signs of consolidation are the most characteristic chest findings (120).

Extrapulmonary Manifestations

Psittacosis can also involve organs other than the lungs (Table 20-3). In nonfatal cases there have been reports of clinical and electrocardiographic evidence suggesting myocarditis (131). Endocarditis, pericarditis, and pericardial effusion occasionally occur (72,94). Psittacosis has also been implicated as a cause of acquired valvular heart disease (132).

Encephalitis is a well-known manifestation of psittacosis. Only rarely is a case reported in the literature without mention of severe headache, sometimes with restlessness or stupor. Delirium and transient meningeal or focal neurologic signs can also be seen. Rarely, a patient presents with seizures or even status epilepticus accompanied by electroencephalographic changes consistent with diffuse cerebral dysfunction. Pathologic changes in the central nervous system are nonspecific and include meningeal and cerebral congestion, perivascular hemorrhages in the brain and spinal cord, and lymphocytic infiltrates.

TABLE 20–3. *Extrapulmonary manifestations of psittacosis*

Cardiac:	Myocarditis, pericarditis, endocarditis, and acquired valvular heart disease
Neurologic:	Encephalitis, seizures, focal neurologic signs, lymphocytic meningitis
Hematologic:	Severe anemia, hemolytic anemia, positive Coombs' test, disseminated intravascular coagulation
Gastrointestinal:	Hepatitis, pancreatitis
Renal:	Proteinuria, oliguria, acute renal failure, nephritis
Miscellaneous:	Splenomegaly, exudative tonsillitis, thyroiditis, fever of unknown origin

From Murray and Tuazon (88).

Hematologic abnormalities have been reported in patients with psittacosis: anemia can develop, sometimes requiring transfusion (116); and hemolysis can occur, usually with negative cold agglutinins. Rarely, the Coombs' test is positive and persists for several months. More recently, disseminated intravascular coagulation has been reported in fulminant cases (9).

Hepatitis and pancreatitis can complicate psittacosis. Pathologic studies have shown areas of focal hepatic necrosis in patients dying of psittacosis, but otherwise jaundice is unusual. Acute pancreatitis has been reported in two fulminant cases (9).

Renal involvement has been manifested with proteinuria and oliguria. In an outbreak in 1930, pathologic studies reported cloudy swelling of renal parenchyma, glomerular congestion, and epithelial degeneration (97). Nephritis can also be secondary to subacute endocarditis (72). The patient with psittacosis can occasionally present with acute renal failure; two patients developed acute tubular necrosis (9). Renal damage was attributed to a possible direct toxic effect of the virulent chlamydial infection, although organisms were not documented in kidney tissue.

Polyarthritis has been reported in patients with *C. psittaci* infection presenting with symptoms resembling those of acute rheumatic fever, Reiter's syndrome, and even rheumatoid arthritis. The last responded to long-term steroid treatment (19).

Patients with psittacosis commonly have splenomegaly, considered by some as a most helpful diagnostic sign both pathologically and clinically (75). Furthermore, in experimental psittacosis, spleens are enlarged and involved pathologically. Psittacosis can also present as fever of unknown origin (54). Unusual presentation of psittacosis bacteremia in a setting of familial sarcoidosis has been described (55).

Laboratory and Roentgenographic Manifestations

There are no laboratory or radiologic abnormalities specifically associated with psittacosis. The leukocyte count is usually normal (116,138). Sputum examination shows predominantly mononuclear cells, and no etiologic agents are recovered on culture. Other abnormalities include elevated transaminases, occasional increases in serum bilirubin levels, and proteinuria.

Radiographic examination of the chest shows striking variability in the extent and character of infiltrates, although they are generally bronchopneumonic in type. In one study 28% of cases showed no radiographic abnormality (21). Chest films usually show patchy reticular infiltrates radiating out from the hilar areas or involving the basilar lung segments (116). Because the chest examination is often unimpressive in patients with psittacosis, clinicians are often surprised by the extent of roentgenographic involvement.

Radiographic clearance occurred more slowly compared with *Mycoplasma* pneumonia. Ninety-six percent cleared at 8 weeks, whereas only 50% of psittacosis cases resolved radiographically at 7 weeks (21).

Diagnosis

The protean manifestations of psittacosis make secure diagnosis difficult on clinical grounds alone. A history of direct exposure to birds is an important clue to elicit, especially if such occurred within the 1- to 2-week incubation period. The diagnosis is confirmed by the isolation of *C. psittaci* from sputum, tissue, or exudates. Because the isolation studies require laboratory expertise and are quite hazardous, serologic testing is the diagnostic method of choice. Antibodies to *C. psittaci* can be detected as early as the end of the first week of illness, but usually 3 weeks are needed for the antibody to appear. The serological method most often used is the direct complement fixation test, which detects antibodies against a heat-stable group antigen prepared from *C. psittaci*. A paired serum sample with a fourfold or greater rise in titer is considered diagnostic. A titer of 1:16 during an acute pneumonic illness is presumptive evidence of disease. In untreated cases, antibody titers usually peak approximately 21 days after the onset of illness. Cross-reactions of *C. psittaci* with *Brucella* and *Coxiella burnetii* can occur and thus give false-positive complement-fixation tests.

Pulmonary infections caused by *M. pneumoniae, Coxiella burnetii, Francisella tularensis,* and *Legionella pneumophila,* and by some viruses and fungi, can mimic psittacosis. If pulmonary symptoms are less prominent or overshadowed, systemic febrile illnesses such as typhoid fever, brucellosis, mononucleosis syndromes, infectious hepatitis, endocarditis, rheumatic fever, occult carcinoma, and sarcoidosis should be considered.

Thus, the diagnostic of psittacosis is usually based on an epidemiologic history of contact with avian species (patients should be carefully and repeatedly questioned), a clinical syndrome of high fever, severe headache, and relative bradycardia with nonbacterial pneumonia symptoms, and a fourfold rise in specific complement fixation titer.

Treatment and Prevention

Although *C. psittaci* is sensitive to tetracycline, and, to a lesser degree, to chloramphenicol and penicillin (54), it has been difficult to measure the true efficacy of antibiotic therapy. Laboratory evidence and clinical experience, however, suggest that tetracycline is effective in the treatment of psittacosis. In some cases, response to tetracycline treatment is slow; thus, therapeutic trials with tetracycline cannot be relied on as a diagnostic maneuver (116). Also, relapse can occur. Tetracycline (2 to

3 g per day) should be continued for 10 to 14 days after defervescence. Doxycycline 100 mg twice a day for 14 days has been recommended in a recent review (139). Limited clinical experience suggests that erythromycin can be active against *C. psittaci* (52). Before effective therapy was available the mortality rate was 20 to 40%, but recently it has declined to as low as 1% (115).

Problems in the prevention of psittacosis still exist. Historically, efforts to control psittacosis in humans emphasize administrative procedures such as embargoes or bans on shipment of avian species. As a result of pressures from bird fanciers and the pet industry, importation of exotic birds has been reopened with the proviso that the birds be treated. Chlortetracycline-impregnated millet seeds are commercially available for the treatment of chlamydial infection in parakeets. Liquid vehicles have been developed for nectar-feeding birds, and the medicated mash has been formulated for the treatment of larger psittacines such as parrots. These medicated feeds may be used therapeutically or prophylactically to eradicate latent chlamydial infection. In addition, the United States Public Health Service regulations require that important psittacine species receive a 30-day course of chlortetracycline in a quarantine center licensed by the United States Department of Agriculture before being released for sale (112). Smuggled birds, however, evade such measures.

Despite the above precautions, there has recently been a small increase in the number of human psittacosis infections (21). Most of these were associated with contact in the commercial flow of the pet bird industry. However, the potential for point-source outbreaks in pet stores and department stores has been clearly documented. The absence of adequate monitoring could be a flaw in the current regulations concerning treatment of imported psittacines. The regulations specify methods of treatment but contain no provision for monitoring the efficacy of these procedures (112).

CHLAMYDIA PNEUMONIAE (TWAR)

Initially classified as *C. psittaci* (48,111), *Chlamydia pneumoniae* (TWAR) is a new, third species of *Chlamydia*. The name TWAR is derived from the first two human isolates—TW-183, from the eye of a Taiwanese child with conjunctivitis, and AR 39, from the respiratory tract of a college student with pharyngitis—in the United States (44). In contrast to *C. psittaci* respiratory infections, no avian transmission has been detected in outbreaks caused by *C. pneumoniae*.

The Organism

Initially, the TWAR organism was considered to be *C. psittaci;* subsequent studies, however, have identified these organisms as separate species of *Chlamydia* (15,47). Using quantitative DNA homology studies, *C. pneumoniae* isolates ≥94% homology with each other but <10% with *C. psittaci* and *C. trachomatis* isolates (11,22). By electron microscopy, the elementary body of *C. pneumoniae* is pear-shaped with a large periplasmic space, as contrasted with the typically round elementary bodies of *C. psittaci* and *C. trachomatis* (15,67). Electron-dense bodies were also demonstrated in the periplasmic space of the elementary bodies of *C. pneumoniae*.

Epidemiology

Both epidemic and endemic infections have been described in North America and Nordic countries, e.g., Finland, Denmark, Norway, and Sweden (49,65,104). It has been reported as a cause of community-acquired pneumonia in the elderly population in Nova Scotia (79) and as a cause of acute respiratory disease among students in Seattle, Washington (48). Population prevalence antibody studies suggest that *C. pneumoniae* is worldwide in distribution and that 40–60% are infected and reinfected during their lifetime. Infection is common in people of all ages except those under 5 years old in temperate-zone countries. Interestingly, nearly 10% of Filipino children under 5 years of age who present with lower respiratory tract infection have either acute or chronic antibody to *C. pneumoniae* (103). The age curve of antibody prevalence with most of the infection after school age and the higher prevalence in men suggest that the phase of infection is more often outside the household (44). No evidence of seasonal periodicity has been reported in studies.

Transmission is mainly human to human without bird or animal transmission. It is still not known what the mode and place of transmission is, what the incubation period is, and the infectiousness of the organisms (43).

Pathogenesis

C. pneumoniae strain TWAR has been established as an important cause of respiratory infections. Recently, it has been associated with atherosclerosis and coronary artery disease (68,125). No information is available on the pathology of *C. pneumoniae* infections in humans. An experimental mouse model of *C. pneumoniae* has been evaluated by intranasal inoculation of the organism (136). A prolonged course of infection was induced. The lung pathology was characterized by patchy interstitial pneumonitis with predominance of polymorphonuclear leukocytes in the early stage and mononuclear cell infiltration in the later stage. Serum IgG response was observed in the mice and correlated with the decrease in the number of organisms recoverable from the lungs.

Clinical Features

Infection with *C. pneumoniae* can manifest with a wide variety of clinical presentations that are not unique to this particular organism. It is estimated that it accounts for about 10% of pneumonias in both outpatient settings and hospitalized patients (43). Pneumonia is usually mild and self-limited, but severe illness can occur in the elderly, in patients with chronic diseases, or in patients with concurrent bacterial infections. Reactivation of latent infection has also been suggested in cases of hospital-acquired *C. pneumoniae* infections in critically ill patients. In some patients, persistent infection can follow an acute infection and persist for many months (53). Infection can be biphasic with prolonged upper respiratory symptoms manifested by pharyngitis and hoarseness followed by onset of cough and malaise.

Severe pharyngitis and hoarseness is frequently reported in *C. pneumoniae* infection with up to 80% of those infected presenting with sore throat (43). Sinusitis has been consistently reported in studies of *C. pneumoniae* infections and estimated to account for about 5% of primary sinusitis in young adults. Otitis is less common with *C. pneumoniae* infection. Although the first isolate of *C. pneumoniae* was from a conjunctival swab, no further association with ocular disease has been reported (115).

Other syndromes that have been reported include fever of undetermined origin and influenza-like illness associated with *C. pneumoniae* infection. An association between serologic evidence of acute *C. pneumoniae* and airway reactivity in adults with lower respiratory tract infection has been reported (51).

C. pneumoniae has been suggested as a causative agent of myocarditis and endocarditis as isolated infections or in association with pneumonia (125). Recently a serologic association of *C. pneumoniae* with coronary artery disease as well as sarcoidosis (102,125) has been reported. In other studies using immunocytochemistry, and by polymerase chain reaction, *C. pneumoniae* was detected in coronary artery atheromas. Electron microscopy revealed typical pear-shaped elementary bodies in 6 of 21 atheromatous plaques (68).

Diagnosis

Data indicate that clinical differentiation of TWAR and *M. pneumoniae* infections is difficult. Laboratory and radiographic findings are likewise nondiagnostic. White blood count is usually normal, and mild increase in sedimentation rate can be seen. Chest roentgenograms usually reveal a single lesion involving one lobe, round, and measuring 2–3 cm in size (79). The more extensive infiltrates usually present with sequential consolidation. Density is described as either homogenous or heterogenous, and there is no particular anatomic distribution of the lesion. Resolution of infiltrates usually occurs within 4 to 6 weeks after the initial chest roentgenogram.

C. pneumoniae is a fastidious organism. It can be isolated using yolk sac of embryonated chicken eggs and HeLa 229 cell cultures. Yolk sac smears are stained with a modified Macchiavello method and direct fluorescent antibody technique using TWAR monoclonal antibody. Isolation of *C. pneumoniae* has been hampered by low sensitivity of existing culture systems; however, laboratories with experience in doing chlamydial cultures should be successful in isolating *C. pneumoniae* (10). Recently, *C. pneumoniae* has been grown and isolated more readily in HL cells, a human cell line used to isolate respiratory syncytial virus (18). Enzyme immunoassay techniques for chlamydial antigen detection has low sensitivity compared with culture. DNA amplification using polymerase chain reaction had a higher sensitivity and specificity compared with culture (59).

Diagnosis can be confirmed by a rise in the serologic titer. Both complement-fixation test and the microimmunofluorescence test with IgM and IgG conjugates have been used. Two patterns of antibody response are observed in patients with TWAR infection (79). The first, usually seen in younger persons with primary infection, is an early rise of the complement-fixation test and a slower response in the microimmunofluorescent test. Diagnostic titers in the serum IgM fraction are usually seen 3 weeks after onset of disease, and IgG antibody usually appears 6 weeks after onset of symptoms (44). The second antibody response is that observed in older persons and presumed to be associated with secondary infection or reinfection. Microimmunofluorescent antibody to TWAR in the IgG fraction appears sooner, and the complement-fixation antibody is usually not observed. IgM antibody titer, if present, tends to be at low titer.

Treatment

Limited data suggest that tetracycline or erythromycin is the antibiotic of choice for treating *C. pneumoniae* infection. Current recommended therapy is either tetracycline or erythromycin 2 grams/day in divided doses for 10 to 14 days or 1 gram daily for 3 weeks.

There are no controlled studies evaluating clinical efficacy of treatment regimens against *C. pneumoniae* infections. Recent *in vitro* studies have demonstrated efficacy of azithromycin, clarithromycin, and quinolones against *C. pneumoniae*. Clarithromycin appears to be the most active drug *in vitro* compared to other macrolides, such as tetracycline and ciprofloxacin (16,133). A limited clinical study of four patients with *C. pneumoniae* lower respiratory tract infections has shown that ofloxacin could be an effective alternative antibiotic (73).

CHLAMYDIA TRACHOMATIS

C. trachomatis strains are human pathogens with man as the sole natural host, in contrast to *C. psittaci* strains, which involve human diseases only as zoonoses. *C. trachomatis* strains are antigenically related and represent a spectrum of immunologic reaction. Different serotypes cause the various disease syndromes: L_1–L_3 are the three serotypes of lymphogranuloma venereum; A–C serotypes cause trachoma; and serotypes D–K are agents of conjunctivitis, genital infections, and pneumonia of newborns (110).

Recently, *C. trachomatis* has been recovered from nasopharyngeal and tracheobronchial aspirates of infants with a distinctive pneumonic syndrome (3). Clinical symptoms were cough and congestion, tachypnea, and diffuse pulmonary infiltrate on chest x-ray. The infant is usually afebrile. The disease is characteristically chronic, lasting a month or longer. No fatalities were reported. The ages of affected infants were 4 to 24 weeks. Elevated serum Ig and IgM levels were noted, and some infants had a slight eosinophilia. Ninety percent (18/20) of infants with the syndrome yielded chlamydia from the tracheal aspirates. Eleven of the 20 infants had conjunctivitis by either history or examination. However, chlamydiae were also recovered from the nasopharynx of 10 of 12 infants with inclusion conjunctivitis but without respiratory manifestations. The infants with respiratory disease differed from those with inclusion conjunctivitis alone in having significantly higher levels of antibody to chlamydiae. Thus, it appears that chlamydiae might be an important cause of respiratory disease in infants. Support for this hypothesis has come from a recent report of the isolation of chlamydia from an open lung biopsy of a child with similar disease (41). Although newly recognized, chlamydia may account for up to 30% of pneumonitis in hospitalized infants (56). A recent serodiagnostic study of 30 infants with suspected chlamydial pneumonitis concluded that enzymes immunoassay (EIA) using the major outer membrane protein (MOMP) is specific and sensitive and can be useful in screening children under 6 months of age with respiratory tract symptoms and IgM antibodies to chlamydia (98).

The incidence of *C. trachomatis*–associated respiratory disease in adults is unknown. *C. trachomatis* was isolated from the lower respiratory tract of six immunosuppressed adult patients who had pulmonary infection, the severity varying from acute bronchitis to severe diffuse interstitial pneumonia. The severity of *C. trachomatis*–associated pulmonary disease in adults seemed to correlate with the degree of immunosuppression; this observation could explain the occurrence of the disease in infants in whom the immune system is not yet fully competent. Concomitant infection with cytomegalovirus was demonstrated in three patients by culture of blood, bronchial washings, and lung tissue obtained at necropsy. Two patients seemed to respond to treatment with doxycycline and erythromycin, both drugs having recognized activity against *C. trachomatis* (7).

It is unclear whether infection in this group of patients represented a primary infection or reactivation of latent infection. In addition, the role of other synergistic organisms and optimum therapy remain unclear. Further studies are necessary to determine the importance of *C. trachomatis* as a cause of respiratory tract infection in the adult and to clarify how the disease develops.

Q FEVER PNEUMONIA

In the United States, except for farming and rural communities, Q fever is a medical curiosity. It rarely occurs in urban areas, and seldom do its signs or symptoms specifically raise the suspicion of the diagnosis. Still, it is certainly capable of causing the atypical pneumonia syndrome.

Q fever was first described in 1935 in Australia (25). An unidentified organism was recovered from the urine and blood of nine Australian abattoir workers. "Q" stood for query because the etiology of the illness was unknown. The causative agent was subsequently isolated by Davis and Cox from ticks in Montana and was identified as rickettsia-like by Burnet and Freeman. The organism, which has a worldwide distribution, was first named *Rickettsia burnetii* but is most often referred to as *Coxiella burnetii*.

The Organism

C. burnetii is an obligate intracellular organism which differs in several major respects from the other members of genus *Rickettsia*. It fails to evoke cross-reacting serum agglutinins to *Proteus* X strains (Weil-Felix reaction), is not associated with a typical rickettsial rash, and does not require an arthropod vector to maintain itself in nature (93). *C. burnetii* is extremely infectious for humans and animals. In guinea pigs, a single inhaled organism is sufficient to initiate infection (127). The organism is highly resistant to physical and chemical agents such as toxic levels of heat, formaldehyde, and phenol. *C. burnetii* has been recovered in dry tick feces after 18 months; in dry animal blood, clay, or sand for 4 to 6 months; and in tap water or milk for 30 to 42 months (93).

The recent discovery of plasmids in *C. burnetii* could provide some insight into the different clinical manifestations of Q fever. Isolates from patients with acute self-limited illness can be distinguished from those from patients with endocarditis by their plasmid type and by restriction endonuclease analysis of plasmid DNA (107). The organism exists in 2 phases, phase 1 and phase 2, and the plasmids are present regardless of existence in phase 1 or 2. Recent studies suggest that variation in phase 1 lipopolysaccharide (LPS) affects pathogenicity in that isolates from patients with endocarditis have a benign LPS (50,106).

Epidemiology

The organism infects a wide variety of insects, rodents, and large domestic and wild animals. The disease is usually maintained in nature by animal-to-animal spread. In transmission to man, the infected milk, feces, urine, placentas, and uterine discharges of sheep, goats, and cattle are most often implicated. Most recently, Q fever outbreaks have been associated with infected parturient cats and with skinning wild rabbits (69,80,96). *C. burnetii's* resistance to drying allows the dust in sheep pens and cattle sheds to become heavily contaminated, and, usually following inhalation, human infection results. The association with livestock need not be intimate. Outbreaks have occurred in wool and felt processing plants and tanneries and have been related to contaminated clothing and dusty straw used for packing (93) and spreading in a university hospital environment where research with sheep was being conducted (81). Infection can also occur in laboratory workers; the handling of infected egg cultures or animals inoculated with the organism must always be considered hazardous (113). Rarely, transmission of Q fever from person to person within a family has been reported (77). Some cases have been attributed to travel to a country where the disease is endemic (74). Urban outbreaks of Q fever among persons living near the road traveled by animals and vehicles have been reported (14,105).

Transmission by tick bite probably occurs as well. There is also evidence to suggest that Q fever can develop following the organism's penetration of skin abrasions or the conjunctivae or injection of contaminated raw milk.

Pathogenesis

The incubation period of Q fever is 2 to 4 weeks. After inhalation, organisms multiply in the lung (or other sites of entry), followed by hematogenous spread to other organs. Later they may be excreted in the urine (93). Q fever is most often a benign illness, so few patients have come to autopsy. In fatal cases, the lung resembles that seen in pneumococcal pneumonia. However, a mononuclear exudate distinguishes the process from a bacterial infection. Alveolar walls are thickened by infiltration with macrophages, lymphocytes, and plasma cells; septal necrosis can be present. Alveolar exudates are mostly comprised of macrophages; polymorphonuclear leukocytes are conspicuously absent. The bronchiolar mucosa can be necrotic (93). Widespread lesions have been noted in the pericardium, spleen, liver, brain, kidney, and testis, and *C. burnetii* has been observed lying free within macrophages in various organs. Biopsies of liver and bone marrow demonstrate typical granulomatous and nongranulomatous changes in response to *C. burnetii* infections (124). In Q fever endocarditis, organisms can be isolated from or observed in valvular tissue and vegetations (63,93).

Clinical Features

Pneumonia

The occurrence of pulmonary involvement in patients with Q fever is highly variable and has ranged from 0 to 90% in several studies (17,78). The onset of illness is typically abrupt, with high fever, shaking chills, and malaise. Headache and neck stiffness can be severe and sometimes overshadows other complaints. Anorexia, abdominal pain, vomiting, myalgias, and sore throat also occur. Diaphoresis can be marked. Over half of patients develop a dry cough that is not as prominent as in *M. pneumoniae* pneumonia. Chest pain, occasionally pleuritic, is present in less than 20% of cases.

Clinical signs include an acutely ill appearance and pulse-temperature dissociation. Aside from fine rales, chest findings are usually modest or absent and signs of pulmonary consolidation are rare. Hepatosplenomegaly occurs in a few cases. Nuchal rigidity can be prominent. Although cutaneous manifestations typical of other rickettsial infections are absent in Q fever, some patients develop mild erythema or a transient maculopapular rash (75,80).

In most cases, Q fever pneumonia is a benign, self-limited illness, which resolves within 1 or 2 weeks with or without treatment. Although fever can persist for up to 3 months in atypical cases, patients are usually afebrile by the second week of illness. Sometimes, however, Q fever is complicated by extrapulmonary lesions, persistence of symptoms, or relapse despite treatment. On occasion, the syndrome of chronic Q fever develops with endocarditis the prominent feature. It should also be pointed out that *C. burnetii* infections can be asymptomatic, detected only by fortuitous serum antibody testing.

Extrapulmonary Manifestations

Although pneumonia is the most common clinical presentation, Q fever is a true systemic infection which can produce disease in other organs (Table 20-4). Q fever hepatitis can present with an infectious hepatitis-like picture, as a cause of fever of unknown origin with characteristic granulomas on liver biopsy, and as a finding in a patient with acute Q fever (78). Hepatitis can be mild or can be associated with jaundice and marked transaminase elevation and, rarely, death. Pathologic studies have revealed minimal to widespread parenchymal inflammation, necrosis, and granulomata. Organisms have been isolated in the liver. Vascular complications include thrombophlebitis with pulmonary embolism, arteritis, and thromboangiitis obliterans. Cardiovascular involvement with pleuropericarditis, pericardial effusion, myocarditis, and endocarditis has also been reported (129). The latter is usually a mani-

TABLE 20–4. *Nonrespiratory manifestations of Q fever*

Gastrointestinal:	Hepatitis
Vascular:	Thrombophlebitis, arteritis
Cardiac:	Pericarditis, pericardial effusion, myocarditis, endocarditis
Ocular:	Uveitis, iritis, optic neuritis
Neurologic:	Meningitis, neuropathy
Miscellaneous:	Otitis, arthritis, epididymitis, abortion, congenital malformations, fever of unknown origin

From Murray and Tuazon (88).

festation of chronic Q fever and represents one of the causes of culture-negative endocarditis.

The signs of endocarditis are frequently not apparent until months or years (up to 20 years) after the original infection (63). Because blood cultures are often negative, the diagnosis is by serology, isolation, or histologic demonstration of the organism from valve tissue or vegetation. The aortic valve is most often involved, although in a recent series the mitral valve was involved often; and some cases have occurred in prosthetic valves (132). Embolic episodes are not uncommon, and thrombocytopenia, purpuric rashes, hepatitis, nephritis, and venous thrombosis can be complications (93). Response to antibiotic therapy is usually poor, and valve replacement is probably required for cure.

Additional nonrespiratory manifestations of Q fever have included ocular disease (uveitis, iritis, optic neuritis), arthritis, bone marrow granulomata, neurologic involvement (meningitis, neuropathy), otitis, epididymitis, abortion, and congenital malformations. A few patients with documented Q fever fail to fully recover their general health and experience prolonged weakness, fatigue, weight loss, and vague aches.

Laboratory and Roentgenographic Manifestations

Routine studies yield little helpful information. The white blood cell count is typically normal, with a slight shift to the left. Liver function tests are often abnormal; in a series of 111 cases 85% had abnormalities (123). The serum transaminase can be elevated. The gram stain of the sputum shows predominantly mononuclear leukocytes. Although headache and nuchal rigidity are often present, lumbar punctures are usually unremarkable.

Chest film abnormalities generally resemble viral and mycoplasmal pneumonias with patchy infiltrates, often as single, rounded segmental opacities having a ground-glass appearance. Lower lobe involvement and linear atelectasis are common. The absence of vascular engorgement and tendency to produce lobar consolidation have been used to suggest the diagnosis of Q fever in patients with the atypical pneumonia syndrome (83). Pleural effusions occur in less than 10% of cases, and hilar adenopathy is rare. Infiltrates can take up to 10 weeks to resolve, but resolution in most cases is complete by 3 to 4 weeks (109).

Diagnosis

A history of direct or indirect exposure to livestock, ticks, or an ill patient with atypical pneumonia should arouse suspicion of Q fever. Moreover, one must be aware that Q fever can be a hazard of tourism. Patients might have visited an endemic area and become infected before returning home (74). Medical centers engaged in research with pregnant sheep should be alert to the risk of Q fever (81).

The diagnosis of Q fever is established either by isolation of *C. burnetii* or by demonstration of a significant rise in specific antibody titer. *C. burnetii* has been recovered from blood, sputum, urine, spinal and pleural fluids, and tissue obtained at biopsy or postmortem. Rickettsemia is most often documented in the acute phase of the illness. Clinical materials can be inoculated into guinea pigs, hamsters, mice, or embryonated eggs (93). Animals are examined 4 to 6 weeks later for the presence of specific antibody. All isolation procedures are extremely hazardous, and adequate safeguards must be enforced (130).

Serologic diagnostic methods are simpler and safer. Specific antibodies, identified by complement fixation, microagglutination, and microimmunofluorescence, appear in man 2 to 4 weeks after the onset of illness and are most often used to establish the diagnosis. The most commonly used serologic methods are the complement-fixation (CF) and indirect fluorescent antibody (IFA) techniques (27). IFA reached peak levels 4–8 weeks after onset of disease and CF titers peak during the 12-week period (95). Both titers gradually decrease over the succeeding 12 months. In addition, IgM IFA can distinguish recent Q fever infections.

C. burnetii has antigenic phase variations (phase 1 to phase 2). Phase II antibodies predominate in acute, self-limited Q fever infections; whereas phase 1 antibodies are prominent only in patients with chronic Q-fever (109). Phase I *C. burnetii* antigen should be used in the serologic diagnosis of Q fever endocarditis (63). Immunity is apparently lifelong. Direct identification of *C. burnetii* in tissue may be accomplished by a fluorescent antibody technique (93).

Treatment and Prevention

Despite *in vitro* sensitivity of *C. burnetii* to tetracycline and chloramphenicol, it is not clear if antibiotics alter the clinical course of Q fever. In clinical practice patients who are acutely ill or those with persistent symptoms or relapses are treated with antibiotics. Tetracycline (2 g per day) is the drug of choice because of few adverse reactions. Doxycycline 100 mg twice daily is an alternative regimen. Chloramphenicol also appears effective. Erythromycin has been reported to be beneficial in some cases; others have reported failures despite maximal dosages (24,78). In patients with endocarditis trimethoprim-sulfamethoxazole and rifampin have also been employed (63). Quinolones have been shown to be active *in vitro* against *C. burnetii* (137).

Measures to reduce the likelihood of infection in areas where Q fever is enzootic in domestic livestock are desirable. Milk should be boiled or pasteurized at high temperatures. Although the possibility of man-to-man transmission is not sufficient to warrant quarantine procedures, sputum, blood, urine, and other infected specimens, clothing, and autopsy material should be handled carefully.

Q fever vaccine trials in humans have been recently reported (2). The duration of protection and the markers that best correlate with protection after vaccination are not known with certainty (109). There are suggestions that immunity can be long-lasting. In institutions that use sheep for research, vaccination of these animals has been considered a strategy for minimizing transmission of *C. burnetii* to humans (101). Veterinary Q fever vaccine and human Q fever vaccine can be obtained under IND status.

HANTAVIRUS PNEUMONIA

See Chapter 24 for a full discussion.

REFERENCES

1. Abramovitz, P., Schvartzman, P., Harel, D., Lis, I., and Naot, Y. (1987): Direct invasion of the central nervous system by *Mycoplasma pneumoniae:* a report of two cases. *J. Infect. Dis.,* 155(3):482–487.
2. Ascher, M.S., Berman, M.A., and Ruppanner, R. (1983): Initial clinical and immunologic evaluation of a new phase 1 Q fever vaccine and skin test in humans. *J. Infect. Dis.,* 148:214–222.
3. Beem, M.O., and Saxon, E.M. (1977): Respiratory tract colonization and a distinctive pneumonia syndrome in infants infected with *Chlamydia trachomatis. N. Engl. J. Med.,* 196:306–310.
4. Berkel, M.V., Dik, H., Van Der Meer, J., et al. (1985): Acute respiratory insufficiency from psittacosis. *Br. Med. J.,* 290:1503.
5. Bibenfeld, G., and Norberg, R. (1974): Circulating immune complexes in mycoplasma infection. *J. Immunol.,* 112:413–415.
6. Biberfield, G., Stenbeck, J., and Johnson, T. (1968): *Mycoplasma pneumoniae* infection in hospitalized patients with acute respiratory illness. *Acta Pathol. Microbiol. Scand.* [A], 74:287.
7. Blackman, H.J., Yoneda, C., Dawson, C.R., and Schacter, J. (1977): Antibiotic susceptibility of *Chlamydia trachomatis. Antimicrob. Agents Chemother.,* 12:673–677.
8. Brolin, I., and Wernstedt, L. (1978): Radiologic appearance of mycoplasma pneumonia. *Scand. J. Respir. Dis.,* 59:179–189.
9. Byrom, N.P., Walls, J., and Mair, H.J. (1979): Fulminant psittacosis. *Lancet,* 1:353–356.
10. Campbell, J.E., Barnes, R.C., Kozarsky, P.E., and Spika, J.S. (1991): Culture-confirmed pneumonia due to *Chlamydia pneumoniae. J. Infect. Dis.,* 164:411–413.
11. Campbell, L.A., Kuo, C.C., and Grayston, J.T. (1990): Structural antigenic analysis of *Chlamydia pneumoniae. Infect. Immunol.,* 58:93–97.
12. Cassell, G.H., and Cole, B.C. (1981): Mycoplasmas as agents of human disease. *N. Engl. J. Med.,* 304:80.
13. Cassell, G.H., Lerner, J., Waites, K.B., Pate, M.S., Duffy, L.B., Watson, H.L., and McIntosh, J.C. (1991): Efficacy of clarithromycin against *Mycoplasma pneumoniae. J. Antimicrob. Chemother.,* 27(Suppl. A):47–59.
14. Centers for Disease Control. (1984): Q fever outbreak—Switzerland. *M.M.W.R.,* 33:355–356, 361.
15. Chi, E.Y., Kuo, C.C., and Grayston, J.T. (1987): Unique ultrastructure in the elementary body of *Chlamydia* sp. strain TWAR. *J. Bacteriol.,* 169:3757–3763.
16. Chirgwin, K., Roblin, P.M., and Hammerschlag, M.R. (1989): *In vitro* susceptibilities of *Chlamydia pneumoniae* (Chlamydia sp. strain TWAR). *Antimicrob. Agents Chemother.,* 33:1634–1635.
17. Clark, W.H., Lennette, E.H., and Railsbach, O.C. (1951): Q fever in California: clinical features in one hundred eighty cases. *Arch. Intern. Med.,* 88:155–167.
18. Cleal, D., and Stamm, W.E. (1990): Use of HL cells for improved isolation and passage of *Chlamydia pneumoniae. J. Clin. Microbiol.,* 28:934–940.
19. Cooper, S.M., and Ferriar, J.A. (1986): Reactive arthritis and psittacosis. *Am. J. Med.,* 81:555–557.
20. Couch, R.B. (1990): Mycoplasma pneumoniae (primary atypical pneumonia). In: *Principles and Practice of Infectious Diseases,* edited by G.L. Mandell, R.G. Douglas, and J.E. Bennett, pp. 1447–1458. Churchill Livingstone, New York.
21. Coutts, H., MacKenzie, S., and White, R.J. (1985): Clinical and radiographic features of psittacosis infections. *Thorax,* 40:530.
22. Cox, R.L., Kuo, C.C., Grayston, J.T., and Campbell, L.A. (1988): Deoxyribonucleic acid relatedness of *Chlamydia* sp. strain TWAR to *Chlamydia trachomatis* and *Chlamydia psittaci. Int. J. Syst. Bacteriol.,* 38:265–268.
23. Dallo, S.F., Su, C.J., Horton, J.R., and Baseman, J.B. (1988): Identification of P_1 gene domain containing epitope(s) mediating *Mycoplasma pneumoniae* cytoadherence. *J. Exp. Med.,* 167(2):718–723.
24. D'Angelo, L.J., and Hetherington, R. (1979): Q fever treated with erythromycin. *Br. Med. J.,* 2:305–306.
25. Derrick, E.H. (1937): Q fever, new fever entity: clinical features, diagnosis and laboratory investigation. *Med. J. Aust.,* 2:281–299.
26. Devos, M., VanNimmen, L., and Baele, G. (1974): Disseminated intravascular coagulation during fatal *Mycoplasma pneumoniae* infection. *Acta Hematol.,* 52:120–125.
27. Dupuis, G., Peter, O., Peacock, M., Burgdorfer, W., and Haller, E. (1985): Immunoglobulin responses in acute Q fever. *J. Clin. Microbiol.,* 22:484–487.
28. Durfee, P.T. (1975): Psittacosis in humans in the United States. *J. Infect. Dis.,* 132:604–605.
29. Durfee, P.T., Pullen, M.M., Currier, R.W., and Parker, R.L. (1975): Human psittacosis associated with commercial processing of turkeys. *J. Am. Vet. Med. Assoc.,* 167:804–808.

30. Feizi, T. (1967): Cold agglutinins, the direct Coomb's test and serum immunoglobulins in *Mycoplasma pneumoniae* infections. *Ann. NY Acad. Sci.,* 143:801–812.
31. Feizi, T., Maclean, H., Sommerville, R.G., and Selwyn, J.G. (1967): Studies on an epidemic of respiratory disease caused by *Mycoplasma pneumoniae*. *Br. Med. J.,* 1:457.
32. Fernald, G.W. (1969): Immunologic aspects of experimental *Mycoplasma pneumoniae* infection. *J. Infect. Dis.,* 119:255–266.
33. Fine, N.L., Smith, L.R., and Sheedy, P.F. (1970): Frequency of pleural effusions in *Mycoplasma* and viral pneumonias. *N. Engl. J. Med.,* 283:790–793.·
34. Fleischhauer, P., Huben, U., Mertens, H., Sethi, K.K., and Thurmann, D. (1972): Nachweis von *M. pneumoniae* im Liquor bei akuter Polyneuritis. *Dtsch Med. Wochenschr.,* 97:678–782.
35. Forsyth, B.R., and Chanock, R.M. (1966): Mycoplasma pneumonia. *Ann. Rev. Med.,* 17:371–382.
36. Foy, H.M., Kenny, G.E., Cooney, M.K., Allan, I.D., and Van Belle, G. (1983): Naturally acquired immunity to pneumonia due to *Mycoplasma pneumonia*. *J. Infect. Dis.,* 147:967–973.
37. Foy, H.M., Kenny, G.E., McMahan, R., Kaiser, G., and Grayston, J.T. (1971): *Mycoplasma pneumoniae* in the community. *Am. J. Epidemiol.,* 93:55–67.
38. Foy, H.M., Nugent, C.G., Kenny, G.E., McMahan, R., and Grayston, J.T. (1971): Repeated *Mycoplasma pneumoniae* pneumonia after 4 1/2 years. *J.A.M.A.* 216:671–672.
39. Foy, H.M., Ochs, H., Davis, S.D., Kenny, G.E., and Luce, R.R. (1973): *Mycoplasma pneumoniae* infections in patients with immunodeficiency syndromes: report of four cases. *J. Infect. Dis.,* 127:388–393.
40. Francis, D.A., Brown, A., Miller, D.H., Wiles, C.M., Bennett, E.D., and Leigh, N. (1988): MRI appearances of the CNS manifestations of *Mycoplasma pneumoniae:* a report of two cases. *J. Neurol.,* 235(7):441–443.
41. Frommell, G.T., Bruhn, W.F., and Schwartzman, J.D. (1977): Isolation of *Chlamydia trachomatis* from infant lung tissue. *N. Engl. J. Med.,* 296:1150–1152.
42. George, R.B., Aizkind, M.M., Rasch, J.R., and Mogabbab, W.J. (1977): Mycoplasma and adenovirus pneumonia. *Ann. Intern. Med.,* 65:931.
43. Grayston, J.T. (1989): *Chlamydia pneumoniae,* strain TWAR. *Chest,* 95:664–669.
44. Grayston, J.T., Campbell, L.A., Kuo, C.C., Mordhorst, C.H., Saikku, P., Thom, D.H., and Wang, S.P. (1990): A new respiratory tract pathogen: *Chlamydia pneumoniae* strain TWAR. *J. Infect. Dis.,* 161:618–625.
45. Grayston, J.T., Foy, H.M., and Kenny, G.E. (1967): Mycoplasms (PPLO) in human disease. *DM,* December.
46. Grayston, J.T., Kenny, G.E., Foy, H.M., Kronmal, R.A., and Alexander, E.R. (1967): Epidemiological studies of *Mycoplasma pneumoniae* infections in civilians. *Ann. NY Acad. Sci.,* 143:436–446.
47. Grayston, J.T., Kuo, C.C., Campbell, L.A., et al. (1989): *Chlamydia pneumoniae* sp. nov. for Chlamydia sp. strain TWAR. *Int. J. Syst. Bacteriol.,* 39:88.
48. Grayston, J.T., Kuo, C.C., Wang, S.P., and Altman, J. (1986): A new *Chlamydia psittaci* strain, TWAR isolated in acute respiratory tract infections. *N. Engl. J. Med.,* 351:161–164.
49. Grayston, J.T., Mordhorst, C., Bruu, A.L., Vene, S., and Wang, S.P. (1989): Countrywide epidemics of *Chlamydia pneumoniae,* strain TWAR, in Scandinavia, 1981–1983. *J. Infect. Dis.,* 159:1111–1114.
50. Hackstadt, T. (1986): Antigenic variation in the phase I lipopolysaccharide of *Coxiella burnetii* isolates. *Infect. Immun.,* 52:337–340.
51. Hahn, D.L., Dodge, R.W., and Galubjatrikor, R. (1991): Association of *Chlamydia pneumoniae* (strain TWAR) infection with wheezing, asthmatic bronchitis and adult-onset asthma. *J.A.M.A.,* 266:225–230.
52. Hammers-Berggren, S., Gramath, F., Judander, I., and Kalin, M. (1991): Erythromycin for treatment of ornithosis. *Scand. J. Infect. Dis.,* 23(2):159–162.
53. Hammerschlag, M.R., Chigwin, K., Roblin, P.M., Gelling, M., Dumornay, W., Mandel, L., Smith, P., and Schacter, J. (1992): Persistent infection with *Chlamydia pneumoniae* following acute respiratory illness. *Clin. Infect. Dis.* 14:178–182.
54. Harding, H.B. (1970): The bacteria-like chlamydia of ornithosis and the diseases they cause. *CRC Crit. Rev. Clin. Lab. Sci.,* 1:451–469.
55. Harris, A.A., Pottage, J.C., Ressler, H.A., et al. (1984): Psittacosis bacteremia in a patient with sarcoidosis. *Ann. Intern. Med.,* 101:502.
56. Harrison, H.R., English, M.G., Lee, C.K., and Alexander, E.R. (1978): *Chlamydia trachomatis* infant pneumonitis—comparison with matched controls and other infant pneumonitis. *N. Engl. J. Med.,* 298:703–708.
57. Hernandez, L.A., Urquhard, G.E.D., and Dick, W.G. (1977): Mycoplasma infection and arthritis in man. *Br. Med. J.,* 2:14–16.
58. Hodges, G.R., Fass, R.J., and Saslaw, S. (1972): Central nervous system disease associated with *Mycoplasma pneumoniae* infection. *Arch. Intern. Med.,* 130:277–282.

59. Holland, S.M., Gaydos, C.A., and Quinn, T.C. (1990): Detection and differentiation of *Chlamydia trachomatis, Chlamydia psittaci,* and *Chlamydia pneumoniae* by DNA amplification. *J. Infect. Dis.,* 162:984–987.

60. Holt, S., Ryan, W.F., and Epstein, E.J. (1977): Severe *Mycoplasma pneumoniae. Thorax,* 32:112–115.

61. Jacobs, E., Rock, R., and Dalehite, L. (1990): A B cell–T cell–linked epitope located on the adhesion of *Mycoplasma pneumoniae. Infect. Immunol.,* 58(8):2464–2469.

62. Jastremski, M.S. (1979): Adult respiratory distress syndrome due to *Mycoplasma pneumoniae. Chest,* 75:529.

63. Kimbrough, R.C., Ormsbee, R.A., and Peacock, M. (1979): Q fever endocarditis in the United States. *Ann. Intern. Med.,* 91:400–402.

64. Kingston, J.R., Chanock, R.M., and Mufson, M.A. (1961): Eaton agent pneumonia. *J.A.M.A.,* 176:118–123.

65. Kleemola, M., Saikku, P., Visakorpi, R., Wang, S.P., and Grayston, J.T. (1988): Evaluation of pneumonia caused by TWAR: a new chlamydia organism in military trainees in Finland. *J. Infect. Dis.,* 157:230–236.

66. Kleemola, S.R., Karjahainen, J.E., and Raty, R.K. (1990): Rapid diagnosis of *Mycoplasma pneumoniae* infection: clinical evaluation of a commercial probe test. *J. Infect. Dis.,* 162(1): 70–75.

67. Kuo, C.C., Chi, E.Y., and Grayston, J.T. (1988): Ultrastructural study of entry of *Chlamydia* strain TWAR into HeLa cells. *Infect. Immunol.,* 56(6):1668–1672.

68. Kuo, C.C., Shor, A., Campbell, L.A., et al. (1993): Demonstration of *Chlamydia pneumoniae* in atherosclerotic lesions of coronary arteries. *J. Infect. Dis.,* 167:841–849.

69. Langley, J.M., Marrie, T.J., Covert, A., Wang, D.M., and Williams, J.C. (1988): Poker Players' Pneumonia: an urban outbreak of Q fever following exposure to a parturient cat. *N. Engl. J. Med.,* 319:354–356.

70. Lerer, R.J., and Kalavsky, S.M. (1973): Central nervous system disease associated with *Mycoplasma pneumoniae* infection: report of five cases and review of the literature. *Pediatrics* 52:658–668.

71. Levine, D.P., and Lerner, A.M. (1978): The clinical spectrum of *Mycoplasma pneumoniae* infections. *Med. Clin. No. Amer.,* 62:961–978.

72. Levison, D.A., Guthrie, W., Ward, C., Green, D.M., and Robertson, P.G.C. (1971): Infective endocarditis as part of psittacosis. *Lancet,* 2:844–846.

73. Lipsky, B.A., Tack, K.J., Kuo, C., Wang, S.P., and Grayston, J.T. (1990): Ofloxacin treatment of *Chlamydia pneumoniae* (strain TWAR) lower respiratory tract infections. *Am. J. Med.,* 89:722–724.

74. Lumio, J., Penttinen, K., and Petterson, T. (1981): Q fever in Finland: clinical, immunological and epidemiological findings. *Scand. J. Infect. Dis.,* 13:17–21.

75. Machlachlan, W.W.G., Crum, G.E., Kleinschmidt, R.E., and Wehrle, P.F. (1953): Psittacosis. *Am. J. Med. Sci.,* 226:157–163.

76. Madsen, R.D., Weiner, L.B., McMillan, J.A., Saeed, F.A., North, J.A., and Coates, S.R. (1988): Direct detection of *Mycoplasma pneumoniae* antigen in clinical specimens by a monoclonal antibody immunoblot assay. *Am. J. Clin. Pathol.,* 89(1):95–99.

77. Mann, J.S., Douglas, J.G., Inglis, J.M., and Leitsch, A.G. (1986): Q fever: person to person transmission within a family. *Thorax,* 41:974–975.

78. Marrie, T.J. (1990): *Coxiella burnetii.* In: *Principles and Practice of Infectious Diseases,* 3rd Edition, edited by G.L. Mandell and R.G. Douglas, pp. 1472–1476. Churchill Livingstone, New York.

79. Marrie, T.J., Grayston, J.T., Wang, S.P., and Kuo, C.C. (1987): Pneumonia associated with the TWAR strain of Chlamydia. *Ann. Intern. Med.,* 106:507–511.

80. Marrie, T.J., Schlech, W.F., III, Williams, J.C., and Yates, L. (1986): Q fever pneumonia associated with exposure to wild rabbits. *Lancet,* 1:427–429.

81. Meiklejohn, G., Reimer, L.G., Graves, P.S., and Helmick, C. (1981): Cryptic epidemic of Q fever in a medical school. *J. Infect. Dis.,* 144:107–113.

82. Meyer, K.F. (1942): The ecology of psittacosis and ornithosis. *Medicine,* 21:175–206.

83. Millar, J.K. (1978): The chest film findings in "Q" fever—a series of 35 cases. *Clin. Radiol.,* 29:371–375.

84. Mizutani, H., and Mizutani, H. (1986): Immunoglobulin rheumatoid factor in patients with mycoplasmal pneumoniae. *Am. Rev. Respir. Dis.,* 134(6);1237–1240.

85. Morgan, H.R., and Bader, J.P. (1957): Latent viral infection of cells in tissue culture. IV. Latent infection of cells with psittacosis virus. *J. Exp. Med.,* 106:39.

86. Mufson, M.A., Manko, M.A., Kingston, J.R., and Chanock, R.M. (1961): Eaton agent pneumonia: clinical features: *J.A.M.A.,* 178:369.

87. Murray, H.W., Masur, H., Senterfit, L.B., and Roberts, R.B. (1975): The protean manifestation of *Mycoplasma pneumoniae* infections in adults. *Am. J. Med.,* 58:229–242.

88. Murray, H.W., and Tuazon, C.U. (1980): Atypical pneumonias. *Med. Clin. No. Amer.,* 64:507.
89. Naftalin, J.M., Wellisch, G., Kahana, Z., and Diengott, D. (1974): Mycoplasma septicemia. *J.A.M.A.,* 228:565.
90. Nakao, T., Orii, T., and Umetsu, M. (1971): *Mycoplasma pneumoniae* pneumonia with pleural effusion with special reference to isolation of *Mycoplasma pneumoniae* from pleural fluid. *Tohoku J. Exp. Med.,* 104:13–18.
91. Noriega, E.R., Simberkoff, M.S., Gilroy, F.J., et al. (1974): Life-threatening *Mycoplasma pneumoniae* pneumonia. *J.A.M.A.,* 229:1471–1472.
92. Olson, B.J., and Truling, W.L. (1944): An epidemic of severe pneumonitis in the Bayou region of Louisiana. Public Health Report. *J. Epidemiol. Study.,* 59:1299–1311.
93. Ormsbee, R.A. (1965): Q fever rickettsia. In: *Viral and Rickettsial Infection of Man,* 4th Edition, edited by F.L. Horsfall and E.I. Tamm, Chapter 52. J.B. Lippincott, Philadelphia.
94. Page, S.R., Stewart, J.T., and Bernstein, J.J. (1988): A progressive pericardial effusion caused by psittacosis. *Br. Heart J.,* 60:87.
95. Peter, O., Dubruis, G., Burgdorfer, W., and Peacock, M. (1985): Evaluation of the complement fixation and indirect immunofluorescence tests in the early diagnosis of primary Q fever. *Eur. J. Clin. Microbiol.,* 4:394–396.
96. Pinsky, R.L., Fishbein, D.B., Greene, C.R., and Gensheimer, K.F. (1991): An outbreak of cat-associated Q Fever in the United States. *J.Infect. Dis.,* 164:202–204.
97. Polayes, S.H., and Lederer, M. (1932): Psittacosis with results of postmortem examination in a case including studies of the spinal cord. *Arch. Intern. Med.,* 49:253–269.
98. Puolakkainen, M., Saikku, P., Leinonen, M., Nurminen, M., Vaananen, and Makela, P.H. (1984): Chlamydial pneumonitis and its serodiagnosis in infants. *J. Infect. Dis.,* 149:598–604.
99. Rasch, J.R., and Mogabgab, W.J. (1965): Therapeutic effect of erythromycin on *Mycoplasma pneumoniae* pneumonia. *Antimicrob. Agents Chemother.,* 5:683–699.
100. Rifkind, D., Chanock, R., Kravetz, H., Johnson, K., and Knight, V. (1962): Ear involvement (myringitis) and primary atypical pneumonia following inoculation of volunteers with Eaton's agent. *Am. Rev. Respir. Dis.,* 85:479–489.
101. Ruppanner, R., Brooks, D., Franti, C.E., Behymer, D.E., Morrish, D., and Spinelli, J. (1982): Q fever hazards from sheep and goats used in research. *Arch. Environ. Health,* 37:103–110.
102. Saikku, P., Leinonen, M., Tenkanen, L., et al. (1992): Chronic *Chlamydia pneumoniae* infection as a risk factor for coronary heart disease in the Helsinki Heart Study. *Ann. Intern. Med.,* 116:273–278.
103. Saikku, P., Ruutu, P., Leinonen, M., et al. (1988): Acute lower respiratory tract infection associated with chlamydial TWAR antibody in Filipino children. *J. Infect. Dis.,* 158:1095–1097.
104. Saikku, P., Wang, S.P., Kleemola, M., Brandes, E., Rusasen, E., et al. (1985): An epidemic of mild pneumonia due to an unusual strain of *Chlamydia psittaci. J. Infect. Dis.,* 151:832–839.
105. Salmon, M.M., Howells, B., Glencross. E.J.G., Evans, A.D., and Palmer, S.R. (1982): Q fever in an urban area. *Lancet,* 1:1002–1004.
106. Samuel, J.E., Frazier, M.E., Kahn, M.L., Thomashow, L.S., and Mallavia, L.P. (1983): Isolation and characterization of plasmid from phase 1 *Coxiella burnetti. Infect Immunol.,* 41:488–493.
107. Samuel, J.E., Frazier, M.E., and Mallavia, L.P. (1985): Correlation of plasmid type and disease caused by *Coxiella burnetii. Infect. Immunol.,* 49:775–779.
108. Sands, M.J., Satz, J.E., Turner, W.E., and Soloff, L.A. (1977): Pericarditis and myopericarditis associated with active *Mycoplasma pneumoniae* infection. *Ann. Intern. Med.,* 86:544–548.
109. Sawyer, L.A., Fishbein, D.B., and McDade, J.E. Q fever: current concepts. *Rev. Infect. Dis.,* 9:935–946.
110. Schachter, J. (1978): Chlamydial infections. *N. Engl. J. Med.,* 298:428–435.
111. Schacter, J. (1986): *Chlamydia psittaci:* "reemergence" of a forgotten pathogen. *N. Engl. J. Med.,* 315:189.
112. Schacter, J., Sugg, N., and Sung, M. (1978): Psittacosis: the reservoir persists. *J. Infect. Dis.,* 137:44–49.
113. Schacter, J., Sung, M., and Meyer, K.F. (1971): Potential danger of Q fever in a university hospital environment. *J. Infect. Dis.,* 123:301–304.
114. Schaffner, W. (1990): *Chlamydia psittaci* (psittacosis). In: *Principles and Practice of Infectious Diseases,* 3rd Edition, edited by G.L. Mandell, R.G. Douglas, and J.E. Bennett, p. 1440. Churchill Livingstone, New York.
115. Schaffner, W. (1990): TWAR. In: *Principles and Practice of Infectious Diseases,* 3rd Edition, edited by G.L. Mandell, R.G. Douglas, and J.E. Bennett, pp. 1443–1444. Churchill Livingstone, New York.
116. Schaffner, W., Drutz, D.J., Duncan, G.W., and Koenig, M.G. (1967): The clinical spectrum of endemic psittacosis. *Arch. Intern. Med.,* 119:433–443.
117. Schonwald, S., Gunjaca, M., Kolaony-Babio, L., Car, V., and Gosev, M. (1990): Comparison of azithromycin and erythromycin in the treatment of atypical pneumonias. *J. Antimicrob. Chemother.,* 25(Suppl. A):123–126.

118. Seggev, J.S., Lis, I., Siman-Tov, R., Gutman, R., Abu Samara, H., Schey, G., and Naot, Y. (1986): *Mycoplasma pneumoniae* is a frequent cause of exacerbation of bronchial asthma in adults. *Ann. Allergy*, 57(4):263–265.

119. Shames, J.M., George, R.B., Holliday, W.B., Rasch, J.R., and Mogabgoab, W.J. (1970): Comparison of antibiotics in the treatment of mycoplasmal pneumonia. *Arch. Intern. Med.*, 125:680–684.

120. Siebert, R.H., Jordan, W.S., and Dingle, J.H. (1956): Clinical variations in the diagnosis of psittacosis. *N. Engl. J. Med.*, 254:928–930.

121. Slotkin, R.I., Clyde, W.A., and Denny, F.W. (1967): The effects of antibiotics on *Mycoplasma pneumoniae in vitro* and *in vivo*. *Am. J. Epidemiol.*, 86:225–237.

122. Solanki, D.L., and Bordoff, R.L. (1979): Severe mycoplasma pneumonia with pleural effusions in a patient with sickle cell-hemaglobin C (SC) disease. *Am. J. Med.*, 66:707–710.

123. Spelman, D.W. (1982): Q fever: a study of 111 consecutive cases. *Med. J. Aust.*, 1:547–553.

124. Srigley, J.R., Velland, H., Palmer, N., Phillips, M.J., Geddie, W.R., Van Nostrand, A.W.P., and Edwards, V.D. (1985): Q fever: the liver and bone marrow pathology. *Am. J. Surg. Pathol.*, 9:752–758.

125. Thom, D.H., Grayston, J.T., Siscovick, D.S., Wang, S.P., Weiss, N.S., and Daling, J.R. (1992): Association of prior infection with *Chlamydia pneumoniae* and angiographically demonstrated coronary artery disease. *J.A.M.A.*, 268:68–72.

126. Thomas, M., Jones, M., and Ray, S. (1975): *Mycoplasma pneumoniae* in a tubo-ovarian abscess. *Lancet*, 2:774–775.

127. Tigertt, W.D., Benenson, A.S., and Gochenaur, W.S. (1961): Airborne Q fever. *Bacteriol. Rev.*, 25:285–293.

128. Tilton, R.C., Dias, F., Kidd, H., and Ryan, R.W. (1988): DNA probe versus culture for detection of *Mycoplasma pneumoniae* in clinical specimens. *Diag. Microbiol. Infect. Dis.*, 10(2):109–112.

129. Tobin, M.J., Cahill, N., Gearty, G., Maurer, B., Blake, S., Dealy, K., and Hone, R. (1982): Q fever endocarditis. *Am. J. Med.*, 72:396–400.

130. Tully, J.C., Whitcomb, R.F., Clark, H.F., and Williamson, D.L. (1977): Pathogenic mycoplasmas: cultivation and vertebrate pathogenicity of a new spiroplasma. *Science*, 195:892–894.

131. Vosti, G.J., and Roffward, H. (1961): Myocarditis and encephalitis in a case of unsuspected psittacosis. *Ann. Intern. Med.*, 54:764–776.

132. Ward, C., and Ward, A.M. (1974): Acquired valvular heart disease in patients who keep pet birds. *Lancet*, 2:734–736.

133. Welsh, L.A., Gaydos, C.A., and Quinn, T.C. (1992): *In vitro* evaluation of activities of azithromycin, erythromycin and tetracycline against *Chlamydia trachomatis* and *Chlamydia pneumoniae*. *Antimicrob. Agents Chemother.*, 36:291–294.,

134. Wenzel, R.P., Hendley, J.O., Dodd, W.K., and Gwaltney, J.M. (1976): Comparison of josamycin and erythromycin in the therapy of *Mycoplasma pneumoniae*. *Antimicrob Agents Chemother.*, 10:899–901.

135. Wiernik, A., Jarstrand, C., and Tunevall, G. (1978): The value of immunoelectroosmophoresis (IEOP) for etiologic diagnosis of acute respiratory tract infections due to pneumococci and *Mycoplasma pneumoniae*. *Scand. J. Infect. Dis.*, 10:173–197.

136. Yang, Z.P., Kuo, C.C., and Grayston, J.T. (1993): A mouse model of *Chlamydia pneumoniae* strain TWAR pneumonitis. *Infect. Immunol.*, 61:2037–2040.

137. Yeaman, M.R., Roman, M.J., and Baca, O.G. (1989): Antibiotic susceptibilities of two *Coxiella burnetii* isolates implicated in distinct clinical syndromes. *Infect. Immunol.*, 37:1052–1057.

138. Yow, E.M., Brennan, J.C., Preston, J., and Levy, S. (1959): The pathology of psittacosis. *Am. J. Med.*, 27:739–749.

139. Yung, A.P., and Grayson, M.L. (1988): Psittacosis: a review of 135 cases. *Med. J. Aust.*, 148:228–233.

Respiratory Infections: Diagnosis and Management, 3d ed.,
edited by James E. Pennington.
Raven Press, Ltd., New York © 1994

21

Hemophilus influenzae Pneumonia

Arnold L. Smith

*Department of Pediatrics, University of Washington and Children's Hospital and
Medical Center, 4800 Sand Point Way N.E., Seattle, Washington, 98105*

Longitudinal studies of children (32,39) demonstrate a progressive and ultimately near-ubiquitous acquisition of *Hemophilus influenzae* in the nose or throat. By 5 years of age, 90% of all children harbor the organism; with selective isolation techniques, the prevalence could be even higher. In pediatric studies, 95% (or more) of these strains are unencapsulated (2,51,89). During epidemics of viral respiratory tract disease, the rate of isolation appears to increase, and in one study the proportion that are capsulated increased (51). This phenomenon was probably responsible for Pfeiffer erroneously concluding that the influenzae syndrome was due to this bacterium, hence the designation "influenzae bacillus."

The same problem, verifying that *H. influenzae* is the etiologic agent in a patient with pneumonia, is present today. Sputum easily becomes contaminated with *H. influenzae* during expectoration (42,44); bacteremia is uncommon, and invasive diagnostic procedures are rarely performed. Cases clearly identified as caused by *H. influenzae* are considered here; the organism was isolated from blood, pleural fluid, or lung tissue. Cases in which it was the sole organism isolated from microscopically purulent sputum, or was present in densities exceeding 10^5 bacteria per ml, are also included. On the basis of data tabulated from such cases and knowledge of the biology of the organism, a clinical diagnosis can be made with certainty.

CULTURE AND MORPHOLOGY

T.M. Rivers, in classifying the organisms isolated from the lungs of individuals dying during the 1918 influenzae pandemic, identified one genera as blood-loving. With that observation, and noting that two factors present in blood were necessary for growth (77), Pfeiffer's bacillus was named *H. influenzae* (55,95). Current criteria require that the organism be gram-negative and have an absolute requirement for "X factor" (heme, i.e., protoporphyrin IX with iron) for aerobic growth and "V factor" β-nicotinamide adenine dinucleotide (NAD^+) (81). The organism is pleomorphic when infected cerebrospinal fluid (CSF) is examined, but strains cultured in the laboratory show only coccobacillary forms on gram stain. Pathogenic isolates will grow on many readily available media (e.g., trypticase soy, Mueller-Hinton, chocolate blood agar, Levinthal, brain heart infusion) provided that heme and NAD^+ are supplied; 10 µg/ml of each usually ensures growth. It is a facultative anaerobe, and growth in that environment does not require added heme; bacterial division is stimulated by carbon dioxide. The organism will grow at temperatures between 35 and 40°C, appearing as small, gray colonies on most media.

Encapsulated strains can be recognized on clear media by their iridescence in oblique natural or ultraviolet light. There are six encapsulated types (designated a through f), but 95% of all invasive infections (such as bacteremia) are caused by type b. The type b capsule is unique, as it is a pentose polymer of ribose linked to ribitol through 3'–5' phosphodiester bonds. All other capsules are hexose polymers. Type f, the third most prevalent isolate from the nasopharynx and the least common isolated from children's CSF, is the second most common cause of bacteremic *H. influenzae* pneumonia in adults (70). Type d, also a rare meningeal pathogen, has also been isolated from adults with bacteremic pneumonia (29).

VIRULENCE

Role of Capsule

All *H. influenzae* strains are potentially pathogenic; that is, they possess the capacity to cause disease. However, in most individuals with functional host defenses, only capsulated strains have the capacity to cause bacteremia and metastatic tissue infections. Thus, strains isolated from blood, CSF, tissue aspirates, or abscesses of children are invariably capsulated. Inoculation of a single type b organism (intraperitoneally) into a young adult rat will lead to bacteremia, which will be sustained for several days at the density of 10^3 cfu/ml. In contrast, an identical intraperitoneal inoculation of 10^8 unencapsulated (or rough, on the basis of colonial morphology) organisms produces only a transitory (4 hr) bacteremia (94). Other routes of inoculation (intranasal, subcutaneous, intravenous) also indicate that the capsulated organisms evade bacterial clearance mechanisms, making them more virulent. In immunocompetent children an infection with an unencapsulated (and therefore untypeable) *H. influenzae* is always a mucosal surface infection (otitis media, sinusitis, bronchitis). The occurrence of bacteremic *H. influenzae* pneumonia with unencapsulated strains in adults suggests an age-related loss of immunity to this usually commensal organism. Capsulation is thought to promote "virulence" by resisting clearance by fixed macrophages; it is clear, however, that other bacterial surface structures are also necessary for systemic infection (65).

Immunity

Because of the striking age-dependent susceptibility of children to invasive *H. influenzae* infection (most commonly, meningitis), the blood of infants has been repeatedly compared with that of adults (in whom the disease is extremely rare) to identify the basis of "natural immunity." One factor possessed by most adults and absent in most susceptible children is anticapsular antibody; serum from a normal adult has an average of 358 ng/ml (range 192 to 666), whereas children in the age group with the highest attack rate (5 to 12 months) have an average of 14 ng/ml (range 7 to 26). Anticapsular antibody is opsonic and, under certain assay conditions, bactericidal. Anticapsular antibodies protect against *H. influenzae* type b bacteremia by promoting bacterial clearance through phagocytosis by fixed macrophages of the reticuloendothelial system. Current vaccines administered to children are conjugates of the type b capsule with various proteins. These proteins, which include tetanus toxoid, diphtheria toxoid, an inactive mutant diphtheria toxin, and the major outer membrane proteins from group B meningococcus, make the carbohydrate capsule T-cell dependent and immunogenic in young infants. Since the introduction of conjugate vaccines which evoke antibodies against *H. influenzae,* the incidence of the most common form of invasive disease, meningitis, has decreased dramatically. The antibody evoked by the conjugate vaccine is IgG and would be expected to function in the alveoli. Thus, the incidence of bacteremic *H. influenzae* pneumonia in infants is also expected to decrease (71).

The sera of adults with chronic bronchitis usually contain precipitins against *H. influenzae.* These antibodies protect against a lethal inoculum of capsulated organisms and promote reticuloendothelial clearance of both type b and unencapsulated organisms in model infections (94). These antibodies, when present, are in higher concentration than those directed against the capsule and are directed against six immunologically distinct somatic antigens (85). An increase in precipitin titer occurs with an exacerbation of chronic obstructive pulmonary disease associated with the isolation of *H. influenzae* from sputum (85). The role of these antibodies in protection against invasive human disease is unknown.

PATHOGENESIS

H. influenzae pneumonia represents a failure of host defense. A natural (as in children) or acquired deficiency of immunity to capsulated strains leads to tissue invasion; this form of illness is accompanied by a high frequency of bacteremia and metastatic infections. Failure of local pulmonary defense (as in pneumoconiosis, diabetes mellitus, alcoholism) leads to bronchopneumonia with noncapsulated strains in which bacteremia is rare and secondary foci even rarer.

In all experimental studies of pneumonia, an implicit assumption is that bacteria reach the lower respiratory tract from the upper airway. Thus, organisms are introduced through endotracheal tubes, or inoculated transtracheally. Experimental pneumonia has been induced in mice by direct intratracheal inoculation (16). Once bacteria enter alveoli an acute inflammatory response occurs; polymorphonuclear leukocytes fill the airspaces, the capillaries are congested, and the alveolar septa contain mononuclear cells. With most bacteria (staphylococci are probably an exception) the damage to the lung is superficial, limited to focal degeneration of alveolar epithelium and capillary endothelium (56,96).

In humans, *H. influenzae* presumably gain access to the alveoli at a time when the cough mechanism is inoperative, and in sufficient numbers to divide at a rate greater than local clearance mechanisms. Pulmonary parenchyma invasion is most often recognized in the portion of the lung that is most dependent during sleep: the right lower, right middle, and left lower lobe in adults; and the right upper and right middle lobe in infants. If opsonizing IgG is absent, the type b strains are not phagocytosed by alveolar macrophages (26). Untypeable strains do not appear to need specific antibody to be phagocytosed; therefore, their mechanism of evading host defenses in adults is unclear. Both capsulated type b and unencapsulated strains are cleared from the lungs of mice by polymorphonuclear leukocyte recruitment (83). In adults, local bacterial growth "spills" into adjacent alveoli through the pores of Kohn and the canals of Lambert (76). In infants, these collateral pathways are less well developed, leading to more collapse but a smaller magnitude of involvement of lung parenchyma.

In adults with chronic surface infection of their lower respiratory tract, an increase in bacterial replication or lapse of local alveolar defense would permit pneumonia to occur (27). Preceding viral infection increases the density of colonization of the upper airway with gram-negative bacilli (60); it is not known whether this is also true with *H. influenzae*. In animal models, antecedent infection with parainfluenzae virus increases susceptibility to *H. influenzae* pneumonia by decreasing ciliary clearance (12). This observation could explain, in part, the basis for the "common cold" progressing to pneumonia.

ANTIBIOTIC RESISTANCE

H. influenzae is unique in several aspects of antibiotic resistance. Streptomycin resistance occurs by chromosomal mutation at high frequency. When streptomycin was used alone for treatment of meningitis, 50% of the patients had a bacteriologic relapse with streptomycin-resistant strains. Once a strain is streptomycin-resistant, the property remains stable, is readily passed to progeny, and can be introduced into susceptible strains by transformation with chromosomal DNA.

Ampicillin resistance was not detected until the drug had been used for 9 years for both minor (otitis media) and life-threatening *H. influenzae* infections (meningitis). A TEM β-lactamase produced by these strains is immunologically identical to the enzyme-produced *E. coli;* and, not surprisingly, the DNA segment encoding for the enzyme (a transposon, TnA) is virtually homologous with plasmid DNA encoding for β-lactamase commonly found in enteric gram-negative bacilli. Production of this enzyme is responsible for more than 95% of the ampicillin resistance in enteric gram-negative bacilli, yet up to 10% of ampicillin-resistant *H. influenzae* do not have detectable β-lactamase. The national prevalence of ampicillin resistance in *H. influenzae* in 1986 was 30%: regional variation is great—as high as 55% in Washington, D.C., but only 5% in Omaha, Nebraska. A recent multicenter national study of the antibiotic susceptibility of *H. influenzae* isolated from adults older than 50 years found that 16.5% were resistant to ampicillin and amoxicillin, 2.1% to tetracycline, 0.7% to trimethoprim-sulfamethoxazole, 1.1% to cefaclor, and 0.2% to cefuroxime and the combination amoxicillin-clavulanate (36). Importantly, the incidence of β-lactamase production was lowest in nontypeable strains (15%), those most commonly causing pneumonia in adults. Ampicillin resistance is associated with failure of that agent in the treatment of meningitis, but is of uncertain importance in the treatment of pneumonia.

Chloramphenicol resistance occurs in *H. influenzae*. Like ampicillin resistance, it is primarily plasmid-mediated; the transposon encodes for the production of chloramphenicol acetyltransferase. This enzyme inactivates the antibiotic through acetylation of the essential 3′ hydroxyl group. Similar to ampicillin resistance, there is the existence of nonenzymatic, chromosomally mediated chloramphenicol resistance. A little-recognized feature of the chloramphenicol-resistant isolates is that 90% are also tetracycline-resistant (68); tetracycline is often used for *Hemophilus* bronchial infections. Trimethoprim (TMP) resistance is chromosomally mediated, but its exact prevalence is unknown. Rich media required for the isolation of *H. influenzae* antagonizes the bioactivity of TMP, falsely identifying the strains as susceptible.

A shortcoming of all of the surveys of antibiotic resistance is that they have almost exclusively examined pediatric isolates, and almost exclusively capsulated organisms. The significance of antibiotic resistance in pneumonia was thought to be less important than in sepsis and meningitis. "Inappropriate" antibiotics are often efficacious in *H. influenzae* pneumonia for reasons that are not clear. However, the capacity of the organism to evolve a variety of resistance mechanisms portends a dismal future for new antibacterial agents active against *Hemophilus*.

PNEUMONIA IN CHILDREN

Clinical Features

The true incidence of *H. influenzae* pneumonia in children is only estimated (58). More seriously ill children are more likely to undergo invasive diagnostic tests that unequivocally establish the diagnosis: blood culture, pleural fluid culture, or culture of lung aspirate. Even when these procedures are performed, the cultivation conditions might not be optimal for *H. influenzae*. Ravitch and Fein (61) found that 6.4% of the cases of empyema (complicating pneumonia) in 1944 were due to *H. influenzae*, but none were found in subsequent years. In a Chilean study of pediatric pneumonia 2.2% of lung punctures yielded *H. influenzae* (21,52). A seasonal distribution has not been noted. In fact, Jacobs and Harris (33) noted that only 4 of 34 children with *H. influenzae* pneumonia had an antecedent clinical syndrome consistent with a viral lower respiratory tract disease, militating against the concept (75) that this bacterium is a secondary invader.

The median age of a child with *H. influenzae* is 11 months; the range is 2 days through adolescence, and the overall male to female ratio is 1.5 : 1. Table 21-1 depicts the age-specific attack rate in intervals.

Diagnosis

In contrast to the Jacobs and Harris study (33), in virtually every reported case of *H. influenza* pneumonia, coryza preceded the symptoms. Its duration is from 5 to 21 days and is associated with low-grade (38°C) fever without systemic signs or symptoms. This "cold" insidiously worsens with the onset of cough, higher daily temperatures, and increasing subjective systemic complaints (anorexia, malaise, fussiness). Usually the failure to improve and the recognition of tachypnea prompts medical evaluation. In one-third of cases, the transition from "a URI" to pneumonia will be abrupt, with pleuritic chest pain, productive cough, and rigors. Ten percent have a chronic course, often with symptoms of cough for 3 or more weeks before diagnosis. The temperature at diagnosis, degree of leukocytosis, and clinical presentation is surprisingly variable. Infants can be dyspneic with minimal fever and leukocytosis and have a segmental or lobar infiltrate on chest radiograph. The diagnosis will be apparent only if appropriate diagnostic procedures are pursued: blood culture, antigen detection, and examination of pleural fluid if indicated. Table 21-2 depicts the distribution of patients by course, the temperature on admission, and initial

TABLE 21–1. *Age-specific attack rate of* H. influenzae *pneumonia*

Age	Percent of total	
0–6 months	11	
6–12 months	28	
18–24 months	11	
2–4 years	13	
4–6 years	7	
6–8 years	7	
8–10 years	1	
10–12 years	0.5	
12–14 years	0.5	
>14 years	1.0[a]	(2.3 cases/10,000 VA admissions)

[a]The annual incidence of *H. influenzae* pneumonia in adults in Sweden was found to be 1.1 cases/100,000 population. (Tabulated from references 3, 4, 5, 11, 19, 21, 31, 34, 49, 54, 57, 73, 82, and 88.)

granulocyte count. The reported range of total leukocyte count on admission was 5,000 to 42,000 leukocytes/μl; the mean percentage of granulocytes, including immature forms, is 75%. The magnitude of the granulocytosis is not of prognostic significance and does not correlate with rapidity of onset or the degree of pulmonary parenchymal involvement. In contrast, virtually all children who were admitted with granulocytopenia (defined as <2,000 cells/μl) had a fatal outcome.

Bacteriology

Unequivocal diagnosis is established by the isolation of *H. influenzae* from blood, pleural fluid, or lung parenchyma. Identification of *H. influenzae* in the sputum alone is of little value because of the ubiquity of commensal carriage in the throat and nasopharynx (2,51). If a sputum isolate from a child with pneumonia is type b, then

TABLE 21–2. *Patient distribution as to pace of illness, admission temperature, and admission granulocyte count for children with pneumonia*

Course	Percent of total
Acute	32
Subacute	57
Chronic	11
Temperature (°F)	
≤99	5
100–101	23
101–103	61
≥103	11
Granulocytes/μl × 10³	
>25	3
18–25	29
12–18	59
8–12	7
<8	2

Tabulated from references 3, 4, 5, 6, 13, 21, 31, 34, 54, 62, 74, 82, and 88.

it can be considered suggestive evidence of pneumonia due to *H. influenzae,* as the carriage rate in infants is 0.5 to 5.0%. Isolation rates by anatomic location in children ultimately proven to have *H. influenzae* pneumonia are depicted in Table 21-3.

Antigen Detection

A useful adjunct to the diagnosis of *H. influenzae* pneumonia is the detection of type b capsular polysaccharide in serum or fluid from the infectious focus. The key factor in the reliability of antigen detection is the reagent antibody. All commercially available reagents contain serum that has been harvested after immunization of animals with formalinized whole type b organisms. Because most invasive pediatric infections are due to capsular type b, the antisera used should be high in titer to type b capsular carbohydrate. A serious limitation of this approach is the variability in titer, degree of contamination with other cross-reacting antibodies, and specificity of the reagent antibody. Methods of detecting type b capsular antigen include immunoelectrophoresis (CIE) (87), latex particle agglutination LPA (93), coagglutination of staphylococci bound to antibody (CoA), and enzyme-linked immunosorbent assay (ELISA); only the former two have been used in the diagnosis of pneumonia. In the available studies other diagnostic procedures were not always performed, precluding calculation of the accuracy of the method. LPA will detect as little as 7 ng of capsular polysaccharide in 1 ml of serum, whereas the sensitivity of CIE is approximately tenfold lower. Use of the LPA method to diagnose type b pneumonia by testing serum has an accuracy and specificity exceeding 90% (1). Urine is also a reliable source of type b antigen, provided care is taken to exclude other compounds which will agglutinate the particles (50). Pleural fluid obtained from children with *H. influenzae* pneumonia contains approximately 800 ng/ml, whereas serum from the same patients contains (on average) 20 ng of the capsular carbohydrate (23,93). Antigenic capsular carbohydrate can be detected with LPA if the sample is first deproteinized to remove those serum proteins that cause nonspecific agglutination. This can be easily accomplished by boiling the sample for 3–5 min; low-speed centrifugation will permit recovery of supernatant which contains the heat-stable carbohydrate. This same manipulation can be applied to urine, serum, or pleural fluid. With a less-sensitive technique (i.e., detecting concentrations >50 ng/ml), only one of five children with bacteremic *H. influenzae* pneumonia had detectable anigenemia (30,87). Eventually the use of specific monoclonal antibodies will place antigen detection (including noncapsular bacterial components) on a surer footing for diagnostic purposes.

TABLE 21–3. *Rate of isolation of* H. influenzae *from various anatomic locations from children with pneumonia*

Source of specimen	Percent
Blood	93
Pleural fluid	50
Lung abscess	100
Lung aspirate	100

Tabulated from references 3, 4, 5, 11, 19, 21, 31, 34, 37, 54, 62, 73, 82, and 88. In certain patients, the organism was cultured from more than one location.

Radiographic Appearance

There is only one consistent radiographic finding: early pleural reaction/effusion. It is noted in 50% of the reported cases, but when specifically sought, it is present in every case (Fig. 21-1). Often, after an effusion is obvious, the early increase in density of the pleural line will be noted retrospectively. The frequencies of specific radiographic findings are depicted in Table 21-4.

Typically, the radiograph is interpreted as being consistent with (segmental) pneumonococcal pneumonia. In infants younger than 9 months old, probably because they are recumbent, the infiltrate is usually in the right upper lobe. Pneumatoceles have not been reported, but abscess is not infrequently recognized.

Treatment

Increasing severity of disease (i.e., greater anatomic involvement and increasing oxygen requirement) often occurs when treatment is with an antibiotic to which *H. influenzae* is resistant *in vitro*. Most commonly, an ampicillin-resistant organism is isolated and ampicillin (at a daily dose of 200 to 400 mg/kg) is being administered (66,73). This response is not unexpected. Surprisingly, however, there is often prompt improvement (by objective criteria) even though an antibiotic that is not

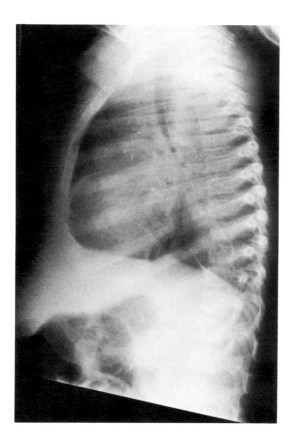

FIG. 21–1. An upright lateral radiograph of a 14-month-old male in which bilateral pleural effusion is apparent. A spine film revealed a minimal left upper lobe infiltrate.

TABLE 21–4. *Radiographic appearance in* H. influenzae *pneumonia in children*

Appearance	Percent
Segmental infiltrate	62
Lobar pneumonia	28
Bilateral lobular pneumonia	5
Diffuse bronchopneumonia	4
Interstitial pneumonia	1

Summarized from references 3, 23, 31, 82, 88, and 89.

thought of as efficacious for *H. influenzae* disease is being administered, for example, erythromycin. Most commonly, penicillin G (in various formulations) is administered for clinical "pneumococcal pneumonia"; 24 hours later, after defervescence and marked improvement, *H. influenzae* can be recovered from a pretreatment blood culture. Twenty-five percent of the reported pediatric cases have been treated effectively with penicillin G, an antibiotic uniformly ineffective in *H. influenzae* meningitis. In addition to penicillin G, methicillin, sulfonamides, erythromycin, and streptomycin have been used successfully for single-drug treatment of *H. influenzae* pneumonia. The reason for the apparent efficacy of these agents in *H. influenzae* pneumonia, in contrast with their failure in meningitis, osteomyelitis, septic arthritis, and so forth, is unknown. In spite of the apparent "ease" with which *H. influenzae* can be treated with a variety of antibiotics, drug choice should be based on the susceptibility of the recovered organism. Secondary infectious foci (most commonly, meningitis) occur in approximately 5% of the cases: it would be tragic to effectively treat pneumonia and have the infant suffer the sequelae of meningitis.

Parenteral antibiotics are usually administered for 7 to 10 days for type b *H. influenzae* pneumonia. The rationale for this approach recognizes the high frequency of bacteremia and the desire to eradicate organisms in silent, distant foci. In uncomplicated cases, the average duration of fever is 3.5 days, but the chest radiograph is abnormal for 7 to 44 days (3,4,31,82,88).

Supportive therapy (such as oxygen administration, intravenous fluids, and chest physical therapy) appears less important than in other pediatric pneumonias. Studies critically examining the importance of supportive treatment relative to specific antibiotic therapy are not available. The best approach uses supportive treatment for the patient who is tachypneic and fatigued.

The reported fatality rate is 5%; of these, 90% have multisystem disease, usually meningitis or epiglottitis. In these cases, the exact role of pneumonia in causing death is not clear (3,4,31).

PNEUMONIA IN ADULTS

Two studies have estimated the incidence of *H. influenzae* pneumonia (78,80). In three years in Finland there were seven cases of type b pneumonia; these comprised 23% of all the cases of invasive disease whose overall rate was 0.22 per 100,000 population. This prevalence was lower than that found with active surveillance in San Francisco where the overall incidence of invasive disease was 2.8 per 100,000 population, with 23% of the cases having pneumonia. In a Veterans Administration Hospital, there were eight cases of bacteremic disease over a 5-year period ending in 1974 (24,700 admissions) (46). Serial tabulations of the incidence of *H. influenzae*

pneumonia in adults are not available; it is being reported more often in the literature. Whether this is increased recognition, better culture techniques, or a true increase in incidence in disease is unknown. In all the reported cases of bacteremic
H. influenzae pneumonia, the male : female ratio was 1 : 1; if known, immunosuppressed non-HIV-infected patients are excluded from the tabulation, and the
male : female ratio becomes 1 : 3. When HIV-infected individuals are considered,
the demographics of *H. influenzae* pneumonia reflects that of HIV infection: two-
thirds are males. HIV-infected patients most commonly have *H. influenzae* bacteremia (two-thirds), with approximately 25% having pneumonia (7). At the Veterans
Administration Hospital in Seattle, Washington, *H. influenzae* pneumonia was diagnosed 15 times between June 1975 and October 1982; 11 of these cases were recognized in the last 22 months of surveillance. One-half were bacteremic, and one-
half of those were nontypeable. Only one of the 15 was ampicillin-resistant (personal
communication, Dr. J. Plorde). The bronchopneumonia form is by far the most commonly diagnosed *H. influenzae* pneumonia and is most common in patients with
chronic obstructive pulmonary disease (Table 21-5).

Relationship to Chronic Bronchitis

As noted, adults with chronic bronchitis are at increased risk for *H. influenzae*
pneumonia. In certain populations, *H. influenzae* is the bacterium present in the
sputum in greatest density (72,45). The presence of high densities of *H. influenzae*
evokes a local IgA response as well as a systemic IgG response (24). In spite of the
intense immune response to *Hemophilus* antigens, bacteria persist. This suggests a
defect in bacterial clearance mechanisms, even though there is some antigenic drift
in the immunodominant epitopes of two major outer membrane proteins: P2, ~40
kDa and P5, ~38 kDa (25). Because some patients with chronic bronchitis develop
bacteremic *H. influenzae* pneumonia, and improvement occurs when antimicrobial
therapy is directed against *H. influenzae,* the same organism that colonizes the respiratory tract is thought to cause the pneumonia. Oral immunization with killed *H.
influenzae,* which appears to recruit mucosal cellular immunity, decreases the incidence of exacerbations of bronchitis but has no effect on the incidence of pneumonia
(8,45).

TABLE 21–5. *Clinical features of* H. influenzae *pneumonia in adults*

	Type of pneumonia	
	Segmental (%)	Bronchopneumonia (%)
Male : female ratio	2:1	5:1
Bacteremia	72	28
Type b isolated	65	24
COPD[a]	37	73
Metastatic infections	54	15
Alcoholism	50	50
Underlying disease[a]	85	85
Pleural reaction	66	17

[a]Most commonly a malignancy; however, certain patients also had COPD.

Clinical Features

Assuming that immunity to type b organisms is mediated by IgG that is functional in the alveoli, adults with humoral immune deficiency would be predicted to have the "pediatric form" of pneumonia, that is, segmental or lobar involvement with bacteremia. Adults with local host defense dysfunction, but with intact humoral immunity, would be more likely to have bronchopneumonia. Clinical observations tend to confirm these predictions.

The patient with segmental lung disease (about 15% of the total) has 1 to 4 days of coryza with slight cough and sudden onset of pleuritic chest pain and fever (Fig. 21-2). They are usually younger adults (<40 years old) and complain of sore throat and myalgias. In the remaining patients, increasing productive cough appears more prominent than fever or constitutional symptoms (10).

Bronchopneumonia is most commonly thought to be an exacerbation of chronic bronchitis (41,47). Excessive tachypnea and increasing constitutional symptoms prompt a chest radiograph. The temperature ranges from 36.8 to 38.5°C, in contrast with that reported with segmental disease (38.3 to 42.3°). However, many of the patients with segmental disease were subjects of case reports emphasizing bacteremia or systemic complications, factors that would favor a bias toward reporting of patients with higher temperatures. If all cases of *H. influenzae* pneumonia in adults are summarized, the typical case is a 55-year-old man who smokes and has a history of alcohol abuse and who has cough, fever, and the sudden onset of pleuritic chest pain. A pleural effusion/reaction will be seen during the illness, but abscess formation is rare.

Twenty-four strains isolated from the blood or CSF of adults with pneumonia were examined in detail by Wallace et al. (91). Of these, 9 were type b, 3 were type f, and 12 were not typeable. Biotyping (15) was performed with 23 of the 24 strains; 11, biotype I; 8, II; 2, III; and 2, V, a distribution similar to that seen with type b strains isolated from children (57). Capsular type f *H. influenzae,* a type responsible for only 0.5% of all pediatric infections caused by encapsulated strains, is more common in elderly men and more often fatal (14,18,22,67,79). Type d strains have also been associated with bacteremic bronchopneumonia (29).

Diagnosis

Leukocytosis

Most reports have not noted a difference in the magnitude of leukocytosis and the percent of circulating immature granulocytes from that found in patients with other bacterial pneumonias (Table 21-6).

Although culture of transtracheal aspirates has been used to diagnose *H. influenzae* pneumonia, this procedure is reliable only in individuals without chronic obstructive pulmonary disease. Laurenzi and coworkers (44) found that *H. influenzae* could be cultured from adults without signs and symptoms of pneumonia with nonbacterial chronic lower respiratory tract diseases (e.g., carcinoma). Thus, the presence of *H. influenzae* on transtracheal aspirate does not confirm the diagnosis of pneumonia caused by that organism, particularly in patients with chronic obstructive pulmonary disease (COPD) (42).

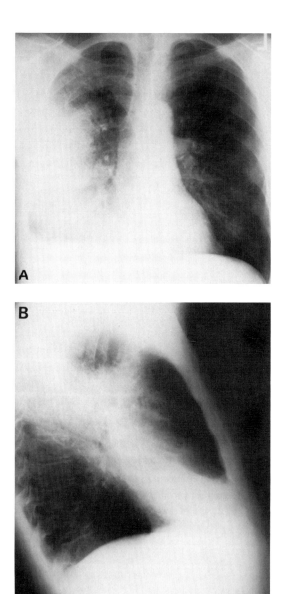

FIG. 21–2. A: Upright PA radiograph of a 55-year-old white male alcoholic admitted to the Seattle V.A. Medical Center with a 3-day history of subjective fever, productive cough, and right-sided pleuritic chest pain. **B:** Lateral film shows infiltrate in lower posterior portion of right upper lobe.

Levin et al. (46) reported that 12 of 16 bacteremic cases had a predominance of gram-negative coccobacillary forms present on gram stain of sputum. Only one of five patients with bacteremic *H. influenzae* pneumonia reported by Quintiliani and Hymans (59) had the organism identified on sputum gram stain; all had other bacteria identified; most often the gram stain was interpreted as "mixed flora." It is not clear

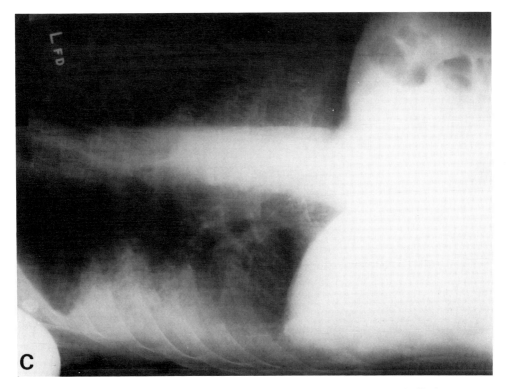

FIG. 21–2. *(continued)* **C:** Lateral decubitus reveals a large pleural effusion.

whether this represents an inability to culture *H. influenzae* from sputum containing other bacteria or a sampling bias in those with bacteremic disease.

Blood cultures are likely to yield the organism in patients with segmental parenchymal disease; however, because this form is less common, most patients with *H. influenzae* pneumonia will have sterile blood cultures. Douglas and Devitt (13) reported three adults (one with segmental and two with bronchopneumonia) who had *H. influenzae* in cultures of lung aspirate and sputum; none had the organism recovered from blood culture.

Examination of pleural fluid, serum, or a urine concentrate for type b antigen had not been pursued in adults suspected to have *H. influenzae* pneumonia (23). The majority of *H. influenzae* pneumonia in adults appears to be caused by non-type b strains, so somatic antigen detection could be more productive.

TABLE 21–6. *Leukocyte count for adults on admission*

Leukocytes/μl × 10³	Percent
<5	8
5–10	18
10–15	37
15–20	21
>20	16

Radiographic Appearance

As is seen in children, an early pleural reaction is the only consistent roentgeno-graphic feature of *H. influenzae* pneumonia seen in adult cases. It is present in one-half of the cases regardless of the form of the disease. A bulging or sagging fissure, as seen in *Klebsiella pneumonia,* has also been reported (20,74,86).

Treatment

Although there is less experience in adults in comparison with children, qualita-tively similar data exist; patients can have a clinical response to a variety of anti-biotics including penicillin G, erythromycin, chloramphenicol, cefamandole, genta-micin, and streptomycin (40,43). Nevertheless, *H. influenzae*–specific antibiotics (e.g., ampicillin, second generation cephalosporins) should be employed when this pathogen is suspected or proved to cause pneumonia. Past studies suggest that the incidence of ampicillin resistance in strains isolated from pneumonia patients is lower than that found in children. Two studies have reported a 2% to 3% incidence (68,91). In contrast, sputum *H. influenzae* isolates from adults with chronic bron-chitis have a higher prevalence of resistance (ampicillin, 5%, and tetracycline, 6% [38]); in one report, isolates from adults with chronic lung disease demonstrated 12.5% ampicillin resistance (92). Chloramphenicol resistance has not been reported in strains isolated from adults (38,68,72,91).

NOSOCOMIAL HEMOPHILUS PNEUMONIA

Nosocomial *Hemophilus* pneumonia is becoming increasingly recognized. Most often the patient is an adult who has chronic mild bronchitis and is hospitalized with an acute, nonpulmonary illness. Intubation often becomes necessary to manage acute hypotension or cardiac arrest. Following intubation and stabilization 5 to 12 days later, the patient is found to have pneumonia. Bronchial brushing or tracheal aspirate reveals nontypeable *H. influenzae*. In one study of risk factors for this dis-ease, the absence of prior antibiotic administration was the only variable that had statistical significance (63). Because most oropharyngeal *H. influenzae* are suscep-tible to many antibiotics, the flora reaching the lower airway is the indigenous bac-teria, rather than the gram-negative bacilli found in patients who receive prophylac-tic antibodies.

COMPLICATIONS

Empyema

If the term *empyema* (3,19,42,48,61,62,64,67,82) is defined as an opaque fluid con-taining leukocytes and semisolid material, then it is a relatively common complica-tion of segmental *H. influenzae* pneumonia. This form of pneumonia is primarily a disease of children, and so available literature only describes pediatric cases. Em-pyema appears during later stages of *H. influenzae* pneumonia and is relatively com-mon; 10% of children with *H. influenzae* pneumonia have empyema; and 6.4% of pediatric empyema is caused by this organism. Most often it is first recognized as a "loculated" or "immobile" pleural effusion in a nontoxic child. Thoracentesis yields empyema fluid early in the disease, but later (most patients are diagnosed 3 weeks after onset of symptoms) the inflammatory exudate coagulates into a semisolid mass (described as chicken fat) that cannot be drained by aspiration, tube thoracostomy, or thoracotomy. Children with a coagulated empyema are relatively asymptomatic with a daily low-grade fever (38.0 to 38.5°C) that can persist for 3 to 4 weeks with appropriate antibiotic therapy. Most patients are treated until their temperature is normal for 5 days. The chest radiograph does not appear normal in 75% of patients until 6 months after the onset of symptoms. On pulmonary function testing, there is restrictive dysfunction for 12 to 18 months (69).

Except for the report of Tillotson and Lerner (82), who noted an 18% incidence, empyema is rarely mentioned as a complication of *H. influenzae* pneumonia in adults. Management in a fashion similar to that with children seems appropriate, but documentation of the efficacy of a conservative, nonsurgical approach is not available.

Abscess

Approximately 5% of children ultimately proven to have *H. influenzae* pneumonia develop lung abscess. This complication appears to be an alternative pathway (rather than coagulated empyema) in the natural evolution of the disease, particularly after partial antibiotic treatment. A pleural reaction is invariably present, and an air-fluid level is apparent. The presentation can be confused with cavitary tuberculosis (a rare disease in children) because of the paucity of symptoms; low-grade fever, slight cough, malaise, and failure to gain weight. In all reported cases, *H. influenzae* was isolated from the abscess fluid. Smaller abscesses are usually drained by thoracentesis. The usual practice is to place thoracostomy tubes for the larger ones (i.e., >5 cm diameter). Antibiotics, usually amoxicillin for susceptible organisms, are administered for 2 to 3 months. Lung abscess after *H. influenzae* pneumonia in adults has been reported (46,79,90). If an abscess is suspected, a thoracic CT is necessary to document its presence and size.

Metastatic Foci

As many as 79% of children with *H. influenzae* pneumonia will have an associated focus. The most common site is otitis media (50%); however, meningitis (20%), pericarditis, and septic arthritis have all been described. In such patients, the pneumonia is often not the admitting diagnosis. Conversely, children with *H. influenzae* pneumonia should be repeatedly examined for an additional infectious focus.

In adults with *H. influenzae* pneumonia, a 24% incidence of meningitis has been reported in some series (46,79). If meningitis is present, it is invariably in those patients with bacteremia (28,39,46,53,70,77).

FATALITY RATE

The reported case fatality rate for *H. influenzae* pneumonia ranges from zero to 75% (18,35,90). In some cases the illness can be fulminant. Such patients have the usual risk factors for *Hemophilus* pneumonia; clinical features that permit anticipation of such a fulminant course are not available (17). The rate is dependent on age, approximately 30% in adults over 50 years old, and is related to underlying disease if present. The cause of death in adults with *H. influenzae* pneumonia has not been investigated. Presumably it is similar to pneumococcal pneumonia in which a failure to increase cardiac output cannot correct pulmonary volume expansion (9).

REFERENCES

1. Ajello, G.W., Bolan, G.A., Hayes, P.S., Lehmann, D., et al. (1987): Commercial latex agglutination tests for detection of *Haemophilus influenzae* type b and streptococcus pneumoniae antigens in patients with bacteremic pneumonia. *J. Clin. Micobiol.*, 25:1388–1391.
2. Alexander, H.E., Craig, J.R., Shirley, R.G., and Ellis, C. (1941): Validity of etiological diagnosis of pneumonia in children by rapid typing from nasopharyngeal mucus. *J. Pediatr.*, 18:31–35.
3. Asmar, B.I., Slovis, T.L., Reed, J.O., and Dajani, A.S. (1978): *Hemophilus influenzae* type b pneumonia in 43 children. *J. Pediatr.*, 93:389–393.
4. Bale, J.F., and Watkins, M. (1978): Fulminant neonatal *Haemophilus influenzae* pneumonia and sepsis. *J. Pediatr.*, 92:233–234.
5. Benjamin, E.L. (1931): Case of influenzal bacteremia in child eight months old. *Arch. Pediatr.*, 48:340–342.
6. Berk, S.L., Holtsclaw, S.A., Wiener, S.L., and Smith, J.K. (1982): Nontypeable *Haemophilus influenzae* in the elderly. *Arch. Intern. Med.*, 145:537–539.
7. Casadevall, A., Dobroszycki, J., Small, C., and Pirofski, L.A. (1992): *Hemophilus influenzae* type b bacteremia in adults with AIDS and at risk for AIDS. Comment in: *Am. J. Med.*, 92(6):583–586, 587–590.
8. Clancy, R.L., and Cripps, A.W. (1992): Specific protection against acute bronchitis associated with nontypeable *Hemophilus influenzae*. *J. Infect. Dis.*, 165(Suppl. 1):S194–S195.
9. Cooligan, T., Light, R.B., Wood, L.D.H., and Mink, S.N. (1981): Plasma volume expansion in canine pneumococcal pneumonia. *Am. Rev. Respir. Dis.*, 126:86–91.
10. Crowe, H.M., and Levitz, R.E. (1987): Invasive *Haemophilus influenzae* disease in adults. *Arch. Intern. Med.*, 147:241–244.
11. Crowell, J., and Loube, S.D. (1954): Primary *Hemophilus influenzae* pneumonia. *Arch. Intern. Med.*, 93:921–927.
12. Degré, M. (1971): Synergistic effect in viral-bacterial infection. *Acta Pathol. Microbiol. Scand.*, 79:137–141.
13. Douglas, R.M., and Devitt, L. (1973): Pneumonia in New Guinea: I. Bacteriologic findings in 632 adults with particular reference to *Haemophilus influenzae*. *Med. J. Aust.*, 1:42–48.
14. Dworzack, D.L., Blessing, L.D., Hodges, G.R., and Barnes, W.G. (1978): Case Report. *Hemophilus influenzae* type F pneumonia in adults. *Am. J. Med. Sci.*, 275:87–91.
15. Eng, R.H.K., Corrado, M.L., Cleri, D., and Sierra, M.F. (1980): Non-type b *Haemophilus influenzae* infections in adults with reference to biotype. *J. Clin. Microbiol.*, 11:669–671.
16. Esposito, A.L., and Pennington, J.E. (1984): Experimental pneumonia due to *Haemophilus influenzae*: Observations on pathogenesis and treatment. *J. Infect. Dis.*, 149:728–734.
17. Eveloff, S.E., and Braman, S.S. (1990): Acute respiratory failure and death caused by fulminant *Hemophilus influenzae* pneumonia. *Am. J. Med.*, 88(6):683–685.
18. Everett, E.D., Rahm, A.E., Jr., and Adaniya, M.R. (1977): *Haemophilus influenzae* pneumonia in adults. *J.A.M.A.*, 238:319–321.
19. Faden, H.S., and Overall, J.C., Jr. (1976): *Haemophilus influenzae* empyema: two cases. *Clin. Pediatr.*, 15:1143–1145.
20. Francis, J.B., and Francis, P.B. (1978): Bulging (sagging) fissure sign in *Hemophilus influenzae* lobar pneumonia. *South Med. J.*, 71:1452–1453.
21. Garcia do Olarti, D., Trujillo, H.S., Uribe, P.A., and Agudelo, N. (1971): Lung puncture-aspiration as a bacteriologic diagnostic procedure in acute pneumonias in infants and children. *Clin. Pediatr.*, 19:346–356.
22. Goldstein, E., Daly, A.K., and Seamans, C. (1967): *Haemophilus influenzae* as a cause of adult pneumonia. *Ann. Intern. Med.*, 66:35–40.
23. Granoff, D.M., Covgeni, B., Baker, R., Ogra, P., and Nankervis, G.A. (1977): Counter-current immunoelectrophoresis in the diagnosis of *Haemophilus influenzae* type b infection: relationship of detection of capsular antigen to age, antibody response and therapy. *Am. J. Dis. Child.*, 131: 1357–1362.
24. Groeneveld, K., Eijk, P.P., van Alphen, L., Jansen, H.M., and Zanen, H.C. (1990): *Hemophilus*

influenzae infections in patients with chronic obstructive pulmonary disease despite specific antibodies in serum and sputum. *Am. Rev. Respir. Dis.*, 141(5, Pt. 1):1316–1321.

25. Groeneveld, K., van Alphen, L., Voorter, C., Eijk, P.P., Jansen, H.M., and Zanen, H.C. (1989): Antigenic drift of *Hemophilus influenzae* in patients with chronic obstructive pulmonary disease. *Infect. Immunol.*, 57(10):3038–3044.

26. Hand, W.L., and Canty, J.R. (1974): Antibacterial mechanisms of the lower respiratory tract: I. Immunoglobulin synthesis and secretion. *J. Clin. Invest.*, 53:354–364.

27. Hirschmann, J.V., and Everett, E.D. (1979): *Haemophilus influenzae* infections in adults: report of nine cases and a review of the literature. *Medicine*, 58:80–94.

28. Holdsworth, P.E. (1960): *Hemophilus influenzae* meningitis in an adult. *Arch. Intern. Med.*, 106: 653–656.

29. Holmes, R.L., and Kozinn, W.P. (1983): Pneumonia and bacteremia associated with *Haemophilus influenzae* serotype d. *J. Clin. Microbiol.*, 18:730–732.

30. Holsclaw, D.S., Jr., and Schaeffer, D.A. (1980): Counterimmunoelectrophoresis in the diagnosis of *Hemophilus influenzae* pleural effusion. *Chest*, 78:867–869.

31. Honig, P.J., Pasquariello, P.S. Jr., and Stool, S.E. (1973): *H. influenzae* pneumonia in infants and children. *J. Pediatr.*, 82:215–219.

32. Huntington, R.W., Jr. (1935): On the behavior of *Hemophilus influenzae* in certain diseases of children. *J. Clin. Invest.*, 14:459–464.

33. Jacobs, N.M., and Harris, V.J. (1979): Acute *Haemophilus* pneumonia in childhood. *Am. J. Dis. Child.*, 133:603–605.

34. Jenkins, R.R., Smith, D.D., and White, P.L. (1979): *Hemophilus influenzae* pneumonia in an adolescent. *Clin. Pediatr.*, 18:571–575.

35. Johnson, W.D., Kaye, D., and Hook, E.W. (1968): *Hemophilus influenzae* pneumonia in the adult. *Am. Rev. Respir. Dis.*, 133:603–605.

36. Jorgensen, J.H., Doern, G.V., Maher, L.A., Howell, A.W., and Redding, J.S. (1990): Antimicrobial resistance among respiratory isolates of *Hemophilus influenzae, Moraxella catarrhalis,* and *Streptococcus pneumoniae* in the United States. *Antimicrob. Agents Chemother.*, 34(11):2075–2080.

37. Kaplan, N.M., and Braude, A.I. (1958): *Hemophilus influenzae* infection in adults. *Arch. Intern. Med.*, 101:515–523.

38. Kauffman, C.A., Bergman, A.G., and Hertz, C.S. (1979): Antimicrobial resistance of *Hemophilus* species in patients with chronic bronchitis. *Am. Rev. Respir. Dis.*, 120:1382–1385.

39. Kaufmann, J.A. (1960): Report of a case of proven fulminating hemophilus influenzae pneumonia in an adult with recovery. *Dis. Chest*, 38:199–201.

40. Keefer, C.S., and Remmelkamp, C.H. (1942): Case report. *Hemophilus influenzae* bacteremia: report of two cases recovering following sulfathiazole and sulfapyridine. *Ann. Intern. Med.*, 16:1221–1227.

41. Keith, T.A., and Shreiner, A.W. (1962): *Hemophilus influenzae* in adult bronchopulmonary infection. *Ann. Intern. Med.*, 56:27–38.

42. Lapinski, E.M., Flakos, E.D., and Taylor, B.C. (1964): An evaluation of some methods for culturing sputum from patients with bronchitis and emphysema. *Am. Rev. Respir. Dis.*, 89:760–763.

43. Lauermann, M., Barza, M., and Tally, F.P. (1979): Cefamandole in the treatment of *Hemophilus influenzae* and other pneumonias and lung abscess. *Curr. Ther. Res.*, 25:573–583.

44. Laurenzi, G. (1961): Bacteriologic flora of the lower respiratory tract. *N. Engl. J. Med.*, 265:1273–1278.

45. Lehmann, D., Coakley, K.J., Coakley, C.A., Spooner, V., Montgomery, J.M., Michael, A., Riley, I.D., Smith, T., Clancy, R.L., and Cripps, A.W. (1991): Reduction in the incidence of acute bronchitis by an oral *Hemophilus influenzae* vaccine in patients with chronic bronchitis in the highlands of Papua, New Guinea. *Am. Rev. Respir. Dis.*, 144(2):324–330.

46. Levin, D.C., Schwarz, M.I., Matthay, R.A., and LaForce, F.M. (1977): Bacteremia *Hemophilus influenzae* pneumonia in adults: a report of 24 cases and a review of the literature. *Am. J. Med.*, 62:219–226.

47. Lowe, M.B. (1964): *Haemophilus influenzae* type-C bronchopneumonia. *J. Pathol. Bacteriol.*, 88:315–316.

48. Lundstrom, R. (1955): Purulent pericarditis and empyema caused by *Hemophilus influenzae,* type B. *Am. Heart J.*, 49:108–115.

49. Marraro, R.V., McCleskey, F.K., and Mitchell, J.L. (1977): Pneumonia due to *Haemophilus influenzae* (H. aegyptius) biotype 3. *J. Clin. Microbiol.*, 6:172–173.

50. Martin, S.J., Hoganson, D.A., and Thomas, E.T. (1987): Detection of *Streptococcus pneumoniae* and *Haemophilus influenzae* type b antigens in acute nonbacteremic pneumonia. *J. Clin. Microbiol.*, 25:248–250.

51. Michaels, R.H., Poxinisk, C.S., Stonebraker, F.E., and Norden, C.W. (1976): Factors affecting pharyngeal *Haemophilus influenzae* type b colonization rates in children. *J. Clin. Microbiol.*, 4: 413–417.

52. Mimica, I., Donoso, E., Howard, J.E., and Ledermann, G.W. (1971): Lung puncture in the etiological diagnosis of pneumonia. *Am. J. Dis. Child.*, 122:278–282.
53. Nasou, J.P., Romansky, M.J., and Barr, J.F. (1953–1954): The treatment of *Hemophilus influenzae,* type b bacteremia, and pneumonia with erythromycin. In: *Antibiotic Annual* 1953–1954, pp. 470-474. Medical Encyclopedia Publishers, New York.
54. Nyhan, W.L., Rectanus, D.R., and Fousek, J.D. (1955): *Hemophilus influenzae* type b pneumonia. *Pediatrics,* 16:31–41.
55. Pfeiffer, R. (1893): Die Aetiologic der Influenzae. *J. Hyg. Infektionskr.,* 13:357–386.
56. Pine, J.H., Richter, W.R., and Esterly, J.R. (1973): Experimental lung injury. *Am. J. Pathol.,* 73:115–130.
57. Plouffe, J.F., and Powell, D.A. (1981): Serious infections in adults exposed to children with *Haemophilus influenzae* type b meningitis. *Ann. Intern. Med.,* 94:785–786.
58. Potter, A.R., and Fischer, G.W. (1977): *Haemophilus influenzae,* The predominant cause of bacterial pneumoniae in Hawaii. *Pediatr. Res.* (Baltimore), 11:504.
59. Quintiliani, R., and Humans, P.J. (1971): The association of bacteremic *Haemophilus influenzae* pneumonia in adults with typable strains. *Am. J. Med.,* 50:781–786.
60. Ramierz-Ronda, C.H., Fuxench-Lopez, A., and Nevarez, M. (1981): Increased pharyngeal bacterial colonization during viral illness. *Arch. Internal Med.,* 141:1599–1603.
61. Ravitch, M.M., and Fein, R. (1961): The changing picture of pneumonia and empyema in infants and children: A review of the experience at the Harriet Lane Home from 1934 through 1958. *J.A.M.A.,* 17:1039–1044.
62. Reddy, C.M. (1979): *Haemophilus influenzae* type d pneumonia. *Am. J. Dis. Child.,* 133:96.
63. Rello, J., Ricart, M., Ausina, V., Net, A., and Prats, G. (1992): Pneumonia due to *Hemophilus influenzae* among mechanically ventilated patients: incidence, outcome, and risk factors. *Chest,* 102(5):1562–1565.
64. Riley, H.D., Jr., and Bracken, E.C. (1965): Epyema due to *Hemophilus influenzae* in infants and children. *Am. J. Dis. Child.,* 110:24–28.
65. Roberts, M.C., Stull, T., and Smith, A.L. (1981): Comparative virulence of *H. influenzae* bearing the type b or type d capsule. *Infect. Immun.,* 32:518–524.
66. Rubenstein, E., Lederman, B., Bogokowsky, B., and Altmann, G. (1975): Ampicillin-resistant *Haemophilus influenzae* pneumonia and empyema in an infant. *Israel J. Med. Sci.,* 11:1121–1123.
67. Rusthoven, J., and Kabins, S.A. (1978): *Hemophilus influenzae* f cellulitis with bacteremia, peritonitis, and pleuritis in an adult with nephrotic syndrome. *South. Med. J.,* 71:1433–1434.
68. Saginur, R., and Bartlett, J.G. (1980): Antimicrobial drug susceptibility of respiratory isolates of *Hemophilus influenzae* from adults. *Am. Rev. Respir. Dis.,* 122:61–64.
69. Santosham, M., Chipps, B.E., Strife, J.L., and Moxon, E.R. (1979): Sequelae of *H. influenzae* type b empyema. *J. Pediatr.,* 95:160–161.
70. Schwimmer, R. (1959): Primary *H. influenzae* pneumonia in an adult with extreme hyperpyrexia. *Am. J. Med. Sci.,* 238:713–719.
71. Smith, A.L. (1981): *Haemophilus influenzae.* In: *Textbook of Pediatric Infectious Diseases,* edited by R. Feigin and J. Cherry, pp. 858–871. W.B. Saunders, Philadelphia.
72. Smith, C.B., Golden, C.A., Kanner, R.E., and Renzetti, A. (1976): *Haemophilus influenzae* and *Haemophilus parainfluenzae* in chronic obstructive pulmonary disease. *Lancet,* 1:1253–1261.
73. Soto, E., and Silverio, J. (1976): Report of five children with *Haemophilus influenzae* pneumonia (resistance to ampicillin must always be looked for). *Clin. Pediatr.,* 15:419–421.
74. Sproul, J.M. (1969): Spherical pneumonia due to *Hemophilus influenzae* (a definitive study by transtracheal aspiration). *Am. Rev. Respir. Dis.,* 100:67–69.
75. Stadel, B.V., Foy, H.M., Nuckolls, J.W., and Kenny, G.E. (1975): Mycoplasma pneumoniae infection followed by *Haemophilus influenzae* pneumonia and bacteremia. *Am. Rev. Respir. Dis.,* 112:131–133.
76. Stanger, P., Lucas, R.V., and Edwards, J.E. (1969): Anatomic factors causing respiratory distress in acyanotic congenital heart disease. *Pediatrics,* 43:760–769.
77. Stein, J.A., DeRossi, R., and Neu, H.C. (1969): Adult *Hemophilus influenzae* meningitis: associated with disseminated intravascular coagulation. *NY J. Med.,* 69:1760–1766.
78. Steinhart, R., Reingold, A.L., Taylor, F., Anderson, G., and Wenger, J.D. (1992): Invasive *Hemophilus influenzae* infections in men with HIV infection. *J.A.M.A.,* 268(23):3350–3352.
79. Stratton, C.W., Hawley, H.B., Horsman, T.A., Tu, K.K., Ackley, A., Fernando, K., and Weinstein, M.D. (1980): *Hemophilus influenzae* pneumonia in adults: report of five cases caused by ampicillin-resistant strains. *Am. Rev. Respir. Dis.,* 121:595–598.
80. Takala, A.K., Eskola, J., and van Alphen, L. (1990): Spectrum of invasive *Hemophilus influenzae* type b disease in adults. *Arch. Intern. Med.,* 150(12):2573–2576.
81. Thjotta, T., and Avery, O.T. (1921): Studies on bacterial nutrition: II. Growth accessory substances in the cultivation of hemophilic bacilli. *J. Exp. Med.,* 34:97–113.
82. Tillotson, J.R., and Lerner, A.M. (1968): *Hemophilus influenzae:* bronchopneumonia in adults. *Arch. Intern. Med.,* 121:428–432.

83. Toews, G.B., Viroslav, S., Hart, D.A., and Hansen, E.J. (1984): Pulmonary clearance of encapsulated and unencapsulated *Haemophilus influenzae* strains. *Infect. Immun.*, 45:437–442.
84. Trollfors, B., Claesson, B., Lagergard, T., and Sandberg, T. (1984): Incidence, predisposing factors and manifestations of invasive *Haemophilus influenzae* infections in adults. *Eur. J. Clin. Microbiol.*, 3:180–184.
85. Tunevall, G. (1953): Studies on *Haemophilus influenzae*. *Acta Pathol. Microbiol. Sand.*, 32:193–197.
86. Vinik, M., Altman, D.H., and Parks, R.E. (1966): Experience with *Hemophilus influenzae*. *Radiology*, 86:701–706.
87. Wald, E.R., and Levine, M.M. (1976): Frequency of detection of *Hemophilus influenzae* type b capsular polysaccharide in infants and children with pneumonia. *Pediatrics*, 57:266–268.
88. Wald, E.R., and Levine, M.M. (1978): *Haemophilus influenzae* type b pneumonia. *Arch. Dis. Child.*, 53:316–318.
89. Walker, E.R., and Levin, M.M. (1978): The respiratory manifestations of systemic *Hemophilus influenzae* infection. *J. Pediatr.*, 62:386–390.
90. Wallace, R.J., Jr., Musher, D.M., and Martin, R.R. (1978): *Hemophilus influenzae* pneumonia in adults. *Am. J. Med.*, 64:87–93.
91. Wallace, R.J., Jr., Musher, D.M., Septimus, E.J., McGowan, J.E., Quinones, F.J., Wiss, K., Vance, P.H., and Trier, P.A. (1981): *Haemophilus influenzae* infections in adults: characterization of strains by serotypes, biotypes, and β-lactamase production. *J. Infect. Dis.*, 144:101–105.
92. Wallace, R.J., Steele, L.C., Brooks, D.L., Forrester, G.D., Garcia, J.G.N., Luman, J.I., Wilson, R.W., Shepherd, S., and McLarty, J. (1988): Ampicillin, tetracycline, and chloramphenical resistant *Hemophilus influenzae* in adults with chronic lung disease. *Am. Rev. Respir. Dis.*, 137:695–699.
93. Ward, J.I., Siber, G.R., Scheifele, D.W., and Smith, D.H. (1978): Rapid diagnosis of *Haemophilus influenzae* type b infections by latex particle agglutination and counterimmunoelectrophoresis. *J. Pediatr.*, 93:37–42.
94. Weller, P.F., Smith, A.L., Smith, D.H., and Anderson, P. (1978): The role of immunity in the clearance of *H. influenzae* bacteremia. *J. Infect. Dis.*, 138:427–436.
95. Winslow, C.E.A., Broadhurst, J., Buchanan, R.E., Krumwiede, C., Rogers, L.A., and Smith, G.H. (1920): The family and genera of the bacteria. Final report of the Society of American Bacteriologists on characterization and classification of bacterial types. *J. Bacteriol.*, 5:101–236.
96. Woodsell, S.H., and Shapiro, J.L. (1960): Interstitial pneumonitis induced by experimental infection with *Hemophilus influenzae*. *Am. J. Dis. Child.*, 100:16–22.

Respiratory Infections: Diagnosis and Management, 3d ed.,
edited by James E. Pennington.
Raven Press, Ltd., New York © 1994

22

Legionella Pneumonias

Paul H. Edelstein and Richard D. Meyer

*Departments of Pathology and Laboratory Medicine, Hospital of the University of
Pennsylvania, University of Pennsylvania School of Medicine, Philadelphia,
Pennsylvania 19104-4283; and Division of Infectious Diseases, Department
of Medicine, Cedars-Sinai Medical Center, School of Medicine,
8700 Beverly Boulevard, Los Angeles, California 90048*

The discovery of the "new pneumonias" has led to some confusion in terminology. Legionnaires' disease is a pneumonic illness with systemic manifestations caused by the gram-negative bacillus *Legionella pneumophila*. The term *legionellosis* has been used in different fashions by many to denote infections other than pneumonia caused by *L. pneumophila,* or infections caused by the other species of *Legionella,* or infections caused by any *Legionella* sp regardless of clinical manifestations. We, however, prefer to use more specific appellations such as *L. pneumophila* pneumonia.

An outbreak of pneumonia in Philadelphia in July 1976 at an American Legion convention led to recognition of the clinical entity of Legionnaires' disease (LD), and eventually to isolation and identification of the etiologic agent (41,85,133). Subsequent to the identification of *L. pneumophila* as the etiologic agent of LD, it was discovered that outbreaks of the illness had occurred as long ago as 1957 and sporadic cases even earlier (9). A mild nonpneumonic form of the illness was also discovered to have occurred in 1968 (33,113), and seroprevalence studies have demonstrated that 5–10% of the general population could have significant antibody directed against *L. pneumophila* (33,98), although these tests are not necessarily specific. This is thus neither a new nor an unusual disease. The issue has been further illuminated by the discovery of more than 14 serogroups of *L. pneumophila* based on surface antigens (9,31,150), and over 30 other *Legionella* sp, many of which have been shown to be responsible for pneumonia or associated with disease (Table 22-1) (17,31,42,95,100,171,175–179,184,191–193). Some of these "new" species have been causing disease for at least the last several decades (9,180). Some have been isolated first from the environment and later from immunosuppressed patients, and others have been found first in immunosuppressed patients and then other patients. Additional species thus far isolated only from the environment are likely to be associated with human disease in the future (18,19,26,174,184,189).

ETIOLOGY

The *Legionella* sp (see Table 22-1) are fastidious gram-negative bacilli that are strict aerobes. They are unusual in that they will not grow on routine bacteriologic media, such as MacConkey or blood agars, that are commonly used in most clinical microbiology laboratories; growth does occur on supplemented charcoal yeast ex-

TABLE 22–1. Legionella *species and serogroups*

Species	No. serogroups	Clinical isolates?
L. adelaidensis	1	No
L. anisa	1	Yes
L. birminghamensis	1	Yes
L. bozemanii	2	Yes
L. brunensis	1	No
L. cherrii	1	No
L. cincinnatiensis	1	Yes
L. dumoffii	1	Yes
L. erythra	1	No
L. fairfieldensis	1	No
L. feeleii	2	Yes
L. gormanii	1	Yes
L. gratiana	1	No
L. hackeliae	2	Yes
L. israelensis	1	No
L. jamestowniensis	1	No
L. jordanis	1	Yes
L. lansingensis	1	Yes
L. longbeachae	2	Yes
L. maceachernii	1	Yes
L. micdadei	1	Yes
L. moravica	1	No
L. oakridgensis	1	Yes[a]
L. parisiensis	1	No
L. pneumophila	15	Yes
L. quinlivanii	1	No
L. rubrilucens	1	No
L. sainthelensi	2	Yes
L. santicrucis	1	No
L. shakespearei	1	No
L. spiritensis	2	No
L. steigerwaltii	1	No
L. tucsonensis	1	Yes
L. wadsworthii	1	Yes

[a] By DFA test only.

tract (BCYEα) medium (111). BCYEα medium is commercially available; its preparation is not beyond any competent microbiology laboratory. Semiselective BCYEα media are also used (58). All species grow well in humidified air at 35°C; some species grow better in 2.5 to 3.0% CO_2. The average incubation time required for first growth is 3 days, with a range of 1 to 10 days.

Once isolated on a culture medium, *Legionella* sp are relatively easy to identify to the genus level. This is based on characteristic colonial morphology, growth requirement for 1-cysteine, and serotyping (111). Also helpful in differentiation are characteristic branched-chain cellular fatty acid and ubiquinone compositions, and failure to produce acid from carbohydrates. Because of the antigenic complexity of legionellae, it is impossible to serologically distinguish several of the species. Combined with a paucity of other useful phenotypic characteristics, this means that identification to the species level can be very difficult, except for extremely sophisticated research laboratories. However, all laboratories should be able to identify *L. pneumophila,* and other legionellae to the genus level.

Microscopic morphology of the organisms depends on growth conditions. They are usually very faintly staining small coccobacilli in lung and sputum, and often long and filamentous bacilli when taken from a culture plate. Although colonies growing on artificial media stain well with gram stain (especially if basic fuchsin rather than safranin is used as the counterstain), the bacteria are exceptionally difficult to visualize using this stain on fixed lung specimens, and often with fresh tissues and fluids also. The Gimenez stain is a more effective method to examine tissues, and is much simpler and more sensitive than the previously touted Dieterle silver impregnation stain (111).

At least 15 serogroups and several subserogroups have been identified for *L. pneumophila* (9,71,134); 33 other *Legionella* species have been characterized. The nomenclature is confusing, as some strains are named after cities, some after states, and others from initials of patients. *L. pneumophila* serogroups 1, 4, and 6 appear to be the most common causes of infection, with about 80% of cases caused by serogroup 1, and 5 to 10% each caused by the other two groups. Infections caused by legionellae other than *L. pneumophila* are uncommon, constituting perhaps 20 to 30% of infections. Of these, infections caused by *L. micdadei, L. longbeachae, L. dumoffii,* and *L. bozemanii* appear to be most common, in that order.

The natural reservoir for legionellae is our aqueous environment, where they are ubiquitous, especially in warm water. There is substantial evidence that these bacteria exist in nature by growing in free-living amoebae such as *Acanthamoeba, Hartmannella,* and *Naegleria.*

PATHOGENESIS AND IMMUNITY

Legionnaires' disease is caused by inhalation, or perhaps aspiration, of virulent *Legionella* sp (12,13,33,127,128). Rarely, disease is caused by direct inoculation of *Legionella* sp into a wound or the skin (122,183,186). Devices that aerosolize *Legionella*-contaminated water serve as disseminators of the disease. Such devices have included cooling towers, humidifiers, respiratory therapy equipment, an ultrasonic nebulizer used to mist vegetables, shower heads, faucets, and industrial cooling sprays.

Once the bacteria gain entrance to the lung, whether by aerosol or aspiration, they are phagocytosed by alveolar macrophages (57,102). Because of their ability to grow and survive in macrophages, the *Legionella* bacteria multiply in the lung. The bacteria are toxic to the macrophages, eventually causing their death and resulting in release of large numbers of bacteria extracellularly. This cycle starts again in other, uninfected macrophages, which serves to greatly amplify bacterial concentrations within the lungs. *L. pneumophila* attains concentrations in the lung as high as 10^{11} bacteria/gram, in a guinea pig model of Legionnaires' disease. Extrapulmonary spread of bacteria occurs experimentally, and in at least some humans with Legionnaires' disease; it is probable that hematogenous spread is facilitated by the circulation of *Legionella*-infected monocytes (50,51). Activation of alveolar macrophages by interferon gamma, and probably other cytokines, greatly slows bacterial growth *in vitro,* and probably has a similar effect in humans (36,37,103).

Several important *L. pneumophila* virulence determinants have been described, although the molecular pathogenesis of infection is still incompletely understood (43,57,102). A bacterial protein, called MIP (macrophage infectivity potentiator), is important for bacterial entry into cells (44,45). Macrophage complement receptors can serve as ligands for *L. pneumophila,* although this is controversial, as is the role of serum complement in the uptake of the bacterium into the macrophage. Several different exotoxins, as well as a weakly active endotoxin, have been described for *L. pneumophila*. One of the most interesting is a protease that can be important in the pathogenesis of *L. pneumophila* infections, at least in animals (15,48,157). Several toxins that inhibit white blood cell function or integrity have been characterized, including a cytotoxin, a phospholipase, an inhibitor of oxidative metabolism and intracellular killing, and an inhibitor of chemotaxis (8,121,154). Similar findings have been made for *L. micdadei*. Virtually nothing is known about the virulence factors of other *Legionella* species.

The systemic manifestations of the disease are likely caused by toxin elaboration by the bacterium rather than by extrapulmonary infection. However, extrapulmonary infection involving the brain, intestine, lymph nodes, kidneys, liver, spleen, peritoneum, bone marrow, myocardium, pericardium, and the blood stream itself have been documented (49,56,82,145,194).

The cellular immune system is most important for immunity to Legionnaires' disease; most particularly macrophages, monocytes, and probably lymphocytes. Polymorphonuclear leukocytes appear to play little role in protective immunity, as evidenced by the paucity of Legionnaires' disease cases in patients with neutropenia but intact macrophage function. There is little evidence that antibodies play a protective role, and no evidence at all that antibody formation is required for recovery from disease. The implications of this are that medical therapies or underlying diseases that reduce systemic or local cellular immunity greatly increase the risk of Legionnaires' disease. Because of the ability of *Legionella* sp to evade extracellular host defenses, relapses of disease are seen after short courses of antimicrobials, or with renewed immunosuppression.

The pathogenesis of Pontiac fever is not understood, and has not been studied thoroughly. The leading hypotheses include inhalation of *Legionella* and other bacterial toxins, self-limited pulmonary infection caused by *Legionella* strains that are able to infect macrophages but not multiply within them, and an infectious or toxic disease caused by microorganisms coexisting with *Legionella* in contaminated waters.

PATHOLOGY

Consistent pathologic findings are usually limited to the chest cavity. Lobar or, less commonly, segmental consolidations are constant findings. Abnormalities are usually confined to the alveoli and respiratory bronchioles, with dense infiltration of intra-alveolar polymorphonuclear leukocytes and macrophages; microabscesses are not uncommon. The larger airways and alveolar septa are spared. Pleural inflammation can occur. Organisms have been seen in hilar lymph nodes rarely (194).

Extrapulmonary *L. pneumophila* has been detected in kidney, lymph nodes, muscle, skin, brain, spleen, bone marrow, liver, blood, peritoneum, intestine, pericardium, and myocardium. Pathologic findings in large series do not, however, reveal consistent changes in these organs (194). It can only be concluded that in extraordinary cases, particularly in immunosuppressed patients, extrapulmonary dissemination can occur. Microabscess formation has been demonstrated in association with *L. pneumophila* infection of multiple extrapulmonary organs of a severely immunosuppressed child (49). Infection of nonpulmonary organs, in the absence of pneumonia, has been documented to occur of prosthetic heart valves, of respiratory sinuses, of the pleural space, of skin and muscle, and of wounds. These extrapulmonary infections are caused either by bacteremia during open heart surgery without subsequent pneumonia or by direct seeding of susceptible tissues by *Legionella*-contaminated water.

Usual tissue stains do not show bacteria. These include hematoxylin and eosin, Brown-Brenn, and methenamine silver stains. Mycobacterial stains do not show organisms, except for the Kinyoun acid-fast stain, which demonstrates a minority of *L. micdadei* organisms present (196). The best nonimmunologic method of demonstrating bacilli from lung is a Gimenez stain of a tissue imprint; this can be either fresh or fixed tissue. Once the tissue is embedded in paraffin, the Dieterle silver impregnation stain or a modified Gimenez stain can be used (111). These methods are nonspecific and probably relatively insensitive. Direct immunofluorescence examination is the most specific and sensitive means of visualizing *Legionella* in tissues and body fluids and is also suitable for Formalinized specimens (68,111). A monoclonal antibody (Genetic Systems, Seattle, Wash.), widely used for examination of nonfixed clinical specimens, cannot be used for Formalin-fixed tissues; commercially available polyvalent reagents should be used instead (63). All of the immunologic techniques have the major drawback of being species- and serogroup-specific, and may therefore lead to a false-negative diagnosis if the wrong serogroup or species conjugate is used. *Legionella*-specific DNA probes have been used to demonstrate the bacteria in tissues (74). Culture of tissue and respiratory secretions is a sensitive and specific method (see below).

EPIDEMIOLOGY

L. pneumophila is a water organism and is widely distributed. Legionellae are associated in natural water sources with free-living amoebae, and *L. pneumophila* has been found with amoeba in at least one outbreak of disease (30,143,159). Centers for Disease Control (CDC) workers showed that *Legionella* inoculated into water survived for prolonged periods of time (9). *L. pneumophila* within amoebae is protected from high levels of chlorine, which makes eradication of the organism from the environment difficult, and fosters its presence in treated waters (11,115).

After some of the early outbreaks had occurred, *L. pneumophila* was found in water from cooling towers and evaporative condensers, from thermal effluent, and from fresh-water lakes not known to be associated with disease (9,81,194). Almost all cases are associated not with these natural sources but rather from conditions that amplify and spread the bacilli. These include heat-exchange apparatuses and distribution systems for potable water in large buildings. Isolations of legionellae, including species other than *L. pneumophila,* have been made from cooling-tower water, evaporative condensers, air from ventilation ducts, and the evaporative air-conditioning system on a bus (18,19,194).

Legionnaires' disease exists both in outbreaks and as sporadic cases. Over 30 nosocomial outbreaks and a smaller number of building-associated outbreaks have been reported. Sporadic cases likely outnumber cases associated with defined outbreaks.

Transmission usually results from inhalation of aerosols (12,13,33). Aspiration is a possible mode of transmission in hospitalized patients (127,128). Rarely, wound infections follow irrigation with contaminated water, as has been reported for sternal wound and pleural infections (122,183).

Outbreaks associated with spread from heat-exchange apparatuses include those in a Memphis, Tennessee, hospital (55), in a Pontiac, Michigan, building (33,113), at a country club in Atlanta, Georgia (33), in a hospital in Staffordshire, England (120), in a Rhode Island hospital (90), a Burlington, Vermont, hospital (110,118), in a British power station, where cooling-tower water had not been decontaminated (139), in a Los Angeles retirement hotel (29), and in a wide community area in Glasgow, Scotland. In Glasgow some sporadic (nonoutbreak, nontravel) cases were shown to have been associated with proximity of a patient's home to a cooling tower and probably resulted from it (20–22). Another notable community-based outbreak associated with a cooling tower is the London Broadcasting House (BBC) outbreak in 1988 (89).

In another recent community-based outbreak with a large number of cases ($\geq$33), an ultrasonic mist machine which was supplied with potable water produced aerosols in a grocery store that caused LD in shoppers (126).

One community-acquired outbreak that was not associated with either potable water or heat-exchange apparatuses but was linked to recent grounds excavation recently occurred in Barcelona (138). Recent excavation has been associated with several other outbreaks but no clear transmission has been documented.

Clear demonstrations of the role of air-conditioning apparatuses in nosocomial transmission of LD have been shown by the Memphis outbreak in 1978, by the Staffordshire outbreak, and, especially convincing, by the Los Angeles retirement hotel outbreak. In Memphis a cluster of 19 confirmed and 14 presumptive cases were found to have occurred both inside and outside a hospital. Risk was related to position relative to a temporary auxiliary water tower; *L. pneumophila* was recovered from it. Contaminated aerosols probably reached the air intakes for the ventilation system. There were no further cases found after return to use of the standard cooling tower (55). In Staffordshire disease temporally followed use of untreated pond water in a heat-exchange apparatus (7,120). Many cases occurred in patients who had visited and been exposed in the clinics and then returned to the community, and so the source was not immediately apparent. In the Los Angeles retirement hotel outbreak, *L. pneumophila* was found both in an evaporative condenser and in potable water, but results of a case-control study, air sampling, and monoclonal antibody subtyping of isolates supported the evaporative condenser as the source (29).

That legionellae are distributed in potable water, particularly after heating and subsequent distribution as hot water, was elucidated first in Oxford. English workers showed a link between cases and finding the organism in shower heads in an Oxford outbreak (181). Later the legionellae were found in shower water and/or tap water in other hospitals with cases. Some notable examples include hospitals in Pittsburgh, Los Angeles; Columbus, Ohio; Iowa City; Kingston, England; and Palo Alto, California; one each in South Dakota, Leiden, and Brussels; and in Paris (9,30,70, 80,99,135,144,153,165,168,170,183). Shower heads and hot water faucets have been shown to spread aerosol particles with *Legionella* (23). Thus, tap water aerosols from faucets can likely transmit LD in the absence of shower or nebulizer use, for example, in an intensive care unit. Similarly, hot water faucet use was postulated as a source for cases in a cardiac transplantation unit (170). A difference in attack rates between subtypes of serogroups of *L. pneumophila* defined by monoclonal typing has been shown with isolates from potable water, as has dissociation between environmental and clinical isolates (110,153,170). Stagnation of flow of water and a reduction in hot water temperature are factors associated with risk of transmission of *Legionella* from potable water (46,147).

A smaller series of outbreaks of disease due to *L. pneumophila* and *L. dumoffii* have also been associated with use of contaminated tap water or nonsterile distilled water to fill or clean respiratory therapy devices, for example, nebulizers (5,109,131). Likelihood of recovery of *L. pneumophila* from hot tap-water systems in apartments and houses has been associated with temperatures of <60°C; isolation was not associated with history of pneumonia. Generally, the level of contamination, when found, was low ($\leq 10^4$ organisms/ml[6]). Electric water heaters, city residence, and temperature <48.8°C were associated with isolation of *L. pneumophila* in several studies (2,107,108,119). On the other hand, monoclonal antibody subtyping of clinical isolates from apparently sporadic cases of LD and then from water sources indicates that, in some cases, disease is associated with or caused by environmental contamination, including household water systems in multidwelling residences (169). Outbreaks of *L. micdadei* infection in Charlottesville, Virginia, and *L. bozemanii* in Stamford, Connecticut, without clear sources defined at either site, have also been reported (142,148); and *L. longbeachae* contamination of Australian potting soil made with composted wood products (not peat) has been linked to clusters of cases (166,167).

Philadelphia Outbreak and Discovery of Etiology—Historical Note

The first outbreak discovered was in Philadelphia in the summer of 1976. It centered about people at four meetings at a Philadelphia hotel, or people who had entered the hotel; the State Delegation of the American Legion was the most noteworthy meeting. Clinical criteria were development of fever (temperature 38.9°C) and cough, or fever and radiographic evidence of pneumonia. One hundred and eighty-two patients fulfilled epidemiologic and clinical criteria; 29 of these died. Milder nonpneumonic illnesses also occurred. A separate group of patients who fulfilled the clinical criteria and were within one block of the hotel during the epidemic period were designated as Broad Street pneumonia patients; five of these 39 patients died. The attack rates for persons at the American Legion Convention were 9.0% for those in the hotel and 4.0% overall. Time spent in the lobby of the hotel and drinking hotel water were correlated with risk of acquisition of disease in visitors, but no conclusions were made then about the latter finding. Male sex, older age groups, and underlying disease increased the risk of acquisition of cases of both Legionnaires' disease and Broad Street pneumonia (85).

The epidemic curve suggested an incubation period of 2 to 10 days and a common source outbreak. Case control studies also showed no person-to-person transmission. Airborne spread, which was postulated as likely, is consistent with subsequent knowledge of aerosol spread (85). There is no evidence now to support drinking of water as a mode of transmission.

In January 1977, *L. pneumophila* was isolated from four cases by inoculating autopsy lung tissue intraperitoneally into guinea pigs and then into yolk sacs of embryonated hens' eggs. This led to development of antigens for use in the indirect fluorescent antibody (FA) test and to antibody for the direct FA test (133). The CDC then retrospectively identified *L. pneumophila* as the cause of other sporadic cases of severe pneumonia, and of unsolved outbreaks of respiratory tract disease in 1968 (33,113) and nosocomial pneumonia in 1965 in Washington, D.C. (173). Likewise, five other cases of confirmed or presumptive LD in Philadelphia not related to the hotel were identified (87). Subsequently, the CDC showed that there had been an outbreak of LD with a lower attack rate at the same hotel in 1974 at an Odd Fellows convention (33).

LD has also been linked to other hotels, for example, in an outbreak initially among Scottish tourists who had stayed in a hotel in Benidorm, Spain, and died with pneumonias in 1973. Cases occurred at the hotel for almost a decade before control was brought about (14,96). It is noteworthy that outbreaks occurred later in hotels in Garda, Como, and Lido di Savio (all in Italy) and in a motel in Eau Claire, Wisconsin (10,52,158), as well as in 1985 at a Michigan hotel. Travel-related cases with a recent stay in a hotel continue to be recognized; one example among several is the cluster in travelers with exposure to thermal baths and hotel water on the Island of Ischia (40).

Nosocomial and Community Clusters and Outbreaks

In Burlington, Vermont, 69 cases of LD with 17 deaths occurred between May and December 1977. Immunocompromised hosts were at particular risk (including chronic dialysis patients). Ownership of a home air-conditioner was found to be a risk factor for a community-acquired group of cases (9,16). Additional cases of LD subsequently occurred and accounted for 11.6% of nosocomial pneumonias at the Medical College of Vermont hospital in Burlington (9,91). Most occurred in patients receiving corticosteroids or who were otherwise immunosuppressed. In the Pittsburgh V.A. Hospital, *L. pneumophila* was shown to cause 18% of nosocomial pneumonias (34). On the other hand, *Legionella* infection has occurred in conspicuously low frequency in another hospital where search was made (93).

Between May 1977 and November 1981, over 220 cases of LD were confirmed at the V.A. Wadsworth Medical Center in Los Angeles, the site of probably the longest and largest outbreak (9,70,165). The first group of cases was recognized primarily in renal transplant recipients. All cases were associated with exposure to the hospital as inpatients, recently discharged patients, clinic visitors, or employees. Duration of hospitalization was a risk factor, except for immunosuppressed patients, who also had a ninefold greater risk of acquisition of LD. Compromised immunity was a significant risk factor (p ≤ 0.01). The major underlying predispositions were, in order of frequency, immunosuppressive therapy, cardiac disease, malignancy, pulmonary disease, and renal disease (9). Postoperative surgical patients were also at especial risk (164). A 3-month prospective cohort study at Wadsworth V.A. of 1,658 consecutive admissions revealed that the attack rate was 0.5% for all new admissions and that asymptomatic seroconversion occurred in 0.8%. It is not known how many of the latter might have been due to the nonspecific nature of serologic testing; Legionnaires' disease accounted for 8 of 73 cases of nosocomial pneumonia and for 4 of 14 nosocomial pneumonia deaths (9). Hyperchlorination of the cooling towers had no effect on the problem. In 1980, *L. pneumophila* was isolated from shower and tap water, and subsequent changing of shower heads and hyperchlorination of the potable water led to a dramatic decrease in cases and control of the problem (165).

Although multiple strains of *Legionella* were isolated from potable water, only one strain accounted for most of the culture-proven cases (70).

Data from the 1970s indicated that *Legionella* accounted for up to 10% of nosocomial pneumonias, although the distribution was spotty, and more in an outbreak. Current estimates are considerably lower because of maintenance measures on heat-exchange apparatuses and maintenance both of higher hot water temperatures in distribution systems and of the systems themselves; but outbreaks and clusters can and do still occur in the era of supposed control measures. This is exemplified by the aforementioned Staffordshire experience (7,120) as well as by others, including a 1991 California office building outbreak which was also linked to a cooling tower source (197).

Sporadic Cases and Prevalence

Most of the first 1,005 sporadic cases of LD reported to the Centers for Disease Control were found in the Northeast and Middle West between June and October. The age range in affected individuals was 16 months to 89 years. The risk for males was 2.6 to 1. Age ≥ 50 years, male sex, chronic bronchitis, and smoking were predisposing factors (72). In another study from Barcelona, alcohol use and smoking history were risk factors (75). Sporadic LD has been recognized almost worldwide.

Immunosuppressed patients, as noted in aforementioned outbreaks, are at particular risk for acquiring LD in the presence of disordered T-cell function. Examples include not only kidney transplant recipients but also heart, heart-lung, and liver transplant recipients; these include patients receiving cyclosporine A and/or OK-T3 monoclonal antibody (32,155,182). Curiously, *Legionella* infections probably occur no more commonly in human immunodeficiency virus (HIV)–infected individuals and AIDS patients than in others with no additional risk factors (114,163,198).

Serological studies showed that LD has accounted for 1% of community-acquired pneumonias in adults who did not require hospitalization (84); fewer than 0.4% of pneumonia cases treated at home in an area previously endemic for LD were recently shown to be LD (200). Legionellae were previously thought to cause from 5 to 15% of pneumonias in patients admitted to hospital and 6.7% in a more recent study (9,76,125). These latter estimates are based on serological studies fraught with cross-reactions and/or presumptive cases with a single, elevated convalescent antibody reaction, so the estimates are likely high. A more realistic current estimation of the frequency of LD as a cause of community-acquired pneumonia in patients requiring hospitalization is 2.3% (129). Nonetheless, in another earlier study, it accounted for about 10 to 15% of so-called atypical pneumonias serologically diagnosed (9). Legionella infections in children occur but are rare in the absence of underlying predisposing disease (28,38,47,73).

Description of Pontiac Fever

In July 1968, an illness with a shorter incubation period (mean of 36 hours) and more upper respiratory tract and neurologic symptoms but no pneumonia occurred in a new county health department building in Pontiac, Michigan (Pontiac fever). Excavation, rains, hot weather, and use of the air-conditioning system preceded the outbreak. This was an explosive outbreak characterized by fever, headache, myalgia, and malaise. The attack rate was 95% for employees and 29% for visitors, and the episode involved at least 144 patients. Unlike patients with LD, the affected people had been healthy. A self-limited airborne infection was suggested; acquisition of disease was related to use of the air-conditioner in the building. Re-exposure resulted in a much lower symptomatic attack rate. The evaporative condenser discharge units of the air-conditioner leaked into the air ducts. No cases occurred after repairs were made, and the building was reopened (33,113). *L. pneumophila* serogroup I was recovered from stored lung tissue of guinea pigs that had been placed in the building and from guinea pigs exposed to aerosols of water from the evaporative condenser.

Other known outbreaks of Pontiac fever, all of which are related to aerosols, include one that occurred in 1973 when all ten men who cleaned a steam turbine condenser in James River, Virginia, became ill (all recovered); several related to whirlpool bath use, and one to a heavily contaminated cooling tower (33,88). One in an automobile assembly plant was due to *L. feeleii,* and another spread by water in a fountain in a hotel lobby was due to *L. anisa* (78,100). A sporadic case occurred in another area in a man who cleaned a cooling tower (92). The pathogenesis of this form of *Legionella* infection is unknown, but it could be similar to that of humidifier fever.

CLINICAL FEATURES

After the usual incubation period of 2 to 10 days (which can be shorter, especially in immunosuppressed patients who also usually have more severe disease), most patients develop pneumonia, which often is severe. Infection with *L. pneumophila* can, however, cause many different diseases, some of which could be asymptomatic (9). The finding of elevated antibody levels in the general healthy population indicates that LD could occur as an asymptomatic infection. However, it must be borne in mind that overall estimates of the prevalence of LD based on seroprevalence studies depend on the fact that there is no cross-reaction with other organisms in this test. This is very unlikely (190), and it is possible that the estimated prevalence of LD is lower than that estimated on the basis of currently available seroprevalence studies. Several prospective studies have demonstrated that neither community-acquired nor nosocomial Legionnaires' disease can be differentiated from other common causes of pneumonia, based on clinical, radiographic, or nonspecific laboratory findings (76,94,156,201). We describe the classical presentation of Legionnaires' disease because we believe there is a subset of patients with this disease who do have distinctive symptoms and signs.

Pneumonia

The disease usually has gradual onset, but it can be more abrupt, especially in immunosuppressed patients. First symptoms often are malaise, lethargy, headache, weakness, myalgia, and anorexia; the headache can be severe. Complaints of sore throat or rhinitis are usually absent. The majority of patients have a dry, nonproductive cough, but this is not the usual chief complaint, nor is it as prominent as it is in *Mycoplasma* infections. Moreover, it usually is noted only after a day or two of illness. In about one-half to one-fourth of patients, the sputum can be purulent or bloody; this usually occurs after the illness has progressed for several days. About 75% of patients suffer from recurrent rigors (9,117,199).

Complaints of a systemic nature are common. These include diarrhea, nausea, vomiting, and headache. Diarrhea is usually watery, with three to four bowel movements per day, and occurs in about half the cases. The nausea and vomiting that are often associated with anorexia are seen less commonly (in about one-fourth of patients). Headache, often in association with confusion, is seen frequently. One-fourth to one-third of patients complain of pleuritic pain, which in association with hemoptysis often makes one think of pulmonary infarction. Myalgia and arthralgia can be prominent and lead to consideration of collagen vascular disease. Diaphoresis is sometimes seen (9,117,199).

Elevated temperature greater than 40°C is often striking (e.g., in approximately 50% of patients), even in patients receiving antipyretic agents or corticosteroids. Virtually all patients have fever to some degree; less than 5% of patients have normal temperatures. The fever is a nonremitting, continuous type and is associated in about 60% of cases with relative bradycardia (117).

Examination of the chest usually shows the most impressive physical findings. Early in the course of the disease only scattered rales or evidence of a small pleural effusion are noted. Later in the course of the disease, striking findings of frank consolidation are almost always noted. Findings in the chest are usually proportional to those noted on chest radiograph, as in pneumococcal disease but in contrast with mycoplasmal disease. Friction rubs can be heard (117). Massive pleural effusion and empyema have been noted but are uncommon.

Extrapulmonary Manifestations

Abnormalities of mental status are common and are found in about one-fourth of patients with pneumonia. Findings noted include disorientation, agitation, stupor, confusion, obtundation, coma, hallucinations, ataxia, grand mal seizure, and focal neurologic findings. Nuchal rigidity has occurred but is rare (75,97,117).

Focal visceral abscesses, pancreatitis, peritonitis, pericarditis, myocarditis, leukoencephalitis, cellulitis with myositis, myositis with motor neuropathy, and Henoch-Schönlein purpura have also been separately described (35,124,146,186,187, 194,196). Vasculitis of a hepatic graft and hepatic abscesses were also documented in a liver transplantation patient (182). Many of these cases were serologically documented, but some have had clear demonstration of *Legionella,* either in tissue or by successful cultures (124,146,182,186,187). In a case with pneumonia and exudative pleural effusion, remarkable extensive cellulitis and myositis likely resulted from spread secondary to thoracentesis (186). Transient aplastic anemia in a culture-documented case has also been reported, but medication use confounds conclusion about cause and effect (130).

Disease caused by *Legionella* not involving the lung concurrently has been rarely noted. Aside from Pontiac fever, there have been relatively few well-documented cases of *Legionella* not involving the lung. This includes 13 cases in the original Philadelphia outbreak diagnosed as LD on the basis of epidemiologic criteria despite negative findings on chest radiographs (85). Prosthetic valve endocarditis, peritonitis, and infections of wounds and paranasal sinuses with *Legionella* have been well-documented (4,122,132,163,183). Some of the additional cases that have been reported are those with central nervous system involvement without pneumonia; these include seizures and focal neurologic findings—tremors and ataxia—and peripheral neuropathies or global dysfunction were noted in some cases (87,97,117,151). Pericarditis and the findings of Roth's spots and cotton wool patches in the retina in the same patient have also been associated with putative *Legionella* infection not involving the lung (86). However, these latter cases were documented on the basis of serologic means only, and not by recovery of the organism.

Abnormalities of other systems including hepatic, renal, and musculoskeletal (e.g., myositis or rhabdomyolysis) occur but are usually noted only on laboratory examination. The spectrum of associated renal disease includes interstitial nephritis and, less commonly, acute tubular necrosis, or myoglobinuria or, perhaps, glomerulonephritis (79,188,196). Hemodialysis fistula site infection has followed *Legionella* pneumonia (112).

Other *Legionella* Species Infections

Pneumonia caused by the other *Legionella* species generally seems to be clinically indistinguishable, with a few exceptions, from classic LD. These exceptions are pneumonia caused by *L. micdadei,* the mostly commonly found of the non-*pneumophila Legionella* species, and *L. bozemanii.* Many patients with *L. micdadei* pneumonia (Pittsburgh pneumonia) have been reported to have nodular pulmonary infiltrates of the type commonly seen with septic pulmonary embolism. Some have had less fever than in LD (142). Moreover, pneumonia caused by this agent occurs much more commonly in immunosuppressed than in nonimmunosuppressed patients; there are relatively few well-documented cases of *L. micdadei* pneumonia in nonimmunosuppressed patients. A cutaneous leg abscess due to *L. micdadei* in an immunosuppressed patient has also been noted (3). *L. bozemanii* pneumonia can differ in that most of the cases have occurred in immunosuppressed patients and in a few cases fresh-water near-drowning can be a predisposing factor (148,180). These distinctions are based on analyses of relatively few cases in that cases of pneumonia due to non-*pneumophila* species have been documented perhaps a hundredfold fewer times than has LD. Cerebrospinal fluid (CSF) lymphocytic pleocytosis and brainstem demyelination on magnetic resonance imaging scan were documented in one patient with *L. bozemanii* pneumonia and encephalitis (152). A review article summarizing additional information on these infections is available (77).

Pontiac Fever

Pontiac fever is a nonfatal illness associated with *L. pneumophila* or *L. feeleii;* it is likely an intoxication rather than an infection. There is no lower respiratory tract involvement radiographically documented, although many of the systemic symptoms observed with LD are also seen in Pontiac fever, and some patients have had dry cough; rales have been heard on examination of a minority of patients. Symptoms include chills, fever, headache, dizziness, myalgia, diarrhea, and abdominal pain. Fever tends to be lower than in LD; neurologic complaints were common in one major outbreak but not in others (33,78,88,100,113).

DIAGNOSIS

Clinical Features

The classic presentation of Legionnaires' disease is that of pneumonia, although asymptomatic infection or mild illness can be seen. The combination of consolidating pneumonia, multiorgan involvement, and nonproductive cough should strongly suggest Legionnaires' disease, although these are nonspecific findings. Failure to respond to penicillin, cephalosporins, or aminoglycosides is another clue, but one should consider the diagnosis earlier in many instances.

Radiographic Findings

The finding of alveolar filling patterns with lobar, nodular, patchy, or subsegmental consolidation is characteristic (Figs. 22-1 and 22-2). Pleural effusion can precede other radiographic findings, or appear after the onset of parenchymal infiltration. Interstitial infiltrates can appear early but usually develop into consolidative infiltrates within days. Cavitation and empyema formation occur rarely, as does an obviously bulging interlobar fissure (53,69,116,123). Comparative studies have shown

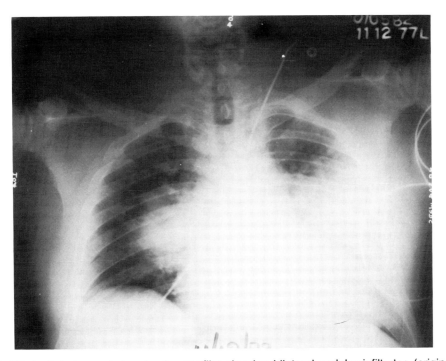

FIG. 22–1. Anterior-posterior chest x-ray film showing bilateral nodular infiltrates (originally alveolar). The patient was a 55-year-old man with chronic renal failure who developed fever, chills, sweats, and confusion. Gentamicin and vancomycin were given without response. Autopsy lung was positive for *L. pneumophila* by direct immunofluorescent examination.

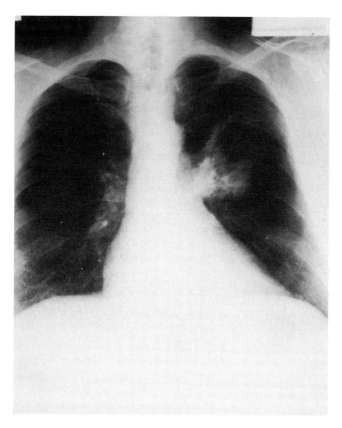

FIG. 22–2. Posterior-anterior chest x-ray film showing left upper lobe posterior-apical alveolar infiltrate. The film was taken on day 9 of illness during erythromycin therapy for Legionnaires' disease. The patient was a 44-year-old asthmatic who developed fever, chills, sweats, myalgia, nausea, and cough while on prednisone therapy.

that there are no radiographic findings that can be used to differentiate Legionnaires' disease from pneumococcal pneumonia (76,94,156,201).

Laboratory Diagnosis: General

A number of nonspecific laboratory abnormalities can occur in Legionnaires' disease. These are abnormal urinalysis with proteinuria and hyaline or granular casts; hypophosphatemia, hyponatremia, and, less commonly, elevations of aldolase or creatine kinase (117). Extreme electrolyte abnormalities related to massive diarrhea occur rarely (83). Renal failure has been reported rarely. The renal failure can occur in conjunction with myositis and/or marked elevations of creatine kinase and aldolase or with myoglobinuria and can represent rhabdomyolysis (87,137). In addition, interstitial nephritis, mesangial proliferative and progressive glomerulonephritis have all been reported (39,79). The white blood cell count is elevated ($>10,000/mm^3$), often with a left shift in about one-half to three-fourths of patients. Leukopenia and thrombocytopenia are observed in severe disease (9). Serum cold agglutinins and even cold agglutinin disease have also been observed in several cases (9). Disseminated intravascular coagulation is observed rarely. Elevations of lactic dehydrogenase, alkaline phosphatase, and aspartate aminotransferase are also common (9,85,87,117). Bilirubin elevation is less common. Hypoxemia is usually in proportion to the degree of pulmonary involvement seen on radiograph (117).

Laboratory Diagnosis: Specific

There are five currently used methods for the laboratory diagnosis of *Legionella* infections (Table 22-2). These are determination of antibody level, demonstration of the bacterium in tissues or body fluids by using immunofluorescent microscopy, actual isolation of the organism on culture media, detection of the bacterium by using a DNA probe, and detection of antigenuria (1,34,60,61,64,111,194).

Estimation of serum antibody to *L. pneumophila* is the most commonly used means of diagnosing Legionnaires' disease (62,111,190). Most laboratories use an indirect immunofluorescent microscopy (IFA) technique to determine antibody concentrations. Antibody to a variety of *Legionella* antigens is measured by different laboratories. About three-quarters of patients with culture-proven Legionnaires' disease caused by *L. pneumophila* serogroup 1 develop a fourfold rise in titer from 1 to 9 weeks after onset of illness. The mean time required for demonstration of seroconversion is about 2 weeks; however, up to 25% of seroconversions are missed unless serum is collected up to 8 weeks after onset of illness (68). Between 5% and 30% of healthy populations sampled have *L. pneumophila* serogroup 1 antibody titers of 1:128 or greater when using a heat-fixed antigen, so only a fourfold rise in titer to 1:128 or greater can be considered significant; significant titers for Formalin-fixed antigen are a rise in titer to 1:32 or greater (9,99). In the face of an outbreak of Legionnaires' disease, a single titer of >1:256 (heat-fixed antigen) in a patient with a compatible clinical illness has been considered significant (111). However, in the sporadic case, such single high titers cannot be interpreted. The specificity of the IFA test in a hospitalized population is not well known; this probably approximates 90% for a fourfold titer rise, although in an epidemic situation in nonhospitalized patients the specificity is close to 100% (68,133). Cross-reactions have been reported in patients with tuberculosis, pneumococcal pneumonia, *Pseudomonas* pneumonia, exacerbations of cystic fibrosis, tularemia, plague, *Bacteroides fragilis* bacteremia, and leptospirosis (25,67). Up to 20% of patients with campylobacter enteritis have been reported to have cross-reactive antibody to *L. pneumophila* (27). Antibody testing is most specific when using *L. pneumophila* serogroup 1 antigen, especially when a Formalin-fixed antigen is used. The specificity of a fourfold antibody rise to the serogroup 1 antigen is at least 99%, whereas test specificity is considerably lower when using antigens from other *L. pneumophila* serogroups, or from other species. Because of this, it is better not to test for antibody to antigens other than *L. pneumophila* serogroup 1, except for epidemiological studies. In addition to the fact that serologic testing is retrospective (and does not influence choice of therapy) and that there is a possibility of cross-reactions, the other major drawback of diagnosing *Legionella* infections using serologic means is that if a patient has infection with a serotype that is not tested for, the test could be negative. Thus, serologic testing in the diagnosis of this disease is much more helpful to epidemiologists than to clinicians caring for individual patients.

TABLE 22–2. *Laboratory diagnosis of Legionnaires' disease*

Test type	Sensitivity (%)	Specificity (%)	Comments
Antibody estimation			
Seroconversion	75	95–99	Optimal sensitivity requires parallel testing of specimens collected acutely and 6–9 weeks later; highest specificity is for *L. pneumophila* serogroup 1; testing for antibodies to other species and serogroups is strongly discouraged.
Single specimen	(unknown)	50–70	
Immunofluorescent detection of antigen			Highest specificity is for a species-specific monoclonal antibody; use of non–*L. pneumophila* antibodies is strongly discouraged; often positive for several days after the start of antibiotic therapy.
Sputum or BAL	25–75	95–99	
Lung biopsy	80–90	99	
Culture			Special media and selective techniques needed for optimal yield; culture is more sensitive than all other methods; often positive after the start of antibiotic therapy, though less sensitive; therapy with third-generation cephalosporins appears to decrease yield.
Sputum or BAL	80–90	100	
Lung biopsy	90–99	100	
Blood	10–30	100	
DNA probe	50–70	95–99	Lower sensitivity for TTA and pleural fluid; can be positive for several days after the start of antibiotic therapy; genus-specific.
Urinary antigen	80–99	99	Specific for *L. pneumophila* serogroup 1; can be positive for weeks to months after completion of therapy.

Immunofluorescent microscopy of respiratory tract secretions, lung, and pleural fluid is one of the rapid test methods available to establish a laboratory diagnosis of Legionnaires' disease (68,111). When this technique is used with an antibody conjugated with a fluorochrome, it is called direct immunofluorescence, or "DFA". About 2 to 3 hours is required to complete the test. This technique has been used very successfully with expectorated sputum, endotracheal suction aspirates, lung biopsies, and transtracheal aspirates. Use of secretions or biopsies obtained by bronchoscopy has not resulted in high yield in our experience, although others have had more success. Pleural fluid examination in patients with Legionnaires' disease usually is unproductive, in terms of both culture and DFA positivity, but has occasionally been helpful (9). The true sensitivity of the DFA test is unknown. About 25 to 70% of patients with culture-proven Legionnaires' disease have positive sputum DFA tests for *L. pneumophila;* test specificity is greater than 99.9%; therefore, a negative result does not rule out disease and a positive result is almost always diagnostic of it (68). A monoclonal antibody DFA reagent which reacts with all serogroups of *L. pneumophila* provides optimal specificity and eliminates the need to use multiple antisera to detect this species (Genetic Systems, Seattle, Wash.) (63). Unlike polyvalent reagents, it does not cross-react with some *Pseudomonas, Flavobacterium-Xanthomonas,* and *Bacteroides* strains; however, it cannot be used to stain tissues fixed in Formalin for prolonged periods (172). Highly specific DFA reagents for use in detection of other *Legionella* sp are not commercially available; use of less-specific available products will result in frequent false-positive tests unless infection caused by the particular species being screened for is common. Exceptional skill is needed to read DFA test slides properly. DFA tests of sputum remain positive for 2 to 4 days after the initiation of specific antibiotic therapy for Legionnaires' disease, and often much longer in cases of cavitary pulmonary disease.

Isolation of *Legionella* from clinical specimens is routinely performed in many laboratories. The medium used, supplemented charcoal yeast extract medium (BCYEα), is easily prepared by any large clinical microbiology laboratory and can be made in a selective form. Use of selective media and specimen decontamination with acid are obligatory for optimal culture yield from normally nonsterile tissues and fluids. Good commercial preparations of the media are available. The organism has been successfully isolated from sputum, transtracheal aspirates, endotracheal suction specimens, blood, lung biopsy, pleural fluid, bronchial lavage, pericardial fluid, peritoneal fluid, wounds, bowel abscesses, prosthetic heart valves, brain abscesses, myocardium, kidney, liver, vascular grafts, and respiratory sinuses (9,68, 117,163). Like all other tests for Legionnaires' disease, the true sensitivity of culture is unknown; however, it is more sensitive than other available tests.

A commercially produced DNA probe can be used to rapidly detect legionellae in clinical specimens; assay time is less than 3 hours (64). The product is much less sensitive than is culture, and probably about as specific as is DFA testing (149). Although the probe reacts with other *Legionella* species, experience with the probe for detection of legionellae other than *L. pneumophila* is very limited. Non–respiratory tract specimens, pleural fluids, and transtracheal aspirates should not be tested with the probe, as it appears to be very insensitive for testing these specimens. One apparent advantage of the DNA probe test over that of DFA testing is that it can remain positive a day or two longer after the initiation of specific antibiotic therapy. Also, it is more broadly reactive than is the DFA test. The polymerase chain reaction has been used to diagnose Legionnaires' disease, but this test is still regarded as a research tool (105).

L. pneumophila serogroup 1 antigenuria can be detected using a commercial radioimmunoassay (1,161). Cross-reactions between serogroups are uncommon, somewhat limiting the usefulness of this test. This is a rapid test with extraordinary specificity; we have never documented a false-positive test. Test sensitivity has been 95% in culture-proven disease, and about 80% in serologically proven disease. We have observed many instances of positive urine antigen tests with negative sputum cultures, probably because testing has been done after more than 5 days of specific antibiotic therapy. One minor drawback of this test is that it can remain positive for weeks to months after recovery from pneumonia.

DIFFERENTIAL DIAGNOSIS

Clinical diagnosis of *Legionella* infections in a nonepidemic setting can be difficult. Any patient who has a pneumonic illness with multisystem abnormalities, and who is responding poorly to therapy with penicillin, cephalosporin, and/or an aminoglycoside or clindamycin, should be suspected of having *Legionella* infection, but this may be a late clue. Nonetheless, this observation is especially true if the patient has a nonremitting, progressively rising fever, recurrent rigors, nonproductive cough, relative bradycardia, and severe prostration. It should be stressed that a patient with consolidating pneumonia almost always has production of large amounts of purulent sputum; in the absence of sputum production the clinician should be alerted to alternative diagnoses. Most patients with LD produce little sputum early in the disease; when produced, it is rarely grossly purulent.

Pneumococcal pneumonia differs from *Legionella* infection in that the patients with pneumococcal infection usually have the single rigor, produce purulent sputum, and respond favorably to penicillin. Pneumococcal bronchopneumonia, especially in the older patient, can more closely mimic LD, despite an accompanying pneumococcal bacteremia. The chief complaint of most people with *Mycoplasma pneumoniae* pneumonia is that of a persistent dry, hacking cough. Although patients with *Legionella* infections often have a nonproductive cough, it is unusual for the cough to be their primary complaint early in the disease. Moreover, it is very unusual for *Mycoplasma pneumoniae* pneumonia to produce systemic manifestations and severe disease, although this can occur in patients with hemoglobinopathies and those being treated with immunosuppressive drugs.

Psittacosis and Q fever can mimic LD very closely. Up to 25% of patients with psittacosis have no history of bird exposure, and although psittacosis usually produces a nonconsolidating pneumonia, it can produce disease indistinguishable from LD. The same is true of Q fever, which is endemic in Southern California. *Chlamydia pneumoniae* pneumonia appears to have some nonspecific features similar to LD, but it is a more common occurrence in a younger age group, and the findings of pharyngitis, laryngitis, and a normal WBC differ from LD. Early coccidioidomycosis, histoplasmosis, typhoid fever, and tularemia are additional possibilities. A superinfected viral pneumonia can also be confused with LD. In trying to rule in or out any of these diseases, it is helpful to remember that sputum bacteriology is notoriously unreliable in establishing the etiology of pneumonia, and that dual infections can occur, especially in hospitalized patients.

THERAPY

Supportive therapy for hypotension and respiratory failure is sometimes needed in patients with *Legionella* infection. Although thrombocytopenia can occur, we have never documented bleeding abnormalities associated with this. Immunosuppressive agents should be stopped or dosage reduced, if at all possible. Corticosteroids have absolutely no role in the treatment of LD itself, except in the face of adrenal insufficiency.

Erythromycin remains the drug of choice in the treatment of *Legionella* infections (9,85,117,136). This is based chiefly, no doubt, on retrospective reviews of therapy of LD, as unfortunately no prospective comparative study of antimicrobial therapy of LD has been performed. In the Philadelphia epidemic of LD in 1976, the case fatality rate was lower with erythromycin therapy than with tetracycline, and highest in those patients treated with cephalothin (85). In retrospective reviews of other outbreaks of LD, erythromycin appears to be an effective antimicrobial agent, capable of lowering the case fatality rate approximately three- to fourfold over that of patients given no therapy (9,16,75,117). Resistance to erythromycin among *L. pneumophila* has been elicited by *in vitro* selection but is clinically unknown.

Drawbacks for use of erythromycin include bacteriostatic action, drug toxicity, and drug interactions with warfarin, theophylline, cyclosporine A, and disopyramide, as well as problems in iv or po administration. Nonetheless, erythromycin alone or with rifampin remains the drug of choice. Newer macrolides, including roxithromycin, clarithromycin, and azithromycin, deserve further evaluation in this area (66,136). None of these newer macrolides are available in an intravenous preparation in the United States, limiting their use in patients unable to absorb oral medications; clarithromycin is available in intravenous as well as oral preparations in several countries other than the United States.

Results of therapy with tetracycline have been variable in that there have been several clear-cut failures in patients treated with tetracycline. On the other hand, there are reports of patients responding favorably to tetracycline (117). It is clear, however, that penicillins, cephalosporins, cefamycins (cefoxitin and cefotetan), and aminoglycosides have no influence on progression of LD. Likewise, imipenem, a carbapenem, should not be used. Clavulanic acid is active *in vitro*. In animal models of infection, therapy with amoxicillin-clavulanate has been effective; nonetheless it failed in one clinical case, and a related agent, ampicillin/sulbactam, did not halt progressive infection in another (101,186). Co-trimoxazole in high dose has been used successfully in a small number of cases, particularly to treat *L. micdadei* infection, and it is possible but certainly not proven that it may be an effective drug (136).

Use of *in vitro* susceptibility testing to predict clinical response in Legionnaires' disease can be very misleading. For example, all aminoglycosides and cefoxitin inhibit *Legionella* at low concentrations. However, these drugs do not work clinically. The reason for this is, in part, likely the ability of some antimicrobials to enter the alveolar macrophage. Erythromycin, other macrolides, and tetracycline enter the alveolar macrophage quite readily, and in fact are concentrated in it; whereas the penicillin drugs do not achieve significant levels within macrophages (106). The fluoroquinolones also penetrate monocyte-derived cells well. Use of animal models of infection can lead to better prediction of efficacy of antimicrobials in LD therapy (195). Agents active in experimental *Legionella* pneumonia include erythromycin, rifampin, doxycycline, co-trimoxazole, ofloxacin, ciprofloxacin, fleroxacin, pefloxacin, and sparfloxacin (65,136,160).

Erythromycin should be given in a dose of 2 to 4 gms per day for at least 3 weeks' time. We prefer to give the drug intravenously (iv) to moderately or severely ill patients for the first several days of therapy, or until the patient has a clinical response. If the drug is given *per os* (po), patients cannot generally tolerate more than 2 gms per day because of gastrointestinal side effects. Rifampin in a dose of 600 mg given twice per day, iv or po, should be considered as an adjunct to erythromycin if the patient is critically ill or in patients with pulmonary cavities; it should not be given alone because of the possibility of emergence of resistance. Cavitary pulmonary disease or *empyema thoracis* generally requires prolonged therapy.

Because of its greater lipid solubility, doxycycline is the preferred tetracycline drug if erythromycin cannot be given. Doxycycline is given iv or po in a dose of 200 mg initially, then 100 mg in 12 hours and then 100 mg daily thereafter. Information about the efficacy of tetracycline in LD is limited, so we prefer to give rifampin with the doxycycline at least for the first week of therapy in moderately severe to severely ill patients.

Results with quinolone therapy are quite promising, although published clinical data on the treatment of culture-proven *Legionella* infections are few. Reported successes of therapy in patients with serologically documented infections include some immunosuppressed patients and some who had failed therapy with erythromycin and/or rifampin; eight of ten patients treated with ciprofloxacin responded, including one who required two courses of ciprofloxacin therapy. Other successes include treatment of *Legionella* infections in two patients receiving cyclosporine A. Ciprofloxacin has less of an effect on cyclosporine A levels than does erythromycin. Not surprisingly, failures of ciprofloxacin treatment of legionellosis have also been reported (136).

At a dose of 800 mg given iv or po, pefloxacin alone or combined with either rifampin or erythromycin has been used in patients in intensive care or bone marrow transplantation units and appears to have been efficacious. Ofloxacin alone at a dose of 200 mg po tid or 400 mg bid in serologically confirmed cases of legionellosis has likewise been successful. Ofloxacin in reduced doses was successful in therapy of three cases of *Legionella* infections in renal transplant recipients receiving cyclosporine A (136). Ofloxacin has no adverse drug interaction with cyclosporine A. More studies of fluoroquinolone therapy are needed; nonetheless, for the patient with documented *Legionella* infection who is intolerant of or has failed standard therapy, either ciprofloxacin in doses of 750 mg po or 300 to 400 mg iv given bid, or pefloxacin in doses of 400 mg po or iv given bid, or ofloxacin 400 mg po or iv given bid is an alternative therapeutic regimen (136).

The clinical response to erythromycin therapy is usually prompt. Within 12 to 48 hours after initiation of therapy, many patients begin to feel better and usually have a decrease in temperature. Pulmonary infiltrates can continue to progress, as well as signs of pulmonary consolidation, while the patient is manifesting a clinical response. Therefore, it is important to monitor the patient for such subjective findings as appetite, chest pain, shortness of breath, and sense of well being (117). It is exceptionally unusual for a patient to have persistent fever, leukopenia, and confusion after more than 3 to 4 days of erythromycin therapy, although we have observed this in patients with coexisting lymphoma. If this occurs, the diagnosis should be questioned and superinfection considered.

PROGNOSIS, MORTALITY, AND SEQUELAE

Prognosis and case fatality rates are affected by underlying disease and antimicrobials administered. The case fatality rate in otherwise well patients not receiving erythromycin therapy is about 20 to 30%, whereas patients who are immunosuppressed who do not receive erythromycin therapy have a case fatality rate of about 80%. Treated nonimmunosuppressed patients have a case fatality rate of about 5% versus 24% in treated immunosuppressed patients. These rather high rates were observed mostly in seriously ill hospitalized patients (9,117). Overall mortality rates in sporadic cases have been about 19%, and as low as 10% in those receiving erythromycin (71,75).

Some patients complain of persistent fatigue and weakness for several months after completion of therapy. In patients who develop respiratory failure during the course of their disease, there is anecdotal evidence that restrictive lung disease can develop. Bronchiolitis obliterans following antibiotic therapy for LD has also been reported, but the diagnosis of LD in this single case was based only on rise in serum antibody titers (162). Similarly, corticosteroid-responsive fibrosing alveolitis has been associated with serologic evidence of Legionnaires' disease in two patients; whether these patients truly had Legionnaires' disease is unclear (104). Chest radiographs usually show resolution of infiltrates from 3 weeks to 3 months after initiation of therapy, although some at 3 months show residual scarring or volume loss (54).

CASE INVESTIGATIONS AND CONTROL MEASURES

No person-to-person transmission of Legionnaires' disease has been documented; therefore there is no need for patient isolation. The finding of a nosocomially acquired case or cases should prompt the search for other cases, including search in the autopsy files. The most efficient means of case finding is to perform respiratory tract cultures for *Legionella* from patients with nosocomial pneumonia; serosurveys have been no more sensitive in more than one nosocomial outbreak, and have been far less specific (R.D. Meyer and P.H. Edelstein, unpublished data, 1980; 128). There is no published experience with the use of bacterial antigen detection for case finding in nosocomial Legionnaires' disease, but this should be as effective as culture if *L. pneumophila* serogroup 1 is the etiologic agent. The best means of detecting the presence of nosocomial Legionnaires' disease at an institution not known to have this disease is to focus on immunosuppressed patients, who have been the sentinel guinea pigs in most outbreaks. Cases of community-acquired Legionnaires' disease should be reported promptly to local public health authorities so that a search for other such cases can be undertaken. If an outbreak is documented, then epidemiologic studies should be performed to determine the source, extent of outbreak, and risk factors.

Opinion is divided on the proper course of action if only a single case of Legionnaires' disease is discovered. Many hospital infection control officers would undertake environmental studies if a single nosocomial case of Legionnaires' disease is discovered, because it is common for more such cases to occur with time. For single community-acquired cases affecting immunosuppressed patients, environmental investigation of the home and work environment might be indicated, to prevent reinfection. Opinion is also divided on the advisability of hospital environmental culturing in the absence of documented nosocomial Legionnaires' disease. This is because of the common finding of legionellae in the aqueous environment; 30 to 80% of all hospital cooling towers or potable water supplies are contaminated with *Legionella*. Many would rather focus on the institution of routine maintenance schedules and installation of drift eliminators for cooling towers, and on the strict avoidance of use of tap water for respiratory therapy, including washing tubing or nebulizers without subsequent sterilization. However, many view the presence of *Legionella*-contaminated water or cooling towers as a medical liability that is remediable, albeit at high cost.

We suggest that hospitals ascertain that the water and air supplying wards containing highly immunosuppressed patients be *Legionella*-free if possible. There appears to be little to no correlation with the concentrations of *L. pneumophila* in environmental sites and the likelihood of Legionnaires' disease, so it is difficult to base any decision regarding remediation solely on organism concentration alone. Most would agree, however, that *L. pneumophila* concentrations greater than 10^8 CFU per liter represent more of a hazard than do lower concentrations. The percentage of positive sites has been demonstrated to be predictive of nosocomial transmission at one hospital.

Remediation of *Legionella*-contaminated cooling towers and potable water systems can be exceptionally difficult and expensive. Approaches that have been successful include chlorination, pasteurization, and modification of plumbing to eliminate blind loops and heating of cold water (55,80,113,140,141,165). It might be advisable for cooling tower maintenance workers to wear respirators when using high-pressure equipment to clean cooling towers. Almost always, engineering expertise is required for successful remediation.

Several techniques can be used to isolate legionellae from water. In almost all cases, except for the most grossly contaminated water specimens, isolation of legionellae can be done using selective media; the yield for potable water specimens is better with selective media than with animal inoculation (24,59,185).

REFERENCES

1. Aguero-Rosenfeld, M.E., and Edelstein, P.H. (1988): Retrospective evaluation of the Du Pont radioimmunoassay kit for detection of *Legionella pneumophila* serogroup 1 antigenuria in humans. *J. Clin. Microbiol.*, 26:1775–1778.
2. Alary, M., and Joly, J.R. (1991): Risk factors for contamination of domestic hot water systems by *Legionellae*. *Appl. Environ. Microbiol.*, 57:2360–2367.
3. Ampel, N.M., Ruben, F.L., and Norden, C.W. (1985): Cutaneous abscess caused by *Legionella micdadei* in an immunosuppressed patient. *Ann. Intern. Med.*, 102:630–632.
4. Arnouts, P.J., Ramael, M.R., Ysebaert, D.K., et al. (1991): *Legionella pneumophila* peritonitis in a kidney transplant patient. *Scand. J. Infect. Dis.*, 23:119–122.
5. Arnow, P.M., Chou, T., Weil, D., Shapiro, E.N., and Kretzschmar, C. (1982): Nosocomial Legionnaires' disease caused by aerosolized tap water from respiratory devices. *J. Infect. Dis.*, 146:460–467.
6. Arnow, P.M., Weil, D., Para, M.F. (1985): Prevalence and significance of *Legionella pneumophila* contamination of residential hot tap water systems. *J. Infect. Dis.*, 152:145–151.
7. Badenoch, J. (1986): *First Report of the Committee of Inquiry into the Outbreak of Legionnaires' Disease in Stafford in April 1985.* Her Majesty's Stationery Office, London.
8. Baine, W.B. (1985): Cytolytic and phospholipase C activity in *Legionella* species. *J. Gen. Microbiol.*, 131:1383–1391.
9. Balows, A., and Fraser, D.W. (Editors) (1979): International symposium on Legionnaires' disease. *Ann. Intern. Med.*, 90:481–714.
10. Band, J.D., LaVenture, M., Davis, J.P., et al. (1981): Epidemic Legionnaires' disease: airborne transmission down a chimney. *J.A.M.A.*, 245:2404–2407.

11. Barker, J., Brown, M.R., Collier, P.J., Farrell, I., and Gilbert, P. (1992): Relationship between *Legionella pneumophila* and *Acanthamoeba polyphaga:* physiological status and susceptibility to chemical inactivation. *Appl. Environ. Microbiol.*, 58:2420–2425.

12. Bartlett, C.L.R. (1981): *Facts and Theories on Legionnaires' Disease*. Secretariat, Industrial Water Society, Tamworth, England.

13. Bartlett, C.L.R., Macrae, A.D., and Macfarlane, J.T. (1986): Legionella *Infections*, pp. 1–163. E. Arnold, Baltimore, Md.

14. Bartlett, C.L.R., Swann, R.A., Casal, J., Canada Royo, L., and Taylor, A.G. (1984): Recurrent Legionnaires' disease from a hotel water system. In: *Legionella,* edited by C. Thornsberry, A. Balows, J.C. Feeley, and W. Jakubowski, pp. 237–239. Proceedings of the 2nd International Symposium, American Society for Microbiology, Washington, D.C.

15. Baskerville, A., Conlan, J.W., Ashworth, L.A., and Dowsett, A.B. (1986): Pulmonary damage caused by a protease from *Legionella pneumophila*. *Br. J. Exp. Pathol.*, 67:527–536.

16. Beaty, H.N., Miller, A.A., Broome, C.V., Goings, S., and Phillips, C.A. (1978): Legionnaires' disease in Vermont, May to October 1977. *J.A.M.A.*, 240:127–131.

17. Benson, R.F., Thacker, W.L., Fang, F.C., Kanter, B., Mayberry, W.R., and Brenner, D.J. (1990): *Legionella sainthelensi* serogroup 2 isolated from patients with pneumonia. *Res. Microbiol.*, 141:453–463.

18. Benson, R.F., Thacker, W.L., Lanser, J.A., Sangster, N., Mayberry, W.R., and Brenner, D.J. (1991): *Legionella adelaidensis*, a new species isolated from cooling tower water. *J. Clin. Microbiol.*, 29:1004–1006.

19. Benson, R.F., Thacker, W.L., Waters, R.P., et al. (1989): *Legionella quinlivanii* sp. nov. isolated from water. *Curr. Microbiol.*, 18:195–197.

20. Bhopal, R.S., Diggle, P., and Rowlingson, B. (1992): Pinpointing clusters of apparently sporadic cases of Legionnaires' disease. *Br. Med. J.*, 304:1022–1027.

21. Bhopal, R.S., and Fallon, R.J. (1991): Variation in time and space of non-outbreak Legionnaires' disease in Scotland. *Epidemiol. Infect.*, 106:45–61.

22. Bhopal, R.S., Fallon, R.J., Buist, E.C., Black, R.J., and Urquhart, J.D. (1991): Proximity of the home to a cooling tower and risk of non-outbreak Legionnaires' disease. *Br. Med. J.*, 302:378–383.

23. Bollin, G.E., Plouffe, J.F., Para, M.F., and Hackman, B. (1985): Aerosols containing *Legionella pneumophila* generated by shower heads and hot-water faucets. *Appl. Environ. Microbiol.*, 50:1128–1131.

24. Bopp, C.A., Sumner, J.W., Morris, G.K., and Wells, J.G. (1981): Isolation of *Legionella* spp from environmental water samples by low-pH treatment and use of a selective medium. *J. Clin. Microbiol.*, 13:714–719.

25. Bornstein, N., Janin, N., Bourguignon, G., Surgot, M., and Fleurette, J. (1987): Prevalence of anti-*Legionella* antibodies in a healthy population and in patients with tuberculosis or pneumonia. *Pathol. Biol.* (Paris), 35:353–356.

26. Bornstein, N., Marmet, D., Surgot, M., et al. (1989): *Legionella gratiana* sp. nov. isolated from French spa water. *Res. Microbiol.*, 140:541–552.

27. Boswell, T.C., and Kudesia, G. (1992): Serological cross-reaction between *Legionella pneumophila* and campylobacter in the indirect fluorescent antibody test. *Epidemiol. Infect.*, 109:291–295.

28. Brady, M.T. (1989): Nosocomial Legionnaires' disease in a children's hospital. *J. Pediatr.*, 115:46–50.

29. Breiman, R.F., Cozen, W., Fields, B.S., et al. (1990): Role of air sampling in investigation of an outbreak of Legionnaires' disease associated with exposure to aerosols from an evaporative condenser. *J. Infect. Dis.* 161:1257–1261.

30. Breiman, R.F., Fields, B.S., Sanden, G.N., Volmer, L., Meier, A., and Spika, J.S. (1990): Association of shower use with Legionnaires' disease. Possible role of amoebae. *J.A.M.A.*, 263:2924–2926.

31. Brenner, D.J., Steigerwalt, A.G., Gorman, G.W., et al. (1985): Ten new species of *Legionella*. *Int. J. Syst. Bacteriol.*, 35:50–59.

32. Brooks, R.G., Hofflin, J.M., Jamieson, S.W., Stinson, E.B., and Remington, J.S. (1985): Infectious complications in heart-lung transplant recipients. *Am. J. Med.*, 79:412–422.

33. Broome, C.V., and Fraser, D.W. (1979): Epidemiologic aspects of legionellosis. *Epidemiol. Rev.*, 1:1–16.

34. Brown, A., Yu, V.L., Elder, E.M., Magnussen, M.H., and Kroboth, F. (1980): Nosocomial outbreak of Legionnaire's disease at the Pittsburgh Veterans Administration Medical Center. *Trans. Assoc. Am. Physicians*, 93:52–59.

35. Bull, P.W., Scott, J.T., and Breathnach, S.M. (1987): Henoch-Schonlein purpura associated with Legionnaires' disease. *Br. Med. J. (Clin. Res. Ed.)*, 294:220.

36. Byrd, T.F., and Horwitz, M.A. (1989): Interferon gamma-activated human monocytes downregulate transferrin receptors and inhibit the intracellular multiplication of *Legionella pneumophila* by limiting the availability of iron. *J. Clin. Invest.*, 83:1457–1465.

37. Byrd, T.F., and Horwitz, M.A. (1991): Lactoferrin inhibits or promotes *Legionella pneumophila* intracellular multiplication in nonactivated and interferon gamma–activated human monocytes depending upon its degree of iron saturation. Iron-lactoferrin and nonphysiologic iron chelates reverse monocyte activation against *Legionella pneumophila*. *J. Clin. Invest.*, 88:1103–1112.

38. Carlson, N.C., Kuskie, M.R., Dobyns, E.L., Wheeler, M.C., Roe, M.H., and Abzug, M.J. (1990): Legionellosis in children: an expanding spectrum. *Pediatr. Infect. Dis. J.*, 9:133–137.

39. Cases, A., Ferrer, A., Montoliu, J., Torres, A., and Torras, A. (1987): Insuficiencia renal aguda en el enfermedad del legionario. Descripcion de 2 casos y revision de la literatura. *Enferm. Infec. Microbiol. Clin.*, 5:296–300.

40. Castellani Pastoris, M., Benedetti, P., Greco, D., et al. (1992): Six cases of travel-associated Legionnaires' disease in Ischia involving four countries. *Infection*, 20:73–77.

41. Chandler, F.W., Hicklin, M.D., and Blackmon, J.A. (1977): Demonstration of the agent of Legionnaires' disease in tissue. *N. Engl. J. Med.*, 297:1218–1220.

42. Chereshsky, A.Y., and Bettelheim, K.A. (1986): Infections due to *Legionella sainthelensi* in New Zealand [letter]. *N.Z. Med. J.*, 99:335.

43. Cianciotto, N., Eisenstein, B.I., Engleberg, N.C., and Shuman, H. (1989): Genetics and molecular pathogenesis of *Legionella pneumophila*, an intracellular parasite of macrophages. *Mol. Biol. Med.*, 6:409–424.

44. Cianciotto, N.P., Eisenstein, B.I., Mody, C.H., and Engleberg, N.C. (1990): A mutation in the mip gene results in an attenuation of *Legionella pneumophila* virulence. *J. Infect. Dis.*, 162:121–126.

45. Cianciotto, N.P., Eisenstein, B.I., Mody, C.H., Toews, G.B., and Engleberg, N.C. (1989): A *Legionella pneumophila* gene encoding a species-specific surface protein potentiates initiation of intracellular infection. *Infect. Immun.*, 57:1255–1262.

46. Ciesielski, C.A., Blaser, M.J., and Wang, W.L. (1984): Role of stagnation and obstruction of water flow in isolation of *Legionella pneumophila* from hospital plumbing. *Appl. Environ. Microbiol.*, 48:984–987.

47. Claesson, B.A., Trollfors, B., Brolin, I., et al. (1989): Etiology of community-acquired pneumonia in children based on antibody responses to bacterial and viral antigens. *Pediatr. Infect. Dis. J.*, 8:856–862.

48. Conlan, J.W., Baskerville, A., and Ashworth, L.A. (1986): Separation of *Legionella pneumophila* proteases and purification of a protease which produces lesions like those of Legionnaires' disease in guinea pig lung. *J. Gen. Microbiol.*, 132:1565–1574.

49. Cutz, E., Thorner, P.S., Rao, C.P., Toma, S., Gold, R., and Gelfand, E.W. (1982): Disseminated *Legionella pneumophila* infection in an infant with severe combined immunodeficiency. *J. Pediatr.*, 100:760–762.

50. Davis, G.S., Winn, W.C., Jr., Gump, D.W., and Beaty, H.N. (1983): The kinetics of early inflammatory events during experimental pneumonia due to *Legionella pneumophila* in guinea pigs. *J. Infect. Dis.*, 148:823–835.

51. Davis, G.S., Winn, W.C., Jr., Gump, D.W., Craighead, J.E., and Beaty, H.N. (1982): Legionnaires' pneumonia after aerosol exposure in guinea pigs and rats. *Am. Rev. Respir. Dis.*, 126:1050–1057.

52. de Lalla, F., Rossini, G., Giannattasio, G., Giura, R., Nessi, G., and Santoro, D. (1980): Legionnaires' disease in an Italian hotel [letter]. *Lancet*, 2:1187.

53. Dietrich, P.A., Johnson, R.D., Fairbank, J.T., and Walke, J.S. (1978): The chest radiograph in Legionnaires' disease. *Radiology*, 127:577–582.

54. Domingo, C., Roig, J., Planas, F., Bechini, J., Tenesa, M., and Morera, J. (1991): Radiographic appearance of nosocomial Legionnaires' disease after erythromycin treatment. *Thorax*, 46:663–666.

55. Dondero, T.J., Jr., Rendtorff, R.C., Mallison, G.F., et al. (1980): An outbreak of Legionnaires' disease associated with a contaminated air-conditioning cooling tower. *N. Engl. J. Med.*, 302:365–370.

56. Dournon, E., Bure, A., Kemeny, J.L., Pourriat, J.L., and Valeyre, D. (1982): *Legionella pneumophila* peritonitis [letter]. *Lancet*, 1:1363.

57. Dowling, J.N., Saha, A.K., and Glew, R.H. (1992): Virulence factors of the family Legionellaceae. *Microbiol. Rev.*, 56:32–60.

58. Edelstein, P.H. (1981): Improved semiselective medium for isolation of *Legionella pneumophila* from contaminated clinical and environmental specimens. *J. Clin. Microbiol.*, 14:298–303.

59. Edelstein, P.H. (1982): Comparative study of selective media for isolation of *Legionella pneumophila* from potable water. *J. Clin. Microbiol.*, 16:697–699.

60. Edelstein, P.H. (1987): The laboratory diagnosis of Legionnaires' disease. *Sem. Respir. Infect.*, 2:235–241.

61. Edelstein, P.H. (1990): Use of DNA probes for the diagnosis of infections caused by *Mycoplasma pneumoniae* and Legionellae: a review. *Adv. Exp. Med. Biol.*, 263:57–69.

62. Edelstein, P.H. (1992): Detection of antibodies to *Legionella*. In: *Manual of Clinical Laboratory*

Immunology, 4th Edition, edited by N.R. Rose, E.C. de Macario, J.L. Fahey, H. Friedman, and G.M. Penn, pp. 459–466. American Society for Microbiology, Washington, D.C.

63. Edelstein, P.H., Beer, K.B., Sturge, J.C., Watson, A.J., and Goldstein, L.C. (1985): Clinical utility of a monoclonal direct fluorescent reagent specific for *Legionella pneumophila:* comparative study with other reagents. *J. Clin. Microbiol.,* 22:419–421.

64. Edelstein, P.H., Bryan, R.N., Enns, R.K., Kohne, D.E., and Kacian, D.L. (1987): Retrospective study of Gen-Probe rapid diagnostic system for detection of legionellae in frozen clinical respiratory tract samples. *J. Clin. Microbiol.,* 25:1022–1026.

65. Edelstein, P.H., Calarco, K., and Yasui, V.K. (1984): Antimicrobial therapy of experimentally induced Legionnaires' disease in guinea pigs. *Am. Rev. Respir. Dis.,* 130:849–856.

66. Edelstein, P.H., and Edelstein, M.A. (1991): *In vitro* activity of azithromycin against clinical isolates of *Legionella* species. *Antimicrob. Agents Chemother.,* 35:180–181.

67. Edelstein, P.H., McKinney, R.M., Meyer, R.D., Edelstein, M.A., Krause, C.J., and Finegold, S.M. (1980): Immunologic diagnosis of Legionnaires' disease: cross-reactions with anaerobic and microaerophilic organisms and infections caused by them. *J. Infect. Dis.,* 141:652–655.

68. Edelstein, P.H., Meyer, R.D., and Finegold, S.M. (1980): Laboratory diagnosis of Legionnaires' disease. *Am. Rev. Respir. Dis.,* 121:317–327.

69. Edelstein, P.H., Meyer, R.D., and Finegold, S.M. (1981): Long-term follow-up of two patients with pulmonary cavitation caused by *Legionella pneumophila. Am. Rev. Respir. Dis.,* 124:90–93.

70. Edelstein, P.H., Nakahama, C., Tobin, J.O., et al. (1986): Paleoepidemiologic investigation of Legionnaires' disease at Wadsworth Veterans Administration Hospital by using three typing methods for comparison of legionellae from clinical and environmental sources. *J. Clin. Microbiol.,* 23:1121–1126.

71. England, A.C., Fraser, D.W., Plikaytis, B.D., Tsai, T.F., Storch, G., and Broome, C.V. (1981): Sporadic legionellosis in the United States: the first thousand cases. *Ann. Intern. Med.,* 94:164–170.

72. England, A.C., McKinney, R.M., Skaliy, P., and Gorman, G.W. (1980): A fifth serogroup of *Legionella pneumophila. Ann. Intern. Med.,* 93:58–59.

73. Ephros, M., Engelhard, D., Maayan, S., Bercovier, H., Avital, A., and Yatsiv, I. (1989): *Legionella gormanii* pneumonia in a child with chronic granulomatous disease. *Pediatr. Infect. Dis. J.,* 8:726–727.

74. Fain, J.S., Bryan, R.N., Cheng, L., Lewin, K.J., Porter, D.D., and Grody, W.W. (1991): Rapid diagnosis of *Legionella* infection by a nonisotopic *in situ* hybridization method. *Am. J. Clin. Pathol.,* 95:719–724.

75. Falcó, V., Fernández de Sevilla, T., Alegre, J., Ferrer, A., and Martínez, V. (1991): *Legionella pneumophila:* a cause of severe community-acquired pneumonia. *Chest,* 100:1007–1011.

76. Fang, G.D., Fine, M., Orloff, J., et al. (1990): New and emerging etiologies for community-acquired pneumonia with implications for therapy: a prospective multicenter study of 359 cases. *Medicine* (Baltimore), 69:307–316.

77. Fang, G.D., Yu, V.L., and Vickers, R.M. (1989): Disease due to the Legionellaceae (other than *Legionella pneumophila*): historical, microbiological, clinical, and epidemiological review. *Medicine* (Baltimore), 68:116–132 [published erratum appears in *Medicine* (Baltimore), 68(4)(July 1989):209].

78. Fenstersheib, M.D., Miller, M., Diggins, C., et al. (1990): Outbreak of Pontiac fever due to *Legionella anisa. Lancet,* 336:35–37.

79. Fenves, A.Z. (1985): Legionnaires' disease associated with acute renal failure: a report of two cases and review of the literature. *Clin. Nephrol.,* 23:96–100.

80. Fisher-Hoch, S.P., Bartlett, C.L., Tobin, J.O., et al. (1981): Investigation and control of an outbreak of Legionnaires' disease in a district general hospital. *Lancet,* 1:932–936.

81. Fliermans, C.B., Cherry, W.B., Orrison, L.H., Smith, S.J., Tison, D.L., and Pope, D.H. (1981): Ecological distribution of *Legionella pneumophila. Appl. Environ. Microbiol.,* 41:9–16.

82. Fogliani, J., Domenget, J.F., Hohn, B., Merignargues, G., and Bornstein, N. (1982): Maladie des légionnaires avec localisation digestive: une observation. *Nouv. Presse. Med.,* 11:2699–2702.

83. Foltzer, M.A., and Reese, R.E. (1985): Massive diarrhea in *Legionella micdadei* pneumonitis. *J. Clin. Gastroenterol.,* 7:525–527.

84. Foy, H.M., Broome, C.V., Hayes, P.S., Allan, I., Cooney, M.K., and Tobe, R. (1979): Legionnaires' disease in a prepaid medical-care group in Seattle, 1963–1975. *Lancet,* 1:767–770.

85. Fraser, D.W., Tsai, T.R., Orenstein, W., et al. (1977): Legionnaires' disease: description of an epidemic of pneumonia. *N. Engl. J. Med.,* 297:1189–1197.

86. Friedland, L., Snydman, D.R., Weingarden, A.S., Hedges, T.R., Brown, R., and Busky, M. (1984): Ocular and pericardial involvement in Legionnaires' disease. *Am. J. Med.,* 77:1105–1107.

87. Friedman, H.M. (1978): Legionnaires' disease in non-Legionnaires: a report of five cases. *Ann. Intern. Med.,* 88:294–302.

88. Friedman, S., Spitalny, K., Barbaree, J., Faur, Y., and McKinney, R. (1987): Pontiac fever outbreak associated with a cooling tower. *Am. J. Public Health*, 77:568–572.
89. Gabbay, J. (1988): *Broadcasting House Legionnaires' Disease. Report of the Westminster Action Committee Convened to Co-ordinate the Investigation and Control of the Outbreak of Legionnaires' Disease Associated with Portland Place, London W1 in April/May 1988.* Department of Public Health, Parkside District Health Authority, London.
90. Garbe, P.L., Davis, B.J., Weisfeld, J.S., et al. (1985): Nosocomial Legionnaires' disease: epidemiologic demonstration of cooling towers as a source. *J.A.M.A.*, 254:521–524.
91. Gerber, J.E., Casey, C.A., Martin, P., and Winn, W.C., Jr. (1981): Legionnaires' disease in Vermont, 1972–1976. *Am. J. Clin. Pathol.*, 76:816–818.
92. Girod, J.C., Reichman, R.C., Winn, W.C., Jr., Klaucke, D.N., Vogt, R.L., and Dolin, R. (1982): Pneumonic and nonpneumonic forms of legionellosis: the result of a common-source exposure to *Legionella pneumophila*. *Arch. Intern. Med.*, 142:545–547.
93. Goldstein, J.D., Keller, J.L., Winn, W.C., Jr., and Myerowitz, R.L. (1982): Sporadic Legionellaceae pneumonia in renal transplant recipients: a survey of 70 autopsies, 1964 to 1979. *Arch. Pathol. Lab. Med.*, 106:108–111.
94. Granados, A., Podzamczer, D., Gudiol, F., and Manresa, F. (1989): Pneumonia due to *Legionella pneumophila* and pneumococcal pneumonia: similarities and differences on presentation. *Eur. Respir. J.*, 2:130–134.
95. Griffith, M.E., Lindquist, D.S., Benson, R.F., Thacker, W.L., Brenner, D.J., and Wilkinson, H.W. (1988): First isolation of *Legionella gormanii* from human disease. *J. Clin. Microbiol.*, 26:380–381.
96. Grist, N.R., Reid, D., and Najera, R. (1979): Legionnaires' disease and the traveller. *Ann. Intern. Med.*, 90:563–564.
97. Harris, L.F. (1981): Legionnaires' disease associated with acute encephalomyelitis. *Arch. Neurol.*, 38:462–463.
98. Hedlund, K.W. (1981): *Legionella* toxin. *Pharmacol. Ther.* 15:123–130.
99. Helms, C.M., Massanari, R.M., Zeitler, R., et al. (1983): Legionnaires' disease associated with a hospital water system: a cluster of 24 nosocomial cases. *Ann. Intern. Med.*, 99:172–178.
100. Herwaldt, L.A., Gorman, G.W., McGrath, T., et al. (1984): A new *Legionella* species, *Legionella feeleii* species nova, causes Pontiac fever in an automobile plant. *Ann. Intern. Med.* 100:333–338.
101. Hohl, P., Buser, U., and Frei, R. (1992): Fatal *Legionella pneumophila* pneumonia: treatment failure despite early sequential oral-parenteral amoxicillin-clavulanic acid therapy. *Infection*, 20:99–100.
102. Horwitz, M.A. (1992): Interactions between macrophages and *Legionella pneumophila*. *Curr. Top. Microbiol. Immunol.*, 181:265–282.
103. Horwitz, M.A., and Silverstein, S.C. (1981): Activated human monocytes inhibit the intracellular multiplication of Legionnaires' disease bacteria. *J. Exp. Med.* 154:1618–1635.
104. Hürter, T., Rumpelt, H.J., and Ferlinz, R. (1992): Fibrosing alveolitis responsive to corticosteroids following Legionnaires' disease pneumonia. *Chest*, 101:281–283.
105. Jaulhac, B., Nowicki, M., Bornstein, N., et al. (1992): Detection of *Legionella* spp in bronchoalveolar lavage fluids by DNA amplification. *J. Clin. Microbiol.*, 30:920–924.
106. Johnson, J.D., Hand, W.L. Francis, J.B., King-Thompson, N., and Corwin, R.W. (1980): Antibiotic uptake by alveolar macrophages. *J. Lab. Clin. Med.*, 95:429–439.
107. Joly, J. (1985): *Legionella* and domestic water heaters in the Quebec City area. *Can. Med. Assoc. J.* 132:160.
108. Joly, J.R., Boissinot, M., Duchaine, J., et al. (1984): Ecological distribution of Legionellaceae in the Quebec City area. *Can. J. Microbiol.*, 30:63–67.
109. Joly, J.R., Déry, P., Gauvreau, L., Coté, L., and Trépanier, C. (1986): Legionnaires' disease caused by *Legionella dumoffii* in distilled water. *Can. Med. Assoc. J.*, 135:1274–1277.
110. Joly, J.R., and Winn, W.C. (1984): Correlation of subtypes of *Legionella pneumophila* defined by monoclonal antibodies with epidemiological classification of cases and environmental sources. *J. Infect. Dis.*, 150:667–671.
111. Jones, G.L., and Hébert, G.A. (1978): *"Legionnaires': The Disease, the Bacterium, and Methodology*, pp. 1–25. Centers for Disease Control, Atlanta, Ga.
112. Kalweit, W.H., Winn, W.C., Jr., Rocco, T.A., Jr., and Girod, J.C. (1982): Hemodialysis fistula infections caused by *Legionella pneumophila*. *Ann. Intern. Med.*, 96:173–175.
113. Kaufmann, A.F., McDade, J.E., Patton, C.M., et al. (1981): Pontiac fever: isolation of the etiologic agent *(Legionella pneumophila)* and demonstration of its mode of transmission. *Am. J. Epidemiol.*, 114:337–347.
114. Khardori, N., Haron, E., and Rolston, K. (1987): *Legionella micdadei* pneumonia in the acquired immune deficiency syndrome [letter]. *Am. J. Med.*, 83:600–601.
115. Kilvington, S., and Price, J. (1990): Survival of *Legionella pneumophila* within cysts of *Acanthamoeba polyphaga* following chlorine exposure. *J. Appl. Bacteriol.*, 68:519–525.

116. Kirby, B.D., Peck, H., and Meyer, R.D. (1979): Radiographic features of Legionnaires' disease. *Chest,* 76:562–565.

117. Kirby, B.D., Snyder, K.M., Meyer, R.D., and Finegold, S.M. (1980): Legionnaires' disease: report of sixty-five nosocomially acquired cases, review of the literature. *Medicine* (Baltimore), 59:188–205.

118. Klaucke, D.N., Vogt, R.L., LaRue, D., et al. (1984): Legionnaires' disease: the epidemiology of two outbreaks in Burlington, Vermont, 1980. *Am. J. Epidemiol.,* 119:382–391.

119. Lee, T.C., Stout, J.E., and Yu, V.L. (1988): Factors predisposing to *Legionella pneumophila* colonization in residential water systems. *Arch. Environ. Health,* 43:59–62.

120. Lessons from Stafford [editorial] (1986): *Lancet,* 1:1363–1364.

121. Lochner, J.E., Bigley, R.H., and Iglewski, B.H. (1985): Defective triggering of polymorphonuclear leukocyte oxidative metabolism by *Legionella pneumophila* toxin. *J. Infect. Dis.,* 151:42–46.

122. Lowry, P.W., Blankenship, R.J., Gridley, W., Troup, N.J., and Tompkins, L.S. (1991): A cluster of *Legionella* sternal-wound infections due to postoperative topical exposure to contaminated tap water. *N. Engl. J. Med.,* 324:109–113.

123. Lucas, R.S., Kuzmowych, T.V., and Spagnolo, S.V. (1991): *Legionella* pneumonia presenting as a bulging fissure on chest roentgenogram. *Chest,* 100:567–568.

124. Lück, P.C., Helbig, J.H., Wunderlich, E., et al. (1989): Isolation of *Legionella pneumophila* serogroup 3 from pericardial fluid in a case of pericarditis. *Infection,* 17:388–390.

125. Macfarlane, J.T., Finch, R.G., Ward, M.J., and Macrae, A.D. (1982): Hospital study of adult community-acquired pneumonia. *Lancet,* 2:255–258.

126. Mahoney, F.J., Hoge, C.W., Farley, T.A., et al. (1992): Communitywide outbreak of Legionnaires' disease associated with a grocery store mist machine. *J. Infect. Dis.,* 165:736–739.

127. Marrie, T.J., Haldane, D., MacDonald, S., et al. (1991): Control of endemic nosocomial Legionnaires' disease by using sterile potable water for high-risk patients. *Epidemiol. Infect.,* 107:591–605.

128. Marrie, T.J., MacDonald, S., Clarke, K., and Haldane, D. (1991): Nosocomial Legionnaires' disease: lessons from a four-year prospective study. *Am. J. Infect. Control,* 19:79–85.

129. Marston, B., Plouffe, J., Breiman, R., et al. (1992): Findings of a community-based pneumonia incidence study through November 1991. *Program and Abstracts of the 1992 International Symposium on Legionella,* January 26–29, 1992, Orlando, Florida. American Society for Microbiology, Washington, D.C. [Abstract 7].

130. Martinez, E., Domingo, P., and Ruiz, D. (1991): Transient aplastic anaemia associated with Legionnaires' disease [letter]. *Lancet,* 338:264.

131. Mastro, T.D., Fields, B.S., Breiman, R.F., Campbell, J., Plikaytis, B.D., and Spika, J.S. (1991): Nosocomial Legionnaires' disease and use of medication nebulizers. *J. Infect. Dis.,* 163:667–671.

132. McCabe, R.E., Baldwin, J.C., McGregor, C.A., Miller, D.C., and Vosti, K.L. (1984): Prosthetic valve endocarditis caused by *Legionella pneumophila.* *Ann. Intern. Med.* 100:525–527.

133. McDade, J.E., Shepard, C.C., Fraser, D.W., Tsai, T.R., Redus, M.A., and Dowdle, W.R. (1977): Legionnaires' disease: isolation of a bacterium and demonstration of its role in other respiratory disease. *N. Engl. J. Med.,* 297:1197–1203.

134. McKinney, R.M., Wilkinson, H.W., Sommers, H.M., et al. (1980): *Legionella pneumophila* serogroup six: isolation from cases of legionellosis, identification by immunofluorescence staining, and immunological response to infection. *J. Clin. Microbiol.,* 12:395–401.

135. Meenhorst, P.L., Reingold, A.L., Groothuis, D.G., et al. (1985): Water-related nosocomial pneumonia caused by *Legionella pneumophila* serogroups 1 and 10. *J. Infect. Dis.,* 152:356–364.

136. Meyer, R.D. (1991): Role of the quinolones in the treatment of legionellosis [editorial]. *J. Antimicrob. Chemother.,* 28:623–625.

137. Meyer, R.D., Edelstein, P.H., Kirby, B.D., et al. (1980): Legionnaires' disease: unusual clinical and laboratory features. *Ann. Intern. Med.* 93:240–243.

138. Monforte, R., Cayla, J., Sala, M., et al. (1989): Community outbreak of Legionnaires' disease in Barcelona [letter]. *Lancet,* 1:1011.

139. Morton, S., Bartlett, C.L., Bibby, L.F., Hutchinson, D.N., Dyer, J.V., and Dennis, P.J. (1986): Outbreak of Legionnaires' disease from a cooling water system in a power station. *Br. J. Ind. Med.,* 43:630–635.

140. Muraca, P.W., Stout, J.E., Yu, V.L., and Yee, Y.C. (1988): Legionnaires' disease in the work environment: implications for environmental health. *Am. Ind. Hyg. Assoc. J.,* 49:584–590.

141. Muraca, P.W., Yu, V.L., and Goetz, A. (1990): Disinfection of water distribution systems for *Legionella:* a review of application procedures and methodologies. *Infect. Control Hosp. Epidemiol.,* 11:79–88.

142. Myerowitz, R.L., Pasculle, A.W., Dowling, J.N., et al. (1979): Opportunistic lung infection due to "Pittsburgh pneumonia agent." *N. Engl. J. Med.,* 301:953–958.

143. Nahapetian, K., Challemel, O., Beurtin, D., Dubrou, S., Gounon, P., and Squinazi, F. (1991):

The intracellular multiplication of *Legionella pneumophila* in protozoa from hospital plumbing systems. *Res. Microbiol.*, 142:677–685.

144. Neill, M.A., Gorman, G.W., Gibert, C., et al. (1985): Nosocomial legionellosis, Paris, France: evidence for transmission by potable water. *Am. J. Med.*, 78:581–588.

145. Nelson, D.P., Rensimer, E.R., and Raffin, T.A. (1985): *Legionella pneumophila* pericarditis without pneumonia. *Arch. Intern. Med.* 145:926.

146. Nomura, S., Hatta, K., Iwata, T., and Aihara, M. (1989): *Legionella pneumophila* isolated in pure culture from the ascites of a patient with systemic lupus erythematosus. *Am. J. Med.*, 86: 833–834.

147. Palmer, S.R., Zamiri, I., Ribeiro, C.D., and Gajewska, A. (1986): Legionnaires' disease cluster and reduction in hospital hot water temperatures. *Br. Med. J. (Clin. Res. Ed.)*, 292:1494–1495.

148. Parry, M.F., Stampleman, L., Hutchinson, J.H., Folta, D., Steinberg, M.G., and Krasnogor, L.J. (1985): Waterborne *Legionella bozemanii* and nosocomial pneumonia in immunosuppressed patients. *Ann. Intern. Med.*, 103:205–210.

149. Pasculle, A.W., Veto, G.E., Krystofiak, S., McKelvey, K., and Vrsalovic, K. (1989): Laboratory and clinical evaluation of a commercial DNA probe for the detection of *Legionella* spp. *J. Clin. Microbiol.*, 27:2350–2358.

150. Pastoris, M.C., Berchicci, C., and Pallonari, G. (1992): Isolation of *Legionella pneumophila* serogroup 14 from a human source. *J. Clin. Pathol.* 45:627–628.

151. Peliowski, A., and Finer, N.N. (1986): Intractable seizures in Legionnaires disease. *J. Pediatr.*, 109:657–658.

152. Platzeck, C., Foerster, E.C., Schneider, M.U., et al. (1990): Enzephalitis bei *Legionella-bozemanii*-pneumonie. *Dtsch. Med. Wochenschr.*, 115:1956–1959.

153. Plouffc, J.F., Para, M.F, Maher, W.E., Hackman, B., and Webster, L. (1983): Subtypes of *Legionella pneumophila* serogroup 1 associated with different attack rates. *Lancet*, 2:649–650.

154. Rechnitzer, C., Kharazmi, A., and Nielsen, H. (1986): Effects of *Legionella pneumophila* sonicate on human neutrophil granulocyte and monocyte chemotaxis. *Eur. J. Clin. Invest.*, 16:368–375.

155. Redd, S.C., Schuster, D.M., Quan, J., Plikaytis, B.D., Spika, J.S., and Cohen, M.L. (1988): Legionellosis in cardiac transplant recipients: results of a nationwide survey [letter]. *J. Infect. Dis.*, 158:651–653.

156. Roig, J., Aguilar, X., Ruiz, J., et al. (1991): Comparative study of *Legionella pneumophila* and other nosocomial-acquired pneumonias. *Chest*, 99:344–350.

157. Rosenfeld, J.S., Kueppers, F., Newkirk, T., Tamada, R., Meissler, J.J., Jr., and Eisenstein, T.K. (1986): A protease from *Legionella pneumophila* with cytotoxic and dermal ulcerative activity. *FEMS Microbiol. Letters*, 37:51–58.

158. Rosmini, F., Castellani-Pastoris, M., Mazzotti, M.F., et al. (1984): Febrile illness in successive cohorts of tourists at a hotel on the Italian Adriatic coast: evidence for a persistent focus of *Legionella* infection. Am. J. Epidemiol., 119:124–134.

159. Rowbotham, T.J. (1986): Current views on the relationships between amoebae, legionellae and man. *Isr. J. Med. Sci.*, 22:678–689.

160. Saito, A., Koga, H., Shigeno, H., et al. (1986): The antimicrobial activity of ciprofloxacin against *Legionella* species and the treatment of experimental *Legionella* pneumonia in guinea pigs. *J. Antimicrob. Chemother.*, 18:251–260.

161. Sathapatayavongs, B., Kohler, R.B., Wheat, L.J., et al. (1982): Rapid diagnosis of Legionnaires' disease by urinary antigen detection. Comparison of ELISA and radioimmunoassay. *Am. J. Med.*, 72:576–582.

162. Sato, P., Madtes, D.K., Thorning, D., and Albert, R.K. (1985): Bronchiolitis obliterans caused by *Legionella pneumophila*. *Chest*, 87:840–842.

163. Schlanger, G., Lutwick, L.I., Kurzman, M., Hoch, B., and Chandler, F.W. (1984): Sinusitis caused by *Legionella pneumophila* in a patient with the acquired immune deficiency syndrome. *Am. J. Med.*, 77:957–960.

164. Serota, A.I., Meyer, R.D., Wilson, S.E., Edelstein, P.H., and Finegold, S.M. (1981): Legionnaires' disease in the postoperative patient. *J. Surg. Res.*, 30:417–427.

165. Shands, K.N., Ho, J.L., Meyer, R.D., et al. (1985): Potable water as a source of Legionnaires' disease. *J.A.M.A.*, 253:1412–1416.

166. Steele, T.W., Lanser, J., and Sangster, N. (1990): Isolation of *Legionella longbeachae* serogroup 1 from potting mixes. *Appl. Environ. Microbiol.*, 56:49–53.

167. Steele, T.W., Moore, C.V., and Sangster, N. (1990): Distribution of *Legionella longbeachae* serogroup 1 and other legionellae in potting soils in Australia. *Appl. Environ. Microbiol.*, 56: 2984–2988.

168. Stout, J., Yu, V.L., Vickers, R.M., and Shonnard, J. (1982): Potable water supply as the hosptial reservoir for Pittsburgh pneumonia agent. *Lancet*, 1:471–472.

169. Stout, J.E., Yu, V.L., Muraca, P., Joly, J., Troup, N., and Tompkins, L.S. (1992): Potable water as a cause of sporadic cases of community-acquired Legionnaires' disease. *N. Engl. J. Med.*, 326:151–155.

170. Struelens, M.J., Maes, N., Rost, F., et al. (1992): Genotypic and phenotypic methods for the investigation of a nosocomial *Legionella pneumophila* outbreak and efficacy of control measures. *J. Infect. Dis.,* 166:22–30.

171. Tang, P.W., Toma, S., and MacMillan, L.G. (1985): *Legionella oakridgensis:* laboratory diagnosis of a human infection. *J. Clin. Microbiol.,* 21:462–463.

172. Tenover, F.C., Edelstein, P.H., Goldstein, L.C., Sturge, J.C., and Plorde, J.J. (1986): Comparison of cross-staining reactions by *Pseudomonas* spp and fluorescein-labeled polyclonal and monoclonal antibodies directed against *Legionella pneumophila. J. Clin. Microbiol.,* 23: 647–649.

173. Thacker, S.B., Bennett, J.V., Tsai, T.F., et al. (1978): An outbreak in 1965 of severe respiratory illness caused by the Legionnaires' disease bacterium. *J. Infect. Dis.,* 138:512–519.

174. Thacker, W.L., Benson, R.F., Hawes, L., et al. (1991): *Legionella fairfieldensis* sp nov. isolated from cooling tower waters in Australia. *J. Clin. Microbiol.,* 29:475–478.

175. Thacker, W.L., Benson, R.F., Schifman, R.B., et al. (1989): *Legionella tucsonensis* sp nov. isolated from a renal transplant recipient. *J. Clin. Microbiol.,* 27:1831–1834.

176. Thacker, W.L., Benson, R.F., Staneck, J.L., et al. (1988): *Legionella cincinnatiensis* sp nov. isolated from a patient with pneumonia. *J. Clin. Microbiol.,* 26:418–420.

177. Thacker, W.L., Dyke, J.W., Benson, R.F., et al. (1992): *Legionella lansingensis* sp nov. isolated from a patient with pneumonia and underlying chronic lymphocytic leukemia. *J. Clin. Microbiol.,* 30:2398–2401.

178. Thacker, W.L., Wilkinson, H.W., Benson, R.F., and Brenner, D.J. (1987): *Legionella pneumophila* serogroup 12 isolated from human and environmental sources. *J. Clin. Microbiol.,* 25:569–570.

179. Thacker, W.L., Wilkinson, H.W., Benson, R.F., Edberg, S.C., and Brenner, D.J. (1988): *Legionella jordanis* isolated from a patient with fatal pneumonia. *J. Clin. Microbiol.,* 26:1400–1401.

180. Thomason, B.M., Harris, P.P., Hicklin, M.D., Blackmon, J.A., Moss, W., and Matthews, F. (1979): A *Legionella*-like bacterium related to WIGA in a fatal case of pneumonia. *Ann. Intern. Med.,* 91:673–676.

181. Tobin, J.O., Beare, J., Dunnill, M.S., et al. (1980): Legionnaires' disease in a transplant unit: isolation of the causative agent from shower baths. *Lancet,* 2:118–121.

182. Tokunaga, Y., Concepcion, W., Berquist, W.E., et al. (1992): Graft involvement by *Legionella* in a liver transplant recipient. *Arch. Surg.,* 127:475–477.

183. Tompkins, L.S., Roessler, B.J., Redd, S.C., Markowitz, L.E., and Cohen, M.L. *Legionella* prosthetic-valve endocarditis. *N. Engl. J. Med.,* 318:530–535.

184. Verma, U.K., Brenner, D.J., Thacker, W.L., et al. *Legionella shakespearei* sp nov., isolated from cooling tower water. *Int. J. Syst. Bacteriol.,* 42:404–407.

185. Wadowsky, R.M., and Yee, R.B. (1981): Glycine-containing selective medium for isolation of Legionellaceae from environmental specimens. *Appl. Environ. Microbiol.,* 42:768–772.

186. Waldor, M.K., Wilson, B., and Swartz, M. (1993): Cellulitis caused by *Legionella pneumophila. Clin. Infect. Dis.,* 16:51–53.

187. Warner, C.L., Fayad, P.B., and Heffner, R.R., Jr. (1991): *Legionella* myositis. *Neurology,* 41:750–752.

188. Wegmüller, E., Weidmann, P., Hess, T., and Reubi, F.C. (1985): Rapidly progressive glomerulonephritis accompanying Legionnaires' disease. *Arch. Intern. Med.,* 145:1711–1713.

189. Wilkinson, H.W., Drasar, V., Thacker, W.L., et al. (1988): *Legionella moravica* sp nov. and *Legionella brunensis* sp nov. isolated from cooling tower water. *Ann. Inst. Pasteur. Microbiol.,* 139:393–402.

190. Wilkinson, H.W., Farshy, C.E., Fikes, B.J., Cruce, D.D., and Yealy, L.P. (1979): Measure of immunoglobulin G-, M-, and A-specific titers against *Legionella pneumophila* and inhibition of titers against nonspecific, gram-negative bacterial antigens in the indirect immunofluorescence test for legionellosis. *J. Clin. Microbiol.,* 10:685–689.

191. Wilkinson, H.W., Thacker, W.L., Benson, R.F., et al. (1987): *Legionella birminghamensis* sp nov. isolated from a cardiac transplant recipient. *J. Clin. Microbiol.,* 25:2120–2122.

192. Wilkinson, H.W., Thacker, W.L., Brenner, D.J., and Ryan, K.J. (1985): Fatal *Legionella maceachernii* pneumonia. *J. Clin. Microbiol.,* 22:1055.

193. Wilkinson, H.W., Thacker, W.L., Steigerwalt, A.G., Brenner, D.J., Ampel, N.M., and Wing, E.J. (1985): Second serogroup of *Legionella hackeliae* isolated from a patient with pneumonia. *J. Clin. Microbiol.,* 22:488–489.

194. Winn, W.C., Jr. (1985): *Legionella* and Legionnaires' disease: a review with emphasis on environmental studies and laboratory diagnosis. *Crit. Rev. Clin. Lab. Sci.,* 21:323–381.

195. Winn, W.C., Jr., Davis, G.S., Gump, D.W., Craighead, J.E., and Beaty, H.N. (1982): Legionnaires' pneumonia after intratracheal inoculation of guinea pigs and rats. *Lab. Invest.,* 47:568–578.

196. Winn, W.C., Jr., and Myerowitz, R.L. (1981): The pathology of the *Legionella* pneumonias: a review of 74 cases and the literature. *Human Pathol.,* 12:401–422.

197. Wise, F., Crane, C., Taylor, S., and Weilerstein, R. (1991): Outbreak of Legionnaires' disease in an office building, Richmond, California, 1991. *Calif. Morbid.,* 15–16.
198. Witt, D.J., Craven, D.E., and McCabe, W.R. (1987): Bacterial infections in adult patients with the acquired immune deficiency syndrome (AIDS) and AIDS-related complex. *Am. J. Med.,* 82:900–906.
199. Woodhead, M.A., and Macfarlane, J.T. (1986): Legionnaires' disease: a review of 79 community-acquired cases in Nottingham. *Thorax,* 41:635–640.
200. Woodhead, M.A., Macfarlane, J.T., McCracken, J.S., Rose, D.H., and Finch, R.G. (1987): Prospective study of the aetiology and outcome of pneumonia in the community. *Lancet,* 1:671–674.
201. Yu, V.L., Kroboth, F.J., Shonnard, J., Brown, A, McDearman, S., and Magnussen, M. (1982): Legionnaires' disease: new clinical perspective from a prospective pneumonia study. *Am. J. Med.,* 73:357–361.

Respiratory Infections: Diagnosis and Management, 3d ed.,
edited by James E. Pennington.
Raven Press, Ltd., New York © 1994

23

Unusual Bacterial Pneumonias Caused by Human Commensal, Environmental, and Animal-Associated Pathogens

Arnold N. Weinberg and Howard M. Heller

*Harvard Medical School and Massachusetts Institute of Technology,
77 Massachusetts Avenue, Cambridge, Massachusetts 02139; and Harvard Medical
School and Massachusetts General Hospital, Boston, Massachusetts 02114*

The lower respiratory tract can be infected by many bacterial species via several routes. The pathophysiologic mechanisms, clinical presentations, and pathology of the diseases produced are limited and predictable. A discussion of pneumonias caused by "unusual bacteria" will, therefore, stress the unique properties of the pathogens including ecologic and epidemiologic characteristics. In this chapter pneumonias caused by *Bacillus anthracis* (anthrax), *Brucella* sp, *Francisella tularensis* (tularemia), *Moraxella (Branhamella) catarrhalis*, *Neisseria meningitidis*, *Pasteurella multocida*, *Pseudomonas pseudomallei* (melioidosis), *Rhodococcus equi,* and *Yersinia pestis* (plague) will be reviewed, with emphasis on their special features.

This group of organisms illustrates the diversity of ecological niches where bacteria that could be pathogens in humans reside. *M. catarrhalis* and *N. meningitidis* stand apart as obligate human parasites that often are commensal or transient members of the normal nasopharyngeal flora. Their importance as pathogens in pneumonia has emerged especially during the past decade. Melioidosis caused by the soil resident *P. pseudomallei* is indigenous to Southeast Asia, and the AIDS epidemic has alerted us to the importance of *R. equi,* a microbe with a predilection for horses, livestock, and their immediate environment. *P. multocida* is a zoonotic pathogen that inhabits the oral cavity of cats and dogs, and thus is closely related to humans via the association of pets with people. The remaining zoonotic organisms rarely cause human disease in the United States. Historically, however, respiratory diseases such as inhalation anthrax ("Woolsorter's Disease") and pneumonic plague (the "Black Death" of medieval times) were important manifestations of epidemic and endemic infections in humans. Worldwide, they still occur sporadically. A death attributable to pneumonic plague after exposure to an infected domestic cat occurred in the United States in August 1992.

PNEUMONIA CAUSED BY OBLIGATE HUMAN COMMENSALS

The majority of bacterial pneumonias are caused by obligate human parasites that are relatively easy to identify morphologically in stained smears from sputum and

485

grow well on appropriate bacteriologic media. Among the less common commensals causing pneumonia, *Neisseria meningitidis* and *Moraxella* (formerly *Branhamella*) *catarrhalis* are pathogens or opportunists that often escape identification in the mixed flora of the respiratory tract and therefore present problems in precise diagnosis and in therapy.

NEISSERIA MENINGITIDIS PNEUMONIA

Definition and Historical Background

Respiratory infections caused by *N. meningitidis* usually occur as acute bronchitis or bronchopneumonia, often complicating an antecedent viral process. Although meningococcal infections were probably first described in the early 1800s as epidemic meningitis with a hemorrhagic rash, there are no specific references to pulmonary disease until 1907. The recognition of the meningococcus as a respiratory pathogen became firmly established during the influenza pandemic of 1918–1919, when hundreds of cases were described in American soldiers in the United States and Europe (41). After World War I few references to the meningococcus occurred, and the medical literature of bacterial pneumonias emphasized the importance of *Streptococcus pneumoniae, Hemophilus influenzae,* and *Staphylococcus aureus*. However, the report by Putsch et al. (73) in 1970 firmly established in the modern literature a respiratory pathogenic role for *N. meningitidis*. Over 100 cases have been reported in the last decade in the United States, reflecting increased awareness or a true increase in incidence of this unusual cause of pneumonia (95). In a recent report from the Netherlands, in a single general district hospital, 46 isolates were obtained from patients with pneumonia or acute exacerbations of chronic bronchitis (16). Kerttula and colleagues (47) studied 162 cases of pneumonia in Finland and found six that were caused by *N. meningitidis*.

Bacteriology and Immunology

N. meningitidis is an aerobic gram-negative organism that grows as kidney-shaped diplococci. It is very fastidious, not surviving long in droplets or on surfaces, and is rapidly killed by drying or cold temperatures. Humans are the only hosts, and meningococci reside with a wide variety of other organisms, including nonpathogenic *Neisseria,* in the nasopharynx and oral pharynx.

Growth *in vitro* is optimal on enriched solid media, such as chocolate agar, in an atmosphere of 6% CO_2, at 35 to 37% C and approximately 50% humidity. *N. meningitidis* can grow slower than competing flora in mixed specimens, such as expectorated sputum, and will be overgrown and therefore often overlooked if cultured routinely. Modified Thayer-Martin agar (containing vancomycin, colistin, and nystatin) is especially useful for culturing sputum that has characteristic gram-negative diplococci on smear, as competing "normal respiratory flora" will be inhibited by this selective medium. On the basis of specific capsular polysaccharides, the meningococci can be divided into at least 13 chemically defined serogroups, of which A, B, C, D, X, Y, Z, W-135, and 29E are most important clinically.

Natural immunity to meningococcal infections is complex but appears to be mediated by serum bactericidal immune lysis and phagocytosis facilitated via the terminal complement components C5-8 (31,32). Congenital or acquired deficiency of one of these late components has been associated with recurrent meningococcal disease in some individuals (21). In addition, antibodies are made to capsular polysaccharides and to outer membrane noncapsular protein antigens and possibly lipopolysaccharides. Bactericidal antibody is present in the newborn as a maternal contribution, disappears by 6 to 9 months of age, and subsequently increases with subclinical (the carrier state) and clinical exposures to *N. meningitidis* and to nonpathogenic *Neisseria*. In addition, organisms such as *Escherichia coli* capsular types K_1 and K_{92} have cross-reacting envelope antigens shared with *N. meningitidis*, which may confer immunity to some capsular groups. Individuals lacking bactericidal antibody to a specific serogroup are susceptible to colonization and disease caused by that serogroup. There is evidence that the protective effects of group-specific bactericidal antibody may be "blocked" by high titers of circulating IgA in some individuals, making them susceptible to invasive disease (35).

Epidemiology

Five to fifteen percent of all healthy individuals are transient nasopharyngeal carriers of meningococci. Rates of carriage vary for different seasons and are influenced by circumstances such as crowding. In the military experience of the 1960s, for example, these rates approached 100%, associated with epidemic disease in some camps (29). Carriage rates and clinical disease can be drastically reduced by modifying crowded living conditions.

These obligate human parasites probably spread via droplet aerosol during close contact, hence the increased colonization rates with crowding. A carrier can remain subclinically colonized for more than a year or can develop acute infection within days of acquiring a new capsular group. In addition to sporadic civilian cases, minor epidemics of respiratory infection have occurred in military camps (50,78), and nosocomial spread has been identified in hospital units (15). Cases of meningitis and septicemia have also occurred in day care centers, but as yet respiratory infections have not been reported in that setting. Serogroups Y and W-135 have been frequently identified as respiratory pathogens, which could reflect less natural immunity to these serogroups or unique properties that permit their attachment and survival within the respiratory tract (28,50). As is true for other respiratory pathogens, influenza and adenoviral infections can predispose to meningococcal pneumonia.

Pathogenesis and Pathophysiology

The respiratory tract is usually involved directly, via aspiration or inhalation of droplet particles. A viral infection, resulting in excessive airway secretions and damage to mucous membranes, often precedes meningococcal pneumonia (100). In nonimmune individuals these encapsulated organisms resist phagocytosis. Filamentous pili can facilitate surface attachment, leading to rapid multiplication of organisms in the lower respiratory tract. In addition, the elaboration of IgA protease, which inactivates secretory IgA on mucous membrane surfaces, can enhance attachment, multiplication, and invasion of local tissues (51).

Bacteremia rarely complicates meningococcal pneumonia, and secondary bacteremic respiratory infections are unusual (50). The absence of diffuse intravascular coagulation (DIC), cutaneous petechiae, and "shock lung" in most respiratory cases supports the thesis that an aspiration mechanism, not bacteremia, is the common initiating event in pneumonia. An occasional patient with septicemic meningococcal infection will develop noninfectious acute respiratory failure, so-called shock lung, which can be confused with pneumonia.

Although there are numerous pathologic studies of pneumococcal infections, as well as experimental animal subjects, no experimental models of meningococcal pneumonia exist and few contemporary patients have died. The postmortem material from 1918 to 1919 cases confirmed that meningococcal pneumonia is a typical pyogenic exudative process, usually with an alveolar or bronchoalveolar distribution, rarely lobar or multilobar. Unlike the benign tissue effects in the usual case of pneumococcal disease necrosis, alveolar septal destruction and abscess formation do occur in meningococcal infections.

Clinical and Radiologic Features

Following an antecedent viral illness that could be common to a number of individuals in the immediate environment, chills, fever, productive cough, and pleuritic pain herald the onset of meningococcal pneumonia. Rales and consolidation are present, but pleural rubs, hemoptysis, cutaneous petechial rash, and signs of shock and septicemia are rare (50). The presence of multiple cases in military, school, hospital, or day care facilities should alert physicians to the possibility of meningococcal pneumonia, especially if there has been influenza or other viral disease in the community.

Radiologic findings consistent with patchy lower lobe airspace disease is usually noted, but lobar consolidation also occurs. An effusion is present in approximately 20% of cases. Some of the radiologic features could be due to the accompanying or preceding viral infection, in addition to bacterial pneumonia.

Laboratory Findings and Diagnosis

Isolation of *N. meningitidis* from a carefully collected sputum specimen, in the absence of other potential respiratory pathogens, is the major means of diagnosing the disease. The typical features of meningococcemia and meningitis are usually absent, so the direct gram-stained sputum examination is especially critical. If microscopic study indicates that gram-negative *Neisseria*-like organisms are present, in association with abundant polymorphonuclear leukocytes, then the sputum must also be cultured on a selective medium such as Thayer-Martin agar. Failure to use selective media or to incubate the specimens in an enriched CO_2 atmosphere can lead to false-negative results, even when the gram stain shows typical gram-negative diplococci. In our experience the morphology is as important as the staining characteristics in raising the possibility of *N. meningitidis* (see Table 23-1).

Some authors advise that meningococcal pneumonia should only be diagnosed from specimens obtained by methods that avoid pharyngeal contamination, like transtracheal aspiration, percutaneous lung puncture, and direct bronchial-pulmonary brushing (20). These procedures are not without risk, however, and should be resorted to only if adequate expectorated specimens are not obtainable.

TABLE 23–1. *Diagnosis of meningococcal pneumonia*

Single or multiple cases in community or hospital
Antecedent viral respiratory infection
Purulent or pulmonary edema-like sputum
Kidney-shaped gram-negative diplococci associated with polymorphs
Consider the diagnosis
    Culture on modified Thayer-Martin medium
    Incubate at 37°C, CO_2 enrichment

Blood cultures are rarely positive in this disease but should be obtained prior to treatment. In a recent case that we treated the blood culture results were the earliest documentation of the etiology of a postviral acute lobar pneumonia. Alternative methods to identify *N. meningitidis* in sputum include the capsular swelling technique (Quellung reaction), latex bead coagglutination, and fluorescent antibody staining. These methods are not widely available and at the present time are only useful in identifying group A or C organisms.

Differential Diagnosis

The diagnosis of meningococcal pneumonia depends on the availability and careful observation and interpretation of the stained sputum and selective cultures. Other pathogens, including morphologically similar *M. catarrhalis,* can produce a similar pulmonary infection, and the following diagnostic alternatives need to be considered.

Viral Pneumonia

A respiratory illness affecting a number of individuals, especially under institutional conditions, often is caused by an agent such as influenza A or B or an adenovirus. Examination of sputum usually reveals mononuclear cells without a predominant bacterial flora. The diagnosis can be confirmed by culture, but a rising antibody titer in sera taken acutely and during convalescence is usually confirmatory.

Mycoplasma Pneumonia

Sputum is nondiagnostic but may contain polymorphonuclear leukocytes and monocytes, as well as a mixture of mouth organisms. Multiple cases in young adults, in military or civilian circumstances, can mimic the epidemiologic characteristics of meningococcal or viral pneumonias. Mycoplasma infections are usually sporadic and sequential, rather than being multiple simultaneous cases. Antibody elevations or a cold agglutinin titer of 1:32 or greater can help establish the correct diagnosis.

Pyogenic Pneumonia

Aspiration of mouth organisms or disease caused by pyogenic bacteria such as the pneumococcus or *S. aureus* can complicate a viral respiratory infection. Hospitalized patients on respirators, exposed to selective antibiotics and the hospital flora, can develop pneumonia with organisms that can be confused with *Neisseria* on smear, such as *Moraxella, Hemophilus,* or *Acinetobacter.*

Rocky Mountain Spotted Fever

The petechial rash of rocky mountain spotted fever (RMSF) involves the distal parts of the extremities. The rash of *N. meningitidis,* rare in pneumonia, is diffuse when it occurs. Respiratory disease in RMSF is usually caused by small pulmonary vessel involvement or the adult respiratory distress syndrome, and the sputum is nondiagnostic. The season of the year, history of tick exposure, and the radiologic picture of a diffuse process, such as acute pulmonary edema, can help distinguish the respiratory symptoms in RMSF from meningococcal pneumonia.

Treatment

Prior to the early 1960s the sulfonamides were uniformly effective against clinical strains of *N. meningitidis* and were the drugs of choice. During the ensuing decade sulfa resistance required a new therapeutic strategy, and penicillin emerged as the most potent antimicrobial. From the limited experience available it appears that low doses of penicillin are adequate for most uncomplicated respiratory infections, but higher doses (6 million units or more) should be instituted if empyema or systemic involvement is present or suspected. Chloramphenicol is an effective alternative drug in patients allergic to penicillin. Usually 3 to 4 g are given in 4 to 6 divided doses, intravenously. Of the cephalosporins, ceftriaxone and cefotaxime have been proved to be useful.

The pendulum has begun to swing back in recent years, and the majority of meningococcal strains, including most group Y isolates, are now sulfa-susceptible. Unless resistance to penicillin becomes a problem, the sulfa drugs can continue to be used as alternative agents, guided by sensitivity testing of clinical isolates.

Prevention

Military and civilian experience confirms that meningococci spread via aerosol to susceptible individuals in close proximity. For this reason, in contrast with the general practice in mixed aspiration of pneumococcal pneumonia, patients with suspected meningococcal respiratory infection should be isolated for the initial 48 hours of treatment.

Rifampin was found to be an able substitute for sulfonamides and is the accepted first-line agent for chemoprophylaxis of meningococcal disease. The effectiveness of rifampin is probably attributable to its appearance, in high concentrations, in oral and respiratory secretions (40). The usual dosage is 600 mg orally, twice daily for 2 days. Another useful prophylactic antibiotic is minocycline, which also reaches high concentrations in oral secretions (13). Unfortunately, labyrinthitis is a frequent toxic effect that prevents its wider use as an alternative to rifampin. Recent clinical experience with the quinolone ciprofloxacin has been favorable and can require only a single day's prophylactic treatment (72).

The efficacy of prophylaxis for meningococcal meningitis and septicemia is well documented in military and civilian settings. There are no comparable studies for prevention of respiratory infections. Well-documented secondary cases of pneumonia, however, including hospital-acquired disease, support the need for preventive antimicrobials such as rifampin, as well as strict isolation procedures.

A previously available bivalent vaccine (30) has been replaced by a quadrivalent polysaccharide vaccine, comparable to the pneumonococcal product, and offers protection against infection by serogroups A, C, Y, and W-135 (55). Immunoprophylaxis has been most useful when given systematically to a large at-risk population, as in military installations and day care centers, or in geographic areas experiencing epidemics of meningitis (3). Children below age 2 years respond poorly or unpredictably to the vaccine, and reliance must be placed on chemoprophylaxis for this age group.

MORAXELLA (BRANHAMELLA) CATARRHALIS RESPIRATORY INFECTIONS

Definition and Historical Background

Long considered a harmless commensal of the oropharynx, *M. catarrhalis* has aroused renewed interest as a frequent pathogen responsible for primary middle ear and maxillary sinus infections in children and as an opportunist causing acute purulent bronchitis and bronchopneumonia in older individuals, especially those with chronic lung disease (18,36,88).

Bacteriology

Moraxella are kidney-shaped gram-negative diplococci that resemble *Neisseria* on stained smears. Their shaky and often changing tononomic status has now been clarified through DNA homology studies and biochemical reactions. *Branhamella* are officially called *Moraxella* in the newest edition of *Bergey's Manual of Systemic Microbiology*. In contemporary medical literature, *Branhamella* often persists, so in this section the popular nomenclature will be included. The organism is not fastidious, readily multiplying on nonselective media like blood or chocolate agar. *Moraxella* fail to utilize a variety of sugars and often grow poorly or unpredictably on the classic selective medium used to identify *Neisseria* sp, Modified Thayer-Martin (MTM). The majority of clinical isolates produce beta-lactamases and are therefore resistant to penicillin and ampicillin.

Epidemiology

M. catarrhalis is an inconstant member of the microflora of the pharynx and is present in increasing amounts, along with other commensals, in the respiratory secretions of individuals with chronic lung disease, especially during colder months of the year. There is recent evidence of human-to-human transmission in nosocomial settings (67). Many cases of respiratory infection occur in hospitalized patients, related to underlying problems, exposure to antimicrobial agents, and opportunities for aspiration. In normal children and adults, disease probably follows direct spread to contiguous structures and to aspiration. This view is supported by the frequent association of *Moraxella* with other upper airway residents like *H. influenzae* and *Streptococcus pneumoniae* (36,76).

Pathogenesis and Pathophysiology

Moraxella lack antiphagocytic capsules and IgA protease, but some strains possess pili that can facilitate attachment to mucosal surfaces. In most strains no specific pathogenic factors have been identified, and the endotoxin component appears to have little potency from clinical observations made in septicemic patients (12). There is often a history of a previous viral respiratory illness. The mechanism of initiation of respiratory infection appears to be aspiration of upper airway secretions, almost exclusively in individuals who suffer from chronic bronchitis, obstructive pulmonary disease, bronchiectasis, or pulmonary neoplasm. Invasive disease is rare, although empyema, septicemia, and meningitis have been observed. Beta-lactam antibiotics and chronic bronchopulmonary disease appear to heighten the likelihood of adherence of *M. catarrhalis* to oropharyngeal surfaces (88). There is also evidence that resistance to penicillins could be a predisposing factor for invasive disease (19).

Clinical and Radiologic Features

Patients are usually chronically ill and elderly, averaging 65 years. In addition to some form of respiratory disease, other conditions like diabetes, alcoholism, or corticosteroid usage are often present. Following an intercurrent viral infection or during a sojourn in a hospital, over a 2–3 day period, patients develop a productive cough, worsening bronchospasm, and other symptoms of acute bronchitis (98). Respiratory failure, if present, is usually due to the added insult in someone with borderline function. Hemoptysis, pleurisy, and significant temperature elevation are rarely observed. Physical findings relate to the underlying disease, usually complicated by large airway secretions, bronchospasm, and occasionally fine rales. A primary laryngitis can occur in normal adults, and a nonproductive cough syndrome has been reported in healthy children.

Aside from chronic changes, the radiologic abnormalities are usually minimal to absent when purulent bronchitis is present. Scattered bronchopneumonic infiltrates are described, but cavitation, necrotizing or lobar pneumonia, and pleural effusions are extremely rare.

Laboratory Findings and Diagnosis

A provisional diagnosis often rests upon the presence of characteristic gram-negative kidney-shaped diplococci in association with polymorphonuclear leucocytes in an expectorated sputum. Organisms can decolorize poorly or partially, but the kidney shape should help in avoiding confusion with lancet-shaped pneumococci. The organism grows well on blood or chocolate agar, but unpredictably on inhibitory media like MTM. Blood cultures should be obtained prior to instituting antimicrobial therapy, and any pleural effusion should be aspirated and examined bacteriologically. The white blood count is usually mildly elevated but can remain normal (see Table 23-2).

TABLE 23–2. *Diagnosis of* Moraxella *respiratory infection*

Chronic lung disease in the elderly
Underlying immunocompromising conditions
History of viral infection or aspiration
Kidney-shaped gram-negative diplococci on smear
Grows well on nonselective media like blood agar
Growth uncertain on selective Modified Thayer-Martin media
CO_2 not essential for growth
Firm colonies, nonmucoid, slide on blood agar

Differential Diagnosis

The contribution of accompanying isolates, like *S. pneumoniae,* to the overall process might not be clear in patients with chronic lung disease. Although coccobacillary microorganisms like *Brucella* or *Pasteurella* may resemble *Moraxella,* major confusion is with *N. meningitidis.* Meningococcal pneumonia is a rare disease that begins more abruptly with chills and fever in a patient who is usually acutely ill and without a background of chronic lung disease.

Treatment

The majority (75 to 85%) of clinical isolates produce a beta-lactamase and are, therefore, resistant to the penicillins. Many treatment failures have been described, attesting to the clinical significance of this observation. Therapy should be initiated with amoxicillin-clavulanate (Augmentin), a second- or third-generation cephalosporin, ampicillin-sulbactam (Unasyn), or trimethoprim-sulfamethoxazole. The macrolides (erythromycin, clarithromycin, and azithromycin) are also effective as are fluoroquinolones such as ciprofloxacin and ofloxacin (86,88,91). Supportive measures are essential, including optimal hydration, bronchodilators, and efforts to improve pulmonary function.

PSEUDOMONAS PSEUDOMALLEI PNEUMONIA: AN IMPORTED ENVIRONMENTAL INFECTION

Definition and Historical Background

Melioidosis is a disease that has its principal effects in the respiratory tract, where it can mimic tuberculosis, necrotizing pneumonia, or lung abscess. *P. pseudomallei* infection has been seen in the United States almost exclusively in military personnel returning from Southeast Asia, often after a latent period of months to years (54). More recently, refugees from endemic areas have resettled in many parts of the Western world and undoubtedly will bring with them unrecognized and potentially recurrent infection. The disease was initially described from Rangoon in 1912 by Whitmore and Kreshnosivami and was reminiscent of another Pseudomonad-caused disease called "glanders." Originally referred to as Whitmore's disease, the name "melioidosis" was introduced in 1921 in recognition of the Greek word for glanders, *melis.* An extensive review from Thailand provides an excellent update on all aspects of the disease (54).

Bacteriology and Immunology

The organism is a motile, aerobic, gram-negative pseudomonad, without a true capsule. Colonies produce a typical musty, fruity odor, like *Pseudomonas aeruginosa,* but blue-green pyocyanin or other pigments are not elaborated. Morphology is variable, but after several days rough, wrinkled, cream-to-orange-colored colonies emerge that are characteristic. The organism grows well on blood, MacConkey, or mineral-base media. Glucose is the sole carbon source. Identification is confirmed by a battery of biochemical tests, agglutination, or fluorescent-antibody procedures.

There is little information available on the role of humoral antibody and cellular immunity in melioidosis. Natural exposure to relatively avirulent strains can induce immunity. IgG antibodies persist for long periods following inapparent disease, but IgM-immunofluorescent antibody tends to disappear within 3 to 6 months after appropriate therapy. The striking resemblance of chronic melioidosis to tuberculosis and respiratory fungal diseases is noteworthy (24). Latency, and activation following viral infection, various stressful situations, or administration of steroids suggest that cellular immunity is essential for protection. The formation of characteristic granulomas also indicates that a cellular immune mechanism is operative.

Epidemiology

Like many other pseudomonads, *P. pseudomallei* occupies an environmental niche that includes moist soils, stream beds, and stagnant water. The distribution of the organism appears to be tropical to subtropical, especially in Southeast Asia and Australia and rarely in the Western hemisphere. Humans as well as wild and domestic animals residing in the areas subtended by latitude 20° north to 20° south have evidence of subclinical and clinical disease (42). Likewise, individuals who travel to, through, and reside in endemic areas are susceptible to infection. As many as 10 to 30% of natives have indirect hemagglutinin titers. One to two percent of healthy soldiers and up to 9% of wounded individuals who served in Vietnam are serologically positive. The approximately 3 million American soldiers who traveled and lived in that region include a significant number with latent infection. Active disease has emerged even 25 years after leaving an endemic area.

Transmission to humans appears to be mainly by direct contact with contaminated soil or water through either minor abrasions or major wounds occurring especially during the wet seasons. Common-source outbreaks have also been recorded. Ingestion and inhalation are less-frequent modes of spread. There is no confirmation that human-to-human or animal-to-human respiratory disease occurs. Lack of previous exposure to the pathogen and underlying debilitating conditions, such as malnutrition and diabetes, can increase susceptibility to infection. There have been a few reports of nosocomial spread via instruments, catheters, and even antiseptic and intravenous solutions (4,54). Sexual transmission and laboratory acquisition via inhalation have also been documented (54,61,77).

Pathogenesis and Pathophysiology

The disease can be acute and fulminating, with a skin lesion at the site of inoculation from contaminated soil or water (93). The lung is most often the organ of involvement, usually via bacteremic spread from a subclinical or clinical peripheral focus but occasionally following inhalation. In nonimmune individuals, acute disease begins as multiple small regions of microabscesses, with necrosis and coalescence of smaller lesions leading to larger areas of suppuration. A modified slime capsular layer as well as soluble toxic components of the organism can be responsible for resisting phagocytosis and causing local cytotoxic effects. Endotoxic manifestations can also play a role, but are probably less important than in Enterobacteriaceae or neisserial infections.

In the subacute and more chronic forms of melioidosis the lung lesions are often in an upper lobe, resembling tuberculosis in location and with propensity for granuloma formation and cavitation (69).

A clinically important feature of pathogenesis in melioidosis is activation of disease after a latent period of months to many years (75). This activation can follow influenza viral disease and other infections, acute stress (trauma, thermal burns, surgery, etc.), or administration of immunosuppressive drugs such as corticosteroids. The specific mechanism of activation is unknown in melioidosis, just as in most other bacterial disease, including tuberculosis.

Clinical and Radiologic Features

Acute respiratory disease can be a manifestation of the syndrome of fulminating septicemia, dominated by high fever and toxicity. A local skin lesion can be present, with cellulitis and lymphangitis, and this can represent the initial area of entry of organisms after minor trauma. Respiratory features include dyspnea and cough, pleuritic pain, and purulent, bloody sputum. Prognosis is very grave in this form of acute systemic disease, which is rarely seen in the West (49,93).

Milder types of subacute and chronic pneumonia are more frequently seen in patients developing clinical illness after leaving an endemic area. Fever, productive cough, and pleuritic pain are dominant findings together with marked weight loss. The respiratory disease resembles classic pyogenic bacterial pneumonia in the acute form and tuberculosis or pulmonary fungal infections in the subacute and chronic phases (80). Physical findings are nondiagnostic and include rales, consolidation, bronchial airway changes, and pleural friction rubs. Manifestations of disease in other organ systems such as the skin, subcutaneous tissues, and lymph nodes can dominate the clinical findings.

X-ray changes vary with the pace of the respiratory disease (85). In acute pneumonia there may be little evidence of airspace involvement, or there may be miliary nodules throughout the lungs. In subacute infections subapically located soft nodules are most common, progressing to diffuse airspace disease. The upper lobe location argues for an inhalation mechanism, as bacteremic spread should localize in basilar regions where the blood flow is greatest. In chronic disease the upper lobe lesions are fibronodular and often cavitate with evidence of surrounding fibrosis. This form of melioidosis especially resembles tuberculosis.

Laboratory Findings and Diagnosis

The diagnosis should be *seriously considered if a history of prior residence in an endemic area is obtained.* Careful examination of sputum for *P. pseudomallei* should be requested; bipolar staining, gram-negative bacilli can be present in expectorated sputum in more acute cases. Routine culture on blood agar, subculture to differential media, and serology testing can be rapidly diagnostic. Quickly alerting the bacteriology laboratory is essential, to accelerate identification of the organism; it could prove to be life-saving (see Table 23-3).

In addition to sputum, local skin or subcutaneous lesions and blood should be cultured. In most cases of pneumonia, except those that are acute fulminating infections, blood cultures are negative. Serologic studies, including a specific IgM immunofluorescence test, can help to confirm the diagnosis of clinically active disease. The indirect hemagglutination assay is also a valuable diagnostic aid, but a single elevated titer is not as useful as a fourfold or greater rise with paired specimens. There is an urgent need for rapid and specific diagnosis if the patient is to receive optimal antibiotic therapy.

Occasionally a lung, pleural, or node biopsy for culture and histopathology might be necessary, especially in chronic cases. Tissue-staining procedures are not helpful in melioidosis, except when a touch prep of removed material is gram stained in the routine manner. Histopathology can reveal focal necrotizing suppuration or granuloma formation, the two major tissue reactions to *P. pseudomallei*.

Differential Diagnosis

Chronic forms of melioidosis resemble pulmonary tuberculosis and respiratory fungal infections such as histoplasmosis, blastomycosis, and coccidioidomycosis. A careful history, including travel and residence in endemic areas, and occupational and hobby activities, assists in diagnostic investigations. Skin testing and acid-fast staining of sputum can confirm tuberculosis. Serologic titers and occasionally biopsy material are essential to establish a fungal etiology.

Other acute bacterial pneumonias caused by organisms that are endemic in tropical areas of Southeast Asia include plague caused by *Yersinia pestis* and tularemia caused by *Francisella tularensis* (see below).

Treatment

Results of therapy in acute forms of melioidosis have been disappointing, even when large-to-enormous doses of theoretically effective antibiotics are administered. In subacute and chronic pneumonia, results are favorable. Antibiotics should be administered for prolonged periods, up to 6 to 12 months, and sometimes combined with extensive pulmonary resection.

TABLE 23–3. *Diagnosis of melioidosis pneumonia*

Exposure to rural Southeast Asia, Australia, or other endemic regions (latitudes 20°N to 20°S)
Potentially long latent period like tuberculosis
Activation by viral illness, stress, steroids, etc.
Consider the diagnosis—alert the bacteriology lab
  Nodular upper lobe lesions, including cavities
  Usually a subacute or chronic illness in USA
  Bipolar staining gram-negative bacilli
  Rapid growth on routine media—blood or minimal agar

Since the mid-1970s a number of encouraging case reports have described the use of trimethoprim-sulfamethoxazole (TMP-SMX) for treating pneumonia, prostatitis, and other tissue infections caused by *P. pseudomallei* (27,44,64). Frequently, however, strains from some geographic areas are resistant to TMP-SMX. A recent study of clinical isolates from Thailand demonstrated an 81% resistance rate among approximately 200 clinical isolates tested (79). With widespread use of TMP-SMX in most parts of the world, significant rates of resistance can become more common. Susceptibility testing of the clinical isolate should therefore be used to guide the choice of antimicrobial therapy. The recommended dose is 240 mg of trimethoprim and 1,200 mg of sulfamethoxazole every 6 hours. The duration of treatment and modification of dosage with improvement are aspects of management that await further experience and study. High doses should be maintained until clinical improvement and radiological healing are apparent.

Doxycycline (4 mg per kg per day) remains a useful alternative antibiotic. It has a favorable *in vitro* spectrum and some clinical success. Chloramphenicol (6 to 8 grams per day) and kanamycin (but *not* the other aminoglycosides) are effective for some strains and can be combined with doxycycline in appropriate cases.

Among the cephalosporins the third-generation drug ceftazidime appears to have significant potency for *P. pseudomallei* (97). Ceftazidime in doses of 2 to 3 gm every 8 hours combined with TMP-SMX can be recommended in acute disease. Imipenem, amoxicillin-clavulanate (Augmentin), and ticarcillin-clavulanate (Timentin) have good activity *in vitro,* but clinical experience with the drugs is limited. Quinolones are not active against most strains of *P. pseudomallei* at levels achievable in serum (79).

Prevention

There are no prophylactic antimicrobial studies available, and a vaccine has not been developed. At the present time individuals traveling, working, or living in endemic regions, especially Southeast Asia, should be made aware of this soil-and-water-dwelling organism. These individuals should use care and caution to avoid traumatic injuries and assiduously clean wounds contaminated with soil or stagnant water.

RHODOCOCCUS EQUI PNEUMONIA: AN ORGANISM WITH ENVIRONMENTAL AND ANIMAL ASSOCIATIONS

Definition and Historical Background

Rhodococcus equi, formerly known as *Corynabacterium equi,* was first isolated by Magnussen in 1923 and identified as a cause of suppurative pneumonia in foals. It was later shown to be a frequent pathogen in horses, cattle, and swine. First described as a pathogen in humans in 1967 (33), it has been reported most commonly as causing pneumonia in immunocompromised hosts (5,57,87), especially those receiving corticosteroid therapy (39). In recent years the majority of reported cases of *R. equi* disease have been patients infected with the human immunodeficiency virus (22,38) (Fig. 23-1).

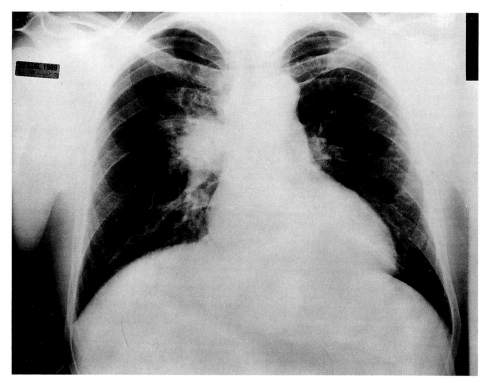

FIG. 23–1. *R. equi* pneumonia in a patient with AIDS. A right middle lobe cavitating nodular lesion with surrounding infiltrate and an upper lobe cavity is present.

Bacteriology and Immunology

Rhodococcus is a pleomorphic gram-positive bacillus in the order Actinomycetales. It grows well on most media aerobically, at 37°C, as mucoid pale-pink or salmon-pink-colored colonies that are usually observed by 48 hours incubation. *R. equi* has a high cell wall mycolic acid content and as a result is weakly acid-fast, similar to *Nocardia* species and Mycobacteriaceae. Some strains will ferment glucose but most will not ferment carbohydrates; most produce catalase and hydrogen sulfide. Beta-lactamase is present in some strains (see Table 23-4).

Epidemiology

Most of the reported cases occurring in humans without HIV infection have been patients who had significant contact with livestock or with soil and environment heavily contaminated with livestock waste. In contrast, HIV-related *Rhodococcus* disease appears to occur in patients who do not have any particular environmental exposure history, implying a wide distribution of the organism. There is no geographic endemicity.

History of exposure to horses, cattle, or their environment
Immunocompromised host: malignancy, steroids, HIV
Cavitary or nodular infiltrates on radiograph
Gram-positive pleomorphic bacilli
Acid-fast
Pale-pink or salmon-pink mucoid colonies
Grows rapidly, aerobically on most media
Differential diagnosis includes *Nocardia* sp, *Mycobacteria*

Pathogenesis and Pathophysiology

R. equi usually enters the body by direct inhalation, although soft tissue infections after cutaneous inoculation can occur. It is an intracellular pathogen and causes disease in patients with impaired cell-mediated immunity and defects in phagocytic processing of organisms.

Involved tissue usually shows a necrotizing granulomatous reaction with histiocytes and macrophages that frequently contain bacteria. Unlike lesions infected with *Mycobacterium tuberculosis* and systemic fungi, there is usually a prominent infiltration of neutrophils in the involved areas.

Clinical and Radiographic Features

Patients often present with indolent symptoms of fever, nonproductive cough, and dyspnea. Typically there is a paucity of findings on physical examination of the chest, but signs of consolidation and pleural friction rubs can be present. Patients with HIV infection generally present in a manner similar to patients without HIV infection, although pleuritic chest pain might be more common. In HIV-infected patients *R. equi* disease tends to occur after there has been significant deterioration in their immune systems with CD-4 lymphocyte counts below 200 cells/mm^3. It is frequently found concurrent with other pulmonary infections. Extrapulmonary dissemination occurs in both HIV-infected and non-HIV-infected patients, but there is a significantly greater rate of recovery of the organism from blood cultures in HIV patients. The central nervous system appears to be a common site of metastatic infection, similar to *Nocardia* sp (65).

The most common radiographic abnormalities are lobar infiltrates which usually evolve into nodular or cavitating lesions within weeks or months. There is no predilection for involvement of any particular lobe. Pleural effusions are common, occurring in up to 40% of HIV patients with pulmonary *R. equi* infection. Significant hilar adenopathy is unusual.

Differential Diagnosis

Rhodococci share many microbiological features with *Mycobacteria* and *Nocardia,* and this may account for similarities in the subacute to chronic evolution of the disease. The high mycolic acid content of their cell walls results in their acid-fast staining properties and could play a role in their similar clinical and pathological manifestations. *R. equi, Nocardia* sp, and *Mycobacterium tuberculosis,* as well as nontuberculous *Mycobacteria,* must be considered in the differential diagnosis of nodular or cavitating pulmonary lesions in immunocompromised patients, especially when acid-fast organisms are found in clinical specimens.

Other considerations in the differential diagnosis of nodular or cavitating pulmonary lesions include malignancy, fungal infection such as *Cryptococcus neoformans,* anaerobic lung abscess, or necrotizing pneumonia caused by facultative bacteria like *Staphylococcus aureus* or *Klebsiella pneumoniae.*

Laboratory Findings and Diagnosis

R. equi can usually be cultured from sputum, bronchial lavage, pleural fluid or other infected tissue, and often from blood. Because the organisms stain as gram-positive bacilli, grow readily on most media, and are usually catalase producers, they can be mistaken for "diphtheroid" or "Coryneform" contaminants unless further testing is done. It is therefore important for the clinician to alert the microbiology staff if the possibility of *R. equi* is entertained.

Treatment

Antibiotic therapy alone is usually adequate to achieve cure. Like mycobacterial infections, a multidrug regimen and prolonged therapy of 2 to 6 months' duration might be needed. Erythromycin, rifampin, ciprofloxacin and other quinolones, chloramphenicol, sulfonamides, and aminoglycosides are active against most isolates. *R. equi* is an intracellular pathogen capable of multiplying in phagocytes, so antibiotics that are capable of achieving high intracellular levels, such as erythromycin and the newer macrolides, rifampin and quinolones, are preferred. In some patients surgical resection of a nodular or cavitating lesion might be needed to achieve cure.

PNEUMONIAS CAUSED BY ANIMAL-ASSOCIATED BACTERIA: ZOONOTIC INFECTIONS

Bacteria associated with domestic and wild animals are often capable of colonizing and producing disease in humans. Spread can be by direct contact, inhalation, ingestion, or via animal bites or arthropod intermediates. Some of these microorganisms, such as *Pasteurella multocida* and *Francisella tularensis,* are widely distributed geographically and are found in a large number of different animal hosts. Others, such as *Yersinia pestis,* the cause of plague, are local and infect a limited number of animal species, including domestic cats. *Bacillus anthracis* has an even narrower ecological niche, and humans contact the pathogen mainly in occupational encounters, as in the hide-hair industry.

This brief introduction should alert physicians to the vital importance of including a careful history of travel, occupation, hobbies, contact with animals and insects, and knowledge of other persons similarly afflicted. These zoonotic bacterial infections have few unique characteristics that distinguish the etiologic agent. Many of the pathogens are difficult to isolate from sputum. The diagnosis is often first considered from a provocative history, and this can initiate appropriate bacteriologic and serologic studies and provisional therapy.

In this section the important features of five zoonotic bacterial pneumonias will be reviewed. Each is a rare cause of respiratory infection in the United States at present. A few, like anthrax ("Woolsorter's Disease") and plague, have a history of causing significant numbers of infections and worldwide epidemics. The diseases are anthrax, brucellosis, pasteurellosis, plague, and tularemia. The pathogens responsible for these pneumonias cause more frequent and uniquely characteristic infections in extrarespiratory foci, but the emphasis here is on pulmonary disease (see Table 23-5).

Anthrax Caused by *Bacillus anthracis*

Infection is initiated in susceptible individuals by inhalation of spores from animal hides, hair, or wool, or from other contaminated products or soil. In the 19th century it was a frequently noted disease, especially in towns like Bradford, England, where mohair and alpaca wools were brought to be processed. "Woolsorter's Disease" and "Bradford Disease" were synonymous with acute inhalation anthrax (52). Today, most imported animal hides have been steam sterilized, thus reducing the density of contaminating spores to which workers in the hide-hair industry are exposed.

Since the early 1900s this form of pneumonia has become very rare, with fewer than 50 new cases reported in the Western literature. Five patients were described in 1960 in a single epidemic in New Hampshire (70), and a home craftsman working with yarn imported from Pakistan died of inhalation anthrax in 1976 (81). Approximately three to five cases of cutaneous anthrax have been reported yearly in the United States for the past decade. They occur in persons working in the animal hide-hair industry while providing ancillary services, or working with contaminated materials in crafts or other projects. Worldwide, the disease is much more prevalent and almost certainly underreported. Epidemic ingestion anthrax, a devastating enteric and systemic disease, was reported from the former Soviet Union in the 1970s (90).

Bacillus anthracis is a large, square-ended, gram-positive bacillus which forms spores under adverse environmental conditions such as drying. The spores can persist in wool and other hair, and in soil and fertilizer products, thus contaminating food and other products. The organism grows well on blood agar under ambient atmospheric conditions, forming irregular ground-glass colonies with comma-shaped outgrowths. It is easily recognized in the laboratory.

Respiratory disease is initiated by inhalation of spores. The organism possesses a polyglutamic acid capsule that impedes phagocytosis. A potent exotoxin is secreted that causes local edema and necrosis (56). The disease can appear in the paranasal sinuses but usually there is a proximal bronchitis. The hilar and mediastinal structures, including the lymph nodes, become involved when spore-laden macrophages migrate via the lymphatics to these nodes. Edema interferes with airflow and gas exchange, and asphyxia results from obstruction rather than parenchymal disease. Organisms spread via the blood to many organs, including liver, spleen, and the central nervous system (89).

The clinical manifestations usually begin insidiously with fever, nonproductive cough, and malaise, approximately 4 days after an inhalation exposure. This is fol-

TABLE 23–5. *Comparative aspects of zoonotic bacterial pneumonias*

Disease	Gram-stain morphology	Culture methods	Identifying tests	Distribution	Animal habitat
Anthrax *Bacillus anthracis*	Large gram-positive rods Central spores	Blood agar Blood cultures	Colony morphology Fluorescent Ab	Worldwide Warmer regions	Hairs and hides, especially goats Bone meal fertilizer
Brucellosis *Brucella* sp	Small gram-negative coccobacilli	Enriched media, serum, $CO_2 + O_2$	Rise in agglutinating antibodies	Worldwide	Animal products Meat packing and processing
Pasteurellosis *Pasteurella multocida*	Small gram-negative coccobacilli with bipolar staining	Blood agar with CO_2	Biochemical tests	Worldwide	Oral flora of domestic cats, dogs; many wild animals
Plague *Yersinia pestis*	Gram-negative bacilli with bipolar staining	Blood and MacConkey agar Blood cultures	Biochemical tests, fluorescent antibody	Worldwide Southwest USA	Ground rodents such as prairie dogs; fleas, cat
Tularemia *Francisella tularensis*	Tiny bipolar staining gram-negative bacilli	Media with serum, and cystine	Rise in agglutinating antibodies Immunofluorescent stain	North America Europe Asia	Rabbits, squirrels, aquatic mammals; arthropods Many wild animals and birds

Disease	Epidemiologic spread	Characteristics of pneumonia	Therapy[a]
Anthrax *Bacillus anthracis*	Inhalation spores in industry or home hobbies	Mediastinal and hilar involvement primarily	P: Penicillin G A: Erythromycin or Chloramphenicol
Brucellosis *Brucella sp*	Contact Ingestion of unpasteurized daily products ? Inhalation Slaughter house	Isolated nodules frequently in basal segments	P: Doxycycline and Rifampin A: Doxycycline and Streptomycin Trimethoprim-Sulfamethoxazole
Pasteurellosis *Pasteurella multocida*	Uncertain but probably contact	Underlying lung disease Single or multiple infiltrates sparing upper lobes	P: Penicillin G or Ampicillin A: 3rd-generation Cephalosporin (Ceftriaxone) or Chloramphenicol
Plague *Yershinia pestis*	Flea bite Contact Inhalation from animal or human case of pneumonia	Airspace lower lobe infiltrates, miliary nodules, bilateral diffuse disease	P: Streptomycin and Tetracycline A: Chloramphenicol (CNS)
Tularemia *Francisella tularensis*	Inhalation Contact Ingestion Tick or deerfly bite	Bronchopneumonia with hilar adenopathy and frequent pleural involvement	P: Gentamicin or Streptomycin A: Tetracycline

P, primary; A, alternates.
[a]See individual sections for dosage and discussion.

lowed by acute deterioration that features severe dyspnea, stridor, hypoxic confusion, and usually death within 24 hours of the worsening phase. Physical findings can include edema of the neck and anterior chest, stridor and wheezing with intercostal retractions, and evidence of mediastinal widening. A widened mediastinum and bilateral pleural effusions are frequently seen radiologically. Although the lung fields are often clear, prominent lung marking secondary to peribronchial edema and hemorrhage occur (70).

Diagnosis depends on a careful history of an appropriate inhalation exposure to animal hide products. Examination of blood-tinged sputum with gram stain is sometimes positive, but the organisms are frequently sequestered in macrophages and lymph tissues and might not be present in expectorated secretions. Blood cultures can be positive, and if the central nervous system is involved organisms can be seen in the typically hemorrhagic spinal fluid. A fluorescent antibody test is available, but it is rarely necessary to make a correct diagnosis.

Chest wall and neck edema associated with breathing difficulties might suggest a number of other diagnoses, including diphtheria or a neck space abscess. The lack of upper respiratory inflammatory complaints such as pharyngitis and a history of diphtheria immunization are helpful in ruling out these possibilities. Acute Group A streptococcal pneumonia can cause hilar inflammation and bilateral pleural effusions, but pharyngitis frequently is present and gram-positive chains of cocci are often seen in pleural fluid. Acute epiglottitis is usually a disease of young children. The examining physician sees an enlarged epiglottis or can be helped by a lateral x-ray of the neck, revealing the local soft tissue swelling. Lymphoproliferative and other neoplasms can produce local edema, respiratory symptoms, and radiologic changes of hilar and mediastinal swelling, but the pace of these diseases is slower and usually without constitutional symptoms of inflammation.

Intravenously administered penicillin in doses of 1 to 2 million units every 4 hours is the treatment of choice. Rare instances of resistance to penicillin have been reported, and erythromycin or chloramphenicol are effective substitutes in penicillin-allergic patients. In the presence of meningitis the penicillin dose should be 2 million units every 2 hours, and chloramphenicol is the alternative drug, 1 gm intravenously every 4 to 6 hours. Respiratory support is essential, including aspiration of significant pleural effusions (see Table 23-5 for comparison with other zoonotic pneumonias).

An effective vaccine is currently available, and a number of alternative vaccines and routes of administration, including nasal insufflation, are being tested. Veterinarians and animal industry employees working with hides and hair products from regions such as the Indian subcontinent and the Near East should be immunized. Unfortunately, home textile craftsmen using natural fibers and individuals providing services to the animal product industries, such as ventilation specialists, rarely are immunized.

Brucellosis Pneumonia Due to *Brucella* Species

Approximately 200 cases of brucellosis are reported in the United States yearly, mostly in persons working in the meat processing or livestock industries, in veterinarians, and in individuals consuming unpasteurized dairy products from endemic regions such as Mexico and Italy (26). Although acute cases are diagnosed each year, the majority are subacute to chronic, and respiratory disease is usually recognized when a chest x-ray pattern raises the differential diagnosis of tumor versus inflammatory granuloma.

Involvement of the lung in brucellosis has not stimulated an extensive literature, and, on the basis of surveys from this country, it is probably a rare clinical entity. The experience abroad is different. In a prospective study of 400 cases from Kuwait, 16% of patients developed a nonproductive cough, but documented parenchymal disease occurred in only 1% (58). The pulmonary disease appears to be via bacteremic spread to basal segments or to hilar nodes. Occasionally pleurisy with an effusion is present (68). Single or multiple nodules resembling typical "coin lesions" are most often asymptomatic when discovered (14).

Brucella are small coccobacillary, gram-negative, nonmotile aerobes that can be separated into four major species: *B. abortus, B. melitensis, B. suis,* and *B. canis.* They grow well in a CO_2 atmosphere, on medium enriched with vitamins and serum. Organisms are speciated by a battery of biochemical tests and serologic agglutinin reactions. In general, the animal species infected corresponds to the bacterial species involved, that is, *B. suis* in pigs, *B. abortus* in cattle, and so on.

The epidemiology of brucellosis is the association of susceptible individuals with animals and animal products, bacteriology technicians, veterinarians, farmers, and those ingesting unpasteurized imported dairy products. There are a number of cases occurring in rural settings or among dog fanciers without specific details of transmission. The organisms are usually acquired through ingestion or, rarely, contact. Epidemiologic studies in abattoirs in the United States provide evidence for aerosol spread among workers in the killing rooms. These individuals exhibit significantly higher sero-conversion rates than people who work in other areas (46). No human-to-human transmission has been reported (26).

After ingestion, inhalation, or skin penetration the reticuloendothelial system and lymph nodes are involved, followed by bacteremic spread to many organs. Like tuberculosis, the major host defense is cellular immunity. A race between the growth of organisms and the development of cell-mediated immunity ensues. The end result is often containment in granulomas that can become fibrotic and calcify. The lung is usually involved via bacteremic spread, and the nodular lesions are usually located in basal segments which are exposed to the highest blood flow.

The clinical expression of brucellosis usually is dominated by a variety of nonspecific constitutional manifestations, including relapsing fever and headache. Cough has been described from 16 to 25% in two large series of cases (58,68). Other respiratory symptoms or signs, including productive sputum and pleurisy, are rarely noted (9). There have been isolated reports of "coin lesions," granulomata, pleural effusions, and patchy bronchopneumonias, but many of these cases are poorly documented and therefore suspect.

In Greer's major study of 59 patients with pulmonary complaints only 27 were well described (34). With the exception of fever and other constitutional symptoms, cough (40%), dyspnea (10%), and chest pain (8%) were the major respiratory findings. The most characteristic radiologic changes, evident in 17 and 13 patients, respectively, were perihilar thickening and peribronchial infiltrates. Nodular lesions were noted in 8 patients, miliary patterns in 4 patients, and a variety of airspace infiltrates and vague changes in occasional patients.

Unfortunately, there are no data on sputum exam and culture although purulent and bloody expectoration are occasionally described. Blood cultures are occasionally positive in more acute cases. Biopsy specimens of granulomas are frequently culture-positive, and the brucella agglutination tests are almost always confirmatory (94). In negative-reacting patients, "inhibitory" or blocking antibodies can be present (the so-called prozone phenomenon). Further dilution of the specimen can lower the concentration of inhibitor sufficiently for a positive agglutination to occur.

The differential diagnosis includes pulmonary fungal disease, especially histoplasmosis, with hilar and peribronchial involvement. Other fungi, tuberculosis, sarcoidosis, diseases that produce "coin lesions" like the dog heartworm *Dirofilaria immitis,* and pulmonary neoplasms should be considered.

The combination of doxycycline 100 mg twice per day combined with rifampin 300 mg twice per day orally for 1 month is considered the most effective form of antibiotic therapy with the fewest relapses. Alternative therapies include TMP-SMX (480 mg TMP + 2.4 gm SMX divided in 3 doses) combined with rifampin, or streptomycin 1.0 gm daily combined with rifampin. Fluoroquinolones are inhibitory but not bactericidal for *Brucella* sp. There have been limited reports of successful therapy with ofloxacin (1), but treatment failures with ciprofloxacin in both humans and animals have been described (53). No preventive vaccines for humans are currently available. Immunization of dairy herds, destruction of diseased animals, ventilation protection in meat industry killing rooms, caution in working with animal products, and use of protective ventilation hoods in microbiology laboratory practice are essential to avoid infection.

Pasteurella multocida Respiratory Infections

The agent of fowl cholera and epidemic disease in a variety of domestic and wild animals and birds, *P. multocida,* is a frequent cause of cat- and dog-bite cellulitis in humans. Respiratory disease is rarely reported, although sputum is the most common source of isolates after animal-bite cellulitis (43). Approximately 20 cases of pneumonia and 15 of empyema have been described during the past 30 years (92).

P. multocida is a small, gram-negative, bipolar-staining coccobacillary organism that can pair or chain. It grows well on blood agar in a CO_2 atmosphere, but growth is inhibited on MacConkey media. The organism produces a capsule that interferes with phagocytosis. There are lipopolysaccharide (endotoxin) components in the cell envelope, but no other toxins have been identified.

Most human cases of pneumonia occur in individuals with chronic respiratory disease, including bronchiectasis, emphysema, chronic obstructive pulmonary disease, and carcinoma (92). Spread to humans is probably via animals, but in only half the cases is there a positive exposure history. Bites precede almost 100% of *P. multocida* cellulitis, but in many of the cases of respiratory disease there are no clues to the method of spread although a cat is often present in the home. It is also recognized that the organism can be asymptomatically carried by individuals with chronic lung disease for long periods of time.

Lung involvement is probably initiated by aspiration of upper airway flora in an individual with chronic respiratory disease. Encapsulated organisms avoid phagocytosis, and tissue invasion and airspace disease follow. Spread to the pleura and to the bloodstream can complicate pneumonia. Necrotizing properties of the organism can occasionally lead to abscess formation. Fever and airspace disease aggravate the underlying pulmonary process, dyspnea is frequent, and productive cough is often present. Radiologic changes include lobar, multilobar, or diffuse patchy infiltrates engrafted onto the basic lung abnormalities. The upper lobes tend to be spared. Pleural effusions were found in approximately 20% of cases in one series. Empyema associated with pneumonia is less frequent than as a primary and dominant problem, probably from spread of a subpleural focus following local necrotizing pneumonitis.

Diagnosis depends on isolating the organism from sputum, pleural fluid, or blood. The ease of growing *P. multocida* makes culture an excellent way to identify the etiologic agent, especially because history and findings usually do not help define this pathogen. The sputum is purulent and usually contains bipolar-staining, gram-negative rods.

P. multocida can resemble *Brucella* sp, *Yersinia pestis, Francisella tularensis, Moraxella* sp, or *Hemophilus influenzae* in gram-stained smears of sputum. The history can help exclude some possibilities, and cultures usually confirm the specific pathogen.

Treatment with penicillin is indicated, and the majority of strains are exquisitely sensitive (17). Ampicillin is often begun initially based on the *H. influenza*–like appearance of the gram-negative coccobacillary organisms seen. Tetracycline and chloramphenicol are also effective and can be used in penicillin-allergic patients. The third-generation cephalosporin ceftriaxone is effective *in vitro* and is useful clinically (92). Fluoroquinolones are very active *in vitro* (71), and although they have been used successfully in animals with *Pasteurella* pneumonia, there have been no reports of their use in treating the disease in humans. Empyema is treated with closed tube drainage if the material is viscous, but repeated aspirations of thin effusions, coupled with 6 to 12 million units of penicillin daily, will often obviate the need for a chest tube. No effective preventive measures are known.

Plague Pneumonia Due to *Yersinia pestis*

Yersinia pestis was not isolated and characterized until the late 19th century, but this organism's indelible mark on humanity is obvious from ancient writing. Three major pandemics are known, beginning with the 6th century A.D., and from the 14th and the late 19th centuries. Epidemics were characterized by skin and node disease, that is, bubonic plague, but bacteremic pneumonia ("Black Death") and primary aerosol spread from patient to patient probably accounted for the rapid spread and high mortality rates.

The organism is a gram-negative bacillus, related to *E. coli* and other enteric bacteria. It often stains bipolar and grows well on blood agar and MacConkey media. Identification is by differential biochemical testing, agglutination reactions, or fluorescent antibody staining.

This zoonotic microorganism is associated with a variety of rodents and spreads among rock squirrels, prairie dogs, and other ground animals via the rodent flea (59). Low-grade infections occur, so-called enzootics, and occasional animals succumb. At times epizootic (epidemic) spread can erupt and wipe out large numbers of colonial animals, such as prairie dogs. At these times a larger number of infected fleas might be searching for blood meals. Any susceptible human in the area can be bitten, and the disease that follows frequently involves skin and the draining lymph node (45). Fleas can feed on urban rats, and a rat-to-rat cycle can occur. In an urban setting the proximity to humans means that more flea-to-human transmission can occur, sometimes via a domestic cat or dog as intermediate carrier of infected fleas, or directly from diseased pets. The disease can spread via aerosol, from an infected animal alive or dead, wild or domestic, or from one human to another once pneumonia has developed. The pneumonic aerosol dissemination, in crowded circumstances, is potentially a much more efficient and rapid means of spread than flea bites. No human-to-human aerosol transmission has been documented in the United States since 1924. Aerosol spread from a cat with pneumonic plague to a person was described previously (96), and a pulmonary death following contact with a domestic cat with pneumonia was reported by the Centers for Disease Control in October 1992. In the United States the organism is resident in the area west of the Rockies, especially in the Southwest.

Once the organisms enter the body local multiplication is rapid, and spread to regional lymph nodes occurs. The process can become systemic with bacteremic spread to many organs, including the basal lung segments. Y. pestis has a potent endotoxin and diffuse intravascular coagulation (DIC), and renal and pulmonary thrombotic occlusions, suggesting the generalized Shwartzman reaction, have been described (25).

The clinical presentation of pneumonia can follow subclinical or local bubonic (lymph node) disease (66). The patient is febrile and acutely ill, with symptoms that include a hemorrhagic productive cough, pleuritic pain, and dyspnea. There is nothing unique about the respiratory component except that it can follow classic bubonic plague in an individual recently in an endemic area (62). Radiologically, airspace infiltrates in the lower lobes (blood borne) can be present, and in association with bubonic plague should be considered early secondary pneumonia for purposes of patient isolation and prognosis. Other respiratory patterns include pulmonary nodules, adult respiratory distress syndrome, hilar adenopathy, nodular lesions evolving to alveolar exudates, and pleural effusions (2).

The organism can be cultured from sputum on basic media used to grow E. coli. Fluorescent antibody staining of expectorated material can provide rapid diagnosis. Evidence of hypoxia, venous shunting, adult respiratory distress syndrome, and renal failure can be present.

Therapy includes streptomycin 2.0 g intramuscularly daily and either tetracycline 2.0 g orally or, if meningitis is present, chloramphenicol 3.0 g daily intravenously for 2 weeks. A vaccine is available for persons with intense exposure to this microorganism, such as laboratory personnel who work with the agent (11). Prevention is also possible by careful surveillance of ground rodent populations, watching for die-offs, spraying for flea control in local regions, advising people to wear protective clothing and repellants, and using publicity to warn people against entering an epizootic area.

Tularemic Pneumonia Due to *Francisella tularensis*

Acute bacterial pneumonia caused by *F. tularensis* can mimic many other respiratory infections. There are unique epidemiologic features associated with acquiring the disease, through handling infected animals, or from tick or deerfly bites (6,7). The ulceroglandular form of tularemia was described in 1907, but the pleuropneumonic disease was not reported until 1924. Sporadic cases and occasionally minor epidemics of pneumonia have been idenitifed (84). The overall incidence of tularemia is approximately 150 cases per year in the United States with the lungs involved in 10–15% of cases (23).

F. tularensis is a tiny, gram-negative, pleomorphic coccobacillary organism that grows poorly on artificial media unless fortified with serum, glucose, and cystine. Because of the potential for laboratory-acquired infection, routine isolation is not recommended except in special reference laboratories.

The organism is found in nature endemically, between 30° and 70° north latitude, associated with a large number of wild animals and birds, but especially squirrels and rabbits. Spread among animals is via deerflies or ticks, or by bites. The organism is very hardy and can live in water or mud for long periods (99). Most human cases are acquired from tick or deerfly exposure or from contact with infected animals. Human-to-human transmission is not known, in contrast with pneumonic plague (see above).

Transmission to humans can occur through arthropod penetration, skin or mucous membrane defects, via inhalation, or after ingestion of contaminated meat. Local growth often leads to an ulcerated eschar followed by lymph node involvement. After ingestion pharyngitis or gastrointestinal (typhoidal) disease can occur. Bacteremia can complicate node spread but is most prevalent in association with the typhoidal form of diseases. The organism has an endotoxic cell envelope component that probably is responsible for pathogenesis, but very little is known about specific toxic properties. The reticuloendothelial system and macrophages are colonized, and microbes can persist inside nonsensitized cells for prolonged periods. The organism causes necrosis, granuloma formation, and local abscesses. Protective immunity is primarily cell mediated, with a minor contribution of humoral antibody (83).

Respiratory disease can begin with a poorly productive cough, chest pain, and dyspnea. This can accompany local ulceroglandular disesae or occur *de novo* in association with bactermic spread to the lungs (63). A second and perhaps more frequent presentation in recently reported cases is via inhalation (37,84). Radiologic changes characteristically include evidence of parenchymal and pleural disease. The pattern is diffuse bronchopneumonia, often with hilar adenopathy. Pleural effusions are not unusual. Although a central oval density was described as especially characteristic in the early literature, it has rarely been reported in recent cases (74).

The diagnosis should be considered in any patient who has had animal or arthropod exposure in an endemic region (63). Ulceroglandular or glandular disease can be present. Sputum is rarely positive, so the serologic agglutinin rise in paired sera is often essential for diagnosis. Blood cultures can be positive in association with pulmonary disease spread via the bacteremic route. Recent reports have described elevated creatine phosphokinase and rhabdomyolysis in association with bacteremic and pneumonic tularemia (48). An immunofluorescent technique offers rapid diagnosis, but is not readily available, and only rarely will organisms be seen on gram stain of sputum or lymph nodes. A skin test is available that produces a typical delayed hypersensitivity reaction, becomes positive in about a week after onset of disease, and like tuberculosis remains positive for years. Skin testing does not stimulate an antibody response (8).

Other entities that are confused with this rare form of bacterial pneumonia include the various nonbacterial pneumonias (psittacosis, Q fever, mycoplasma), bacterial pneumonias including plague (see above), tuberculosis, and systemic fungi.

Optimal therapy consists of an aminoglycoside such as gentamicin in doses of 1.5 mg/kg every 8 hours intramuscularly (60). Streptomycin 2.5 gm intramuscularly for 3 days, then 1.0 gm per day for an additional 4 to 7 days, is also effective. Tetracycline or chloramphenicol are additional agents useful in patients who cannot tolerate an aminoglycoside. The fluoroquinolones norfloxacin and ciprofloxacin are also effective (82).

Immunoprophylaxis has been only partially successful for prevention, but a recently developed attenuated strain could prove beneficial in high-risk patients, including laboratory personnel who work with this pathogen (10,83). Handling animal carcasses with rubber gloves and cooking rabbit and other wild animal meat thoroughly are ways of avoiding contact and ingestion exposures.

Concluding Remarks on Zoonotic Pneumonias

Respiratory infections caused by the five microorganisms discussed in this section can be severe, life-threatening, contagious (for *Y. pestis*), and an indicator of a potentially serious epidemiologic risk. All of these diseases are diagnosed by a careful history and use of selective cultures and/or serologic studies. The development of immunofluorescent techniques, utilizing biopsy material and sputum, will help in making rapid and accurate diagnoses and will ensure earlier therapy and isolation of selected patients. It cannot be emphasized enough that all of these sophisticated studies and efforts depend upon the accuracy of the history, which will then result in essential diagnostic confirmatory procedures and appropriate therapies.

REFERENCES

1. Akalin, H.E., Firat, M., and Serin, A. (1989): *In vitro* activity and clinical efficacy of ofloxacin in infections due to *Brucella melitensis*. *Rev. Infect. Dis.,* 11(Suppl. 5):S993–S994.
2. Alsofrom, D.J., Mettler, F.A., and Mann, J.M. (1981): Radiographic manifestations of plague in New Mexico, 1975–1980. *Radiology,* 139:561–565.
3. Artenstein, M.S. (1975): Prophylaxis for meningococcal diseases. *J.A.M.A.,* 231:1035–1037.
4. Ashdown, L.R. (1979): Nosocomial infection due to *Pseudomonas pseudomallei:* two cases and an epidemiologic study. *Rev. Infect. Dis.,* 1:891–894.
5. Berg, R., Chmel, H., Mayo, J., and Armstrong, D. (1977): *Corynebacterium equi* infection complicating neoplastic disease. *A.J.C.P.,* 68(1):73–77.
6. Boyce, J.M. (1975): Recent trends in the epidemiology of tularemia in the United States. *CEC News,* 131:197–198.
7. Brooks, G.F., and Buchanan, T.M. (1970): Tularemia in the United States: epidemiologic aspects in the 1960s and follow-up of the outbreak of tularemia in Vermont. *J. Infect. Dis.,* 121:357–359.
8. Buchanan, T.M., Brooks, G.F., and Brachman, P.S. (1971): The tularemia skin test. 325 skin tests in 210 persons: serologic correlation and review of the literature. *Ann. Intern. Med.,* 74:336–343.
9. Buchanan, T.M., Faber, L.C., and Feldman, R.A. (1974): Brucellosis in the United States 1960–72. An abattoir-associated disease. *Medicine,* 53:403–413.
10. Burke, D.S. (1977): Immunization against tularemia: analysis of the effectiveness of live *Francisella tularensis* vaccine in prevention of laboratory-acquired tularemia. *J. Infect. Dis.,* 135:55–60.
11. Burmeister, R.W., Tigertt, W.D., and Overhold, E.L. (1962): Laboratory-acquired pneumonic plague: report of a case and review of previous cases. *Ann. Intern. Med.,* 56:789–800.
12. Catlin, B.W. (1990): *Branhamella catarrhalis:* an organism gaining respect as a pathogen. *Clin. Microb. Rev.,* 3:293–320.
13. Centers for Disease Control (1976): Vestibular reactions to minocycline. *M.M.W.R.,* 25:31.
14. Chavez, C.A., and Veach, G.E. (1976): Localized pulmonary nodule due to *Brucella suis. J. Kansas Med. Soc.,* 76:434–437.
15. Cohen, M.S., Steere, A.C., Baltimore, R., von Graevnitz, A., Pantelick, E., Camp, B., and Root, R.K. (1979): Possible nosocomial transmission of group Y. *Neisseria meningitidis* among oncology patients. *Ann. Intern. Med.,* 91:7–12.
16. Davies, B.I., Spangaard, L., and Dankert, J. (1991): Meningococcal chest infections in a general hospital. *Eur. J. Clin. Micro. ID,* 10:399–404.

17. Dibb, W.L., and Digranes, A. (1981): Characteristics of 20 human pasteurella isolates from animal bite wounds. *Acta Microbiol. Scand.* (B), 89:137–141.
18. Doern, G.V. (1986): *Branhamella catarrhalis:* an emerging human pathogen. *Diag. Microb. Infect. Dis.*, 4:191–201.
19. Doern, G.V. (1990): *Branhamella catarrhalis:* phenotypic characteristics. *Am. J. Med.*, 88 (5A):33S–35S.
20. Ellenbogen, C., Graybill, J.R., Silva, J., Jr., and Homme, P.J. (1974): Bacterial pneumonia complicating adenoviral pneumonia. *Am. J. Med.*, 56:169–178.
21. Ellison, R.T., Kohler, P.F., et al, (1983): Prevalence of congenital or acquired complement deficiency in patients with sporadic meningococcal disease. *N. Engl. J. Med.*, 308:913–916.
22. Emmons, W., Reichwein, B., and Winslow, D.L. (1991): *Rhodococcus equi* infection in the patient with AIDS: literature review and report on an unusual case. *Rev. Infect. Dis.*, 13(1):91–96.
23. Evans, M.E., Gregory, D.W., Schaffner, W., and McGee, Z.A. (1985): Tularemia: a 30-year experience with 88 cases. *Medicine*, 64:251–269.
24. Everett, E.D., and Nelson, R.A. (1975): Pulmonary melioidosis: observations in thirty-nine cases. *Am. Rev. Respir. Dis.*, 112:331–340.
25. Finegold, M.J. (1968): Pathogenesis of plague: a review of plague deaths in the United States during the last decade. *Am. J. Med.*, 45:549–554.
26. Fox, M.D., and Kaufman, A.F. (1977): From the Centers for Disease Control: brucellosis in the United States, 1965–1974. *J. Infect. Dis.*, 136:312–316.
27. Fuller, P.B., Fisk, D.E., Byrd, R.B., Griggs, G.A., and Smith, M.R. (1978): Treatment of pulmonary melioidosis with combination of trimethoprim and sulfamethoxazole. *Chest*, 74: 222–224.
28. Galaid, E.I., Cherubin, C.E., Marr, J.S., Schaefler, S., Barone, J., and Lee, W. (1980): Meningococcal disease in New York City, 1973 to 1978: recognition of groups Y and W-135 as frequent pathogens. *J.A.M.A.*, 244:2167–2171.
29. Gauld, J.R., Nitz, R.E., Hunter, D.H., Rust, J.H., and Gauld, R.L. (1965): Epidemiology of meningococcal meningitis at Ford Ord. *Am. J. Epidemiol.*, 82:56–72.
30. Gold, R., Lepow, M.L., Goldschneider, I., Draper, T.L., and Gotschlich, E.C. (1975): Clinical evaluation of group A and group C meningococcal polysaccharide vaccines in infants. *J. Clin. Invest.*, 56:1536–1547.
31. Goldschneider, I., Gotschlich, E.C., and Artenstein, M.S. (1969): Human immunity to the meningococcus. I. The role of humoral antibodies. *J. Exp. Med.*, 129:1307–1326.
32. Goldschneider, I., Gotschlich, E.C., and Artenstein, M.S. (1969): Human immunity to the meningococcus. II. Development of natural immunity. *J. Exp. Med.*, 129:1327–1348.
33. Golub, B., Falk, G., and Spink, W.W. (1967): Lung abscess due to *Corynbacterium equi:* report of first human infection. *Ann. Int. Med.*, 66(6):1174–1177.
34. Greer, A.E. (1956): Pulmonary brucellosis. *Dis. Chest*, 29:508–519.
35. Griffiss, J.M., and Bertram, M.A. (1977): Immunoepidemiology of meningococcal disease in military recruits. II. Blocking of serum bactericidal activity by circulating IgA early in the course of invasive disease. *J. Infect. Dis.*, 136:733–739.
36. Hager, H., Verghese, A., Alvarez, S., and Berk, S.L. (1987): *Branhamella catarrhalis* respiratory infections. *Rev. Inf. Dis.*, 9:1140–1149.
37. Halsted, C.C., and Kulasinghe, H.P. (1978): Tularemia pneumonia in urban children. *Pediatrics*, 61:660–662.
38. Harvey, R.L., and Sunstrum, J.C. (1991): *Rhodococcus equi* infection in patients with and without human immunodeficiency virus infection. *Rev. Infect. Dis.*, 13(1):139–145.
39. Hilderdal, G., Riesenfeldt-Orn, I., Pedersen, A., and Ivanovica, E. (1988): Infection with *Rhodococcus equi* in a patient with sarcoidosis treated with corticosteroids. *Scand. J. Infect. Dis.*, 20:673–677.
40. Hoeprich, P.D. (1971): Prediction of anti-meningococcal chemoprophylactic efficacy. *J. Infect. Dis.*, 123:125–133.
41. Holm, M.L., and Davison, W.C. (1919): Meningococcus pneumonia. I. Occurrence of post-influenzal pneumonia in which the diplococcus intracellularis meningitidis was isolated. *Bull. Johns Hopkins Hosp.*, 30:324–329.
42. Howe, C., Sampath, A., and Spotnitz, M. (1971): The pseudomallei group: a review. *J. Infect. Dis.*, 124:598–606.
43. Hubbert, W.T., and Rosen, M.N. (1970): II. *Pasteurella multocida* infection in man unrelated to animal bites. *Am. J. Publ. Health*, 60:1109–1117.
44. John, J.F. (1976): Trimethoprim-sulfamethoxazole therapy of pulmonary melioidosis. *Am. Rev. Respir. Dis.*, 114:1021–1025.
45. Kaufman, A.F., Boyce, J.M., and Martone, W.J. (1980): From the Centers for Disease Control: trends in human plague in the United States. *J. Infect. Dis.*, 141:522–524.
46. Kaufman, A.G., Fox, M.D., Boyce, J.M., et al. (1980): Airborne spread of brucellosis. *Ann. NY Acad. Sci.*, 353:105–114.

47. Kerttula, Y., Leinonen, M., et al. (1987): The etiology of pneumonia: application of bacterial serology and basic laboratory methods. *J. Infect.*, 14:21–30.
48. Klotz, S.A., Penn, R.L., and Provenza, J.M. (1987): The unusual presentation of tularemia. *Arch. Intern. Med.*, 147:214.
49. Koponen, M.A., Zlock, D., et al. (1991): Melioidosis: forgotten, but not gone. *Arch. Intern. Med.*, 151:605–608.
50. Koppes, G.M., Ellenbogen, C., and Gebhart, R.J. (1977): Group Y meningococcal disease in United States Air Force recuits. *Am. J. Med.*, 62:661–666.
51. Kornfeld, S.F., and Plaut, A.G. (1981): Secretory immunity and the bacterial IgA proteases. *Rev. Infect. Dis.*, 3:521–534.
52. Laforce, F.M. (1978): Woolsorter's disease in England. *Bull. NY Acad. Med.*, 54:956–963.
53. Lang, R., Raz, R., Sacks, T., Michel, J., and Shapira, M. (1988): Failure of prolonged treatment of ciprofloxacin in acute brucellosis. 1988 Program abstr., 28th Intersci. Conf. *Antimicrob. Agents Chemother.* [abstract 368].
54. Leelarasamee, A., and Bovornkitti, S. (1989): Melioidosis: review and update. *Rev. Infect. Dis.*, 11:413–425.
55. Lepow, M.L., Beeler, J., et al., (1986): Reactogenicity and immunogenicity of a quadrivalent combined meningococcal vaccine in children. *J. Infect. Dis.*, 154:1033–1036.
56. Leppela, S.H. (1982): Anthrax toxin edema factor: a bacterial adenylate cyclase that increases cyclic AMP concentrations in eukaryotic cells. *Proc. Natl. Acad. Sci. USA*, 79:3162–3166.
57. Lipsky, B.A., Goldberger, A.C., Tompkins, L.S., and Plorde, J.J. (1982): Infections caused by nondiphtheria Corynebacteria. *Rev. Inf. Dis.*, 4(6):1220–1235.
58. Lulu, A.R., Araj, G.F., et al. (1988): Human brucellosis in Kuwait: a prospective study of 400 cases. *Q. J. Med.*, 66:39–54.
59. Mann, J.M., Martone, W.J., Boyce, J.M., Kaufmann, A.R., Barnes, A.M., and Weber, N.S. (1979): Endemic human plague in New Mexico: risk factors associated with infection. *J. Infect. Dis.*, 140:397–401.
60. Mason, W.L., Eigelsbach, H.T., Little, S.F., and Bates, J.H. (1980): Treatment of tularemia including pulmonary tularemia, with gentamicin. *Am. Rev. Respir. Dis.*, 121:39–45.
61. McCormick, J.B., Sexton, D.J., McMurray, J.G., Carey, E., Hayes, P., and Feldman, R.A. (1975): Human-to-human transmission of *Pseudomonas pseudomallei*. *Ann. Int. Med.*, 83:512–513.
62. Meyer, K.F. (1961): Pneumonic plague. *Bact. Rev.*, 25:249–261.
63. Miller, R.P., and Bates, J.H. (1969): Pleuropulmonary tularemia: a review of 29 patients. *Am. Rev. Respir. Dis.*, 99:31–41.
64. Morrison, R.E., Young, E.J., Harper, W.K., and Maldonado, L. (1979): Chronic prostatic melioidosis treated with trimethoprim-sulfamethoxazole. *J.A.M.A.*, 241:500–501.
65. Obana, W.G., Scanell, K.A., Jacobs, R., Greco, C., and Rosenblum, M.L. (1991): A case of *Rhodococcus equi* brain abscess. *Surg. Neurol.*, 35:321–324.
66. Palmer, D.L., Kisch, A.L., Williams, R.C., Jr., and Reed, W.P. (1971): Clinical features of plague in the United States: the 1969–1970 epidemic. *J. Infect. Dis.*, 124:367–371.
67. Patterson, T.F., Patterson, J.E., et al. (1988): A nosocomial outbreak of *Branhamella catarrhalis* confirmed by restriction endonuclease analysis. *J. Infect. Dis.*, 157:996–1001.
68. Pfischner, W.C.E., Jr., Ishak, K.G., et al. (1957): Brucellosis in Egypt. *Am. J. Med.*, 22:915–919.
69. Piggott, J.A., and Hochholzer, L. (1970): Human melioidosis: a histopathologic study of acute and chronic melioidosis. *Arch. Pathol.*, 90:101–111.
70. Plotkin, S.A., Brachman, P.S., Utell, M., Bumford, F.H., and Atchinson, M.M. (1960): An epidemic of inhalation anthrax, the first in the twentieth century. *Am. J. Med.*, 29:992–1001.
71. Prescott, J.F., and Yielding, K.M. (1990): *In vitro* susceptibility of selected veterinary bacterial pathogens to ciprofloxacin, enrofloxacin and norfloxacin. *Can. J. Vet. Res.*, 54:195–197.
72. Pugsley, M.P., Dworzaack, D.I., et al. (1987): Efficacy of ciprofloxacin in treatment of nasopharyngeal carriers of *Neisseria meningitidis*. *J. Infect. Dis.*, 156:211–213.
73. Putsch, R.W., Hamilton, J.D., and Wolinsky, E. (1970): *Neisseria meningitidis:* a respiratory pathogen? *J. Infect. Dis.*, 121:48–54.
74. Rubin, S.A. (1978): Radiographic spectrum of pleuropulmonary tularemia. *Am. J. Roentgenol.*, 131:277–281.
75. Sanford, J.P., and Moore, W.L., Jr. (1971): Recrudescent melioidosis: a Southeaset Asian legacy. *Am. Rev. Respir. Dis.*, 104:452–453.
76. Sarubbi, F.A., Myers, J.W., et al. (1990): Respiratory infections caused by *Branhamella catarrhalis:* selected epidemiologic features. *Am. J. Med.*, 88(5A):9S–14S.
77. Schlech, W.F., III, Turchik, J.B., et al. (1981): Laboratory-acquired infection with *Pseudomonas pseudomallei* (melioidosis). *N. Engl. J. Med.*, 305:1133–1135.
78. Smilack, J.D. (1974): Group-Y meningococcal disease: twelve cases at an Army training center. *Ann. Intern. Med.*, 81:740–745.

79. Sookpranee, T., Sookpranee, M., Mellencamp, M.A., and Preheim, L.C. (1991): *Pseudomonas pseudomallei,* a common pathogen in Thailand that is resistant to bactericidal effects of many antibiotics. *Antimicrob. Agents Chemother.,* 35(3):484–489.
80. Spotnitz, M., Rudnitzky, J., and Rambaud, J.J. (1967): Melioidosis pneumonitis: analysis of nine cases of a benign form of melioidosis. *J.A.M.A.,* 202:126–130.
81. Suffin, S.C., Carnes, W.H., and Kaufmann, A.F. (1978): Inhalation anthrax in a home craftsman. *Human Pathol.,* 9:594–597.
82. Syrjala, H., Schildt, R., and Raisainen, S. (1991): *In vitro* susceptibility of *Francisella tularensis* to fluoroquinolones and treatment of tularemia with norfloxacin and ciprofloxacin. *Eur. J. Clin. Microbiol. Infect. Dis.,* 10:68–70.
83. Tarnvik, A. (1989): Nature of protective immunity to *Francisella tularensis. Rev. Inf. Dis.,* 11:440–451.
84. Teutsch, S.M., Martone, W.J., Brink, E.W., Potter, M.E., Eliot, G., Hoxsie, R., Craven, R.B., and Kaufmann, A.F. (1979): Pneumonia tularemia on Martha's Vineyard. *N. Engl. J. Med.,* 301:826–828.
85. Thin, R.N.T., Brown, M., Stewart, J.B., and Garrett, C.J. (1970): Melioidosis: a report of ten cases. *Q. J. Med.,* New Series, 39:115–127.
86. Thys, J.P., Jacobs, F., and Motte, S. (1989): Quinolones in the treatment of lower respiratory tract infections. *Rev. Infect. Dis.,* 11(Suppl. 5):S1212–S1219.
87. Van Ette, L.L., Filice, G.A., Ferguson, R.M., and Gerdin, D.N. (1983): *Corynebacterium equi:* a review of 12 cases of human infection. *Rev. Inf. Dis.,* 5(6):1012–1018.
88. Verghese, A., and Berk, S.L. (1991): *Moraxella (Branhamella) Catarrhalis.* In: *Infectious Disease Clinics of North America,* vol. 5, edited by R.J. Wallace, Jr., pp. 523–538. W.B. Saunders, Philadelphia.
89. Vessal, K., Yeganehdoust, J., Dutz, W., and Kohout, E. (1975): Radiological changes in inhalation anthrax: a report of radiological and pathological correlation in two cases. *Clin. Radiol.,* 26:471–474.
90. Wade, N. (1980): Death at Sverdlovsk: a critical diagnosis. *Science,* 209:1501–1502.
91. Wallace, R.J., Jr., Nash, D.R., and Steingrube, V.A. (1990): Antibiotic susceptibilities and drug resistance in *Moraxella (Branhamella) catarrhalis. Am. J. Med.,* 88(5A):46S–50S.
92. Weber, D.J., Wolfson, J.S., Swartz, M.N., and Hooper, D.C. (1984): *Pasteurella multocida* infections. *Medicine,* 63:133–154.
93. Weber, D.R., Douglass, L.E., Brundage, W.G., and Stallkampk, T.C. (1969): Acute varieties of melioidosis occurring in U.S. soldiers in Vietnam. *Am. J. Med.,* 46:234–244.
94. Weed, L.A., Sloss, P.T., and Clagett, O.T. (1956): Chronic localized pulmonary brucellosis. *J.A.M.A.,* 161:1044–1047.
95. Weinberg, A.N. (1983): Pneumonias due to *Neisseria meningitidis.* In: *Seminars in Infectious Diseases,* vol. 8, edited by L. Weinstein and B.N. Fields, pp. 147–158. Thieme-Stratton, New York.
96. Werner, S.B., Weidner, C.E., et al. (1984): Primary plague pneumonia contracted from a domestic cat at South Lake Tahoe, California. *J.A.M.A.,* 251:929–931.
97. White, N.J., Chavwagul, W., et al. (1989): Halving of mortality of severe melioidosis by ceftazidime. *Lancet,* 2:698–700.
98. Wright, P.W., Wallace, R.J., Jr., and Shepherd, J.R. (1990): A descriptive study of 42 cases of *Branhamella catarrhalis* pneumonia. *Am. J. Med.,* 88(5A):2S–8S.
99. Young, L.S., Bicknell, D.S., Archer, B.G., Clinton, J.M., Leavens, L.J., Feeley, J.C., and Brachman, P.S. (1969): Tularemia epidemic, Vermont 1968: forty-seven cases linked to contact with muskrats. *N. Engl. J. Med.,* 280:1253–1260.
100. Young, L.S., LaForce, F.M., Head, J.J., Feeley, J.C., and Bennett, J.V. (1972): A simultaneous outbreak of meningococcal and influenza infections. *N. Engl. J. Med.,* 287:5–9.

Respiratory Infections: Diagnosis and Management, 3d ed.,
edited by James E. Pennington.
Raven Press, Ltd., New York © 1994

24

Viral Pneumonia

Robert S. Kauffman

Department of Medicine, Stanford University School of Medicine,
Stanford, California 94305

Viruses cause most pneumonias in infants and children, whereas in adults, viral pneumonia is uncommon. However, viral pneumonias have the potential for producing devastating respiratory failure and death, even among previously healthy adults; more chronic sequelae such as bronchiectasis and altered airway reactivity can also occur after the acute episode has resolved.

Viral lower respiratory tract disease in adults is usually considered a possible diagnosis when a nonlobar infiltrate is noted on chest roentgenogram in association with a dry cough or with production of nonpurulent sputum and in the absence of positive cultures for a bacterial pathogen. There are often prominent extrapulmonary symptoms such as myalgias, arthralgias, headache, and rhinorrhea, in addition to fever, in this symptom complex. In children, in whom viral pneumonias are relatively common, the diagnosis of a viral pneumonia is based more often on the clinical presentation and epidemiologic setting, as well as by exclusion of bacterial pathogens by negative routine cultures. In both age groups, however, establishing a definitive diagnosis is often difficult, and in a large number of cases a specific etiologic agent is not identified. Many organisms can produce this clinical syndrome aside from viruses, including *Mycoplasma pneumoniae, Legionella species, Rickettsia,* especially *Coxiella burnetii,* and *Chlamydia* (*C. psittaci* and *C. pneumoniae* (TWAR) [28,56]).

This chapter is divided into several general introductory sections on the incidence and epidemiology, diagnostic criteria, radiographic appearance, and pathophysiology and pathologic changes in viral pneumonias. These are followed by a discussion of the diagnostic and distinguishing features of the individual agents producing disease in both children and adults, followed by a discussion of management and complications, including the chemotherapeutic agents available for treatment of viral pneumonias.

INCIDENCE AND EPIDEMIOLOGY

Most of the studies of viral pneumonias, particularly in adults, are based on data derived from hospitalized patients and patients in military training centers. In addition, in case reports, generally only the most severe cases or those in which a specific pathogen has been isolated are reported. Therefore, the clinical features and spectrum of disease presented for a given agent can represent a biased sample of the general pattern of illness, likely more severe, produced by that virus. In addition, because larger numbers of cases are available for study during epidemics, or in closed population groups, other elements of bias could be introduced by these factors.

Many factors influence the incidence and epidemiology of viral pneumonias. Although the groups of agents producing disease in adults and children overlap, the relative proportions produced by each virus vary markedly in these two age groups. In addition to age, the season of the year, and particularly the presence of influenza in the community, as well as the specific setting—such as military base, nursing home, or day care center—alter the proportion of cases caused by particular viruses. Immunosuppressed patients, whether by congenital or acquired illness, or as a result of medical treatment, can develop pneumonia caused by viruses that do not usually cause pneumonia in otherwise normal patients, or by viruses that rarely cause pneumonia in that age group. In addition, such patients can develop a more severe syndrome caused by usual respiratory tract pathogens.

Age

Viruses are by far the most common agents producing pneumonia in infants and young children (27,41), whereas *M. pneumoniae* infections become more prominent in children above age 5 years (27). In infants, respiratory syncytial virus (RSV) accounts for about 40 to 60% of cases, with the remainder of cases produced by parainfluenza virus type 3, and a smaller number by adenoviruses. Influenza type A and parainfluenza types 1 and 2 produce upper respiratory tract disease more often than pneumonia in children (27,41,64,91). In most studies, a specific agent is identified in only about half the cases of presumed viral pneumonia (6,27,41), so other agents could be involved as well. RSV, however, is clearly the dominant agent in terms of incidence and severity in this age group.

In adults, influenza A is the most common cause of viral pneumonia in the civilian population (6,23,51), whereas adenoviruses produce most of the pneumonias reported in military trainees (19). Adenoviruses are also a common cause of sporadic severe viral pneumonias in adults, often ending in respiratory failure and death. Parainfluenza type 3 and RSV produce only a small proportion of viral pneumonias in adults. Rhinoviruses have also been implicated in a small number of cases (26). Associated with the increased incidence of measles in the United States has come increased reports of measles pneumonia in children and adults (4,10,69). Overall, viral pneumonias comprise less than 10% of pneumonias in civilian adults (23,60). Of note is that varicella pneumonia is seen virtually exclusively in adults (80,81), as is the pneumonia of atypical measles (58).

Season of the Year

All respiratory tract infections including viral pneumonias occur more commonly in the winter. Glezen and Denny (27), in a study of lower respiratory tract disease in children, noted a distinct periodicity of most respiratory tract infections with a peak in mid-winter and early spring. When the data were analyzed by specific agent, however, parainfluenza type 3, in contrast to all the other agents, was found to be endemic throughout most of the year, a pattern corroborated by other investigators (64). In contrast, those unusual cases of enterovirus respiratory tract disease are more often noted during periods of peak enterovirus activity in the late summer and fall (11).

Epidemiologic Setting

Closed population groups, such as trainees at military bases, provide the ideal setting for the spread of respiratory viruses and have led to the enhanced recognition of cases of viral pneumonia in this group of patients. In the civilian adult population, influenza is the most common cause of viral pneumonias, whereas adenovirus pneumonia occurs only sporadically. In military training centers, however, adenovirus pneumonias are much more common (19,20). Reports have also demonstrated outbreaks of measles (29) and parainfluenza pneumonias (83) in military centers. In hospitals, transmission of RSV from child to child (31) and from children to adults (31,37) has been documented, as has transmission of adenovirus in a respiratory intensive care unit (67). An outbreak of RSV pneumonia has been reported from a nursing home (72), whereas sporadic cases of RSV pneumonia among adults are very rare. Thus, closed population groups provide for greater spread of respiratory viruses, and increased recognition of viral pneumonias.

Host Factors

Adult patients with underlying cardiac disease, particularly valvular heart disease, appear to have a greater likelihood of developing influenza pneumonia (51,57). Smoking also appears to be a risk factor for influenza infection (43). RSV pneumonia in children is more severe in the presence of underlying heart disease (52) and in immunosuppressed children (35), but it does not appear that the incidence of disease is increased in this group of patients. In immunosuppressed adults, particularly recipients of renal or bone marrow transplants and adult patients with acquired immune deficiency syndrome (AIDS) (49), cytomegalovirus (CMV) pneumonia occurs at a much greater rate than in the general population (1,8,66); up to 50% of diffuse pulmonary infiltrates in bone marrow recipients are caused by CMV (88), with a mortality rate of about 50%. Rarely, patients with burns and leukemia develop herpes simplex virus (HSV) pneumonia as a complication of herpetic infection of the upper respiratory tract (87). Severe combined immunodeficiency disease in children has been associated with fatal parainfluenza (16,42) and measles (22) pneumonia. Immunosuppressed adults are also at increased risk of severe RSV, parainfluenza virus (84), and measles pneumonias (4,69).

DIAGNOSTIC CRITERIA

The clinical illnesses produced by respiratory viruses are sufficiently variable and overlap to such a degree among themselves and among nonviral respiratory pathogens that an etiologic diagnosis cannot confidently be made on clinical grounds alone. Establishing the presence of viral pneumonia and identification of the causative agent during the acute phase of the illness can be difficult. During known outbreaks, a presumptive diagnosis can often be made on the basis of the clinical presentation and epidemiologic setting. However, virus isolation or seroconversion, preferably both, are necessary for definitive diagnosis.

Successful virus isolation in tissue culture depends on transport of an appropriate specimen to the laboratory in proper condition (generally on ice or frozen at $-70°C$ in viral transport medium) and as quickly as possible. Specimens should be obtained as early in the illness as possible, during the period of greatest viral excretion. Nasopharyngeal washings and swabs, nasal washings, throat washings, transtracheal aspirates, and lung aspirates or biopsies have all been used to isolate respiratory viruses (48); nasopharyngeal washings or swabs and throat washings have been the most widely used. Detection of viral cytopathic effect or viral-induced hemadsorption is noted within the first 4 days of culture in most cases, but can take 7 days or more (18). Cultures are negative in up to 40% of patients with acute viral respiratory tract disease (27,41), so that failure to isolate a virus cannot be taken as evidence against the diagnosis of viral pneumonia. On the contrary, it is well established that certain latent viruses such as HSV, CMV, and adenovirus can be shed from the respiratory tract and certain other sites such as urine or stool in the presence of nonviral illness, causing misleading false-positive culture results. A similar phenomenon can occur with viruses such as RSV that are excreted from the respiratory tract for prolonged periods after acute infection. Simultaneous infection with two viruses has also been noted (59).

Immunofluorescence studies of exfoliated cells from the nasopharynx collected on a swab or by washings have been shown to provide rapid, specific diagnosis of RSV infections in infants (44), providing results the same day the sample was taken. This technique has been adapted to other respiratory viruses and can provide rapid viral diagnosis in a large number of cases. Viral antigen detection in respiratory tract secretions by solid-phase assay is also being used increasingly for rapid diagnosis (18,48).

Serologic tests of a number of types, including complement fixation, hemagglutination-inhibition, neutralization, and, more recently, enzyme-linked solid-phase assays (ELISA) have been used in the diagnosis of viral infection (48). A fourfold rise in titer between acute- and convalescent-phase sera tested simultaneously is accepted as a significant change for diagnostic purposes. The detection of a single elevated convalescent-phase titer is much less specific because another illness can nonspecifically elevate the titer in patients with preexisting immunity. However, the presence of specific IgM in a single sample during the acute phase of illness is usually diagnostic of infection with a particular agent. Activation of a latent virus such as HSV by acute illness or recent asymptomatic infection by another virus can also cause confusion in serologic diagnosis of viral diseases. Serologic tests are generally more reliable for diagnosis during widespread outbreaks than in sporadic cases because the number of false-positive results would be much lower.

Histologic evidence of infection in biopsy or postmortem specimens is often helpful in diagnosis. However, it can be difficult in some cases to distinguish the inclusions of some viruses from others, such as the intranuclear inclusion of herpes viruses and adenoviruses. In general, finding inclusions is less sensitive than viral culture, because a smaller portion of the specimen is being directly examined. For example, in one study, typical CMV "owl eye" intranuclear inclusions were found in postmortem lung tissue of infected patients, but detection was 6 times less sensitive than simultaneous viral culture of the same specimen (77). Nevertheless, in the absence of a positive culture, presence of viral inclusion bodies can often be of diagnostic significance.

RADIOGRAPHIC APPEARANCE

The radiographic appearance of viral pneumonia is nonspecific, and differentiation from bacterial pneumonia cannot be confidently made on roentgenographic pattern alone (53). In a retrospective review of 123 children with presumed viral infection of the lower respiratory tract, however, several general features were identified (63). Bronchial wall thickening, peribronchial shadowing, and, less commonly, perihilar linearity were noted. Involvement of multiple areas of lung and patchy involvement of a portion of a lobe (63), with shifting of infiltrates from one region to another, have been noted for a variety of viral pneumonias in both children and adults. In children, air trapping and areas of hyperinflation and atelectasis have been seen most often with RSV pneumonia (63), but also with other agents as well. Hilar adenopathy with a fine reticulonodular infiltrate has been noted in measles pneumonia (29). In severe influenza and adenovirus pneumonias in adults, diffuse bilateral infiltrates similar to those described in the adult respiratory distress syndrome have been reported. Pleural effusions, occasionally massive, can occur in adenovirus (12) and parainfluenza pneumonias (83). Varicella pneumonia in adults can result in diffuse, punctate, pulmonary calcifications during the postconvalescent phase (80). Pulmonary nodules, some persisting for as long as 5 months after the acute illness, have been seen in atypical measles (47,58,75).

PATHOPHYSIOLOGY AND PATHOLOGIC CHANGES

The pathologic changes occurring in the lower airways and lungs of patients with viral pneumonia are histologically similar for all the primary respiratory viruses. Occasionally, intracellular inclusions can provide a clue to the etiologic agent, but confirmation must come from viral isolation or serology.

For the usual respiratory viruses including RSV, adenovirus, influenza, and parainfluenza viruses, the mechanism of pulmonary infection appears to be a progressive downward spread of the infective process from the larger bronchi to the bronchioles and alveoli. In virtually all cases of viral pneumonia, infection of the lung parenchyma is accompanied by a viral bronchiolitis of varying severity, with extension of the infective process into adjacent pulmonary interstitium and alveoli (2). An exception to this pattern appears to occur in CMV pneumonia in immunocompromised patients, where virus appears to reach the lung by hematogenous spread, producing a widespread miliary pattern of involvement of alveoli without a significant component of infection in the airways (8).

The pathologic changes seen in the lung include necrosis and sloughing of the bronchial and bronchiolar epithelium, resulting in a denuded mucosa. Enhanced mucous formation along with the sloughed mucosa leads to plugging of the bronchioles with necrotic debris. The muscularis and cartilage of the airways are not affected in the absence of bacterial superinfection. In later stages there is both a peribronchiolar lymphocytic infiltrate and an interstitial round cell infiltrate in the alveolar ducts and alveolar walls. In severe cases, an intraalveolar round cell infiltrate, often with hyaline membrane formation, occurs along with intraalveolar hemorrhage in some cases of RSV, influenza, and adenovirus pneumonia (15,19,61). Multinucleated giant cells are seen in the bronchioles and alveoli of patients infected both with measles (22) and parainfluenza virus (16,42). The major radiographic features of viral pneumonia can be understood in light of the pathologic changes that occur, consisting of airways plugged with necrotic debris, resulting in atelectasis due to underaeration of pulmonary lobules, as well as hyperinflation due to a "ball-valve" effect of the bronchiolar debris producing obstruction during expiration (2,7).

The sequelae of viral pneumonia can be severe and long lasting. In several series, bronchiectasis has been described in a significant proportion of infants who have recovered from adenovirus pneumonia. In 25 children studied after an outbreak of adenovirus type 21 pneumonia in New Zealand, 5 developed bronchiectasis within 5 years (7), whereas 16 had residual lung changes on roentgenogram. In a group of 22 children studied 10 years after an outbreak of type 7 adenovirus pneumonia, 12 had abnormal chest roentgenograms, and of these, 6 had bronchiectasis. Six of the 10 children with normal chest roentgenograms and 10 of 12 with abnormal roentgenograms had abnormal pulmonary function tests, usually with a restrictive pattern (76).

It appears that RSV and measles infection in children and adults can exacerbate underlying asthma and lead to prolonged changes in airway reactivity (37,82). These effects can be mediated by IgE produced in the respiratory tract during and after infection (82). In adults, the radiographic and in some cases pathologic appearance of interstitial pulmonary fibrosis has been reported in survivors of influenza pneumonia (89), whereas in other series, recovery has been complete (62,67). There have been no large series of patients followed over a long period of time after an episode of viral pneumonia to determine accurately the extent of sequelae. In addition, many of these patients are critically ill and are tested with numerous drugs, as well as with mechanical ventilation with high inspired O_2 concentrations. Thus, allocating the contributions of the original infection and treatment to the production of sequelae can be difficult.

SPECIFIC AGENTS IN ADULTS AND CHILDREN: DIAGNOSTIC AND DISTINGUISHING FEATURES

Primary Respiratory Pathogens

Influenza

In the adult civilian population, influenza is the most common cause of viral pneumonia, whereas in children, influenza is more commonly responsible for febrile upper respiratory tract infections, although pneumonia has been recognized during outbreaks of influenza (91). Pneumonia is reported in the literature more often during epidemic or pandemic years, although pneumonia is not confined to these periods but can occur any time influenza infection is present in a community. As a result of their prevalence, influenza and adenovirus pneumonias are the best-studied viral lower respiratory tract infections of adults.

Louria et al. (51) studied 33 patients during the 1958–1959 Asian flu epidemic and divided influenza lower respiratory infections into four types. Twenty percent of the patients were thought to have primary viral pneumonia without bacterial superinfection. All of these patients had heart disease, particularly rheumatic valvular disease. The clinical signs included typical flu symptoms followed 24 hours later by relentlessly increasing dyspnea, high fever, cyanosis, and wheezing. Bloody sputum was produced by about half the patients. Although there were no signs of consolidation on examination of the chest, a bilateral diffuse perihilar infiltrate was seen in all the cases. None had purulent sputum nor pathogenic bacteria cultured from the sputum, but the white blood cell count was elevated in all patients to the 13,000 to 19,000 range with a left shift. Five of the six patients in this group died of respiratory failure.

Two groups of patients with bacterial infection were also described: those with simultaneous influenza and bacterial pneumonia; and those with bacterial superinfection and evidence of recent influenza but without active influenza at the time of presentation. In both of these groups there was a variable period of apparent improvement before sudden worsening, marked by the production of purulent sputum, return of fever, and development of signs of pulmonary consolidation. Pathogenic bacteria were cultured from the sputum at this time. In the patients with simultaneous viral and bacterial pneumonia, influenza virus was recovered successfully only if cultures were taken before the fifth day of the illness. Patients with bacterial superinfection without active influenza represented nearly half the total cases; *S. pneumoniae, S. aureus,* and *H. influenzae* were cultured from nine, six, and two patients, respectively. The second (bacterial) phase of the illness in this series occurred an average of 3.8 days from first onset of symptoms. Other authors have not observed such a clear-cut separation of the phases of the illness (57). Bronchiolitis without pneumonia, the fourth pattern of illness, was identified on clinical grounds in 10% of patients. These patients had rales and wheezes along with physical signs and symptoms of lower respiratory tract involvement including dry cough, dyspnea, high fever, and pleuritic chest pain, but without infiltrates on chest x-ray. This illness lasted from 3 days to several weeks.

Diagnosis of influenza pneumonia is made by culture of the virus from respiratory secretions, serologic techniques (hemagglutination inhibition), and in one reported case by culture of virus from open lung biopsy (61). Rapid diagnosis using immunofluorescence on exfoliated nasopharyngeal cells is also possible. The role of chemotherapeutic agents in treatment of influenza is discussed in a later section.

Respiratory Syncytial Virus

RSV is the most common cause of pneumonia in the United States in children from 6 months to 3 years of age. Approximately 40 to 60% of pneumonias in this age group are due to this agent (27,41), and 50% of RSV pneumonias occur in children under 2 years of age (27). RSV infection usually occurs in the winter and early spring, often in local outbreaks. Transmission in day care centers occurs readily (39), as does spread within families (32), and in the hospital, where adults are often infected (31,37). The disease produced by RSV varies from a benign upper respiratory tract infection (the pattern most often seen in adults) to bronchiolitis and pneumonia with wheezing and severe respiratory distress. Symptoms and signs of RSV pneumonia are similar to those of bronchiolitis, with prominent wheezing, pulmonary infiltrates, and areas of atelectasis and hyperinflation seen on chest x-ray. More severe and prolonged symptoms occur in children with underlying cardiac disease, especially those with pulmonary hypertension (52). Children receiving antineoplastic chemotherapy and those with immunodeficiency experience more severe RSV infections and have a higher mortality rate (35). Children receiving corticosteroids shed the virus for a longer period but have disease of normal severity (35).

Whereas infection with RSV is universal by 3 years of age, immunity is not fully protective, and repeated attacks occur, although each is less severe than the preceding one (39). RSV pneumonia can occur in adults, although with much lower frequency than in children (23,60,72). A fatal case of RSV pneumonia, probably community acquired, has been reported in an adult patient with leukemia and Hodgkin's disease (15), and an outbreak of RSV infection, including pneumonia, has been reported among bone marrow transplant recipients (38). High mortality was reported with pneumonia in these patients. RSV infection in both adults and children can result in increased airway reactivity and airway resistance which can persist for months (37,82).

The virus can be readily cultured from nasal washings, although rapid transport to the laboratory is essential for efficient recovery of the virus (18,48). An indirect immunofluorescence test on exfoliated nasopharyngeal epithelial cells can provide a specific diagnosis within hours (44).

Adenoviruses

Adenoviruses are responsible for about 3% of pneumonias in children (27,41) and a variable proportion in adults—up to 80% of cases in military training centers (20), to sporadic cases in civilian adults (25,65,90). Transmission within a respiratory intensive care unit has also been documented (67). Adenoviruses produce pneumonia in both normal and immunocompromised hosts (46,90,93); in the latter group several new serotypes have been identified (92). Usually there are no extrapulmonary manifestations of adenovirus infection, such as conjunctivitis, to allow a specific diagnosis in the absence of positive cultures or serology. Serotypes 4, 7, and 21 have been associated with most cases (7,12,19,76). Clinical features are the same as for other viral pneumonias, except that, even in the most severe cases, onset of illness is often gradual, over several days to a week, unlike *Mycoplasma* or influenza (19). Massive pleural effusion with isolation of virus from pleural fluid has been reported in children (12). Rhabdomyolysis and myoglobinuria with adenovirus type 21 pneumonia has been reported (90); similar muscle necrosis has also been associated with cases of influenza A and Coxsackie virus infection. Bronchiectasis and restrictive lung disease have been noted in children followed for several years after acute adenovirus infection (7,76). Fatal cases of adenovirus pneumonia rarely occur, even in previously healthy young people (19).

Parainfluenza Virus

Parainfluenza virus infection is associated more often with tracheobronchitis and croup (generally types 1 and 2) than with pneumonia (usually type 3, most often in infants under 6 months of age). In children, parainfluenza virus is second only to RSV in being responsible for hospitalization for acute respiratory disease, although croup rather than pneumonia accounts for most of these hospitalizations (27,41,64). The pneumonia is usually mild, but fatal cases after a prolonged course with persistent viral shedding have been reported with severe combined immunodeficiency disease (16,42). In adults, case reports of parainfluenza pneumonia are few (60,83), and overall, parainfluenza virus is associated with only a few percent of cases of pneumonias. The disease in adults is usually mild and rarely requires hospitalization (83).

Pneumonia as Part of the Disease Syndrome Produced by Systemic Viral Infections

Pneumonia that occurs during the course of a systemic viral disease is rarely a diagnostic problem, as the systemic disease usually presents a characteristic clinical pattern that is easily recognized. Although CMV and HSV can produce pneumonia in neonates and immunocompromised patients, measles (especially atypical measles) and varicella account for most of the pneumonias occurring during systemic viral infections in adults. Epstein-Barr virus pneumonia during the course of infectious mononucleosis is also seen in a small proportion of adults (3,24).

Measles

The true prevalence of viral pneumonia in measles is difficult to determine accurately, as respiratory symptoms are nearly universal in this illness and a chest x-ray might be performed only in those with more severe symptoms. Reports ranging from an 81% prevalence during an epidemic of measles in Greenland in 1957 to an average value of 3.8% have been cited (78). A prevalence of 3.3% was found during a military outbreak in 1976–1979 (29). In that study, of the cases of measles pneumonia, 87% had a fine reticulonodular infiltrate on chest roentgenogram, whereas nodular infiltrates were more common in those with atypical measles. Eighty-five percent of the patients with pneumonia had rales and 17% had wheezing, with significant hypoxemia detected in those in whom arterial blood gasses were measured. Measles pneumonia can be severe, and fatal cases in previously healthy adults have been reported (4,10,78). In immunocompromised patients, fatal measles pneumonia with giant cell formation in the absence of a rash (Hecht's giant cell pneumonia) is a well-described entity (22). Pregnancy may be an additional risk factor for severe pneumonia, and may result in an adverse fetal outcome (4).

Pneumonia is a central feature of "atypical measles" that occurs during natural infection with measles virus in individuals previously immunized with inactivated measles virus vaccine (36,58). This vaccine was withdrawn from use in 1968 because of the recognition of this syndrome. Atypical measles is marked clinically by high fever and a skin rash that typically begins on the extremities and spreads centripetally; the rash is commonly petechial, pustular, or vesicular, as well as morbilliform, and involves the palms and soles. Koplick's spots are uniformly absent, but mucous membrane involvement is common, including a "strawberry tongue" often mistaken for that of scarlet fever. Pneumonia is nearly universal, and usually consists of a diffuse or segmental nodular infiltrate associated with dyspnea and a nonproductive cough. The clinical syndrome usually resolves over 1 to 2 weeks; both chest x-ray abnormalities (47,58,75) and abnormalities of pulmonary function (36,58) can persist for months. There have been no fatalities associated with atypical measles, but severe respiratory compromise is occasionally seen.

Varicella-Zoster

Pneumonia is a well-described complication of both varicella and disseminated zoster. The incidence of viral pneumonia in varicella is age-related; in late adolescence and in adults pneumonia can be present in as many as 10 to 20% of all cases of varicella (80,81), whereas it is rare in children. The pneumonia can produce fatal respiratory failure in older patients (81) and in pregnant women. Smoking appears to be a risk factor for development of varicella pneumonia (30). Pneumonia usually occurs in those most severely affected by chicken pox, and the pneumonia is most severe at the time of maximum skin involvement. Pneumonia without rash has not been reported. Wheezing, obstruction to outflow of air, and cyanosis, along with pleuritic pain and pleural effusions, are not uncommon. Most patients begin to recover within several days, but often residual changes on chest x-ray can be seen for months. Punctate diffuse pulmonary calcifications are sometimes a residuum of varicella pneumonia (80). Pathologically, the disease is similar to other viral pneumonias, with bronchial and bronchiolar involvement accompanying the interstitial pneumonitis (80). Diagnosis is straightforward on the basis of the characteristic skin eruption. Bacterial superinfection can occur, accompanied by purulent sputum production and culture of pathogenic bacteria from the sputum.

Cytomegalovirus

This member of the herpes virus group has been implicated as an important pathogen in immunocompromised patients, particularly those recipients of renal or bone marrow transplants (66,70,87,88), and in patients with acquired immune deficiency syndrome (AIDS) (49). Immunologically intact patients rarely develop CMV pneumonia (45). Pulmonary involvement with CMV, although often part of a mixed infection (66,70), can be severe, and often fatal. Although the incidence of pneumonia varies with the patient population studied, up to 50% of bone marrow transplant recipients develop diffuse interstitial pneumonias, of which about half are attributable to CMV (88); about half of the CMV-associated cases are fatal. Among renal transplant recipients in one series, about 30% developed overt CMV disease, of whom 42% developed pneumonia; again, about half the cases were fatal (66). In AIDS, CMV pulmonary infection frequently coexists with *Pneumocystis carinii* or atypical mycobacteria (49). CMV pneumonia is also seen in neonates infected shortly after birth (85).

Clinical signs include systemic symptoms such as fever, myalgias, arthralgias, and fatigue followed by dry cough and tachypnea. Diffuse pulmonary infiltrates were noted in 96% of renal transplant patients with CMV pneumonia in one series (66), whereas in other series, several cases showed focal consolidation more suggestive of fungal or bacterial infection; rarely, pulmonary nodules were seen (70). Histologically, two distinct patterns of infection occur. In fatal cases of pneumonia in bone marrow transplant recipients, a miliary pattern of involvement with focal areas of infiltrate including cytomegaly with surrounding normal lung was seen, in contrast to those less severe cases in which only diffuse involvement occurred. The so-called miliary pattern was associated with a fulminant course and fatal outcome resulting from respiratory failure (8). Viremia was present in each of these patients, all of whom had no CMV antibodies at the time of transplant and, thus, were undergoing a "primary" infection. It was postulated that this clinical and histologic pattern of involvement resulted from bloodstream dissemination of virus. Up to half of CMV pulmonary infections in these patients were accompanied by bacterial, fungal, or protozoan superinfection; these combined infections were highly lethal.

Definitive diagnosis of CMV pneumonia is difficult, as CMV produces a persistent viral infection with either continuous or intermittent viral shedding; patients often have preexisting positive serologic tests, so that a positive or rising titer is not diagnostic of acute infection. A combination of histologic (demonstration of viral inclusions in infected tissue), virologic (culture of virus from infected tissue or blood), and serologic tests offer the most reliable basis for definitive diagnosis (1,66,70,87).

Epstein-Barr Virus

Pneumonia has been reported to occur in 5 to 7% of cases of infectious mononucleosis (24). The pneumonitis is usually benign and self-limited, although the infiltrates, and occasionally pleural effusions, can be present for several weeks after diagnosis (24). Bacterial superinfection occurs and must be differentiated from the uncomplicated viral pneumonia.

MANAGEMENT AND COMPLICATIONS

Several antiviral agents are currently in use for treatment of respiratory and systemic viral infections. Rapid developments are occurring in this area; new agents and new indications and formulations for use of the currently licensed agents are expected.

Amantadine hydrochloride (Symmetrel) has been shown to be useful for prophylaxis against influenza A infections (40). Amantadine is ineffective against influenza B infections. Several studies of prophylaxis in both communitywide outbreaks and among hospital personnel exposed to influenza have shown an average effectiveness of 60% in preventing clinical disease and a 50% effectiveness in preventing influenza infection (40). If given within the first 24 to 48 hours of clinical illness, amantadine can be useful in the treatment of influenza A infections, by shortening the period of clinical illness by 1 to 2 days, and decreasing the degree of fever. In one uncontrolled study in which large doses (400 to 500 mg per day for 7 days) were used in 11 patients with influenza pneumonia, improvement was seen in two patients; four survived but had no improvement that could be attributed to the drug, and five patients died (14). In another placebo-controlled study of influenza not complicated by pneumonia (all patients had a normal chest roentgenogram), both clinical improvement and improvement in airflow were noted in an amantadine-treated group (50). Thus, if given early in the course of the illness, amantadine can produce some improvement in influenza pneumonia. Adverse effects of amantadine include hallucinations, mental confusion, insomnia, and anxiety in about 3 to 7% of treated patients (40). The usual dosage is 100 mg orally every 12 hours. A dosage reduction is necessary if renal impairment is present.

Adenosine arabinoside (Vidarabine) has been used to treat disseminated zoster, resulting in a shorter period of viral shedding and a somewhat more rapid crusting of skin lesions (86). There have been no reports of the use of this drug specifically in varicella pneumonia or the pulmonary involvement of disseminated zoster. Its use for nearly all its indications has been supplanted by acyclovir (Zovirax), a much more potent anti–herpes virus agent.

Acyclovir has clinical activity against both herpes simplex virus (HSV) and varicella zoster virus (VZV) (17). It is available in both oral and intravenous form. For severe infections, the intravenous form is preferred, especially for VZV infections, where higher blood levels are necessary. There is no published data on the use of acyclovir in the rare cases of HSV pneumonia, but the drug is highly active and the toxicity is low, so its use can be justified in this severe infection. In disseminated zoster, acyclovir reduces the period of viral shedding and of healing of skin lesions (74), and can prevent dissemination from localized zoster in immunocompromised patients (5). A similar effect in varicella has been observed in immunocompromised children (68). In a retrospective controlled study, treatment with acyclovir significantly reduced the duration of fever, the respiratory rate, and improved oxygenation (30) in patients with varicella pneumonia. Early treatment, within 36 hours of onset of disease, resulted in a better outcome. The use of acyclovir in these patients can be justified by the low toxicity of the drug (primarily minor hematologic and central nervous system alterations and impairment of renal function) and potential severity of the illness. As with all antiviral agents, treatment as early in the course of illness as possible is advisable. The dose of intravenous acyclovir for herpes simplex infection is 250 mg/m^2 every 8 hours or 5 mg/kg every 8 hours, and for herpes zoster, 500 mg/m^2 every 8 hours (17).

Ribavirin (Virazole) is a synthetic triazole nucleoside analogue that has been licensed for use in the United States in an aerosol form for treatment of severe respiratory syncytial virus disease in children (33,34). Because of the requirement for aerosol generation, use is restricted to the hospital setting. Several placebo-controlled studies in infants with bronchiolitis and pneumonia have demonstrated more rapid improvement in blood gas values and decreased viral shedding in treated patients (34), including those with risk factors for more severe RSV disease such as congenital heart disease (33). Aerosolized ribavirin has also been studied in young adults with influenza B virus infection and has resulted in more rapid defervescence, more rapid decrease in viral shedding, and improvement in clinical symptoms than a placebo group (54). Thus, this agent might be useful for treating severe cases of both RSV and influenza pneumonia. Although the oral form has been effective in treatment of Lassa fever (55), use of oral ribavirin in respiratory infections appears less efficacious. Use of the aerosolized drug in patients requiring mechanical ventilation is possible but must be monitored closely.

Gancyclovir (9-(1,3-dihydroxy-2-propoxy-methyl) guanine, DHPG) is an antiviral drug with activity against cytomegalovirus (13). It has been used in immunocompromised patients with disseminated CMV disease, including those with pneumonia (13,73). Clinical improvement has been noted in CMV retinitis and bowel disease; pneumonia, however, has been more refractory to treatment with this agent alone (73). However, recent studies suggest that the combination of gancyclovir and intravenous immunoglobulin results in improved outcome for patients with CMV pneumonia (21,71).

Respiratory failure resembling the adult respiratory distress syndrome (ARDS) can occur in severe viral pneumonia, usually in cases of influenza, adenovirus, and, more rarely, varicella and CMV infections. Progression to respiratory failure is often precipitous, within 24 to 48 hours after clinical symptoms develop. Severe hypoxemia, increased alveolar-arterial oxygen difference, and high pulmonary inflation pressures often necessitate intubation with mechanical ventilation and the addition of positive end-expiratory pressure to maintain small airway and alveolar patency and promote gas exchange (25). Continuous positive airway pressure (CPAP) without intubation has also been effective in some cases (79). Many patients recover within several days so that intensive support of this nature is indicated. The role of corticosteroid treatment is uncertain and controversial; there have been no controlled studies to evaluate their effectiveness and complications. Doses as high as 500 mg of methylprednisolone every 6 hours have been used (25).

Bacterial superinfection of the lung accompanying or following viral respiratory tract infections are often more common than pure viral pneumonia (51,57). However, only influenza has been clearly shown to be the precursor of bacterial pneumonia, when all patients with bacterial pneumonia have been studied for evidence of preceding viral infection (23). The role of viral pneumonia in the development of bronchiectasis has been described in previous sections. Destruction and desquamation of the respiratory mucosa, as well as adverse effects of viral infection on alveolar macrophages, ciliary function (9), and other host defenses, are the major factors contributing to the development of bacterial superinfection. Staphylococcal and *H. influenzae* pneumonia were deadly complications of influenza during the 1918 pandemic and have continued to complicate influenza infections since then (51,57). In a number of series studying the complications of influenza, *S. pneumoniae, S. aureus,* and *H. influenzae* have been the most common secondary invaders (20,51,57). Diagnosis of superinfection is established by the development of purulent sputum with organisms seen on sputum gram stain, culture of pathogenic organisms from the sputum or blood, the presence of lobar pulmonary involvement, or the development of new infiltrates after a period of clinical improvement. Antibiotics appropriate for the organism present should be administered after cultures have been taken. There is no evidence that prophylactic antibiotics are of use in viral pneumonia (20), and could predispose to superinfection by more resistant organisms.

HANTAVIRUS PNEUMONIA

A newly described, life threatening form of atypical pneumonia has been linked to a hantavirus. The June 11, 1993 issue of *Morbidity and Mortality Weekly Report* (59a) described several cases of acute febrile respiratory illness, all occurring in the Southwestern United States. American Indians were prominently affected, and most of these early cases occurred in or near New Mexico. Since this initial report, cases have been reported from several other western and southern states, and as far east as Louisiana. The clue that a common causal agent may be involved was the May, 1993 occurrence of two previously healthy members of the same household dying of an acute and similar febrile respiratory illness within five days of each other.

The illness is characterized by sudden onset of fever, headache, myalgias, and dry cough. Rapidly progressive respiratory failure ensues, with a syndrome resembling ARDS. All cultures remain negative and laboratory data are non-specific. Mortality to date has been reported to be about 50 percent, although many less severe and non-fatal cases have probably not been reported.

Using antibody screening for viral and other atypical respiratory pathogens, a consistent pattern of reactivity to the hantavirus has been found in most cases. There are four known members of the genus hantavirus (Hantaan, Puumala, Seoul, and

Prospect Hill), which is a member of the family Bunyaviridae. The current outbreak strain appears to be a previously unidentified member of this genus, which has been labelled Muer-to-Canyon virus (MCV). Hantavirus-associated disease has not previously been described in the Western Hemisphere, having occurred mainly in Korea and Europe. Rodents are the natural host for hantavirus and human disease is thought to result from contact with rodent excreta or its aerosol. Testing of rodent populations in the Southwest states has identified the deer mouse (*Peromyscus maniculatus*) as the most common source of hantavirus (9a). Other rodent species also may be involved.

Currently, bedside diagnosis is dependent upon clinical suspicion in the proper setting. Fulminant atypical pneumonia in a patient known to be exposed to rodents should alert the clinician. Diagnosis may be confirmed by ELISA antibody testing at the Centers for Disease Control and Prevention, either by a scroconversion, or by a single high immunoglobulin M titer, indicative of recent infection. Immunohistochemistry on formalin fixed lung tissues, or PCR amplification of hantavirus nucleotide sequences from frozen tissues also may be useful.

The only therapeutic agent available for treatment is intravenous ribavirin. Ribavirin treatment has not been evaluated systematically in this outbreak, but has proven effective in a controlled trial as therapy for a different form of hantavirus infection (40a). A case of successful treatment of hantavirus pneumonia with ribavirin has recently been described in detail (68a). Intravenous ribavirin is not licensed for general use in the United States but may be obtained by contacting the Centers for Disease Control and Prevention in Atlanta. In endemic areas, local public health offices may have stock on hand.

Prevention of hantavirus pneumonia relies upon avoidance of rodent excreta. Sweeping, dusting, cleaning, moving, and other activities in rodent-infested areas may lead to disease. Rodent control programs also may be useful.

REFERENCES

1. Abdallah, P.S., Mark, J.B.D., and Merigan, T.C. (1976): Diangosis of cytomegalovirus pneumonia in compromised hosts. *Am. J. Med.,* 61:326–332.
2. Aherne, W., Bird, T., Court, S.D.M., Gardner, P.S., and McQuillin, J. (1970): Pathologic changes in virus infections of the lower respiratory tract in children. *J. Clin. Pathol.,* 23:7–18.
3. Andiman, W.A., McCarthy, P., Markowitz, R.I., Cormier, D., and Horstmann, D.M. (1981): Clinical virologic and serologic evidence of Epstein-Barr virus infection in association with childhood pneumonia. *J. Pediatr.,* 99:880–886.
4. Atmar, R.L., Englund, J.A., and Hammill, H. (1992): Complications of measles during pregnancy. *Clin. Inf. Dis.,* 14:217–226.
5. Balfour, H.H., Jr., Bean, B., Laskin, O.L., Ambinder, R.F., Meyers, J.D., Wade, J.C., Zaia, J.A., Aeppli, D., Kirk, L.E., Segreti, A.C., Keeney, R.E., and the Burroughs Wellcome Collaborative Acyclovir Study Group. (1983): Acyclovir halts progression of herpes zoster in immunocompromised patients. *N. Engl. J. Med.,* 308:1448–1453.
6. Balfour, H.H., Jr., and Burke, B.A. (1975): Viral and mycoplasma pneumonias. *Postgrad. Med.,* 59(7):48–55.
7. Becroft, D.M.O. (1971): Bronchiolitis obliterans, bronchiectasis, and other sequelae of adenovirus type 21 infection in young children. *J. Clin. Pathol.,* 24:72–82.
8. Beschorner, W.E., Hutchins, G.M., Burns, W.H., Saral, R., Tutschka, P.J., and Santos, G.W. (1980): Cytomegalovirus pneumonia in bone marrow transplant recipients: miliary and diffuse patterns. *Am. Rev. Respir. Dis.,* 122:107–114.
9. Carson, J.L., Collier, A.M., and Hu, S.-C.S. (1985): Acquired ciliary defects in nasal epithelium of children with acute viral upper respiratory infections. *N. Engl. J. Med.,* 312:463–468.
9a. Centers for Disease Control and Prevention. Outbreak, hantavirus infection–southwestern United States, 1993. *J.A.M.A.* 270:27.
10. Chapnick, E.K., Gradon, J.D., Kim, Y.D., Narvios, A., Gerard, P., Till, M., and Sepkowitz, D.V.

(1992): Fatal measles pneumonia in an immunocompetent patient: case report. *Clin. Inf. Dis.,* 15:377–379.

11. Cheesman, S.H., Hirsch, M.S., Keller, E.W., and Keim, D.E. (1977): Fatal neonatal pneumonia caused by echovirus type 9. *Am. J. Dis. Child.,* 1331:1169–1172.

12. Cho, C.T., Hiatt, W.O., and Behbehani, A.M. (1973): Pneumonia and massive pleural effusion associated with adenovirus type 7. *Am. J. Dis. Child.,* 126:92–94.

13. Collaborative DHPG Treatment Study Group. (1986): Treatment of serious cytomegalovirus infections with 9-(1,3-dihydroxy-2-propoxymethyl) guanine in patients with AIDS and other immunodeficiencies. *N. Engl. J. Med.,* 314:801–805.

14. Couch, R.B., and Jackson, G.G. (1976): Antiviral agents in influenza: summary of influenza workshop VIII. *J. Infect. Dis.,* 134:516–527.

15. Crane, L.R., Kish, J.A., Ratanatharathorn, V., Merline, J.R., and Raval, M.F. (1981): Fatal syncytial virus pneumonia in a laminar airflow room. *J.A.M.A.,* 246:366–367.

16. Delage, G., Brochu, P., Pelletier, M., Jasmin, G., and Lapointe, N. (1979): Giant-cell pneumonia caused by parainfluenza virus. *J. Pediatr.,* 94:426–429.

17. Dorsky, D.I., and Crumpacker, C.S. (1987): Acyclovir. *Ann. Intern. Med.,* 107:859–874.

18. Drew, W.L. (1986): Controversies in viral diagnosis. *Rev. Inf. Dis.,* 8:814–824.

19. Dudding, B.A., Wagner, S.C., Zeller, J.A., Gmelich, J.T., French, G.R., and Top, F.H., Jr. (1972): Fatal pneumonia associated with adenovirus type 7 in three military trainees. *N. Engl. J. Med.,* 286:1289–1292.

20. Ellenbogen, C., Graybill, J.R., Silva J. Jr., and Homme, P.J. (1974): Bacterial pneumonia complicating adenoviral pneumonia: a comparison of respiratory tract bacterial culture sources and effectiveness of chemoprophylaxis against bacterial pneumonia. *Am. J. Med.,* 56:169–178.

21. Emanuel, D., Cunningham, I., Jules-Elysee, K., Brochstein, J.A., Kernan, N.A., Laver, J., Stover, D., White, D.A., Fels, A., Polsky, B., Castro-Malaspina, H., Peppard, J.R., Bartus̀, P., Hammerling, U., and O'Reilly, R.J. (1988): Cytomegalovirus pneumonia after bone marrow transplantation successfully treated with the combination of ganciclovir and high-dose intravenous immune globulin. *Ann. Intern. Med.,* 109:777–782.

22. Enders, J.F., McCarthy, K., Mitus, A., and Cheatham, W.J. (1959): Isolation of measles virus at autopsy in cases of giant cell pneumonia without rash. *N. Engl. J. Med.,* 261:875–880.

23. Fekety, F.R., Jr., Caldwell, J., Gump, D., Johnson, J.E., Maxson, W., Mulholland, J., and Thoburn, R. (1971): Bacteria, viruses, and mycoplasma in acute pneumonias in adults. *Am. Rev. Respir. Dis.,* 104:499–507.

24. Fermaglich, D.R. (1975): Pulmonary involvement in infectious mononucleosis. *J. Pediatr.,* 86: 93–95.

25. Ferstenfeld, J.E., Schlueter, D.P., Rytel, M.W., and Molloy, R.P. (1975): Recognition and treatment of adult respiratory distress syndrome secondary to viral interstitial pneumonia. *Am. J. Med.,* 58:709–718.

26. George, R.B., and Mogabgab, W.J. (1969): Atypical pneumonia in young men with rhinovirus infection. *Ann. Intern. Med.,* 71:1073–1078.

27. Glezen, W.P., and Denny, F.W. (1973): Epidemiology of acute lower respiratory disease in children. *N. Engl. J. Med.,* 288:498–505.

28. Grayston, J.T., Kuo, C-C., Wang, S-P., and Altman, J. (1986): A new *Chlamydia psittaci* strain, TWAR, isolated in acute respiratory tract infections. *N. Engl. J. Med.,* 315:161–168.

29. Gremillion, D.H., and Crawford, G.E. (1981): Measles pneumonia in young adults: an analysis of 106 cases. *Am. J. Med.,* 71:539–542.

30. Haake, D.A., Zakowski, P.C., Haake, D.L., and Bryson, Y. (1990): Early treatment with acyclovir for varicella pneumonia in otherwise healthy adults: retrospective controlled study and review. *Rev. Inf. Dis.,* 12:788–798.

31. Hall, C.B., Douglas, R.G., Jr., Geiman, J.M., and Messner, M.K. (1975): Nosocomial respiratory syncytial virus infections. *N. Engl. J. Med.,* 293:1343–1346.

32. Hall, C.B., Geiman, J.M., Biggar, R., Kotok, D.I., Hogan, P.M., and Douglas, R.G., Jr. (1976): Respiratory syncytial virus infections within families. *N. Engl. J. Med.,* 294:414–419.

33. Hall, C.B., McBride, J.T., Gala, C.L., Hildreth, S.W., and Schnabel, K.C. (1985): Ribavirin treatment of respiratory syncytial viral infection in infants with underlying cardiopulmonary disease. *J.A.M.A.,* 254:3047–3051.

34. Hall, C.B., McBride, J.T., Walsh, E.E., Bell, D.M., Gala, C.L., Hildreth, S., Teneyck, L.G., and Hall, W.J. (1983): Aerosolized ribavirin treatment of infants with respiratory syncytial virus infection. *N. Engl. J. Med.,* 308:1443–1447.

35. Hall, C.B., Powell, K.R., MacDonald, N.E., Gala, C.L., Menegus, M.E., Suffin, S.C., and Cohen, H.J. (1986): Respiratory syncytial virus infection in children with compromised immune function. *N. Engl. J. Med.,* 315:77–81.

36. Hall, W.J., and Hall, C.B. (1979): Atypical measles in adolescents: evaluation of clinical and pulmonary function. *Ann. Intern. Med.,* 90:882–886.

37. Hall, W.J., Hall, C.B., and Speers, D.M. (1978): Respiratory syncytial virus infection in adults. *Ann. Intern. Med.,* 88:203–205.

38. Harrington, R.D., Hooten, T.M., Hackman, R.C., Storch, G.A., Osborne, B., Gleaves, C.A., Benson, A., and Myers, J.D. (1992): An outbreak of respiratory syncytial virus in a bone marrow transplant center. *J. Inf. Dis.,* 165:987–993.
39. Henderson, F.W., Collier, A.M., Clyde, W.A., Jr., and Denny, F.W., Jr. (1979): Respiratory syncytial virus infections, reinfections, and immunity: a prospective longitudinal study in young children. *N. Engl. J. Med.,* 300:530–534.
40. Hirsch, M.S., and Swartz, M.N. (1980): Antiviral agents. *N. Engl. J. Med.,* 302:903–907, 949–953.
40a.Huggins, J.W., Hsiang, C.M., Cosgriff, T.M., Guang, M.Y., Smith, J.I., Wu, Z.O., LeDuc, J.W., Zheng, Z.M., Meegan, J.M., Wang, Q.N., Oland, D.D., Gui, X.E., Gibbs, P.H., Yuan, G.H., Zhang, T.M. (1991): Prospective, double blind concurrent, placebo-controlled clinical trial of intravenous ribavirin. Therapy of hemorrhagic fever with renal syndrome. *J. Infect. Dis.,* 164:1119–1127.
41. Jacobs, J.W., Peacock, D.B., Corner, B.D., Caul, E.O., and Clarke, S.K.R. (1971): Respiratory syncytial and other viruses associated with respiratory disease in infants. *Lancet,* 1:871–876.
42. Jarvis, W.R., Middleton, P.J., and Gelfand, E.W. (1979): Parainfluenza pneumonia in severe combined immunodeficiency disease. *J. Pediatr.,* 94:423–426.
43. Kark, J.D., Lebiush, M., and Rannon, L. (1982): Cigarette smoking as a risk factor for epidemic A (H_1N_1) influenza in young men. *N. Engl. J. Med.,* 307:1042–1046.
44. Kaul, A., Scott, R., Gallagher, M., Scott, M., Clement, J., and Ogra, P.L. (1978): Respiratory syncytial virus infection: rapid diagnosis in children by use of indirect immunofluorescence. *Am. J. Dis. Child.,* 132:1088–1090.
45. Klemola, E., Stenstrom, R., and vonEssen, R. (1972): Pneumonia as a clinical manifestation of cytomegalovirus infection in previously healthy adults. *Scand. J. Infect. Dis.,* 4:7–10.
46. Komshian, S.V., Chandrasekar, P.H., and Levine, D.P. (1987): Adenovirus pneumonia in healthy adults. *Heart Lung,* 16:146–150.
47. Laptook, A., Wind, E., Nussbaum, M., and Shenker, I.R. (1978): Pulmonary lesions in atypical measles. *Pediatrics,* 62:42–46.
48. Lennette, D.A., Melnick, J.L., and Jahrling, P.B. (1980): Clinical virology: introduction to methods. In: *Manual of Clinical Microbiology,* edited by E.H. Lenette, A. Balows, W.H. Hausler, Jr., and J.P. Truant, pp. 760–771. American Society for Microbiology, Washington, D.C.
49. Lerner, C.W., and Tapper, M.L. (1984): Opportunistic infection complicating acquired immune deficiency syndrome: clinical features of 25 cases. *Medicine* (Baltimore), 63:155–164.
50. Little, J.W., Hall, W.J., Douglas, R.G., Jr., Hyde, R.W., and Speers, D.M. (1976): Amantadine effect on peripheral airways abnormalities in influenza: a study of 15 students with natural influenza A infection. *Ann. Intern. Med.,* 85:177–182.
51. Louria, D.B., Blumenfeld, H.L., Ellis, J.T., Kilbourne, E.D., and Rogers, D.E. (1959): Studies on influenza in the pandemic of 1957–58. II. Pulmonary complications of influenza. *J. Clin. Invest.,* 38:213–265.
52. MacDonald, N.E., Hall, C.B., Suffin, S.C., Alexson, C., Harris, P.J., and Manning, J.A. (1982): Respiratory syncytial viral infection in infants with congenital heart disease. *N. Engl. J. Med.,* 307:397–400.
53. McCarthy, P.L., Spiesel, S.Z., Stashwick, C.A., Ablow, R.C., Masters, S.J., and Dolan, T.F., Jr. (1981): Radiographic findings and etiologic diagnosis in ambulatory childhood pneumonias. *Clin. Pediatr.,* 20:686–691.
54. McClung, H.W., Knight, V., Gilbert, B.E., Wilson, S.Z., Quarles, J.M., and Divine, G.W. (1983): Ribavirin aerosol treatment of influenza B virus infection. *J.A.M.A.,* 249:2671–2674.
55. McCormick, J.B., King, I.J., Webb, P.A., Scribner, C.L., Craven, R.B., Johnson, K.M., Elliott, L.H., and Belmont-Williams, R. (1986): Lassa fever: effective therapy with ribavirin. *N. Engl. J. Med.,* 314:20–26.
56. Marrie, T.J., Grayston, J.T., Want, S-P., and Kuo, C-C. (1987): Pneumonia associated with the TWAR strain of *Chlamydia. Ann. Intern. Med.,* 106:507–511.
57. Martin, C.M., Kunin, C.M., Gottlieb, L.S., Barnes, M.W., Liu, C., and Finland, M. (1959): Asian influenza A in Boston, 1957–58. I. Observations in 32 influenza-associated fatal cases. *Arch. Intern. Med.,* 103:515–523.
58. Martin, D.B., Weiner, L.B., Nieburg, P.I., and Blair, D.C. (1979): Atypical measles in adolescents and young adults. *Ann. Intern. Med.,* 90:877–881.
59. Mathur, U., Bentley, D.W., and Hall, C.B. (1980): Concurrent respiratory syncytial virus and influenza A infections in the institutionalized elderly and chronically ill. *Ann. Intern. Med.,* 93:49–52.
59a.Outbreak of acute illness–southwestern United States, (1993): *Morb. Mortal. Wkly. Rep.* 42:421–424.
60. Mufson, M.A., Chang, V., Gill, V., Wood, S.C., Romansky, M.J., and Chanock, R.M. (1967): The role of viruses, mycoplasmas, and bacteria in acute pneumonia in civilian adults. *Am. J. Epidemiol.,* 86:526–532.

61. Noble, R.L., Lillington, G.A., and Kempson, R.L. (1973): Fatal diffuse influenzal pneumonia: premortem diagnosis by lung biopsy. *Chest*, 63:644–647.
62. O'Brien, T.G., and Sweeney, D.F. (1973): Interstitial viral pneumonitis complicated by severe respiratory failure. *Chest*, 63:314–322.
63. Osborne, D. (1978): Radiologic appearance of viral disease of the lower respiratory tract in infants and children. *Am. J. Roentgenol.*, 130:29–33.
64. Parrott, R.H., Vargasko, A.J., Kim, H.W., Bell, J.A., and Chanock, R.M. (1962): Myxovirus: parainfluenzae. *Am. J. Pub. Health*, 52:907–917.
65. Pearson, R.D., Hall, W.J., Menegus, M.A., and Douglas, R.G., Jr. (1980): Diffuse pneumonitis due to adenovirus type 21 in a civilian. *Chest*, 78:107–109.
66. Peterson, P.K., Balfour, H.H., Jr., Marker, S.C., Fryd, D.S., Howard, R.J., and Simmons, R.L. (1980): Cytomegalovirus disease in renal allograft recipients: a prospective study of the clinical features, risk factors, and impact on renal transplantation. *Medicine*, 59:283–300.
67. Pingleton, S.K., Pingleton, W.W., Hill, R.H., Dixon, A., Sobonya, R.E., and Gertzen, J. (1978): Type 3 adenoviral pneumonia occurring in a respiratory intensive care unit. *Chest*, 73:554–555.
68. Prober, C.G., Kirk, L.E., and Keeney, R.E. (1982): Acyclovir therapy of chickenpox in immunosuppressed children—a collaborative study. *J. Pediatr.*, 101:622–625.
68a. Prochoda, K., Mostow, S.R., Greenberg, K. (1993): Hantavirus-associated acute respiratory failure. *N. Eng. J. Med.* 329:1744.
69. Radoycich, G.R., Zuppan, C.W., Weeks, D.A., Krous, H.F., and Langston C. (1992): Patterns of measles pneumonitis. *Pediatr. Pathol.*, 12:773–786.
70. Ramsay, P.G., Rubin, R.H., Tolkoff-Rubin, N.E., Cosimi, A.B., Russell, P.S., and Greene, R. (1980): The renal transplant patient with fever and pulmonary infiltrates. Etiology, clinical manifestations, and management. *Medicine* (Baltimore), 59:206–222.
71. Reed, E.C., Bowden, R.A., Dandliker, P.S., Lilleby, K.E., and Meyers, J.D. (1988): Treatment of cytomegalovirus pneumonia with ganciclovir and intravenous cytomegalovirus immunoglobulin in patients with bone marrow transplants. *Ann. Intern. Med.*, 109:783–788.
72. Respiratory syncytial virus-Missouri. (1977): *Morbid. Mortal. Week. Rep.*, 26:351–352.
73. Shepp, D.H., Dandliker, P.S., deMiranda, P., Burnette, T.C., Cederberg, D.M., Kirk, L.E., and Meyers, J.D. (1985): Activity of 9-[2-hydroxy-1(hydroxy-methyl)ethoxymethyl]guanine in the treatment of cytomegalovirus pneumonia. *Ann. Int. Med.*, 103:368–373.
74. Shepp, D.H., Dandliker, P.S., and Meyers, J.D. (1986): Treatment of varicella-zoster virus infections in severely immunocompromised patients. *N. Engl. J. Med.*, 314:208–212.
75. Sherkow, L. (1980): Pulmonary residuum 14 months after skin rash and pneumonia. *J.A.M.A.*, 243:65–66.
76. Simila, S., Linna, O., Lanning, P., Heikkinen, E., and Ala-Houhala, M. (1981): Chronic lung damage caused by adenovirus type 7: a ten-year follow-up study. *Chest*, 80:127–131.
77. Smith, T.F., Holley, K.E., Keys, T.F., and Macasaet, F.F. (1975): Cytomegalovirus studies of autopsy tissue. I. Virus isolation. *Am. J. Clin. Pathol.*, 63:854–858.
78. Sobonya, R.E., Hiller, C., Pingleton, W., and Watanabe, I. (1978): Fatal measles (rubeola) pneumonia in adults. *Arch. Pathol. Lab. Med.*, 102:366–371.
79. Taylor, G.J., Brenner, W., and Summer, W.R. (1976): Severe viral pneumonia in young adults. *Chest*, 69:722–728.
80. Triebwasser, J.H., Harris, R.E., Bryant, R.E., and Rhoades, E.R. (1967): Varicella pneumonia in adults. Report of seven cases and a review of literature. *Medicine*, 46:409–423.
81. Weinstein, L., and Meade, R.H. (1956): Respiratory manifestations of chickenpox. *Arch. Intern. Med.*, 98:91–102.
82. Welliver, R.C., Kaul, T.N., and Ogra, P.L. (1980): The appearance of cell-bound IgE in respiratory tract epithelium after respiratory-syncytial-virus infection. *N. Engl. J. Med.*, 303:1198–1202.
83. Wenzel, R.P., McCormick, D.P., and Beam, W.E., Jr. (1972): Parinfluenza pneumonia in adults. *J.A.M.A.*, 221:294–295.
84. Whimbey, E., and Bodey, G.P. (1992): Viral pneumonia in the immunocompromised host with neoplastic disease: the role of common community respiratory viruses. *Sem. Respir. Infect.*, 7:122–131.
85. Whitley, R.J., Brasfield, D., Reynolds, D.W., Stagno, S., Tiller, R.E., and Alford, C.A. (1976): Protracted pneumonitis in young infants associated with perinatally acquired cytomegaloviral infection. *J. Pediatr.*, 89:16–22.
86. Whitley, R.J., Ch'ien, L.T., Dolin, R., Galasso, G.J., and Alford, C.A., editors, and the Collaborative Study group. (1976): Adenine arabinoside therapy of herpes zoster in the immunosuppressed. *N. Engl. J. Med.*, 294:1193–1199.
87. Williams, D.M., Krick, J.A., and Remington, J.S. (1976): Pulmonary infection in the compromised host. Part II. *Am. Rev. Respir. Dis.*, 114:593–627.
88. Winston, D.J., Gale, R.P., Meyer, D.V., and Young, L.S. (1979): Infectious complication of human bone marrow transplantation. *Medicine* (Baltimore), 58:1–31.
89. Winterbauer, R.H., Ludwig, W.R., and Hammar, S.P. (1977): Clinical course, management, and

long-term sequelae of respiratory failure due to influenza viral pneumonia. *Johns Hopkins Med. J.*, 141:148–155.

90. Wright, J., Couchonnal, G., and Hodges, G.R. (1979): Adenovirus type 21 infection: occurrence with pneumonia, rhabdomyolysis, and myoglobinuria in an adult. *J.A.M.A.*, 241:2420–2421.

91. Wright, P.F., Ross, K.B., Thompson, J., and Karzon, D.T. (1977): Influenza A infections in young children. Primary natural infection and protective efficacy of live-vaccine-induced or naturally acquired immunity. *N. Engl. J. Med.*, 296:829–834.

92. Zahradnik, J.M., Spencer, M.J., and Porter, D.D. (1980): Adenovirus infection in the immuno-compromised patient. *Am. J. Med.*, 68:725–732.

93. Zarraga, A.L., Kerns, F.T., and Kitchen, L.W. (1992): Adenovirus pneumonia with severe sequelae in an immunocompetent adult. *Clin. Infect. Dis.*, 15:712–713.

Respiratory Infections: Diagnosis and Management, 3d ed.,
edited by James E. Pennington.
Raven Press, Ltd., New York © 1994

25

Opportunistic Fungal Pneumonias: *Aspergillus, Mucor, Candida, Torulopsis*

James E. Pennington

University of California, San Francisco, California 94143

Fungi are ubiquitous in nature, and their constant aerosol exposure to respiratory tissues is inevitable. It is not surprising, therefore, that the lung is a major target organ for fungal infections. "Pathogenic fungi," such as *Coccidioides immitis* or *Histoplasma capsulatum,* usually infect immunologically normal individuals. However, a separate group of potential fungal pathogens generally infect only those patients with abnormal host defenses to infection. These so-called opportunistic fungi, which include *Aspergillus* sp, the Phycomycetes *(Mucor, Rhizopus, Absidia), Candida* sp, and *Torulopsis glabrata,* are discussed in this chapter. *Cryptococcus neoformans* is another fungal pathogen that can invade the compromised host; however, this infectious agent can also infect normal individuals, and is discussed elsewhere in this text.

ASPERGILLUS LUNG INFECTION

Aspergillus species are molds spread by aerosols of spores. The most common involved in human lung diseases are *A. fumigatus, A. flavus,* and *A. niger. Aspergillus* sp are interesting pulmonary pathogens. This ubiquitous mold can act as an allergen, causing a variety of hypersensitivity lung diseases: asthma, extrinsic allergic alveolitis, allergic bronchopulmonary aspergillosis. *Aspergillus* can also act as a saprophyte, quietly coexisting for years with the human host, usually in old pulmonary cavities (mycetoma). In the immunocompromised patient, *Aspergillus* can produce a fulminant invasive pulmonary infection. Of great interest is the paradox that glucocorticosteroids can be therapeutic when *Aspergillus* is an allergen and causative when *Aspergillus* is an invasive infectious agent. Most fascinating of all is that these clinical syndromes can overlap in some patients. For example, patients with mycetoma can develop a bronchopulmonary aspergillosis component to their disease (35). Likewise, rapidly invasive pneumonia can suddenly arrest and manifest as a mycetoma (28,70,78,103). Furthermore, a chronic mycetoma can suddenly break down and become a rapidly invasive pulmonary infection (70).

In summary, the occurrence and type of lung disease caused by *Aspergillus* is determined both by the frequency and the extent of respiratory exposure. This section covers both noninvasive and invasive pulmonary *Aspergillus* infections. The reader is referred to previous reviews for a full discussion of *Aspergillus* hypersensitivity lung disease (85,87,104).

Noninvasive

Incidence and Pathogenesis

Chronic and asymptomatic growth of *Aspergillus* in human lung is well known. The most common form of this growth is called aspergilloma or mycetoma ("fungus ball") and involves a mass of mycelia, located within a chronic lung cavity. Such lesions can be discovered incidentally at autopsy, or by a routine radiographic examination, revealing a rounded mass inside a lung cavity, with a crescent of air shadow around the mass. The French term this finding *grelot,* meaning bell-like image with a clapper inside a bell. Fungi other than *Aspergillus,* particularly *Mucor* species, can occasionally cause pulmonary mycetoma, but *Aspergillus* is by far the most common etiologic agent (56). The major clinical concern for a patient with aspergilloma is to determine whether this is truly saprophytic and needs no specific attention or represents a clinically important lesion, requiring therapy.

The incidence of aspergilloma in the general population is unknown. In reviewing 60,000 chest films, MacPherson (72) found an incidence of 0.01% in Great Britain. In this country, Varkey and Rose (112) noted an incidence of 0.017% in their medical center. A large, multicentered study in Great Britain surveyed 544 patients with healed tuberculous cavities on chest films, measuring 2.5 cm in diameter or greater (18). In that study, 25% had precipitins to *Aspergillus* in serum, and 11% had radiologic evidence for aspergilloma. Aspergillomas occurred as frequently in patients with recently healed tuberculosis as in those with inactive disease for long periods. A follow-up study of this group, 3 years after the first survey, revealed an increase in incidence of aspergilloma to 17% (17). The new aspergilloma cases were generally patients who had only serum precipitins during the first survey.

Although most aspergilloma are discovered long after their initial phase, there is growing evidence that in some cases, a subacute, suppurative process could have initiated this more chronic form of lung infection (13). Rarely, mycetomas can develop within several weeks after acute necrotizing lung infections (36). In any event, the most common predisposing factor to the formation of an aspergilloma appears to be the presence of a preexisting lung cavity. Aspergillomas have been identified in cavities associated with a wide array of lung diseases, including tuberculosis, histoplasmosis, sarcoidosis, bronchial cysts, asbestosis, ankylosing spondylitis, bronchiectasis, and malignant disease (56). Most observers consider this fungal growth to be the consequence of a saprophytic fungus growing in a poorly drained lung space. Although mycelia are frequently seen growing into the walls of these cavities, the fungus does not generally invade surrounding lung parenchyma or spread via the blood (112). Under unusual circumstances, however, the behavior of an aspergilloma can change from that of a chronic, benign lesion into an invasive, life-threatening infection (70,97).

The natural history of an aspergilloma is highly variable. These lesions are often well formed when first diagnosed and can remain stable, increase in size, or spontaneously resolve without treatment in about 7 to 10% of cases (47,112). Several observers have described several stages in the "life cycle" of aspergillomata (89,113). In the early phase of formation, *Aspergillus* mycelia grow inside a lung cavity. This eventually leads to a radiologically evident mass, which on histologic examination reveals both living and dead fungus. This is the fully developed stage, and the eventual course of the fungus ball is apparently determined by the predominance of living or dead organisms. If local conditions favor death, the fungus ball will usually liquefy and be expectorated in sputum. Less usual is calcification of a residual mass of dead fungus.

Clinical Features

Although an aspergilloma can exist for years without clinical symptomatology, in the majority of cases, some symptoms will eventually occur (56). The most common symptom associated with an aspergilloma is hemoptysis, with estimates of frequency ranging from 50 to 90% of patients (48,56). Hemoptysis can be infrequent and minimal in amount; however, it can also be severe, with a fatal outcome reported in some cases (34,56,105). The cause of hemoptysis in association with aspergilloma is uncertain and has variously been ascribed to mechanical friction of the mycetoma (89), an endotoxin with hemolytic properties, and an anticoagulant factor derived from aspergillus (23). Local vascular invasion in cavitary wall vessels is also a likely factor. Patients with aspergilloma also can have a chronic cough (17,18), and, rarely, weight loss (29). Fever is exceedingly rare, unless a superimposed bacterial infection occurs. The latter can be in association with bronchial obstruction by the fungus ball. Although progressive dyspnea has been reported (29), presumably from local pleural thickening, this is rare.

Diagnosis

Most aspergilloma are discovered in one of two ways: either by routine or unrelated radiographic examination of the chest, with the incidental finding of a classic mycetoma lesion (see above); or during an evaluation for unexplained hemoptysis. Lung cavities containing aspergilloma are usually present in upper lobes and can have thick walls. Differential diagnoses include hematoma, neoplasm, abscess, and hydatid cyst. The ability to observe movement of the mass inside the cavity on changing the patient's position is variable and not a reliable diagnostic finding.

Sputum cultures can confirm the presence of aspergillus, but in some cases they are negative. Serologic evaluation has been helpful in the latter situation. Close to 100% of patients with aspergilloma have positive serum precipitins for *Aspergillus* (18,20). Precipitins can be positive but only for the species of *Aspergillus* infecting the patient; in some instances, unusual *Aspergillus* sp are involved (66). In such a case, the usual commercially available antigen testing kit will not include the correct antigen, and a false-negative test will occur. Normal controls have routinely had a 1% or less incidence of serum precipitins to *Aspergillus* (80); thus, serum precipitins appear to be both sensitive and specific in the setting of a radiologically suspicious lesion (18). Skin testing has been much less helpful in the evaluation of patients with aspergilloma (22% positive) than in allergic bronchopulmonary aspergillosis (99% positive) (20).

In some cases bronchoscopy is carried out to confirm the location of hemoptysis. In addition, intrabronchial washings, brushing, or forceps biopsy can help to isolate *Aspergillus* by microbiologic or histologic techniques. If cavitary lesions are located

near a pleural surface, percutaneous transthoracic needle aspiration is often a diagnostically useful approach. Finally, in some cases, particularly those with intractable
hemoptysis, thoracotomy can be carried out and surgical resection will reveal the
characteristic lesion of an aspergilloma.

Treatment

The natural history of aspergilloma is highly variable, and considerable controversy has accumulated regarding the proper therapeutic approach to this lesion. The
basic controversy involves the advisability of either observing the patient with no
therapy, treating with medical therapy alone, or surgically resecting the lesions. Although a few cases of aspergilloma have been reported to respond to medical therapy
alone (13,93), most observers agree that systemic antimicrobials, such as amphotericin B, are ineffective in treating this lesion (40,50,55,60,81). It is likely that the
medical failures with aspergillomata are partially attributable to the high concentrations of amphotericin B (54,119) and 5-fluorocytosine (106) required to inhibit this
organism, and partially to the inability of systemically administered drugs to penetrate into the site of infection. The latter problem has led to several attempts at direct
endobronchial intracavitary instillations of antifungal compounds. In one case (54),
local amphotericin B was well tolerated, but after an initial response to therapy the
fungus ball recurred. Others have had more success with local therapy using pastes
of nystatin and amphotericin B (63). Local instillations of amphotericin B and sodium iodide have been used in two patients (91), and sodium iodide appeared more
effective in clearing sputum of *Aspergillus*. In a recent report (49), six patients with
symptomatic aspergillomas were treated with percutaneous instillations of intracavitary amphotericin B, with clinical improvement noted in four. In this report, amphotericin B was mixed in 5% dextrose water, and instilled in concentrations up to
2.5 mg/ml. Dosages were given several times per week, and cumulative amounts of
500 mg were achieved in several patients. Only one patient experienced systemic
reactions to this local therapy. This experience is encouraging and suggests a nonsurgical alternative for therapy in poor surgical candidates. However, efforts to duplicate this methodology at our own institution in one patient resulted in profound
bronchospasm. Thus, considerable caution is advised when attempting such local
instillations.

Surgical resection of an aspergilloma is the only certain method of cure, and this
approach has been advocated by a number of investigators (12,34,93,105). It must
be pointed out, however, that most patients with aspergilloma have preexisting
chronic lung disease and are poor surgical candidates. It should also be noted that
studies recommending routine surgical removal of aspergilloma have generally been
based on rather small personal series in which life-threatening hemoptysis, with an
occasional fatality, has occurred. Many such experiences have occurred on surgical
services in which particularly bothersome cases of aspergilloma were selected out
for care. Thus, the high incidence of severe hemoptysis seen in these series might
not truly reflect the overall population of patients with aspergilloma. Indeed, others
have noted no difference in eventual outcome for unselected patients with aspergilloma, whether or not they were treated (48,112). Even the presence of hemoptysis
did not appear necessarily to dictate a need for surgery, as a number of such patients
resolved their symptoms without therapy (112). In this latter series, it appeared that

the severity of underlying disease (e.g., chronic lung disease) was a more important determinant of eventual outcome and that surgical resection of aspergillomata should not be routinely recommended (112).

Thus, management of the patient with aspergilloma must be individualized. In some cases, the severity of underlying lung disease precludes surgical resection, even in the presence of life-threatening hemoptysis. It does not appear that amphotericin B alone can be relied on to help such patients (48). It is possible that the combination of amphotericin B and 5-fluorocytosine could be of some benefit (13). In surgical candidates with severe hemoptysis, resection of the aspergilloma is appropriate. Perioperative coverage with systemic amphotericin B can reduce postsurgical complications such as bronchopleural fistula or empyema (34,56,93). Patients without symptoms or with mild, infrequent hemoptysis can be carefully observed without therapy (48,106).

Suppurative Bronchitis

Aspergillomas are by far the most common form of noninvasive pulmonary aspergillus infection, yet it is evident that an occasional pneumonitis or lung abscess could be primarily caused by *Aspergillus* infection (13). These infections are either self-limited or predecessors of a more chronic lung infection with *Aspergillus* (13). In some cases an aspergilloma will eventuate (13). In addition to these primary infections, *Aspergillus* infection can complicate preexisting bronchiectasis, chronic bronchitis, or lung cysts (13,48,71). In these cases, the fungus can be saprophytic or can greatly increase the suppurative process. Whether or not these suppurative, noninvasive forms of pulmonary aspergillosis respond to medical therapy is controversial (48), but in some cases they appear to have benefited from antifungal medications (13).

Invasive

Incidence and Pathogenesis

Invasive and rapidly advancing pneumonia caused by aspergillosis is almost exclusively a disease of immuno- and myelosuppressed patients (57,68,84,117,119). Nevertheless, an occasional immunocompetent individual might also develop this form of *Aspergillus* lung infection (12,19,27,53,57,59). Myelosuppression appears to be the greatest risk factor for invasive pulmonary aspergillosis (42,115), and patients with acute leukemia experience an incidence 20 times greater than do lymphoma or organ transplant patients (68). A report by Sherertz et al. (101) emphasized the particular risk of invasive aspergillosis in bone marrow transplantation patients. Among various patient groups, the incidence of invasive aspergillosis was: 1.1% renal transplant; 1.8% acute leukemia; 1.8% burned patients; and 19% for bone marrow transplant patients housed outside of laminar airflow protection units. For bone marrow transplant patients housed in laminar airflow units, however, the incidence was 0% (0/39).

The importance of chemotherapy-induced myelosuppression as a risk factor for invasive aspergillosis has been further emphasized in a report documenting a high risk of recurrent aspergillosis in patients requiring multiple courses of chemotherapy for treatment of acute nonlymphocytic leukemia (95). Among 15 patients with one episode of fungal pneumonia (predominantly *Aspergillus*), 12 underwent further courses of chemotherapy. Additional fungal pneumonias (usually *Aspergillus*) developed in 9 (75%) of these patients.

In vitro studies support the critical role of phagocytic cells in host defense against aspergillus (32). Nevertheless, other factors are likely important as well. Glucocorticosteroids and immunosuppressing drugs such as azathioprine also appear to predispose to invasive *Aspergillosis* (25,46,107). This implies that a component of lymphocyte-directed, cell-mediated immunity could also be involved. The role of humoral antibodies to aspergillosis is unclear. Immunosuppressed patients with invasive aspergillosis usually do not have detectable *Aspergillus* antibodies (118), yet this infection is not particularly common in patients with dysgammaglobulinemia or hypogammaglobulinemia. It has become apparent that heavy aerosol exposure of immuno- and myelosuppressed patients to *Aspergillus* spores increases their chance of developing pneumonia (2,9,10,101). Accordingly, every effort to remove such patients from areas of excavation, construction, or contaminated air circulating systems should be made.

Clinical Features

Acute, invasive *Aspergillus* pneumonia is a dramatic disease. In many ways, the presentation of this illness mimics an acute bacterial pneumonia. The typical patient is granulocytopenic and often has been receiving broad-spectrum antibiotics for unexplained fever (41). Occasionally the white cell count is normal, particularly in organ transplant recipients receiving glucocorticosteroids. Cough, usually unproductive, and fever are the most frequent presenting symptoms. Dyspnea could be prominent. Pleuritic chest pain is common, and pleural friction rub is not unusual. A clinical "scorecard" that incorporates many of the features described above has recently been described by Gerson et al. (41). A prospective evaluation of this scorecard was applied to 49 adult leukemia patients, and cases of invasive *Aspergillosis* could be predicted accurately a mean of 4.1 days prior to clinical recognition by usual diagnostic methods (41).

Radiographs of the chest can reveal virtually any infiltrative pattern with invasive pulmonary *Aspergillosis*. Although lobar involvement (119) and a miliary pattern (86) are occasionally seen, the most common initial finding is a patchy bronchopneumonia. Multiple focal sites are common, and lesions tend to be peripheral in distribution. In addition to chest roentgenography, one report has described the usefulness of pulmonary CT examination (64). Pulmonary CT sometimes reveals a characteristic finding called the "halo sign" (64).

Pathologic examination of lung tissues has revealed that in some cases these local areas of consolidation represent areas of pulmonary infarction secondary to vascular invasion by *Aspergillus* leading to thrombosis and distal necrosis. Thus, in some cases, the clinical presentation resembles acute pulmonary embolus and infarction (103). As infection continues, cavitation is often seen in areas of lung infiltrate. In a recent report, progression to cavitation and hemoptysis were associated with recovery of bone marrow function (7). Others have reported the acute formation of mycetomas in these cavities (103).

Diagnosis

The traditional diagnostic maneuvers for pneumonia are often unhelpful in this disease. Sputum is generally absent. If available, cultures for *Aspergillus* are only positive in 8 to 34% (117) of cases. Also, some consider a positive sputum culture for *Aspergillus* a likely contaminant (38). However, clinical experience has shown that the presence of *Aspergillus* in sputum, or even nasal scrapings (1,65), in the proper clinical setting, as described above, is likely of diagnostic importance. It should also be kept in mind that a positive nasal culture for *Aspergillus* in the febrile neutropenic host could be indicative of underlying invasive *Aspergillus* rhinosinusitis, a condition that warrants aggressive diagnostic and therapeutic interventions (43,108). Two reports emphasize the importance of positive sputum cultures in appropriate settings. In one study, positive cultures from patients with leukemia and neutropenia were highly predictive of lung infection, whereas in mildly or nonimmunosuppressed patients, positive sputum cultures generally were contaminants (120). In another report, the significance of the positive sputum culture increased dramatically if obtained on two or more occasions (110). Blood cultures are routinely negative for *Aspergillus*.

Because noninvasive microbiologic methods are often negative, many cases of *Aspergillus* pneumonia are not discovered until autopsy (78,117). Interest in earlier diagnosis in hopes of instituting appropriate therapy has led to several other approaches, including the aggressive use of lung aspirates or lung biopsies (4,6,78,86). Although these invasive techniques have been successful in reaching early and specific diagnoses in this setting, it must be noted that a considerable number of immuno- and particularly myelosuppressed patients are poor candidates for such invasive diagnostic maneuvers. Accordingly, great interest in rapid and specific serologic detection of invasive aspergillosis has developed (Table 25-1). In contrast with the high degree of sensitivity and specificity in bronchopulmonary aspergillosis and in aspergilloma, however, poor sensitivity has plagued serologic detection among immunocompromised patients (44,118). In addition, false-positive results occasionally occur (Table 25-1). Recent experience with solid-phase radioimmunoassays (73), counterimmunoelectrophoresis, and enzyme-linked immunosorbent assay (ELISA) (51) has greatly increased the sensitivity for detecting *Aspergillus* antibodies in this patient population. In addition, detection of circulating *Aspergillus*

TABLE 25–1. *Serologic tests for* Aspergillus *infection in immunosuppressed patients*

Series	Tests[a]	False-positive (%)	False-negative (%)
Young, 1971 (117)	ID, CF, IFA	0	100
Schaefer, 1976 (98)	ID (concentrated sera)	Uncertain	30
Marier, 1979 (73)	RIA	8	21
	ID	5	74
	CIE	5	79
Holmberg, 1980 (51)	CIE	0	30
	ELISA	8	20

[a]Abbreviations for serologic tests: ID, immunodiffusion; CF, complement fixation; IFA, indirect fluorescent antibody; RIA, radioimmunoassay; CIE, counterimmunoelectropheresis; ELISA, enzyme-linked immunosorbent assay.

antigens (100,114), or antigens in bronchoalveolar lavage specimens (8) in suspect patients, is also under investigation.

In one recent report, radioimmunoassay for *Aspergillus fumigatus* serum antigen was validated by screening sera from 79 hospitalized hematology patients (109). The sensitivity of the assay was 74% and specificity 90%, and the assay was positive prior to traditional clinical diagnosis (pathology, microbiology) in 46% of hospital admissions. Others have found that detection of *Aspergillus galactomannan* antigen in urine might be a more sensitive test than detection in sera (33). To date, however, reliable serologic tests for guiding therapeutic decisions in this disease are not widely available.

Treatment

Early reports described *Aspergillus* pneumonia in the immunocompromised host as uniformly fatal (84). This assumption was based on a large experience in which the correct diagnosis was obtained terminally or at autopsy. It is now well known that early and aggressive therapy can result in cure of certain patients with invasive *Aspergillus* pneumonia (4,22,40,78,82,83,107). In one series, a mortality of 64% was associated with groups receiving early therapy (38). Furthermore, recovery of bone marrow function is associated with markedly improved prognosis (7,95). Nevertheless, mortality exceeding 80% is reported in many series (4,7,83).

There are indications from more recent reports that outcome from invasive aspergillosis might be improving. In one report, use of high-dose amphotericin B 1.0–1.5 mg/kg per day alone (n = 4) or with 5 fluorocytosine (n = 10) was successful in 13 of 14 neutropenic patients (21). Treatment was initiated early (within 2 days of symptoms), and in successfully treated cases, amphotericin B was continued for an average of 1 month after bone marrow recovery. In a published review of the literature regarding outcome for patients treated for invasive pulmonary aspergillosis, among 75 cases in neutropenic patients 51 survived (68%) (31). In most cases, amphotericin B alone was employed.

Amphotericin B is the drug of choice for invasive *Aspergillus* pneumonia. If this diagnosis is established or seriously considered, amphotericin B should be rapidly escalated to full therapeutic dosages. Generally, an adult should be receiving 0.6 mg/kg i.v. per day, within 2 days of starting therapy. Experience suggests that attempts to escalate doses up to 1.0 mg/kg or more per day might be worthwhile (21). However, renal toxicity at this dosage might be a limiting factor, particularly in the elderly. The proper duration of therapy is unknown. Cumulative doses that have been associated with success have ranged from 100 mg to 4000 mg (4,22,31,40,82,83,107). Our policy is to give at least 1.8 g cumulative dose, generally over a month or more. Empiric trials of amphotericin B are occasionally carried out in patients who are suspected of having *Aspergillus* pneumonia but who are unable to tolerate invasive diagnostic procedures (83,85,95). In this setting, we have utilized a 7-day trial period, and if no clinical improvement occurs we discontinue the empiric amphotericin B.

Synergism of amphotericin B with 5-fluorocytosine (5FC) for *Aspergillus* has been described (11,13,21,31,67,103). However, the myelosuppressive effects of 5FC preclude its usefulness in immunosuppressed patients unless serum levels can be monitored. Likewise, there are *in vitro* and animal data that describe synergism of rifampin with amphotericin B (67,76). However, the potential hepatotoxic and immunosuppressive potential for rifampin must also be considered. Clinical data establishing the usefulness of rifampin in this setting are not available. Roles of miconazole or ketoconazole for pulmonary aspergillosis have not been established. However, the oral azole, itraconazole, has been used successfully in some cases of pulmonary aspergillosis (30,31). The use of itraconazole is not well described for myelosuppressed patients with invasive aspergillosis; however, it has been used with some success for prophylaxis in myelosuppressed patients (111). Finally, the successful use of high-dose amphotericin B plus 5FC as prophylaxis in patients with prior episodes of *Aspergillus* pneumonia who again must receive chemotherapy has been reported (58). Nine patients with prior episodes of invasive pulmonary aspergillosis were begun on amphotericin B (1.0 gm/kg/day) plus 5FC 48 hours prior to beginning chemotherapy, and continuing until resolution of neutropenia. Only two patients developed clinical evidence of recurrent *Aspergillus* lung infection, and no patient died from aspergillosis infection.

Occasionally, a patient with acute invasive aspergillosis will develop cavitary disease and evidence for mycetoma (70,78,103). These lesions are generally regarded with greater caution than the chronic mycetomas already described. It is also clear that these lesions can be quiescent for periods of time and then break down with further invasive disease when host defenses falter (70). Thus, surgical resection has generally been recommended for such lesions in the compromised host. Despite these concerns, a recent report (103) describes nine patients with leukemia and acute pulmonary aspergillosis, in six of whom mycetoma developed. None of these patients underwent surgery, and six of the nine patients, including several with mycetoma, were treated successfully with medical therapy alone. Thus, surgical resection of *Aspergillus* mycetoma in the compromised host might not be routinely required.

Finally, some have advocated a role for adjunctive therapy with granulocyte transfusions (40,103). The report of an increase in toxic pulmonary reactions in patients receiving combinations of amphotericin B with granulocyte transfusions (116), however, argues for extreme caution when using granulocyte transfusions in this setting.

Pulmonary Aspergillosis in Patients with Acquired Immunodeficiency Syndrome (AIDS)

Pulmonary aspergillosis has been rare among patients with AIDS (88). Until recently, only 12 cases of invasive disease had been reported, as well as one patient with an aspergilloma (reviewed in 30). Recently, ten more cases of invasive lung infection were described, along with three cases of obstructing bronchial *Aspergillus* infections (30). The latter condition appears to be a form of fungal tracheobronchitis (see below). In general, *Aspergillus* lung infections were late complications, and among the ten patients with invasive disease, eight died and one was lost to follow-up.

More recently, two reports from New York City describe retrospective attempts to identify the incidence and outcome of cases of invasive pulmonary aspergillosis in AIDS patients. In one report (79), 18 cases were identified over a 9-year period. In contrast to the report by Denning et al. (30), these cases occurred relatively soon after diagnosis of AIDS, with an average length of time from diagnosis of AIDS to onset of aspergillosis of 10 months. Only one survivor was reported in this series. In the other report (90), 972 patients with AIDS were assessed for aspergillosis over a 10-year period. Although *Aspergillus* was isolated from respiratory specimens in 45 patients, only five of these patients had evidence (autopsy or clinical) of actual infection. In these cases, *Aspergillus* pneumonia occurred in the terminal stages of illness. Thus, although AIDS patients do not appear to be at high risk for aspergillosis, it can occur, particularly in later stages of disease.

Chronic Necrotizing Aspergillosis

An indolent form of invasive aspergillosis, termed *chronic necrotizing pulmonary aspergillosis* (15), or "semi-invasive" pulmonary aspergillosis (39), has been described. This infection occurs in mildly immunocompromised hosts (e.g., diabetes mellitus, low-dosage glucocorticoids) and often progresses slowly, usually over a several-month period. The hallmarks of this infection are slowly evolving infiltrates with radiographic evidence of lung cavitation. Mycetoma usually develops in these cavities. Patients generally have fever and productive cough. Lung pathology demonstrates *Aspergillus* invading the tissues adjacent to the cavities, leading to tissue necrosis. In contrast to patients with acute invasive pulmonary aspergillosis, patients with chronic necrotizing aspergillosis generally develop positive serum precipitins for aspergillosis, and *Aspergillus* is often cultured from their sputum. Antifungal chemotherapy has been useful in treating this infection (39). A role for surgical drainage and resection of mycetoma has also been demonstrated. Although this condition is considered by some to represent a distinct *Aspergillus* syndrome, it is clear that the chronic, suppurative *Aspergillus* infections described by others (see Noninvasive section, above) resemble chronic necrotizing aspergillosis in many ways.

Aspergillus *Tracheobronchitis*

Recently, several reports have described an unusual but clinically important form of *Aspergillus* lung infection called *Aspergillus* tracheobronchitis (26), obstructing bronchial aspergillosis (30), or ulcerative tracheobronchitis (62). In one report, nine cases of fungal tracheobronchitis were described (26). *Aspergillus* was the sole pathogen in six cases and was present in association with *Candida* in another case. Five of the seven patients with *Aspergillus* tracheobronchitis were immunocompromised by neutropenia and/or corticosteroids. However, in two cases, the only risk factors identified were diabetes mellitus and antibiotic therapy. In a separate report, infection occurred as a late complication of AIDS (30). Very recently, six cases of aspergillosis localized to large airways were described in patients with lung transplants (62). In two unilateral lung transplant cases, the infection was limited to the airways on the transplanted side.

The pathology of *Aspergillus* tracheobronchitis could be that of circumferential infection of bronchi with pseudomembrane formation. Plugging and airway obstruction can occur in some cases. A less common form of infection is local plaque formation, with elements of peribronchial invasion and microabscesses. Local blood vessel invasion by *Aspergillus* is common, resulting in blood-streaked bronchial secretions in many cases. Deep mucosal ulceration and local cartilage invasion has also been described.

Patients with *Aspergillus* tracheobronchitis generally experience increasing dyspnea, with or without other clinical signs or symptoms of lung infection. Hemoptysis can occur, and plugs of purulent sputum could be expectorated. These plugs can be filled with hyphae and are usually culture-positive for *Aspergillus*. Chest roentgenography might show infiltrates; if so, these infiltrates likely represent areas of atelectasis. Diagnosis when made premortem is usually by cultures of sputum or bronchoscopy specimens in patients at risk for opportunistic infection. In one series, three of three patients received treatment and two of three survived (30). In another series, only two of seven cases received antifungal therapy, and there was only one survivor (26). Each of the fatal cases was complex in nature, and *Aspergillus* tracheobronchitis was believed to have contributed to the fatal outcome in several instances. In a recent report, two of six cases of *Aspergillus* tracheobronchitis in lung transplant patients experienced late dissemination and fatal outcome (62).

The optimal therapy for *Aspergillus* tracheobronchitis is unknown. However, some promising results have been reported with oral itraconazole (30). In another case, surgical excision of an involved lobe of lung was curative (26). Amphotericin B still should be considered as the first-line agent for these infections, however.

LUNG INFECTION WITH MUCORACEAE

The family Mucoraceae is clinically the most important among the order of Mucorales. This order is characterized by molds with broad nonseptate hyphae, often branching at 90° angles. The most frequent genera within the family to cause human infection are *Mucor, Absidia,* and *Rhizopus,* with *Mucor* the most commonly involved (mucormycosis). Although rhinocerebral mucormycosis in diabetic patients is perhaps the best described infectious syndrome with *Mucor,* an increasing incidence of invasive pulmonary infection among immunosuppressed patients has been reported for these genera (68,77). Other groups also at increased risk for pulmonary mucormycosis are patients with diabetes mellitus, renal failure, and burns (68). Acute pulmonary mucormycosis resembles acute invasive aspergillosis in its predilection for neutropenic hosts (77). Also like *Aspergillus,* this pathogen has the propensity for blood vessel invasion which results in massive tissue necrosis.

Clinically, pulmonary infection with *Mucor* can be chronic, such as a mycetoma (68), or acute. The latter illness has many of the clinical features described for acute *Aspergillus* pneumonia. In particular, sputum and blood cultures are almost always negative. Likewise, serologies are not clinically useful. Thus, acute pulmonary mucormycosis must be included in the differential diagnosis of unexplained pneumonia in the myelosuppressed patient. The diagnosis rests on demonstration of the typical broad, nonseptate hyphae in lung tissues obtained by biopsy, aspirate, or autopsy. Treatment with amphotericin B is recommended, but survival from acute pneumonia in the compromised host is rare.

CANDIDA LUNG INFECTION

Primary candidal pneumonia is exceedingly rare. In one recent report, 1,506 bone marrow transplant patients were surveyed over a 6-year period for invasive candidal infection (45). Among 171 documented cases, only 18 were of pulmonary origin. In a separate report, 135 cases of candidemia were evaluated in a general hospital setting, and in only three cases was the lung considered the site of origin (61). Nevertheless, sputum cultures frequently are positive for *Candida,* particularly in individuals receiving antibiotics. This paradox has led to widespread confusion regarding the incidence of candidal pneumonia and the necessity to offer treatment to patients harboring *Candida* in the respiratory tract. It is now evident that *Candida* is a normal inhabitant of the mouth and can be recovered from sputum of 20 to 55% of normal humans (14). Chakravarty (24) cultured 487 sputum cultures from patients treated with antibiotics and glucocorticosteroids and found *Candida* present in 41.6% of cultures. Many of the patients had underlying pulmonary disease. Thus, the presence of *Candida* in sputum, even in a patient with pneumonia, offers no diagnostic assurance of the etiology. To establish that *Candida* is a primary lung pathogen, the only certain method is to demonstrate yeast or pseudohyphae in a lung biopsy specimen. Even direct examination of lung tissues might not provide precise diagnostic information (52). Like *Aspergillus,* serologic tests for invasive candidiasis in the compromised host have been exceedingly unreliable (37,75,94). Tests for circulating *Candida* antigens appear to hold more promise (69,75,94), but are not yet widely available.

A small number of cases of *Candida* pneumonia originating from the airway have been described (92,96,99). However, dissemination of *Candida* from blood to lungs appears to be the more common cause of clinically significant pneumonias. This generally occurs in immunocompromised patients suffering from disseminated candidiasis and is usually a preterminal event (102). Even among immunosuppressed patients, however, *Candida* pneumonia is rarely of clinical significance. In one series reported by Masur et al. (74), 30 patients, mainly with neoplastic diseases, were found to have histologic evidence for *Candida* in lung tissues. All but one case was found at autopsy. In only three cases, however, was the candidal infection thought to have been a significant clinical factor. For the most part, small pulmonary foci of *Candida* appeared to result from terminal events in the patient's illness.

In summary, primary candidal pneumonia is exceedingly rare and cannot be assumed from positive sputum cultures, even in the face of otherwise unexplained pneumonia.

TORULOPSIS

Torulopsis glabrata is a yeast-like organism, normally present as a commensal in the human vagina. Several reports have documented the occurrence of *T. glabrata* pneumonia in myelosuppressed patients with neoplasia (5,16). In one report (5), three patients with pneumonia were described in whom torulopsis was cultured in pure growth from transtracheal or transbronchial aspirations. In one case, lung infection progressed despite amphotericin B, and torulopsis was still present in lungs at the time of autopsy. In the other two cases, the apparent lung infection regressed with no specific treatment, coincident with bone marrow recovery. The true incidence of *T. glabrata* pneumonia appears to be low, but could be increasing in certain medical centers (3).

REFERENCES

1. Aisner, J., Murillo, J., Schimpff, S.C., and Steere, A.C. (1972): Invasive aspergillosis in acute leukemia: correlation with nose cultures and antibiotic use. *Ann. Intern. Med.,* 90:4–9.
2. Aisner, J., Schimpff, J., Bennett, J.E., Young, V.M., and Wiernick, P.H. (1976): Aspergillus infections in cancer patients: association with fireproofing in a new hospital. *J.A.M.A.,* 235:411–412.

3. Aisner, J., Schimpff, S.C., Sutherland, J., et al. (1976): *Torulopsis glabrata* infections in patients with cancer: increasing incidence and relationship to colonization. *Am. J. Med.*, 61:23–28.
4. Aisner, J., Schimpff, S.C., and Wiernik, P.H. (1977): Treatment of invasive aspergillosis: relation of early diagnosis and treatment to response. *Ann. Intern. Med.*, 86:539–543.
5. Aisner, J., Sickles, E.A., Schimpff, S.C., et al. (1974): *Torulopsis glabrata* pneumonitis in patients with cancer: report of three cases. *J.A.M.A.*, 230:584–585.
6. Albelda, S.M., Talbot, G.H., Gerson, S.L., Miller, W.T., and Cassileth, P.A. (1984): Role of fiberoptic bronchoscopy in the diagnosis of invasive pulmonary aspergillosis in patients with acute leukemia. *Am. J. Med.*, 76:1027–1034.
7. Albelda, S.M., Talbot, F.H., Gerson, S.L., Miller, W.T., and Cassileth, P.A. (1985): Pulmonary cavitation and massive hemoptysis in invasive pulmonary aspergillosis: influence of bone marrow recovery in patients with acute leukemia. *Am. Rev. Respir. Dis.*, 131:115–120.
8. Andrews, C.P., and Weiner, M.H. (1982): *Aspergillus* antigen detection in bronchoalveolar lavage fluid from patients with invasive aspergillosis and aspergillomas. *Am. J. Med.*, 73:372–380.
9. Arnow, P.M., Anderson, R.L., Mainous, P.D., and Smith, E.J. (1978): Pulmonary aspergillosis during hospital renovation. *Am. Rev. Respir. Dis.*, 118:49–53.
10. Arnow, P.M., Sadigh, M., Costas, C., Weil, D., and Chudy, R. (1991): Endemic and epidemic aspergillosis associated with in-hospital replication of *Aspergillus* organisms. *J. Infect. Dis.*, 164:998–1002.
11. Arroyo, J., Medoff, G., and Kobayasi, G.S. (1977): Therapy of murine aspergillosis with amphotericin B in combination with rifampin of 5-fluorocytosine. *Antimicrob. Agents Chemother.*, 11:21.
12. Aslam, P.A., Eastridge, C.E., and Hughest, F.A. (1971): Aspergillosis of the lung: an 18-year experience. *Chest*, 59:28–32.
13. Atkinson, G.W., and Israel, H.L. (1977): 5-Fluorocytosine treatment of meningeal and pulmonary aspergillosis. *Am. J. Med.*, 55:496–504.
14. Baum, G.L. (1960): The significance of *Candida albicans* in human sputum. *N. Engl. J. Med.*, 263:70–73.
15. Binder, R.E., Faling, J., Pugatch, R.D., Mahasaen, C., and Snider, G.L. (1982): Chronic necrotizing pulmonary aspergillosis: a discrete entity. *Medicine*, 61:109–124.
16. Bodey, G.P., Powell, R.D., Hersch, E.M., et al. (1966): Pulmonary complications of acute leukemia. *Cancer*, 19:781–793.
17. British Thoracic and Tuberculosis Association (1970): Aspergilloma and residual tuberculous cavities: the results of a resurvey. *Tubercle*, 51:227–245.
18. British Tuberculosis Association (1968): *Aspergillus* in persistent lung cavities after tuberculosis. *Tubercle*, 49:1–11.
19. Brown, E., Freedman, S., Arbeit, R., and Come, S. (1980): Invasive pulmonary aspergillosis in an apparently non-immunocompromised host. *Am. J. Med.*, 69:624–628.
20. Buechner, H.A., Seaburg, J.H., Campbell, C.C., Georg, L.K., Kaufman, L., and Kaplan, N. (1973): The current status of serologic, immunologic and skin tests in the diagnosis of pulmonary mycoses. *Chest*, 63:259–270.
21. Burch, P.A., Karp, J.E., Merz, W.G., Kuhlman, J.E., and Fishman, E.K. (1987): Favorable outcome of invasive aspergillosis in patients with acute leukemia. *J. Clin. Oncol.*, 5:1985–1993.
22. Burton, J.R., Zachery, J.B., Bessin, R., et al. (1972): Aspergillosis in four renal transplant recipients; diagnosis and effective treatment with amphotericin B. *Ann. Intern. Med.*, 77:383–388.
23. Campbell, M.J., and Clayton, Y.M. (1976): Bronchopulmonary aspergillosis: a correlation of the clinical and laboratory findings in 272 patients investigated for bronchopulmonary aspergillosis. *Am. Rev. Respir. Dis.*, 89:186.
24. Chakravarty, S.C. (1964): Incidence and significance of fungi in sputum in bronchopulmonary diseases. *Acta Tuberc. Scand.*, 45:295–300.
25. Chung, C., Lord, P.L., and Krumpe, P.E. (1978): Diagnosis of invasive pulmonary aspergillosis by fiberoptic transbronchial lung biopsy. *J.A.M.A.*, 239:749–750.
26. Clarke, A., Skelton, J., and Fraser, R.S. (1991): Fungal tracheobronchitis: report of 9 cases and review of the literature. *Medicine*, 70:1–14.
27. Cook, D.J., Achong, M.R., and King, D.E.L. (1990): Disseminated aspergillosis in an apparently healthy patient. *Am. J. Med.*, 88:74–76.
28. Curtis, A., Smith, G.J.W., and Ravin, C.E. (1977): Air crescent sign of invasive aspergillosis. *Radiology*, 133:17–21.
29. Davies, D., and Sommer, A.R. (1972): Pulmonary aspergillosis treated with corticosteroids. *Thorax*, 27:156–162.
30. Denning, D.W., Follansbee, S.E., Scolaro, M., Norris, A., Edelstein, H., and Stevens, D.A. (1991): Pulmonary aspergillosis in the acquired immunodeficiency syndrome. *N. Engl. J. Med.*, 324:654–662.
31. Denning, D.W., and Stevens, D.A. (1990): Antifungal and surgical treatment of invasive aspergillosis: review of 2,121 published cases. *Rev. Infect. Dis.*, 12:1147–1201.

32. Diamond, R.D., Krzesicki, R., Esptein, B., et al. (1978): Damage to hyphal forms of fungi by human leukocytes *in vitro. Am. J. Pathol.,* 91:313–328.
33. Dupont, B., Huber, M., Kim, S.J., and Bennett, J.E. (1987): Galactomannan antigenemia and antigenuria in aspergillosis: studies in patients and experimentally infected rabbits. *J. Infect. Dis.,* 155:1–11.
34. Edge, J.R., Stansfield, D., and Fletcher, D.E. (1971): Pulmonary aspergillosis in an unselected hospital population. *Chest,* 59:407–413.
35. Ein, M.E., Wallace, R.J., and Williams, T.W. (1979): Allergic bronchopulmonary aspergillosis-like syndrome consequent to aspergilloma. *Am. Rev. Respir. Dis.,* 119:811–820.
36. Fahey, P.J., Utell, M.J., and Hyde, R.W. (1980): Spontaneous lysis of mycetomas after acute cavitating lung disease. *Am. Rev. Respir. Dis.,* 123:336–339.
37. Filice, G., Yu, B., and Armstrong, D. (1977): Immunodiffusion and agglutination tests for *Candida* in patients with neoplastic disease: inconsistent correlation of results with invasive infections. *J. Infect. Dis.,* 135:349–357.
38. Fisher, B.D., Armstong, D., Yu, B., and Gold, J.W.M. (1981): Invasive aspergillosis: progress in early diagnosis and treatment. *Am. J. Med.,* 71:571–577.
39. Gefter, W.B., Weingrad, T.R., Epstein, D.M., Ochs, R.H., and Miller, W.T. (1981): "Semi-invasive" pulmonary aspergillosis: a new look at the spectrum of *Aspergillus* infections of the lung. *Radiology,* 140:313–321.
40. Gercovich, F.G., Richman, S.P., Rodriguez, V., et al. (1975): Successful control of systemic *Aspergillus niger* infections in two patients with acute leukemia. *Cancer,* 36:2271–2276.
41. Gerson, S.L., Talbot, G.H., Hurwitz, S., Lusk, E.J., Strom, B.L., and Cassileth, P.A. (1985): Discriminant scorecard for diagnosis of invasive pulmonary aspergillosis in patients with acute leukemia. *Am. J. Med.,* 79:57–64.
42. Gerson, S.L., Talbot, G.H., Hurwitz, S., Strom, B.L., Lusk, E.J., and Cassileth, P.A. (1984): Prolonged granulocytopenia: the major risk factor for invasive pulmonary aspergillosis in patients with acute leukemia. *Ann. Int. Med.,* 100:345–351.
43. Goering, P., Berlinger, N.T., and Weisdorf, D.J. (1988): Aggressive combined modality treatment of progressive sinonasal fungal infections in immunocompromised patients. *Amer. J. Med.,* 85:619–623.
44. Gold, J.W.M., Fisher, B., Yu, B., Chein, N., and Armstrong, D. (1980): Diagnosis of invasive aspergillosis by passive hemagglutination assay of antibody. *J. Infect. Dis.,* 142:87–94.
45. Goodrich, J.M., Reed, E.C., Mori, M., Fisher, L.D., Skerrett, S., Dandliker, P.S., Klis, B., Counts, G.W., and Meyers, J.D. (1991): Clinical features and analysis of risk factors for invasive candidal infection after marrow transplantation. *J. Infect. Dis.,* 164:731–740.
46. Gustafson, T.L., Schaffner, W., Lavely, G.B., Stratton, C.W., Johnson, H.K., and Hutchesons, R.H., Jr. (1983): Invasive aspergillosis in renal transplant recipients: correlation with corticosteroid therapy. *J. Infect. Dis.,* 148:230–238.
47. Hammerman, K.J., Christianson, C.S., Huntington, I., et al. (1973): Spontaneous lysis of aspergillomata. *Chest,* 64:697–699.
48. Hammerman, K.J., Sarosi, G.A., and Tosh, F.E. (1974): Amphotericin B in the treatment of saprophytic forms of pulmonary aspergillosis. *Am. Rev. Respir. Dis.,* 109:57–62.
49. Hargis, J.L., Bone, R.C., Stewart, J., Rector, N., and Hiller, F.C. (1980): Intracavitary amphotericin B in the treatment of symptomatic pulmonary aspergillomas. *Am. J. Med.,* 68:389–394.
50. Henderson, A.H., English, M.P., and Vecht, R.J. (1968): Pulmonary aspergillosis: a survey of its occurrence in patients with chronic lung disease and a discussion of the significance of diagnostic tests. *Thorax,* 23:513–518.
51. Holmberg, K., Berdischewsky, M., and Young, L.S. (1980): Serologic immunodiagnosis of invasive aspergillosis. *J. Infect. Dis.,* 141:656–664.
52. Humphrey, D.M., and Weiner, M.H. (1983): Candidal antigen detection in pulmonary candidiasis. *Am. J. Med.,* 74:630–640.
53. Hunter, R.V.P., and Collins, H.S. (1962): The occurrence of opportunistic fungus infections in a cancer hospital. *Lab. Invest. (Part 2),* 11:1035–1048.
54. Ikemoto, H. (1965): Treatment of pulmonary aspergilloma with amphotericin B. *Arch. Intern. Med.,* 115:598–601.
55. Israel, H.L., and Astrow, A. (1969): Sarcoidosis and aspergilloma. *Am. J. Med.,* 47:243–250.
56. Joynson, D.H.M. (1977): Pulmonary aspergilloma. *Br. J. Clin. Pract.,* 31:207.
57. Karam, G.H., and Griffin, F.M., Jr. (1986): Invasive pulmonary aspergillosis in nonimmunocompromised, nonneutropenic hosts. *Rev. Infect. Dis.,* 8:357–363.
58. Karp, J.E., Burch, P.A., and Merz, W.G. (1988): An approach to intensive antileukemia therapy in patients with previous invasive aspergillosis. *Am. J. Med.,* 85:203–206.
59. Kennedy, W.D.U., Malone, D.N., and Blyth, W. (1970): Necrotizing pulmonary aspergillosis. *Thorax,* 25:691–701.

60. Kilman, J.W., Ahn, C., Andrews, N.C., et al. (1969): Surgery for pulmonary aspergillosis. *J. Thorac. Cardiovasc. Surg.,* 57:642–647.
61. Komshian, S.V., Uwaydah, A.K., Sobel, J.D., and Crane, L.R. (1989): Fungemia caused by *Candida* species and *Torulopsis glabrata* in the hospitalized patient: frequency, characteristics, and evaluation of factors influencing outcome. *Rev. Infect. Dis.,* 11:379–390.
62. Kramer, M.R., Denning, D.W., Marshall, S.E., Ross, D.J., Berry, G., Lewiston, J., Stevens, D.A., and Theodore, J. (1991): Ulcerative tracheobronchitis after lung transplantation. *Am. Rev. Respir. Dis.,* 144:552–556.
63. Krakowka, P., Traczyk, K., Walczak, J., et al. (1970): Local treatment of aspergilloma with a paste containing nystatin or amphotericin B. *Tubercle,* 51:184–191.
64. Kuhlman, J.E., Fishman, E.K., and Siegelman, S.S. (1985): Invasive pulmonary aspergillosis in acute leukemia: characteristic findings in CT, and CT halo sign, and the role of CT in early diagnosis. *Radiology,* 157:611–614.
65. Kusne, S., Torre-Cisneros, J., Mañez, R., Irish, W., Martin, M., Fung, J., Simmons, R.L., and Starzl, T.E. (1992): Factors associated with invasive lung aspergillosis and the significance of positive *Aspergillus* culture after liver transplantation. *J. Infect. Dis.,* 166:1379–1383.
66. Laham, M.N., and Carpenter, J.L. (1982): *Aspergillus terreus,* a pathogen capable of causing infective endocarditis, pulmonary mycetoma, and allergic bronchopulmonary aspergillosis. *Am. Rev. Respir. Dis.,* 125:769–772.
67. Laskey, W., and Sarosi, G.A. (1978): Endogenous activation in blastomycosis. *Ann. Intern. Med.,* 88:50–52.
68. Leher, R.I., Howard, D.H., Sypherd, P.S., Edwards, J.E., et al. (1980): Mucormycosis. *Ann. Intern. Med. (Part 1),* 93:93–108.
69. Lew, M.A., Siber, G.R., Donahue, D.M., and Maiorca, F. (1982): Enhanced detection with an enzyme-linked immunosorbent assay of *Candida mannan* in antibody-containing serum after heat extraction. *J. Infect. Dis.,* 145:45–56.
70. Lipinski, J.K., Weisbrod, G.L., and Sanders, D.E. (1978): Unusual manifestations of pulmonary aspergillosis. *J. Can. Assoc. Radiol.,* 29:216–220.
71. Louira, D.B., and Collins, H.S. (1964): Some aspects of pulmonary mycotic infections. *Tuberculology* (Denver), 21:76.
72. MacPherson, P. (1965): Pulmonary aspergillosis in Argyll. *Br. J. Dis. Chest,* 59:148–157.
73. Marier, R., Smith, W., Jansen, M., and Andriole, V.T. (1979): A solid phase radioimmunoassay for the measurement of antibody to *Aspergillus* in invasive aspergillosis. *J. Infect. Dis.,* 140:771–779.
74. Masur, H., Rosen, P.P., and Armstrong, D. (1977): Pulmonary disease caused by *Candida* species. *Am. J. Med.,* 63:914–925.
75. Meckstroth, K.L., Reiss, E., Keller, J.W., and Kaufman, L. (1981): Detection of antibodies and antigenemia in leukemic patients with candidiasis by enzyme-linked immunosorbent assay. *J. Infect. Dis.,* 144:24–32.
76. Medoff, G., and Kobayashi, G.S. (1980): Strategies in the treatment of systemic fungal infections. *N. Engl. J. Med.,* 302:145–155.
77. Meyer, R.D., Rosen, P., and Armstrong, D. (1972): Phycomycosis complicating leukemia and lymphoma. *Ann. Intern. Med.,* 77:871–879.
78. Meyer, R.D., Young, L.S., Armstrong, D., and Yu, B. (1973): Aspergillosis complicating neoplastic disease. *Am. J. Med. Sci.,* 4:6–15.
79. Minamoto, G.Y., Barlam, T.F., and Vander Els, N.J. (1992): Invasive aspergillosis in patients with AIDS. *Clin. Infect. Dis.,* 14:66–74.
80. Muchmore, H.G., McKown, B.A., and Mohr, J.A. (1971): *Aspergillus precipitins* in hospitalized and non-hospitalized subjects. *Bacteriol. Proc. Abstracts of 71st ASM Meeting,* p. 120.
81. Parker, J.D., Sarosi, G.A., Doto, I.L., et al. (1970): Pulmonary aspergillosis in sanitoriums in the South Central United States. *Am. Rev. Respir. Dis.,* 101:551–557.
82. Pennington, J.E. (1976): Successful treatment of *Aspergillus* pneumonia in hematologic neoplasia. *N. Engl. J. Med.,* 295:426–427.
83. Pennington, J.E. (1977): *Aspergillus* pneumonia in hematologic malignancy: improvements in diagnosis and therapy. *Arch. Intern. Med.,* 137:769–771.
84. Pennington, J.E. (1978): Infection in the compromised host: recent advances and future directions. *Semin. Infect. Dis.,* 1:142–168.
85. Pennington, J.E. (1980): *Aspergillus* lung disease. *Med. Clin. No. Amer.,* 64:475–490.
86. Pennington, J.E., and Feldman, N.T. (1977): Pulmonary infiltrates and fever in patients with hematologic malignancy. *Am. J. Med.,* 62:581–587.
87. Pepys, J., Jenkins, P.A., Fesenstein, G.H., et al. (1963): Farmer's lung: thermophilic actinomycetes as a source of farmer's lung hay antigens. *Lancet,* 2:607–611.
88. Pervez, N.K., Kleinerman, J., Kattan, M., Freed, J.A., Harris, M.B., Rosen, M.J., and Schwartz, I.S. (1985): Pseudomembranous necrotizing bronchial aspergillosis: a variant of in-

vasive aspergillosis in a patient with hemophilia and acquired immune deficiency syndrome. *Am. Rev. Respir. Dis.*, 131:961–963.

89. Pimental, J.C. (1966): Pulmonary calcification in the tumor-like form of aspergilloma. *Am. Rev. Respir. Dis.*, 94:208–216.

90. Pursell, K.J., Telzak, E.E., and Armstrong, D. (1992): *Aspergillus* species colonization and invasive disease in patients with AIDS. *Clin. Infect. Dis.*, 14:141–148.

91. Ramirez, R.J. (1964): Pulmonary aspergilloma: endobronchial treatment. *N. Engl. J. Med.*, 291:1281–1285.

92. Ramirez, G., Schuster, M., Kozub, W., and Pribor, H.C. (1967): Fatal acute *Candida albicans* bronchopneumonia: report of a case. *J.A.M.A.*, 119:118–120.

93. Reddy, P.A., Christianson, C.S., Brasher, C.A., et al. (1970): Comparison of treated and untreated aspergilloma: an analysis of 16 cases. *Am. Rev. Respir. Dis.*, 101:928–934.

94. Repentigny, L., and Reiss, E. (1984): Current trends in immunodiagnosis of candidiasis and aspergillosis. *Rev. Infect. Dis.*, 6:301–312.

95. Robertson, M.J., and Larson, R.A. (1988): Recurrent fungal pneumonias in patients with acute nonlymphocytic leukemia undergoing multiple courses of intensive chemotherapy. *Am. J. Med.*, 84:233–239.

96. Rosenbaum, R.B., Barber, J.V., and Stevens, D.A. (1974): *Candida albicans* pneumonia: diagnosis by pulmonary aspiration, recovery without treatment. *Am. Rev. Respir. Dis.*, 109:373–378.

97. Rosenberg, R.S., Creviston, S.A., and Schonfeld, A.J. (1982): Invasive aspergillosis complicating resection of a pulmonary aspergilloma in a nonimmunocompromised host. *Am. Rev. Respir. Dis.*, 126:1113–1115.

98. Schaefer, J.C., Yu, B., and Armstrong, D. (1976): An *Aspergillus* immunodiffusion test in the early diagnosis of aspergillosis in adult leukemia patients. *Am. Rev. Respir. Dis.*, 113:325–329.

99. Schiffman, R.L., Johnson, R.S., Weinberger, S.E., Weiss, S.T., and Schwartz, A. (1982): *Candida* lung abscess: Successful treatment with amphotericin B and 5-flucytosine. *Am. Rev. Respir. Dis.*, 125:766–768.

100. Shaffer, P.J., Medoff, G., and Kobayashi, G.S. (1979): Demonstration of antigenemia by radioimmunoassay in rabbits experimentally infected with *Aspergillus*. *J. Infect. Dis.*, 139:313–319.

101. Sherertz, R.J., Belani, A., Kramer, B.S., Elfenbein, G.J., Weiner, R.S., Sullivan, M.L., Thomas, R.G., and Samsa, G.P. (1987): Impact of air filtration on nosocomial *Aspergillus* infections. *Am. J. Med.*, 83:709–718.

102. Sickles, E.A., Young, V.M., Greene, W.H., et al. (1973): Pneumonia in acute leukemia. *Ann. Intern. Med.*, 79:528–534.

103. Sinclair, A.J., Rosoff, A.H., and Coltman, C.A. (1978): Recognition and successful management in pulmonary aspergillosis in leukemia. *Cancer,* 42:2019–2024.

104. Slavin, R.G. (1976): Immunologically mediated lung diseases: extrinsic allergic alveolitis and allergic bronchopulmonary aspergillosis. *Postgrad. Med.*, 59:137–141.

105. Solit, R.W., McKeown, J.J., Smullens, S., et al. (1971): The surgical implications of intracavitary mycetomas (fungus balls). *J. Thorac. Cardiovasc. Surg.*, 62:411–422.

106. Steer, P.L., Marks, M.I., Klite, P.D., et al. (1972): 5-Fluorocytosine, an oral and antifungal compound: a report on clinical and laboratory experience. *Ann. Intern. Med.*, 76:15–22.

107. Stinson, E.B., Bielier, C.C., Griepp, R.B., et al. (1971): Infectious complications after cardiac transplantation in man. *Ann. Intern. Med.*, 74:22–36.

108. Talbot, G.H., Huang, A., and Provencher, M. (1991): Invasive aspergillus rhinosinusitis in patients with acute leukemia. *Rev. Infect. Dis.*, 13:219–232.

109. Talbot, G.H., Weiner, M.H., Gerson, S.L., Provencher, M., and Hurwitz, S. (1987): Serodiagnosis of invasive aspergillosis in patients with hematologic malignancy: validation of the *Aspergillus fumigatus* antigen. *J. Infect. Dis.*, 155:12–27.

110. Treger, R.T., Visscher, D.W., Bartlett, M.S., and Smith, J.W. (1985): Diagnosis of pulmonary infection caused by *Aspergillus:* usefulness of respiratory cultures. *J. Infect. Dis.*, 152:572–576.

111. Tricot, G., Joosten, E., Boogaerts, M.A., Pitte, J.V., and Cauwenbergh, G. (1987): Ketoconazole vs. itraconazole for antifungal prophylaxis in patients with severe granulocytopenia: preliminary results of two nonrandomized studies. *Rev. Infect. Dis.*, 9(Suppl. 1):S94–S99.

112. Varkey, B., and Rose, H.D. (1967): Pulmonary aspergilloma: a rational approach to treatment. *Am. J. Med.*, 61:626–631.

113. Villar, T.G., Pimental, J.C., and Avila, R. (1967): Some aspects of pulmonary aspergilloma in Portugal. *Dis. Chest*, 51:402–405.

114. Weiner, M.H., Talbot, G.H., Gerson, S.L., Filice, G., and Cassileth, P.A. (1983): Antigen detection in the diagnosis of invasive aspergillosis. *Ann. Int. Med.*, 99:777–782.

115. Wingard, J.R., Beals, S.U., and Santos, G.W., (1987): Aspergillus infections in bone marrow transplant recipients. *Bone Marrow Transplantation*, 2:175–181.

116. Wright, D.G., Robichaud, K.J., Pizzo, P.A., and Deisseroth, A.B. (1981): Lethal pulmonary

reactions associated with the combined use of amphotericin B and leukocyte transfusions. *N. Engl. J. Med.*, 304:1185–1190.

117. Young, R.C., and Bennett, J.E. (1971): Invasive aspergillosis: absence of detectable antibody response. *Am. Rev. Respir. Dis.*, 104:710–715.

118. Young, R.C., Bennett, J.E., Vogel, C.L., et al. (1970): Aspergillosis: the spectrum of the disease in 98 patients. *Medicine*, 49:147–173.

119. Young, R.C., Vogel, C.L., and DeVita, V.T. (1969): Aspergillus lobar pneumonia. *J.A.M.A.*, 208:1156–1162.

120. Yu, V.L., Muder, R.R., and Poorsattar, A. (1986): Significance of isolation of aspergillus from the respiratory tract in diagnosis of invasive pulmonary aspergillosis. *Amer. J. Med.*, 81:249–254.

Respiratory Infections: Diagnosis and Management, 3d ed.,
edited by James E. Pennington.
Raven Press, Ltd., New York © 1994

26

Cryptococcus neoformans Pneumonia

Richard D. Diamond and Stuart M. Levitz

*Boston University School of Medicine, 88 East Newton Street,
Boston, Massachusetts 02118-2393*

Cryptococcosis is a systemic fungus infection caused by *Cryptococcus neoformans,* an encapsulated yeast-like fungus that reproduces by budding. Although this mycosis most commonly involves the central nervous system, almost all infections presumably are initiated by inhalation, followed by subclinical or symptomatic pulmonary involvement. Thereafter, dissemination to other sites beyond the lung might or might not occur.

Four different serotypes of *C. neoformans* (A, B, C, and D) have been described on the basis of antigenic specificity of the capsular polysaccharide (69,123). Isolates of serotypes A and D differ from serotypes B and C biochemically as well as in the morphology of their perfect (sexual) states that exist in mycelial phase (6), so that *C. neoformans* types A and D have been classified as *C. neoformans* var. *neoformans,* as opposed to *C. neoformans* var. *gattii* for serotypes B and C (66,69). There are two mating types of *C. neoformans* from which the sexual or perfect state *(Filobasidiella neoformans)* can be derived; however, one of the mating types predominates over the others, with a 30 to 40% higher frequency in natural and clinical isolates (63). Differences in clinical manifestations related to serotypes or mating types have not been described, although in a small study there was a suggestion that infections due to *C. neoformans* var. *gattii* might be more difficult to treat than those due to *C. neoformans* var. *neoformans* (54).

Unfortunately, the necessity for consistency in microbiology has dictated a rationale for all too frequent changes in nomenclature of organisms. A brief review of the history of cryptococcosis should serve to at least partially dispel the often repeated speculation about overt desires of mycologists to confound and confuse clinicians. The organism now known as *C. neoformans* was isolated from peach juice by Sanfelice in 1894 and named *Saccharomyces neoformans.* At about the same time, Busse and Buschke described the first clinical case of cryptococcosis in a patient with bone and skin lesions, naming the causative organism *Saccharomyces hominis.* The first case of pulmonary cryptococcosis was recorded by Frothingham in 1902 (in a horse). Postmortem evidence of central nervous system involvement was first noted in 1905, but a living patient with cryptococcal meningitis was not noted until 1914. In an otherwise useful monograph published by Stoddard and Cutler in 1916, the causative organism was renamed *Torula histolytica* because clear spaces seen in histologic sections were attributed erroneously to tissue lysis in areas of infection. It is now known that these spaces represent unstained cryptococcal polysaccharide.

Because nomenclature for the genus *Torula* was inconsistent with established taxonomic rules for classification of fungi, the name did not last long. Not until 1935 did Benham clearly separate and distinguish between causative agents of cryptococcosis and North American blastomycosis. Thus, many clinical descriptions of the disease refer to cryptococcosis as "torulosis," "blastomycosis," or "European blastomycosis."

INCIDENCE AND EPIDEMIOLOGY

Unlike many other fungi that are predominantly restricted to certain well-defined endemic areas, *C. neoformans* has a worldwide distribution. It exists as a saprophyte in nature. Since Emmons (38) noted the association of cryptococci with pigeon manure and soil in 1955, many other workers have isolated the organism from pigeon nesting places and aged pigeon droppings, although the birds themselves do not develop invasive cryptococcal infections (75). The fungus is commonly found in soil that has been contaminated by feces of pigeons or other birds. In contrast with nonpathogenic species of the genus *Cryptococcus*, *C. neoformans* is isolated less commonly from fruits and natural sites other than bird manure or soil (111). Except in very unusual circumstances, such as transplantation of infected tissue, neither human-to-human nor animal-to-human transmission of cryptococcosis occurs (69). Rather, it appears that cryptococcal infections are initiated by inhalation of aerosolized yeasts from environmental sources. Although well-encapsulated organisms can be as large as 30 μm or more in diameter, cryptococci in nature more often are poorly encapsulated. Thus, organisms with a size range (from 0.6 to 3.5 μm) compatible with alveolar deposition can be readily isolated from natural sites including pigeon excreta or aerosolized soil (93,97,102).

The central role of the pigeon and other birds as vehicles for dispersal of cryptococci is supported by the increased rates of reactivity of delayed skin tests to cryptococcal antigens seen in pigeon fanciers (92). However, the epidemiology of cryptococcosis differs from that of other respiratory mycoses, as clustered outbreaks of cryptococcosis rarely occur, occupational predisposition to clinically apparent disease is not apparent, and histories of heavy exposure to pigeons and dust are not helpful clinically. Only *C. neoformans* var. *neoformans* is found in isolates obtained from pigeon droppings. In contrast, *C. neoformans* var. *gattii* has been isolated from material collected under the canopies of certain species of *Eucalyptus* trees (36). Consistent with these data, infections due to *C. neoformans* var. *neoformans* are seen worldwide, whereas those due to *C. neoformans* var. *gattii* are prevalent only in tropical and subtropical regions (where *Eucalyptus* trees are found) (64,69). Nevertheless, knowledge about how *C. neoformans* infections are acquired remains incomplete, and it remains possible that sources of *C. neoformans* other than pigeons and *Eucalyptus* trees serve as major vectors. In AIDS patients, *C. neoformans* var. *neoformans* predominates, even in tropical and subtropical regions (69,108,115).

The process of sorting out epidemiologic factors that are critical in initiating cryptococcosis is undoubtedly complicated by the likelihood that host factors could be the critical determinants for significant infections. Presumably, exposure to *C. neoformans* is common because the organism is ubiquitous (38). Surveys involving delayed skin testing of normal subjects support this concept (1,92). However, clinically apparent cases are relatively rare in patients without obvious immunocompromise, possibly approximating 300 per year in the United States. Moreover, neither laboratory-acquired pulmonary nor disseminated cryptococcosis has been reported, yet most workers in such laboratories are exposed to aerosols of organisms often enough to convert their delayed skin tests to cryptococcal antigen (1). Even when clinical manifestations of cryptococcosis are present, findings related to the central nervous system usually predominate, and neither historical nor roentgenographic evidence of pulmonary involvement are usually apparent. Nevertheless, the presence in autopsied humans of small pulmonary lesions apparently consistent with clinically inapparent primary subpleural nodules supports the notion of a pulmonary portal of entry for cryptococcosis. Thus, the concept emerges that common exposure to this saprophytic organism can often lead to subclinical infections, but only rarely is the combination of exposure and host factors sufficient to result in clinically apparent disease.

PATHOGENESIS

Invasion of tissues by *C. neoformans* stimulates an inflammatory response that ranges from minimal to strong, depending on the location of lesions within the patient and the patient's overall immunocompetence (26). For instance, within the brain (and in other tissues as well in some patients), lesions are comprised of cystic clusters of encapsulated yeasts with little or no surrounding inflammatory response. Cortical gray matter and basal ganglia are often heavily involved by diffuse or, occasionally, focal lesions, so that the disease would be better termed a meningoencephalitis rather than meningitis. In contrast with involvement of brain, lesions in the meninges and outside the central nervous system often are moderately to heavily infiltrated by inflammatory cells. Cryptococci are usually seen within or adjacent to macrophages and giant cells. Plasma cells and lymphocytes are generally present, but without well-formed epithelioid granulomas. A neutrophilic response rarely predominates. Long-term involvement of tissues seldom leads to hemorrhage, necrosis, calcification, or extensive fibrosis. Thus, because *C. neoformans* does not produce exotoxins and is apt to incite a less pronounced inflammatory response than that seen with many other infectious agents, organ dysfunction occurs largely by virtue of displacement of tissues by masses of growing organisms. As would be expected, these effects are most pronounced intracranially, where space for brain expansion is limited. With this in mind, it is apparent why cryptococcosis could be quite chronic, with significant functional impairment of tissues occurring only late in the clinical course of the disease, unless the infecting load of organisms is unusually heavy. Within the lungs, focal lesions predominate, although immunosuppressed patients in particular can, rarely, develop diffuse lesions that can progress rapidly and impair pulmonary function (40,47,91). A review of 36 autopsy cases of pulmonary cryptococcosis in patients without AIDS defined four basic morphologic patterns: (i) peripheral pulmonary granulomas (7 patients); (ii) granulomatous pneumonia with intraalveolar proliferating organisms and varying degrees of inflammatory response (19 patients); (iii) diffuse pneumonia with organisms present within alveolar capillaries and interstitial tissues (7 patients); and (iv) massive pneumonia with large numbers of intraalveolar and intravascular organisms present (3 patients) (82).

It has been suggested that ubiquitous *C. neoformans* yeast-like particles are commonly inhaled, producing self-limited, asymptomatic pulmonary lesions in almost all exposed subjects. Careful examination of tissues at autopsies has revealed small, subpleural nodules containing cryptococci, sometimes with involved hilar nodes as well (2,105) in some patients, implying that primary pulmonary foci exist even when clinically inapparent in disseminated infections. However, although this provides an appealing and consistent explanation for the pathogenesis of cryptococcosis, the documentation of primary pulmonary foci of infections in all cases is not so well established for cryptococcosis as it is for histoplasmosis, coccidioidomycosis, or tuberculosis.

Experimental studies suggest that potent cellular host defense mechanisms are responsible for the strong natural resistance against cryptococcosis. Within lungs of animals challenged with cryptococci, neutrophils rapidly appear, clear most of the organisms, and are replaced by monocytes in later lesions (42). Human neutrophils and monocytes can ingest and kill cryptococci (30). Acquired resistance to cryptococcosis appears to depend on cell-mediated immunity (44), presumably with sensitized T-cells inducing activated macrophages, perhaps by the release of lymphokines (e.g., interferon-γ), with increased microbicidal capacity (55,70). Macrophages can inhibit cryptococcal growth and kill at least some of the organisms *in vitro* (70,87,119). The HIV-1 envelope protein (gp120) reduces the anticryptococcal activity of human bronchoalveolar macrophages (118). Encapsulated cryptococci may be too large to be ingested by phagocytic cells, but several potential cellular mechanisms have been described that might control such organisms. Several phagocytic cells together may form rings surrounding uningested cryptococci and kill that fungi (55). Nonphagocytic, antibody-dependent killing of cryptococci mediated by human neutrophils, monocytes, or lymphocytes also has been reported (28). In addition, both natural killer cells active against tumor cell lines (89) and sensitized T-cells (41,71,74) can inhibit cryptococcal growth. Thus, several types of host cells might be active in controlling cryptococcosis, and experimental studies suggest that the outcome of these infections may well be determined primarily by the quantity of the inflammatory response in infectious foci (25).

A number of abnormalities in various aspects of immune function have been described in association with cases of cryptococcosis in humans. These abnormalities occur even in patients who are not receiving immunosuppressive drugs and have no apparent factors predisposing them to cryptococcal infections, although some of the patients studied could have had unrecognized immune defects such as idiopathic CD4+ T-lymphocytopenia (34). Responses to cryptococcal antigens (and sometimes unrelated antigens as well) are often depressed, as evidenced by cutaneous anergy, as well as impaired *in vitro* responses in assays of lymphocyte transformation or production of migration inhibitory factor (29,85,106,112). It is unclear whether such defects represent factors that predispose to cryptococcosis or, alternatively, result from the disease itself. However, at least some of these defects can persist for years after the disease is cured, even in the absence of immunosuppressive therapy (29,53).

One factor that may have great effects on host immune responses is the capsular polysaccharide (8). This gelatinous material surrounds the organisms, often conferring a characteristic appearance on gross and histologic cryptococcal lesions. In addition, polysaccharide sloughed from the surfaces of organisms dissolves and circulates during infections in measurable levels in blood, cerebrospinal fluid, and various inflammatory exudates, where interaction with host cells can occur. Cryptococcal polysaccharide can impair phagocytosis and suppress antibody and cell-mediated immune responses (14,72,83,90).

Presumably, such cellular defects predispose certain groups of patients to clinically apparent cryptococcosis. The incidence of cryptococcosis is increased in patients with AIDS whose CD4 lymphocyte counts are below 200–250/mm³ (81), idiopathic CD4+ T-lymphocytopenia (34), lymphoreticular malignancy (especially Hodgkin's disease), patients receiving therapeutic doses of corticosteroids, and patients with sarcoidosis in the absence of corticosteroid therapy (26,69). Diabetes mellitus has been noted in many patients with cryptococcosis (75), but its role as a predisposing factor is not as certain (26,69). Transplant recipients who develop cryptococcosis most often have received corticosteroid therapy. In most series from the pre-AIDS era, men have predominated over women in ratios approximating 3 : 1, and the disease is more commonly seen in white than in black races (26,69,75). Whether this is related to likelihood of heavy exposure to organisms or to immunologic differences has not been definitely established. Among patients with AIDS in the United States, cryptococcosis occurs with increased frequency among blacks, intravenous drug users, and residents of southern states immediately east of the Mississippi River (69). Despite the clear association of some cases of cryptococcosis with conditions that are known to impair cell-mediated immunity, reviews of large series of patients, prior to the AIDS epidemic, indicated that 50% or more of those who had developed cryptococcosis had no apparent predisposing factors (26).

CLINICAL MANIFESTATIONS

Pulmonary involvement (as defined by positive roentgenographic findings) can occur with a subacute or chronic course (75), sometimes lasting for several years (48), with or without concomitant extrapulmonary lesions involving brain, meninges, skin, bone, or multiple other organs and tissues (75). In one series, 45% of autopsied patients with central nervous system cryptococcosis had obvious cryptococcal pulmonary disease as well (73). Presenting symptoms of pulmonary cryptococcosis are usually minimal and nonspecific. At least a third of patients are completely asymptomatic, whereas others can have cough (usually nonproductive, but occasionally with some mucoid sputum), pleuritic or nonpleuritic chest pain, weight loss, low-grade fever, and malaise. Dyspnea is unusual in patients without AIDS, and night sweats or hemoptysis are rare findings. Most often, single or multiple nodular masses are observed on chest x-ray films without conspicuous hilar adenopathy (47, 60,75,76). Lower lobe lung involvement was said to be more common (17,76), but a later series reported a preponderance of upper lobe lesions (47). Total segmental or lobar consolidation can occur occasionally (47,78), and Pancoast's syndrome with a right upper lobe consolidation, axillary and supraclavicular adenopathy, and Horner's syndrome have been noted (86). Fibrosis and calcification are typically minimal, and cavitation is rare (76), occurring in 10% or less of cases (47,75). Cavities that do form can become secondarily colonized to form aspergillomas (101). Obvious lymphadenitis rarely can extend to involve mediastinal structures (116). Epipleural lesions have been reported in the absence of obvious parenchymal lung involvement (77), and unilateral or bilateral minimal to massive pleural effusions can accompany focal or diffuse pulmonary cryptococcosis and can recur over months or years (48). In such cases, pleural fluid usually is consistent with an exudate, with mononuclear cells predominating, although cultures of fluid yield the fungus in less than half the cases (124). Occasionally, cryptococcal pleural effusions are noted with no discernible parenchymal pulmonary infiltrates. Especially in patients with underlying disease (e.g., AIDS, lymphoma, or other predisposing factors that compromise the immune response), pulmonary cryptococcosis can be more diffuse, with peribronchial, interstitial, or miliary pneumonic lesions (40,47,75). Adult respiratory distress syndrome has complicated a few such cases (109). A rare diffuse presentation of pulmonary cryptococcosis, bronchiolitis obliterans–organizing pneumonia, was described in an HIV-negative patient with no obvious predisposing immunocompromise (18).

Up to half of patients with AIDS and cryptococcosis have evidence of pulmonary involvement (16,19,21,43,61,80,121,125), although in one recent large series, only 4% of such patients had clinically apparent pneumonia (20). However, based on retrospective studies, it has been suggested that unrecognized pulmonary cryptococcosis frequently occurs in the 4 months prior to the development of cryptococcal meningitis in patients with AIDS (33). In most cases of pulmonary cryptococcosis seen in patients with AIDS, involvement of the central nervous system and/or other organ systems is also seen. Many of these patients have concurrent pulmonary infection with other opportunistic organisms, especially *Pneumocystis carinii*, although cryptococcal lung involvement can be indistinguishable clinically (16,19, 43,125). However, cryptococcosis, by itself, particularly in patients with AIDS, can present with clinical and x-ray findings that are indistinguishable from those associated with diffuse pneumonias caused by *P. carinii* or other opportunistic pathogens. These patients most often present with interstitial infiltrates on chest roentgenogram which can be accompanied by a productive cough and respiratory distress, especially later in the course of the infection (21). Pathologically, there tends to be an abundance of cryptococci with an interstitial pattern of dissemination. Alveolar and occasionally capillary and lymphatic distribution of yeasts can also be seen. As with other infections in this group of patients, there is usually a minimal cellular infiltrate (43). Generally, this form of pulmonary cryptococcosis is associated with widespread dissemination. In one series of HIV-positive patients with cryptococcal pneumonia, there was a 42% mortality during the acute phase (16). Extensive central nervous system involvement in AIDS patients can be present despite the total absence of clinical signs and symptoms, or abnormalities in cerebrospinal fluid (except for the readily apparent presence of large numbers of yeasts on microscopic examination). Even within this category of extensive, diffuse pulmonary infections which can cause mild to severe hypoxemia, massive pulmonary collapse is rare (76,89). However, death owing to cryptococcal lung disease occasionally occurs in the absence of central nervous system involvement, in patients both with and without AIDS (75).

Patients who have predisposing factors are also far more likely to have disseminated, extrapulmonary cryptococcosis either coexisting with or developing later in the course of pulmonary cryptococcosis (16,60,121). Thus, the prognosis of patients with pulmonary cryptococcosis depends on the presence or absence of both extrapulmonary cryptococcal lesions and predisposing factors that can compromise the immune response. Localized, focal lesions in patients without underlying disease are usually self-limited, carrying a low risk of local progression and systemic dissemination (60,75). In patients who are immunosuppressed by chemotherapeutic agents (e.g., patients receiving corticosteroids), decreasing immunosuppression improves the likelihood of successful antifungal therapy (26,114).

Diagnosis of pulmonary cryptococcosis is complicated by the fact that, except in patients with AIDS (61,125), positive sputum cultures for the organisms are seen most often in the absence of x-ray evidence of cryptococcal lesions. In patients with central nervous system involvement, this combination of findings is a bad prognostic sign compared with patients who have definite pulmonary lesions on x-ray (26). In one series, only 19 of 101 patients with cryptococcal pulmonary lesions by x-ray (with or without disseminated disease) had positive sputum cultures (17). However, patients with AIDS, in keeping with the large numbers of organisms combined with the absent inflammatory response in lungs, usually have positive cultures if any sputum can be produced, or likely will yield the organism upon culture of bronchoalveolar lavage specimens (13,16,19,80,121).

Interpretation of sputum cultures is further complicated by the occurrence of saprophytic colonization of the respiratory tree by cryptococci, especially in patients with underlying pulmonary disease due to other causes. As many as 0.5 to 1.0% of patients with underlying bronchopulmonary disorders have carried *C. neoformans* in their sputa without tissue invasion (51) for documented periods as long as 10 months to 3 1/2 years (118). Associated conditions include pulmonary neoplasms, chronic obstructive pulmonary disease, chronic bronchitis, tuberculosis, asthma, and allergic bronchopulmonary aspergillosis (35,99,120). Occasional patients have no obvious pulmonary disorders (118), although many have some other potential predisposing factor, such as uremia. Thus, rather than signifying tissue invasive lesions of cryptococcosis, a positive sputum culture for *C. neoformans* could be a reflection of the presence of an unrelated pulmonary problem.

DIAGNOSIS

Identification of the organism by specific histopathology in lung tissue with positive cultures is generally a prerequisite for definitive diagnosis of pulmonary cryptococcosis. However, a rapid presumptive diagnosis can be made using smears or serology. As is the case with other fungi, cryptococci are best seen in sputum or specimens of tissue fluids using wet mounts, with or without alkaline digestion (by mixture on the slide with 10% sodium or potassium hydroxide and gentle heating). Gram stains are likely to obscure internal morphology of the organism and lead to misidentification of artifacts as yeasts. Care must be taken that stains, other solutions, slides, or the specimens themselves are not contaminated by fungi from the environment, including nonpathogenic cryptococci. To delineate the capsule that differentiates cryptococci (both pathogenic and nonpathogenic) from other budding yeasts, a drop of the specimen is mixed with an equal amount of India ink or nigrosin. To avoid overinterpretation, specific criteria are used to define cryptococci: round or oval cells that measure 2 to 10 μm in diameter with refractile cytoplasmic inclusions and thick (doubly refractile) cell walls surrounded by distinctly outlined capsules that are 1 to 30 μm or more in diameter. Thus, whether or not budding is observed, careful observation can separate cryptococci from artifacts (96). Sometimes cryptococci are seen in cytology preparations (104), but cryptococci can be difficult to distinguish from other yeasts. Occasionally, nonencapsulated or pseudohyphal forms of cryptococci are observed in lesions (116), and can be confused with other fungi. Most important, because presence of organisms in sputa (or bronchial washings) might not reflect tissue-invasive cryptococcosis, smears made from tissues or other specimens (pleural or cerebrospinal fluid), if positive, are more likely to be helpful.

With the use of special stains, cryptococcosis can be specifically diagnosed from examination of histologic sections of pulmonary tissues. On routine hematoxylin and eosin stains the organisms are generally difficult to see, with barely visible eosinophilic cell walls and colorless cytoplasm. Somewhat refractile, unstained capsular material generally surrounds extracellular organisms, creating the appearance of multiple cystic clusters (Fig. 26-1). The reactive inflammatory response is variable, most often moderate, with macrophages and giant cells (some with intracellular organisms) predominating, without well-formed granulomas or necrosis. Sometimes, a neutrophilic or mixed cellular response will be seen, or leukocytic infiltration might be minimal or absent. Definitive identification of the organism as yeasts with characteristic size and shape is achieved using silver or periodic acid-Schiff stains that delineate fungal walls. Generally, extracellular *C. neoformans* can be differentiated

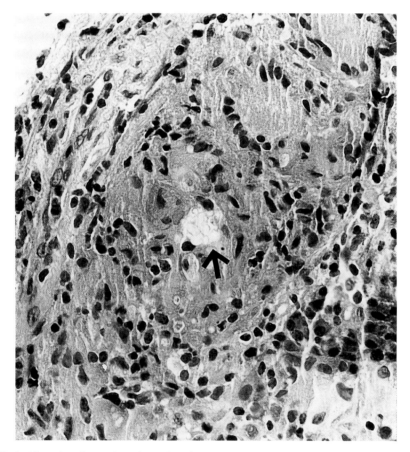

FIG. 26–1. Hematoxylin and eosin stain of a lung biopsy specimen from a patient without known immunocompromise who presented with cavitary pulmonary cryptococcosis. Note the cluster of poorly staining *C. neoformans* (*arrow*) within a granuloma. (Photomicrograph courtesy of Dr. Lucia Shuger.)

from *Blastomyces dermatitidis* yeasts of similar size, by the presence of narrow-based buds in the former as opposed to broad-based buds in the latter. Especially when poorly encapsulated forms of cryptococci predominate, as is often the case with AIDS patients (11,43), clusters of organisms within macrophages and granulomas can appear similar to *Histoplasma capsulatum.* Mayer's mucicarmine stain colors the cryptococcal capsule rose red but does not stain other fungi that share a similar morphology, making it possible to distinguish *C. neoformans* definitively from other yeasts as well as artifacts.

The Masson-Fontana stain also permits distinction of cryptococci from other yeasts, such as *Candida,* by staining melanin present in the cryptococcal cell wall dark brown (Fig. 26-2) (65). This stain has proved especially useful in determining the presence of cryptococci within lesions of patients with AIDS, who can also have extensive mucocutaneous candidiasis, especially when poorly encapsulated and/or pseudohyphal forms of *C. neoformans* are present within lesions.

All specimens should be cultured. In patients who do not produce sputum, stool cultures can be positive (26). Bronchoalveolar lavage can yield organisms, especially

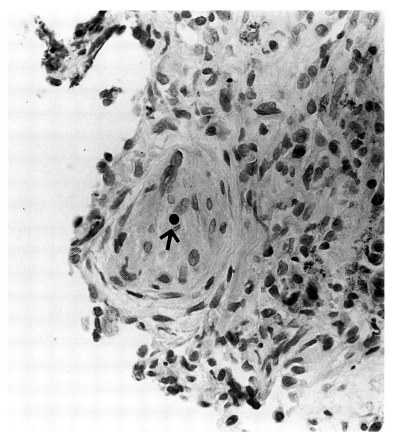

FIG. 26–2. Masson-Fontana stain of the same lung biopsy specimen as in Figure 26-1. A darkly staining *C. neoformans* cell (*arrow*) can be seen within a granuloma. (Photomicrograph courtesy of Dr. Lucia Shuger.)

in patients with AIDS (13,43). In patients with subpleural cryptococcal lesions, percutaneous ultrasound or CT-guided lung aspiration has been reported to have a diagnostic yield greater than that of bronchoscopy (68). In addition to specimens related to pulmonary lesions, extrapulmonary dissemination must be ruled out by cultures of large volumes (5 to 10 ml or more) of cerebrospinal fluid, as well as urine, skin lesions (88), and material from any other suspected sites of infection (26). Negative cultures do not necessarily rule out disseminated cryptococcosis, so that multiple specimens (especially of spinal fluid and urine) should be tested. Urine cultures are often positive, even though renal parenchymal involvement is unusual. Blood cultures, when positive, often signify the presence of extensive infection (26,94). AIDS patients commonly have positive blood cultures.

Cultures must be performed on media that do not contain cycloheximde (Actidone), an ingredient, often incorporated in fungal growth media (especially for isolation of dermatophytes) to suppress nonpathogens, that also inhibits growth of *C. neoformans*. Although *C. neoformans* characteristically grows at 37°C, primary isolation at lower temperatures (room temperature of 30°C) is preferred because the latter promotes more rapid growth. For most specimens, modified Sabouraud agar (with antibiotics for contaminated materials such as sputum) or a comparable medium is used for primary isolation. Use of the lysis-centrifugation technique appears to increase the sensitivity of blood cultures for detection of *C. neoformans*. Sometimes, cryptococci can be recovered from culture for mycobacteria if digestion of sputa with sodium hydroxide has not been performed (22). Digestion of sputum specimens with N-acetyl cysteine dithiothreitol and trypsin, followed by concentration by centrifugation, has been said to increase the yield of *C. neoformans* (45).

On solid culture media, cryptococci form smooth, sometimes quite mucoid, convex, yellow or tan colonies. Agar containing birdseed *(Guizotia abyssinica)* or chemical substitutes (phenol and diaminobenzene compounds such as caffeic acid or dihydroxyphenylalanine) can be used to rapidly differentiate *C. neoformans* from encapsulated, nonpathogenic cryptococci or other yeasts. Unlike other yeasts, *C. neoformans* has a phenol oxidase that forms melanin pigment from these compounds, producing brown colonies. These culture media can be especially useful for direct identification of cryptococci in sputum samples which also contain large numbers of *Candida* (69). Other characteristics of *C. neoformans*, such as growth at 37°C, lack of formation of pseudomycelia on cornmeal agar, hydrolysis of urea, and assimilation and fermentation patterns, facilitate microbiological identification (69). Rarely, particularly in compromised hosts, usually nonpathogenic species of *Cryptococcus* (e.g., *laurentii, albidus*) have been reported to cause clinically apparent illness (49,62,79).

Numerous immunologic tests have been described for cryptococcosis. Delayed skin testing has been performed with a variety of different antigens and is experimental, useful only for epidemiologic and immunologic studies. Although antibodies to cryptococcosis are detectable in serum of many patients and can signal a good prognosis when central nervous system involvement is present (26), they are often detected in healthy, normal subjects (9), so are not useful in diagnosis. Only tests to detect the specific cryptococcal capsular polysaccharide antigen (10) are clinically useful. A commercially available latex agglutination test is generally employed. Rheumatoid factor nonspecifically agglutinates the antibody-coated latex particles, so controls for this must be performed with all samples (4). Rheumatoid factor is eliminated from specimens, permitting testing of such samples, by reduction with dithiothreitol or mercaptoethanol (46), or by addition of ethylenediaminetetraacetic acid (EDTA) or pronase (39). Pronase treatment of serum samples can be of particular benefit because it appears to eliminate false-negative results from a prozone-like reaction (50). Although detection of an antigenic product of an organism is theoretically specific, variation in quality and relative sensitivity of different commercial kits (50,98) and in practices of personnel performing the tests makes it necessary to confirm results with cultural and histopathologic identification of the organism because false-positive reactions canoccur, especially if titers are low (<1:8) (56). Due to antigenic cross-reactivity, some patients with *Trichosporon beigelii* infections have positive latex agglutination tests for cryptococcal antigen (84). Enzyme-linked immunoadsorbent assays (107) are sensitive, specific, and can prove to be less labor intensive than latex agglutination tests in laboratories processing large numbers of samples, although experience with this test is limited.

Whereas cryptococcal antigen is detectable in spinal fluid and/or serum of more than 90% of patients with central nervous system cryptococcosis (37), isolated pulmonary or other localized cryptococcal lesions far less often produce sufficient antigen to be detectable in serum. For example, in one series, 14 of 15 cases of pulmonary or cutaneous cryptococcosis had no detectable cryptococcal antigen in serum (98). Immunocompromised patients with more diffuse pulmonary infiltrates, such as interstitial pneumonia, can be more likely to have positive serum antigen tests (40,58,59). When effusions are present, cryptococcal antigen can be detectable in pleural fluid (124). In a recent prospective study of 220 immunocompromised patients undergoing bronchoalveolar lavage for suspected pulmonary infection, all eight patients eventually diagnosed with cryptococcal pneumonia had positive titers (3). However, definitive diagnosis of isolated pulmonary cryptococcosis still must rest on histopathology and confirmatory positive cultures from suitable clinical specimens.

Pulmonary cryptococcosis, especially when it presents with chronic, focal lesions, must be distinguished from neoplasm, bronchiectasis, lung abscess, pneumoconiosis, sarcoidosis, tuberculosis, and other systemic mycoses (52). In fact, it has been suggested that focal pulmonary lesions on x-ray film combined with cryptococci cultured from sputum can be more likely to represent a primary lung tumor with saprophytic colonization by fungi rather than invasive cryptococcosis (35). In immunosuppressed patients with diffuse, rapidly progressive pulmonary cryptococcosis, the differential diagnosis must include infections due to gram-positive or gram-negative bacteria, viruses (especially cytomegalovirus), *Pneumocystis carinii,* and other fungi (40).

TREATMENT

Although extrapulmonary cryptococcosis requires systemic antifungal chemotherapy, not all cases of isolated pulmonary cryptococcosis require specific drug treatment (51,57,60). First, it is necessary to exclude the presence of disease that has disseminated outside the lungs. All patients should have a complete physical examination with particular attention paid to the presence of skin lesions. The possibility of bone involvement should be considered, and cerebrospinal fluid should be examined for cell count, fungal culture, and cryptococcal antigen. Serology for human immunodeficiency virus (HIV) should be performed. If no such dissemination is present, most cases of focal cryptococcal lesions in patients without predisposing factors (lymphoreticular malignancy, corticosteroid therapy, AIDS, idiopathic CD4+ T-lymphocytopenia) resolve spontaneously without specific antimycotic therapy, with minimal risk of late dissemination (51,57,60). This appears to be true as long as lesions are unilateral and do not progress, although such patients should be followed with cultures, serial chest x-rays, and serology to check for dissemination (5,95). Surgery is not required as a part of therapy for pulmonary cryptococcosis, although focal pulmonary lesions may be partially or completely resected as a part of a patient's diagnostic evaluation. Surgical manipulation by itself does not appear to increase the likelihood of extrapulmonary dissemination (95,110). In a cooperative study, 3 of 92 patients developed meningitis following surgical resection, although specific details of efforts to rule out dissemination prior to surgery in those patients are unclear (51).

Patients with more diffuse pulmonary lesions and those in whom lesions progress, as well as those who are immunocompromised, require systemic antifungal therapy. This is because late extrapulmonary dissemination is much more likely in such patients (60). A multicenter cooperative study of cryptococcal meningitis established that intravenous amphotericin B (0.3 mg/kg body weight/day or 0.6 mg/kg on alternate days) combined with oral flucytosine (25–37.5 mg/kg every 6 hr in patients with normal renal function) given for 6 weeks is the treatment of choice (5). For some patients, it appears that a 4-week course of combined therapy is adequate (31), although it is unclear at this time how such a subgroup can be identified reliably in a prospective evaluation. Amphotericin B alone (0.4 to 0.6 mg/kg/day, or double doses on alternate days) for 1 to 3 months or more is a second choice. Although based on anecdotal experience, some experts prefer higher doses of amphotericin B (up to 1 mg/kg/day), but this increases the likelihood of renal impairment, thereby increasing the likelihood of flucytosine accumulation and toxicity. Patients with profound immunocompromise or extensive disease could require longer or more intensive therapy (31).

Flucytosine alone can be effective, but resistance to this drug frequently emerges during therapy of cryptococcosis in this situation. The imidazole agents miconazole and ketoconazole inhibit cryptococci *in vitro,* but clinical experience is limited, and they have been replaced largely by apparently more effective and less toxic triazole derivatives (30). In a large, randomized trial of AIDS patients with cryptococcosis, fluconazole at a dose of 200 mg/day was compared with amphotericin B with or without flucytosine (103). Overall outcome was similar in both groups, although there was a trend toward earlier sterilization of the cerebrospinal fluid and fewer deaths during the first 2 weeks of therapy among patients given amphotericin B. In a smaller randomized study, 8 of 14 patients receiving fluconazole failed therapy versus none of 6 receiving amphotericin B (67). Fluconazole is usually used in 400 mg daily doses, and higher doses up to 800 mg/day can be more efficacious, especially in patients who have failed initial therapy (7). The experience with itraconazole for treatment of cryptococcosis is mostly anecdotal or uncontrolled (23,24), although in one small series of AIDS patients, amphotericin B plus flucytosine appeared superior to itraconazole (24). Until further studies are completed, initial therapy of patients with cryptococcosis should probably be individualized. The patient and physician must weigh the convenience, decreased toxicity, and decreased expense of triazoles with the greater experience and (possibly) increased efficacy of amphotericin B. For moderately and severely ill patients, we recommend amphotericin B as initial therapy, followed by fluconazole 400 mg/day once the patient has stabilized. Other patients can be treated, cautiously, with fluconazole (400 mg/day) alone. It should be noted that there is only limited experience using triazoles in patients with cryptococcosis who do not have AIDS.

Clinical experience with treatment of isolated pulmonary cryptococcosis is limited, but when systemic drugs are required, it seems reasonable to choose those regimens known to be effective against cryptococcal meningitis. Patients receiving amphotericin B can develop acute toxic reactions to infusions characterized by chills, high fevers, nausea, anorexia, and occasionally hypotension. Should they occur, hydrocortisone (25–50 mg by intravenous push or incorporated into infusion bags) will help control most of the reactions, and meperidine (50–75 mg given slowly, intravenously) can ameliorate severe chills (15). Acute azotemia can develop, and the daily dose of amphotericin B should be reduced if the serum creatinine rises above 3.0 to 3.5 mg/dl, although it should be noted that levels of amphotericin B in blood do not rise in renal failure, as there is no appreciable renal clearance of the drug. Hypokalemia and a reversible anemia can also occur. Azotemia induced by amphotericin B can also cause blood levels of flucytosine to rise into a toxic range, because the latter drug is cleared primarily by the kidney. Therefore, if flucytosine is used, blood levels should be closely monitored, especially during periods of minimal changes in serum creatinine (between serum creatinine levels of 1.0 and 2.0 mg/dl), because dosages recommended by nomograms can be significant overestimations. In most cases, flucytosine should be started at doses no higher than 25 mg/kg every 6 hours and blood levels monitored frequently to keep concentrations at about 40–80 µg/ml to minimize the risk of thrombocytopenia and leukopenia. Reactions to flucytosine are generally reversible but can be severe and life-threatening, including leukopenia and diarrhea. At least in HIV-negative patients, it is generally agreed that combination therapy permits use of a lower dose of amphotericin B and thus reduces toxicity and appears to prevent emergence of resistance to flucytosine (5). Based on experience with ketoconazole, hepatitis is rare but can be serious and even fatal, especially if the drug is not stopped when signs or symptoms of hepatitis first appear. The likelihood of serious hepatitis with the newer triazoles still must be determined. Gastrointestinal side effects occur less often with fluconazole or itraconazole than with ketoconazole. Like ketoconazole, the absorption of itraconazole is reduced by antacids or cimetidine, but fluconazole bioavailability is unaffected. Interactions between azoles and other drugs is common. Cyclosporine concentrations increase in patients receiving ketoconazole or, sometimes, fluconazole or itraconazole. Fluconazole slows metabolic inactivation of phenytoin, oral hypoglycemic drugs, or warfarin. Itraconazole similarly affects phenytoin, but metabolic changes affecting antidiabetic drugs or anticoagulants are less certain. However, itraconazole usage has been associated with rises in blood digoxin levels. Concomitant use of itraconazole or ketoconazole and newer antihistamines (terfenadine, astemizole) should be avoided as potentially fatal arrhythmias or QT interval prolongation have been reported. Rifampin, carbamazipine, phenytoin, or phenobarbital can cause reduction in blood levels of itraconazole or ketoconazole (117).

The minimally sufficient duration of therapy for pulmonary cryptococcosis remains to be established. As is the case with cryptococcal meningitis (26), immunosuppressive agents should be withdrawn during and after antifungal therapy whenever feasible (114).

Like most opportunistic infections in AIDS patients, cryptococcosis is often slow to respond to therapy. Moreover, relapse following treatment is extremely common unless suppressive (maintenance) therapy, administered indefinitely, is given (12). Several studies have demonstrated the efficacy of oral fluconazole, given at a dose of 200 mg/day, to prevent relapse (12,113). Based on retrospective, uncontrolled data, ketoconazole (200 mg/day) has been suggested as a potentially effective, less expensive alternative to fluconazole for prevention of relapse (20), but the drug is poorly absorbed by AIDS patients, and this limited experience should be confirmed before such a regimen is recommended. Intravenous amphotericin B, given once to 3 times weekly, is also efficacious (61,125). However, due to its toxicity and inconvenience of administration, amphotericin B suppressive therapy should be reserved for rare patients who fail or cannot tolerate azole therapy.

In summary, decisions about the therapy and projections about the prognosis of pulmonary cryptococcosis depend on the extent of the infection and the overall immunocompetence of the patient. As long as cerebrospinal fluid appears normal, cultures of that fluid and urine are negative, no other extrapulmonary lesions are evident in skin or elsewhere, pulmonary lesions are small and stable or decreasing in size, and predisposing factors (AIDS, lymphoreticular malignancy, corticosteroid therapy) are absent, patients can be observed closely for 3 to 6 months. Where doubts arise or definite indications exist, a course of antifungal chemotherapy is in order.

REFERENCES

1. Atkinson, A.J., Jr., and Bennett, J.E., (1968): Experience with a new skin test antigen prepared from *Cryptococcus neoformans. Am. Rev. Respir. Dis.*, 97:637–643.
2. Baker, R.D. (1976): The primary pulmonary lymph node complex of cryptococcosis. *Am. J. Clin. Pathol.*, 65:83–92.
3. Baughman, R.P., Rhodes, J.C., Dohn, M.N., Henderson, H., and Frame, P.T. (1992): Detection of cryptococcal antigen in bronchoalveolar lavage fluid: a prospective study of diagnostic utility. *Am. Rev. Respir. Dis.*, 145:1226–1229.
4. Bennett, J.E., and Bailey, J.W. (1971): Control for rheumatoid factor in the latex test for cryptococcosis. *Am. J. Clin. Pathol.*, 56:360–365.
5. Bennett, J.E., Dismukes, W.E., Duma, R.J., et al. (1979): A comparison of amphotericin B alone and combined with flucytosine in the treatment of cryptococcal meningitis. *N. Engl. J. Med.*, 301:126–131.
6. Bennett, J.E., Kwon-Chung, K.J., and Theodore, T.S. (1978): Biochemical differences between serotypes of *Cryptococcus neoformans. Sabouraudia*, 16:167–174.
7. Berry, A.J., Rinaldi, M.G., and Graybill, J.R. (1992): Use of high-dose fluconazole as salvage therapy for cryptococcal meningitis in patients with AIDS. *Antimicrob. Agents Chemother.*, 36:690–692.
8. Bhattacharjee, A.K., Bennett, J.E., and Glaudemans, C.P.J. (1984): Capsular polysaccharides of *Cryptococcus neoformans. Rev. Infect. Dis.*, 6:619–624.
9. Bindschadler, D.D., and Bennett, J.E. (1968): Serology of human cryptococcosis. *Ann. Intern. Med.*, 69:45–52.
10. Bloomfield, N., Gordon, M.A., and Elmendorf, D.F., Jr. (1963): Detection of *Cryptococcus neoformans* antigen in body fluids by latex particle agglutination. *Proc. Soc. Exp. Biol. Med.*, 114:64–67.
11. Bottone, E.J., Toma, M., Johansson, B.E., and Wormser, G.P. (1986): Poorly encapsulated *Cryptococcus neoformans* from patients with AIDS: I. Preliminary observations. *AIDS Res.*, 2:211–218.
12. Bozzette, S.A., Larsen, R.A., Chiu, J., et al. (1991): A placebo-controlled trial of maintenance therapy with fluconazole after treatment of cryptococcal meningitis in the acquired immunodeficiency syndrome. *N. Engl. J. Med.*, 324:580–584.
13. Broaddus, C., Dake, M.D., Stulbarg, M.S., et al. (1985): Bronchoalveolar lavage and transbronchial biopsy for the diagnosis of pulmonary infections in the acquired immunodeficiency syndrome. *Ann. Int. Med.*, 102:747–752.

14. Bulmer, G.S., and Sans, M.D. (1968): *Cryptococcus neoformans:* III. Inhibition of phagocytosis. *J. Bacteriol.,* 95:5–8.

15. Burks, L.C., Aisner, J., Fortner, C.L., and Wiernik, P.H. (1980): Meperidine for the treatment of shaking chills and fever. *Arch. Intern. Med.,* 140:483–484.

16. Cameron, M.L., Bartlett, J.A., Gallis, H.A., and Waskin, H.A., (1991): Manifestations of pulmonary cryptococcosis in patients with acquired immunodeficiency syndrome. *Rev. Infect. Dis.,* 13:64–67.

17. Campbell, G.D. (1966): Primary pulmonary cryptococcosis. *Am. Rev. Respir. Dis.,* 94:236–243.

18. Carey, C.F., Mueller, L., Fotopoulos, C.L., and Dall, L. (1991): Bronchiolitis obliterans–organizing pneumonia associated with *Cryptococcus neoformans* infection. *Rev. Infect. Dis.,* 131:253–254.

19. Chechani, V., and Kamholz, S.L. (1990): Pulmonary manifestations of disseminated cryptococcosis in patients with AIDS. *Chest,* 98:1060–1066.

20. Chuck, S.T., and Sande, M.A. (1989): Infections with *Cryptococcus neoformans* in the acquired immunodeficiency syndrome. *N. Engl. J. Med.,* 321:794–799.

21. Clark, R.A., Greer, D., Atkinson, W., Valainis, G.T., and Hyslop, N. (1990): Spectrum of *Cryptococcus neoformans* infection in 68 patients infected with human immunodeficiency virus. *Rev. Infect. Dis.,* 12:768–777.

22. Damsker, B., and Bottone, E.J. (1975): Recovery of *Cryptococcus neoformans* from modified Dubos liquid medium utilized for isolation of mycobacteria. *J. Clin. Microbiol.,* 1:393–395.

23. de Gans, J., Portegies, P., Tiessens, G., et al. (1992): Itraconazole compared with amphotericin B plus flucytosine in AIDS patients with cryptococcal meningitis *AIDS,* 6:185–190.

24. Denning, D.W., Tucker, R.M., Hanson, L.H., Hamilton, J.R., and Stevens, D.A. (1989): Itraconazole therapy for cryptococcal meningitis and cryptococcosis. *Arch. Intern. Med.,* 149:2301–2308.

25. Diamond, R.D. (1977): Effects of stimulation and suppression of cell-mediated immunity on experimental cryptococcosis. *Infect. Immun.,* 17:187–194.

26. Diamond, R.D. (1990): *Cryptococcus neoformans.* In: *Principles and Practice of Infectious Diseases,* 3rd Edition, edited by G.L. Mandell, R.G. Douglas, and J.E. Bennett, pp. 1980–1989. Churchill Livingstone, New York.

27. Diamond, R.D., and Allison, A.C. (1976): Nature of the effector cells responsible for antibody-dependent cell-mediated killing of *Cryptococcus neoformans. Infect. Immun.,* 14:716–720.

28. Diamond, R.D., and Bennett, J.E. (1973): Disseminated cryptococcosis in man: decreased lymphocyte transformation in response to *Cryptococcus neoformans. J. Infect. Dis.,* 127:694–697.

29. Diamond, R.D., and Bennett, J.E. (1974): Prognostic factors in cryptococcal meningitis: a study of 111 cases. *Ann. Intern. Med.,* 80:176–181.

30. Diamond, R.D., Root, R.K., and Bennett, J.E. (1972): Factors influencing killing of *Cryptococcus neoformans* by human leukocytes *in vitro. J. Infect. Dis.,* 125:367–376.

31. Dismukes, W.E., Cloud, G., Gallis, H.A., et al. (1987): Treatment of cryptococcal meningitis with combination amphotericin B and flucytosine for four as compared with six weeks. *N. Engl. J. Med.,* 317:334–341.

32. Dismukes, W.E., Stamm, A.M., Graybill, J.R., et al. (1983): Treatment of systemic mycoses with ketoconazole: emphasis on toxicity and clinical response in 52 patients. *Ann. Intern. Med.,* 98:13–20.

33. Driver, J.A., Saunders, C.A., Heinze-Lacey, B., and Sugar, A.M. (1994): Cryptococcal pneumonia in AIDS: Is cryptococcal meningitis preceded by clinically recognizable pneumonia? Submitted for publication.

34. Duncan, R.A., von Reyn, C.F., Alliegro, G.M., Toossi, Z., Sugar, A.M., and Levitz, S.M. (1993): Idiopathic CD4+ T-lymphocytopenia: four patients with opportunistic infections and no evidence of HIV infection. *N. Engl. J. Med.,* 328:393–398.

35. Duperval, R., Hermans, P.E., Brewer, N.S., and Roberts, G.D. (1977): Cryptococcosis with emphasis on the significance of isolation of *Cryptococcus neoformans* from the respiratory tract. *Chest,* 72:13–19.

36. Ellis, D.H., and Pfeiffer, T.J. (1990): Natural habitat of *Cryptococcus neoformans* var. *gattii. J. Clin. Microbiol.,* 28:1642–1644.

37. Ellner, J.J., and Bennett, J.E. (1976): Chronic meningitis. *Medicine,* 55:341–369.

38. Emmons, C.W. (1955): Saprophytic sources of *Cryptococcus neoformans* associated with the pigeon (Columbia livia). *Am. J. Hygiene,* 62:227–232.

39. Eng, R.H.K., and Person, A. (1981): Serum cryptococcal antigen determination in the presence of rheumatoid factor. *J. Clin. Microbiol.,* 14:700–702.

40. Fisher, B.D., and Armstrong, D. (1977): Cryptococcal interstitial pneumonia: value of antigen determination. *N. Engl. J. Med.,* 297:1440–1441.

41. Fung, P.Y.S., and Murphy, J.W. (1982): *In vitro* interactions of immune lymphocytes and *Cryptococcus neoformans. Infect. Immun.,* 36:1128–1138.

42. Gadebusch, H.H. (1972): Mechanisms of native and acquired resistance to infection with *Cryptococcus neoformans*. *CRC Crit. Rev. Microbiol.*, 1:311–320.
43. Gal, A.A., Koss, M.N., Hawkins, J., Evans, S., and Einstein, H. (1986): The pathology of pulmonary cryptococcal infections in the acquired immunodeficiency syndrome. *Arch. Pathol. Lab. Med.*, 110:502–507.
44. Gentry, L.O., and Remington, J.S. (1971): Resistance against *Cryptococcus* conferred by intracellular bacteria and protozoa. *J. Infect. Dis.*, 123:22–31.
45. Gervasi, J.P., and Miller, N.G. (1975): Recovery of *Cryptococcus neoformans* from sputum using new techniques for the isolation of fungi from sputum. *Am. J. Clin. Pathol.*, 63:916–920.
46. Gordon, M.A., and Lapa, E.W. (1974): Elimination of rheumatoid factor in the latex test for cryptococcosis. *Am. J. Clin. Pathol.*, 61:488–494.
47. Gordonson, J., Birnbaum, W., Jacobson, G., and Sargent, E.N. (1974): Pulmonary cryptococcosis. *Radiology,* 112:557–561.
48. Grosse, G., Niedobitek, F., l'Age, M., and Staib, F. (1981): Chronische lungenkryptokokkose: ein kasuistischer Beitrag zur Diagnostik der Kryptokokkose des Menschen aus pathologisch-anatomischer Sicht. *Deutsche Med. Wochenschr.* 106:1035–1037.
49. Gutierrez, F., Fu, Y.S., and Lurie, H.I. (1975): Cryptococcosis histologically resembling histoplasmosis. *Arch. Pathol.,* 99:347–352.
50. Hamilton, J.R., Noble, A., Denning, D.W., and Stevens, D.A. (1991): Performance of *Cryptococcus* antigen latex agglutination kits on serum and cerebrospinal fluid specimens of AIDS patients before and after pronase treatment. *J. Clin. Microbiol.,* 29:333–339.
51. Hammerman, K.J., Powell, K.E., and Christianson, C.S. (1973): Pulmonary cryptococcosis: forms and treatment. A Centers for Disease Control Cooperative Mycoses Study. *Am. Rev. Respir. Dis.,* 108:1116–1123.
52. Hatcher, C.P., Sehdeva, J., Waters, W.C., III, et al. (1971): Primary pulmonary cryptococcosis. *J. Thoracic Cardiovasc. Surg.,* 61:39–48.
53. Henderson, D.K., Bennett, J.E., and Huber, M.A. (1982): Long-lasting specific immunologic unresponsiveness associated with cryptococcal meningitis. *J. Clin. Invest.,* 69:1185–1190.
54. Henderson, D.K., Edwards, J.E., Dismukes, W.E., and Bennett, J.E. (1981): Meningitis produced by different serotypes of *Cryptococcus neoformans*. [Abstract]. In: *Proceedings of the Annual Meeting of the American Society for Microbiology*. American Society for Microbiology, Washington D.C.
55. Hill, J.O. (1992): CD4+ T cells cause multinucleated giant cells to form around *Cryptococcus neoformans* and confine the yeast within the primary site of infection in the respiratory tract. *J. Exp. Med.,* 175:1685–1695.
56. Hopfer, R.L., Perry, E.V., and Fainstein, V. (1982): Diagnostic value of cryptococcal antigen in the cerebrospinal fluid of patients with malignant disease. *J. Infect. Dis.,* 145:915.
57. Houk, V.N., and Moser, K.M. (1965): Pulmonary cryptococcosis: must all receive treatment? *Ann. Intern. Med.,* 63:583–596.
58. Jenkins, C., and Breslin, A.B.X. (1982): Pulmonary cryptococcosis: atypical results in the serum test for cryptococcal antigen. *Aust. NZ J. Med.,* 12:527–530.
59. Jensen, W.A., Rose, R.M., Hammer, S.M., and Karchmer, A.W. (1985): Serologic diagnosis of focal pneumonia caused by *Cryptococcus neoformans*. *Am. Rev. Respir. Dis.,* 132:189–191.
60. Kerkering, T.M., Duma, R.J., and Shadomy, S. (1981): The evolution of pulmonary cryptococcosis: clinical implications from a study of 41 patients with and without compromising host factors. *Ann. Intern. Med.,* 94:611–616.
61. Kovacs, J.A., Kovacs, A.A., Polis, M., et al. (1985): Cryptococcosis in the acquired immunodeficiency syndrome. *Ann. Intern. Med.,* 103:533–538.
62. Krumholz, R.A., (1972): Pulmonary cryptococcosis: a case due to *Cryptococcus albidus*. *Am. Rev. Respir. Dis.,* 105:421–424.
63. Kwon-Chung, K.J., and Bennett, J.E. (1978): Distribution of α and mating types of *Cryptococcus neoformans* among natural and clinical isolates. *Am. J. Epidemiol.,* 108:337–340.
64. Kwon-Chung, K.J., and Bennett, J.E. (1984): Epidemiologic differences between the two varieties of *Cryptococcus neoformans*. *Am. J. Epid.,* 120:123–130.
65. Kwon-Chung, K.J., Hill, W.B., and Bennett, J.E. (1981): New special stain for histopathological diagnosis of cryptococcosis. *J. Clin. Microbiol.,* 13:383–387.
66. Kwon-Chung, K.J., Polacheck, I., and Bennett, J.E. (1982): Improved diagnostic medium for separation of *Cryptococcus neoformans* var. *neoformans* (serotypes A and D) and *Cryptococcus neoformans* var. *gatti* (serotypes B and C). *J. Clin. Microbiol.,* 15:535–537.
67. Larsen, R.A., Leal, M.A.E., and Chan, L.S. (1990): Fluconazole compared with amphotericin B plus flucytosine for cryptococcal meningitis in AIDS: a randomized trial. *Ann. Intern. Med.,* 113:183–187.
68. Lee, L.N., Yang, P.C., Kuo, S.H., Luh, K.T., Chang, D.B., and Yu, C.J. (1983): Diagnosis of pulmonary cryptococcosis by ultrasound-guided percutaneous aspiration. *Thorax,* 48:75–78.

69. Levitz, S.M. (1991): The ecology of *Cryptococcus neoformans* and the epidemiology of crypto-coccosis. *Rev. Infect. Dis.*, 13:1163–1169.
70. Levitz, S.M., and DiBenedetto, D.J. (1988): Differential stimulation of murine resident perito-neal cells by selectively opsonized encapsulated and acapsular *Cryptococcus neoformans*. *Infect. Immun.*, 56:2544–2551.
71. Levitz, S.M., and Dupont, M.P., (1993): Phenotypic and functional characterization of human lymphocytes activated by interleukin-2 to directly inhibit growth of *Cryptococcus neoformans in vitro*. *J. Clin. Invest.*, 91:1490–1498.
72. Levitz, S.M., Farrell, T.P., and Maziarz, R.T. (1991): Killing of *Cryptococcus neoformans* by human peripheral blood mononuclear cells stimulated in culture. *J. Infect. Dis.*, 163:1108–1113.
73. Lewis, J.L., and Rabinovich, S. (1972): The wide spectrum of cryptococcal infections. *Am. J. Med.*, 53:315–322.
74. Lim, T.S., and Murphy, J.W. (1980): Transfer of immunity to cryptococcosis by T-enriched splenic lymphocytes from *Cryptococcus neoformans*–sensitized mice. *Infect. Immun.*, 30:5–11.
75. Littman, M.L., and Walter, J.E. (1968): Cryptococcosis: current status. *Am. J. Med.*, 45:922–932.
76. Littman, M.L., and Zimmerman, L.E. (1956): *Cryptococcosis*. Grune and Stratton, New York.
77. Lomvardias, S., and Lurie, H.I. (1972): Epipleural cryptococcosis in a patient with Hodgkin's disease: a case report. *Sabouraudia*, 10:256–259.
78. Long, R.F., Berens, S.V., and Shambhag, G.R. (1972): An unusual manifestation of pulmonary cryptococcosis. *Br. J. Radiol.*, 45:757–759.
79. Lynch, J.P., III, Schaberg, D.R., Kissner, D.G., and Kauffman, C.A. (1981): *Cryptococcus laurentii* lung abscess. *Am. Rev. Respir. Dis.*, 123:135–138.
80. Malabonga, V.M., Basti, J., and Kamholz, S.L. (1991): Utility of bronchoscopic sampling tech-niques for cryptococcal disease in AIDS. *Chest*, 99:370–372.
81. Masur, H., Ognibene, F.P., Yarchoan, R., et al. (1991): CD4 counts as predictors of opportunistic pneumonias in human immunodeficiency virus (HIV) infection. *Ann. Int. Med.*, 111:223–231.
82. McDonnell, J.M., and Hutchins, G.M. (1985): Pulmonary cryptococcosis. *Human Pathol.*, 16:121–128.
83. McGaw, T.G., and Kozel, T.R. (1979): Opsonization of *Cryptococcus neoformans* by human immunoglobulin G: masking of immunoglobulin G by cryptococcal polysaccharide. *Infect. Immun*, 25:262–267.
84. McManus, E.J., Bozdech, M.J., and Jones, J.M. (1985): Role of the latex agglutination test for cryptococcal antigen in diagnosing disseminated infections with *Trichosporon beigelii*. *J. Infect. Dis.*, 151:1167–1169.
85. Miller, G.P.G., and Puck, J. (1984): *In vitro* human lymphocyte responses to *Cryptococcus neoformans:* evidence for primary and secondary responses in normals and infected subjects. *J. Immunol.*, 133:166–172.
86. Mitchell, D.H., and Sorrell, T.C. (1992): Pancoast's syndrome due to pulmonary infection with *Cryptococcus neoformans* variety *gattii*. *Clin. Infect. Dis.*, 14:1142–1144.
87. Mitchell, T.G., and Friedman, L. (1972): *In vitro* phagocytosis and intracellular fate of variously encapsulated strains of *Cryptococcus neoformans*. *Infect. Immun.*, 5:491–498.
88. Moore, M. (1957): Cryptococcosis with cutaneous manifestations. *J. Invest. Dermatol.*, 28:159–182.
89. Murphy, J.W., and McDaniel, D.O. (1982): *In vitro* reactivity of natural killer (NK) cells against *Cryptococcus neoformans*. *J. Immunol.*, 128:1577–1583.
90. Murphy, J.W., and Moorhead, J.W. (1982): Regulation of cell-mediated immunity in cryptococ-cosis: induction of specific afferent T suppressor cells by cryptococcal antigen. *J. Immunol.*, 128:276–282.
91. Murray, R.J., Becker, P., Furth, P., and Criner, G.J. (1988): Recovery from cryptococcemia and the adult respiratory distress syndrome in the acquired immunodeficiency syndrome. *Chest*, 93:1304–1306.
92. Newberry, W.M., Jr., Walter, J.E., Chandler, J.W., and Tosh, F.E. (1967): Epidemiologic study of *Cryptococcus neoformans*. *Ann. Intern. Med.*, 67:724–732.
93. Nielson, J.B., Fromtling, R.A., and Bulmer, G.S. (1977): *Cryptococcus neoformans:* size range of infectious particles from aerosolized soil. *Infect. Immun.*, 17:634–638.
94. Perfect, J.R., Durack, D.T., and Gailis, H.A. (1983): Cryptococcemia. *Medicine*, 62:98–109.
95. Perkins, W. (1969): Pulmonary cryptococcosis: report on the treatment of 9 cases. *Dis. Chest*, 56:389–394.
96. Portnoy, D., and Richards, G.K. (1981): Cryptococcal meningitis: misdiagnosis with India ink. *Can. Med. Assoc. J.*, 124:891–892.
97. Powell, K.E., Dahl, B.A., Weeks, R.J., and Tosh, F.E. (1972): Airborne *Cryptococcus neoformans:* particles from pigeon excreta compatible with alveolar deposition. *J. Infect. Dis.*, 125:412–415.

98. Prevost, E., and Newell, R. (1978): Commercial cryptococcal latex kit: clinical evaluation in a medical center hospital. *J. Clin. Microbiol.,* 8:529–533.

99. Randhawa, H.S., and Pal, M. (1977): Occurrence and significance of *Cryptococcus neoformans* in the respiratory tract of patients with bronchopulmonary disorders. *J. Clin. Microbiol.,* 5:5–8.

100. Rinaldi, M.G., Drutz, D.J., Howell, A., Sande, M.A., Wofsy, C.B., and Hadley, W.K. (1986): Serotypes of *Cryptococcus neoformans* in patients with AIDS. *J. Infect. Dis.,* 153:642.

101. Rosenheim, S.H., and Schwarz, J. (1975): Cavitary pulmonary cryptococcosis complicated by aspergilloma. *Am. Rev. Respir. Dis.,* 111:549–553.

102. Ruiz, A., Fromtling, R.A., and Bulmer, G.S. (1981): Distribution of *Cryptococcus neoformans* in a natural site. *Infect. Immun.,* 31:560–563.

103. Saag, M.S., Powderly, W.G., Cloud, G.A., et al. (1992): Comparison of amphotericin B with fluconazole in the treatment of actue AIDS-associated cryptococcal meningitis. *N. Engl. J. Med.,* 326:83–89.

104. Saigo, P., Rosen, P.P., Kaplan, M.H., Solan, G., and Melamed, M.R. (1977): Identification of *Cryptococcus neoformans* in cytologic preparation of cerebrospinal fluid. *Am. J. Clin. Pathol.,* 67:141–145.

105. Salyer, W.R., (1974): Primary complex of *Cryptococcus* and pulmonary lymph nodes. *J. Infect. Dis.,* 130:74–77.

106. Schimpff, S.C., and Bennett, J.E. (1975): Abnormalities in cell-mediated immunity in patients with *Cryptococcus neoformans* infections. *J. Allergy Clin. Immunol.,* 55:430–441.

107. Scott, E.N., Muchmore, H.G., and Felton, F.G. (1980): Comparison of enzyme immunoassay and latex agglutination methods for detection of *Cryptococcus neoformans* antigen. *Am. J. Clin. Pathol.,* 73:790–794.

108. Shimizu, R.Y., Howard, D.H., and Clancy, M.X. (1986): The variety of *Cryptococcus neoformans* in patients with AIDS. *J. Infect. Dis.,* 154:1042.

109. Similowski, T., Datry, A., Jais, P., Katlama, C., Rosenheim, M., and Gentilini, M. (1989): AIDS-associated cryptococcosis causing adult respiratory distress syndrome. *Respir. Med.,* 83:513–515.

110. Smith, F.E.S., Gibsons, P., Nicholls, T.A.T., and Simpson, J.E.A. (1976): Pulmonary resection for localized lesions of cryptococcosis (torulosis): a review of eight cases. *Thorax,* 31:121–126.

111. Staib, F., Grave, B., Altmann, L., Mishra, S.K., Abel, T., and Blisse, A. (1978): Epidemiology of *Cryptococcus neoformans. Mycopathologia,* 65:73–76.

112. Stobo, J.D. (1977): Immunosuppression in man: suppression by macrophages can be mediated by interactions with regulatory T cells. *J. Immunol.,* 119:918–924.

113. Sugar, A.M., and Saunders, C. (1988): Suppressive therapy of disseminated cryptococcosis in patients with acquired immunodeficiency syndrome (AIDS) with oral fluconazole. *Am. J. Med.,* 85:481–489.

114. Swenson, R.S., Kountz, S.L., Blank, N., and Merigan, T.C. (1969): Successful renal allograft in a patient with pulmonary cryptococcosis. *Arch. Intern. Med.,* 124:502–506.

115. Swinne, D., Nkurikiyinfura, J.B., and Muyembe, T.L. (1986): Clinical isolates of *Cryptococcus neoformans* from Zaire. *Eur. J. Clin. Microbiol.,* 5:50–51.

116. Talerman, A., Bradley, J.M., and Woodland, B. (1970): Cryptococcal lymphadenitis. *J. Med. Microbiol.,* 3:633–638.

117. Terrell, C.L., and Hughes, C.E. (1992): Antifungal agents used for deep-seated mycotic infections. *Mayo Clin. Proc.,* 67:69–91.

118. Tynes, B., Mason, K.N., Jennings, A.E., and Bennett, J.E. (1968): Variant forms of pulmonary cryptococcosis. *Ann. Intern. Med.,* 69:1117–1125.

119. Wagner, R.P., Levitz, S.M., Tabuni, A., and Kornfeld, H. (1992): HIV-1 envelope protein (gp120) inhibits the activity of human bronchoalveolar macrophages against *Cryptococcus neoformans. Am. Rev. Respir. Dis.,* 146:1434–1438.

120. Warr, W., Bates, J.H., and Stone, A. (1968): The spectrum of pulmonary cryptococcosis. *Ann. Intern. Med.,* 69:1109–1116.

121. Wasser, L., and Talavera, W. (1987): Pulmonary cryptococcosis in AIDS. *Chest,* 92:692–695.

122. White, M., Cirrincione, C., Blevins, A., and Armstrong, D. (1992): Cryptococcal meningitis: outcome in patients with AIDS and patients with neoplastic disease. *J. Infect. Dis.,* 165:960–963.

123. Wilson, D.E., Bennett, J.E., and Bailey, W. (1968): Serologic grouping of *Cryptococcus neoformans. Proc. Soc. Exp. Biol. Med.,* 127:820–823.

124. Young, E.J., Hirsh, D.D., Fainstein, V., and Williams, T.W. (1980): Pleural effusions due to *Cryptococcus neoformans:* a review of the literature and report of two cases with cryptococcal antigen determinations. *Am. Rev. Respir. Dis.,* 121:743–747.

125. Zuger, A., Louie, E., Holzman, R.S., Simberkoff, M.S., and Rahal, J.J. (1986): Cryptococcal disease in patients with the acquired immunodeficiency syndrome. *Ann. Intern. Med.,* 104:234–240.

Respiratory Infections: Diagnosis and Management, 3d ed.,
edited by James E. Pennington.
Raven Press, Ltd., New York © 1994

27

Coccidioidal Pneumonia

David J. Drutz

*Department of Microbiology and Immunology, Temple University School of Medicine,
Philadelphia, Pennsylvania, and Daiichi Pharmaceutical Corporation,
1 Parker Place, Ft. Lee, New Jersey 07024*

ETIOLOGY

Coccidioides immitis, the etiologic agent of coccidioidomycosis, is a biphasic fungus that exists as a mycelium (mold) in its natural environmental habitat, and as a unique endosporulating spherule in the infected host. Dissolution of alternating cells in the segmented mycelium frees the intervening arthroconidia that are easily dispersed by air currents. When inhaled, the arthroconidia (2×5 μm in their rectangular dimensions) undergo progressive enlargement to produce spherical cells (spherules) that may reach 30 to 80 μm in diameter. Segmentation of the spherule cytoplasm results in the production of hundreds of endospores that are released when each spherule ruptures. Each endospore then develops into a new spherule. This morphogenic cycle is unique to *C. immitis;* there is no yeast-like stage (29).

EPIDEMIOLOGY

Geography-Related

Coccidioidomycosis is unique to the Western Hemisphere. Fifty to 100,000 cases occur yearly in the Southwestern United States (especially Arizona, California, and Texas) and contiguous areas of Mexico. Coccidioidomycosis was first described in Argentina, and occurs in other parts of South and Central America as well (29).

C. immitis exists as a soil saprophyte (mycelial phase) principally in semiarid surroundings that receive short periods of intense rainfall. The microorganism is probably destroyed in the uppermost layers of the soil by direct summer sunlight, but survives at deeper levels (e.g., within rodent burrows). With rainfall, the microorganism percolates to the surface. With soil drying, arthroconidia are set free to be wafted about by air currents, or carried by animals to new habitats. A current epidemic of coccidioidomycosis in California may be attributable to the fact that intense rainfall has ended a drought of approximately 5 years. Mycelia that have accumulated for years in the depths of the soil might have thus been washed to the surface where they are now germinating and releasing arthroconidia (32).

The precise soil conditions that are necessary for *C. immitis* to thrive are not known. However, they seem to be quite specific because *C. immitis* may be found in high numbers in one location, yet be absent from another site several yards away. *C. immitis* tends to disappear from soil that has come under agricultural use and regular irrigation, perhaps because competing microorganisms are given a selective advantage (29).

Although *C. immitis* is traditionally associated with semidesert conditions (e.g., the Phoenix and Tucson areas of Arizona, or the San Joaquin Valley of California), the distribution of the fungus is actually not that restricted. For example, *C. immitis* has been found in cool, moist, sandy soil (San Diego, California); in frankly tropical areas (Colima, Michoacan, and Guerrero states, Mexico); and in mediterranean woodland areas of northern California (29).

Acquisition of coccidioidomycosis is traditionally associated with outdoor activities such as farming, ranching, military maneuvers, and excavation—including at archeological sites. However, driving through an endemic area on a windy day or merely visiting a highly endemic area can be sufficient to allow exposure to the arthroconidia. (Experimental animals can often be infected with fewer than 10 inhaled arthroconidia.) Modern tourism provides the opportunity for the disease to present to physicians thousands of miles from the site of the original infection, raising serious problems in diagnosis (56). Hence, the travel history must be taken with some care if coccidioidomycosis is to be included in the differential diagnosis. In 1977, a dust storm in California produced the first documented modern epidemic of coccidioidomycosis when arthroconidia were carried hundreds of miles to nonendemic areas. The incidence of coccidioidomycosis quadrupled in California in 1978, and increased 20-fold in the San Joaquin Valley (32). Rare cases of coccidioidomycosis have occurred in clearly nonendemic areas where material from an endemic area was handled (e.g., cotton shipped from the San Joaquin Valley being unloaded in Italy).

Although nearly all cases of coccidioidomycosis are acquired via the respiratory route, rare instances of percutaneous inoculation have been recorded.

Neither animals nor humans appear to be important for the survival of *C. immitis* in nature. Thus, it is unclear what advantage accrues to the fungus by infecting mammals, especially when a totally unique developmental cycle is required to do so.

Host-Related

Although rates of disease acquisition are related predominantly to environmental exposure, a number of host-determined factors influence the subsequent course of events (29).

Race

On the basis of the results of clinical and autopsy series, blacks are approximately 10 to 15 times as likely as whites to experience extrapulmonary coccidioidal dissemination. This appears to be true even under identical conditions of exposure (e.g., in military trainees). The explanation is obscure; there is no regular association with genetic markers. Increased "racial" susceptibility of Filipinos, Orientals, Native Americans, and Hispanics is based on less firm epidemiologic data (29,52).

Sex

Under ordinary circumstances, men are more likely to experience coccidioidal dissemination than women. The explanation is uncertain.

Pregnancy

The second and third trimesters of pregnancy have been considered a period of extreme risk for the dissemination of newly acquired coccidioidomycosis. Possible explanations include the state of relative immunologic tolerance associated with pregnancy (81), antigen-specific immune suppression (10), and the presence of sex hormone receptors in *C. immitis* that could mediate fungal growth stimulation in the enhanced hormonal milieu of pregnancy (30). Coccidioidomycosis in pregnancy may be less common and less often associated with maternal mortality than previously reported (87). It is possible that the high maternal mortality reported in the older literature is related less to the pregnant state than to associated racial or socioeconomic factors.

Age

Carefully conducted studies in Native American populations living in the endemic zone of Arizona suggest that the very young and the very old are more susceptible to coccidioidal dissemination. In the case of the young, this might relate to greater opportunities for direct soil exposure afforded by outside play. The explanation for increased dissemination in the very old could be reduced immunocompetence or intercurrent debilitating disease.

Immunosuppression

Intact cell-mediated immunity (CMI) appears to be essential for containment of *C. immitis* infection. Patients with depressed CMI (24,47), and especially those with acquired immune deficiency syndrome (AIDS) (4,5,19,35,59) are more susceptible to coccidioidal dissemination. Corticosteroid therapy, used as concomitant therapy for *Pneumocystis carinii* pneumonia, can result in dissemination of unrecognized, simultaneous *C. immitis* infection (59). Reactivation of prior infection has been documented in the setting of AIDS or transplant-related immunodepression (4).

IMMUNOLOGY

Because *C. immitis* is a complex microorganism, the host must be prepared to deal with arthroconidia, followed by spherules and endospores (30). Each presents unique problems for host defenses. Arthroconidia possess a surface component (the hyphal outer wall layer) that is antiphagocytic and antiproliferative for lymphocytes (30). The *C. immitis* cell wall activates suppressor cells that down-regulate host immunity (20). Even when ingested by phagocytes present in the blood and/or lung [e.g., polymorphonuclear neutrophils (PMNs), mononuclear phagocytes, and alveolar macrophages], arthroconidia are killed inefficiently (2). Spherules reach extraordinary sizes (30 to 80 μm diameter) and possess an antiphagocytic extracellular fibrillar matrix (36). The joint activity of PMNs and macrophages appears necessary for their destruction *in vitro,* but their vulnerability to these cells *in vivo* is uncertain. Spherules release endospores by the hundreds, taxing immunologic reserves. Young endospores, freshly released from spherules, are bound together by a fibrillar matrix that appears difficult for phagocytes to penetrate. By the time the matrix has dissipated, the endospores are already young spherules, with thick cell walls. Proteolytic enzymes that facilitate spherule rupture and endospore release could also mediate tissue destruction by their collagenolytic and elastinolytic activities.

It is generally considered that cell-mediated immunity (i.e., macrophages, lymphocytes, and cytokines) constitutes the principal host defense mechanism in coccidioidomycosis (3,42). Although endospores are ingested by monocytes and macrophages, they do not appear to be killed unless appropriate cytokines are present (14). Early *in vitro* studies suggested that complement-fixing antibody might be opsonic for *C. immitis,* but this observation has never been confirmed. The immunity associated with coccidioidin (or spherulin) skin test positivity is ordinarily considered to be solid. However, patients with AIDS can disseminate their infections despite well-documented positive skin tests (4). Reinfection is likewise rare except under conditions of heavy arthroconidial reexposure (e.g., in a laboratory accident) or profound immunoincompetence (e.g., AIDS) (4).

CLINICAL MANIFESTATIONS

Primary Coccidioidomycosis

More than 60% of cases of coccidioidomycosis are acquired asymptomatically. Under these conditions, the occurrence of infection can be inferred by the demonstration of coccidioidin or spherulin skin test positivity, or by a suitably elevated antibody titer. Undoubtedly many of these patients would have pulmonary roentgenographic changes, but these are missed unless a chest roentgenogram happens to be taken for other reasons. Either cavitary pulmonary disease or extrapulmonary dissemination can follow an asymptomatic primary pulmonary infection.

In the approximately 40% of patients who experience symptoms, the majority have nonspecific complaints that are difficult to differentiate from a variety of other respiratory infectious diseases (53). These include fever (80%), chest pain that is substernal or pleuritic in type (70 to 80%), cough (sometimes mildly productive, with or without minor hemoptysis) (60 to 70%), malaise (40 to 50%), anorexia (30%), and chills or chilly sensations (10%). In many circumstances, patients attribute such symptoms to "the flu," and medical attention is sometimes not sought. Even when the patient is seen by a physician, disease can be attributed to common nonfungal respiratory pathogens. In some cases, the occurrence of cutaneous hypersensitivity phenomena 1 to 2 weeks later may prompt medical consultation when the original respiratory symptoms were not severe enough to do so (see below).

Pulmonary Manifestations

Coccidioidal infection can begin as an endobronchial process; both mucosal hyperemia and bronchial ulceration have been reported at bronchoscopy. The most common roentgenographic manifestation of primary infection is a pulmonary infiltrate that may be peribronchial, subsegmental, segmental, or sometimes even lobar in distribution (11,45). Occasionally there can be multiple discrete areas of infiltration. Parenchymal infiltrates are commonly seen in association with hilar. Paratracheal and superior mediastinal adenopathy, however, are not usually considered part of the primary complex and may signal dissemination (32). Rarely, there may be bilateral hilar adenopathy in the absence of apparent pulmonary disease, raising the possibility of sarcoidosis or lymphoma in the differential diagnosis. In accordance with the frequency of pleuritic pain as an initial symptom, pleural fluid can be demonstrated in up to 20% of patients (11). As a rule, a pulmonary infiltrate will be demonstrable near the pleura, on the same side as the effusion. Massive pleural effusions have been reported (57).

Smaller coccidioidal pulmonary infiltrates characteristically evolve with rapidity, often disappearing entirely in days to weeks. However, areas of dense infiltration can take months to clear. The central portions of some infiltrates can "shell out," resulting in one or more cavities, usually without contained fluid. The frequency with which such cavitation occurs is not well documented but can range from 5 to 11% (50) and could be more common in diabetics (11,31,32). In most cases, cavities identified in the first few weeks of infection are only transient ("will-o-the-wisp") (90). They can often be seen to fill in and contract, resulting in the formation of nodules, or leaving no apparent residua at all. Occasionally, cavities fill and empty several times before nodule formation is secure. Some cavities, especially in diabetics, persist to result in more chronic cavitation (72). In addition, diabetics commonly have multiple lesions, and a significant rate of cavitary recurrence after resection (31). The relationship between acute cavities and later chronic cavitary disease is not well defined. Rarely, acute cavities can perforate into the pleural space with the result that the first manifestation of otherwise unsuspected primary pulmonary coccidioidomycosis is pyopneumothorax with empyema and bronchopleural fistula formation (31).

Acute respiratory failure can occur as a rare complication of primary pulmonary coccidioidomycosis, most commonly in association with underlying immunosuppression (e.g., steroid therapy, AIDS) or the inhalation of a large fungal inoculum (55). In such patients, there is commonly evidence of an overwhelming, hematogenously disseminated infection with miliary pulmonary lesions. The clinical presentation can resemble septic shock (58).

Concomitant Phenomena

In a variable proportion of patients with primary coccidioidal infection, the disease is announced by a variety of immunologic phenomena, the basis of which is uncertain (29).

Toxic erythema. The development of a diffuse erythematous exanthem, commonly confused with drug eruption, measles, or scarlet fever, has been reported as an initial manifestation of coccidioidal infection in men and women, children and adults. The rash, which can be macular, urticarial, or vesicular, apparently occurs within the early days following fungal exposure, well before the 2 to 3 weeks necessary for the development of CMI, and it fades spontaneously. Its etiology is obscure.

Valley fever, desert rheumatism, desert fever, "the bumps." Approximately 25% of women and 4% of men experience erythema nodosum and/or erythema multiforme, in the presence or absence of nonspecific arthralgias and conjunctivitis, as a manifestation of primary coccidioidal infection. Often it is the frightening aspect of the cutaneous eruption, and not respiratory symptoms, that leads to medical consultation. The lesions of erythema nodosum are hot, red, and tender nodules that occur predominantly, but by no means exclusively, on the shins. These cutaneous phenomena coincide with the development of coccidioidin skin test reactivity (i.e., 2 to 3 weeks postexposure) and are therefore considered to relate somehow to the acquisition of CMI. If a coccidioidal skin test is actually applied during such an episode, a violent cutaneous response can result. Conversely, a negative coccidioidin or spherulin skin test in a person experiencing erythema nodosum or multiforme is considered to eliminate coccidioidomycosis as a diagnostic possibility.

The occurrence of erythema nodosum has been rather uncritically considered to signal a favorable outcome of infection. However, because those persons who most frequently experience erythema nodosum (i.e., white women) normally have an excellent prognosis for spontaneous recovery, the significance of this association is uncertain. Moreover, it is clear that some persons with erythema nodosum or multiforme do go on to develop extrapulmonary disseminated infection.

The manifestations of "valley fever" complex are not unique to coccidioidomycosis but have, in fact, been described in patients with histoplasmosis, blastomycosis, tuberculosis, and sarcoidosis (Lofgren syndrome).

Eosinophilia. Moderate degrees of peripheral blood eosinophilia (10 to 20%) are often encountered in patients with primary coccidioidomycosis, and eosinophilia in the cerebrospinal fluid can signal the presence of coccidioidal meningitis (68). Tissue eosinophilia is also well documented, but the role that these cells play in coccidioidal host defense is unknown. There is no particular association of eosinophilia with the "valley fever" syndrome. Eosinophilia tends to clear spontaneously. Its persistence can be associated with a poor prognosis.

Persistent Pneumonia

Particularly in immunocompromised patients, symptoms and roentgenographic abnormalities can persist beyond 6 to 8 weeks. These patients are considered to have persistent coccidioidal pneumonia (29). They are often quite ill, with fever, chest pain, productive cough, and hemoptysis. Infiltrates can be extensive, and clear only slowly. Striking cavitation can be present. *C. immitis* can multiply within and damage the bronchi. Subsequent endobronchial spread of infection can involve previously uninfected areas. The dominant histologic response in coccidioidal pneumonia can be suppurative or granulomatous. Microabscess formation in the midst of granulomas is characteristic.

Simultaneous extrapulmonary dissemination of infection is the rule, but the organs that are commonly involved tend not to give rise to clinically apparent phenomena (miliary lesions are most often demonstrable in the liver, spleen, kidneys, and myocardium). However, the lungs can be secondarily reinvaded by the miliary process, and death from respiratory failure has been documented.

Miliary Coccidioidomycosis

Miliary pulmonary coccidioidomycosis is a manifestation of hematogenously disseminated infection and is encountered most commonly in patients with impaired host defenses, particularly those with AIDS or immunosuppression for organ transplantation (5). Despite the widespread nature of the infection, clinical manifestations of pulmonary involvement can dominate, leading to shocklike syndromes with respiratory failure (55,58). Chest roentgenograms commonly show diffuse reticulonodular pulmonary infiltrates (4,5,19,39,59). Blood cultures can be positive for *C. immitis* (5). In patients with AIDS, CD4 cell counts are commonly below 250 per cmm when this presentation occurs (4).

Miliary involvement of the lungs can also occur in a more leisurely manner, with no threat of imminent fatal outcome, even in those with AIDS (35). Presumably, these patients have retained a relatively greater extent of cell-mediated immunity (16). The presence of a miliary infiltrate signals the likelihood of disseminated disease (especially meningitis), and appropriate evaluation and therapy should ensue.

Chronic Pulmonary Coccidioidal Lesions

In approximately 5% of patients infected with *C. immitis*, whether symptomatic or not at the time of disease acquisition, chronic pulmonary coccidioidal lesions will develop (29,50,77,79,89,90). Although less widely appreciated as a problem than extrapulmonary dissemination, residual pulmonary disease poses a major clinical management problem in its own right. Unfortunately, the natural history of many of the pulmonary processes to be described has not been clearly defined. Thus, the relative roles of medical and surgical management under some circumstances are difficult, if not impossible, to ascertain.

Chronic pulmonary coccidioidal lesions include "thin-walled" residual cavities; nodules (coccidioidomas), with or without central necrosis, and abscess formation; chronic progressive coccidioidal pneumonia (CPCP); and bronchiectasis. Residual calcifications are less common than in histoplasmosis or tuberculosis.

Cavities

It has become traditional to consider chronic coccidioidal cavities in two categories, based on the apparent thickness of the cavity wall on chest roentgenograph, and perceived differences in their pathophysiology (61,90). Those with a wall measuring 3 mm or less in thickness are considered "thin-walled cavities" and are commonly referred to as "residual cavities" (Fig. 27-1). They are cystic in appearance, usually contain no fluid, and have little surrounding pulmonary infiltrate. They are thought to arise from foci of necrotizing bronchitis or bronchiolitis, and tend to pursue a relatively indolent course. The other major category is the thick-walled cavity or abscess (Fig. 27-2). These lesions are thought to arise from central necrosis of residual coccidioidal nodules ("abscessing nodule"; see below) and may contain fluid or semisolid material. They are often considered to pursue a more aggressive course.

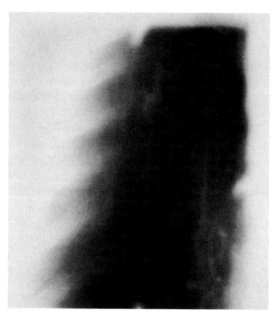

FIG. 27–1. Residual cavity in a young woman with recent primary coccidioidomycosis. This lesion evolved from a much thicker-walled lesion that had formed within an original infiltrate (tomogram; 6.5 cm).

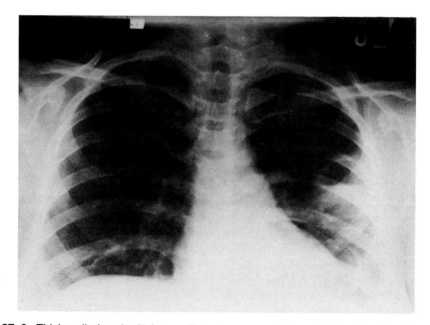

FIG. 27–2. Thick-walled cavity ("abscess") in close association with the pleural surface. The patient also has a right lower lobe infiltrate with a nodular component established by tomography. The cavitary lesion underwent spontaneous contraction; pleural perforation did not occur.

Whether there are true differences in the pathogenesis and pathophysiology of these lesions is problematical. They share many features, including a propensity to involve peripheral areas, in contiguity with the pleura. Thus, pleural extension with rupture and pyopneumothorax (bronchopleural fistula formation) is always a potential complication. Location at pleural interfaces also helps to explain the tendency of coccidioidal cavities to cross fissure lines ("fissure jumpers"), with consequent bilobar involvement—an issue of potential importance when planning surgical resection. Either type of cavity can be surrounded by satellite lesions ("daughter granulomas"), with their own potential to undergo cavitation. Again, this issue is of importance in planning resectional surgery, and in understanding complications that can arise when segmental resection of an apparently isolated cavity is undertaken. Even when a lobectomy is carried out, previously quiescent granulomas can undergo reactivation with formation of cavities in areas of the lung that were apparently roentgenographically normal (Fig. 27-3). This complication was reported in 18% of patients in one series (50). Thus, surgery may act, on occasion, as a destabilizing event.

Despite the distinction that is often made between thin-walled residual cavities and thick-walled abscesses on chest x-ray, it is difficult to be convinced of major differences in their clinical behavior, as summarized in Table 27-1. Patients with either type of cavitary lesion come to medical attention either because of the presence of symptoms (typically hemoptysis and cough; less frequently, chest pain, fatigue, or fever) or because of coincidental discovery on routine chest roentgenogram. Thus, coccidioidal cavities are not necessarily symptomatic. The frequency with which asymptomatic cavitation occurs is a direct function of the frequency with which routine chest roentgenograms are obtained. In populations subjected to x-rays on a regular, routine basis (e.g., military populations in California during WWII), up to 60% of cavities have been found in persons with no symptoms of pulmonary disease. Among civilian populations with less frequent x-ray tests, only about 25% of cavities have been found in persons without symptoms.

There are four principal complications of coccidioidal cavities (29).

Hemorrhage. Hemoptysis, sometimes as a result of secondary bacterial infection, can occur in 25 to 50% of patients with coccidioidal cavities (9). This is seldom much more than blood-streaked sputum; antibiotic therapy and/or reassurance may be all that is necessary. However, severe hemoptysis can complicate occasional cases and require surgical intervention.

Pyopneumothorax. Despite the largely peripheral location of coccidioidal pulmonary lesions, spontaneous rupture into the pleural space appears to be an uncommon event. In several series, including a total of more than 1,000 patients, the incidence was only 1 to 3%. Cavitary ruptures usually occur in young people who engage in vigorous physical activities or heavy physical work, or in incidences of severe g force or atmospheric pressure change such as those encountered by skiers or scuba divers (31). Pyopneumothorax can also complicate excisional pulmonary surgical procedures.

Expansion. Thin-walled cavities, in particular, can occasionally expand progressively and encroach on surrounding normal lung parenchyma (Fig. 27-4). Whether this activity is attributable to a ball-valve effect with air trapping or to actual progressive infection is not clear.

Secondary infection. Occasionally cavities become obstructed, with the result that upper respiratory flora initiate local infection. This can result in hemoptysis (9),

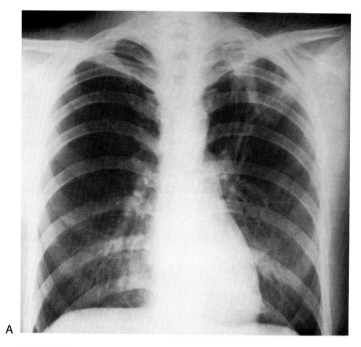

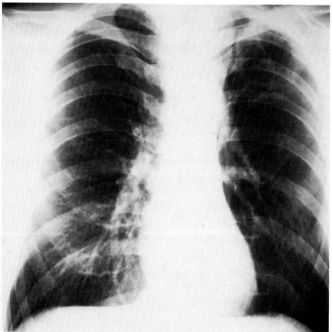

FIG. 27–3. A: Extensive left upper lobe cavitary disease in a 41-year-old man who also has peribronchial alveolar disease in the superior segment of the left lower lobe. Approximately 6 months later the left upper lobe was removed; the left lower lobe disease had apparently cleared. **B:** Fifteen years later there is cavitary and infiltrative disease in the left subapical area with evidence of contraction. The cavitary disease has apparently arisen from the old area of left lower lobe peribronchial infiltration.

TABLE 27–1. *Comparative features of thin-walled residual cavities and thick-walled abscesses (% positive for a given feature)*

	Residual cavities (%)	Abscesses (%)
Single lesions[a]	80–90	80–90
Upper lobe location[a]	65	60
Diameter[a] <2 cm	20	37
2–4 cm	62	51
4–6 cm	10	12
>6 cm	8	—
Formed within the 1st 3 months following primary infection	33	25
Not formed until 2 years or more following primary infection	11	18
Manifestations[b]		
Hemoptysis	51	37
Cough	43	26
Chest pain	25	26
Fatigue	24	15
Fever	14	7
Weight loss	15	12
Spontaneous pneumothorax	1	3
Asymptomatic	25	41

[a]Denominator: 222 residual cavities; 83 abscesses.
[b]Denominator: 215 patients with residual cavities; 73 patients with abscesses.
Modified from Winn (90).

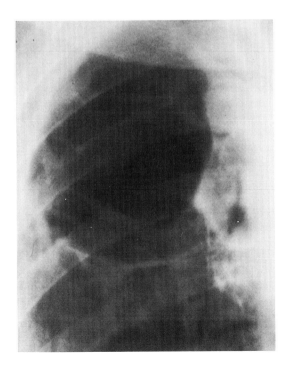

FIG. 27–4. Giant right upper lobe cavity in an elderly man. The lesion is in intimate contact with the pleura. Medical considerations precluded a surgical approach. Ketoconazole therapy had no effect on the pulmonary lesion. Pleural perforation has not occurred.

cavitary expansion, and development of acute symptoms. Rarely, there can be a secondary colonization by *Aspergillus* species with the occurrence of aspergilloma.

Between 25 and 50% of all cavities are said to close spontaneously within 2 to 4 years. Closure is particularly likely when the cavity diameter is 2 to 4 cm or less. Unfortunately, the authors of these figures have failed to provide any indication of potential differences between residual cavities and thick-walled abscesses in this regard. This issue is in need of further study, because a clear idea of the likelihood of spontaneous closure would have a profound effect on considerations regarding the proper role for surgery.

Nodules (Coccidioidomas, Coccidiomas, Coccidioidal Residual Granulomas)

Coccidioidal nodules represent the culmination of dynamic events, including pneumonia and cavitation (23). Although smaller lesions can calcify and appear completely healed, those greater than 1.5 to 2 cm in diameter (often biopsied or surgically resected as "coin lesions" in an attempt to rule out malignancy) are commonly found to have necrotic caseous centers that contain viable fungi. Not only spherules, but on occasion hyphal elements (saprobic cycle) can be demonstrated. In general, coccidioidal nodules are found to occur in relationship to a bronchus. Marked bronchitis or bronchiolitis is commonly demonstrable by microscopic examination in areas that are adjacent to the principal lesion. With bronchial patency, and contact with air passages, nodules can "reactivate," shelling out to form cavities ("abscessing nodules"). In some cases, these lesions actually represent bronchiectatic cavities. Neither the cavity nor the nodular stage is necessarily stable; a single lesion can be a cavity, solid nodule, and cavity again as it fills and empties. Nodule formation can be more apparent than real as inspissated material builds up in a cavity following obstruction of a communicating bronchus. As this material undergoes dissolution or is expectorated, a cavity reappears.

Coccidioidal nodules usually occur singly, sharply demarcated from adjacent lung parenchyma. In 80% of cases, satellite granulomas are present, generally in close contiguity to the coccidioidoma. These lesions can be too small to visualize on chest x-ray, but can be detectable by computerized tomography. Rupture of a coccidioidoma into the pericardium can result in the occurrence of *C. immitis* pericarditis (6).

Coccidioidomas are most conveniently diagnosed by transthoracic needle aspiration, a procedure that often obviates the need for exploratory thoracotomy (67).

Bronchiectasis

Bronchial involvement is common in pulmonary coccidioidomycosis, and spherules have been found in the walls of bronchiectatic cavities. Although rare, coccidioidal bronchiectasis can cause chronic productive cough, hemoptysis, fever, and recurring respiratory infection.

Chronic Progressive Coccidioidal Pneumonia (CPCP)

This process has also been termed "chronic progressive coccidioidal pneumonitis" (12,13), "chronic pulmonary coccidioidomycosis" (74), "chronic coccidioidal pneumonitis" (33), and "chronic fibrocaseocavernous disease" (71).

The presentation of CPCP is similar to that of chronic pulmonary histoplasmosis or chronic tuberculosis, but it is apparently a much less common process, accounting for less than 5% of all the chronic pulmonary manifestations of coccidioidomycosis. Although the disease process apparently evolves by a steady progression of primary pulmonary infection, there is excellent documentation of its development years after the acquisition and subsequent arrest of primary infection. In many cases, CPCP has apparently arisen from reactivation of chronic cavities or nodules. The unique features of CPCP are cavitation, extension, and fibrosis.

Chest roentgenograms of patients with CPCP generally show soft, confluent infiltrates with single or multiple radiolucent areas or frank cavities, most frequently located in apical or subapical areas. As the disease progresses, fibrosis and retraction become prominent. Most patients appear chronically ill with cough, weight loss, fever, chest pain, dyspnea, and hemoptysis. However, the disease process can also be extremely indolent, with few symptoms and only slow progression of pulmonary destruction. Predisposing factors for CPCP seem uncertain. Some report a higher incidence in diabetics, or those of "dark-skinned ethnic background" (prominently blacks, Native Americans, or Hispanics). However, these associations are by no means clear. Although one might expect CPCP to occur more commonly in chronic smokers or those with chronic obstructive pulmonary disease, as is the case with chronic pulmonary histoplasmosis, there is no evidence that such an association has been specifically sought in the limited analyses published to date. Because some patients with apparent CPCP have also had concomitant pulmonary tuberculosis, the latter diagnosis must be firmly ruled out before a diagnosis of CPCP can be considered established.

Extrapulmonary Dissemination

Primary pulmonary coccidioidomycosis is probably routinely associated with transient fungemia and hematogenous extrapulmonary dissemination of fungi. However, in patients with intact CMI, most systemically distributed fungi are apparently eliminated without clinical sequelae. They almost never give rise to metastatic calcifications (e.g., in the spleen or liver) that might attest to the occurrence of earlier arrested infection. Patients with persistent coccidioidal pneumonia that is severe enough to result in death commonly have disseminated lesions demonstrable at autopsy. Patients with chronic lung cavities, including CPCP, occasionally manifest evidence of extrapulmonary involvement, such as coccidioidouria (65). However, clinically apparent extrapulmonary disease in the presence of chronic cavitary pulmonary coccidioidomycosis is distinctly unusual and has given rise to the impression that cavitary lung disease provides an almost mystical protection against extrapulmonary dissemination. There are sufficient published case reports, however, to indicate that this is not true. The crux of the issue is that the factors that influence persistent pulmonary infection (cavity formation; bronchial obstruction; disordered pulmonary anatomy) are not the same as those that predispose to extrapulmonary dissemination (race; pregnancy; depressed CMI). Even if organisms from the damaged, infected lung were to be distributed hematogenously to distant sites, development of progressive distal disease would not be expected if CMI remained intact. However, with AIDS or initiation of immunosuppressive drug therapy, extrapulmonary disease of clinical significance might be expected to occur in patients with chronic cavitary pulmonary infection.

In most patients who develop clinically significant extrapulmonary coccidioidal dissemination, the disease becomes apparent soon after the primary infection. Dissemination at more than 1 year following primary infection is uncommon, except in immunosuppressed patients in whom dissemination may follow reactivation of a latent focus of infection. In immune-intact patients, the incidence of dissemination ranges from 1 in 500 white men to 3 in 100 black men, whether or not symptoms of primary infection were present. White women are less susceptible to dissemination than white men, but they have been reported to experience dissemination with a frequency near that for black men when infection occurs during the second or third trimesters of pregnancy.

Coccidioidal dissemination can involve any organ of the body, with the general exception of the gastrointestinal tract. However, certain organs are more commonly associated with clinically significant disease than others (29). Among these are the skin and soft tissues; the bones and joints; and the meninges. Except in the case of meningitis, which is ordinarily fatal within 2 years if left untreated (86), the natural history of infection in other sites includes considerable exacerbation and remission. As a result it is extremely difficult to evaluate the role of therapeutic modalities in many forms of extrapulmonary infection.

Skin and Subcutaneous Tissues

The skin is eventually involved in nearly all cases of disseminated coccidioidomycosis except those in which immunosuppression or meningitis leads to an early death. Major categories of skin lesions are as follows:

Verrucous granulomas. These lesions begin as epithelial thickenings with little inflammation. Eventually they resemble common warts with papillomatous excrescences. Verrucous granulomas can heal, or they can progress, disseminate, and coalesce to result in disfigurement. Verrucae located on the nasolabial fold often signal the presence of meningeal spread of infection.

Subcutaneous abscesses. These lesions can be single or multiple and are often located on the back or hip. Heat, tenderness, and erythema are minimal; thus they behave as "cold abscesses."

Indolent ulcers. These lesions often represent the cutaneous extension of sinus tracts originating in subcutaneous tissue, bone, or viscera. Sometimes large areas of skin are undermined by a labyrinth of discharging sinuses. Sinus tracts can extend for extraordinary distances; a bronchogluteal sinus tract has even been reported.

Plaques, pustules, and cellulitis. These can be manifestations of disseminated coccidioidomycosis in patients with AIDS (66).

Bones and Joints

Bones. Osteomyelitis occurs in 10 to 50% of all cases of coccidioidal dissemination and is second only to skin involvement as a manifestation of extrapulmonary spread. Bone scans commonly detect foci of infection that are not demonstrable clinically or by standard roentgenography. Lesions can be single or multiple and occur in approximately the following order: vertebrae, skull, and ribs > tibia, femur, and pelvis > radius, humerus, and fibula > metacarpals and metatarsals > others. Lesions are particularly likely to occur at sites of ligament or tendon insertion (malleoli; tibial tubercle; patella, acromion and coracoid processes of the scapula; etc.). Paravertebral abscess formation commonly complicates vertebral involvement.

Joints. Joints can become involved by perforation from an adjacent bony lesion or by direct hematogenous spread. Involvement of the knees and ankles is particularly common. The typical pathologic picture is that of villonodular granulomatous synovitis. *C. immitis* is rarely found in the synovial fluid, but can be seen in or recovered from excised synovium.

Tenosynovitis. Direct tendon sheath invasion by *C. immitis* occurs occasionally and has been responsible for several reported instances of carpal tunnel syndrome.

Meninges. Meningitis occurs in one-third to one-half of all patients with coccidioidal dissemination, often as the sole site of extrapulmonary involvement. Its onset is extremely subtle, with headache, personality changes, confusion, and lethargy. In this regard it resembles tuberculous and cryptococcal meningitis. Because of the nonspecificity of clinical findings, it is essential that lumbar puncture be considered routine in the evaluation of a patient with suspected coccidioidal dissemination. If coccidioidal meningitis proceeds unchecked, obstruction of the aqueduct of Sylvius and the foramina of the fourth ventricle can occur, with resultant hydrocephalus. In some cases, involvement of the cerebrospinal fluid (CSF) resorptive surfaces adds an element of communicating hydrocephalus. Patients must be watched carefully for evidence of obstructed CSF flow (ventricular dilatation on CT or MRI scan; radionuclide CSF flow studies; mental changes; papilledema) so that shunting procedures can be appropriately timed. In some cases, vasculitis and encephalitis lead to cerebral, cerebellar, or pontine infarction and neurologic findings resembling a stroke (88,91).

The CSF picture in coccidioidal meningitis is typical of that for any chronic granulomatous meningitis: elevated protein; pleocytosis (lymphocytes dominant; occasionally with elevated neutrophils or eosinophils); and hypoglycorrhachia (CSF glucose ≤ 60% of simultaneous blood glucose). *C. immitis* can be cultured from the CSF in only 20 to 40% of cases. However, the presence of complement-fixing antibody in the CSF is virtually diagnostic of coccidioidal meningitis. Occasionally a positive CF titer in the CSF can represent a contiguous bony focus of infection (e.g., skull) without frank meningeal infection.

Other Major Loci

Genitourinary tract. In 35 to 60% of cases that come to autopsy, miliary renal granulomas are demonstrable. These lesions are seldom of clinical importance, but coccidioidouria may lead to recognition of otherwise unsuspected extrapulmonary dissemination. As an isolated finding, coccidioidouria does not always indicate the need for therapy (22). Occasional instances of prostatic, epididymal, testicular, uterine, and tuboovarian disease have been reported. Rarely, tuboovarian disease can lead to peritonitis.

Liver and spleen. Disseminated coccidioidomycosis is found at autopsy to involve the liver and spleen in 50 to 70% of instances. There are few clinical manifestations of involvement of either organ. In immunocompromised patients with suspected miliary coccidioidomycosis, liver biopsy has sometimes led to the correct diagnosis. Serial sectioning of the biopsy specimen is often required to demonstrate fungi. Fungi can also be demonstrable in the bone marrow, another reticuloendothelial organ.

Adrenal. Although the adrenals can harbor coccidioidal lesions in 30 to 40% of fatal cases, clinically significant adrenal impairment is rare. In this regard, coccidioidomycosis resembles blastomycosis, as opposed to histoplasmosis, paracoccidioidomycosis, or tuberculosis, in which adrenal involvement is commonly complicated by adrenal insufficiency.

Pericardium. Pericarditis can occur when a contiguous infected, necrotic area of lung or lymph node ulcerates into the pericardium (6). Alternately, pericardial disease can result from direct hematogenous seeding. In the former instance, pericarditis is often considered a complication of primary coccidioidal pneumonia; in the latter, a manifestation of extrapulmonary dissemination.

Peritoneum. Peritoneal coccidioidomycosis has been reported in a number of patients with AIDS or continuous ambulatory peritoneal dialysis (CAPD), sometimes as the principal manifestation of infection (16,51).

DIAGNOSIS

Stains and Culture

The most reliable method for diagnosing coccidioidomycosis is to demonstrate the characteristic endosporulating spherules within secretions or infected tissues, or to recover the fungus by culture. Sputum, pus, gastric secretions, and exudates from cutaneous lesions can be screened for spherules by examining wet mounts in 10% potassium hydroxide under subdued lighting. Occasionally, elm pollen or fat globules bear a superficial resemblance to spherules. In tissue sections, the Grocott-Gomori methenamine silver stain is clearly superior to hematoxylin-eosin, and appears to give better results than the Hotchkiss-McManus periodic acid-Schiff or the Gridley stain. In addition, fluorescent antibody techniques have been utilized for specific identification of the fungi in tissues. Although spherules are the characteristic tissue infective form of *C. immitis,* mycelial elements are occasionally found within pulmonary cavities, coccidioidomas, or empyema fluid (27).

C. immitis is not fastidious, and can be recovered on a variety of culture media. Growth seldom requires more than 5 to 7 days. However, colonial and sporulation patterns are atypical in up to 25% of cases, and the fungi can be confused with saprophytes. If fungi grown on solid media are handled carelessly in the diagnostic laboratory, arthroconidia are often dispersed by air currents with infection of laboratory personnel. Hence, it is essential that cultures of unidentified fungi be opened only in a safety hood. Any fungus that grows on cycloheximide-containing media should be considered *C. immitis* until proven otherwise, especially if alternating arthroconidia are demonstrable. However, definitive identification of a mycelial fungus such as *C. immitis* requires its conversion to the diagnostic endosporulating spherule phase. This can be accomplished either in special media (Converse medium cultured at 40°C), or by animal inoculation. A far simpler and safer method is to detect characteristic antigens of the mycelial phase of *C. immitis* in liquid medium using immunodiffusion methodology (exoantigen test). This method has the advantage of rapidity and safety because mycelia and arthroconidia are suspended in the medium that is directly tested for marker antigens.

C. immitis can be recovered in cultures of sputum, bronchoalveolar lavage fluid

(78), blood, exudates, and tissue aspirates (76) or biopsies (67). In the diagnosis of pleural or joint disease, pleural and synovial tissue biopsies are more likely to reveal fungi than pleural and synovial fluid.

Skin Tests

There are two skin test preparations for detecting delayed hypersensitivity to *C. immitis* (29). Coccidioidin is prepared from culture filtrates of the mycelial-arthroconidial phase; spherulin represents the soluble fraction from lysed *C. immitis* spherules. Although most of the classic epidemiologic studies of coccidioidomycosis were conducted with coccidioidin, either preparation is considered acceptable for diagnostic purposes. Coccidioidin is ordinarily used in a dilution of 1 : 100; the equivalent concentration of spherulin is referred to as "usual skin test strength." The criterion for positivity with either test is a 5 × 5 mm area of induration and erythema.

In general, patients with primary pulmonary coccidioidomycosis develop sensitivity to coccidioidin within 3 days to 3 weeks of the onset of symptoms. If the exact time of arthroconidial exposure can be established (e.g., laboratory accident), coccidioidin reactivity can become detectable as early as 10 to 12 days later.

Patients with an established diagnosis of coccidioidomycosis and a negative coccidioidin or spherulin skin test are considered to be manifesting a poor immune response to infection. A proportion of such patients can respond to tenfold more concentrated preparations of coccidioidin or spherulin, or to undiluted skin test material. In this way, the extent of anergy can be titrated.

Repeated skin testing can elicit skin test positivity based on primary sensitization or a "boosting" of immunity from latent infection (4).

Serology

Precipitin Test (28,38,63)

Precipitating antibody is detected by mixing serum and coccidioidin in a test tube (tube precipitin test; TP), by latex particle agglutination (LPA), or, most satisfactorily, by immunodiffusion (IDTP). Because there can be 10% or more false-positive results with the LPA technique, this test should be regarded only as an indicator of need for further serologic evaluation. In contrast, the TP and IDTP tests appear to be specific for coccidioidomycosis. Precipitins are IgM class antibodies and occur early in the course of infection: using the TP method, 53% of sera are positive during the first week of illness; 91% during the second and third weeks; and 86% during the fourth week. Thereafter rates of positivity diminish quickly. In patients who develop infection in the absence of symptoms (asymptomatic skin test converters), the precipitin test might never become positive. In patients with mild disease, a positive precipitin test might not be followed by a positive complement-fixation (CF) antibody response.

Tests for precipitins are reported as either "positive" or "negative"; quantification has not been found to be of value. Measurement of precipitins in the CSF is without diagnostic value.

Complement-Fixation Test (28,38,63)

CF antibody can be measured either by classical hemolytic assays or, far more conveniently, by immunodiffusion methodology (IDCF). There is some variation in CF titers from laboratory to laboratory, so that noncritical attempts at comparison can be misleading. Obtaining coccoidiodial serologies outside the endemic region requires special attention, and consideration should be given to using a laboratory with specialized expertise (39).

In asymptomatic skin test converters, the CF antibody response might never develop. When CF antibody does develop in patients with primary coccidioidomycosis, it characteristically follows the precipitin response (as IgG follows IgM). CF titers seldom exceed 1 : 16 in uncomplicated primary infections and usually decrease shortly after recovery. However, antibody can persist in the serum in low titers (1 : 2 to 1 : 8) for many years.

Properly performed, the CF test can be a valuable guide to diagnosis (conversion from negative to positive or documentation of a fourfold titer increase during a current illness), and especially to prognosis. High or rapidly increasing CF titers (especially in association with negative skin tests) are generally associated with extrapulmonary dissemination, whereas a significant decrease in the CF titer during therapy (especially with maintenance of recovery of skin test positivity) is generally associated with a favorable prognosis.

There is no single CF titer that indicates extrapulmonary dissemination of infection. Indeed, it is not widely appreciated that a continuum of CF titers exists in patients with disseminated infection—the lowest titers in those with a single extrapulmonary lesion, and the highest titers in those with extensive multisystem dissemination. Thus, 60% of patients with a single extrapulmonary lesion, 30% of those with meningitis (some with other loci of infection; some not), and 5 to 10% of those with extensive dissemination have titers of 1 : 8 or less.

Patients with nodular or cavitary pulmonary coccidioidal residuals seldom have CF antibody titers in excess of 1 : 8. However, patients with CPCP or extensive pneumonia can have titers that exceed 1 : 64, with or without a positive skin test. These patients seldom have clinical evidence of extrapulmonary dissemination.

The above data indicate that although marked CF titer elevation is suggestive of dissemination and a poor prognosis, such an assessment is not always accurate. Conversely, a low CF titer provides no assurance that dissemination has not occurred. In general, a titer of 1 : 16–1 : 32, especially in association with a negative skin test, should raise the likelihood of dissemination, and an appropriate clinical evaluation should ensue. Patients with AIDS appear to manifest the expected serologic concomitants of infection (4,19,35). However, negative serologies, despite widespread dissemination, have been reported (7).

CF antibody can be detected not only in serum but also in peritoneal and pleural fluid, joint fluid, cord blood, and CSF. As a rule CF titers in body fluids are one or two dilutions lower than in the serum. Except for rare instances of vertebral or skull infection in direct contiguity with the meninges, the detection of CF antibody in the CSF is considered diagnostic of coccidioidal meningitis. By using an overnight binding method, the percent positivity of CF antibody tests in CSF is raised from 75% (standard hemolytic assay) to 95%.

Antigen Detection

Sera from patients with various forms of coccidioidomycosis, and bronchoalveolar lavage specimens from experimentally infected animals, have been shown to contain antigens apparently unique to *C. immitis*. These tests are not available commercially (38).

MEDICAL THERAPY

Therapeutic Agents

Amphotericin B

Amphotericin B is the mainstay of treatment in life-threatening coccidioidomycosis (32,39,62). Its mechanism of action involves binding to ergosterol, the principal structural membrane sterol of fungi. The resulting steric reorientation of the cell membrane causes enhanced fungal permeability with loss of critical intracellular constituents. In addition, amphotericin B undergoes autooxidation with consequent oxidative damage to the fungus. Because amphotericin B is not reliably fungicidal at achievable serum concentrations, host immunity is of considerable importance in recovery from infection.

Treatment with amphotericin B is limited by its innate toxicity. Toxicity is of two major types: acute, variably manifested by fever, chills, headache, nausea, vomiting, anorexia, and thrombophlebitis; and chronic, manifested routinely by anemia (impaired bone marrow red blood cell production), azotemia (impaired glomerular filtration), and hypokalemia (distal renal tubular acidosis). Acute reactions are generally manageable with adjunctive drugs (antipyretics, antiemetics, meperidine [for chills], or corticosteroids). Some have advocated rapid infusion regimens (e.g., total dose delivered in less than 1 hour) in an attempt to curtail acute toxicity (9). The validity of this approach remains uncertain (28,62). Among the chronic toxicities attributable to amphotericin B, only hypokalemia is routinely subject to therapeutic modification. The hematocrit seldom falls below the mid-20s. Azotemia is the major limiting factor in amphotericin B use and necessitates rather frequent dosage adjustments to maintain the serum creatinine at 3 mg/dl or below. Although renal impairment is generally reversible, some degree of permanent damage begins to be documentable at total doses in excess of 2 g. Because some patients require multiple courses of therapy, the issue of cumulative dosage and clinically significant renal impairment could become important. Frank renal failure can seldom be attributed to amphotericin B alone, however.

Three aspects of the pharmacokinetics of amphotericin B have a direct effect on the design of therapeutic regimens: (i) at doses in excess of 30 to 35 mg, a peak serum level of 1.56 to 2.0 μg/ml is achieved that cannot often be exceeded. As a result, serum level measurements are seldom employed as a guide to therapy; (ii) the decline in serum levels following an intravenous dose is sufficiently gradual that amphotericin B can often be administered every other, or every third, day. This is a major advantage in designing long-term outpatient treatment regimens; (iii) intravenously administered amphotericin B does not reach concentrations in the central nervous system adequate to permit cure of coccidioidal meningitis. As a result, intrathecal or intraventricular therapy is essential.

Although there has been some interest in using amphotericin B in combination with other antibiotics (principally rifampin or tetracycline), there is no clinical proof of therapeutic efficacy (62). There are theoretical contraindications to using amphotericin B in combinations with azoles or triazoles because the latter drugs inhibit the synthesis of ergosterol, the binding site for amphotericin B. Whether such putative antagonism is of clinical significance is unknown. Liposomal or other lipid delivery systems can modulate the toxicity of amphotericin B without limiting the efficacy of the parent drug. However, clinical experience is severely limited, and commercial preparations are not currently available in the United States (46).

Amphotericin B is considered to have a faster onset of action than the antifungal azoles or triazoles and to be more nearly fungicidal. It therefore remains the drug of choice for initiation of therapy in patients who are severely ill, especially if immunocompromised. It is becoming increasingly common, however, to substitute azole or triazole therapy, once the disease process has become stabilized. This approach is entirely empirical at this time.

Antifungal Azoles and Triazoles

The antifungal activity of azoles (e.g., miconazole, ketoconazole) and triazoles (e.g., fluconazole, itraconazole) appears to be based on at least three mechanisms: (i) inhibition of sterol C_{14} demethylation in the fungal cell membrane, with accumulation of lanosterol in place of ergosterol (lanosterol-based membranes are intrinsically "leaky"); (ii) attachment to long-chain fatty acids with direct cell membrane damage; and (iii) inhibition of cytochrome c peroxidase and catalase activity, leading to lethal intrafungal accumulations of hydrogen peroxide.

Miconazole

Miconazole is an azole derivative with a broad spectrum of antifungal activity, including *in vitro* and *in vivo* activity against *C. immitis* (80). However, owing to its pharmacokinetics (necessitating every-8-hr intravenous infusions), its vehicle-related toxicities (hyperlipidemia, pruritus, thrombocytosis, anemia, hyponatremia, and thrombophlebitis), and its generally inferior performance relative to amphotericin B, the drug has failed to achieve popularity. It offers no apparent advantages over fluconazole, the only other antifungal of the azole/triazole family that can be administered intravenously. Furthermore, fluconazole is much less toxic than miconazole.

Ketoconazole

This azole drug is absorbable by the oral route (37). It has a broad spectrum of activity, and *C. immitis* is routinely inhibited by achievable serum concentrations. Unfortunately, however, ketoconazole is incapable of killing *C. immitis* in any pharmacologic concentration. As a result, intact host defenses are essential if ketoconazole is to manifest optimal activity. In all situations in which it has been tested, ketoconazole behaves more as a suppressive than as a curative agent. Relapses have been common.

Ketoconazole is soluble at the pH of gastric contents, but in the absence of gastric acid (e.g., gastrectomy, advanced age, AIDS-related gastropathy, therapy with histamine (H_2) antagonists, or antacids) its absorption is impaired. Because absorption is not always predictable, even in patients with apparent normal gastric function, serum levels must be checked to verify absorption. The serum half-life ranges from 2 to 8 hours, and serum levels are maintained for approximately 12 hours. No correlations have been established between serum concentrations and clinical efficacy or between MICs and therapeutic effect.

Ketoconazole is extensively metabolized; little active drug is excreted by any route. Adjustments of dosage are not necessary in the presence of renal failure. Penetration of bones and joints is relatively poor, and penetration into cerebrospinal fluid is limited, with no clear relationship to dose, time after dose, site of CSF sampling, or presence of inflammation. Based upon its broad interactions with cytochrome P-450 enzymes, ketoconazole is subject to a broad variety of adverse drug interactions (e.g., with cyclosporine, methylprednisolone, carbamazepine, phenytoin, rifampin, isoniazid, terfenadine, and possibly theophylline and prednisolone) (8,49,84).

Anorexia, nausea, and vomiting are common side effects that can be ameliorated by giving the medication with meals. Dizziness, drowsiness, lethargy, and headache are also relatively common, but more serious CNS side effects (delusions, paranoia) can be observed with doses in excess of 1500 mg per day. Elevations in serum transaminases are seen in 1 to 10% of patients, but clinical hepatitis is rare, with an estimated incidence of symptomatic liver dysfunction of one in 10,000 to 15,000 patients. Clinical hepatitis is at least 10 times more common in patients receiving long-term therapy (15). Dose- and time-dependent impairment of both adrenal corticosteroid synthesis and testosterone synthesis have been well documented and are apparently based on the capacity of the drug to interfere with steroidogenic pathways. Clinically apparent hypoadrenalism has seldom been reported, but azoospermia, gynecomastia, decreased libido (men), and hair loss can be attributable to impaired testosterone synthesis.

Currently, ketoconazole is the only antifungal azole approved for the therapy of coccidioidomycosis. However, it seems likely that both fluconazole and itraconazole will prove to be superior to ketoconazole in the management of coccidioidomycosis, and with significantly less toxicity. Accordingly, ketoconazole can be viewed as a transitional drug, one that is being rapidly superseded by the triazoles. In patients with AIDS, coccidioidomycosis has actually developed while ketoconazole was being administered for other indications (92).

Fluconazole

Fluconazole is a water-soluble triazole with substantially different pharmacology and pharmacokinetics than ketoconazole or itraconazole. Fluconazole is extremely well absorbed from the GI tract, with little influence by the state of gastric acidity or the presence of food. Its oral bioavailability is nearly the same as when the drug is administered by the intravenous route.

Fluconazole is weakly protein bound (11%) and has a prolonged plasma half-life that offers the possibility of once or twice daily dosing. Fluconazole penetrates well into all body tissues and fluids, including the CSF (>60% of concomitant plasma concentrations, even in the absence of inflammation). In contrast to ketoconazole or itraconazole, fluconazole experiences only limited metabolism, so that >90% of the drug is excreted unchanged in the urine (and feces). Dosage modification is required in renal failure (15).

Fluconazole has relatively selective effects on P-450 enzymes and less propensity than ketoconazole for adverse drug interactions. However, dosage modifications might be necessary when fluconazole is used with rifampin, cyclosporine, anticoagulants, or phenytoin (8). Hepatotoxicity from fluconazole has been reported, but this appears to be quite rare when compared with ketoconazole (15).

The ability of fluconazole to cross the blood-brain barrier has provided a rationale for its use in coccidioidal meningitis, and therapeutic results of oral therapy have been quite promising (40,85).

Itraconazole

Itraconazole is a triazole antifungal agent with high lipid solubility. In this respect, it differs dramatically from fluconazole, which is water soluble. The pharmacologic and pharmacokinetic profiles of itraconazole resemble those of ketoconazole: low plasma concentrations; high (>90%) protein binding; poor penetration into body fluids, such as CSF; and extensive hepatic metabolism (15). However, clinical studies suggest that itraconazole might be superior to ketoconazole for most indications. The absorption of itraconazole from the GI tract depends upon the presence of gastric acidity; absorption may be impaired as a result of antacid therapies, gastric surgery, AIDS gastropathy, or advanced age. Whereas itraconazole has a more favorable drug interaction profile than ketoconazole, significant adverse interactions do occur (e.g., rifampin, phenytoin, carbamazepine, cyclosporine; digoxin [15,70,84]). In addition, like ketoconazole, but unlike fluconazole, itraconazole can influence intrinsic steroid metabolism. At high doses (e.g., 600 mg/d) itraconazole can produce aldosterone-like effects with hypertension and hypokalemia (15).

Itraconazole is showing promise in the treatment of histoplasmosis, blastomycosis, and coccidioidomycosis (26,44), and even in coccidioidal meningitis (83), despite its apparent inability to enter the CSF (15).

Therapeutic Principles and Regimens

Coccidioidomycosis has the reputation of being one of the most difficult mycoses to treat and one of the most likely to relapse when duration or intensity of therapy is inadequate. The explanation is uncertain. *In vitro* susceptibility studies suggest that *C. immitis* is not usually resistant to amphotericin B, azoles, or triazoles. Furthermore, there is no evidence that *C. immitis* is capable of developing significant resistance during the course of treatment with these drugs.

Prior to the advent of azole and triazole therapeutic options, the treatment of coccidioidomycosis tended to be conservative, limited by the undesirable side effects of the intensive regimens of amphotericin B that were required. With the ease of administration of ketoconazole and the strong promise of fluconazole and itraconazole as successors to ketoconazole, forms of disease that were seldom treated in the past (e.g., primary pulmonary infection, asymptomatic cavitary disease) are more apt to be treated now. Whether or not such therapy is necessary, desirable, or effective is uncertain (31,32).

Primary Coccidioidomycosis

In general, patients with uncomplicated pulmonary coccidioidomycosis require no antifungal therapy. However, exceptions must be made when the patient exhibits one of the factors that predispose to extrapulmonary dissemination (race, pregnancy, immunosuppression) or to progressive cavitary lung disease (diabetes mellitus, chronic underlying pulmonary disease). In addition, paratracheal adenopathy or persistent perihilar adenopathy are thought to signal a greater likelihood for dissemination. The goal of therapy in these circumstances is to prevent clinical and radiographic disease progression, to clear *C. immitis* from the sputum, to maintain or restore coccidioidin or spherulin skin test reactivity, and to maintain CF antibody titers in a low and stable range (<1 : 8). No formal therapeutic guidelines exist for these purposes. If amphotericin B is used, a total dose of 1 g will suffice. With ketoconazole or the newer triazoles, treatment (200–400 mg per day) should be given for at least 6 months, especially in immunocompromised patients, subject to modification as more information regarding the performance of these agents becomes available.

Persistent Coccidioidal Pneumonia

The rationale and guidelines for therapy in persistent coccidioidal pneumonia are essentially the same as those described above for primary coccidioidomycosis. However, because many of these patients are immunosuppressed, amphotericin B is the treatment of choice. A cumulative dose of at least 2 g should be administered. With clinical improvement, subsequent long-term ketoconazole or triazole therapy (200–400 mg/day) might be considered. However, it must be emphasized that the performance of azoles and triazoles in this setting has not been fully evaluated, and appropriate dosage and duration are unknown.

Cavitary Disease

Residual pulmonary cavities alone seldom constitute an indication for antifungal therapy because there is no evidence that cavity closure is influenced by medical treatment. However, treatment might logically be of value when symptoms suggesting active infection are present (e.g., fever, cough, purulent sputum), or when cavities are filled with fluid or surrounded by a parenchymal infiltrate. Under these circumstances, the goals for therapy would be reduction of symptoms; clearing of intracavitary contents and pericavitary infiltrates; conversion of sputum cultures to negative, maintenance, or restoration of skin test reactivity; and decrease in CF antibody titer (if elevated) to stable low levels.

Amphotericin B has been used to treat symptomatic cavitary pulmonary disease in the past, generally in a total dose of 1 to 2 grams. Its efficacy has never been proved. The oral azoles and triazoles have appeared as attractive alternatives to amphotericin B, largely because of their ability to be used on an outpatient basis. In the studies of ketoconazole that have been conducted, it appears that symptomatic improvement is common, but objective improvement is not (21,69). Despite treatment lasting almost 2 years, daily doses of 400 to 600 mg of ketoconazole failed to produce consistent changes in chest x-ray films (although isolated infiltrates did improve), sputum cultures, or serology (41). More recent, and more limited, studies with itraconazole (400 mg/day) have shown clinical improvement and sputum conversions in more than 50% of patients, without concomitant serological changes (44). Improvement occurred quite slowly, with the majority of patients achieving remission after more than 9 months of therapy. Although these results provide a rationale for the use of itraconazole in chronic pulmonary coccidioidomycosis, data regarding appropriate duration of therapy are lacking at this time.

Although the presence of cavitary disease on chest x-ray film is alarming, cavities do not in themselves constitute an indication for surgery (34,43,60,61,64,73). As has been pointed out, up to 50% can close spontaneously with time. Indications for surgery include symptomatic mycetoma (aspergilloma) formation; serious, persistent hemoptysis; spontaneous cavity rupture (apparent or inapparent) with bronchopleural fistula formation and empyema; and a rapidly expanding cavity with apparent imminent risk of pleural rupture or cavitary persistence beyond 2 years (31). There is a definite risk of surgical complications.

Both bronchopleural fistula formation and the appearance of new cavities in apparently uninvolved lobes have been discussed. Segmental or subsegmental resection runs the risk of transecting daughter granulomas and inciting another round of cavity formation in the remaining lobar tissue. Even lobectomy can be suboptimal if a lesion has crossed a lung fissure.

The issue of whether or not antifungal "umbrella" therapy should be administered perioperatively has dragged on unresolved for years (29). The problem, once again, is an absence of controlled data. In patients who are to have surgery involving *C. immitis*–infected tissues, it is difficult to imagine why a brief course of pre-, intra-, and postoperative amphotericin B (500 mg) or an azole or triazole should not be provided. Whether or not any drug can actually prevent secondary surgical spread of infection cannot currently be answered.

Nodules (Coccidioidomas)

Coccidioidal nodules, even when manipulated at bronchoscopy or surgery, seldom require drug therapy. In uncertain situations, a short course of azole or triazole therapy might be provided.

CPCP

There are no clear therapeutic guidelines for this form of pulmonary coccidioidomycosis. However, Sarosi and his coworkers have pointed out that amphotericin B (2 to 2.4 g), without surgery, has provided at least some benefit (74). Preliminary studies suggest that ketoconazole can provide subjective improvement and at least transient conversion of sputum cultures.

Extrapulmonary Dissemination

The clearest indication for antifungal therapy in coccidioidomycosis is extrapulmonary dissemination. The ultimate goal of therapy is marked clinical improvement, healing of all apparent lesions, a reduction in CF antibody titers to stable low levels (at least a fourfold titer decline), and maintenance or restoration of skin test reactivity to coccidioidin or spherulin (48).

In acutely ill patients, therapy should be initiated with amphotericin B (29), increasing dosage in a stepwise fashion until up to 40 to 60 mg are being administered each day. Therapy can then be continued on a daily or alternate-day basis, depending on tolerance and renal function. As the illness becomes stabilized (or, at the outset, in patients less seriously ill), the dosage can be decreased to 25 to 50 mg per day (or 50 to 70 mg on alternate days). Patients could require 2 to 4 g of amphotericin B before clinical stabilization is achieved and intermittent therapy thereafter to maintain remission. The exact dose of amphotericin B required is dependent both on site(s) of dissemination and status of host immunity. Azole or triazole therapy can be substituted for amphotericin B once the disease process has become stabilized, but the duration of required therapy with these fungistatic agents is currently uncertain. In patients with AIDS, therapy should be continued indefinitely.

Skin and soft tissue infections resolve much more rapidly than do bone or joint lesions. Some consider early surgery to be desirable for both arthritis (synovectomy) and osteomyelitis (debridement). Surgery is often required to evacuate large collections of pus (e.g., paraspinous abscesses).

In the treatment of meningitis, it has been traditional to initiate therapy with both intravenous and intrathecal amphotericin B. Intrathecal dosage should not ordinarily exceed 0.5 to 1 mg of drug at any one treatment. However, at least one study has recommended doses as high as 1.0 to 1.5 mg of intrathecal amphotericin B mixed with 25 to 50 mg of hydrocortisone, and claimed enhanced survival rates despite more frequent (but transient) CNS side effects (54). Although administration of amphotericin B via the cisterna magna is acceptable and well tolerated, many physicians and neurosurgeons do not feel comfortable using this route. As a result, Ommaya reservoir placement becomes necessary. These devices are often complicated by secondary infection, seizures, or faulty placement. Most meningitis patients also eventually require shunting procedures.

Recent studies suggest that fluconazole can be uniquely useful in the treatment of coccidioidal meningitis and can obviate the need for intrathecal amphotericin B therapy (40,85). This approach has become extremely popular, even though the drug has not yet been approved for this purpose by the FDA. In addition, itraconazole might also prove to be useful in the therapy of coccidioidal meningitis (83).

Approximately two-thirds of patients with soft tissue, bone, or joint disease have improved subjectively and objectively during treatment with ketoconazole (400 to >1,500 mg/day), but few have been cured (17,21,41). Neither optimal dosage nor duration of ketoconazole therapy has been established. Particularly worrisome are repeated instances in which lesions have apparently healed only to reveal viable, cultivable fungi when subsequently biopsied. When treatment is stopped, relapses occur. In high dosage, ketoconazole appears only to suppress meningeal infection. The ultimate role of ketoconazole in coccidioidal dissemination remains to be ascertained. At present it should be regarded as a drug that can maintain remissions as long as it is administered and that can apparently cure isolated cases of infection restricted to skin and soft tissues. There are promising data concerning both itraconazole and fluconazole in the therapy of extrapulmonary manifestations of coccidioidomycosis (18,25,75,82).

Miliary Coccidioidomycosis

The occurrence of miliary pulmonary dissemination reflects the presence of fungemia, signals a failure of host defenses, and indicates the need for treatment, preferably with amphotericin B. Amphotericin B is the drug of choice based upon its more rapid therapeutic effect and its more nearly fungicidal activity when compared with azoles or triazoles. A total dose of 2–4 g of amphotericin B should be preferably administered; follow-up therapy with an azole or triazole can then be given on an empiric basis. Depending upon host immune status and clinical response to amphotericin B, it is possible that azole or triazole therapy might be substituted earlier in the course of therapy. This is a matter of clinical judgment.

In evaluating a patient with miliary pulmonary disease, examination of the cerebrospinal fluid is essential because concomitant coccidioidal meningitis will demand appropriate CNS-directed therapy as well. Fluconazole, and perhaps itraconazole, offer new flexibility in this regard. If other local organ involvement becomes apparent (e.g., osteomyelitis, skin lesions, arthritis), the approach described for extrapulmonary disseminated disease should be pursued (see above).

Prevention

There is no vaccine for coccidioidomycosis at present. However, a multicenter Phase II/III placebo-controlled study of fluconazole for the prevention of coccidioidomycosis in HIV-infected patients is currently under way (1).

REFERENCES

1. American Foundation for AIDS Research (AmFAR) (1993): *AIDS/HIV Treatment Directory*, 6:74, 148.
2. Ampel, N.M., Bejarano, G.C., and Galgiani, J.N. (1992): Killing of *Coccidioides immitis* by human peripheral blood mononuclear cells. *Infect. Immun.*, 60:4200–4204.
3. Ampel, N.M., Bejarano, G.C., Salas, S.D., and Galgiani, J.N. (1992): *In vitro* assessment of cellular immunity in human coccidioidomycosis: relationship between dermal hypersensitivity, lymphocyte transformation, and lymphokine production by peripheral blood mononuclear cells from healthy adults. *J. Infect. Dis.*, 165:710–715.
4. Ampel, N.M., Dols, C.L., and Galgiani, J.N. (1993): Coccidioidomycosis during human immunodeficiency virus infection: results of a prospective study in a coccidioidal endemic area. *Am. J. Med.*, 94:235–240.
5. Ampel, N.M., Ryan, K.J., Carry, P.J., Wieden, M.A., and Schifman, R.B. (1986): Fungemia due to Coccidioides immitis: an analysis of 16 episodes in 15 patients and a review of the literature. *Medicine*, 65:312–321.
6. Amundson, D.E. (1993): Perplexing pericarditis caused by coccidioidomycosis. *South. Med. J.*, 86:694–696.
7. Antoniskis, D., Larsen, R.A., Akil, B., Rarick, M.U., and Leedom, J.M. (1990): Seronegative disseminated coccidioidomycosis in patients with HIV infection. *AIDS*, 4:691–693.
8. Baciewicz, A.M., and Baciewicz, F.A. (1993): Ketoconazole and fluconazole drug interactions. *Arch. Intern. Med.*, 153:1970–1976.
9. Barbee, R.A. (1993): Does a lung cavity always require antifungal therapy? When and how to treat coccidioidomycosis. *J. Respir. Dis.*, 14:818–822.

10. Barbee, R.A., Hicks, M.J., Grosso, D., and Sandel, C. (1991): The maternal immune response in coccidioidomycosis: Is pregnancy a risk factor for serious infection? *Chest,* 100:709–715.
11. Batra, P. (1992): Pulmonary coccidioidomycosis. *J. Thorac. Imaging,* 7:29–38.
12. Bayer, A.S., Yoshikawa, T.T., Galpin, J.E., and Guze, L.B. (1976): Unusual syndromes of coccidioidomycosis: diagnostic and therapeutic considerations. A report of 10 cases and review of the English literature. *Medicine,* 55:131–152.
13. Bayer, A.S., Yoshikawa, T.T., and Guze, L.B. (1979): Chronic progressive coccidioidal pneumonitis: report of 6 cases with clinical, roentgenographic, serologic, and therapeutic features. *Arch. Intern. Med.,* 139:536–540.
14. Beaman, L. (1991): Effects of recombinant gamma interferon and tumor necrosis factor on *in vitro* interactions of human mononuclear phagocytes with *Coccidioides immitis. Infect. Immun.,* 59:4227–4229.
15. Bodey, G.P. (1992): Azole antifungal agents. *Clin. Infec. Dis.,* (Suppl. 1), 14:S161–S169.
16. Byrne, W.R., and Dietrich, R.A. (1989): Disseminated coccidioidomycosis with peritonitis in a patient with acquired immunodeficiency syndrome: prolonged survival associated with positive skin test reactivity to coccidioidin. *Arch. Intern. Med.,* 149:947–948.
17. Catanzaro, A., Einstein, H., Levine, B., Ross, J.B., Schillaci, R., Fierer, J., and Friedman, P.J. (1982): Ketoconazole for treatment of disseminated coccidioidomycosis. *Ann. Intern. Med.,* 96:436–440.
18. Catanzaro, A., Fierer, J., and Friedman, P.J. (1990): Fluconazole in the treatment of persistent coccidioidomycosis. *Chest,* 97:666–669.
19. Cone, L., Woodard, D., Fiala, M., Christopher, S., and Sneider, R. (1990): Epidemiology and immunologic characteristics of symptomatic coccidioidomycosis in patient with HIV/AIDS. *Int. Conf. AIDS,* 6:239[Abstract No. Th.B.470].
20. Cox, R.A. (1988): Immunosuppression by cell wall antigens of *Coccidioides immitis. Rev. Infect. Dis.,* 10(Suppl. 2):S415–S418.
21. DeFelice, R., Galgiani, J.N., Campbell, S.C., Palpant, S.D., Friedman, B.A., Dodge, R.R., Weinberg, M.G., Lincoln, L.J., Tennican, P.O., and Barbee, R.A. (1982): Ketoconazole treatment of nonprimary coccidioidomycosis: evaluation of 60 patients during three years of study. *Am. J. Med.,* 72:681–687.
22. DeFelice, R., Wieden, M.A., and Galgiani, J.N. (1982): The incidence and implications of coccidioidouria. *Am. Rev. Respir. Dis.,* 125:49–52.
23. Deppsich, L.M., and Donowho, E.M. (1972): Pulmonary coccidioidomycosis. *Am. J. Clin. Pathol.,* 58:489–500.
24. Deresinski, S.C., and Stevens, D.A. (1974): Coccidioidomycosis in compromised hosts: experience at Stanford University Hospital. *Medicine,* 54:377–395.
25. Diaz, M., Puente, R., de Hoyos, L.A., and Cruz, S. (1991): Itraconazole in the treatment of coccidioidomycosis. *Chest,* 100:682–684.
26. Dismukes, W.E., Bradsher, R.W., Jr., Cloud, G.C., Kauffman, C.A., Chapman, S.W., George, R.B., Stevens, D.A., Girard, W.M., Saag, M.S., Bowles-Patton, C., and The NIAID-Mycoses Study Group (1992): Itraconazole therapy for blastomycosis and histoplasmosis. *Am. J. Med.,* 93:489–497.
27. Dolan, M.J., Lattuada, C.P., Melcher, G.P., Zellmer, R., Allendoerfer, R., and Rinaldi, M.G. (1992): *Coccidioides immitis* presenting as a mycelial pathogen with empyema and hydropneumothorax. *J. Med. Vet. Mycol.,* 30:249–255.
28. Drutz, D.J. (1992): Rapid infusion of amphotericin B: Is it safe, effective, and wise? *Am. J. Med.,* 93:119–121.
29. Drutz, D.J., and Catanzaro, A. (1978): Coccidioidomycosis (state of the art). *Am. Rev. Respir. Dis.,* 117:559–585, 727–771.
30. Drutz, D.J., and Huppert, M. (1983): Coccidioidomycosis: factors affecting the host-parasite interaction. *J. Infect. Dis.,* 147:372–390.
31. Einstein, H.E., Chia, J.K.S., and Meyer, R.D. (1992): Pulmonary infiltrate and pleural effusion in a diabetic man. (Infectious Disease Rounds) *Clin. Infect. Dis.,* 14:955–960.
32. Einstein, H.E., and Johnson, R.H. (1993): Coccidioidomycosis: new aspects of epidemiology and therapy. *Clin. Infect. Dis.,* 16:349–356.
33. Fiese, M.J. (1958): *Coccidioidomycosis.* Charles C. Thomas, Springfield, Ill.
34. Findlay, F.M., and Melick, D.W. (1967): Treatment of cavitary coccidioidomycosis. In: *Coccidioidomycosis,* edited by L. Ajello, pp. 79–83. University of Arizona Press, Tucson, Ariz.
35. Fish, D.G., Ampel, N.M., Galgiani, J.N., Dols, C.L., Kelly, P.C., Johnson, C.H., Pappagianis, D., Edwards, J.E., Wasserman, R.B., Clark, R.J., Antoniskis, D., Larsen, R.A., Englender, S.J., and Petersen, E.A. (1990): Coccidioidomycosis during human immunodeficiency virus infection: a review of 77 patients. *Medicine,* 69:384–391.
36. Frey, C.L., and Drutz, D.J. (1986): Influence of fungal surface components on the interaction of *Coccidioides immitis* with polymorphonuclear neutrophils. *J. Infect. Dis.,* 153:933–943.
37. Galgiani, J.N. (1983): Ketoconazole in the treatment of coccidioidomycosis. *Drugs,* 26:355–363.

38. Galgiani, J.N. (1992): Coccidioidomycosis: changes in clinical expression, serological diagnosis, and therapeutic options. *Clin. Infect. Dis.*, (Suppl. 1)14:S100–S105.
39. Galgiani, J.N., (1992): Coccidioidomycosis (Mini Review). *Infect. Dis. Clin. Pract.*, 1:357–362.
40. Galgiani, J.N., Catanzaro, A., Cloud, G.A., Higgs, J., Friedman, B.A., Larsen, R.A., Graybill, J.R., and The NIAID-Mycoses Study Group (1993): Fluconazole therapy for coccidioidal meningitis. *Ann. Intern. Med.*, 119:28–35.
41. Galgiani, J.N., Stevens, D.A., Graybill, J.R., Dismukes, W.E., and Cloud, G.A. (1988): Ketoconazole therapy of progressive coccidioidomycosis: comparison of 400- and 800-mg doses and observations at higher doses. *Am. J. Med.*, 84:603–610.
42. Graham, A.R., Sobonya, R.E., Bronnimann, D.A., and Galgiani, J.N. (1988): Quantitative pathology of coccidioidomycosis in acquired immunodeficiency syndrome. *Human Pathol.*, 19:800–806.
43. Grant, A.R., Steinhoff, N.G., and Melick, D.W. (1977): Resectional surgery in pulmonary coccidioidomycosis: a review of 263 cases. In: *Coccidioidomycosis. Current Clinical and Diagnostic Status*, edited by L. Ajello, pp. 209–221. Symposia Specialists, Miami, Fla.
44. Graybill, J.R., Stevens, D.A., Galgiani, J.N., Dismukes, W.E., Cloud, G.A., and The NIAID-Mycoses Study Group (1990): Itraconazole treatment of coccidioidomycosis. *Am. J. Med.*, 89:282–290.
45. Greendyke, W.H., Resnick, D.L., and Harvey, W.C. (1970): The varied roentgen manifestations of primary coccidioidomycosis. *Am. J. Roentgenol. Rad. Ther. Nucl. Med.*, 109:491–499.
46. Gregoriadis, G., and Florence, A.T. (1993): Liposomes in drug delivery: clinical, diagnostic and ophthalmic potential. *Drugs*, 45:15–28.
47. Hall, K.A., Sethi, G.K., Rosado, L.J., Martinez, J.D., Huston, C.L., and Copeland, J.G. (1993): Coccidioidomycosis and heart transplantation. *J. Heart Lung Transplant*, 12:525–526.
48. Hardenbrook, M.H., and Barriere, S.L. (1982): Coccidioidomycosis: evaluation of parameters used to predict outcome with amphotericin B therapy. *Mycopathologia.*, 78:65–71.
49. Honig, P.K., Wortham, D.C., Zamani, K., Conner, D.P., Mullin, J.C., and Cantilena, L.R. (1993): Terfenadine-ketoconazole interaction: pharmacokinetic and electrocardiographic consequences. *J.A.M.A.*, 269:1513–1518.
50. Hyde, L. (1968): Coccidioidal pulmonary cavitation. *Dis. Chest*, 54(Suppl. 1):17–21.
51. Jamidar, P.A., Campbell, D.R., Fishback, J.L., and Klotz, S.A. (1992): Peritoneal coccidioidomycosis associated with human immunodeficiency virus infection. *Gastroenterology*, 102:1054–1058.
52. Johnson, W.M. (1982): Racial factors in coccidioidomycosis: mortality experience in Arizona. *Arizona Med.*, 39:18–24.
53. Kerrick, S.S., Lundergan, L.L., and Galgiani, J.N. (1985): Coccidioidomycosis at a University Health Service. *Am. Rev. Respir. Dis.*, 131:100–102.
54. Labadie, E.L., and Hamilton, R.H. (1986): Survival improvement in coccidioidal meningitis by high dose intrathecal amphotericin B. *Arch. Intern. Med.*, 146:2013–2018.
55. Larsen, R.A., Jacobson, J.A., Morris, A.H., and Benowitz, B.A. (1985): Acute respiratory failure caused by primary pulmonary coccidioidomycosis: two case reports and a review of the literature. *Am. Rev. Respir. Dis.*, 131:797–799.
56. Lefler, E., Weiler-Ravell, D., Merzbach, D., Ben-Izhak, O., and Best, L.A. (1992): Traveller's coccidioidomycosis: case report of pulmonary infection diagnosed in Israel. *J. Clin. Micro.*, 30:1304–1306.
57. Lonky, S.A., Catanzaro, A., Moser, K.M., and Einstein, H. (1976): Acute coccidioidal pleural effusion. *Am. Rev. Respir. Dis.*, 114:681–688.
58. Lopez, A.M., Williams, P.L., and Ampel, N.M. (1993): Acute pulmonary coccidioidomycosis mimicking bacterial pneumonia and septic shock: a report of two cases. *Am. J. Med.*, 95:236–239.
59. Mahaffey, K.W., Hippenmeyer, C.L., Mandel, R., and Ampel, N.M. (1993): Unrecognized coccidioidomycosis complicating *Pneumocystis carinii* pneumonia in patients infected with the human immunodeficiency virus and treated with corticosteroids: a report of two cases. *Arch. Intern. Med.*, 153:1496–1498.
60. Marks, T.S., Spence, W.F., and Baisch, B.F. (1967): Limited resection for pulmonary coccidioidomycosis. In: *Coccidioidomycosis*, edited by L. Ajello, pp. 73–78. University of Arizona Press, Tucson, Ariz.
61. Melick, D.W., and Grant, A.R. (1968): Surgery in primary pulmonary coccidioidomycosis and in the combined diseases of coccidioidomycosis and tuberculosis. *Dis. Chest* (Suppl. 1), 54:22–28.
62. Meyer, R.D. (1992): Current role of therapy with amphotericin B. *Clin. Infect. Dis.*, (Suppl. 1), 14:S154–S160.
63. Pappagianis, D., and Zimmer, B.L. (1990): Serology of coccidioidomycosis. *Clin. Microbiol. Rev.*, 3:247–268.
64. Paulsen, G.A. (1967): Pulmonary surgery in coccidioidal infections. In: *Coccidioidomycosis*, edited by L. Ajello, pp. 69–72. University of Arizona Press, Tucson, Ariz.
65. Petersen, E.A., Friedman, B.A., Crowder, E.D., and Rifkind, D. (1976): Coccidioidouria: clinical significance. *Ann. Intern. Med.*, 85:34–38.

66. Quimby, S.R., Connolly, S.M., Winkelmann, R.K., and Smilack, J.D. (1992): Clinicopathologic spectrum of specific cutaneous lesions of disseminated coccidioidomycosis. *J. Am. Acad. Dermatol.*, 26:79–85.

67. Raab, S.S., Silverman, J.F., and Zimmerman, K.G. (1993): Fine-needle aspiration biopsy of pulmonary coccidioidomycosis: spectrum of cytologic findings in 73 patients. *Am. J. Clin. Pathol.*, 99:582–587.

68. Ragland, A.S., Arsura, E., Ismael, Y., and Johnson, R. (1993): Eosinophilic pleocytosis in coccidioidal meningitis: frequency and significance. *Am. J. Med.*, 95:254–257.

69. Ross, J.B., Levine, B., Catanzaro, A., Einstein, H., Schillaci, R., and Friedman, P.J. (1982): Ketoconazole treatment for chronic pulmonary coccidioidomycosis. *Ann. Intern. Med.*, 96:440–443.

70. Sachs, M.K., Blanchard, L.M., and Green, P.J. (1993): Interaction of itraconazole and digoxin. *Clin. Infect. Dis.*, 16:400–403.

71. Salkin, D. (1967): Clinical examples of reinfection in coccidioidomycosis. In: *Coccidioidomycosis*, edited by L. Ajello, pp. 11–18. University of Arizona Press, Tucson, Ariz.

72. Salkin, D., Birsner, T.W., Tarr, A.D., Johnson, D., and Bitzer, J.W. (1967): Roentgen analysis of coccidioidomycosis pediatric cases in private practice. In: *Coccidioidomycosis*, edited by L. Ajello, pp. 63–67. University of Arizona Press, Tucson, Ariz.

73. Salomon, N.W., Osborne, R., and Copeland, J.G. (1980): Surgical manifestations and results of treatment of pulmonary coccidioidomycosis. *Ann. Thorac. Surg.*, 30:433–438.

74. Sarosi, G.A., Parker, J.D., Doto, I.L., and Tosh, F.E. (1970): Chronic pulmonary coccidioidomycosis. A National Communicable Disease Center Cooperative Mycoses Study. *N. Engl. J. Med.*, 283:325–329.

75. Schwartz, D.N., Fihn, S.D., and Miller, R.A. (1993): Infection of an arterial prosthesis as the presenting manifestation of disseminated coccidioidomycosis: control of disease with fluconazole. *Clin. Infect. Dis.*, 16:486–488.

76. Sherman, M.E., Orr, J.E. Balough, K., and Bardawil, R.G. (1991): Primary diagnosis of disseminated fungal disease by fine-needle aspiration of soft-tissue lesions. *Diagn. Cytopathol.*, 7:536–539.

77. Smith, C.E., Beard, R.R., and Saito, M.T. (1948): Pathogenesis of coccidioidomycosis with special reference to pulmonary cavitation. *Ann. Intern. Med.*, 29:623–655.

78. Sobonya, R.E., Barbee, R.A., Wiens, J., and Trego, D. (1990): Detection of fungi and other pathogens in immunocompromised patients by bronchoalveolar lavage in an area endemic for coccidioidomycosis. *Chest*, 97:1349–1355.

79. Stevens, D.A. (Editor) (1980): *Coccidioidomycosis. A Text.* Plenum Medical Book, New York.

80. Stevens, D.A. (1983): Miconazole in the treatment of coccidioidomycoses. *Drugs*, 26:347–354.

81. Streilin, J.W., and Wegmann, T.G. (1987): Immunologic privilege in the eye and the fetus. *Immunol. Today*, 8:362–366.

82. Tucker, R.M., Denning, D.W., Arathoon, E.G., Rinaldi, M.G., and Stevens, D.A. (1990): Itraconazole therapy for nonmeningeal coccidioidomycosis: clinical and laboratory observations. *J. Am. Acad. Dermatol.*, 23:593–601.

83. Tucker, R.M., Denning, D.W., Dupont, B., and Stevens, D.A. (1990): Itraconazole therapy for chronic coccidioidal meningitis. *Ann. Intern. Med.*, 112:108–112.

84. Tucker, R.M., Denning, D.W., Hanson, L.H., Rinaldi, M.G., Graybill, J.R., Sharkey, P.K., Pappagianis, D., and Stevens, D.A. (1992): Interaction of azoles with rifampin, phenytoin, and carbamazepine: *in vitro* and clinical observations. *Clin. Infect. Dis.*, 14:165–174.

85. Tucker, R.M., Galgiani, J.N., Denning, D.W., Hanson, L.H., Graybill, J.R., Sharkey, K., Eckman, M.R., Salemi, C., Libke, R., Klein, R.A., and Stevens, D.A. (1990): Treatment of coccidioidal meningitis with fluconazole. *Rev. Infect. Dis.*, 3:S380–S389.

86. Vincent, T., Galgiani, J.N., Huppert, M., and Salkin, D. (1993): The natural history of coccidioidal meningitis: VA–Armed Forces Cooperative Studies, 1955–1958. *Clin. Infect. Dis.*, 16:247–254.

87. Wack, E.E., Ampel, N.M., Galgiani, J.N., and Bronnimann, D.A. (1988): Coccidioidomycosis during pregnancy: an analysis of ten cases among 47,120 pregnancies. *Chest*, 94:376–379.

88. Williams, P.L., Johnson, R., Pappagianis, D., Einstein, H., Slager, U., Koster, F.T., Eron, J.J., Morrison, J., Aguet, J., and River, M.E. (1992): Vasculitic and encephalitic complications associated with *Coccidioides immitis* infection of the central nervous system in humans: report of 10 cases and review. *Clin. Infect. Dis.*, 14:673–682.

89. Winn, W.A. (1941): Pulmonary cavitation associated with coccidioidal infection. *Arch. Intern. Med.*, 68:1179–1214.

90. Winn, W.A. (1968): A long-term study of 300 patients with cavitary-abscess lesions of the lung of coccidioidal origin. *Dis. Chest*, 54(Suppl. 1):12–16.

91. Wrobel, C.J., Meyer, S., Johnson, R.H., and Hesselink, J.R. (1992): MR findings in acute and chronic coccidioidomycosis meningitis. *Am. J. Neuroradiol.*, 3:1241–1245.

92. Zar, F.A., and Fernandez, M. (1991): Failure of ketoconazole maintenance therapy for disseminated coccidioidomycosis in AIDS. *J. Infect. Dis.*, 164:824–825.

Respiratory Infections: Diagnosis and Management, 3d ed.,
edited by James E. Pennington.
Raven Press, Ltd., New York © 1994

28

Histoplasma capsulatum Pneumonia

Scott F. Davies

*Department of Medicine, University of Minnesota and Hennepin County Medical
Center, 701 Park Avenue South, Minneapolis, Minnesota 55415*

Histoplasmosis refers to infection by the pathogenic fungus *Histoplasma capsulatum*. Exposure occurs only by inhalation. Although the primary infection is in the lung, there is a strong tendency for invasion of the bloodstream during each primary infection. This fungemia is generally self-limited but results in seeding of reticuloendothelial organs throughout the body. The ability of the organism to cause progressive disease in one or multiple sites results in a wide variety of clinical manifestations.

EPIDEMIOLOGY

H. capsulatum is a thermal dimorphic fungus. At 25°C on Sabouraud's medium it grows as a fluffy white-to-brown septate mycelium that bears microconidia and also the characteristic tuberculate macroconidia. The organism is free-living in soil in the mycelial phase. At 37°C, however, the organism replicates as a small (2 to 4 μm yeast). This yeast form grows in macrophages during mammalian infection.

H. capsulatum has been isolated from the soil in more than 50 countries. It is most common in temperate climates along river valleys and has been found in North, Central, and South America; India; and Southeast Asia. It is also common on the Caribbean Islands of the Western Hemisphere. It is rare in Europe and probably not present in Australia.

Although the fungus has a worldwide distribution, the most heavily endemic area known is the East Central United States bordering the Mississippi and Ohio rivers. The center of disease activity is in Ohio, Kentucky, Indiana, Illinois, Tennessee, Missouri, and Arkansas. Many bordering states have a substantial amount of histoplasmosis, and the endemic area also extends eastward into Virginia and Maryland. Although the organism is widely distributed in these endemic areas, the concentration of the fungus is variable from site to site. Very heavy concentrations are found in excrement of chickens and of pigeons, starlings, and other wild birds.

Infection is almost universal in highly endemic areas. Any disturbance of the soil can scatter the infectious spores (primarily the microconidia) into the air. Over 90% of people living in some areas have had a primary pulmonary histoplasma infection prior to age 20.

PATHOGENESIS OF INFECTION

Fungus-laden soil is most common in rural areas but can also be found in urban or suburban areas where starlings roost. A minor disturbance of contaminated soil can scatter spores into the air. Inhalation of microconidia results in patchy areas of interstitial pneumonitis. The spores are engulfed by macrophages and multiply intracellularly in the yeast phase with a generation time of about 11 hr (7). The draining lymph nodes are quickly involved and hematogenous spread of the organism occurs with clearance by reticuloendothelial cells throughout the body. Specific lymphocyte-mediated cellular immunity develops within 7 to 14 days and results in rapid limitation of infection both in the lung and at distant sites with necrosis and granuloma formation in involved areas. Humoral antibody also develops, but it offers no protection and is not required for recovery.

The histology of the individual lesions depends on the adequacy of the host cellular immune response (5). In overwhelming disseminated infection macrophages can be crowded with organisms and show no tendency to form aggregates. In contrast, the granulomas in the lung and in the reticuloendothelial organs after a normally limited primary spread are well developed with epithelioid histiocytes, giant cells, and central necrosis. Few organisms are seen, even with special stains. Older lesions can be entirely fibrotic or can calcify.

CLINICAL MANIFESTATIONS

Primary Pulmonary Histoplasmosis

If exposure is light, pulmonary histoplasmosis is ordinarily asymptomatic or, at most, minimally symptomatic. Chest roentgenograms, even in asymptomatic cases, can show patchy nonsegmental areas of pneumonitis involving mainly the lower lobes. Hilar adenopathy is common and tends to be more prominent than in primary tuberculosis; pleural effusions are uncommon. Some patients are asymptomatic and have an influenza-like illness with fever, chills, myalgias, and nonproductive cough that follows exposure by 2 weeks.

Regardless of the presence or absence of symptoms, a primary fungemia generally occurs. During the primary infection organisms can, on occasion, be recovered from blood and bone marrow without implying progressive dissemination. The calcified granulomas commonly demonstrated in spleens and livers of patients from endemic areas either radiologically during life or pathologically at postmortem examination result from this primary self-limited fungemia and not from true dissemination.

Following exposure to a large infecting inoculum a more diffuse pulmonary involvement can occur, with an extensive nodular infiltrate on chest roentgenogram. Most of these patients are symptomatic, but they usually recover uneventfully.

The chest roentgenogram often returns to normal after a primary pulmonary infection. However, a variety of residual abnormalities can be seen. Initial soft infiltrates can "harden" and leave one or several nodules. Central necrosis can lead to a dense core of calcium (a "target" lesion), but this is not universal, especially in adults. Infrequently, alternate periods of activity followed by healing can result in characteristic concentric rings of calcium as the nodule slowly enlarges. Lymph node calcification, either in association with a parenchymal nodule or as a solitary finding, is common. Finally, small punctate "buckshot" calcifications can be scattered over both lung fields, a pattern very characteristic of histoplasmosis.

Exposure of small groups to heavy inocula of organisms results in small outbreaks of symptomatic disease. Sources of such exposure include chicken coops, other farm buildings, and, frequently, starling roosts. "Cave fever" caused by inhalation of infected bat guano is a well-known variation on this theme. These small outbreaks are more likely to be both suspected and documented as histoplasmosis than are individual cases of symptomatic primary histoplasmosis, which often are not distinguished from other respiratory illnesses.

Large outbreaks of histoplasmosis have been associated with excavation of infected soil for construction of roads or buildings. The association of erythema nodosum and erythema multiforme with acute histoplasmosis was first noted during study of these epidemics. Careful follow-up studies have revealed that progressive dissemination after a primary respiratory infection is exceedingly rare. Only one case of disseminated disease was seen among more than 6,000 cases in an urban epidemic in Mason City, Iowa.

Primary histoplasmosis has several uncommon local complaints within the chest. Although mediastinal lymph node involvement is common, it usually causes no problem. However, localized mediastinal granulomas can impinge on the superior vena cava (causing the superior vena cava syndrome of head, neck, and upper extremity edema), the esophagus (causing dysphagia), or on major bronchi (causing irritative cough). The prognosis is generally good. A strategically placed node can sometimes be moved surgically (the bulk of the nodal mass is removed with no attempt to dissect the back wall of the node from adjacent structures) with relief of symptoms. Symptoms often improve without therapy. More serious is fibrosing mediastinitis which is an extensive fibrosing process that can entrap and obliterate bronchi, pulmonary arteries, and pulmonary veins. Many patients have hemoptysis. Patients can progress to cor pulmonale and death from pulmonary hypertension, especially if the process is bilateral. Usually nothing can be done surgically, and attempts to bypass obstructed arteries and veins can lead to death. The current concept is that mediastinal granuloma and fibrosing mediastinitis are two different complications of primary histoplasmosis and that the first does not evolve to the second (9). In other rare instances a broncholith can develop when a calcified node erodes through a bronchus. Involvement of the pericardium can result in pericarditis with eventual constriction. Involvement of the esophagus occasionally causes a traction diverticulum.

Chronic Cavitary Histoplasmosis

Upper lobe cavitary histoplasmosis closely resembles reinfection tuberculosis in its roentgenographic appearance. It was first described among sanitorium patients who were thought to have tuberculosis. However, the mechanism of infection is not endogenous reactivation, as it is in tuberculosis. Cavitary histoplasmosis is the direct result of a primary infection in an abnormal lung (6).

Cavitary histoplasmosis occurs most frequently in middle-aged male smokers with centrilobular emphysema. Acute pulmonary histoplasmosis in this setting usually resolves without sequelae, but in a minority of cases infected airspaces persist. A progressive fibrosing cavitary process then develops that may gradually destroy adjacent areas of the lung. Specific antifungal chemotherapy is required. Although bilateral upper lobe involvement is most characteristic, cavitary disease can occur in other parts of the lung.

Chronic cough is a common clinical presentation, although some patients are asymptomatic. Constitutional symptoms increase as the illness progresses. Weight loss is common in far-advanced disease. Fever need not be present. Coexistence of cavitary histoplasmosis with tuberculosis and with bronchogenic carcinoma is not uncommon.

Disseminated Histoplasmosis

Disseminated histoplasmosis refers to any progressive extrapulmonary infection with *H. capsulatum*. It can occur as an overwhelming post-primary spread with no tendency to granuloma formation despite the presence of massive numbers of organisms in all reticuloendothelial tissues. This pattern of dissemination, seen most often in very young children, is called the infantile form and is associated with high fever, lymphadenopathy, hepatosplenomegaly, and pancytopenia. The illness can end in death within weeks. Among adults, dissemination is common in elderly men; adults usually demonstrate more of a granulomatous reaction in involved tissues and can have a smoldering subacute clinical illness of many months' duration. Fever is usually present but can be modest. Skin lesions and mucous membrane lesions are common, and weight loss can be a prominent feature. Adrenal granulomas occur commonly and can cause adrenal insufficiency. Disseminated histoplasmosis also occurs as an opportunistic infection in the immunosuppressed patient; high-dose glucocorticoid therapy is an important predisposing factor (1). The degree of granulomatous response in the immunosuppressed patient can vary from almost none (the "infantile" form) to a considerable amount.

Progressive disseminated histoplasmosis also occurs in patients with acquired immunodeficiency syndrome (AIDS) from areas endemic for histoplasmosis (8). The clinical presentation is a nonspecific febrile illness with lymphadenopathy and hepatosplenomegaly. The chest roentgenogram is either clear or shows diffuse interstitial infiltrates. The illness follows the pattern of the infantile form of disseminated histoplasmosis, not surprising in view of the profound T-cell immunodeficiency. The mechanism of infection can be rapid progression of primary infection while immunosuppressed, as documented in Indianapolis, Indiana. Or it may be late reactivation of latent infection in patients with remote exposure to endemic areas. Most AIDS patients with disseminated histoplasmosis diagnosed in San Francisco have had previous residence in the heavily endemic areas of the central United States. Most AIDS patients with disseminated histoplasmosis diagnosed in New York City have had previous residence in heavily endemic areas in the Caribbean Islands.

Fewer than one-half of patients with disseminated histoplasmosis present with cough, dyspnea, or other pulmonary symptoms. The chest roentgenogram can be normal. Although one-third of nonimmunosuppressed patients will have a localized interstitial infiltrate on chest roentgenogram, such a finding is unusual in the immunosuppressed patient. In these patients there is usually no history of a preceding respiratory illness, and the mechanism of infection can be endogenous reactivation. The chest roentgenogram in immunosuppressed patients sometimes shows a diffuse interstitial pattern suggesting hematogenous spread to the lungs. About 50% of patients with disseminated histoplasmosis have anemia, leukopenia, and thrombocytopenia. A similar percentage have abnormal liver function tests; an elevated alkaline phosphatase is most characteristic, although patients with the infantile form of the disease can have marked elevation of the serum AST (Aspartate aminotransferase). Disseminated intravascular coagulation occurs uncommonly.

The clinical picture of disseminated histoplasmosis is extremely variable and quite nonspecific. Persistent fever is the only finding that is found in almost all patients. Early diagnosis is important because specific therapy is generally effective.

Other cases of progressive extrapulmonary histoplasmosis present with a more localized infection. These include cases of central nervous system histoplasmoma, meningeal histoplasmosis, and isolated gastrointestinal histoplasmosis, usually involving the terminal ileum. Histoplasma endocarditis occurs either as part of general dissemination or as an isolated entity.

DIAGNOSIS

Mycological and Histopathological Methods

The definitive diagnosis of histoplasmosis depends on isolation of the fungus from clinical specimens or its detection in stained histopathological sections.

The organism can sometimes be cultured from the sputum in primary histoplasmosis and is readily recovered from sputum in chronic cavitary histoplasmosis. Sputum is cultured in Sabouraud's agar and on blood agar at 25°C. Colonies that show hyphal growth are subcultured. Formerly the positive identification of *H. capsulatum* required demonstration of characteristic tuberculate macroconidia on the mycelia and conversion of the isolate to the yeast phase while growing on blood agar at 37°C, a process that took several weeks. Today exoantigen testing can confirm histoplasmosis as soon as there is good growth of mycelial colonies, sometimes within 1 to 2 weeks.

Bone marrow aspirates and liver biopsy specimens are usually culture-positive in disseminated histoplasmosis. If there are skin lesions, culture of a skin biopsy is easy and reliable. Tissue is minced and placed directly on Sabouraud's agar and blood agar at 25°C, and isolation of the organism proceeds as for sputum. Blood cultures can also be positive in disseminated histoplasmosis but should be requested specifically for fungal cultures, as they might have to be held for a longer period of time than routine bacterial cultures.

Direct demonstration of the organism offers a quicker diagnosis. Histopathologic specimens that reveal macrophages crowded with small yeast are diagnostic of histoplasmosis. The organisms in such cases are easily seen in routine hematoxylin and eosin sections. With well-developed granulomas, the yeast forms can be rare, larger, and seen only in Gomori methenamine silver-stained sections.

Tissue for histopathological examination can be obtained from the lung, from lymph nodes, from bone marrow or liver biopsy, or from mucocutaneous lesions, depending on the clinical manifestations of this illness. Bone marrow biopsy is positive in a high percentage of cases of disseminated histoplasmosis and can safely and easily be sampled (2). In AIDS patients the density of organisms is so high that they can often be seen directly on stained smears of the buffy coat of the peripheral blood.

Serological Tests

Precipitins to histoplasmin can be detected using an agar gel double-diffusion method. An "M" precipitin line is present in approximately 50% of cases of acute histoplasmosis but is not positive for up to 4 weeks after the onset of clinical illness (3). A positive M band is occasionally found in asymptomatic persons in endemic areas. An "H" band by immunodiffusion is more specific for acute infection but is only found in 10% of acute infections. The immunodiffusion test is positive in 75% of patients with chronic cavitary histoplasmosis but only 30% of immunosuppressed patients with disseminated histoplasmosis.

The complement fixation test is very useful in diagnosis of histoplasmosis. Antigens prepared from both growth forms of histoplasmosis are employed. Higher titers are nearly always present against yeast antigens (HY) than against mycelial antigens (HMy). A fourfold rise in titer is diagnostic of recent infection, and a single titer of 1 : 32 or greater is very suggestive if the patient has a clinical illness compatible with histoplasmosis. CF antibodies are found in 80% of patients with acute histoplasmosis (again, they are not reliably positive until the patient has been ill for several weeks), 90% of patients with chronic cavitary histoplasmosis, and perhaps 50% of immunosuppressed patients with disseminated histoplasmosis (3).

Recently a radioimmunoassay has been developed that detects fungal antigen (histoplasma polysaccharide antigen) directly. Antigen can be detected in serum and also in cerebrospinal fluid, but the test is most sensitive when used on urine specimens (13,14). It has proved very useful to diagnose AIDS patients with progressive disseminated histoplasmosis, to monitor their response to therapy, and to follow them for relapse of infection (11,12). At present the test is available only at Dr. Wheat's laboratory in Indianapolis, Indiana. The urine test for antigen is not useful for diagnosing primary pulmonary histoplasmosis or chronic cavitary histoplasmosis. It is much more sensitive in AIDS patients with progressive disseminated histoplasmosis than in non-AIDS patients with the same form of histoplasmosis because the density of organisms (and thus the quantity of antigen cleared in the urine) is much higher.

Skin Test

Skin testing is performed with histoplasmin, a mycelial antigen. The skin test is generally positive 2 to 3 weeks after a primary pulmonary infection and remains positive for many years. Most inhabitants of an endemic area have a positive skin test. The skin test can be used as an epidemiological tool but should not be used in diagnosis of individual cases because it cannot separate patients with active disease from other residents of endemic areas. Furthermore, skin testing with histoplasmin will boost the CF titer to the HMy antigen, thus creating a potentially confusing situation. To avoid this confusion, blood for CF serologies should be drawn before the skin test is placed.

TREATMENT

Acute histoplasmosis is self-limited and seldom needs treatment. Treatment is necessary for the unusual patient with very severe primary pulmonary infection, for chronic cavitary histoplasmosis that is progressing, and for all cases of disseminated histoplasmosis.

Itraconazole, a new oral imidazole, should be the initial treatment for all patients with nonmeningeal disease who are not critically ill when diagnosed (1). The initial dose should be 200 mg/day for adults. The patient should be reevaluated at 6-week intervals. The drug is given orally once a day. It is probably more potent than ketoconazole which until recently was the oral agent of choice for mild to moderate nonmeningeal histoplasmosis. It is also better tolerated (less nausea and vomiting), better absorbed (less dependent on gastric acidity), and has less toxicity (less hepatitis, lesser tendency to block testosterone and other steroid synthesis).

Patients who are critically ill and all patients with meningeal histoplasmosis should receive intravenous amphotericin B. A total cumulative dose of 2 to 2.5 g is recommended. The usual single dose is 40 to 50 mg and can be administered every other day. This facilitates outpatient treatment regimens after the patient is stable.

Patients with AIDS usually respond to a course of amphotericin B only to relapse after the drug is stopped (8). Itraconazole (200–400 mg/day) can be used after initial improvement from amphotericin B. It must be continued indefinitely because it suppresses but does not cure the infection. In milder cases itraconazole can be used from the start (initial dose = 400 mg/day). Ketoconazole is not effective even to prevent relapse of histoplasmosis. Fluconazole is currently being studied as a maintenance therapy. Once weekly amphotericin B (50–80 mg dose) is also effective to prevent relapse of histoplasmosis in AIDS, but itraconazole has largely replaced weekly amphotericin B for this purpose because it is a convenient oral agent with less toxicity.

Most other immunosuppressed patients with disseminated histoplasmosis, including transplant recipients and patients receiving high-dose glucocorticoids, are usually cured by a course of amphotericin B and do not relapse when it is completed. Patients with lymphoma who have disseminated histoplasmosis are somewhat intermediate. They do have a somewhat higher incidence of relapse following amphotericin B treatment, but relapse is not invariable as it is in AIDS, and maintenance therapy is not required.

Problems with amphotericin B include acute febrile reactions, irritation of veins, depression of glomerular filtration rate, and anemia. In addition, a dose-related renal tubular acidosis develops in most patients, leading to marked potassium wastage (10).

REFERENCES

1. Davies, S.F., Khan, M., and Sarosi, G.A. (1978): Disseminated histoplasmosis in immunologically suppressed patients: occurrence in a non-endemic area. *Am. J. Med.,* 64;94–100.
2. Davies, S.F., McKenna, R.W., and Sarosi, F.A. (1979): Trephine biopsy of the bone marrow in disseminated histoplasmosis. *Am. J. Med.,* 67:617–622.
3. Davies, S.F. (1986): Serodiagnosis of histoplasmosis. *Sem. Respir. Infect.,* 1:9–15.
4. Dismukes, W.E., Bradsher, R.W., Cloud, G.C., Kauffman, C.A., Chapman, S.W., George, R.B., Stevens, D.A., et al. (1992): Itraconazole therapy for blastomycosis and histoplasmosis. *Am. J. Med.,* 93:489–497.
5. Goodwin, R.A., Jr., and DesPrez, R.M. (1978): Histoplasmosis: state of the art. *Am. Rev. Respir. Dis.,* 117:929–956.
6. Goodwin, R.A., Jr., Owens, F.T., Suell, J.D., Hubbard, W.W., Buchanan, R.D., Terry, R.T., and DesPrez, R.M. (1976): Chronic pulmonary histoplasmosis. *Medicine,* 55:413–452.

7. Howard, D.H. (1965): Intracellular growth of *Histoplasma capsulatum*. *J. Bacteriol.*, 89:518–523.
8. Johnson, P.C., Khardori, N., Najjar, A.F., Butt, F., Mansell, P.W.A., and Sarosi, G.A. (1988): Progressive disseminated histoplasmosis in patients with acquired immunodeficiency syndrome. *Am. J. Med.*, 85:152–158.
9. Loyd, J.E., Tillman, B.F., Atkinson, J.B., and DesPrez, R.M. (1988): Mediastinal fibrosis complicating histoplasmosis. *Medicine* (Baltimore), 67:295–310.
10. Utz, J.P., Bennett, J.E., and Brandriss, M.W. (1964): Amphotericin B toxicity. *Ann. Intern. Med.*, 61:334–354.
11. Wheat, L.J., Connolly-Stringfield, P.A. Baker, R.L. (1990): Disseminated histoplasmosis in the acquired immune deficiency syndrome: clinical findings, diagnosis and treatment, and review of the literature. *Medicine* (Baltimore), 69:361–374.
12. Wheat, L.J., Connolly-Stringfield, P.A., Blair, R., Connolly, K., Garringer, T., Katz, B.P., and Gupta, M. (1992): Effect of successful treatment with amphotericin B on *Histoplasma capsulatum* variety *capsulatum* polysaccharide antigen levels in patients with AIDS and histoplasmosis. *Am. J. Med.*, 92:153–160.
13. Wheat, L.J., French, M., Batteiger, B., and Kohler, R. (1989): Significance of *Histoplasma* antigen in the cerebrospinal fluid of patients with meningitis. *Arch. Intern. Med.*, 149:302–304.
14. Wheat, L.J., Kohler, R.B., and Tewari, R.P. (1986): Diagnosis of disseminated histoplasmosis by detection of *Histoplasma capsulatum* antigen in serum and urine specimens. *N. Engl. J. Med.*, 314:83–88.

Respiratory Infections: Diagnosis and Management, 3d ed.,
edited by James E. Pennington.
Raven Press, Ltd., New York © 1994

29

Blastomyces dermatitidis Pneumonia

Scott F. Davies

*Department of Medicine, University of Minnesota and Hennepin County Medical
Center, 701 Park Avenue South, Minneapolis, Minnesota 55415*

Blastomycosis refers to infection by the pathogenic fungus *Blastomyces dermatitidis*. Exposure occurs only by inhalation. Most patients present with a chronic pulmonary illness. A large central inflammatory mass can occur and can mimic carcinoma of the lung. Involvement of skin, bone, and prostate gland are common in disseminated blastomycosis.

EPIDEMIOLOGY

B. dermatitidis is a thermal dimorphic fungus. It grows as a mycelium (branching hyphae) in nature at 25°C *in vitro*. At 37°C *in vitro* and in infected mammalian tissue it converts to a large multinucleated yeast with characteristic broad-based single buds. Unlike *Histoplasma capsulatum*, it is not primarily an intracellular pathogen.

Isolation of *B. dermatitidis* from the soil has been very difficult. The failure of numerous attempts to isolate the fungus from the soil has suggested a restricted ecological niche for the organism. Even attempts to inoculate soil with *B. dermatitidis* have resulted in rapid death of the fungus (7).

Only in 1984 did Klein and associates (5) recover the fungus from nature for the first time in association with an outbreak of human illness. Fifty-one percent of 95 subjects (mostly children) who visited a beaver pond near Eagle River, Wisconsin, were infected. Multiple soil specimens obtained from the beaver lodge were positive. The positive soil samples had a very high organic content (60–70%) and a low pH. Rapidly rising soil temperatures in the few days before exposure apparently favored fungal growth, and rain on the day of exposure apparently wetted the spores, making them release more easily into the air when the site was disturbed. The report gives new insight into the conditions that are favorable for acquiring blastomycosis and helps to explain why previous attempts to culture the fungus have been so difficult. By the time the patient becomes symptomatic, the proper conditions for fungal growth might no longer exist at the site of exposure.

The histoplasmin skin test has enabled precise mapping of endemic areas for histoplasmosis. Confirmation of these findings has been obtained by isolation of *H. capsulatum* from the soil of those areas in which the incidence of positive histoplasmin skin test reactions is high.

In contrast, a reliable skin test has not been developed for blastomycosis. For this reason, and because the fungus is so difficult to isolate from soil, endemic areas can be identified only by recording the location of individual cases of blastomycosis. This is less than ideal, but it does give some indication of areas of disease activity.

B. dermatitidis is co-endemic with histoplasmosis over much of the central United States, including the Mississippi and the Ohio river valleys. The St. Lawrence river valley, where southeastern Canada and the northeastern United States join along a generally southwest/northeast border from the Niagara Falls area of New York State to the northern tip of Maine, also has both fungi, as does the southeastern United States, except Florida. Disease activity for blastomycosis extends farther to the north and the west than for histoplasmosis, across northern Wisconsin, northern Minnesota, eastern North Dakota, and adjacent areas of Canada. It also extends farther southeast to the coastal areas of Virginia, North Carolina, and South Carolina (Fig. 29-1).

Although there have been scattered reports of blastomycosis from many areas of the world, including Central America and Africa, most cases (or at least most cases

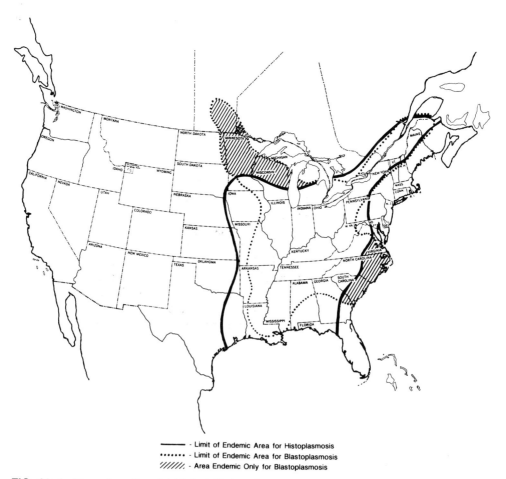

——— - Limit of Endemic Area for Histoplasmosis
•••••• - Limit of Endemic Area for Blastoplasmosis
/////// - Area Endemic Only for Blastoplasmosis

FIG. 29–1. Map of continental United States demonstrates approximate boundaries of endemic areas for histoplasmosis (determined by skin test surveys) and blastomycosis (determined by case reporting).

that have been recognized) come from the United States and Canada. Blastomycosis is not recognized in the Caribbean Islands, unlike histoplasmosis, which is common there.

PATHOGENESIS OF INFECTION

In contrast with histoplasmosis and coccidioidomycosis, direct intimate exposure to an infected site is probably necessary for infection with *B. dermatitidis*. Blastomycosis occurs most frequently in rural areas among individuals with outdoor jobs or interests. Residence near an ecological focus of high disease activity is also a risk factor (1). There is a male predominance of clinical cases, and half of the reported patients are between 20 and 50 years of age. The sex and age distribution could reflect the vocational and recreational activities of this group (11).

When a person is exposed to a contaminated site, microconidia of the fungus can be inhaled into the lung. If infection occurs, an intense neutrophilic response will develop. A specific cell-mediated immunological response occurs within 7 to 14 days. The tissue reaction at the time of diagnosis is of a mixed pyogenic and granulomatous nature.

Acute pulmonary blastomycosis can be symptomatic, but is probably self-limited in the majority of cases. Most investigators believe that the primary infection is less likely to be asymptomatic than is histoplasmosis. However, this is speculation, as there is no skin test to detect a primary infection that has not produced symptoms. A study of forestry workers from northern Minnesota and northern Wisconsin (endemic for blastomycosis but not for histoplasmosis) showed that 30% of this high-risk population demonstrated *in vitro* lymphocyte reactivity to a specific antigen derived from *Blastomyces dermatiditis* (13). This study and information derived from point-source outbreaks suggest that there are subclinical cases, but their frequency relative to histoplasmosis, where the great majority of cases are subclinical, is unknown. Other evidence that asymptomatic primary infection does occur comes from the study of point-source outbreaks. Asymptomatic patients were identified in an outbreak that occurred among a group of persons building a cabin in a wooded area (12). Four cabin builders developed culture-proven blastomycosis. Eight others had abnormal chest radiographs that resolved at around the same time as the proven cases. Three of these eight had symptoms of a mild upper respiratory infection, but the other five were asymptomatic. In the larger Eagle River outbreak, 22 of 48 definite or probable cases (identified by cultures, chest roentgenograms, or immunologic tests) were asymptomatic (5). The observed pattern of reactivation blastomycosis also proves that the primary infection can be asymptomatic. Many patients present with isolated skin lesions and normal chest radiographs. Often they do not recall a previous pneumonic illness. The portal of entry is always the lung, so initial infection in these cases must have been asymptomatic or at least minimally symptomatic.

Of the infections that do produce symptoms, the tendency to healing is probably no so marked as it is with histoplasmosis, and a greater proportion of patients will require specific antifungal therapy.

Seeding of distant sites can occur during primary infections with *B. dermatitidis*. Unlike histoplasmosis, hematogenous spread probably does not occur in all patients. In blastomycosis the commonest sites of spread are the skin, bone, and prostate, rather than the liver, spleen, and bone marrow as seen in histoplasmosis.

Most diagnosed cases of blastomycosis present as a chronic pulmonary process. Symptoms are similar to those seen in tuberculosis, with chronic cough, low-grade fever, malaise, and weight loss.

CLINICAL MANIFESTATIONS

Acute Pulmonary Blastomycosis

Acute pulmonary blastomycosis may or may not be symptomatic. Inhalation of microconidia results in patchy areas of alveolar consolidation as exudation occurs and neutrophils are recruited. Pulmonary involvement can be bilateral, and it is usual for the lower lobes to be affected. The chest roentgenogram is quite variable. Observed patterns include single or multiple nodules, dense consolidation of one or more segments or lobes, and, rarely, diffuse alveolar infiltrates. Blastomycosis can present as a lobar pneumonia similar to pneumococcal pneumonia or as noncardiac pulmonary edema (adult respiratory distress syndrome) similar to that caused by bacteria or by other infectious agents. Hilar adenopathy can occur with primary infection, but pleural effusion and cavitation of infiltrates are uncommon. Symptoms, if present, resemble those of an acute bacterial pneumonia and include high fever, pleuritic chest pain, and myalgias. Cough is usually productive with mucopurulent secretions, reflecting the mixed pyogenic and granulomatous nature of the inflammatory response. Symptoms range from mild to severe and may last from a few days to a few weeks, usually less than 2 weeks. Even if the symptoms resolve rapidly, radiological abnormalities can persist for 3 months or longer.

Some patients with initially focal infiltrates became increasingly toxic. Severe hypoxemia develops as the infiltrates progress to involve both lungs diffusely. This progress probably results from hematogenous spread of infection in most cases but might also reflect bronchogenic spread in a few cases. This spread to involve both lungs diffusely is probably hematogenous in most cases but might also result from bronchogenic spread in some cases. Rapid spread to distant sites can also occur with crops of new skin lesions appearing as gas exchange worsens. Worsening headache can mark meningeal involvement. Rapidly progressive pulmonary and systemic blastomycosis is usually fatal unless treated quickly and aggressively.

Patients who recover spontaneously from symptomatic pulmonary blastomycosis, like patients who have had asymptomatic primary infection, are at some risk of developing late reactivation at distant sites. The chance of reactivation appears highest during the 1 to 2 years immediately following the primary infection (6). Whether or not there is a risk of late reactivation after many years, as in tuberculosis, is uncertain.

Chronic Pulmonary Blastomycosis with or without Involvement of Distant Sites

Most patients with blastomycosis present with the insidious onset of a chronic pulmonary process. They have no history of an antecedent acute pneumonia, but present with chronic respiratory symptoms that have persisted for weeks or even months. Chronic cough, low-grade fever, night sweats, weight loss, and variable dyspnea are the usual manifestations. The chest radiograph might reveal a fibronodular infiltrate with areas of cavitation, similar in all respects to reactivation tuberculosis. Another radiological pattern seen is that of a single large mass, often perihilar, that mimics and can be confused with bronchogenic carcinoma.

Involvement of distant sites is common in chronic pulmonary blastomycosis; one-half of the patients have skin involvement, one-third have bone involvement, and one-fifth have genitourinary tract involvement (14). The occurrence of infection at these sites in association with chronic infiltration on the chest radiograph can be an important diagnostic sign.

Isolated Involvement of Distant Sites

Isolated involvement of skin, bone, or the genitourinary tract can occur in patients with a past history of an apparently self-limited pneumonia, or in patients with no previous history of respiratory tract infection. Such patients can have no pulmonary symptoms and normal chest radiographs when they present with disseminated blastomycosis. These patients had primary pulmonary blastomycosis, either asymptomatic or symptomatic, which eventually resolved completely. However, seeding of distant sites during the primary infection established a situation in which endogenous reactivation of fungal infection could later occur.

Skin disease is common in patients with chronic pulmonary blastomycosis, but can also occur without evidence of infection elsewhere. The characteristic lesions are raised and crusted with irregular borders. They frequently occur on the face or the extremities and can mimic basal cell carcinoma; one distinguishing feature is the finding of small microabscesses at the periphery of the lesions.

Bone is the second most common distant site of infection in blastomycosis. The spine is most frequently involved, followed by the ribs, skull, and long bones. Involvement of the spine mimics tuberculosis with involvement of adjacent vertebrae and destruction of the intervening disc space. Osteolytic and osteoblastic processes can be seen on radiographs. Long bones are involved near the epiphysis, and the infection can extend directly to an adjacent joint space.

Unlike tuberculosis, blastomycosis rarely involves the kidney or ureter. Infection of any part of the female genitourinary tract is uncommon. For unknown reasons there is a marked tendency for infection of the male prostate, epididymis, and, less frequently, the testes. Patients can present with a scrotal or prostatic mass. Hematuria and pyuria are common, and bladder outlet obstruction can be the presenting complaint. Venereal transmission of blastomycosis can result in self-limited genital ulceration or endometritis in the female sexual partner (2). This appears to be the only type of inoculation blastomycosis other than direct surgical inoculation, which also results in a self-limited ulcer.

B. dermatitidis, like *H. dermatitidis,* is a rare cause of chronic meningitis.

Blastomycosis in AIDS

Unlike histoplasmosis, blastomycosis is quite uncommon in patients with AIDS. Possible explanations include lower likelihood of exposure to an infective site while immunosuppressed and/or a smaller reservoir of patients with remote blastomycosis waiting to reactivate. Blastomycosis in AIDS is, as expected, a severe infection with marked tendency to disseminate widely. Four of fifteen patients in one report (combining the experience of ten large medical centers) had diffuse bilateral infiltrates and extensive extrapulmonary involvement including meningitis (9). One patient had diffuse bilateral infiltrates and extensive extrapulmonary involvement without meningitis. Seven patients had isolated pulmonary disease—three focal and four diffuse. One patient each had isolated skin disease and isolated central nervous system diseases. The final patient had focal pneumonia and meningitis. As compared to non-AIDS patients, the incidences of diffuse infiltrates (9 of 15) and of central nervous system involvement (6 of 15) are much higher. AIDS patients present with blastomycosis when severely immunosuppressed. All but one had CD4 count less than 200 cells/mm^3. Five patients were diagnosed outside of the endemic area, including three in New York City, one in Denver, Colorado, and one in Jacksonville, Florida. Four of the five had not lived in an endemic area for at least several years, suggesting reactivation of latent infection.

Outcome was generally poor. Six patients died within a month, including three who died within 3 days, untreated because of the rapidity of their death. Nine patients lived more than a month. At the time of the report seven had died a mean of 11 months after initial presentation and two were still alive on therapy. Five of the seven late deaths were from AIDS-related causes other than blastomycosis. All of the early deaths were due to blastomycosis.

DIAGNOSIS

Mycological and Histopathological Methods

The diagnosis of blastomycosis can often be made by demonstrating the characteristic yeast forms (broad-necked single buds) in the sputum in cases of acute or chronic pulmonary blastomycosis. The fungus can also be demonstrated in aspirates of skin lesions or material massaged from an infected prostate. Organisms can be identified in preparations digested with 10% potassium hydroxide and in cytological specimens treated with the Papanicolaou stain (10).

Histopathological examination of biopsy specimens of infected tissue can also reveal the characteristic yeast forms. The organism is seldom seen in hematoxylin- and eosin-stained sections: Gomori methenamine silver and periodic acid Schiff (PAS) stains are best for diagnosis.

The mycelial form can be isolated from clinical material on Sabouraud's agar or blood agar at 25°C. If a mycelial fungus is isolated, subculture on blood agar at 37°C will yield the characteristic yeast form.

Growth of *B. dermatitidis* on primary isolation can take 1 to 3 or more weeks. The plates must be sealed to prevent drying during the long incubation period. In the yeast phase, and to a lesser degree in the mycelial phase, the organism is sensitive to actidione (cyclohexamide); thus this antibiotic should not be used in the culture medium.

Once good mycelial growth is established, exoantigen testing can provide a positive identification. Formerly, positive identification required conversion of the mycelial isolate to the yeast form, adding one or more weeks to the entire process.

Serological Tests

The complement-fixation test is not sensitive. It is positive in <10% of cases of acute pulmonary blastomycosis and <50% of chronic pulmonary and extrapulmonary infections (3). The test is also not specific. Many patients with histoplasmosis have a positive test.

A more sensitive agar gel double-diffusion test for blastomycosis has been described which is much more useful. It is positive in 30% of patients with acute pulmonary blastomycosis and 70 to 80% of chronic pulmonary and extrapulmonary infections. The test detects antibody against the A antigen and is quite specific. Although a negative test does not exclude blastomycosis, a positive test is suggestive evidence of the infection and should prompt an aggressive diagnostic evaluation aimed at obtaining histopathological or mycological proof of the diagnosis.

A new enzyme immunoassay (also employing antigen A) is even more sensitive than the ID, but is less specific, especially at low titers of 1 : 16 or less.

Skin Test

There is no reliable skin test available for blastomycosis. Blastomycosis and histoplasmosis are coendemic over a wide geographic area, and cross-reaction between skin test preparations limits specificity. No preparation has demonstrated adequate sensitivity. Lack of a reliable skin test has hindered the understanding of the epidemiology of blastomycosis.

TREATMENT

Acute pulmonary blastomycosis (symptoms of acute pneumonia) does not require specific treatment if the disease is very mild or is resolving at the time of diagnosis. Long-term follow-up is indicated because patients can present later with disease at distant sites despite an apparently self-limited primary infection.

All patients with moderate or severe primary infection, chronic pulmonary infection (symptoms resembling tuberculosis), or infection at distant sites require treatment. If the patient is not seriously ill and the disease does not involve the meninges (meningitis is very uncommon), itraconazole can be used for initial treatment (4). The usual dose is 200 mg/day. (Before 1992, ketoconazole was standard oral therapy for non-life-threatening non-meningeal blastomycosis [8], but itraconazole appears to be more potent with less toxicity.) Patients with meningeal or other life-threatening disease should be treated with intravenous amphotericin B to a total dose of 2.0 g in a manner similar to that described for histoplasmosis.

Blastomycosis in AIDS should be treated with amphotericin B initially, especially if the patient is seriously ill. After the patient improves and becomes stable, lifetime suppression can begin, either with itraconazole or perhaps with fluconazole (high doses: 200 to 400 mg daily). Fluconazole has excellent central nervous system penetration. Treatment decisions in AIDS will likely be based on anecdotes and influenced by co-infections. Cases are too rare to conduct formal clinical trials. Itraconazole is the best oral agent and is probably preferred for non-meningeal cases. When the central nervous system is involved, the choice between itraconazole and high-dose fluconazole (the agent is probably less active but has more favorable pharmacokinetics) is less clear, and treatment response will have to be followed closely in individual patients.

REFERENCES

1. Baumgardner, D.J., Buggy, B.P., Mattson, B.J., Burdick, J.S., and Ludwig, D. (1992): Epidemiology of blastomycosis in a region of high endemicity in North Central Wisconsin. *Clin. Infect. Dis.*, 15:629–635.
2. Craig, M.W., Davey, W.N., and Green, R.A. (1970): Conjugal blastomycosis. *Am. Rev. Respir. Dis.*, 102:86–90.
3. Davies, S.F., and Sarosi, G.A. (1986): Role of serodiagnostic tests and skin tests in diagnosis of fungal diseases. *Clin. Chest Med.*, 8:135–146.
4. Dismukes, W.E., Bradsher, R.W., Cloud, G.C., Kauffman, C.A., Chapman, S.W., George, R.B., Stevens, D.A., et al. (1992): Itraconazole therapy for blastomycosis and histoplasmosis. *Am. J. Med.*, 93:489–497.
5. Klein, B.S., Vergeront, J.M., Weeks, R.J., Kumar, U.N., Mathai, G., Varkey, B., Kaufman, L., Bradsher, R.W., Stoebig, J.F., Davis, J.P., and the Investigation Team. (1986): Isolation of *Blastomyces dermatitidis* in soil associated with a large outbreak of blastomycosis in Wisconsin. *N. Engl. J. Med.*, 314:529–534.
6. Laskey, W.L., and Sarosi, G.A. (1978): Endogenous reactivation in blastomycosis. *Ann. Intern. Med.*, 88:50–52.
7. McDonough, E.S., Dubats, J.J., Wisniewski, T.R., Wallenfong, M., and McNamara, W. (1973): Soil streptomycetes and bacteria related to lysis of *Blastomyces dermatitidis. Sabouraudia*, 11:244–245.
8. National Institute of Allergy and Infectious Diseases, Mycoses Study Group. (1985): Treatment of blastomycosis and histoplasmosis with ketoconazole. *Ann. Intern. Med.*, 103:861–872.
9. Pappas, P.G., Pottage, J.C., Powderly, W.G., et al. (1992): Blastomycosis in patients with the acquired immunodeficiency syndrome. *Ann. Intern. Med.*, 116:847–853.
10. Sanders, J.S., Sarosi, G.A., Nollet, D.J., and Thompson, J.I. (1977): Exfoliative cytology in the rapid diagnosis of pulmonary blastomycosis. *Chest*, 72:193–196.
11. Sarosi, G.A., and Davies, S.F. (1979): Blastomycosis: state of the art. *Am. Rev. Respir. Dis.*, 120:911–938.
12. Tosh, F.E., Hammerman, K.J., Weeks, R.J., and Sarosi, G.A. (1974): A common source epidemic of North American blastomycosis. *Am. Rev. Respir. Dis.*, 109:525–529.
13. Vaaler, A.K. Bradsher, R.W., and Davies, S.F. (1990): Evidence of subclinical blastomycosis in forestry workers in northern Minnesota and northern Wisconsin. *Am. J. Med.*, 89:470–476.
14. Witorsch, P., and Utz, J.P. (1968): North American blastomycosis: a study of 40 patients. *Medicine* (Baltimore), 47:169–200.

Respiratory Infections: Diagnosis and Management, 3d ed., edited by James E. Pennington.
Raven Press, Ltd., New York © 1994

30

Pneumonia Due to *Actinomyces,* *Propionibacterium (Arachnia) propionicum,* and *Nocardia*

Phillip I. Lerner

Division of Infectious Diseases, Mount Sinai Medical Center,
1 Mount Sinai Drive, Cleveland, Ohio 44106

The pathogenic actinomycetous bacteria provoke chronic infections not unlike those caused by the true fungi. Not until the 1950s did cell wall analyses establish actinomycetes as slow-growing, gram-positive bacterial filaments, with cell walls containing muramic and diaminopimelic acids (lysine in *Propionibacterium propionicum*), not the chitin or glucans found in fungi. The 1 μm diameter thin bacterial filaments, narrower than fungal hyphae, fragment readily into bacillary forms, although they truly branch and form mycelial-type colonies. Actinomyces are prokaryotic bacteria, Schizomycetes of the order Actinomycetales, families Actinomycetaceae and Nocardiaceae.

Infections produced by Actinomyces, *Propionibacterium propionicum* (formerly *Arachnia propionica*), and *Nocardia* overlap clinically, with each other, and with other chronic pulmonary disorders, infectious (fungal, mycobacterial) and noninfectious, particularly malignancy. Indiscriminate antimicrobial therapy complicates the diagnostic effort because actinomycetes are inhibited by so many antimicrobials, although not by imidazoles or amphotericin B. A positive culture can easily evade the microbiologist not alerted to search for these elusive agents. The clinical spectrum of actinomycosis and nocardiosis is often continuous; to mistake one infection for the other could be disastrous.

ACTINOMYCOSIS

Actinomycosis, a chronic suppurative and fibrosing infection, distinguished by draining sinus tracts which discharge characteristic "sulfur granules," spreads unimpeded by traditional anatomic barriers. Actinomyces and *P. propionicum* are constituents of the normal flora—endogenous oral saprophytes in periodontal pockets and carious teeth, plaque, gingival sulci and tonsillar crypts—which take advantage of infection or injury to penetrate normally intact mucosal barriers and invade adjacent tissues in the head and neck, lungs, or ileocecal regions.

Historical Review and Current Microbiology

Bollinger (1877) first recognized the radially arranged clubbed elements of *Actinomyces bovis* ("ray fungus of the cow") in granules from sarcoma-like masses in cattle with "lumpy jaw" (44). Israel defined actinomycosis in man in 1885; in 1891, he and Wolff grew a filamentous anaerobic organism from human material, named *A. israelii* but thought to represent the same organism (44). Erikson (1940) proved *A. israelii* and *A. bovis* were distinct species (44); the latter does not infect man. Actinomycosis derives from the Greek "Aktino," the ray (radiating) appearance of the organism in the sulfur granule, "mykes," mistakenly designating it a fungus.

Actinomycosis originally designated infection with any pathogenic actinomycete including aerobic strains. In 1943, Waksman and Henrici (111) separated the pathogenic *Actinomycetaceae*. The genus *Actinomyces* included microaerophilic and anaerobic pathogens causing true actinomycosis. Aerobic nocardioform pathogens were placed in the genus *Nocardia*, but are now in a separate family, *Nocardiaceae*.

Human actinomycosis is caused mainly by *A. israelii*. Three other species and one in a related genus, *Propionibacterium* (formerly *Arachnia*), all oral commensals, provoke infections consistent with classic actinomycosis (44); they are, in order of importance, *P. propionicum*, *A. naeslundii*, *A. viscosus*, and *A. odontolyticus*, the latter not as yet associated with pulmonary infection. *A. meyerii* has now been added to the list (2,76,91). Facultative or anaerobic, they grow best under anaerobic conditions at 37°C. Some strains of *A. israelii* are microaerophilic. *A. viscosus* is unique because it grows under microaerophilic or aerobic conditions and produces catalase. *Bifidobacterium adolescentis* (formerly *A. eriksonii*) can also produce an actinomycotic infection.

Direct staining of clinical material by fluorescein isothiocyanate species-specific antiserum rapidly identifies species within granules (even in Formalin-fixed tissues), and permits recognition of mixed species in a granule. Conjugates have been prepared for all four major species of actinomyces and for *P. propionicum* (46,54), but are not readily available.

Pathogenesis and Epidemiology

Infection begins when endogenous *Actinomyces* or *P. propionicum* enters injured tissues following infection, trauma, or surgical manipulation. Thoracic infection follows aspiration of infected oral debris in individuals with lingual or gingivodental infection but seldom complicates cervicofacial infection unless there is direct mediastinal extension from the neck (97). Rarely, thoracic infection derives from retroperitoneal infection, from abdominal infection penetrating the diaphragm, or from a mucosal lesion of the esophagus (11). *Actinomyces* sp are infrequent opportunists in patients on steroids or with leukemia, renal failure, metastatic carcinoma, or AIDS.

All age groups are affected, even infants (31). In one series, patients ranged between 10 and 90 years of age, with two-thirds of subjects between ages 30 and 60; men outnumbered women 4 : 1 (24). In childhood, both sexes appear to be infected equally (2,31,103).

Lesions and sulfur granules almost always contain other bacteria (57). The role of these "associates" in the pathogenesis of actinomycosis is unclear. Mice and hamsters can be infected with pure cultures of *A. israelii* but exhibit differences in pathogenicity among various species (16,44). *Actinobacillus actinomycetemcomitans, Bacteroides* sp, fusobacteria, anaerobic and other streptococci are most frequently recovered, but *Hemophilus* sp, *Eikenella corrodens,* micrococci, or staphylococci also can accompany *Actinomyces* or *Propionibacterium* sp in cervicofacial and thoracic infections. Mixed murine infections provide experimental evidence of mutualism between different pathogens in the lesions (66), supporting Holm (57), who concluded that actinomycosis results from a synergistic interaction between *Actinomyces* and a variety of gram-negative "associates," the latter augmenting the comparatively weak invasive capacities of the former (66,95). Mechanisms of host resistance and immunity to *A. israelii* are unknown.

Clinical and Laboratory Features

Pneumonia caused by *Actinomyces* sp and *P. propionicum* is best considered in the context of thoracic actinomycosis, an infection respecting no anatomic boundaries, commonly involving also the pleural space, mediastinum or chest wall, and occurring in 15–34% of all cases of actinomycosis (33). Without a telltale draining chest wall sinus, the diagnosis is often long delayed. Thoracic infection results from oropharyngeal aspiration, sometimes in association with severe dental disease, abscess or periodontitis, although some patients are edentulous (77,100). Bronchitis, emphysema, and chronic pneumonia or bronchiectasis are common antecedents (24).

The clinical picture mimics tuberculosis or tumor. The correct diagnosis is often uncovered when these two possibilities are being pursued (77) or when an empyema or chest wall fistula leads to proper studies. Constitutional symptoms are nonspecific (weight loss, cough, chest pain, fever), and, indeed, signs of systemic infection might be lacking; fever can be absent, the white blood cell count can be normal, and the patient need not be anemic. Hemoptysis is unusual but occasionally massive (53). A clinical pattern of remission and exacerbation of symptoms, in parallel with initiation and cessation of antibiotic therapy, should raise suspicion of this diagnosis. Hematogenous dissemination can occur in the course of thoracic actinomycosis (25). Skin and subcutaneous lesions suggesting vasculitis on biopsy (119) can herald the infection, with pulmonary lesions uncovered only coincidentally (25).

The classic chest wall sinus discharging granules is rare today because antibiotics limit infection to the lung. Granules can be trapped in gauze placed over the sinus opening or detected by examining closely the side of a tilted tube filled with pus (97). Pleuropulmonary involvement occurs in 1.5% of cases, although small effusions or pleural thickenings are common x-ray findings (37). Massive empyema is rare (77) but does occur (55). *Actinomyces* sp can be but one of several participants in a mixed anaerobic pleuropulmonary infection, where its primacy is less certain, absent characteristic pathology or granules (55).

Radiographic findings are often nonspecific but can be suggestive (37): (i) lung lesions penetrating and exiting the chest wall; (ii) wavy periostitis or frank destruction of ribs, sternum, or shoulder girdle adjacent to a chronic pulmonary process; (iii) involvement of adjacent lobes by extension (transgression) through an interlobar fissure; (iv) characteristic vertebral destruction, extending from mediastinal or retroperitoneal involvement, with erosion of both the body and processes of the affected vertebra as well as the adjacent ribs. Disease confined to the chest wall can even be associated with a normal chest film (88). Periostitis of the ribs is no longer common, and x-rays today frequently demonstrate a mass, suggesting bronchogenic carcinoma (100). Rib abnormalities or destruction can be due to combined carcinoma and actinomycosis (37). One or more small cavities are found in half the cases; large cavities are rare (37). A chronic fibrocavitary process with striking volume contraction can simulate tuberculosis (70), or appear simply as a chronic alveolar infiltrate. A miliary picture has been described in the modern era, and one should be particularly alert to the occasional case of disseminated actinomycosis arising from a pelvic focus secondary to an IUD (85). Less common is mediastinal involvement (103), sometimes with superior vena cava obstruction, tracheo-esophageal fistula, and, rarely, systemic-to-pulmonary artery fistula (78).

Cardiac actinomycosis has been reported in less than 2% of patients with actinomycosis and usually results from the direct extension of thoracic disease, occurring only rarely as a primary infection or by hematogenous spread. It is characterized by involvement of the pericardium, myocardium, and endocardium, in decreasing order of frequency. The pericardium is involved in approximately 70%–80% of cases of cardiac actinomycosis, most often due to contiguous spread from a primary infection of the thorax or mediastinum, but the pericardium can also become involved as the result of direct extension from a primary endocardial or myocardial infection. Pericardial involvement can present as acute pericarditis, purulent pericarditis with effusion, constrictive pericarditis, or acute cardiac tamponade (33,82).

Sulfur granules in sputum cytology specimens can herald the diagnosis (100), but recognition more often follows surgery for presumed carcinoma. The open bronchus sign usually excludes neoplasm, but an actinomycotic mass can at times compress, constrict, enter, or distort a bronchus (9,23,73). Bronchoscopy can reveal irregular granular thickening with partial bronchial obstruction; biopsy can reveal only chronic inflammatory fibrosis (37,100). *Actinomyces* and *Propionibacterium* sp require extended anaerobic or microaerophilic incubation; whenever possible, cultures should be submitted from patients not then receiving antibiotics.

Large lipoid-filled histiocytes and associated bronchiolar and fibrous hyperplasia can be mistaken for malignancy in small-needle aspirations or tiny biopsy specimens (77). As much tissue as can be safely removed should be submitted for thorough pathologic examination. *Actinomyces* sp can colonize devitalized tissue and thus can grow in tumors undergoing necrosis; a positive sputum or aspiration culture requires histopathologic confirmation (100). Actinomycosis and tuberculosis can coexist (11,105). The classic triad of lung infection with empyema and rib or chest wall involvement is seldom a diagnostic problem because involvement of the bony or soft parts of the thoracic cage strongly favors the diagnosis. In reality, actinomycosis should be considered in any chronic lung infiltrate, cavity, or central mass lesion (103,105).

The cellular antigens of *A. israelii* are incompletely defined. Serum agglutinins and complement-fixing antibodies appear in some patients, but cross-precipitating antibodies occur, particularly in tuberculosis (45). Immunoelectrophoresis with monospecific antigen-antibody systems might yet yield a serodiagnostic method (59,60).

Pathology

Gross lesions are single or multiple indurated masses with thick, fibrous walls and soft central purulent loculations. Sinus tracts extend to the skin or into viscera.

Chronic infections tend to localize, but the longer the course, the more likely the formation of sinuses and/or distant spread.

Histopathology reveals suppuration surrounded by acute or chronic fibrosing granulation tissue. Foamy macrophages account for the yellow color. Eosinophils and giant cells are not common; plasma cells, although scarce acutely, increase with chronicity. Fibrosis may be ill-defined, limited, or absent in any early infection. In chronic infection, one typically finds healing by intense, even avascular, fibrosis in one area, with acute suppuration nearby. In the absence of granules or filaments, the biopsy can suggest a noninfectious process, such as Wegener's granulomatosis (vasculitis) (119).

Sulfur granules, conglomerate colonies of the branching filaments, form only *in vivo,* cemented and mineralized by calcium phosphate from host-organism phosphotase activity in response to tissue inflammation. Aggregates of other organisms, including fungi, *Nocardia,* streptomyces, and staphylococci (botryomycosis), can also form similar granules; these imitators lack the characteristic clubbed peripheral fringe (24), which are surface filaments encased in the same polysaccharide-protein complex. Granules can be scarce; multiple blocks of the abscess wall or sinus tract should be fixed and serial sections meticulously examined (24). Granules in early lesions can be loosely aggregated, have poorly developed clubs, and not be surrounded by chronic inflammatory cells; sometimes the organisms appear as free gram-positive filaments. Not all actinomyces provoke granule formation as readily as *A. israelii* (44).

Therapy

Before 1941, death or persistent disease was the end result of all but the most localized infections (11,77). With penicillin, cure became the rule rather than the exception. Peabody and Seabury (84) emphasized the principle of intense and prolonged antibiotic therapy, coupled with appropriate drainage of abscesses or radical excision of sinus tracts. Very high concentrations of penicillin are required to penetrate areas of fibrosis and suppuration and possibly the granules themselves. Occasionally, extensive chronic disease (lungs, pleura, chest wall) responds dramatically and completely to intravenous penicillin alone, either obviating the need for surgery (77) or defining tissue planes more clearly, facilitating subsequent surgery. Intravenous penicillin G, 10–20 million units/day for 4–6 weeks, followed by oral penicillin (e.g., phenoxymethyl penicillin, 2–4 gm/day, to patient tolerance) for 3–6 additional months is an approximate therapeutic goal for most deep-seated infections. Rarely, oral penicillin therapy alone, closely monitored to assure adequate antibiotic absorption, can lead to successful cure of a deep-seated infection (81).

In vitro susceptibility testing is seldom necessary because results are predictable. There are no major species variations in antimicrobial susceptibility among first-line drugs (penicillin, tetracycline, erythromycin, clindamycin), so infection with strains other than *A. israelii* also responds to treatment with penicillin G or any traditional penicillin alternative (74). Some strains of *A. israelii* are inhibited by sulfonamide concentrations attainable in serum (4.0–8.0 mg%). Therefore, proven cases of actinomycosis, not mistaken instances of nocardiosis, might on occasion respond to sulfonamides (74). Parenteral cephalosporins and clindamycin are suitable penicillin alternatives, but oral cephalosporins, the semisynthetic penicillins oxacillin and dicloxacillin, and metronidazole are much less active *in vitro* and should be avoided

(74). Garrod (40) claimed that unsuccessful penicillin treatment might be accompanied by increased *in vitro* resistance; MICs for two strains of *A. israelii* increased from 0.03 U/ml to 0.2 U/ml and >0.5 U/ml, respectively. Actinomyces do not adapt to serial passage in subinhibitory concentrations of penicillin (74); *in vivo* development of acquired penicillin resistance by *Actinomyces* species has not been subsequently reported. When response to penicillin is poor, search for an undrained abscess, although the possibility of a resistant bacterial "associate" cannot be entirely dismissed. Some investigators favor ampicillin (or amoxicillin) for initial therapy because these concomitant bacterial species are less susceptible *in vitro* to penicillin G, or even employ metronidazole or clindamycin as second agents when *Bacteroides* sp are present (95). Imipenem has been used successfully in selected, complicated cases (32). This author has never found penicillin G wanting in any case, unless drug allergy was a problem.

NOCARDIOSIS

Historical Review and Current Microbiology

Nocardiosis is a localized or disseminated infection due to an exogenous aerobic soil actinomycete, usually introduced through the respiratory tract. The pulmonary event can be transient or even subclinical, or provoke an acute or chronic bronchopulmonary process mimicking tuberculous or mycotic infections as well as malignancy. Hematogenous dissemination from the lung spreads particularly to the nervous system and the soft tissues.

Members of the family Nocardiaceae, the aerobic nocardioform actinomycetes, reproduce by fragmenting into bacillary and coccoid elements but are distinguished by a propensity for filamentous growth with true branching. Both vegetative and aerial fragmenting filaments are seen; conidia are absent.

Nocardia asteroides is the predominant pathogen in man; other pathogens include *N. brasiliensis*, *N. otitidiscavarium (caviae)*, and *N. farcinica*, the agent of bovine nocardiosis (58,109). Current tests employed in clinical laboratories do not distinguish *N. farcinica* from *N. asteroides*, but recognition that the formerly controversial species (109) has a specific antibiotic resistance pattern to the newer cephalosporins (vide infra-Therapy) has at last convinced American investigators that the bovine agent also causes significant clinical infection in this country (117) as well as in Denmark and Japan (109). In a survey of nocardial infections 2 decades ago in this country (1972–1974), 83% of isolates were *N. asteroides*, 9% *N. brasiliensis*, 3% *N. caviae*, and 7% were identified only as *Nocardia* sp (14); *N. farcinica* was not considered at that time. The very rare isolate *N. transvalensis* has also been isolated recently from cases of pneumonia (8).

Nocardia sp are not fastidious organisms and grow readily over a wide temperature range on simple laboratory media (Sabouraud's glucose agar, blood agar), but they grow slowly, permitting overgrowth by other microbes. They also grow poorly on inhibitory media commonly used to isolate pathogenic fungi. Colonies can be smooth and moist, or rugate with a velvet surface, due to a rudimentary aerial mycelium. Pigment variations include cream, yellow, pink, coral, orange, and brick red. Whenever possible, specimens for culture should be taken only when the patient is antibiotic-free. Colonies in pure culture can appear in 48 hours, but in clinical material, particularly in respiratory secretions, other more rapidly growing bacteria obscure small *Nocardia* colonies, when routine cultures are held only 24–48 hours (83,84). Characteristic colonies can take several weeks to develop, accounting for a suboptimal recovery rate in many laboratories. Multiple specimens should be submitted because positive smears and cultures occur simultaneously only in a third of cases (123). Employing Modified Thayer-Martin medium and extending the incubation time from the usual 3 days under 10% CO_2 at 35°C to a further 3 weeks at room temperature in a candle jar is an economical and sensitive screening technique to improve the yield of *Nocardia* isolates from routine sputum specimens (4,80). Paraffin baiting also enhances recovery, but it is time-consuming and not readily adaptable to the routine clinical laboratory (4). Buffered charcoal-yeast extract (BCYE) agar can also enhance recovery of *Nocardia* species (68).

Observing delicate, gram-positive, irregularly stained or beaded, branching filaments in a gram-stained specimen is almost pathognomic. Many *Nocardia* sp are acid-fast in tissue or on primary culture, but in comparison to *Mycobacteria* sp they retain fuchsin less tenaciously. Basic fuchsin is not readily removed by aqueous mineral acids, but acid-alcohol solutions usually decolorize *Nocardia* sp. Acid-fastness is quickly lost in older, subcultured strains.

Pathogenesis and Epidemiology

N. asteroides most often enters through the respiratory tract (83). Occasionally the alimentary canal is penetrated (e.g., the appendix); rarely, infection follows a dental injury. Traumatic nocardial wound infections usually remain localized but can disseminate to the lungs (83). *N. brasiliensis* can participate in this latter sequence, or as an opportunistic organism in a compromised host (101). Blood-borne pulmonary infection from intravenous drug abuse has been recorded (110).

Formerly most often a primary pathogen, *Nocardia* now behaves chiefly as an opportunist among a vast array of debilitating diseases, particularly lymphoreticular neoplasms, chronic pulmonary disorders (e.g., alveolar proteinosis), and almost any situation requiring prolonged corticosteroid therapy (14,39,92). Underlying diseases include pemphigus, lupus, asthma, glomerulonephritis, Whipple's disease, vasculitis, Cushing's syndrome, cirrhosis, hemachromatosis, Goodpasture's syndrome, ulcerative colitis, bronchiectasis, bronchopulmonary sequestration, tuberculosis, anthracosilicosis, sarcoidosis, Paget's disease of bone, and even solid tumor malignancy (18,84,123). Individuals with dysgammaglobulinema and chronic granulomatous disease are also at risk (62,64,65), as are alcoholics and, notably, cardiac, renal, and liver transplant recipients (26,38,72,120). The increasing use of immunosuppressive therapy in other disorders such as collagen-vascular diseases can further expand the list of hypersusceptible host diseases (51). Most antecedent disorders display dysfunction of cell-mediated immunity (CMI), but immunoglobulin and leukocyte defects can also be preconditions (65,83). Rarely, *Nocardia* sp invade lung cavities and produce a "fungus-ball." Men outnumber women 3 : 1 (14). Most patients are between the ages of 21 and 50 years, but the age range is broad (3–83 years); infection can occur as early as 4 weeks of age (14,62,64).

Despite the pronounced cellular immunodeficiency associated with HIV infection and AIDS, a relatively modest number of cases of nocardiosis have been reported, to date, among these patients, although the incidence of nocardiosis as a complication of AIDS could well be obscured or underreported, for a variety of reasons, including the common use of trimethoprim-sulfamethoxazole (TMP-SMX) as prophylaxis for and treatment of *P. carinii* pneumonia, and the use of sulfadiazine for treatment of toxoplasmosis (63,69). Nocardiosis in HIV-infected patients typically occurs as an indolent process in the presence of advanced immunodeficiency and is usually disseminated at the time of diagnosis. As might be expected, there is a high incidence of adverse reactions to sulfonamide-containing drugs. Consideration must be given to lifelong maintenance suppressive therapy (63).

There is no evidence for animal-to-man or man-to-man transmission, although reported case clusters suggest the latter possibility (27,107). Nosocomial cases, not clustered, have been recognized (7,83,92). An outbreak in a renal transplant unit found the "epidemic strain" in the dust and air, suggesting the possible need for respiratory isolation for some immunocompromised patients (61,107). Other localized outbreaks support nosocomial acquisition, although "epidemic strains" were less certain (7,56,94). Plasmid analysis is useful in epidemiologic evaluations of outbreaks of nocardiosis (107), or in recurrences in an individual case (65). The role of prophylactic TMP-SMX for the first year after organ transplantation remains to be evaluated in those transplant centers experiencing excess cases of nocardiosis (26).

CLINICAL AND LABORATORY FEATURES

Nocardiosis, an acute, subacute, or chronic suppurative pulmonary infection, most commonly mimics tuberculosis, bronchogenic carcinoma, or lung abscess, but it should also be suspected in high-risk patients when soft-tissue swellings or abscesses and/or signs of brain tumor or abscess develop in conjunction with a current or recent chronic or subacute pulmonary infection. Typically a confluent bronchopneumonia progresses to complete consolidation; necrosis, cavitation, and pleural involvement with empyema are common. Between 25 and 50% of patients have either pleural thickening or pleural fluid at the time of presentation. Clinical findings are nonspecific: anorexia, weight loss, cough, pleurisy, dyspnea, and occasionally hemoptysis (28), particularly from large cavities. Untreated, chronic pulmonary nocardiosis behaves much like tuberculosis, except lower lobe involvement is more common, but the pulmonary infection can also clear spontaneously and therefore obscure the source of subsequent metastatic infection.

Less common clinical presentations include tracheitis, bronchitis, pleuropulmonary fistula, pericarditis (87), endocarditis (natural and prosthetic valves), mediastinitis with superior vena cava obstruction, and a disseminated miliary picture with diffuse organ abscesses (28). Subcutaneous abscesses, single or multiple, generally lack the induration and fistulous tendency of actinomycosis. Vasculitic lesions have been noted and, together with necrotizing pulmonary lesions, can mimic Wegener's granulomatosis (43). Dissemination, via blood or lymphatic channels, can occur from inconspicuous pulmonary lesions (83). Positive blood cultures have been recorded, especially in patients receiving immunosuppressive therapy (39). Central nervous system involvement, seen in a third of cases, can dominate the clinical picture; it occurs more often in the course of disseminated infection. Brain abscess, often multiloculated, is common; meningitis is rare.

X-ray findings include fluffy infiltrates, consolidation, subpleural plaques, nodules (single or multiple), single or multiple abscesses, cavitary pneumonia, miliary lesions, pleural effusions and empyema, and even diffuse alveolar or interstitial infiltrates (10) mimicking adult respiratory distress syndrome (96); calcification is rare. Thick-walled cavities are yet another feature to confuse with malignancy (10). Extension to the chest wall can lead to sinus tract formation. The radiographic appearance of nocardiosis in AIDS patients is variable (71) and includes lobar or multilobar consolidation (52%), solitary masses (24%), reticulonodular infiltrates (33%), and pleural effusion (33%); cavitation is common (62%), and upper lobes are more commonly involved (71%).

The role of the humoral immune response to infection with *Nocardia* sp is not well understood. Serological techniques have never achieved diagnostic utility due to cross-reactions among *Nocardia* sp and also between *Mycobacteria* and *Streptomyces* sp (83). Complement-fixing antibody tests are sensitive, but false-positive reactions occur in leprosy and tuberculosis (98). A recently isolated 55 kilodalton (KDa) protein has apparent specificity for *N. asteroides,* and preliminary results with an enzyme immunoassay suggest antibody titers 1 : 256 or greater, are sensitive and specific, and are "not plagued by broad cross-reactivity to sera from patients infected with *M. tuberculosis*" (3). Further investigations with a similar, partially purified preparation—now 54 KDa by immunoaffinity chromatography—and Western blot measurements of antibody response, confirm the lack of cross-reactivity to sera from patients infected with *M. tuberculosis* and *M. leprae* (closely related to *Nocardia* sp), but did encounter false-positive reactions in sera from patients with mycetoma due to *Rhodococcus rhodochrous* (22). There are no skin tests for demonstrating delayed cutaneous hypersensitivity.

Nocardia sp are distributed widely in nature, so the significance of random sputum isolates continues to be debated (123). Whereas *Nocardia* sp can grow on Lowenstein-Jensen medium and Middlebrook 7H10 agar, it cannot be assumed that all *Nocardia* strains will survive sodium hydroxide decontamination of clinical specimens. Brief digestion (e.g., 4% NaOH for 4 hours) renders a small percentage of *Nocardia*-positive sputa falsely negative; overnight digestion is more uniformly lethal. In fact, even brief periods of exposure (30 min.) to NaOH, N-acetyl-L-cysteine (NAC), or benzalkonium chloride (Zephiran) with tri-sodium phosphate significantly reduce the number of viable *Nocardia* cells in standardized saline suspensions (79).

N. asteroides can be a saprophyte on the skin and in the upper respiratory tract (39,92). Milder infections in man include pharyngitis, bronchitis, or otitis media. Young et al. (123) withheld therapy in seven compromised patients (none on steroids) with fever or upper respiratory tract symptoms, all with sputum *Nocardia* isolates "of uncertain significance"; all recovered. Respiratory colonization occurs in patients with malignancy, tuberculosis, cystic fibrosis, asthma, bronchitis, and allergic aspergillosis (92). Bronchial obstruction or decreased bronchociliary clearance can predispose to colonization; unless steroids are also part of the picture, infection seldom occurs (92).

Pathology and Experimental Infection

Nocardiosis produces suppurative necrosis and abscesses; in the lung, often multiple confluent abscesses with little evidence of encapsulation. Solitary "coin" lesions, miliary patterns, or indolent progressive fibrosis resembling fibronodular tuberculosis can be seen. In contrast to the intense fibrosis of actinomycosis, untreated nocardiosis provokes a poor localizing tissue response, other than an occasional, partial wall of loose granulation tissue or rare bands of fibrous tissue incompletely encircling the lesion. Daughter abscesses are common; peribronchial lymphadenitis can be present. Extension to the pleura or chest wall leads to empyema, subcutaneous abscess, or bone involvement resembling actinomycosis; this pattern can be associated with fibrosis. Sulfur granules are not found in visceral nocardiosis but develop in cutaneous or subcutaneous (mycetoma) infections. *N. asteroides* in tissue section or pus appears as a beaded, branching filament when stained by Gram's method or the Brown-Brenn modification; it is not seen in H & E or PAS preparations.

Host resistance to infection with *N. asteroides* depends on functional phagocytic cells. Initially, neutrophils are mobilized to inhibit but not kill *Nocardia* (34), but they limit spread of infection until the development of cell-mediated immunity (CMI), triggered by "activated macrophages" (34,35,72) and induction of a T-cell population capable of direct lymphocyte-mediated toxicity to *N. asteroides* (34,35); both cells can kill *Nocardia in vitro.*

Immune T-cells clear virulent *Nocardia* from the lung and prevent dissemination (35). Neutrophils predominate in the lesions of nocardiosis, but infections progress unless antimicrobial agents are introduced or CMI takes over. In the presence of an inadequate CMI response, neutrophils might explain the characteristic indolence of human nocardiosis (35). The critical role of phagocyte function is illustrated by the occurrence of *N. asteroides* infection in chronic granulomatous disease, a congenital disorder in which neutrophils and macrophages are unable to generate a burst of oxidative metabolism during phagocytosis, resulting in impaired intracellular killing of catalase-positive bacteria such as *Nocardia* (64). However, *Nocardia* can also be relatively resistant to the metabolites of even a normal oxidative metabolic burst (34).

Filamentous log-phase organisms are more toxic to mouse macrophages and more virulent for mice than are the easily phagocytosed coccoid stationary-phase organisms (12,15), apparently because they resist phagocytosis more effectively (35). Enhanced virulence of log-phase cells correlates with the degree of inhibition of macrophage phagosome-lysosome fusion (29). The route of inoculation (intranasal, intravenous, intraperitoneal, or intracutaneous) also influences the virulence of, and host response to, different strains (15). Lysosomal acid phosphatase is an effective marker of the ability of macrophages to inhibit growth of and kill *N. asteroides;* macrophages isolated from different anatomical sites differ functionally from each other with respect to nocardicidal and acid phosphotase activities (20). Humoral immunity (antibody) can act in concert with the activated macrophage to resist the filamentous form of virulent *Nocardia,* the predominant cell in log-phase growth (12,20). High levels of intracytoplasmic catalase combined with surface-associated and secreted superoxide dismutase (SOD) appear to be mechanisms whereby *N. asteroides* avoids the oxidative killing mechanisms of PMNs; thus, catalase and SOD can represent two important virulence factors for nocardia (13).

Therapy

In the preantibiotic era, 75% of patients with nocardiosis died within 6 months of diagnosis. Currently, 90% of patients with isolated pleuropulmonary disease are cured following prompt administration of appropriate therapy. Sulfonamides are the drugs of choice, in conjunction with appropriate surgery (84). Studies in 1951 emphasized poor correlation of *in vitro* susceptibility testing with protection in experimentally infected mice (93), but this observation might no longer hold true

(50,52,113). Peabody and Seabury (84), in their classic review, recommended sulfadiazine (4–6 gm/day; up to 8–9 gm/day in severely ill patients, to maintain drug levels at 12–15 mg/DL) along with 2 gm/day of chloramphenicol, chlortetracycline, or streptomycin. Since that long-ago empiric recommendation, the value of and need for combined therapy remains an unsettled issue (72). Sulfisoxazole and triple-sulfonamide combinations are probably as effective as sulfadiazine; parenteral sulfonamide preparations are no longer available in this country. Treatment failures with sulfonamides or TMP-SMX, and allergic reactions to these compounds, particularly in patients with AIDS, mandate the routine susceptibility testing of all *Nocardia* isolates in an experienced reference laboratory. The long-recognized variable susceptibility patterns of *Nocardia* isolates may well be accounted for in terms of species differences (116). Routine beta-lactamase testing is no longer recommended, as essentially all strains of *N. asteroides* and *N. brasiliensis* produce the enzyme, and its presence is not predictive of beta-lactam susceptibility (115,117).

In vitro assay systems employing homogeneous nocardial suspensions and agar dilution plates overcome most of the technical difficulties that beset susceptibility testing in the past (6,75,93,115). Older studies suggested that as many as one-third of *Nocardia* isolates would not grow well on Mueller-Hinton agar, but these were primarily laboratory strains stored for years under oil in an inactive metabolic state (115). Recent clinical isolate strains grow 90% of the time; those 10% of isolates that do not grow adequately on unsupplemented Mueller-Hinton agar will grow when 5% sheep's blood is added, or chocolatized M-H agar is used. Disk-diffusion testing is now practical for most antibiotics (115). Many new drugs are available with good activity against *N. asteroides,* although susceptibility to these agents (amikacin, amoxicillin-clavulanic acid, imipenem, and the third-generation cephalosporins) is highly variable, and tests should be carried out only in an experienced reference laboratory (115). TMP-SMX disc testing readily separates sensitive from resistant strains (114). Among the older antimicrobial agents, ampicillin, erythromycin, and minocycline display excellent *in vitro* activity for many strains, but only amikacin and imipenem (among the newer agents tested) appear to be almost uniformly effective *in vitro* (48,49). Ampicillin-resistant strains are often susceptible to amoxicillin-clavulanic acid (47), and β-lactamase is the major mechanism of beta-lactam resistance in *N. brasiliensis* (112). That enzyme is highly susceptible to clavulanic acid, suggesting that the oral combination of amoxicillin and clavulanic acid (Augmentin) might have considerable potential for oral therapy of infections due to this species. However, acquired resistance to the combination, resulting from a mutational change affecting the inhibitor and active site(s) in the beta-lactamase, has already been documented in at least one isolate of *N. brasiliensis* (106). Synergy with erythromycin-ampicillin, ampicillin-sulfonamide, and ampicillin-cloxacillin combinations has been recorded in older studies (5,36). Based on a very small number of cases (90), cycloserine was once recommended as a substitute for or adjunct to sulfonamide therapy, although it exhibits little, if any, *in vitro* activity (30,75). Minocycline continues to accumulate published support for its use as an alternative agent in the treatment of pulmonary nocardiosis (86).

Among newer antimicrobial agents, amikacin demonstrates impressive *in vitro* activity against more than 90% of all strains tested and has already accumulated an impressive clinical record, especially in compromised patients (47,122). It was very effective in reducing mortality in a murine-intraperitoneal infection model (52,113). Several studies confirmed that imipenem and amikacin are the two most consistently active agents on a weight basis against *N. asteroides* (49). In a recent study of pulmonary nocardiosis in immunocompromised mice (given subcutaneous injections of cortisone acetate), amikacin and imipenem were the two most effective single agents tested for ability to reduce the number of CFU per gram of lung tissue (50). Whereas ceftriaxone reduced bacterial counts modestly, sulfadiazine and ciprofloxacin were ineffective. Combination therapy did not enhance the bactericidal activities of the agents tested. Many other new β-lactam antibiotics (cefotaxime, ceftriaxone, and cefuroxime) are active *in vitro* and can also have an ultimate role in therapy (30,47–49,52,67,108). The combinations of amikacin and imipenem with cefotaxime and TMP-SMX display synergy (fourfold or greater reduction in MICs of both drugs) for many strains. Imipenem and cefotaxime results in synergy in 92% of tests; the imipenem-amikacin combination is predominantly additive (49). Synergy is present in 80% of tests with amikacin–TMP-SMX (49). Other combinations shown to act synergistically against susceptible strains of *Nocardia* are amikacin plus cefuroxime and amikacin plus amoxillin-clavulanic acid (47).

TMP-SMX combinations have supplanted sulfonamides as the drugs of choice in the minds of some investigators (102,114), but treatment failures and late relapses have been recorded (42,104); too little TMP may be present in the commercial fixed-dose combination for optimal activity (17); thymidine-free media may be necessary to demonstrate synergy. Only two-thirds of *Nocardia* isolates display synergistic activity when carefully tested against TMP-SMX (1,17,115). The toxicity of the combination is greater than that of sulfonamides alone, especially in patients receiving myelosuppressive therapy (114). Sulfonamide therapy continues to be effective, even in compromised patients (99), but parenteral preparations are no longer available in this country. In patients with AIDS, where prolonged oral therapy with sulfamethoxazole is often needed, serious toxicity to that agent frequently requires alternative therapies (67,108). In general, fluoroquinolones exhibit poor *in vitro* activity against most *Nocardia* strains (19), but selective quinolone therapy can be effective in certain cases (121).

In vitro susceptibility testing of *Nocardia* sp also has taxonomic implications (21,116,117,118). Five major drug resistance patterns have now been identified within the *N. asteroides* group, and all may ultimately correlate with specific taxonomic groups (116,117). *N. farcinica* accounted for 19% of the 200 strains tested in one laboratory and were resistant to third-generation cephalosporins, ciprofloxacin, and all aminoglycosides except amikacin (117). *Nocardia nova* is also emerging as another group with a specific drug-resistance pattern (117).

Optimal duration of therapy is uncertain; treatment is often continued for months after apparent cure because of the pronounced tendency for relapse shortly after treatment is stopped or the appearance of metastatic abscesses (41). In one study of TMP-SMX efficacy, relapse occurred only rarely when patients were treated for longer than 3 months (114). In HIV-infected patients, continuous antinocardial therapy seems prudent.

The late appearance of a metastatic abscess, even during effective therapy, usually represents the evolution of a previously established metastatic infection and not the emergence of a resistant strain (39). Multiple opportunistic pathogens often simultaneously infect a compromised host; therefore, poor response, or the development of new pulmonary lesions, can herald the presence of a second pathogen, such as *M. tuberculosis.* cytomegalovirus. or *Pneumocystis carinii,* rather than resistant or progressive nocardiosis (72).

A retrospective analysis of 147 collected cases of nocardiosis (1945–1968) found increased mortality in patients (i) with acute infection (symptomatic <3 weeks), (ii) receiving corticosteroids or antineoplastic agents, (iii) with Cushing's disease, and (iv) with disseminated disease involving two or more noncontiguous organs or the nervous system (89). Otherwise healthy patients with pulmonary nocardiosis had a mortality rate of 15%. In patients with serious underlying disease but receiving no corticosteroids or antineoplastic agents, mortality in pulmonary nocardiosis was 20%. Corticosteroid therapy appeared to be a significant factor in mortality. Dissemination occurred as frequently in previously healthy patients as in other patient categories; corticosteroids did not influence the incidence of dissemination. Antinocardial therapy did not influence the appearance of extrapulmonary lesions. The issue of chemoprophylaxis for HIV-infected patients has not yet been effectively studied (63).

REFERENCES

1. Adams, H.G., Beeler, B.A., Wann, L.S., Chin, C.K., and Brooks, G.F. (1984): Synergistic action of trimethoprim and sulfamethoxazole for *Nocardia asteroides:* efficacious therapy in five patients. *Am. J. Med. Sci.,* 287:8–12.
2. Allworth, A.M., Ghosh, H.K., and Saltos, N. (1986): A case of *Actinomyces meyeri* pneumonia in a child. *Med. J. Australia.,* 145:33.
3. Angeles, A.M., and Sugar, A.M. (1987): Rapid diagnosis of nocardiosis with an enzyme immunoassay. *J. Infect. Dis.,* 155:292–296.
4. Ashdown, L. (1990): An improved screening technique for isolation of *Nocardia* species from sputum specimens. *Pathology,* 22:157–161.
5. Bach, M.C., Monaco, A.P., and Finland, M. (1973): Pulmonary nocardiosis: therapy with minocycline and with erythromycin plus ampicillin. *J.A.M.A.,* 224:1378–1381.
6. Bach, M.C., Sabath, L.D., and Finland, M. (1973): Susceptibility of *Nocardia asteroides* to 45 antimicrobial agents *in vitro. Antimicrob. Agents Chemother.,* 3:1–8.
7. Baddour, L.M., Baselski, V.S., Herr, M.J., Christensen, G.D., and Bisno, A.L. (1986): Nocardiosis in recipients of renal transplants: evidence for nosocomial acquisition. *Am. J. Infect. Control,* 14:214–219.
8. Baghdadlian, H., Sorger, S., Knowles, K., McNeil, M., and Brown, J. (1989): *Nocardia transvalensis* pneumonia in a child. *Pediatr. Infect. Dis. J.,* 8:470–471.
9. Balikian, J.P., Cheng, T.H., Costello, P., and Herman, P.G. (1978): Pulmonary actinomycosis. *Radiology,* 128:613–616.
10. Balikian, J.P., Herman, P.G., and Kopit, S. (1978): Pulmonary nocardiosis. *Radiology,* 126:569–573.
11. Bates, M., and Cruickshank, G. (1957): Thoracic actinomycosis. *Thorax,* 12:99–124.
12. Beaman, B.J. (1979): Interaction of *Nocardia asteroides* at different phases of growth with *in vitro*–maintained macrophages obtained from the lungs of normal and immunized rabbits. *Infect. Immun.,* 26:355–361.
13. Beaman, B.L., Black, C.M., Doughty, F., and Beaman, L. (1985): Role of superoxide dismutase and catalase as determinants of pathogenicity of *Nocardia asteroides:* importance in resistance to microbicidal activities of human polymorphonuclear neutrophils. *Infect. Immun.,* 47:135–141.
14. Beaman, B.L., Burnside, J., Edwards, B., and Causey, W. (1976): Nocardial infections in the United States. *J. Infect. Dis.,* 134:286–289.
15. Beaman, B.L., Maslan, S., Scates, S., and Rosen, J. (1980): Effect of route of inoculation on host resistance to nocardia. *Infect. Immun.,* 28:185–189.
16. Behbehani, M.J., Heeley, J.D., and Jordan, H.V. (1983): Comparative histopathology of lesions produced by *Actinomyces israelii, Actinomyces naeslundii,* and *Actinomyces viscosus* in mice. *Am. J. Pathol.,* 110:267–274.
17. Bennett, J.E., and Jennings, A.E. (1978): Factors influencing susceptibility of Nocardia species to trimethoprim-sulfamethoxazole. *Antimicrob. Agents Chemother.,* 13:624–627.
18. Berkey, P., and Bodey, G.P. (1989): Nocardial infection in patients with neoplastic disease. *Rev. Infect. Dis.,* 11:407–412.
19. Berkey, P., Moore, D., and Rolston, K. (1988): *In vitro* susceptibility of Nocardia species to newer antimicrobial agents. *Antimicrob. Agents Chemother.,* 32:1078–1079.
20. Black, C.M., Beaman, B.L., Donovan, R.M., and Goldstein, E. (1985): Intracellular acid phos-

photase content and ability of different macrophage populations to kill *Nocardia asteroides. Infect. Immun.,* 47:375–383.

21. Boiron, P., and Provost, F. (1988): In-vitro susceptibility testing of Nocardia spp and its taxonomic implication. *J. Antimicrob. Chemother.,* 22:623–629.

22. Boiron, P., and Provost, F. (1990): Use of partially purified 54-kiladalton antigen for diagnosis of nocardiosis by Western blot (Immunoblot) assay. *J. Clin. Micro.,* 28:328–331.

23. Broquetas, J., Aran, X., and Moreno, A. (1985): Pulmonary actinomycosis with endobronchial involvement. *Eur. J. Clin. Microbiol.,* 4:508.

24. Brown, J.R. (1973): Human actinomycosis: a study of 181 subjects. *Human Pathol.,* 4:319–330.

25. Butas, C.A., Read, S.E., Coleman, R.E., and Abramovitch, H. (1970): Disseminated actinomycosis. *Can. Med. Assoc. J.,* 103:1069–1071.

26. Chapman, S.W., and Wilson, J.P. (1990): Nocardiosis in transplant recipients. *Sem. Respir. Infect.,* 5:74–79.

27. Cox, F., and Hughes, W.T. (1975): Contagious and other aspects of nocardiosis in the compromised host. *Pediatrics,* 55:135–138.

28. Curry, W.A. (1980): Human nocardiosis: a clinical review with selected case reports. *Arch. Intern. Med.,* 140:818–826.

29. Davis-Scibienski, C., and Beaman, B.L. (1980): Interaction of *N. asteroides* with rabbit alveolar macrophages: effect of growth phase and viability on phagosome-lysosome fusion. *Infect. Immun.,* 29:24–29.

30. Dewsnup, D.H., and Wright, D.N. (1984): *In vitro* susceptibility of *Nocardia asteroides* to 25 antimicrobial agents. *Antimicrob. Agents Chemother.,* 25:165–167.

31. Drake, D.P., and Holt, R.J. (1976): Childhood actinomycosis. *Arch. Dis. Child,* 51:979–981.

32. Edelmann, M., Cullmann, W., Nowak, K.H., et al. (1987): Treatment of abdominothoracic actinomycosis with imipenem. *Eur. J. Clin. Micro.,* 6:194–195.

33. Fife, T.D., Finegold, S.M., and Grennan, T. (1991): Pericardial actinomycosis. *Rev. Infect. Dis.,* 13:120–126.

34. Filice, G.A., Beaman, B.L., Krick, J.A., and Remington, J.S. (1984): Defense against *Nocardia asteroides* in man. *Biol. Biochem. Biomed. Aspects Actinomycetes,* 107–118. Academic Press, New York.

35. Filice, G.A., and Niewoehner, D.E. (1987): Contribution of neutrophils and cell-mediated immunity to control of *Nocardia asteroides* in murine lungs. *J. Infect. Dis.,* 156:113–121.

36. Finland, M., Bach, M.C., Garner, C., and Gold, O. (1974): Synergistic action of ampicillin and erythromycin against *N. asteroides:* effect of time of incubation. *Antimicrob. Agents Chemother.,* 5:344–353.

37. Flynn, M.W., and Felson, B. (1970): The roentgen manifestations of thoracic actinomycosis. *Am. J. Roentgenol. Radium. Ther. Nucl. Med.,* 110:707–716.

38. Forbes, G.M., Harvey, F.A.H., Philpott-Howard, J.N., O'Grady, J.G., Jensen, R.D., Sahathevan, M., Casewell, M.W., and Williams, R. (1990): Nocardiosis in liver transplantation: variation in presentation, diagnosis and therapy. *J. Infect.,* 20:11–19.

39. Frazier, A.R., Rosenow, E.C., III, and Roberts, G.D. (1975): Nocardiosis: a review of 25 cases occurring during 24 months. *Mayo Clin. Proc.,* 50:657–663.

40. Garrod, L.P. (1952): The sensitivity of *Actinomyces israelii* to antibiotics. *Br. Med. J.,* 1:1263–1264.

41. Geiseler, P.J., and Andersen, B.R. (1979): Results of therapy in systemic nocardiosis. *Am. J. Med. Sci.,* 278:188–194.

42. Geiseler, P.J., Check, F., Lamothe, F., and Andersen, B.R. (1979): Failure of trimethoprim-sulfamethoxazole in invasive *Nocardia asteroides* infection. *Arch. Intern. Med.,* 139:355–356.

43. Gibb, W., and Williams, A. (1986): Nocardiosis mimicking Wegener's granulomatosis. *Scand. J. Infect. Dis.,* 18:583–585.

44. Georg, L.K. (1974): The agents of human actinomycosis. In: *Anaerobic Bacteria Role in Disease,* edited by A. Balows, R.M. DeHaan, V.R. Dowell, and L.B. Guze, pp. 237–256. Charles C. Thomas, Springfield, Ill.

45. Georg, L.K., Coleman, R.M., and Brown, J.M. (1968): Evaluation of an agar gel precipitin test for the serodiagnosis of actinomycosis. *J. Immunol.,* 100:1288–1292.

46. Gercencser, M.A., and Slack, J.M. (1976): Serological identification of Actinomyces using fluorescent antibody techniques. *J. Dent. Res.,* 55:A184–A191.

47. Goldstein, F.W., Hautefort, B., and Acar, J.F. (1987): Amikacin-containing regimens for treatment of nocardiosis in immunocompromised patients. *Eur. J. Clin. Microbiol.,* 7:198–200.

48. Gombert, M.E. (1982): Susceptibility of *Nocardia asteroides* to various antibiotics, including newer beta-lactams, trimethoprim-sulfamethoxazole, amikacin and n-formimidoyl thienamycin. *Antimicrob. Agents Chemother.,* 21:1011–1012.

49. Gombert, M.E., and Aulicino, T.M. (1983): Synergism of imipenem and amikacin in combination with other antibiotics against *Nocardia asteroides. Antimicrob. Agents Chemother.,* 24:810–814.

50. Gombert, M.E., Berkowitz, L.B., Aulicino, T.M., and DuBouchet, L. (1990): Therapy of pul-

monary nocardiosis in immunocompromised mice. *Antimicrob. Agents Chemother.*, 34:1766–1768.

51. Gruberg, L., Thaler, M., Rozenman, J., Bank, I., and Pras, M. (1991): *Nocardia asteroides* infection complicating rheumatoid arthritis. *J. Rheumatology*, 18:459–461.

52. Guttmann, L., Goldstein, F.W., Kitzis, M.S., Hautefort, B., Darmon, C., and Acar, J.R. (1983): Susceptibility of *Nocardia asteroides* to 46 antibiotics, including 22 beta-lactams. *Antimicrob. Agents Chemother.*, 23:248–251.

53. Hamer, D.H., Schwab, L.E., and Gray, R. (1992): Massive hemoptysis from thoracic actinomycosis successfully treated by embolization. *Chest*, 101:1442–1443.

54. Happonen, R.P., and Viander, M. (1982): Comparison of fluorescent antibody technique and conventional staining methods in diagnosis of cervicofacial actinomycosis. *J. Oral Pathol.*, 11:417–425.

55. Harrison, R.N., and Thomas, D.J.B. (1979): Acute actinomycotic empyema. *Thorax*, 34:406–407.

56. Hellyar, A.G. (1988): Experience with *Nocardia asteroides* in renal transplant recipients. *J. Hosp. Infect.*, 12:13–18.

57. Holm, P. (1950): Studies on the aetiology of human actinomycosis: I. The "other microbes" of actinomycosis and their importance. *Acta. Pathol. Microbiol. Scand.*, 27:736–751.

58. Holm, P. (1975): Seven cases of human nocardiosis caused by *Nocardia farcinica*. *Sabouraudia*, 13:161–169.

59. Holmberg, K. (1981): Immunodiagnosis of human actinomycosis. *Zentralblatt fur Backteriologie, Mikrobiologie und Hygiene. I. Abteilung* (Suppl. 11):259–261.

60. Holmberg, K., Nord, C.E., and Wadstrom, T. (1975): Serological studies of *Actinomyces israelii* by crossed immunoelectrophoresis: taxonomic and diagnostic applications. *Infect. Immun.*, 12:398–403.

61. Houang, E.T., Lovett, I.S., Thompson, F.D., Harrison, A.R., Joekes, A.M., and Goodfellow, M. (1980): *Nocardia asteroides* infection: a transmissible disease. *J. Hosp. Infect.*, 1:31–40.

62. Idriss, Z.H., Cunningham, R.J., and Wilfert, C.M. (1975): Nocardiosis in children: report of three cases and review of the literature. *Pediatrics*, 55:479–484.

63. Javaly, K., Horowitz, H.W., and Wormser, G.P. (1992): Nocardiosis in patients with immunodeficiency virus infection. *Medicine*, 71:128–138.

64. Johnston, H.C., Shigeoka, A.O., Hurley, D.C., and Pysher, T.J. (1989): Nocardia pneumonia in a neonate with chronic granulomatous disease. *Pediatr. Infect. Dis. J.*, 8:526–528.

65. Jonsson, S., Wallace, R.J., Jr., Hull, S.I., and Musher, D.M. (1986): Recurrent nocardia pneumonia in an adult with chronic granulomatous disease. *Am. Rev. Respir. Dis.*, 133:932–934.

66. Jordan, H.V., Kelly, D.M., and Heeley, J.D. (1984): Enhancement of experimental actinomycosis in mice by *Eikenella corrodens*. *Infect. Immun.*, 46:367–371.

67. Joshi, N., and Hamory, B.H. (1991): Drug-resistant *Nocardia asteroides* infection in a patient with acquired immunodeficiency syndrome. *South. Med. J.*, 84:1155–1156.

68. Kerr, E., Snell, H., Black, B.L., Storey, M., and Colby, W.D. (1992): Isolation of *Nocardia asteroides* from respiratory specimens by using selective buffered charcoal-yeast extract agar. *J. Clin. Micro.*, 30:1320–1322.

69. Kim, J., Minamoto, G.Y., and Grieco, M.H. (1991): Nocardial infection as a complication of AIDS: report of six cases and review. *Rev. Infect. Dis.*, 13:624–629.

70. King, J.W., and White, M.C. (1981): Pulmonary actinomycosis: rapid improvement with isoniazid and rifampin. *Arch. Int. Med.*, 141:1234–1235.

71. Kramer, M.R., and Uttamchandani, R.B. (1990): The radiographic appearance of pulmonary nocardiosis associated with AIDS. *Chest*, 98:382–385.

72. Krick, J.A., Stinson, E.B., and Remington, J.B. (1975): Nocardia infection in heart transplant patients. *Ann. Intern. Med.*, 82:18–26.

73. Lee, M., Berger, H.W., Fernandez, N.A., and Tawney, S. (1982): Endobronchial actinomycosis. *Mt. Sinai J. Med.*, 49:136–139.

74. Lerner, P.I. (1974): Susceptibility of pathogenic actinomycetes to antimicrobial compounds. *Antimicrob. Agents Chemother.*, 5:302–309.

75. Lerner, P.I., and Baum, G.L. (1973): Antimicrobial susceptibility of Nocardia species. *Antimicrob. Agents Chemother.*, 4:85–93.

76. Marty, H.U., and Wust, J. (1989): Disseminated actinomycosis caused by *Actinomyces meyerii*. *Infection*, 17:154–155.

77. McQuarrie, D.G., and Hall, W.H. (1968): Actinomycosis of the lung and chest wall. *Surgery*, 64:905–911.

78. Miller, A.R., Robertson, J.M., Nelson, R.J., Castro, C.A., and Dickman, P.S. (1989): Pleuropulmonary actinomycosis associated with a systemic-to-pulmonary artery fistula and contralateral metastatic back mass. *Ann. Thorac. Surg.*, 47:305–307.

79. Murray, P.R., Heeren, R.L., and Niles, A.C. (1987): Effect of decontamination procedures on recovery of *Nocardia* sp. *J. Clin. Micro.* 25:2010–2011.

80. Murray, P.R., Niles, A.C., and Heeren, R.L. (1988): Modified Thayer-Martin medium for recovery of Nocardia species from contaminated specimens. *J. Clin. Micro.,* 26:1219–1220.
81. Nelson, J.D., and Hermann, D.W. (1986): Oral penicillin therapy for thoracic actinomycosis. *Pediatr. Infect. Dis.,* 5:594–595.
82. Orloff, J.J., Fine, M.J., and Rihs, J.D. (1988): Acute cardiac tamponade due to cardiac actinomycosis. *Chest,* 93:661–663.
83. Palmer, D.L., Harvey, R.L., and Wheeler, J.K. (1974): Diagnostic and therapeutic considerations in *Nocardia asteroides* infection. *Medicine,* 53:391–401.
84. Peabody, J.W., and Seabury, J.H. (1960): Actinomycosis and nocardiosis. *Am. J. Med.,* 28:99–115.
85. Perlow, J.H., Wigton, T., Yordan, E.L., Graham, J., Wool, N., and Wilbanks, G.D. (1991): Disseminated pelvic actinomycosis presenting as metastatic carcinoma: association with the Progestasert IUD. *Rev. Infect. Dis.,* 13:1115–1119.
86. Petersen, E.A., Nash, M.L., Mammana, R.B., and Copeland, J.G. (1983): Minocycline treatment of pulmonary nocardiosis. *J.A.M.A.,* 250:930–932.
87. Poland, G.A., Jorgensen, C.R., and Sarosi, G.A. (1990): *Nocardia asteroides* pericarditis: report of a case and review of the literature. *Mayo Clin. Proc.,* 65:819–824.
88. Prather, J.R., Eastridge, C.E., Hughes, F.A., and McCaughan, J.J. (1970): Actinomycosis of the thorax. *Ann. Thorac. Surg.,* 9:307–312.
89. Present, C.A., Wiernik, P.H., and Serpick, A.A. (1973): Factors affecting survival in nocardiosis. *Am. Rev. Respir. Dis.,* 108:1444–1448.
90. Rhodes, E.R., Riley, H.D., and Muchmore, H.G. (1961): Cycloserine in the treatment of human nocardiosis. In: *Antimicrobial Agents and Chemotherapy,* edited by M. Finland and G.M. Savage, pp. 352–358. American Society for Microbiology. Braun-Brumfield, Detroit, Mich.
91. Rose, H.D., Varkey, B., and Kesavan Kutty, C.P. (1982): Thoracic actinomycosis caused by *Actinomyces meyerii. Am. Rev. Respir. Dis.,* 125:251–254.
92. Rosett, W., and Hodges, G.R. (1978): Recent experiences with nocardial infections. *Am. J. Med. Sci.,* 276:279–285.
93. Runyon, E.H. (1951): *Nocardia asteroides:* Studies of its pathogenicity and drug sensitivities. *J. Lab. Clin. Med.,* 37:713–719.
94. Sahathevan, M., Harvey, F.A.H., Forbes, G., O'Grady, J., Gimson, A., Bragman, S., Jensen, R., Philpott-Howard, J., Williams, R., and Casewell, M.W. (1991): Epidemiology, bacteriology and control of an outbreak of *Nocardia asteroides* infection on a liver unit. *J. Hosp. Infect.,* 18(Suppl. A):473–480.
95. Schaal, K.P., and Beaman, B.L. (1983): Clinical significance of actinomycetes. In: *The Biology of the Actinomycetes,* edited by M. Goodfellow, M. Mordarski, and S.T. Williams, pp. 389–424. Academic Press/Harcourt Brace Jovanovich, New York.
96. Schulman, L.L., and Enson, Y. (1987): Case report: *Nocardia pneumonitis* and the adult respiratory distress syndrome. *Am. J. Med. Sci.,* 293:315–319.
97. Schwarz, J., and Baum, G.L. (1970): Actinomycosis. *Sem. Roentgenol.,* 5:58–63.
98. Shainhouse, J.Z., Pier, A.C., and Stevens, D.A. (1978): Complement fixation antibody test for human nocardiosis. *J. Clin. Microbiol.,* 8:516–519.
99. Simpson, G.L., Stinson, E.B., Egger, M.J., and Remington, J.S. (1981): Nocardial infections in the immunocompromised host: a detailed study in a defined population. *Rev. Infect. Dis.,* 3:492–507.
100. Slade, P.R., Slesser, B.V., and Southgate, J. (1973): Thoracic actinomycosis. *Thorax,* 28:73–85.
101. Smego, R.A., and Gallis, H.A. (1984): The clinical spectrum of *Nocardia brasiliensis* infection in the United States. *Rev. Infect. Dis.,* 6:164–180.
102. Smego, R.A., Moeller, M.B., and Gallis, H.A. (1983): Trimethoprim-sulfamethoxazole therapy for nocardia infections. *Arch. Intern. Med.,* 143:711–718.
103. Spinola, S.M., Bell, R.A., and Henderson, F.W. (1981): Actinomycosis: a cause of pulmonary and mediastinal mass lesions in children. *Am. J. Dis. Child.,* 135:336–339.
104. Stamm, A.M., McFall, D.W., and Dismukes, W.E. (1983): Failure of sulfonamides and trimethoprim in the treatment of nocardiosis. *Arch. Intern. Med.,* 143:383–385.
105. Stein, C.A., Ernst, J., Stern, M., Daley, T.J., and Caspe, W.B. (1983): Thoracic actinomycosis in a recent tuberculin converter. *Pediatr. Infect. Dis.,* 2:52–55.
106. Steingrube, V.A., Wallace, R.J., Brown, B.A., Pang, Y., Zeluff, B., Steele, L.C., and Zhang, Y. (1991): Acquired resistance of *Nocardia brasiliensis* to clavulanic acid related to a change in β-lactamase following therapy with amoxicillin-clavulanic acid. *Antimicrob. Agents Chemother.,* 35:524–528.
107. Stevens, D.A., Pier, A.C., Beaman, B.L., Morozumi, P.A., Lovett, I.S., and Houang, E.T. (1981): Laboratory evaluation of an outbreak of nocardiosis in immunocompromised hosts. *Am. J. Med.,* 71:928–934.
108. Telzak, E.E., Hii, J., Polsky, B., Kiehn, T.E., and Armstrong, D. (1989): Nocardia infection in the acquired immunodeficiency syndrome. *Diagn. Microbiol. Infect. Dis.,* 12:517–519.

109. Tsukamura, M. (1982): Nocardiae that recently caused lung infection in Japan: *Nocardia asteroides* and *Nocardia farcinica. Microbiol. Immunol.,* 26:341–345.
110. Vanderstigel, M., Leclercq, R., Brun-Buisson, C., Schaeffer, A., and Duval, J. (1986): Bloodborne pulmonary infection with *Nocardia asteroides* in a heroin addict. *J. Clin. Microbiol.,* 23:175–176.
111. Waksman, S.A., and Henrici, A.T. (1943): The nomenclature and classification of the actinomycetes. *J. Bacteriol.,* 46:337–341.
112. Wallace, R.J., Nash, D.R., Johnson, W.K., Steele, L.C., and Steingrube, V.A. (1987): β-lactam resistance in *Nocardia brasiliensis* is mediated by β-lactam and reversed in the presence of clavulanic acid. *J. Infect. Dis.,* 156:959–966.
113. Wallace, R.J., Septimus, E.J., Musher, D.M., Berger, M.G., and Martin, R.R. (1979): Treatment of nocardiosis in mice: comparison of amikacin and sulfonamide. *J. Infect. Dis.,* 140:244–248.
114. Wallace, R.J., Septimus, E.J., Williams, T.W., Conklin, R.H., Satterwhite, T.K., Bushby, M.B., and Hollowell, D.C. (1982): Use of trimethoprim-sulfamethoxazole for treatment of infections due to *Nocardia. Rev. Infect. Dis.,* 4:315–325.
115. Wallace, R.J., and Steele, L.C. (1988): Susceptibility testing of *Nocardia* species for the clinical laboratory. *Diagn. Microbiol. Infect. Dis.,* 9:155–166.
116. Wallace, R.J., Steele, L.C., Sumter, G., and Smith, J.M. (1988): Antimicrobial susceptibility patterns of *Nocardia asteroides. Antimicrob. Agents Chemother.,* 32:1776–1779.
117. Wallace, R.J., Tsukamura, M., Brown, B.A., Brown, J., Steingrule, V.A., Zhang, Y., and Nash, D.R. (1990): Cefotaxime resistant *Nocardia asteroides* strains are isolates of the controversial species *Nocardia farcinica. J. Clin. Micro.,* 28:2726–2732.
118. Wallace, R.J., Wiss, K., Curvey, R., Vance, P.H., and Steadham, J. (1983): Differences among *Nocardia* sp. in susceptibility to aminoglycosides and beta-lactam antibiotics and their potential use in taxonomy. *Antimicrob. Agents Chemother.,* 23:19–21.
119. Webb, A.K., Howell, R., and Hickman, J.A. (1978): Thoracic actinomycosis presenting with peripheral skin lesions. *Thorax,* 33:818–819.
120. Wilson, J.P., Turner, H.R., Kirchner, K.A., and Chapman, S.W. (1989): Nocardial infections in renal transplant patients. *Medicine,* 68:38–57.
121. Yew, W.W., Wong, P.C., Kwan, S.y.L., Chan, C.Y., and Li, M.S.K. (1991): Two cases of *Nocardia asteroides* sternotomy infection treated with ofloxacin and a review of other active agents. *J. Infection,* 23:297–302.
122. Yogev, R., Greenslade, T., Firlit, C.F., and Lewy, P. (1980): Successful treatment of *Nocardia asteroides* infection with amikacin. *J. Pediatrics,* 96:771–773.
123. Young, L.S., Armstrong, D., Blevins, A., and Lieberman, P. (1971): *Nocardia asteroides* infection complicating neoplastic disease. *Am. J. Med.,* 50:356–367.

Respiratory Infections: Diagnosis and Management, 3d ed.,
edited by James E. Pennington.
Raven Press, Ltd., New York © 1994

31

Pulmonary Tuberculosis

Bonita T. Mangura and Lee B. Reichman

*Department of Medicine, University of Medicine and Dentistry of New Jersey,
65 Bergen Street, Newark, New Jersey 07107-3001*

EPIDEMIOLOGY

Tuberculosis (TB) remains the largest single cause of death from any infectious disease worldwide. One-third of the world's population is infected with the tubercle bacillus (24). In the United States, an annual decline in new cases was interrupted by an ascending trend between 1985 and 1992, marking the first substantial increase in TB morbidity since national reporting was implemented in 1953. As of 1992, 50,000 excess cases are expected over what would have occurred had the decline continued.

The highest incidence of TB cases occurs among the elderly, the urban underprivileged, the immunocompromised, and the foreign born (37). There has also been a shift in predominant incidence of TB cases from children to the adult productive age group of 25–44 years. This phenomenon in the U.S. now matches the proportion in developing countries where the greater proportion of cases (75%) occur in those less than 50 years old. In contrast, 80% of cases in industrialized nations occur in those over 50 years old, representing endogenous reactivation (24).

Co-infection with the HIV virus was recognized as early as 1985; a large portion of TB patients in currently reported cases are co-infected with HIV (37). Moreover, as early as 1990, a new threat arose as outbreaks of multidrug-resistant TB organisms were reported from Florida to New York (7,18).

TRANSMISSION AND PATHOGENESIS

Initial Infection (Primary)

Mycobacterium tuberculosis (MTB) is transmitted in the form of aerosolized droplet nuclei (<5 μm in diameter) from an untreated disease source to a susceptible host resulting in primary infection (4,38). Inhalation is the usual route of transmission. Infection involves the process of a localized, self-limited pneumonia usually occurring in the middle or lower lobes followed 2 to 10 weeks later by the development of a tubercle at the site of localization and by host skin sensitization to the tuberculin antigen. The latter two processes involve a complex interaction of host immune response to the bacillary antigen, namely, cellular mediated immunity (CMI) and delayed-type hypersensitivity (DTH). The host's response is generally successful in activating (e.g., lymphokines) the microbicidal activity of the macrophage. Digestive enzymes as well as reactive oxygen intermediates have been thought to be responsible for this function (13). However, more recently it has been proposed that a combination of factors working in concert with vitamins (calciferol) and cytokines (interferon gamma and tumor necrosis-factor alpha [TNF-α]) retard mycobacterial growth intracellularly (14).

CMI can be considered a beneficial response and DTH nonbeneficial. Factors that tip the balance between these two concurring processes are unclear and continue to be investigated. In the center of all these events is MTB. The mycobacteria is unique in its pathogenicity; its virulence lies in its cell wall (9) and ability in cord formation, its persistence, in its resilience to existing therapies (53).

Tuberculosis Disease

Disease is the progression of the localized pneumonia, possibly because of the failure of the host system to contain the infection (DTH). This results in a stage characterized by the presence of clinical symptoms and demonstration of the bacillus in the lung tissue or in the sputum. From the initial infection, clearance of the viable/ nonviable organism results in blood stream invasion (bacillemia) and localization at sites such as the apical portion (Simon's foci) of the lung. The nature of lung circulation allows clearance and perfusion of the bases better than the apex; thus middle and lower lobe distribution is unusual in the secondary stage. The foci can be dormant for many years. This is the site (apical) at which reactivation TB occurs.

Progression of infection to disease is highest (4–5%) during the first years after infection among the younger age group and specific "high-risk" groups listed in Table 31-1. For the TB-infected individual without risk factors, the risk of developing TB is 10% over his or her lifetime, the risk of disease diminishing with time. However, the untreated tuberculin-reactive cases provide the pool from which more than 90% of reactivation (endogenous) cases will arise. Less than 10% of all new TB cases are believed to be from newly acquired primary infection. This setting is in contrast to the HIV-infected individual. A tuberculin-reactive, HIV-infected person's risk can be at 8% or more per year (46).

TB has low infectivity among casual contacts but is higher among long-term household contacts or closed air system contacts (e.g., air-conditioning and recirculation of ventilation). The mucociliary blanket of the nasopharynx and bronchi is an effective defense in preventing larger clumps of bacilli to be transmitted to the deeper alveoli. In a series of experiments, Wells et al. (52) showed that single organisms transmitted aerodynamically caused more pulmonary TB among rabbits than coarse aerosolized aggregates of up to 10,000 bacilli. Larger aggregates impact on the upper airways and are cleared by the mucociliary blanket. Factors enhancing transmission among human contacts are (i) prolonged contact with an untreated open cavitary case, (ii) poor ventilation such as in a closed system of air recirculation, and (iii) high-velocity activities generating jet moist air, such as singing, coughing, and sneezing of the individual with cavitary disease or laryngeal TB. It has been suggested that a noninfected person has a 50% chance of acquiring infection by inhaling 10,000 cubic feet of air from a person with untreated disease. This usually represents 6 months of 8-hour daily exposure or 2 months of 24-hour daily exposure (1). Thus, persons with close and long-term exposure are at more substantial risk of new infection (1).

TABLE 31–1. *Definition of positive tuberculous infections according to size of turberculin reaction. Clinical picture for prophylaxis (+ risk factor and high incidence)*

+ >5 mm	+ >10 mm
Regardless of age	Regardless of age
Persons with HIV infection	Individuals with medical risk factors for TB[b]
Close contacts of known active TB case	Injection drug users
Persons with abnormal chest films likely to represent healed TB (untreated/ inadequately treated)[a]	Recent skin test converters (within 2 years' period)[c]
	For less than 35 years
	Staff and residents of long-term facilities (prisons, nursing homes, mental institutions, and health care facilities)
	Non–U.S.-born persons from endemic/high prevalence areas (e.g., Asia, Africa, Latin America)
	Indigent or low-income persons including high-risk minorities, especially Blacks, Hispanics, and Native Americans

[a]See text.
[b]Prolonged therapy with corticosteroids; immunosuppressive therapy, hematologic and reticuloen-dothelial disease (e.g., leukemia, Hodgkin's disease, diabetes mellitus, end-stage renal disease), intestinal bypass, post-gastrectomy, chronic malabsorption syndromes, carcinomas of the oropharynx and upper gastrointestinal tract, 10% or more below ideal body weight, and silicosis.
[c]BCG history does not alter guidelines; children, when they are close contacts, are prophylaxed even when PPD is negative at initial investigation; pregnant women are prophylaxed when they are recent converters after first trimester. (Modified from [8].)

Infectiousness can vary with individual cases. Sputum-smear-positive are more infectious than sputum-smear-negative patients and cavitary cases are more likely to be infectious than noncavitary cases.

TB control programs require, first and foremost, effective drug therapy of the host with TB disease and control of environment such as adequate ventilation exchanges or ultraviolet light irradiation (1) of shared air units. In addition, to reduce transmission of disease, covering the nose and mouth of the source case during activities such as coughing or sneezing is very strongly encouraged.

TB infection rates of close contacts have been relatively stable at 29%; other than close contacts are at 15%.

Pathology

The tubercle consists of an aggregation of cells, which might or might not contain the bacilli. At the periphery of this complex are fibroblasts, lymphocytes, and monocytes. Although organization, compactness, and maturity of the predominant cell (35) can help in identifying the mycobacterial granuloma, the histologic form cannot easily be distinguished from the granulomatous reactions resulting from sarcoid, fungal infection and from foreign body. The presence of central necrosis corresponds to the autolysis of the epithelioid center resulting from delayed-type hypersensitivity. The caseous content can liquefy, depending on the intensity of autolysis, and be subsequently expelled, resulting in a cavity. The expressed material is highly infectious until the patient is treated. In the immunosuppressed state of TB and AIDS a non–T-cell-mediated immune response has been proposed (20) as a mechanism for the absence of granuloma. Prior to the AIDS epidemic, a similar event of acute necrosis in the presence of a large number of acid-fast bacilli and intact macrophages was observed in an anergic case. The macrophages were immature and lymphocytes scanty. Because of the spectrum of immunologic response to the mycobacteria, a sequence of events has been suggested, with the succeeding event taking over as the predecessor event fails. Such a sequence is: lymphocytic invasion, granuloma formation, hypersensitivity activation, caseation necrosis, and anergy. In addition, as the trigger is set there is a point of no return in this sequence; beyond that point is immunologic enhancement and behind it is anergy (35).

Lymphohematogenous spread of the mycobacteria to other organs may result in miliary tuberculosis. The latter condition is associated with an x-ray pattern with the appearance of a "shower of millet seeds" over both lungs. Other sites of involvement in miliary tuberculosis include the central nervous system, liver, spleen, bone marrow, kidneys, fallopian tubes, and epididymis. Extrapulmonary TB occurs in high frequency among patients with AIDS or HIV infection.

CLINICAL MANIFESTATIONS

Individuals with infection as opposed to disease are usually completely asymptomatic. Discovery of infection often results from screening and follow-up of household contacts of a known, untreated disease source.

Vague, nonspecific symptoms are common in the individual with tuberculous disease. Most complaints consist of prolonged productive cough over 3 weeks, malaise, headache, and fever. Weight loss and night sweats are variably present. Hemoptysis is an uncommon symptom of TB. TB is responsible for 5–19% of all causes of hemoptysis (33). Conversely, when hemoptysis occurs in massive proportions, TB is the leading cause. With the advent of antituberculous chemotherapy, hemoptysis as a presenting symptom in those who have adequate therapy presents a challenge as to the true cause of bleeding (Rasmussen's aneurysm, aspergilloma, scar cancer, bronchiectasis, or true tuberculous recurrence). History of TB exposure and prior infection (as indicated + tuberculin) or clinical disease should be sought whenever TB is part of differential diagnosis. Recurrence, however, should never be presumed until full diagnostic workup has excluded other causes.

The physical examination of the individual with infection or disease is usually unremarkable. Exceptions to the latter situation occur in the presence of consolidation and pleural effusion; breath sounds can vary from bronchial to crackles at the site of pneumonia. In rare cases of endobronchial extension from direct involvement or lymph node rupture, a localized wheeze (19) can be heard. Prior to chemotherapy, right middle lobe collapse was commonly associated with TB adenopathy. Posttussive crackles have been described in some cases. Laboratory examinations are nonspecific. There can be a normochromic normocytic anemia, leukopenia, or leukemoid reaction and elevated erythrocyte sedimentation rate. Fifteen percent of TB cases present with disease at extrapulmonary sites as the major location of disease.

In the presence of HIV infection, this occurs in over 50%. Physical presentation will vary according to the organ involved. Pleural fluid can reveal an exudative effusion with elevated protein, lymphocytosis, low glucose, low pH, and elevated fluid-to-serum LDH ratio. Early in the course of TB pleural effusion, polymorphonuclear cells can predominate.

The most definitive and diagnostic test for tuberculosis is the isolation of *M. tuberculosis* by culture. Staining of the sputum smear can demonstrate acid-fast organism, but this does not assure the identity as *M. tuberculosis*. In addition to routine acid-fast stains, immunofluorescent stain is often useful. Direct instillation of a specimen into a (7H12) liquid Bactec culture system hastens the recovery of mycobacteria to 7 days, in contrast to 3 weeks on the 7H11 agar media (39). Although growth of MTB can take 3 to 8 weeks on the plain or selective agar media, gene probe technique reduces this time lag to several hours. Mycobacterial probes to DNA have excellent specificity and enhanced sensitivity when applied to mycobacterial RNA (32). Hybridization and use of the polymerase chain reaction (5) can amplify small numbers of mycobacteria but can ultimately prove to be overly sensitive.

Newer techniques like ELISA introduced in 1983 (43) to test sputum have some degree of sensitivity (40–60%) and specificity (80%). Determination of tuberculostearic acid (a component of mycobacterial cell wall) by gas chromatography and mass spectrometry is highly sensitive, but it is expensive as well as nonspecific because tuberculostearic acid is found in actinomycetes and other mycobacteria.

Single morning sputum specimens are preferred to pooling 24-hour specimens because it is more convenient to collect and transport spontaneous specimens and to quantify the bacilli by microscopic examination. Relative infectiousness can be estimated from the number of acid-fast organisms per high-power microscopic field on the smear as well as from the relative effectiveness of therapy ascertained by the reduction in the count (4+ to 3+ to 2+). Induction of sputum might be necessary in some cases by ultrasonic nebulization using heated, aerosolized hypertonic saline. Such induction must be done in a well-ventilated room. Transtracheal aspiration has been described for collection of specimen both percutaneously and endotracheally. Fiberoptic bronchoscopy should be reserved only to collect specimen unobtainable by usual means; when employed for localized infiltrates bronchoalveolar lavage (BAL) yields are likely to be positive (21). Miliary presentations of TB have lower positive yield by BAL than by transbronchial lung biopsy (49,51). BAL can cause extension and spread to the segment or lobe (28,41), so a brush smear or biopsy might be all that is necessary for endobronchial TB. Sputum induction as well as fiberoptic bronchoscopy generates coughing in a patient and can cause an undesirable dissemination of the bacilli. In a survey among graduating Pulmonary and Infectious Disease fellows of cities at risk for TB, there were far more Pulmonary fellows who converted their tuberculin tests than ID fellows. The important variable influencing conversion was bronchoscopy (27). In another hospital setting an outbreak of multidrug-resistant TB (MDRTB) occurred among patients with HIV, and tuberculin skin test conversion among health care workers was reported where pentamidine aerosol was performed in an HIV clinic (7,18). Strict adherence to proper air control and operator protection should be exercised, such as utilizing specially designed collection rooms, air filters in exhaust chambers, and ventilation with adequate air exchanges or ultraviolet light irradiation. Bacteriologic specimens must be handled carefully, in addition to labeling "induced" specimens. Watery appearance of induced sputum can mistakenly lead laboratory personnel to discard the specimen. One protective measure for the patient is covering nose and mouth with tissue while coughing.

Other Specimens

Sputum specimen is more desirable than a nasogastric specimen because saprophytic nontuberculous organisms in the stomach can give an initial false-positive smear for acid-fast bacilli. Depending on organ involvement, other sites and body fluids should be assessed, such as lymph nodes, liver, bone marrow, spinal fluid, pericardial fluid, and urinary tract, as potential sources of specimen. Blood (44,48) and stool cultures can be productive sources. In the patient with pleural effusion, a pleural biopsy will increase the yield of obtaining the diagnosis. Pleural fluid is sent for cell count, glucose, culture, LDH, pH, and protein. Pleural tissue can demonstrate granulomas and acid-fast organisms on staining. Sampling error can affect tissue biopsies; thus, if the first biopsy is nonproductive, a second and even third attempt should be tried. Microscopic examination combined with culture of the pleural tissue and fluid results in over a 75% diagnostic yield (25). Judicious handling of tissue specimens is required to increase the diagnostic yield, that is, specimens for culture must not be placed in formalin, whereas the specimen for pathologic examination should be. There are potential hazards for workers preparing frozen sections. Pathologists have reported conversion of their tuberculin tests by compressed gas freezing (aerosol generation) of lung nodules that turn out to be TB (15).

Skin Testing

Tuberculin testing is a major diagnostic tool in the diagnosis of tuberculous infection (12,34). The Mantoux test is the standard against which all other available techniques are judged. Other techniques are the multipuncture test and its variations, none of which deliver a precise amount of tuberculin; thus, results are difficult to standardize. Their usefulness has been limited to screening large populations, especially infants and children, but even in this situation the Mantoux test is highly preferable. In diagnostic work, the Mantoux technique should always be used. In children in whom TB is a real consideration, the Mantoux test should be used; Tine test can give a false-negative reaction.

In the Mantoux test 0.1 cc of 5 tuberculin units is injected intradermally on the forearm. Later, at 48 to 72 hours, the site is reexamined for reaction. A reaction of 5 mm or more induration is usually considered positive in individuals who are HIV infected, have contacts to active sputum-positive cases, or have abnormal chest x-rays consistent with TB. An induration of 10 mm or more is usually considered positive in others (see Table 31-1). Induration can be measured by approaching the medial and lateral edge of the reaction with a ballpoint pen. The distance between the two points at which the induration stops the rolling point is measured as the size of the reaction ($\rightarrow$ $\leftarrow$). Two similar points can be made above and below the reaction at a direction parallel to the forearm if desired (23).

Tuberculin reading is based on using standard strength 5 TU of purified protein derivative (PPD), Tween-stabilized tuberculin. First-strength (1 TU) PPD has not been standardized; second-strength PPD (250 TU), on the other hand, is so potent that it can give a large reaction from a cross-reacting, clinically insignificant, non-tuberculous mycobacterial infection (past or present). Skin test conversion is defined as an increase of 6 mm or more in reaction size from less than 10 mm to greater than 10 mm to the same strength of antigen.

Certain individuals with infection or disease do not produce positive reaction to tuberculin skin testing. Reasons for this false-negative reaction or anergy are impairment in T-cell function, viral illness, neoplastic disease, immunosuppressive therapy, HIV infection, severe malnutrition, and overwhelming disseminated disease. In addition, individuals without existing disease but who are in the early incubation period (in the presence of a positive contact history) can show a negative reaction. Elderly patients with infection can show a negative reaction at initial skin testing; a repeat skin test should be done within 10 days of the first to rule out the booster phenomenon. The booster effect is a negative first reaction to tuberculin and positive reaction on the second of a series of skin tests of as little as a week apart (17). The booster effect often represents old infection, whereas true conversion represents a newly acquired infection. If one tests personnel annually, an apparent conversion could be either a true (new) infection or the booster effect (old infection). This phenomenon can occur at any age but is most often seen in the elderly. If repeated skin testing is necessary, as in surveillance of health personnel, it might be advisable to carry out a two-step skin test. An initial tuberculin screening of negative reactors, the two-step skin test distinguishes better between a true conversion and a booster phenomenon (see Fig. 31-1). In Figure 31-1, situation A could represent boosting or true conversion (from 4 to 14 mm). By testing at 1 week, positive reaction (situation C) would be unlikely to represent new infection in 1 week (from 4 to 12 mm), so it is diagnostic of boosting (i.e., the subject likely had old infection). In situation B, the 1-week test was negative (2 mm). The test done at 1 year was positive (14 mm); thus, this would represent true (new) infection.

It must be remembered that although a positive Mantoux skin test confirms tuberculous infection, a negative reaction never rules out TB.

Chest Radiograph

Chest x-rays are important in the diagnostic workup of pulmonary TB. Although chest x-ray had previously been used to follow extent of disease and monitor re-

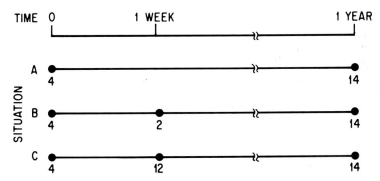

FIG. 31–1. Schema of possible serial skin testing situations and how two-step testing helps interpretation (see text).

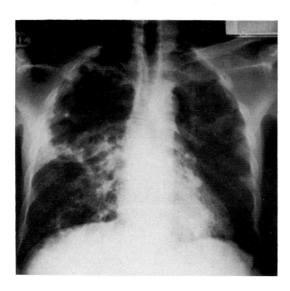

FIG. 31–2. Initial chest x-ray film of a 55-year-old severe diabetic, alcoholic, previously noncompliant patient prior to start of treatment.

sponse to therapy, such practice has proved to be costly and nonproductive and should be abandoned, as clinical measures and bacteriology are easier, cheaper, and more meaningful (26,40). A baseline and end-of-therapy chest x-ray is usually enough.

Posteroanterior and lateral projections are standard films for all cases at the start of diagnosis and treatment; when a change in the clinical course occurs, they can be repeated. Occasionally, lordotic view of the apices are necessary to delineate uncertain shadows in the collar area; the lordotic view can also provide a useful and better outline of shadows in the middle lobe. Oblique views are done when indicated.

Patterns of densities can be variable. The most common sites of involvement are the apical and posterior segments of the upper lobes and the superior segments of the lower lobes. Densities can range from a single nodule (tuberculoma) to clustered multiple nodules to a segmental infiltrate to a diffuse acinar infiltrate (as in tuberculous pneumonia). Ghon's complex refers to the presence of an enlarged or calcified node at the hilum ipsilateral to the site of primary infection in the middle lobe. Calcification and/or cavitation might be present in the densities described (Fig. 31-2). Tomography can still be useful in demonstrating cavitations and delineating mycetomas (fungus balls) within treated residual cavitations. Tuberculous cavities frequently appear empty; however, the cavities can fill up and develop a fluid level during hemoptysis and aspiration.

Computed tomograph (CT scan) of the chest is a very useful technique. Potential application in TB can be extended to complicated cases where better definition of structures is needed to plan for diagnostic or surgical interventions.

SPECIAL PROCEDURES

Fiberoptic bronchoscopy is usually not necessary to diagnose TB. When bronchoscopy is done, specimens obtained, such as bronchial aspirates or brush smears, should be collected for staining and culture of MTB. Aerosolization of mycobacteria during such procedure can be hazardous. Fiberoptic bronchoscopy has been used to localize sites of significant bleeding in both treated and untreated cases. When hemoptysis is massive, rigid bronchoscopy with the surgical team in the operating room might be advisable. Embolization of feeding vessels have been used to reduce bleeding in nonoperable cases (42).

Pleural biopsy can most often be done by the closed technique (Cope or Abrams needles) or, if necessary (rarely), by open surgical technique. In biopsy done of any suspected or unsuspected case of pulmonary or extrapulmonary TB, culture of tissue should be planned and carried out so that tissue is not inadvertently put in Formalin. Pleuroscopy to guide biopsy is currently being utilized in some centers.

Tuberculosis and Human Immune Deficiency Virus (HIV) Infection

HIV infection and AIDS are largely responsible for the resurgence of tuberculosis in U.S. cities where large increases in TB cases have been observed. Important risk factors include injection drug use, homosexuality, and birth in a pattern II country (heterosexual transmission of HIV). Pulmonary involvement is relatively unusual, whereas extrapulmonary involvement is frequent (40–75%). Extrapulmonary TB can concurrently occur with pulmonary involvement. The stage of TB in which the disease presents in the HIV infected is inversely related to the level of immunosuppression by the virus. Thus, at earlier and less severe levels of immunosuppression by HIV infection, TB presents in the traditional manner (as in immunocompetent individuals), such as reactivation pulmonary TB, preceding other infectious diseases (3). Conversely, at a later and more severe level of immunosuppression from HIV, the patient presents in a more primitive manner, such as miliary TB, lymphatic TB, and TB of middle and lower lobes of the lung. The latter situation can account for the better yield of blood cultures for MTB in AIDS (bacillemia of TB). Pulmonary TB in AIDS is indistinguishable from other infectious pulmonary diseases that affect the HIV+ population. *Pneumocystis carinii* pneumonia is an important differential in interstitial lung presentations. Depending on the locality (e.g., Florida, New Jersey), hilar adenopathy can be an important marker for granulomatous lung disease such as TB, but it might not be of help in the presence of multiple opportunistic infections. Delayed diagnosis has resulted in increased mortality (16,50). Some experts suggest empiric treatment in all HIV-infected patients in endemic areas in whom radiologic and clinical presentations are suggestive of TB. Although confirmative workup might be under way, without culture confirmation, it is difficult to follow or terminate therapy when complications arise from medications among patients so empirically treated.

The local response to a tuberculin skin test in an HIV-infected individual follows the same course as the systemic (see above) response. Prior to a diagnosis of AIDS, 71% of cases respond to tuberculin with induration, whereas only 33% respond after the diagnosis of AIDS (36). HIV infection strategically affects the same CD_4 (T-cells) and macrophage systems that are crucial in antimycobacterial defense (31). Anergy characterized by absence of response to DTH testing has also been associated with lower CD_4 counts, although the association is not consistent and low CD_4 does not predict anergy (29). Because of the extremely high risk of active TB in the HIV-seropositive injection drug user, prophylaxis for dual infection (HIV + and TB) has been recommended even for the anergic (PPD −) seropositive individual (22,47). The length of prophylaxis is controversial. Current recommendations are 12 months (see Table 31-1), and some groups consider lifetime coverage. 5 mm induration is considered a positive reaction for the HIV-seropositive individual (8). Clinical disease occurs very rapidly (less than 6 months) in AIDS.

Therapy for disease in the HIV infected consists of daily doses of 3 or 4 drugs (isoniazid, rifampin, pyrazinamide) for 2 months followed by isoniazid and rifampin for 6–7 months (total duration minimum 9 months) beyond documented culture conversion. If drug resistance or disseminated and CNS TB are suspected, ethambutol or streptomycin are added during the first 2 months. Therapy is extended to 12–18 months after culture conversion if either rifampin or isoniazid are not included in the latter phase of treatment. Extrapulmonary TB is treated in the same manner (2).

DISEASE TREATMENT

Preventive Therapy

The current preventive therapy regimen is 6–12 months of daily isoniazid (10 mg/kg up to 300 mg/day) by mouth. Table 31-1 enumerates the groups in whom prophylaxis for infection (PPD positive/x-ray negative) is indicated (8). As shown in the table, >5 mm is the cut-off for PPD reaction among adult close contacts, those with radiologic fibrotic lesions, and the HIV infected. Risk is defined as presence of HIV infection, contact exposure, recent conversion of skin test (within 2 years), abnormal chest x-ray, injection drug use, and specific medical indications described in footnotes of Table 31-1. Low-risk population when skin tested are considered for INH prophylaxis if PPD is more than 15 mm. 10 or 15 mm cut-off can be used in low-risk population depending on the relative prevalence of MTB. Generally, a person's risk of developing TB disease is weighed against his or her risk of INH toxicity (11). The risk of hepatic injury occurs only during the period of treatment, whereas the benefit of treatment is lifelong. The objective of preventive therapy is reduction in the actual bacterial population of "healed" or radiologically unseen lesions. PPD-reactive fibrotic lesions consistent with untreated old TB and silicosis are currently treated with a single (INH) regimen for 6 months (from Table 31-1) (2,8). However, there are recommendations suggesting full antituberculosis (3–4 drugs) regimen for 4 months in some of these patients.

Baseline clinical interview and laboratory tests to include serum aminotransferase, bilirubin (for INH), creatinine (aminoglycoside), uric acid (pyrazinamide), complete blood count, and platelet count should be drawn to screen patients before starting therapy. Monthly monitoring of symptoms for adverse drug reactions is recommended. Isoniazid is discontinued when there is intolerance and aminotransferase levels are 5 times baseline. Persons over 35 years of age and especially the elderly should be carefully monitored. Aminotransferase levels should be done only when symptoms arise. Isoniazid should be promptly discontinued when gastrointestinal symptoms occur in the elderly.

Alternative forms of prophylaxis are not backed by sufficient clinical data for efficacy, although they can be effective. Studies are ongoing.

For close contacts of isoniazid-(I) resistant cases, rifampin (R) is recommended for 6 months in adults, 9 months in children. Combination with ethambutol (EMB) can be used. For those with resistance to both isoniazid and rifampin, the current recommendation is to observe and not treat; high-risk groups such as the immunosuppressed and HIV infected might be covered for 6 months with ethambutol and pyrazinamide (PZA). If a patient's isolate is resistant to I, R, and EMB, then PZA and a quinolone (ofloxacin or ciprofloxacin) might be given for 6 months.

The protection with BCG is variable, and application rarely causes serious complications. It is contraindicated in those with reduced immunity. It is individually recommended (case by case) in the U.S. in infants and children with negative tuberculin who are at high risk of close contact to untreated or ineffectively treated source cases and in those without access to health care. BCG is protective among infants and children from disseminating forms of TB in some studies.

Antituberculosis therapy consists of using two or more drugs at the initiation of therapy. The basis for this intensive approach is the presence of a large number of mycobacteria in tuberculous lesions which favors the emergence of mutant strains resistant to a single drug. In cavitary TB, a cavity of more than 2 cm in size can harbor more than 10^8 bacilli. Mutant strains resistant to isoniazid occur at a frequency of one bacilli in 10^6 (1 in 10^6), and for rifampin the frequency is one mutant in 10^8 bacilli. If both drugs are used, resistant strains would occur at only one in 10^{14}, reducing the likelihood of survival of drug-resistant strains. The emergence of multidrug-resistant strains in the U.S. is initially a result of inappropriate or incomplete therapy and nonadherence. More important, a breakdown in established systems of TB health care follow-up (6) probably contributed to the problem.

Indications for hospitalization in drug-susceptible cases are usually clear-cut; it is rarely an emergency except for tuberculous meningitis, pericarditis, and fulminant pneumonia. The majority of cases can be handled for diagnostic workup and initiation of therapy on an outpatient basis. Isolation of a patient from the family setting is not necessary; however, close household contacts should be screened, monitored with skin testing, and followed up for preventive or disease therapy. Hospitalization should be reserved for severely symptomatic patients who require nursing care.

Respiratory isolation is considered for those with cavitary disease and active coughing. For the HIV infected in an endemic area (TB) in whom complex pulmonary processes can occur together, it has been difficult to triage for bed placement. The most crucial step is to rapidly obtain sputum for AFB staining so the patient does not unnecessarily stay isolated or receive empiric treatment to "rule out TB." Extrapulmonary TB patients are noninfectious unless there is concomitant pulmonary involvement. Although sputum smears can continue to be positive for bacilli for at least 2 months during adequate therapy and cultures for up to 3–4 months, it is unknown when precisely a patient ceases to be infectious while on therapy. With the advent of multidrug resistance, it is important to document effectiveness of therapeutic regimens by diminution of organisms on smear prior to releasing the patient from isolation.

Disease Treatment

1. *6-Month Regimen.* For patients with drug-susceptible organisms, a 6-month regimen consists of initial 2 months of isoniazid, rifampin, and pyrazinamide followed by the continuation phase with isoniazid and rifampin for 4 months. Ethambutol or streptomycin (in children) is added in the initial phase if there is suspicion of (i) drug resistance or (ii) miliary or disseminated and (iii) central nervous system involvement. This regimen applies to HIV- and non-HIV-infected patients. In case

of nonconversion of cultures after the initial 2 months of therapy, the 2-drug regimen of the continuation phase should be extended 6–7 months *after* cultures are negative (2,3). When either rifampin or isoniazid are not part of the regimen, treatment should extend to 18 months total duration or 12 months *after* cultures are negative, whichever is longer. Individual assessment should dictate length of therapy, especially if there is slow therapeutic response despite adequate coverage during the continuation phase.

Extrapulmonary TB is treated in a similar manner and regimen as pulmonary TB, except in children (see below).

2. *9-Month Regimen.* The 9-month regimen is an alternative regimen consisting of isoniazid 300 mg and rifampin 600 mg once daily for those who are unable to take pyrazinamide. Ethambutol or streptomycin (in children) should be added until susceptibility testing shows sensitivity to isoniazid and rifampin. If INH resistance is present, rifampin and ethambutol are continued for a minimum of 12–18 months. The 9-month regimen is clearly inferior as it requires longer treatment and does not adequately protect against resistance to one of the drugs.

Dosages of individual drugs are noted in Tables 31-2 and 31-3. Streptomycin has been used with success as a third drug in initial therapy for the first 2–6 months. A daily dose of 1 g (15–30 mg/kg) can be employed; both ototoxicity and nephrotoxicity are dose-dependent. Employing an injectable drug, such as streptomycin, in a regimen has been used as a "leash" with success to enhance compliance or adherence (30). Intermittent therapy with larger dosing has also been employed to enhance adherence. Currently, directly observed therapy is recommended for all (adults and children), except where patient adherence is well known. The other second-line drugs, capreomycin, kanamycin, ethionamide, cycloserine, and paraaminosalicylic acid are rarely used except in cases of drug resistance or toxicity to the first-line drugs. Such therapy should be given by experienced TB practitioners.

Amikacin, quinolones, rifabutin, rifapentene and clofazimine are potentially effective drugs against TB. However, currently they are not licensed for the treatment of TB in the United States because none of these drugs have been tested in randomized trials for treatment or prophylaxis of TB.

Children

For extrapulmonary TB such as miliary TB, CNS TB, and bone and joint TB in children, duration of therapy is 12 months. There is limited information on whether or not short-course (6–9 month) therapy is effective in children in this setting.

Corticosteroids are indicated for both adults and children in constricting tuberculous pericarditis and tuberculous meningitis. Corticosteroids are particularly important in reducing the neurologic consequences of meningitis, especially when given early in the disease.

TABLE 31–2. *First-line drugs in the initial treatment of tuberculosis*

Drug[a]	Dose — Daily	Dose — Intermittent (twice weekly)	Side effects	Monitoring	Remarks
Isoniazid[b]	5–10 mg/kg up to 300 mg p.o. or i.m.	15 mg/kg p.o. or i.m.	Peripheral neuritis, hepatitis, hypersensitivity	SGOT/SGPT (not routine)	Bactericidal, good for short course
Rifampin[b]	10–20 mg/kg p.o. up to 600 mg	600 mg	Hepatitis, febrile reaction, purpura (rare)	SGOT/SGPT (not routine)	Bactericidal; good for short course; orange urine color benign
Pyrazinamide[b]	15–30 mg/kg up to 2 g p.o.		Hyperuricemia, hepatotoxicity	Uric acid, SGOT/SGPT	Combination of pyrazinamide and aminoglycoside is bactericidal. Kills slowly growing persistent organisms
Streptomycin	15–30 mg/kg up to 1 g i.m.	1 g i.m.	Cranial nerve VIII damage, nephrotoxicity	Vestibular function, audiograms, BUN, creatinine	Use with caution in older patients or those with renal disease. i.m. dose advantage in supervised therapy
Ethambutol	15 mg/kg p.o.	50 mg/kg p.o.	Optic neuritis (reversible with discontinuation of drug; very rare at 15 mg/kg); skin rash	Red-green color, visual activity	Main effect to keep resistant organisms from emerging. Use with caution when eye testing is not feasible

[a] All drugs should be given in a single daily dose to enhance compliance and in fixed-dose combinations where available (e.g., isoniazid-rifampin). Check product labeling for detailed information on dose, contraindications, drug interaction, adverse reactions, and monitoring.
[b] Fixed-dose combination.

TABLE 31–3. *Second-line drugs for the treatment of tuberculosis*

Drug[a]	Daily dose	Side effects	Monitoring	Remarks
Capreomycin	15–30 mg/kg up to 1 g i.m.	Cranial nerve VIII damage, nephrotoxicity	Vestibular function, audiograms, BUN, creatinine	Use with caution in older patients, or those with renal disease, i.m. dose advantage in directly observed therapy
Kanamycin	15–30 mg/kg up to 1 g i.m.	Cranial nerve VIII damage, nephrotoxicity, vestibular toxicity (rare)	Vestibular function, audiograms, BUN, creatinine	Use with caution in older patients, or those with renal disease
Ethionamide	15–30 mg/kg up to 1 g p.o.	Gastrointestinal hepatotoxicity, hypersensitivity	SGOT/SGPT	Divided or hour-of-sleep dose can help gastrointestinal side effects
Para-aminosalicylic acid	150 mg/kg up to 12 g p.o.	Gastrointestinal hypersensitivity, hepatotoxicity, sodium load	SGOT/SGPT	Gastrointestinal side effects very frequent, (50%), making cooperation difficult. Rarely used
Cycloserine	10–20 mg/kg up to 1 g p.o.	Psychosis, personality changes, convulsions, rash	Psychologic testing	Very difficult drug to use. Side effects can be blocked by pyridoxine, ataractic agents, or anticonvulsant drugs

[a]All drugs should be given in a single daily dose to enhance compliance if possible.
[b]Check product labeling for detailed information on dose, contraindications, drug interaction, adverse reactions, and monitoring.

Pregnancy and Lactation

The recommended regimen for pregnant women with TB is isoniazid and rifampin; ethambutol is added if primary isoniazid resistance is suspected. All three drugs cross the placenta and have not been shown to be teratogenic. Breast feeding is not discouraged because levels of the anti-TB medications in breast milk are not enough to cause toxicity. These same levels, moreover, are not adequate to treat TB disease or infection in the infant. Separation of a mother with current disease from her newborn has been recommended until the mother is assessed as noncontagious. The newborn is prophylaxed and monitored with repeat skin testing. In case of a nonadherent mother with active pulmonary TB, BCG has been advocated for the infant.

Smear-Negative, Culture-Negative Pulmonary TB

If drug resistance is absent, a 4-month instead of 6-month antituberculosis drug regimen can be used. Persons with silicosis who are PPD positive and sputum culture negative can receive a 4-month antituberculosis drug regimen. However, current recommendations are for single INH therapy. This 4-month antituberculosis regimen is still under consideration.

Progress of Therapy

Patients on chemotherapy should be followed and supplied with medications (or prescription) on a monthly basis. Symptoms and sputum smears should be monitored. True compliance is reflected by the diminishing number of organisms on smears. Serial chest roentgenograms are unnecessary. Patients can return to work as soon as symptoms subside, usually within less than one month.

Directly Administered Therapy

Directly administered therapy is a program usually devised for the poorly compliant (adherent) group of patients, although it is usually impossible to determine which patients are among the 50% of all patients who are poor compliers. Adherence is not related to age, race, sex, or socioeconomic status. Three or four drugs are given daily for the initial treatment period of 2 months. This is then followed by larger dose, two-drug regimens on a twice- or thrice-a-week basis if the patient's isolate is susceptible to the medications. The twice-a-week therapy is not adequate if the patient misses a visit; the thrice-a-week therapy allows for a once-a-week missed visit so that at the end of the treatment period the patient is still effectively treated. Whereas the isoniazid-rifampin combination would be effective in 9 months, a full 18-month period is advised if isoniazid-streptomycin or isoniazid-ethambutol combinations are used. Two-drug combinations should almost *never* be used because of the specter of resistance. An injectable drug provides a "leash" to the nonadherent patient, enhancing compliance. It is our practice in very recalcitrant patients to give 5-times-weekly dosage, allowing even more flexibility in missed appointments (see Figs. 31-2 and 31-3).

Treatment failure is defined as failure to convert culture-positive sputums after 5–6 months of treatment. Relapse is defined as occurrence of TB after completion of

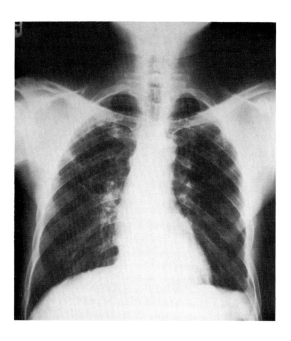

FIG. 31–3. Follow-up film of patient in Fig. 31–2 after 6 months' outpatient supervised treatment with prescribed 5-times-weekly streptomycin (the "leash") and daily isoniazid-rifampin combination capsules (patient's average clinic attendance was twice weekly).

regimen containing isoniazid and rifampin (organisms were susceptible to I & R at the start of therapy).

Known causes for treatment failures are poor patient adherence and inappropriate drug therapy. Drug-resistant organisms are likely to occur in patients who have been treated previously and experience reappearance of disease. Primary drug resistance is less than 4% for each drug except in areas of known high levels of drug resistance.

Treatment failure should be suspected if (i) the patient remains symptomatic, (ii) the sputum cultures do not revert in 3 to 4 months despite adequate therapy, and (iii) the chest roentgenogram shows progression of disease. New patients with prior histories of antituberculous drug treatment should be interviewed closely regarding the duration, type, and frequency of previous treatment. Old records from previous treatment programs should be obtained to determine exactly which drugs were used by the patient and for how long. Susceptibility studies can be included in those past records that could be vital or contributory to management of these patients.

Drug susceptibility studies should be done on all retreatment cases before initiation of a retreatment program. There is sometimes a delay before culture reports are returned, so therapy can be started after specimens have been obtained. Two courses of action can be taken: (i) initiate the same previous combination, not adding any new drug to the regimen until culture and susceptibility patterns return; or (ii) in addition to the old regimen, start at least two new drugs that the patient has never had in the previous treatment. The first course can be used, especially in treatment failures, where the interval from start of therapy has been short (as in patients who voluntarily discontinued their treatment after 2 months). Patients who have absconded from isoniazid-rifampin regimens are usually drug susceptible.

Multidrug-Resistant Tuberculosis

Resistance to antimycobacterial drugs can be primary or secondary. Initial or primary resistance refers to patients who have not had previous treatment; secondary refers to patients who have been treated in the past. Poor treatment programs enable the development of resistant strains in inadequately treated patients and secondary resistance ensues; these resistant organisms can then be transmitted to a new contact, and the organisms can occur in a "primary" setting. In the past, primary resistance to isoniazid occurred in <4% in the United States. After the recent outbreak of multidrug-resistant organisms, resistance to two to four drugs has been observed (18). At least two antimycobacterial drugs with known organism susceptibility should be used until bacteriologic conversion, followed by an additional 12 months of therapy using the two-drug regimen after sputum conversion is observed. A total of up to 24 months of empiric therapy has been recommended. It is advisable that before all therapy is started (i) drug susceptibility of the source case be known if the new patient is a contact; (ii) drug resistance patterns of the U.S. cities or countries of origin be identified; and, most especially, (iii) drug resistance patterns be identified for hospitals (if in the U.S.) where the patient has been located. Patients with suspected TB should be isolated. They should not be removed from isolation until there is evidence (diminished cough, fewer organisms on smear, clinical response) that the antibiotics are working against the patient's organisms.

Drug resistance does not occur if patients take multiple drugs as prescribed. Currently available fixed-dose combinations of isoniazid plus rifampin ensure that patients cannot take either drug without the other. Fixed-dose combinations with pyrazinamide are available internationally and will soon be available in the U.S. (10).

Bacteriologic studies should include niacin and catalase activity determination. *M. tuberculosis* resistant to isoniazid have impaired catalase activity, whereas nontuberculous mycobacteria, which have primary drug resistance, produce niacin poorly. Deletion of an MTB gene (katG) from the chromosome of two patient MTB isolates was associated with INH resistance. This gene encoded both catalase and peroxidase activity for MTB (53).

The most important thing to remember is that a single new, potentially effective drug should never be added alone to a failing or failed regimen unless the susceptibility patterns of the organisms are known. This, if adhered to, would keep retreatment cases to a minimum. In the presence of overwhelming disease and unavailability of historical data, five- to seven-drug regimens might be necessary with modification as indicated by the acquisition of new information.

TB is a very straightforward, relatively easy condition to treat. If the guidelines suggested in this chapter were adhered to, its incidence would diminish markedly. Unfortunately, physicians' own compliance to new guidelines and therapy often match their patients' (45).

REFERENCES

1. ATS, and CDC. (1992): Control of tuberculosis in the U.S. *Am. Rev. Respir. Dis.,* 146(6):1623–1633.
2. ATS, CDC. [Official statement] (1994): Treatment of tuberculosis and tuberculosis infection in adults and children. ATS, medical section of American Lung Association. *Am J. Resp. Crit. Care. Med.* 149:(4): (In press).
3. Barnes, P.F., Bloch, A.B., Davidson, P.T., and Snider, D.E. (1991): Tuberculosis in patients with human immunodeficiency virus infection. *N. Engl. J. Med.,* 324(23):1644–1650.
4. Bass, J.B., Farer, L.S., Hopewell, P.C., Jacobs, R.F., and Snider, D.E. (1990): American Thoracic Society diagnostic standards and classification of tuberculosis. *Am. Rev. Respir. Dis.,* 142:725–735.
5. Brisson-Noel, A., Gicquel, B., Lecossier, D., et al. (1989): Rapid diagnosis of tuberculosis by amplification of mycobacterial DNA in clinical samples. *Lancet,* 2:1069–1071.
6. Brudney, K., and Dobkin, J. (1991): Resurgent tuberculosis in New York City, human immuno-

deficiency virus, homelessness and the decline of tuberculosis control programs. *Am. Rev. Respir. Dis.*, 144:745–749.

7. CDC. (1990): Nosocomial transmission of multidrug resistant tuberculosis to health-care workers and HIV infected patients in an urban hospital—Florida. *M.M.W.R.*, 39(40):718–722.

8. CDC, and ATS. (1991): *National Tuberculosis Training Initiative, Core Curriculum on Tuberculosis,* 2nd Edition, p. 31.

9. Chan, J., Fan, X.D., Hunder, S.W., Brennan, P.J., and Bloom, B.R. (1991): Lipoarabinomannan, a possible virulence factor involved in persistence of mycobacterium tuberculosis within macrophages. *Infect. Immun.*, 59(5):1755–1761.

10. Combs, D.L., O'Brien, R.J., and Geiter, L.F. (1990): USPHS tuberculosis short course chemotherapy trial 21: effectiveness, toxicity and acceptability. *Ann. Intern. Med.*, 112:397–406.

11. Comstock, G.W. (1986): Prevention of tuberculosis among tuberculin reactors: maximizing benefits, minimizing risks. *J.A.M.A.*, 256:2729–2735.

12. Comstock, G.W., Daniel, T.M., Snider, D.E., Edward, P.Q., Hopewell, P.C., and Vandiviere, H.M. (1981): The tuberculin skin test: an official statement of the American Thoracic Society and Centers for Disease Control. *Am. Rev. Respir. Dis.*, 124:356–363.

13. Dannenberg, A.M. (1989): Immune mechanisms in the pathogenesis of pulmonary tuberculosis. *Rev. Infect. Dis.*, 11(2):S369–S389.

14. Denis, M. (1991): Killing of mycobacterium tuberculosis within human monocytes: activation by cytokines and calcitriol. *Clin. Exp. Immuno.*, 84:200–206.

15. Duray, P.H., Flannery, B., and Brown, S. (1981): Tuberculosis infection from preparation of frozen sections. Correspondence. *N. Engl. J. Med.*, 305(3):167.

16. Ellner, J.J. (1990): Tuberculosis in the time of AIDS: the facts and the message. *Chest*, 98(5):1051–1052.

17. Farer, L.S., Thompson, N.J., Glassroth, J.C., and Snider, D.E. (1979): The booster phenomenon in serial tuberculin testing. *Am. Rev. Respir. Dis.*, 119:587–597.

18. Fischl, M.A., Uttamchandani, R.B., Daikos, G.L., et al. (1992): An outbreak of tuberculosis caused by multiple-drug-resistant tubercle bacilli among patients with HIV infection. *Ann. Intern. Med.*, 117:177–183.

19. Ip, S.M.M., So, S.Y., Lam, W.K., et al. (1986): Endobronchial tuberculosis revisited. *Chest,* 89:727–730.

20. Jagadha, V., Andavolu, R.H., and Huang, C.T. (1985): Granulomatous inflammation in the acquired immune deficiency syndrome. *Am. J. Clin. Pathol.*, 84:598–602.

21. Jett, J.R., Cortese, D.A., and Pines, D.E. (1981): The value of bronchoscopy in the diagnosis of mycobacterial disease. *Chest,* 80:575–578.

22. Jordan, T.J., Lewit, E.M., Montgomery, R.L., and Reichman, L.B. (1991): Isoniazid as preventive therapy in HIV-infected intravenous drug abusers (a decision analysis). *J.A.M.A.*, 265(22):2987–2991.

23. Jordan, T.J., Sunderam, G., Thomas, L., and Reichman, L.B. (1987): Comparison of tuberculin reaction size measurement by the pen method as compared to traditional palpation. *Chest,* 92:234–236.

24. Kochi, A. (1991): The global tuberculosis situation and the new control strategy of the World Health Organization. *Tubercle,* 72:1–6.

25. Levine, H., Metzger, W., Lacera, D., et al. (1970): Diagnosis of tuberculous pleurisy by culture of pleural biopsy specimen. *Arch. Intern. Med.*, 126:269–271.

26. Lordi, G.M., and Reichman, L.B. (1985): Tuberculosis: when not to order roentgenograms. *J.A.M.A.*, 253(12):1780–1781.

27. Malasky, C., Jordan, T., Potulski, F., and Reichman, L.B. (1990): Occupational tuberculous infections among pulmonary physicians in training. *Am. Rev. Respir. Dis.*, 142:505–507.

28. Mangura, B.T., Mangura, C.T., and Reichman, L.B. (1991): Tuberculosis and the atypical pneumonia syndrome. *Clin. Chest Med.*, 12(2):349–362.

29. Markowitz, N., Hansen, N.L., Wilcosky, T.C., et al. (1993): Tuberculin and anergy testing among HIV seropositive and HIV seronegative individuals. *Ann. Intern. Med.* 119:185–193.

30. McDonald, R.J., Memon, A.M., and Reichman, L.B. (1982): Successful supervised ambulatory management of tuberculosis treatment. *Ann. Intern. Med.*, 96:297–303.

31. Pantaleo, G., Graziosi, C., and Fauci, A.S. (1993): The immunopathogenesis of human immunodeficiency virus infection. *N. Engl. J. Med.*, 328(5):327–335.

32. Pao, C.C., Lin, S.S., Wu, S.Y., et al. (1988): The detection of mycobacterial DNA sequences in uncultured clinical specimens with cloned mycobacteria tuberculosis DNA as probes. *Tubercle,* 69:27–36.

33. Pursel, S.E., and Lindskag, G.E. (1961): A clinical evaluation of 105 patients examined consecutively on a thoracic surgical service. *Am. Rev. Respir. Dis.*, 84:329–336.

34. Reichman, L.B. (1979): Tuberculin skin testing: the state of the art. *Chest,* 76:764–777.

35. Ridley, D.S. (1983): The histopathological spectrum of the mycobacterioses. *In: Biology of Mycobacteria,* Vol. 2, edited by Ratledge, C. and Stanford, J., pp. 129–171. Academic Press, London.

36. Rieder, H.L., Cauthen, G.M., Block, A.B., et al. (1989): Tuberculosis and acquired immunodeficiency syndrome—Florida. *Arch. Intern. Med.,* 14:1268–1273.
37. Rieder, H.L., Cauthen, G.M., Kelly, G.D., Bloch, A.B., and Snider, D.E. (1989): Tuberculosis in the United States. *J.A.M.A.,* 262:385–389.
38. Riley, R. (1957): Aerial dissemination of tuberculosis. *Am. Rev. Tuberc. Pulmon. Dis.,* 76:931–941.
39. Roberts, G.D., Goodman, N.L., Heifets, L., et al. (1983): Evaluation of the BACTEC radioactive and drug susceptibility testing for mycobacterium tuberculosis for acid-fast smear positive specimens. *J. Clin. Microbiol.,* 18:689–696.
40. Robin, E.D., and Burke, C.M. (1986): Routine chest x-ray examinations. *Chest,* 90(2)1:258–262.
41. Rimmer, J., Gibson, P., and Bryant, D.H. (1988): Extension of pulmonary tuberculosis after fiberoptic bronchoscopy. *Tubercle,* 69:57–61.
42. Russoniello, M., McDonald, R.J., Chakravarty, M., et al. (1983): Successful nonoperative management of massive hemoptysis. *Am. Rev. Respir. Dis.,* 127(Suppl.):124.
43. Sada, E., Ruiz-Palacios, G.M., Vidal, Y.L., et al. (1983): Detection of mycobacterial antigens in cerebrospinal fluid of patients with tuberculous meningitis with enzyme-linked immunosorbent assay. *Lancet,* 2:651–652.
44. Saltzman, B.R., Motyl, M.R., Friedland, G.H., et al. (1986): Mycobacterium tuberculosis bacteremia in the acquired immunodeficiency syndrome. *J.A.M.A.,* 256:390–391.
45. Sbarbaro, J. (1981): The nature of man and physician (editorial). *Am. Rev. Respir. Dis.,* 123:147.
46. Selwyn, P.A., Hartel, D., Lewis, V.A., et al. (1989): A prospective study of the risk of tuberculosis among intravenous drug users with human immunodeficiency virus infection. *N. Engl. J. Med.,* 320:546–550.
47. Selwyn, P.A., Sckell, B.M., Alcabes, P., et al. (1992): High risk of active tuberculosis in HIV-infected drug users with cutaneous anergy. *J.A.M.A.,* 268(4):14–19.
48. Shafer, R.W., Goldberg, R., Sierra, M., and Glatz, A.E. (1989): Frequency of mycobacterium tuberculosis bacteremia in patients with tuberculosis in an area endemic for AIDS. *Am. Rev. Respir. Dis.,* 140:1611–1613.
49. Sharma, S.K., Pande, J.N., and Verma, K. (1988): Bronchoalveolar lavage (BAL) in miliary tuberculosis. *Tubercle,* 69:175–178.
50. Small, P.M., Schecter, G.F., Goodman, P.C., Sande, M.A., Chaisson, R.E., and Hopewell, P.C. (1991): Treatment of tuberculosis in patients with advanced human immunodeficiency virus infection. *N. Engl. J. Med.,* 324(5):289–294.
51. Sunderam, G., McDonald, R.J., Maniatis, T.J., and Reichman, L.B. (1986): Tuberculosis as a manifestation of the acquired immunodeficiency syndrome (AIDS). *J.A.M.A.,* 356:362–366.
52. Wells, W.F., Ratcliffe, H.L., and Crumb, C. (1948): On the mechanics of droplet nuclei infection. *Am. J. Hygiene,* 47:11–28.
53. Zhang, Y., Garcia, M.J., Lathigra, R., et al. (1992): Alterations in the superoxide dismutase gene of an isoniazid-resistant strain of mycobacterium tuberculosis. *Infect Immun.,* 60(6):2160–2165.

Respiratory Infections: Diagnosis and Management, 3d ed.,
edited by James E. Pennington.
Raven Press, Ltd., New York © 1994

32

Lung Disease Caused by Nontuberculous Mycobacteria

David E. Griffith and Richard J. Wallace, Jr.

Department of Medicine, University of Texas Health Center,
P.O. Box 2003, Tyler, Texas 75710

Traditionally, the most important human mycobacterial lung disease has been caused by *Mycobacterium tuberculosis*. A number of other mycobacterial species, however, are capable of producing lung disease in humans. Discussion of disease caused by these nontuberculous mycobacteria has been complicated by several factors. As a group, the species at issue have been labeled anonymous, unclassified, tuberculoid, atypical, environmental, opportunistic, nontuberculous, and MOTT (mycobacteria other than tuberculosis). No single term is ideal, and disagreement persists over which label is most suitable. We have previously encouraged the use of the term *environmental* to describe these organisms because it reflects the fact that the reservoir for these organisms is generally soil or water (22). The American Thoracic Society (ATS) has recently issued a statement in which *nontuberculous* is the preferred term (60). To conform with the ATS statement and to avoid further confusion, nontuberculous mycobacteria (NTM) will be used whenever these species are referred to collectively. The emphasis of this discussion, however, will be on individual species of NTM and their resulting pulmonary disease syndromes, rather than on NTM as a whole. Some of the confusion in the past has also been the result of efforts to group all NTM pulmonary disease syndromes together and then compare them as a group to disease caused by *M. tuberculosis*. This approach has only limited applicability, however, so that clinicians must know the basic elements and characteristics of each NTM associated with pulmonary disease.

Unfortunately, confusing nomenclature extends to specific NTM as well. For instance, within approximately the last 10 years, *M. chelonei* (subspecies *abscessus*) became *M. chelonae* (subspecies *abscessus*) which most recently became *M. abscessus* (32). Some of this confusion is unavoidable as the taxonomic and clinical studies of NTM intensify and evolve with recognition of new NTM pathogens.

There is, additionally, no good working clinical classification of NTM. More than 50 species of NTM are recognized, some since the late 19th century, although the importance of NTM as pathogens was not generally recognized until the 1950s. In 1954, Timpe and Runyon (56) classified the NTM into four groups according to their *in vitro* colony growth characteristics, including rate of growth, morphology, and pigmentation (Table 32-1). The Runyon classification was originally intended as an aid to rapidly identifying NTM. A microbiologist could, pending speciation, presump-

TABLE 32–1. *Runyon's classification of nontuberculous mycobacteria*

Group	Pulmonary pathogen	Colony growth characteristics
I		
Photochromogens	M. kansasii	Yellow colonies when exposed to light
	M. simiae	
II		
Scotochromogens	M. xenopi	Orange colonies whether or not exposed to light
	M. szulgai	
III		
Nonphotochromogens	M. avium complex	Little or no colony pigmentation
	M. malmoense	
IV		
Rapid growers	M. abscessus	Little or no colony pigmentation
	M. fortuitum	Growth of visible colonies in less than 7 days
	M. chelonae	

tively identify an NTM by its Runyon classification characteristics. A major limitation of the Runyon classification is that there is no correlation between mycobacterial growth characteristics and specific clinical NTM disease syndromes. Pulmonary pathogens occur in each Runyon group, and no clinical information about a specific isolate can be gleaned from the Runyon classification. Current use of commercial DNA probes by most laboratories now allows for one-day identification once colonies are visible on agar plates or in broth, so descriptive grouping is rapidly being replaced by species identification. Some familiarity with the Runyon classification is useful so that a clinician can presumptively identify a potential NTM pulmonary pathogen from preliminary culture results when DNA probes are not readily avail-

TABLE 32–2. *Classification of nontuberculous mycobacteria recovery from humans based on principal site of involvement*

Pulmonary disease	Lymphadenitis
M. avium complex	M. avium complex
M. kansasii	M. scrofulaceum
M. abscessus	M. fortuitum
M. xenopi	M. chelonae
M. szulgai	M. abscessus
M. malmoense	M. kansasii
M. simiae	

Disseminated disease	Cutaneous disease
M. avium complex	M. marinum
M. kansasii	M. fortuitum
M. abscessus	M. chelonae
M. chelonae	M. abscessus
M. hemophilum	M. ulcerans
M. fortuitum	M. avium complex
M. xenopi	M. kansasii
M. genavense	M. nonchromogenicum
	M. smegmatis

able. For instance, a clinician should be aware that the isolation from sputum of a Runyon Group I organism likely means *M. kansasii* in the appropriate clinical setting. Alternatively, knowing that a pigmented Group IV organism has been isolated suggests a contaminant rather than a true pathogen. Knowledge of mycobacterial growth characteristics can also reassure a clinician that an isolate is not *M. tuberculosis*. Because of the availability of DNA probes, it is likely the Runyon classification will soon be of historical interest only.

A more appropriate organization scheme for NTM based on the type of clinical disease an NTM species produces has been proposed by the ATS (60) (Table 32-2). Only a few NTM are commonly associated with pulmonary disease, so clinicians can and should be familiar with individual NTM disease syndromes.

EPIDEMIOLOGY

Because the NTM associated with pulmonary disease can be recovered from a variety of environmental sources, it is likely that these pathogens enter the human respiratory tract from the environment, although the exact mode of transmission is poorly understood. In one study, at least, one species of NTM was isolated from 86% of soil samples collected from the eastern United States (65); to date, there is no convincing evidence of animal-to-human or human-to-human transmission of NTM. Clusters or groupings of NTM pulmonary infection, even infections proved by DNA fingerprinting to be due to the same organism, at this point are believed to be related to a common source for the organism. Whatever the source, because many people are presumed exposed but few develop clinical disease, it is also likely that host susceptibility factors are very important in determining which individual will develop clinical NTM pulmonary disease. It is also not currently known whether NTM disease develops soon after infection or, like tuberculosis, develops after a period of latent infection.

M. avium complex (MAC) is probably the most ubiquitous NTM in the environment and has been recovered from soil, fresh and brackish water, house dust, birds, animals, and foods. The southeast U.S. is a particularly likely area to find MAC in the environment as MAC along with *M. scrofulaceum* have been recovered from approximately one-third of aquatic environmental samples in the southeastern U.S. (18). It is not surprising that the geographic area of greatest environmental recovery of MAC is the area of highest prevalence of skin test reactivity to MAC-purified protein derivative and the area of greatest recovery of human MAC isolates (31). Further support for the environment as the source of MAC disease comes from matching serotypes of MAC from soil and from patients living in areas where the soil was sampled (38,50). MAC strains with plasmids, possibly associated with virulence, are preferentially aerosolized, which might be one mechanism for airborne transmission of the organism (39).

Unlike MAC, *M. kansasii* is only rarely recovered from the natural environment. There has been no isolation of *M. kansasii* from the soil and only rare isolation from fresh water, such as municipal water supplies, water treatment plants, domestic water supply systems, aquaria, and tap water sources. These sites of isolation are compatible with the general urban pattern of clinical disease with *M. kansasii*. In spite of limited recovery of the organism in the environment and more frequent disease in the urban setting, there is still no good evidence for human-to-human transmission of this organism.

Rapidly growing mycobacteria (RGM), especially *M. abscessus* and *M. fortuitum*, have been recovered from soil and water supplies as well as nosocomial sources including surgical cleaning solutions. Nosocomial transmission of RGM skin and soft tissue infections are thought to be the result of such contaminated sources (61). *M. xenopi* has been recovered almost exclusively from hot water systems, including hospital water supplies.

The prevalence and incidence of NTM lung disease is difficult to quantitate accurately, for several reasons. Infections due to NTM infrequently cause death directly, so that NTM rarely appear as the cause of death in state death registries. NTM lung disease is also not routinely reported to public health departments. In addition, assumptions about NTM disease are largely based on, or extrapolated from, the number of NTM isolates referred to state laboratories. There might be no correlation between the presence of disease and the recovery of these isolates. Therefore, estimates of NTM on this basis might overestimate the true incidence of NTM lung disease. Alternatively, private laboratories might isolate these organisms without referring them to state health departments for further identification, which could result in a lack of documentation of cases.

In spite of these limitations, two national surveys from 1982 and 1987 have helped define the extent of NTM infection in the U.S. Using combined data from these studies, the prevalence of NTM disease has been estimated to be 1.8 cases per 100,000 population in the U.S., of which MAC accounts for approximately 1.1 cases per 100,000 population (19,41). The next most common NTM isolates are RGM and *M. kansasii*.

We believe, overall, that there has been an important shift in recovery of mycobacterial isolates. In the early 1980s, NTM accounted for approximately one-third of all mycobacteria isolated by state laboratories, with MAC comprising the majority of these isolates (19,41). A more recent study has found that NTM, most commonly MAC, are now the more frequently identified mycobacterial species (42). Our experience (unpublished data from the Texas State Department of Health) also suggests that NTM isolates, again primarily MAC, are now more common than *M. tuberculosis* isolates. This trend is likely due to several factors, including a better appreciation of disease caused by NTM, more careful handling of NTM isolates by microbiology laboratories, the perspective from a state with high endemnicity for MAC, and the increasing prevalence of human immunodeficiency virus–related disease.

LABORATORY EVALUATION

Specimen Collection and Processing

The usual methods for obtaining respiratory specimens for *Mycobacterium tuberculosis* (MTB) appears adequate for the NTM responsible for lung disease (60). These include routine expectorated sputum, induced sputums, and bronchoalveolar lavage (BAL). The standard method for bacterial decontamination of respiratory samples for *M. tuberculosis* utilizes 1% sodium hydroxide and is generally satisfactory for the NTM. It should be recognized, however, that some NTM are more sensitive to this decontamination procedure, which can result in reduced NTM colony counts, especially RGM and *M. abscessus*.

Acid-Fast Staining

Routine methods of acid-fast staining used for *M. tuberculosis* have proved satisfactory for most species of NTM (60). In general, however, NTM are less acid-fast than MTB and hence more easily missed on stain evaluation. This applies to stains done using carbol fuchsin (Ziehl-Neelson or Kinyoun method) as well as those with rhodamine and auramine (fluorochrome method). Acid-fast staining can also provide a suggestion that an NTM is present. For instance, isolates of *M. kansasii* typically produce a very long, beaded organism which is rarely if ever associated with MTB. In addition, isolates of MAC can appear as short, even coccobacillary forms by the fluorochrome method. These are not consistent enough findings, however, that laboratories can reliably report that an organism is suggestive of an NTM based on the stain alone.

Culture Methods

The usual culture media used for MTB has proved satisfactory for species of NTM that cause lung disease (60,17). These routine methods include Middlebrook 7H10 or 7H11 agar, Lowenstein-Jensen agar, and Bactec broth. Incubation at 35°C is satisfactory for MTB as well as most pulmonary NTM. However, it should be remembered that some rare lung pathogens such as *M. chelonae*, *M. hemophilum*, and *M. genavense* grow better at lower temperatures (i.e., 30°C). In addition, some rare pathogens require special media for growth, including *M. hemophilum* which requires iron or hemin to grow and *M. genavense* which often grows well only in Bactec broth (13). When acid-fast, smear-positive respiratory samples are encountered from a patient who has not been on prior drug therapy that do not grow, modifications of the media and incubation temperatures should be considered to recover one of these more unusual pathogens.

Identification

The colony morphology of many of the NTM is highly suggestive of the individual species. For example, isolates of MAC produce tiny, translucent, flat fried-egg-like colonies that are seldom mistaken for any other species. The current ready availability of species-specific DNA probes has generally replaced utilization of colony morphology and pigmentation for early presumptive identification of the species. Currently, DNA probes (Accu Probe) are available through the Gen-Probe Company. These probes are available for *M. tuberculosis*, *M. avium*, *M. intracellulare*, *M. kansasii*, and *M. gordonae* and are generally 99% sensitive and 99% specific for the individual species (17,40,64). The equipment is relatively cheap and easily obtained, and species identification from cultured organisms can be obtained in as little as 2 hours.

For the remaining, less frequently encountered species of NTM, DNA probes are not yet available. Hence, they must be identified by standard biochemical methods or by high-performance liquid chromatography (HPLC). Most laboratories utilize standard biochemical techniques for *M. fortuitum*, *M. abscessus*, *M. xenopi*, *M. szulgai*, and *M. malmoense*.

HPLC involves extraction of mycolic acids from whole cells, with subsequent derivatization to bromophenacyl esters (9,10). These long-chain fatty acids are then assessed for their quantity and size by chromatography. Individual species produce reproducible patterns that can be compared to known species patterns. When whole cells are available, this assay can be performed in one day. Limitation for this methodology is the cost of the HPLC system, which has limited the use of this technique to several laboratories around the country.

Recent studies have suggested that polymerase chain reaction (PCR) amplification of selected DNA sequences followed by restriction fragment length polymorphism could allow for rapid diagnosis of all mycobacterial species by a single technique (45). Although no commercial PCR system for rapid mycobacterial identification is currently available, it is only a matter of time until this technique moves from the research lab to the clinical arena.

Susceptibility Testing

Because of the infrequent recovery of NTM from clinical samples, specialized susceptibility testing that applies to each individual species has been slow to develop (23). This observation is important because the current proportion method susceptibility testing done for *M. tuberculosis* generally utilizes only a single drug concentration to determine susceptibility. The single drug concentration that has been chosen for the antituberculous drugs was chosen because it readily separated treated from untreated strains of *M. tuberculosis*. All the species of NTM are more resistant to the antituberculous drugs than *M. tuberculosis,* and for many of them the single drug concentration provides no information about the potential therapeutic usefulness of that drug. This situation is unlike that of bacteria such as *Escherichia coli* where the resistance breakpoint relates to the limits of achievable serum and/or tissue levels of the drug and to the data on clinical responsiveness relative to the amount of the drug required to inhibit the growth of the organism in the laboratory. For convenience reasons, however, these single concentrations of drug chosen for testing *M. tuberculosis* are still generally used for testing NTM by most laboratories (23). Routine susceptibility testing of the antituberculous agents is not recommended for the *M. avium* complex (because of lack of correlation with clinical response) and for the rapidly growing mycobacteria including *M. abscessus* (because these species are all uniformly resistant *in vivo* and *in vitro*). Testing of antituberculous drugs using the critical concentrations for *M. tuberculosis* are still utilized for the remaining pulmonary species of NTM, including *M. kansasii, M. xenopi, M. malmoense,* and *M. szulgai.* Because of the previously mentioned problems, and because drugs are usually given in combinations whereas susceptibility testing is only performed on individual drugs, thereby ignoring potential drug interactions, these susceptibility tests have not generally been good indicators of clinical outcome. The major exception has been rifampin (1 μg/ml) for *M. kansasii,* for which *in vitro* resistance is a good predictor of treatment failure using standard rifampin-containing regimens.

For the RGM, primarily *M. fortuitum* and *M. abscessus,* susceptibility testing to traditional antibacterial agents should be performed. These drugs include amikacin, cefoxitin, imipenem, doxycycline, ciprofloxacin, ofloxacin, sulfonamides, and clarithromycin. A number of methods have been utilized for this testing (23). The best known are agar disk elution, which utilizes commercial susceptibility disks to achieve a specified drug concentration in agar, and broth microdilution with Mueller-

Hinton broth, which is comparable to the standard susceptibility testing done for bacteria with the same drugs. Because of the infrequent character of these tests, only selected reference laboratories currently perform this type of susceptibility testing. However, such testing is essential if antimicrobial therapy is contemplated for the patient with RGM lung disease.

DIAGNOSIS

It is difficult to make generalizations about diagnostic criteria for NTM pulmonary disease. The recovery of some species such as *M. kansasii* from a single culture is highly suggestive, perhaps diagnostic, of clinical disease, whereas the recovery of other species such as *M. fortuitum* from a single sputum culture often is not. General diagnostic guidelines have recently been improved. These are outlined in Table 32-3. Important points about the diagnosis of specific NTM pulmonary syndromes are included in the individual discussions that follow.

The cornerstone of diagnosis of pulmonary disease due to NTM is the isolation of the organism from cultures of respiratory secretions, usually expectorated sputum. Single positive sputum cultures, usually with low numbers of organisms (which are typically associated with negative acid fast bacilli [AFB] smears), can occur as a consequence of transient contamination or colonization of the respiratory tract or even from specimen contamination. Therefore, in general, the diagnosis of NTM lung disease requires more than one positive sputum culture with moderate to heavy growth of the NTM species. A notable exception is recovery of *M. kansasii* from sputum, which usually indicates infection because this organism is rarely a contaminant. Even with *M. kansasii,* a minimum of two positive cultures are preferred. Single sputum cultures positive for *M. abscessus* might, similarly, be reliable indi-

TABLE 32–3. *Recommended diagnostic criteria for pulmonary disease caused by nontuberculous mycobacteria*

I. For patients with cavitary lung disease
  1. Presence of two or more sputum specimens (or sputum and a bronchial washing) that are acid-fast bacilli smear-positive and/or result in moderate-to-heavy growth of NTM on culture
  2. Other reasonable causes for the disease process have been excluded (e.g., tuberculosis, fungal disease, etc.)
II. For patients with noncavitary lung disease
  1. Presence of two or more sputum specimens (or sputum and a bronchial washing) that are acid-fast bacilli smear-positive and/or produce moderate-to-heavy growth on culture
  2. If the isolate is *M. kansasii* or *M. avium* complex, failure of the sputum cultures to clear with bronchial toilet or within 2 weeks of institution of specific mycobacterial drug therapy (although only studies for these two species, this criterium is probably valid for other species of NTM)
  3. Other reasonable causes for the disease process have been excluded
III. For patients with cavitary or noncavitary lung disease whose sputum evaluation is nondiagnostic, or another disease cannot be excluded
  1. A transbronchial or open lung biopsy yields the organism and shows mycobacterial histopathologic features (i.e., granulomatous inflammation, with or without acid-fast bacilli). No other criteria needed
  2. A transbronchial or open lung biopsy that fails to yield the organism but shows mycobacterial histopathologic features in the absence of a history of other granulomatous or mycobacterial disease, and (i) presence of two or more positive cultures of sputum or bronchial washings and (ii) other reasonable causes for granulomatous disease have been excluded

TABLE 32–4. *Significance of an initial single sputum isolate[a] of selected nontuberculous mycobacteria*

Organism	Probability that isolate is a true pathogen
M. kansasii	Very high probability
M. szulgai[b]	Very high probability
M. abscessus	High probability
M. malmoense[b]	High probability
M. avium complex	Probable
M. xenopi[b]	Probable
M. fortuitum[c]	Possible
M. simiae[b]	Possible
Pigmented rapid grower	Very low
M. chelonae-like organism (MCLO)	Very low

[a]AFB smear-positive and/or moderate-to-heavy growth on culture. In the appropriate setting any of these species can be pathogens. Recovery of any potential pathogen requires careful clinical evaluation to determine significance.
[b]Rare NTM isolate; limited clinical experience.
[c]High probability in the setting of gastroesophageal disorders with chronic vomiting.

cators for the presence of disease, although there is currently not sufficient clinical experience with this organism to make this judgment with certainty. The relative probabilities of clinical disease with the initial isolation of several NTM are listed in Table 32-4. In our opinion, the recovery of an AFB smear-positive specimen with moderate to heavy growth on cultures of an NTM known to be associated with lung disease is usually indicative of significant disease.

It is also our experience that there is a bias that NTM in general are nonpathogenic, which frequently results in long periods between the initial isolation of an NTM and recognition of associated pulmonary disease. In some instances, skepticism is justifiable, whereas, in other situations, delays in therapy can allow a window of opportunity for curative therapy to pass.

Questions also frequently arise about the appropriateness of aggressive diagnostic procedures after recovery of an NTM isolate. As a general guideline, if a clinician is unsure about the significance of an NTM isolate after an appropriate follow-up, then a relatively noninvasive procedure such as bronchoscopy with transbronchial biopsy can be helpful in confirming the presence of disease.

Currently, skin testing is not useful for diagnosing NTM lung disease. Patients with NTM lung disease can react weakly or not at all to intermediate-strength purified protein derivative (PPD), although they can react strongly, in a nonspecific manner, to second-strength PPD. Antigen extracts from NTM are not standardized, not routinely available, and not clinically more useful than standard PPD for distinguishing tuberculosis from NTM lung disease (27).

THERAPY

It is also difficult to make generalizations about therapy for pulmonary NTM syndromes. Some NTM respond to standard antituberculous antibiotics whereas others do not. The importance of specific *in vitro* drug susceptibilities is clear for some organisms and controversial for others. Again, specific therapeutic recommendations are included in the individual NTM discussions. What is sometimes overlooked, however, is that antibiotic therapy is frequently suboptimal and surgical resection potentially curative in selected patients (12,46). For some NTM (MAC, *M. abscessus*) there can be a narrow window of opportunity for surgical resection of limited disease. The alternative is a progressive diffuse process, difficult to treat because of drug resistance, that can lead to respiratory compromise and death. It is apparent that with the current limitations of antibiotic therapy, early diagnosis can be critical for definitive or curative therapy. The discussion of drug therapy for NTM lung disease should also be considered a work-in-progress with few definitive standards. In fact, because of new and evolving drug regimens, the most recent ATS statement on NTM is already out of date with respect to medication recommendations (60). Although there is not yet a large body of data, in our opinion, the newer macrolides clarithromycin or azithromycin should replace isoniazide in many of the current NTM treatment regimens. Similarly, limited data in HIV-positive populations suggest that rifabutin would be preferable to rifampin for treatment of MAC. Also, the newer quinolones, ofloxacin and ciprofloxacin, could become primary drugs for some NTM pulmonary disease. Because definitive or sweeping recommendations are not available, the reader must follow developments in the current literature.

ORGANISMS

Mycobacterium avium Complex (MAC)

The discussion of lung disease caused by MAC in many ways focuses all the controversies, past and present, about NTM lung disease in general. More than any other species of NTM, MAC presents clinically in a heterogeneous fashion. It is in the arena of MAC lung disease that there is the most controversy over what constitutes true infection as opposed to colonization. Significant controversies also exist over optimal therapy for MAC disease and specifically over the importance of *in vitro* drug susceptibilities. Concepts of MAC lung disease are also rapidly changing, spurred to a large degree by interest in disseminated MAC associated with HIV disease. MAC lung disease remains a challenging and difficult problem, although the recent surge in interest is broadening understanding in many areas.

MAC includes several phenotypically similar species: *M. avium, M. intracellulare,* a group of organisms referred to as the "X" strains, *M. paratuberculosis,* and *M. lepraemurium. M. scrofulaceum* is sometimes included in what is referred to as the MAIS complex. Only *M. avium* and *M. intracellulare* are important human pulmonary pathogens. These two species are distinguishable by serologic methods and the use of gene probes, but they cannot be distinguished by routine laboratory biochemical methods. MAC contains at least 28 separate serovars which can be differentiated by seroagglutination. Serotyping is not, however, readily available and has no utility in the evaluation of patients. Commercial DNA probes are currently available that allow rapid and accurate identification of *M. avium* and *M. intracellulare.*

MAC tends to grow best in warm water with low salinity pH and dissolved oxygen. Waters, aerosols, and soils associated with the acidic swamp waters of the southeast U.S. are optimal sources for MAC recovery. In a study of 275,000 Navy recruits, each of whom had resided from birth in a single county, reaction to an MAC skin test (PPD/B) was found in more than 70% of subjects who had lived in coastal states from Virginia to Texas (16).

The typical non–HIV infected patient with pulmonary MAC disease has been described as a middle-aged or older white man from a rural southeast U.S. environment with a history of cigarette abuse and preexisting pulmonary disease (2). Associated preexisting lung diseases include chronic obstructive lung disease, prior tuberculosis, bronchiectasis, pneumoconiosis, bronchogenic carcinoma, pulmonary fibrosis, cystic fibrosis, and chronic aspiration pneumonia. Patients with MAC pulmonary disease typically present with respiratory complaints such as a chronic productive cough, dyspnea, and hemoptysis. These can be associated with nonspecific constitutional symptoms such as malaise and weakness. Fever and weight loss are usually less prominent symptoms than for patients with pulmonary tuberculosis. Because this group of patients has a high incidence of underlying lung disease, it can be difficult to differentiate the symptoms of MAC lung disease from symptoms related to the underlying disorder. Similarly, the preexisting lung disease which can have a high morbidity and mortality makes assessment of the natural history and prognosis of untreated MAC disease difficult to determine. As a rule, disease attributable to MAC is indolent and slowly progressive. However, patients with extensive cavitary MAC disease can demonstrate rapid progression to respiratory failure and death.

It has become apparent, however, that MAC lung disease is broader and more heterogeneous than as described above. Prince and colleagues (47) described pulmonary MAC disease in a subgroup of patients without underlying chronic lung disease. These patients were generally older, nonsmoking women who presented in a manner typical of classical MAC disease with an indolent productive cough and relatively few constitutional symptoms. The distinguishing feature of this group of patients was the radiographic appearance which consisted primarily of multiple discrete small pulmonary nodules (54a). Cavitary disease was present in only a minority of patients. In general, radiographic progression occurred slowly with an increase in the number of patients with cavitary radiographic changes over time. Even in this group with no underlying lung disease, 19% died of progressive and overwhelming MAC pulmonary disease. The greater the initial involvement radiographically, the greater were the chances of progression of disease.

Three other interesting subgroups of patients with MAC disease have also recently been identified. Musculoskeletal abnormalities such as pectus excavatum, abnormally narrowed anterior/posterior thoracic dimension, and thoracic scoliosis appear to be phenotypic markers of patients at increased risk for MAC pulmonary disease (28). The reason for this increased risk is not known, but it is possible that altered lung structure or impaired mucociliary function is involved. Another subgroup of patients has been described with MAC lung disease presenting as an isolated lingular or right middle lobe infiltrate (48). These patients also are usually elderly nonsmoking women with no underlying chronic lung disease. The pathophysiology of this form of MAC disease is also unknown; however, it has been attributed to the habitual voluntary suppression of cough by these patients ("Lady Windermere" syndrome) (49). The third subgroup are patients with cystic fibrosis. Recent studies of both children and young adults with cystic fibrosis have revealed 10 to 20% to be infected with MAC (4,30). A distinct clinical syndrome due to MAC in this setting is difficult to establish given the prominent symptoms of the primary disease. However, some patients have died clearly as a result of progressive mycobacterial disease. It is noteworthy that, aside from the setting of a severe underlying problem such as cystic fibrosis, MAC lung disease specifically, and NTM lung disease in general, rarely occurs in children.

It is clear that MAC lung disease can present in different forms and in a variety of settings. A unifying theme for these different presentations is a generally slow time frame from onset of symptoms to diagnosis. As alluded to earlier, the issue of diagnosing MAC lung disease as opposed to MAC lung colonization remains problematic. The diagnostic guidelines recommended by the ATS not only are applicable to, but to a large extent, were developed with MAC lung disease specifically in mind (60). As is the case with other NTM, MAC lung disease is frequently not diagnosed in a timely fashion because of skepticism about the significance of a single respiratory MAC isolate. Certainly not all patients with a sputum culture positive for MAC need therapy. However, careful follow-up is indicated, especially if the isolate is recovered in the setting of an abnormal chest radiograph. Tsukamura (57) suggests that patients with a new pulmonary cavity with two or more (and perhaps only one) sputum cultures positive for MAC should be considered to have MAC pulmonary disease. This suggestion would allow high sensitivity for diagnosis of MAC but, as yet, unknown specificity. In addition, this approach excludes consideration of subjects with noncavitary MAC disease. If sputum cultures are positive and the chest radiograph shows compatible changes, then, at the very least, careful further clinical evaluation is warranted. If an underlying disease is present, patients should also receive therapy for this underlying disease (such as bronchodilators or broad-spectrum antibiotics and smoking cessation). For patients with significant symptoms and advanced or progressive radiographic disease, an observation period is not needed to establish the need for therapy. The previous recommendations of a trial of chest physiotherapy or short course of antituberculous medication to distinguish disease from colonization are probably not useful (3). Even if the organism is cleared from the sputum expeditiously, radiographic evidence of disease progression can eventually occur. In addition, biopsies of noncavitary infiltrates from patients with MAC in the sputum frequently confirm the presence of invasive mycobacterial disease. Our bias is that MAC disease is both slowly diagnosed and under diagnosed. This concern is not moot, because antibiotic chemotherapy remains inconsistently effective whereas surgical resection of localized disease can be curative (12). If there is doubt about the significance of an MAC isolate from sputum, particularly in the presence of localized disease radiographically, then an invasive procedure such as bronchoscopy might be helpful. In addition, questions about disease versus colonization might be better addressed at referral centers experienced in evaluating MAC disease. Patients who subsequently have a stable clinical picture with minimal symptoms and those whose sputum clears with nonspecific therapy could be observed, although newer, less toxic antimicrobial therapy, including new microlides and quinolones, can reduce the threshold for treating these patients.

There are a number of radiographic patterns associated with MAC lung disease (Fig. 32-1). The classically described pattern involves upper lobe cavities which are sometimes extremely large. This pattern usually occurs in men with a history of cigarette abuse and with underlying chronic pulmonary disease. Other patterns include fibronodular apical infiltrates similar to tuberculosis, infiltrates compatible with bronchiectasis, mixed nodular and reticulonodular infiltrates confined to the right middle and lingula (often associated with bronchiectasis), solitary nodules, and diffuse infiltrates.

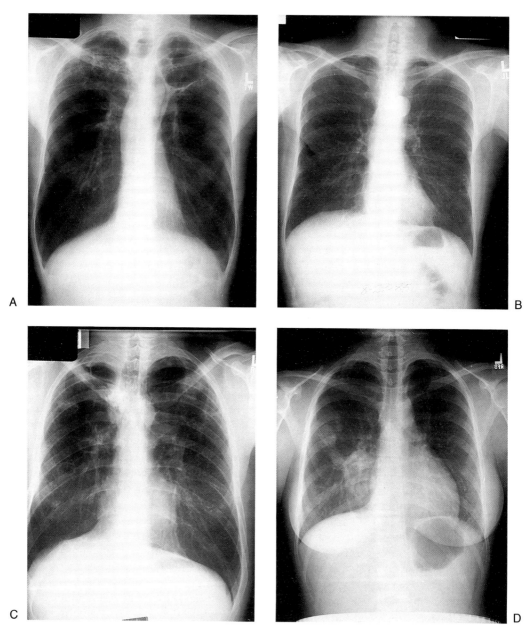

FIG. 32–1. Radiographic presentations of MAC lung disease. **A:** 56-year-old man with chronic obstructive pulmonary disease and bilateral apical cavitary disease due to MAC. **B:** 72-year-old woman, nonsmoker, with bilateral interstitial changes due to MAC. **C:** 34-year-old man with multiple bilateral cavities and infiltrates due to MAC. **D:** 16-year-old woman with consolidation in right middle lobe due to MAC.

Therapy of MAC lung infection is both challenging and frequently frustrating because of the *in vitro* resistance of MAC to first-line antituberculous drugs. The role of *in vitro* drug susceptibility testing itself for MAC disease remains controversial. Although intuitively attractive, the clinical usefulness of *in vitro* drug susceptibility testing (using test concentrations of drugs chosen for their usefulness in treating MTB, not for their usefulness against MAC isolates which are intrinsically much more resistant) for guiding therapy of MAC lung disease has not been established. Treatment approaches guided by *in vitro* drug testing of higher-than-normal drug concentrations or with groups of drugs evaluating synergism against MAC might prove useful at some point. We currently do not think that routine susceptibility testing of MAC should be recommended, as does the ATS, due to a lack of correlation with *in vitro* drug susceptibilities and clinical outcome. Most laboratories have, in fact, stopped performing them. This point is admittedly controversial and other authors do not agree with this approach (24).

In non-AIDS patients with MAC lung disease, the ATS recommends initial therapy with four drugs, that is, INH 300 mg per day, rifampin 600 mg per day, and ethambutol 25 mg per kg for the first 2 months, followed by 15 mg per kg per day with streptomycin (doses adjusted for weight and age) for the initial 3 to 6 months of therapy (60). The optimal length of drug therapy is unknown; however, the usual recommendation is for 18 to 24 months of therapy and for at least 12 months after sputum culture conversion. Several uncontrolled clinical trials using this regimen have shown an initial sputum conversion rate in previously untreated patients of up to 90% (1,48,52). It is clear that multidrug (three to six drugs) regimens are more effective at clearing sputum of MAC than one or two agents alone. Sputum for AFB smear and culture should be collected at least monthly during therapy to assess response. Relapses or progression of disease are unfortunately common, either while on medication or after discontinuation of medication. For these patients, intensive therapy with multiple drugs including cycloserine 250 mg bid, ethionamide 250 mg bid or tid, and prolonged use of an injectable agent such as streptomycin are suggested. Regimens that include these drugs are effective in clearing sputum of MAC but could be quite toxic and difficult to tolerate for prolonged periods (14).

These ATS recommendations antedated the availability of the newer macrolides and rifabutin. The new macrolides, clarithromycin and azithromycin, have striking *in vitro* microbiologic activity against multiple NTM including MAC. Clarithromycin inhibits 90% of strains of MAC at minimum inhibitory concentration (MICs) of 2 to 8 μg/ml (15). Both clarithromycin and azithromycin concentrate well in lung tissue and macrophages and probably remain active in the acid environment of the phagolysosomes. They have proved more active as single agents than any combination of antituberculous drugs in the treatment of disseminated MAC in AIDS patients. Controlled studies of these agents in MAC lung disease are ongoing; therefore, conclusions about their role in MAC lung disease are not yet available. A likely role for the macrolides will be replacement of INH in initial treatment of MAC disease. Rifabutin (ansamycin), a derivative of rifampin, has better *in vitro* activity against MAC than rifampin (25). Rifabutin has also recently been shown to be effective as a prophylactic agent against disseminated MAC in patients with HIV disease (20). Controlled trials with rifabutin in MAC lung disease have not yet been performed, however. The recent release of this drug (January 1993) by the FDA for use in preventing disseminated MAC disease could expedite these studies. The overall impact of these drugs on the most recent ATS recommendations is not clear. It is quite possible, however, that the new macrolides and rifabutin will replace the less active drugs (INH and rifampin) in the initial MAC drug regimen.

Combined medical and surgical therapy should be considered in all patients with radiographically localized disease and adequate cardiopulmonary reserve. A CAT scan of the chest is sometimes necessary to confirm the localized nature of the process. Ideally, patients should be made sputum culture-negative with medications for 2 to 3 months prior to resectional surgery. At this time, surgery is still a very effective therapy for what is otherwise a difficult disease to eradicate (12,46). In the future, the addition of medication such as rifabutin and the new macrolides to standard medication regimens might improve the relapse recurrence rates of MAC disease to a level that would relegate surgery to a very limited role, as has been accomplished with *M. kansasii.* Until that time surgery of limited disease remains an important therapeutic option.

Mycobacterium kansasii

Of the NTM, *M. kansasii* is antigenically most closely related to *M. tuberculosis* and produces pulmonary disease that most closely parallels the clinical disease of *M. tuberculosis.* Infections due to *M. kansasii* occur most commonly in the southern and central United States. The states with the highest incidence of disease include Texas, Louisiana, Illinois, and Florida. Patients with *M. kansasii* lung disease characteristically present in their fifth to seventh decades of life, tend to come from urban environments, and are usually cigarette smokers with one or more underlying pulmonary diseases including chronic obstructive pulmonary disease, lung cancer, prior tuberculosis, bronchiectasis, and pneumoconiosis (2). The majority of patients with *M. kansasii* lung disease are white. However, the ethnic distribution generally corresponds to the area studied. Several series in the past have found a male predominance of *M. kansasii* lung disease. However, a recent series, while confirming a male predominance, also found a relative increase in the percentage of women compared with previous reports (35). These authors suggested that changing smoking patterns in the U.S., with greater numbers of female smokers, might now be impacting the epidemiology of *M. kansasii* lung disease as they have changed the gender pattern of lung cancer. Patients with *M. kansasii* present with cough, sputum production, hemoptysis, chest pain, fever, night sweats, and weight loss. Hepatosplenomegaly and peripheral adenopathy can also be present in association with pulmonary disease (35). Chest radiographic appearance also mimics changes typically associated with *M. tuberculosis,* with apical cavitary fibronodular infiltrates most common. However, infiltrates with pleural scarring are also frequently seen (Fig. 32-2).

As with other NTM, the cornerstone of diagnosis is recovery of the organism on AFB culture. Both sputum culture and cultures of bronchoscopic specimens efficiently recover *M. kansasii.* Although the criteria for diagnosis recommended by the ATS for NTM in general are appropriate for *M. kansasii* specifically, in most circumstances, the isolation of *M. kansasii* from even one respiratory culture is diagnostic of disease. In the setting of apical cavitary lung disease, one respiratory specimen that is culture-positive for *M. kansasii* is especially persuasive. As with other NTM, however, recovery of *M. kansasii* in respiratory specimens can sometimes indicate contamination or colonization without invasive disease, although contamination is less likely than with other NTM because of the difficulty recovering *M. kansasii* from the environment. To be confident that a respiratory isolate of *M. kansasii* is

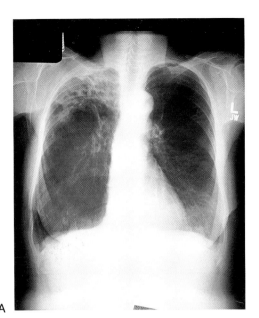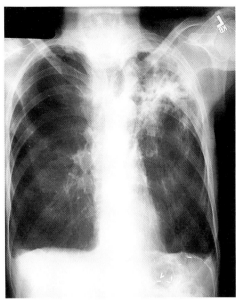

A   B

FIG. 32–2. A: 80-year-old woman with obstructive lung disease and right apical cavitary infiltrate due to *M. kansasii.* **B:** 58-year-old man with obstructive lung disease and extensive left upper lobe cavitary infiltrate due to *M. kansasii.*

not indicative of disease, it should be a single isolate (among multiple sputum specimens) with no radiographic evidence of lung disease. Previous recommendations have also emphasized either early response to antituberculous chemotherapy or clearance of the organism from the sputum with bronchial hygiene as a possible criterion for determining whether or not invasive disease was present (3). In our opinion, these criteria are not pertinent for *M. kansasii* lung disease. The isolation of *M. kansasii* in the face of noncavitary radiographic disease should prompt follow-up according to ATS guidelines with initiation of therapy also according to these guidelines (60). Extreme caution must be exercised before a clinician can feel confident that a respiratory isolate of *M. kansasii* is due to tracheobronchial colonization. Fortunately, *M. kansasii* lung disease is usually slowly progressive and effectively treated by antituberculous chemotherapy; therefore, a brief follow-up period without therapy will usually not have significant adverse consequences.

Multiple drug therapy that includes rifampin is currently the cornerstone of therapy for *M. kansasii.* Although the majority of *M. kansasii* strains are moderately susceptible to most first-line antituberculous drugs, prior to the routine use of rifampin, the 6 months sputum conversion rates for *M. kansasii* lung disease were only 52 to 81% with a 10% relapse rate (29,44). With multidrug therapy using rifampin, virtually all sputum cultures with rifampin-susceptible strains convert within 4 months of initiation of therapy with only a 1% relapse rate (29). Interestingly, *in vitro* drug susceptibilities appear to be important primarily for predicting response to rifampin-containing regimens. Historically, there has been poor correlation between *in vitro* susceptibility to INH and streptomycin and *in vivo* efficacy, with therapeutic results often better than predicted. This observation almost certainly reflects the fact that the test concentrations used (1 μg/ml INH, 2 μg/ml streptomycin) were chosen because those "critical" concentrations separate untreated strains of *M. tuberculosis* from those with mutational drug resistance. These concentrations are well below achievable serum and tissue concentration for these drugs, and are too low to separate treated from untreated strains of *M. kansasii* (10 μg/ml would be a better concentration for both). The treatment of *M. kansasii,* therefore, should be guided by *in vitro* susceptibilities only to rifampin, and *in vitro* resistance to INH (1 μg/ml) and streptomycin (2 μg/ml) should be ignored. The ATS recommendation for therapy for rifampin-susceptible strains is currently INH 300 mg per day, rifampin 600 mg per day, ethambutol 15 mg per kg per day, all for at least 18 months (60).

Wild (untreated) strains of *M. kansasii* are rifampin-susceptible (1 μg/ml). Rifampin resistance develops after treatment with rifampin, usually with inadequate treatment regimens (e.g., rifampin plus INH, or rifampin plus pyrazinamide). In patients who develop rifampin-resistant *M. kansasii* lung disease, long-term sputum conversion can be accomplished with a multidrug regimen including INH 900 mg per day, ethambutol 25 mg/kg per day, trimethoprim sulfamethoxazole 160/800 mg tid, and streptomycin 3 to 5 times per week for 3 to 6 months. Aside from the streptomycin, these medications are administered daily for 18 to 24 months until the patient has been culture negative on therapy at least 12–15 months (58). The newer macrolide clarithromycin has significant *in vitro* activity against both rifampin-susceptible and rifampin-resistant strains of *M. kansasii* with mean MICs ≤ 0.25 μg/ml. Because of its utility in other NTM lung disease, clarithromycin appears to be a reasonable agent for inclusion in future re-treatment (i.e., rifampin-resistant) regimens as a substitute for more toxic agents such as streptomycin that have traditionally been used in these re-treatment regimens.

The effectiveness of antituberculous chemotherapy in *M. kansasii* disease has greatly reduced the role of surgery as therapy. We hope therapeutic agents will also improve for organisms such as MAC and *M. abscessus,* so that a similar reduction in the role of surgical intervention can be attained for these organisms.

The determination of the role of *M. kansasii* in pulmonary morbidity and mortality is sometimes difficult because of the frequent association of *M. kansasii* with other progressive severe lung diseases. Untreated *M. kansasii* disease can remain relatively stable for years. However, our experience, and that of most previous authors, is that patients with *M. kansasii* lung disease all eventually progress clinically and should, therefore, receive drug therapy.

Disseminated disease due to *M. kansasii* occurs exclusively in patients with systemic illnesses who are significantly immunocompromised, usually with hematologic malignancies or while using immunosuppressive medications (35). Disseminated *M. kansasii* affects primarily the lung, reticuloendothelial system, bone, joints, and skin, although most anatomic sites can be affected. Patients with disseminated *M. kansasii* disease present with more pronounced constitutional symptoms and are much more likely to have skin lesions, hepatosplenomegaly, and peripheral adenopathy. As opposed to disseminated MAC, the chest radiograph in disseminated *M. kansasii* is usually abnormal, but it is unlikely to show changes typical for *M. tuberculosis.* Instead, the distribution of pulmonary infiltrates is more variable, and hilar adenopathy and mass lesions are more common. The prognosis in disseminated *M. kansasii* is determined primarily by the severity and course of the underlying problem. The majority of patients die of rapidly fatal underlying disease, although some patients with less aggressive underlying disease respond to standard drug regimens.

M. kansasii infections also occur in patients positive for the human immunodeficiency virus. Compared with *M. tuberculosis* and MAC, there is an absolute and relative paucity of reports of *M. kansasii* infections in HIV-positive patients, even in areas highly endemic for *M. kansasii* (26). It is possible that because isolation of *M. kansasii* from the environment is so much rarer than isolation of MAC, markedly different risks of exposure result in markedly different rates of infection in HIV-positive patients. Infections with *M. kansasii* usually occur late in the course of HIV infection when patients are profoundly immunosuppressed (33). Approximately 50% of patients will have disease localized to the lung, whereas the remainder have disseminated disease (11,33). Therapeutic regimens are no different for the HIV-positive population.

Rapidly Growing Mycobacteria (RGM)

The rapidly growing mycobacteria (RGM) are classified in group IV of the Runyon classification scheme. The major pulmonary pathogens in this group are the nonpigmented species *M. fortuitum* (previously *M. fortuitum* biovariant *fortuitum*) and *M. abscessus* (previously *M. chelonae* subspecies *abscessus*) (32). Pigmented RGM and *M. chelonae*-like organisms, or MCLO, the latter especially common in tap water, almost never cause lung diseases, although they are occasionally seen as single positives in sputum (62). RGM were initially isolated early in this century. However, the first case of pulmonary disease due to RGM was not reported until 1933, and RGM have only recently gained wide acceptance as pulmonary pathogens. To a large degree, the delay in recognition of RGM as pulmonary pathogens is representative of the problem for NTM respiratory isolates as a whole. An impediment specific to RGM has involved the laboratory difficulty in differentiating *M. abscessus* from *M. fortuitum* in the past. Both were previously called "*M. fortuitum* complex."

We have recently reported a large number of cases of RGM lung disease (21). The typical patient with RGM lung disease is a female nonsmoker in her early sixties, although, as with other NTM lung disease syndromes, considerable patient heterogeneity exists. The clinical presentation of patients with RGM lung disease is usually prolonged, with greater than 2 years elapsing between onset of symptoms and the first isolation of RGM. Diagnosis is usually further delayed because the clinician is uncertain about the significance of an RGM respiratory isolate. Cough is the most frequent presenting symptom (71%), although sputum production, fever, and weight loss become more important as the disease progresses; hemoptysis occurs in only a minority of cases (36%). The majority of RGM pulmonary disease cases appear to cluster in southeast U.S. coastal states.

RGM lung disease occurs most commonly in subjects with no known underlying lung disease (32%), although there are some underlying disorders that are associated with RGM lung disease, including esophageal motility disorders with chronic vomiting (primarily achalasia) (6%), cystic fibrosis (6%), previous pulmonary granulomatous disease (usually, treated *M. tuberculosis* or MAC) (18%), and lipoid pneumonia (3%). A rare fulminant presentation with widespread alveolar infiltrates, high fever, and leukocytosis can be seen in patients with underlying gastrointestinal disorders with chronic vomiting. The diagnosis of bronchiectasis is also frequently associated with RGM lung disease but rarely proven. We suspect that, in most cases of "bronchiectasis" and RGM lung disease, either the RGM lung disease is mislabeled as bronchiectasis (because of the similarity in symptoms) or the RGM lung disease was responsible for the development of bronchiectasis. An underlying lung disorder is present in 80% of patients with RGM lung disease under age 40, compared to less than 20% in patients over age 60 (21).

The chest radiograph in RGM lung disease characteristically shows bilateral multi-lobar patchy interstitial or interstitial/alveolar infiltrates (Figure 32.3). The upper lung zones are most frequently involved; however, lower lung zones are also frequently abnormal. Infiltrates can be fleeting, that is, resolve or appear without specific therapy. Pleural effusions occur rarely. In patients with preexisting mycobacterial disease, new infiltrates due to RGM lung disease invariably occur in the area of previous disease. None of these radiographic changes distinguishes RGM lung disease from other mycobacterial disease, although cavitation occurs in only a minority of patients (16%). The majority (82%) of RGM pulmonary isolates are *M. abscessus,* whereas the next most common organism isolated is *M. fortuitum* (13%). *M. abscessus* is the most common cause of RGM lung disease regardless of geographic origin of the isolate or the presence or absence of underlying disease, with one important exception. In patients with gastroesophageal disorders with chronic vomiting, *M. fortuitum* is isolated as frequently as *M. abscessus.*

Once an RGM has been isolated, the diagnosis of disease depends on the species isolated and the clinical circumstance. Our experience has been that the isolation of *M. abscessus* from respiratory secretions is almost always associated with lung disease. However, the diagnostic criteria and recommendations of the ATS are still appropriate (60). At a minimum, the recovery of *M. abscessus* dictates careful clin-

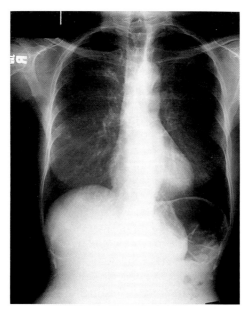

FIG. 32–3. 70-year-old woman, nonsmoker, with bilateral interstitial disease due to *M. abscessus.*

ical follow-up, repeat sputum collection, and consideration of further diagnostic procedures, such as bronchoscopy. In our experience, when *M. abscessus* is repeatedly recovered, invasive diagnostic procedures almost invariably confirm the diagnosis. Interpretation of *M. fortuitum* respiratory isolates are more complicated, but the clinical setting is especially important.

Isolates of *M. fortuitum* and *M. abscessus* are universally resistant to standard antituberculous antibiotics. Isolates of *M. fortuitum* are susceptible *in vitro* to several well-tolerated oral antibiotics, including sulfonamides, the newer fluorinated quinolones (ciprofloxacin, ofloxacin), and, for approximately 50% of isolates, doxycycline and minocycline (8,54). Approximately 80% of isolates are also susceptible to the newer macrolide, clarithromycin (8). *M. fortuitum* isolates are also susceptible *in vitro* to the parenteral agents—amikacin, imipenem, cefoxitin, and cefmetazole. Long-term therapy with oral agents based on *in vitro* susceptibilities has been very successful in treating pulmonary disease caused by *M. fortuitum* (21). Unfortunately, the *M. fortuitum* group produces less than 20% of RGM lung disease.

For patients with more typical RGM lung disease caused by *M. abscessus*, the treatment options are less attractive. In contrast to *M. fortuitum*, *M. abscessus* is generally susceptible *in vitro* only to the parenteral antibiotics amikacin, cefoxitin, and imipenem (59). A small percentage of *M. abscessus* isolates are also susceptible or moderately susceptible *in vitro* to erythromycin (8). *M. abscessus* is more commonly susceptible to the newer macrolides including clarithromycin (8). Patients do not respond favorably to regimens that rely on antibiotics to which the *M. abscessus* shows *in vitro* resistance (e.g., doxycycline or trimethoprim/sulfamethoxazole). Some subjects clinically improve with short courses (2–4 weeks) of parenteral antibiotic therapy, but few patients can tolerate the cost, inconvenience, and toxicity of a prolonged parenteral antibiotic trial. In addition, most patients will have symptomatic relapses following such a therapeutic trial. We are not aware of any documented instances of permanent sputum conversion to culture-negative and permanent symptomatic improvement, utilizing parenteral antibiotic agents alone for *M. abscessus*.

Clinical trials are currently under way to evaluate the efficacy of the newer macrolides, clarithromycin and azithromycin, for *M. abscessus* lung disease. Preliminary results are encouraging; however, it is not clear that these agents alone can produce a clinical and microbiologic cure. At the present time, only surgical resection of localized disease has proved to be effective in producing long-term conversion of sputum cultures to negative and complete and permanent alleviation of symptoms in patients infected with *M. abscessus* (21). Unfortunately, few patients present and are diagnosed at a time when disease is sufficiently well localized for complete surgical resection. Once again, early recognition and diagnosis of disease is critical. In our experience, some patients have been followed for years with multiple positive sputum for *M. abscessus* with no apparent recognition of the role of *M. abscessus* in causing lung disease (21). There is no longer any justification for such a delay in diagnosis.

Disseminated disease due to RGM occurs rarely in immunocompromised patients and typically does not involve the lungs. Although RGM lung disease closely resembles lung disease due to MAC in many respects, MAC is a much more important pathogen in patients with HIV disease, whereas RGM are unusual pathogens in this setting.

Mycobacterium xenopi

In many ways lung disease due to *M. xenopi* closely resembles lung disease due to MAC. This organism was named for the source of its initial isolation: the skin of a toad, *Xenopus laevis*. *M. xenopi* is an uncommon respiratory isolate in the United States, but in areas of Canada it is the second most common NTM respiratory isolate behind MAC, and in southeast England it is the most common (5,53,55). *M. xenopi* respiratory isolates are still viewed suspiciously, the initial assumption being that the organism is a nonpathogenic colonizer with the burden of proof placed on documenting true disease and tissue invasion. Subjects with *M. xenopi* lung disease are typically middle-aged or older men with preexisting lung disease including COPD, previous tuberculosis, and bronchogenic carcinoma. Lung disease presents in a manner almost identical to MAC disease, with chronic cough and sputum production, hemoptysis, and a relative paucity of constitutional symptoms. Radiographic changes include single or multiple upper lobe cavities, nodules, infiltrates, and, rarely, pleural disease (Fig. 32-4). The ATS guidelines are, once again, pertinent for diagnosis of *M. xenopi* lung disease (60). As with MAC lung disease, however, careful clinical follow-up is indicated for subjects with noncavitary infiltrates and sputum isolates of *M. xenopi*. Our impression is that no center has adequate experience and, more importantly, adequate follow-up of a sufficiently large cohort of patients with *M. xenopi* isolates to be confident that an individual patient who is designated as "colonized" does not, in fact, have very slowly progressive invasive disease.

Optimal therapy for *M. xenopi* pulmonary disease is not known, and results of drug therapy are unpredictable. *M. xenopi* isolates have variable *in vitro* susceptibility to first-line antituberculous drugs. As with MAC disease, however, clinical

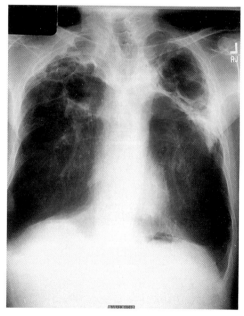

FIG. 32–4. 75-year-old man with severe obstructive lung disease and bilateral apical cavitary disease due to *M. xenopi*.

outcome is not necessarily related to *in vitro* drug susceptibilities (5). Enhanced drug activity has been shown with the combination of rifampin and streptomycin (5). In addition, *M. xenopi* isolates are frequently susceptible to achievable serum and tissue levels of the newer macrolides (clarithromycin) and quinolones (ciprofloxacin and ofloxacin) (34,37). A multidrug regimen including a quinolone, rifampin, ethambutol, and a macrolide seems appropriate for treatment of this disease. Again, there are no controlled studies of these medication regimens to date.

Surgery of limited *M. xenopi* lung disease has been successful in eradicating *M. xenopi* from the lung. In one series, however, surgical intervention, although frequently successful, was also associated with a high (50%) rate of short- and long-term surgical complications including death (43). This study is instructive if only because it demonstrates the variety and severity of postsurgical problems encountered in this typical patient population with NTM lung disease. Although surgery is an important option in a number of NTM pulmonary syndromes, this study offers some important and sobering caveats when considering surgery for an individual patient. Overall, more experience is required to answer important questions about diagnosis and treatment for patients with *M. xenopi* respiratory isolates.

Mycobacterium szulgai

M. szulgai is a rare NTM respiratory isolate from the United States, although it has been reported in various parts of the world. *M. szulgai* can produce a clinical pulmonary syndrome that is essentially indistinguishable from that caused by *M. tuberculosis*. Because isolation of this organism is rare, information about *M. szulgai* lung disease must be gleaned primarily from case reports. There is no single center with extensive experience with this organism and no large published series of cases from a single center.

The source of *M. szulgai* is unknown, although it is also presumably from the environment. The typical patient with *M. szulgai* pulmonary disease is a middle-aged man with symptoms characteristic of mycobacterial disease, including fever, cough, hemoptysis, and weight loss. There is no apparent geographic clustering of cases. The chest radiograph typically shows unilateral or bilateral apical infiltrates which frequently also show cavitation. *M. szulgai* pulmonary disease occurs in patients with no underlying pulmonary disorders, although this disease can also occur in patients with COPD and previous *M. tuberculosis*. Although based on a limited number of cases, isolation of *M. szulgai* from clinical specimens has correlated with evidence of disease and has seldom represented contamination or colonization (36). When isolated from humans, *M. szulgai* should be considered a pathogen (60). Isolation of *M. szulgai* from the sputum, therefore, should prompt aggressive clinical follow-up and probably initiation of therapy.

The *in vitro* drug susceptibility pattern of *M. szulgai* to antituberculous drugs is similar to that of *M. kansasii*. Strains of *M. szulgai* generally show *in vitro* susceptibility to rifampin, higher levels of streptomycin (10 μ/ml), INH, and ethambutol. Selected strains of *M. szulgai* have also been shown to be susceptible *in vitro* to cefoxitin and amikacin. Again, on the basis of very limited experience, it appears that patients receiving three presumably effective drugs have fewer relapses than patients receiving two effective drugs (36). Enhanced activity of rifampin, ethambutol, and streptomycin, when used in combination, has been shown *in vitro*. The optimal duration of therapy is not known, although therapy is recommended for 18 to 24 months.

Mycobacterium malmoense

There is limited clinical experience, and therefore little information, about lung disease caused by *M. malmoense* (6,51). These isolates are particularly unusual in North America, although they are more common in England, Wales, and Northern Europe. It is similar in pathogenicity to MAC in that it causes pulmonary disease in adults and cervical adenitis in children.

M. malmoense pulmonary disease usually occurs in the setting of preexisting disease such as COPD, previous mycobacterial disease, bronchiectasis, and pneumoconiosis. Previous gastrectomy and use of immunosuppressive agents are also sometimes associated with *M. malmoense* lung disease. A significant minority of patients without underlying disorders or medical problems can also develop *M. malmoense* lung disease.

M. malmoense lung disease can be relatively acute or a chronic process more typical of NTM lung disease. Symptoms are characteristic of mycobacterial disease and include cough, sputum production, hemoptysis, and weight loss. Radiographic abnormalities almost universally involve the lung apices with cavitary changes and can be either unilateral or bilateral. *M. malmoense* lung disease is diagnosed according to ATS guidelines; however, a single sputum isolate positive for *M. malmoense* can be indicative of the presence of invasive disease. Any patient with a positive sputum culture isolate of *M. malmoense* warrants careful assessment and close follow-up and will likely require therapy (60).

M. malmoense isolates show almost universal *in vitro* resistance to INH and frequent *in vitro* resistance to rifampin and streptomycin. These isolates are usually susceptible *in vitro* to achievable serum levels of ethambutol and to second-line agents including cycloserine and ethionamide. The most effective drug regimen appears to be a combination of INH, rifampin, and ethambutol administered for 18 to 24 months. *In vitro* susceptibility to rifampin and/or ethambutol appears to correlate with a favorable response, although patients who receive second-line drugs, even guided by *in vitro* susceptibility testing, do poorly (6). The role of *in vitro* susceptibility testing in this disease is therefore unclear, although it is likely less important than compliance with treatment and completion of a prolonged course of therapy. The ATS has suggested the four-drug regimen recommended for MAC for *M. malmoense* lung disease, although the role of streptomycin in this disorder is unclear because patients probably do well with the three-drug regimen outlined above (60). The role of the newer macrolides and quinolones is undefined.

Mycobacterium simiae

M. simiae is a rare cause of NTM pulmonary disease, and, not surprisingly, there is limited clinical experience with this organism (7). *M. simiae* appears to cause disease primarily in patients with underlying lung disease and presents with bilateral interstitial infiltrates, atelectasis, pleural effusion, or apical cavitary infiltrates. *M. simiae* can be isolated from the sputum without evidence of active pulmonary disease and without radiographic progression over time (7). Subjects without invasive disease tend to have episodic recovery of *M. simiae* with smear-negative specimens and low colony counts on culture. As with other NTM, bronchoscopy with transbronchial biopsy can be helpful in determining whether invasive disease is present. Parenthetically, *M. simiae* is the only NTM that is niacin-positive, a biochemical characteristic that can lead to confusion with *M. tuberculosis*.

Isolates of *M. simiae* are uniformly resistant *in vitro* to standard antituberculous drugs. As a result of the small number of cases and drug resistance, the optimal therapy for *M. simiae* lung disease is unknown. The ATS suggests the four-drug regimen recommended for MAC as initial therapy, although the efficacy of this regimen for *M. simiae* is unknown (60). Similarly, the activity of the newer macrolides and quinolones is unknown, although it seems reasonable to include these agents in a therapeutic regimen for *M. simiae*. It is obvious that experience with this disease is lacking.

SUMMARY

Diseases due to NTM have recently generated interest, likely a result of their occurrence in HIV-related disease. It has become clear that the NTM produce heterogeneous lung diseases that are not identical to tuberculosis. Clinicians can no longer approach NTM lung disease in a generic way. Similarly, it has become clear that subjects previously thought to be "colonized" by NTM in fact have slowly progressive invasive disease. The burden of proof is now upon the clinician to prove that an NTM respiratory isolate is not indicative of disease, rather than first assuming that the isolate represents tracheobronchial "colonization." For lung disease due to MAC and *M. abscessus,* particularly early diagnosis is currently the best hope for curative therapy. For most NTM, drug therapy remains problematic, although newer agents, including macrolides and quinolones, offer hope of improved clinical outcome. It is also clear, however, that understanding of epidemiology, disease transmission, host susceptibility factors, definition and diagnosis of disease, and optimal treatment regimens remains inadequate. Any current review of NTM lung disease can, therefore, only be viewed as a work in progress. We hope subsequent reviews will shed more light on all of these unresolved issues.

REFERENCES

1. Ahn, C.H., Ahn, S.S., Anderson, R.A., Murphy, D.T., and Mammo, A. (1986): A four-drug regimen for initial treatment of cavitary disease caused by *Mycobacterium avium* complex. *Am. Rev. Respir. Dis.,* 134:438–441.
2. Ahn, C.H., Lowell, J.R., Onstad, G.D., Shuford, E.H., and Hurst, G.A. (1979): A demographic study of disease due to *Mycobacterium kansasii* or *M. intracellulare-avium* in Texas. *Chest,* 75:120–125.
3. Ahn, C.H., McLarty, J.W., Ahn, S.S., Ahn, S.I., and Hurst, G.A. (1982): Diagnostic criteria for pulmonary disease caused by *Mycobacterium kansasii* and *Mycobacterium intracellulare. Am. Rev. Respir. Dis.,* 125:388–391.
4. Aitken, M.L., Burke, W., McDonald, G., Wallis, C., Ramsey, B., and Nolan, C. (1993): Nontuberculous mycobacterial disease in adult cystic fibrosis patients. *Chest,* 103:1096–1099.
5. Banks, J., Hunter, A.M., Campbell, I.A., Jenkins, P.A., and Smith, A.P. (1984): Pulmonary infection with *Mycobacterium xenopi:* review of treatment response. *Thorax,* 39:376–382.
6. Banks, J., Jenkins, P.A., and Smith, A.P. (1985): Pulmonary infection with *Mycobacterium malmoense:* a review of treatment and response. *Tubercle,* 66:197–203.
7. Bell, R.C., Higuchi, J.H., Donova, W.N., Krasnow, I., and Johanson, W.G., Jr. (1983): *Myco-*

bacterium simiae: clinical features and follow-up of twenty-four patients. *Am. Rev. Respir. Dis.,* 127:35–38.

8. Brown, B.A., Wallace, R.J., Jr., Onyi, G.O., et al. (1992): Activities of four macrolides, including clarithromycin, against *Mycobacterium fortuitum, Mycobacterium chelonae,* and *M. chelonae-like organisms. Antimicrob. Agents Chemother.,* 36:180–184.

9. Butler, W.R., Jost, K.C., Jr., and Kilburn, J.O. (1991): Identification of mycobacteria by high-performance liquid chromatography. *J. Clin. Microb.,* 29:2468–2472.

10. Butler, W.R., Thibert, L., and Kilburn, J.O. (1992): Identification of *Mycobacterium avium* complex strains and some similar species by high-performance liquid chromatography. *J. Clin. Microb.,* 30:2698–2704.

11. Carpenter, J.L., and Parks, J.M. (1990): *Mycobacterium kansasii* infections in patients positive for human immunodeficiency virus. *Rev. Infect. Dis.,* 13:789–796.

12. Corpe, R.F. (1981): Surgical management of pulmonary disease due to *Mycobacterium avium-intracellulare. Rev. Infect. Dis.,* 3:1064–1067.

13. Coyle, M.B., Carlson, L.D.C., Wallis, C.K., Leonard, R.B., Raisys, V.A., Kilburn, J.O., Samadpour, M., and Böttger, E.C. (1992): Laboratory aspects of *"Mycobacterium genavense,"* a proposed species isolated from AIDS patients. *J. Clin. Microb.,* 30:3206–3212.

14. Davidson, P.T., Khanijo, V., Goble, M., and Moulding, T.S. (1981): Treatment of disease due to *Mycobacterium intracellulare. Rev. Infect. Dis.,* 3:1052–1059.

15. deLalla, F., Maserati, R., Scarpellini, P., Marone, P., Nicolin, R., Caccamo F., and Rigoli, R. (1992): Clarithromycin-ciprofloxacin-amikacin for therapy of *Mycobacterium avium–Mycobacterium intracellulare* bacteremia in patients with AIDS. *Antimicrob. Agents Chemother.,* 36:1567–1569.

16. Edwards, L., Aquaviva, F., Livesay, V., Cross, F., and Palmer, C. (1969): An atlas of sensitivity to tuberculin, PPD-B, and histoplasmin in the United States. *Am. Rev. Respir. Dis.,* 99:3–18.

17. Ellner, P.D., Kiehn, T.E., Cammarata, R., and Hosmer, M. (1988): Rapid detection and identification of pathogenic mycobacteria by combining radiometric and nucleic acid probe methods. *J. Clin. Microb.,* 26:1349–1352.

18. Falkinham, J.O., III., Parker, B.C., and Gruft, H. (1980): Epidemiology of infection by nontuberculous mycobacteria: I. Geographic distribution in the eastern United States. *Am. Rev. Respir. Dis.,* 121:931–957.

19. Good, R.C., and Snider, D.E. (1982): Isolation of nontuberculous mycobacteria in the United States. *J. Infect. Dis.,* 146:829–833.

20. Gordin, F., Nightingale, B., and Wynne, D. (1992): Rifabutin monotherapy prevents or delays *Mycobacterium avium* complex (MAC) bacteremia in patients with AIDS. *Prog. Abs. 32nd Interscien. Conf. Antimicrob. Agents Chemother.,* 889:258.

21. Griffith, D.E., Girard, W.M., and Wallace, R.J., Jr. (1993): Clinical features of pulmonary disease caused by rapidly growing mycobacteria: an analysis of 154 patients. *Am. Rev. Respir. Dis.,* 147:1271–1278.

22. Griffith, D.E., and Wallace, R.J., Jr. (1992): Environmental (nontuberculous) mycobacterial disease. *Text. Int. Med.,* 289:1435–1438.

23. Hawkins, J.E., Wallace, R.J., Jr., and Brown, B.A. (1991) Antibacterial susceptibility tests: mycobacteria. In: *Manual of Clinical Microbiology,* Chapter 114, edited by A. Balows, pp. 1138–1152. American Society of Microbiology, Washington, D.C.

24. Heifets, L.B., and Iseman, M.D. (1991): Individualized therapy versus standard regimens in the treatment of *Mycobacterium avium* infections. *Am. Rev. Respir. Dis.,* 144:1–2.

25. Heifets, F., Nightingale, B., and Iseman, M. (1985): Determinations of *in vitro* susceptibility of mycobacteria to ansamycin. *Am. Rev. Respir. Dis.,* 132:710–711.

26. Horsburgh, C.R., and Selik, R.M. (1989): The epidemiology of disseminated nontuberculous mycobacterial infection in the acquired immunodeficiency syndrome (AIDS). *Am. Rev. Respir. Dis.,* 139:4–7.

27. Huebner, R.E., Schein, M.F., Cauthen, G.M., Geiter, L.J., Selin, M.J., Good, R.C., and O'Brien, R.J. (1992): Evaluation of the clinical usefulness of mycobacterial skin test antigens in adults with pulmonary mycobacterioses. *Am. Rev. Respir. Dis.,* 145:1160–1166.

28. Iseman, M.D., Buschman, D.L., and Ackerson, L.E. (1991): Pectus excavatum and scoliosis: thoracic anomalies associated with pulmonary disease caused by *Mycobacterium avium* complex. *Am. Rev. Respir. Dis.,* 144:914–916.

29. Jenkins, D.E., Bahar, D., and Chosnas, I. (1960): Pulmonary disease due to atypical mycobacteria: current concepts. *Trans. 19th Conf. Chemother. TB.,* 224–231.

30. Kilby, J.M., Gilligan, P.H., Yankaskas, J.R., Highsmith, W.E., Jr., Edwards, L.J., and Knowles, M.R. (1992): Nontuberculous mycobacteria in adult patients with cystic fibrosis. *Chest,* 102: 70–75.

31. Kirschner, R.A., Parker, B.C., and Falkinham, J.O., III. (1992): Epidemiology of infection by nontuberculous mycobacteria. *Am. Rev. Respir. Dis.,* 145:271–275.

32. Kusunoki, S., and Ezaki, T. (1992): Proposal of *Mycobacterium peregrinum* sp nov, nom rev, and elevation of *Mycobacterium chelonae* subsp *abscessus* (Kubica et al.) to species status: *Mycobacterium abscessus* comb nov. *Int. J. Syst. Bacteriol.,* 42:240–245.

33. Levine, B., and Chaisson, R.E. (1991): *Mycobacterium kansasii:* a cause of treatable pulmonary disease associated with advanced human immunodeficiency virus (HIV) infection. *Ann. Intern. Med.,* 114:861–868.

34. Leysen, D.C., Haemers, A., and Pattyn, S.R. (1989): Mycobacteria and the new quinolones. *Antimicrob. Agents Chemother.,* 33:1–5.

35. Lillo, M., Orengo, S., Cernoch, P., and Harris, R.L. (1990): Pulmonary and disseminated infection due to *Mycobacterium kansasii:* a decade of experience. *Rev. Infect. Dis.,* 12(5):760–767.

36. Maloney, J.M., Gregg, C.R., Stephens, D.S., Manian, F.A., and Rimland, D. (1987): Infections caused by *Mycobacterium szulgai* in humans. *Rev. Infect. Dis.,* 9(6):1120–1126.

37. Maugein, J., Fourche, J., Mormede, M., and Pelegrin, J.L. (1989): Sensibliite *in vitro* de *Mycobacterium avium* et *Mycobacterium xenopi* a l'erythromycine, roxithromycine et doxycycline. *Pathol. Bio.,* 37:565–567.

38. Meissner, G., and Anz, W. (1977): *Mycobacterium avium* complex infection resulting in human diseases. *Am. Rev. Respir. Dis.,* 116:1057–1064.

39. Meissner, P.S., and Falkinham, J.O., III. (1986): Plasmid DNA profiles as epidemiologic markers for clinical and environmental isolates of *Mycobacterium avium, Mycobacterium intracellulare,* and *Mycobacterium scrofulaceum. J. Infect. Dis.,* 153:325–331.

40. Musial, C.E., Tice, L.S., Stockman, L., and Roberts, G.D. (1988): Identification of mycobacteria from culture by using the gen-probe rapid diagnostic system for *Mycobacterium avium* complex and *Mycobacterium tuberculosis* complex. *J. Clin. Microb.,* 26:2120–2123.

40a. Nightingale, S.D., Cameron, D.W., Gordin, F.M., Sullam, P.M., Cohn, D.L., Chiasson, R.E., Eron, L.J., Sparti, P.D., Bihari, B., Kaufman, D.L., Stern, J.J., Pearce, D.D., Weinberg, W.G., LaMarca, A., and Siegel, F.P. (1993): Two controlled trials of rifabutin prophylaxis against mycobacterium avium complex infection in AIDS. *New. Eng. J. Med.,* 329:828–833.

41. O'Brien, R.J., Geiter, L.J., and Snider, D.E. (1987): The epidemiology of nontuberculous mycobacterial diseases in the United States: results from a national survey. *Am. Rev. Respir. Dis.,* 135:1007–1014.

42. Ostroff, S., Hutwagner, L., and Collin, S. (1992): Mycobacterial species and drug resistance patterns reported by State Laboratories. [Abstract]. *93rd ASM Gen. Meeting,* u-9170.

43. Parrot, R.G., and Grosset, J.H. (1988): Post-surgical outcome of 57 patients with *Mycobacterium xenopi* pulmonary infection. *Tubercle,* 69:47–55.

44. Pezzia, W., Raleigh, J.W., Bailey, M.C., Toth, E.A., and Silverblatt, J. (1981): Treatment of pulmonary disease due to *Mycobacterium kansasii:* recent experience with rifampin. *Rev. Infect. Dis.,* 3:1035–1039.

45. Plikaytis, B.B., Plikaytis, B.D., Yakrus, M.A., Butler, W.R., Woodley, C.L., Silcox, V.A., and Shinnick, T.M. (1992): Differentiation of slowly growing *Mycobacterium* species, including *Mycobacterium tuberculosis,* by gene amplification and restriction fragment length polymorphism analysis. *J. Clin. Microb.,* 30:1815–1822.

46. Pomerantz, M., Madsen, L., Goble, M., and Iseman, M. (1991): Surgical management of resistant mycobacterial tuberculosis and other mycobacterial pulmonary infections. *Ann. Thorac. Surg.,* 52:1108–1112.

47. Prince, D.S., Peterson, D.D., Steiner, R.M., Gottlieb, J.E., Scott, R., Israel, H.L., Figueroa, W.G., and Fish, J.E. (1989): Infection with *Mycobacterium avium* complex in patients without predisposing conditions. *N. Engl. J. Med.,* 321(13):863–868.

48. Reich, J.M., and Johnson, R.E. (1991): *Mycobacterium avium* complex pulmonary disease: incidence, presentation, and response to therapy in a community setting. *Am. Rev. Respir. Dis.,* 143:1381–1385.

49. Reich, J.M., and Johnson, R.E. (1992): *Mycobacterium avium* complex pulmonary disease presenting as an isolated lingular or middle lobe pattern: the Lady Windermere syndrome. *Chest,* 101:1605–1609.

50. Reznikov, M., and Dawson, D.J. (1980): Mycobacteria of the intracellulare-scrofulaceum group in soils from the Adelaide area. *Pathology,* 12:525–528.

51. Roberts, C., Clague, H., and Jenkins, P.A. (1985): Pulmonary infection with *Mycobacterium malmoense:* a report of 4 cases. *Tubercle,* 66:205–209.

52. Seibert, A.F., and Bass, J.B. (1989): Four-drug therapy of pulmonary disease due to *Mycobacterium avium* complex [Abstract]. *Am. Rev. Respir. Dis.,* 139:A399.

53. Simor, A.E., Salit, I.E., and Vellend, H. (1984): The role of *Mycobacterium xenopi* in human disease. *Am. Rev. Respir. Dis.,* 129:435–438.

54. Swenson, J.M., Wallace, R.J., Jr., Silcox V.A., et al. (1985): Antimicrobial susceptibility of five subgroups of *Mycobacterium fortuitum* and *Mycobacterium chelonae. Antimicrob. Agents Chemother.,* 28:807–811.

54a. Swenson, S.J., Hartman, T.E., and Williams, D.E. (1994): Computed tomographic diagnosis of mycobacterium avium-intracellulare complex in patients with brochiectasis. *Chest* 105:49–52.

55. Thomas, P., Liu, F., and Weiser, W. (1988): Characteristics of *Mycobacterium xenopi* disease. *Bult. Intern. Un. Agnst. TB Lung Dis.,* 63(3):12–13.

56. Timpe, A., and Runyon, E.H. (1954): The relationship of "atypical acid-fast" bacteria to human disease: a preliminary report. *J. Lab. Clin. Med.,* 44:202.

57. Tsukamura, M. (1991): Diagnosis of disease caused by *Mycobacterium avium* complex. *Chest,* 99:667–669.
58. Wallace, R.J., Jr., Dunbar, D., Brown, B.A., Onyi, G., Dunlap, R., Ahn, C.H., and Murphy, D.T. (1994): Rifampin-resistant *Mycobacterium kansasii. Clin. Infect. Dis.* (In press).
59. Wallace, R.J., Jr., Brown, B.A., and Onyi, G.O. (1991): Susceptibilities of *Mycobacterium fortuitum* boivar. *fortuitum* and the two subgroups of *Mycobacterium chelonae* to imipenem, cefmetazole, cefoxitin, and amoxicillin-clavulanic acid. *Antimicrob. Agents Chemother.,* 35:773–775.
60. Wallace, R.J., Jr., O'Brien, R., Glassroth, J., Raleigh, J., and Dutt, A. (1990): Diagnosis and treatment of disease caused by nontuberculous mycobacteria. *Am. Rev. Respir. Dis.,* 142:940–953.
61. Wallace, R.J., Jr., Swenson, J.M., Silcox, V.A., Good, R.C., Tschen, J.A., and Stone, M.S. (1983): Spectrum of disease due to rapidly growing mycobacteria. *Rev. Infect. Dis.,* 5:657–679.
62. Wallace, R.J., Jr., Silcox, V.A., Tsukamura, M., Brown, B.A., Kilbum, J.O., Butler, W.R., and Onyi, G. (1993): Clinical significance, biochemical features, and susceptibility patterns of sporadic isolates of the mycobacterium chenolae-like organism. *J Clin Microb,* 31:3231–3239.
63. Wallace, R.J., Jr., Brown, B.A., Griffith, D.E., Girard, W.E., Murphy, D.T., Onyi, G.O., Steingrube, V.A., and Mazurek, G.H. (1994): Initial Clarithromycin monotherapy for *Mycobacterium avium-intracellulare* complex lung disease. *Amer Rev Respir Dis* (In press).

Respiratory Infections: Diagnosis and Management, 3d ed.,
edited by James E. Pennington.
Raven Press, Ltd., New York © 1994

33

Pneumocystis carinii

Lowell S. Young

*Kuzell Institute for Arthritis and Infectious Diseases and Division of Infectious
Diseases, California Pacific Medical Center, and University of California,
San Francisco, California 94115*

Pneumocystis carinii is the accepted taxonomic designation for an infectious agent that is either a fungus or a protozoan parasite that causes diffuse pneumonia in immunosuppressed subjects. Interest in this disease entity has waxed and waned during the last 75 years. Morphologic structures corresponding to the cyst forms of this organism were noted in the lungs of guinea pigs by Chagas and rats by Carini (31,44,48). Following World War II, epidemic "plasma cell interstitial pneumonitis" occurred in the malnourished premature infants housed in orphanages. It was during that period that Jirovec and colleagues convincingly established the presence of cyst forms in the lung as the etiologic agent of diffuse pneumonia. During the 1960s and 1970s considerable attention was focused on this entity as a respiratory pathogen occurring exclusively in patients who were either immunodeficient or recipients of therapeutic immunosuppression (13,40,45).

During the 1980s, the most fascinating manifestation of pneumocystis lung infection was that it was the most common opportunistic infection to define a case of the acquired immunodeficiency syndrome (AIDS). Pneumocystis pneumonia has been the presenting opportunistic infection in more than 70% of patients who are diagnosed with AIDS (3,15,23,27), and recurs frequently. Accordingly, there has been a tremendous amount of new research in efforts to affect the epidemiology, pathogenesis, treatment, and prevention of the infection. Thus, many years after the discovery of this respiratory pathogen much is still unknown.

The current AIDS pandemic has stimulated new investigations of *P. carinii* at both the basic and clinical level. Currently, there is a worldwide effort under way to develop new and more effective means of treating this disease. Despite the fact that *P. carinii* has never really been reliably cultivated *in vitro* for extended passage, we now have improved diagnostic techniques, new chemotherapeutic regimens, several prophylactic options, and supporting evidence for adjunctive use of corticosteroids to improve survival in severely hypoxic patients. Besides benefiting AIDS patients, these advances will without doubt help all immunosuppressed patients who are at risk to develop this disease.

MORPHOLOGY AND ETIOLOGY

In all of the human and animal studies conducted to date, the bases for the identification of *P. carinii* have been morphology and staining characteristics. The agent appears to be a protozoan, for two reasons: (i) light and electron microscopic studies indicate the presence of cyst and trophozoite forms that are analogous to morphologic counterparts among the classic protozoa; and (ii) prevention and treatment of pneumocystis in both animals and humans are successfully achieved using agents that are active against classic protozoan forms.

There is, however, new evidence based on patterns of nucleic acid homology that pneumocystis is more closely related to fungi (saccharomyces) than protozoa (7,42). Epidemiologically, airborne spread of pneumocysts appears similar to spread of yeasts. However, almost all antifungal agents are therapeutically inactive, whereas several agents active against protozoa are clinically effective versus *P. carinii*.

The most readily identified form in infected tissues is a thick-walled cyst form that measures 4 to 6 μm in diameter. This cyst form may contain up to eight so-called oval bodies, intracystic bodies, or sporozoites. The Gomori methenamine silver nitrate stain usually stains the cyst wall structures brown or black, including apparent intracellular structures that appear to be like opposing commas or parentheses. The latter are probably thickened portions of the cyst wall. Silver stains do not stain the intracellular oval bodies. In lung imprints and bronchial washings trophozoite forms can also be identified with the Giemsa stain, which is the preferred method for identification of intracystic bodies by light microscopy. Recognition of pneumocystis in tissues is dependent on experience and the application of appropriate controls. The Giemsa stain can be applied relatively rapidly, but because it can also stain background alveolar structures and cell fragments, a silver stain is considered the definitive procedure for recognition of cyst forms in the lung. It is more time-consuming and is also subject to artifacts, because both red cells and yeast forms can resemble pneumocysts. Furthermore, cysts are not always round. They can be disk-shaped, oval, or crescentic, the latter corresponding to an apparent collapsed form. The positioning of these structures is usually within the intraalveolar spaces tightly bound within a dense "honeycombed" matrix. The major inflammatory response is primarily intraalveolar rather than interstitial. Other cyst stains that can be used are the toluidine blue and gram-weigert methods. Both are more rapid than the silver stain but are not preferable to the silver staining process. Recently, monoclonal antibodies have been prepared which appear to reliably stain pneumocysts and can also be used for rapid identification (29).

A complex life cycle for *P. carinii* has been postulated on the basis of electron microscopic studies (46). Trophozoites are probably derived from intracystic bodies or sporozoites that have escaped through the cyst wall. Trophozoites evolve into larger forms and then "mature" by formation of a classic cyst. The bulk of experimental pneumocystis studies have been carried out in small rodents where the morphologic forms are identical to those seen in human tissue. Nonetheless, there can be major antigenic differences between human and murine forms of the protozoan parasite (46).

EPIDEMIOLOGY

The appearance of human pneumocystis infections in an epidemic form has been a matter of great interest. The first well-documented occurrences of epidemic infantile disease, which initially claimed the largest numbers of victims, occurred in malnourished children, usually under the age of 6 months (31). These epidemics favored the original concept of communicability. It appeared that acquisition of disease in the first few months of life was a fairly common event, and clinical disease appeared in the setting of crowding and malnutrition. In other subjects there have been a few reports of clusters of patients who were "normal" (22) or family contacts of patients who were immunosuppressed. In addition, there have been clusters of infections in some institutions caring for patients with neoplastic disorders. Interpretation of the latter, however, has stimulated some controversy. Clusters of disease in an institution caring for patients with neoplasms might be explained by interpersonal spread. On the other hand, individuals with Hodgkin's disease or lymphatic leukemia seem to be predisposed to pneumocystis infection. The reactivation of latent disease secondary to chemotherapy might create the appearance of an epidemic or a cluster of infections. There is strong evidence from serologic studies that acquisition of low levels of pneumocystis antibody usually occurs in early childhood. Thus, the hypothesis about reactivation under the pressure of or influenced by the circumstances of an acquired immunodeficiency has considerable support.

The recent appearance of epidemic pneumocystis infection in patients with AIDS (giving a history of drug abuse and homosexual or bisexual life style) raises the possibility that the infection can be transmitted by person-to-person contact. On the other hand, if the serologic studies documenting the early acquisition of antibody are correct, a more logical explanation is that the cases of pneumocystis in AIDS also represent reactivation of latent disease.

The mechanism of reactivation appears to be related to the progressive destruction of T-cell–mediated immunity. The etiologic agent of AIDS, human immunodeficiency virus-1, or HIV-1, is a transmissible agent that progressively destroys lymphocytes bearing the CD4 phenotype (T helper cells). This agent appears to be transmitted almost exclusively from person to person via sexual contact or exposure to blood or blood products through transfusions or sharing of contaminated needles. Although the period of latency can be quite long, progression of HIV infection results in an immunologic state analogous to the patient receiving antineoplastic chemotherapy.

Thus, a unifying epidemiologic concept seems to include all of the following: first, clinically inapparent infection is extremely common in the first few years of life and occasionally there are cases of pneumonia in young healthy children that can be attributed to pneumocytis. Second, severe clinical pneumocystis becomes evident primarily in individuals with congenital immunodeficiency or acquired immunodeficiency. Third, after childhood most systematic pneumocystis infection represents reactivation of latent infection. Fourth, groups of cases occurring on a nosocomial basis can result from reactivation of latent infection among individuals with similar underlying diseases who are treated with similar chemotherapeutic protocols or who have a similar type of immunodeficiency, thus giving the appearance of person-to-person disease spread. It is conceivable that a patient who has not acquired an "immune status" as a child could be infected via the person-to-person or airborne route when exposed to an actively infected case, but such examples are rare.

THE HOST AND HOST DEFENSES

Hughes (20) has summarized the distribution of primary diseases associated with pneumocystis infection prior to the appearance of AIDS. Before 1980 more than two-thirds of the observed cases of pneumocystis infection were infants, primarily those studied in the European and Middle Eastern epidemics following World War II. Of interest is that there have been a few scattered cases occurring in orphans from the Vietnamese war who were brought to the United States and developed documented pneumocystis infection after leaving Southeast Asia (4). Some were studied and found to be apparently normal, but others were undernourished. The nutritional deficiency is an important component predisposing to this disease and has been studied in both animals and humans. Children dying with kwashiorkor appear to have a rate of pneumocystis similar to that of immunosuppressed children with neoplasms. At present, the most common group of individuals with pneumocystis infection are those with neoplastic abnormalities of lymphoid cells or disorders of mononuclear cell (T-cell)-mediated host defense function. With the impact of AIDS, patient examples of the latter now predominate in the medical services of hospitals in North America, Australia, and Western Europe.

Malignancies per se might not be as important as the type of immunosuppressive therapy. Corticosteroids, apparently more so than cytotoxic agents, have been more commonly associated with the predisposition to pneumocystis infection. In children undergoing chemotherapy for acute leukemia the most severe pneumocystis infections as well as the highest overall incidence of the disease correlated directly with the intensity of the immunosuppression. In addition, other reports emphasize that a factor such as radiation therapy can predispose to pneumocystis infection. Pneumocystis in individuals who have collagen vascular disease as well as those who have received organ transplants might be related more to the use of corticosteroids than to the underlying disease per se. Before 1980, the highest attack rate in the United States occurred in patients less than 1 year of age, and most patients in that age group have some type of immunodeficiency disorder. Pneumocystis infections have occurred in patients with hypogammaglobulinemia as well as severe combined immunodeficiency and thymic aplasia.

The cortisone-treated rat model has given important information about the pathogenesis of the disease as well as served as a useful model for the evaluation of chemotherapeutic agents (9). Naturally occurring epizootics of pneumocystis have been documented in athymic or nude mice (10). Airborne transmission and close contact have been implicated in experimental mice treated with cortisone and in rats only exposed to room air. The pathogenesis of pneumocystis in the experimental rat can be accelerated by use of corticosteroids, and this process can be further accentuated by giving experimental animals a low protein-containing diet (46). All of these factors therefore correspond to known predisposing factors in human patients, particularly with respect to impaired T helper cell numbers or function.

In vitro studies using cysts harvested from rats as well as antibody from the same species demonstrate that humoral antibody enhances uptake and interiorization by alveolar macrophages. Thus, the findings in humans as well as in experimental animals suggest that intact humoral antibody-synthesizing mechanisms and mononuclear phagocytic cell function are important bulwarks of host defense against pneumocystis infection. Of the two components of host defense, however, T-cell–mononuclear phagocyte function appears to be the most important (46).

PATHOLOGY

There is considerable confusion about the histologic pattern of pneumocystis infection, which probably relates to a discrepancy between what is now commonly seen in immunosuppressed patients and the classic "interstitial plasma cell pneumonitis" of the infantile form. In both forms of the disease, however, routine hematoxylin and eosin stains do *not* recognize the cyst or trophozoite form. In both syndromes, microscopic examination of lung tissue often reveals a foamy eosinophilic, honeycombed material, which represents nonstaining organisms plus inflammatory products, and the exudate is a valuable clue to the presence of pneumocystis infection. In the classic epidemic form of infantile pneumocystis there was pronounced infiltration of the alveoli and interstitial spaces with plasma cells. Immunocompromised children and adults now being seen in tertiary care centers usually have a diffuse intraalveolar inflammation rather than interstitial inflammation. Alveolar lumina are filled with large numbers of organisms that can be in degenerated cyst forms as well as alveolar macrophages. Clearly defined cyst forms are almost exclusively present in the intraalveolar spaces, rather than the interstitium. Furthermore, plasma cells and plasma cell infiltrates are uncommon, although hyaline membranes might be present. The honeycombed intraalveolar material can be stained more brightly with the paraaminosalicyclic acid (PAS) as well as the Giemsa stain. In a few patients without active evidence of pneumonia, cyst forms can occasionally be seen at necropsy. The so-called background recovery rate of cysts in lung tissue has been estimated to be around 5%. Without further evidence of pneumonitis little significance can be attached to the detection of such forms. Pneumocystis infection has been primarily or almost always localized to lung tissue. Well-documented cases have occurred in extrapulmonary sites, as in association with severe immunodeficiency states like AIDS (35). Care must be taken to distinguish pneumocysts from similar staining yeast forms in nonpulmonary sites as well as always to use appropriate control stains (negative controls with red cells and yeasts).

CLINICAL MANIFESTATIONS

The primary clinical manifestations of pneumocystis pneumonia are dyspnea, tachypnea, and nonproductive cough. Although fever is usually present in immunosuppressed children and adults, it might not occur in the epidemic infantile form of the disease. The infantile form has been reported to be insidious in onset, accompanied by nonspecific manifestations such as restlessness, languor, and poor feeding. Eventually tachypnea, fever, and periorbital cyanosis with dyspnea are common, but gross signs of pneumonia can develop slowly. Classic signs of pneumonia such as rales are often absent, but the lung can be hyperexpanded. Cases occurring in immunosuppressed patients can have a more fulminant course. Many of these patients have fever, prodromal agitation, increased respiratory rate, and episodes of coughing and dyspnea for days or weeks. Nonetheless, as the disease progresses, dyspnea becomes associated with more severe hypoxia and tachypnea. Of some 80 cases of pneumocystis infection studied by Hughes (20), almost all patients had fever, tachypnea, and an abnormal roentgenogram. Less common findings were cough, cyanosis, and nasal flaring. Arterial hypoxemia was observed in all cases by the time pneumonitis was evident by roentgenogram. Usually the blood gas pattern is that of an uncompensated alkalosis, but the terminal events as determined by the blood gas studies are right to left shunting, venous admixture, increased hypoxia, and decreased diffusion capacity. The terminal events can be associated with severe respiratory acidosis. Pleural effusion and hemoptysis are seen only rarely. Whereas it is clear that immunosuppressive medications such as corticosteroids predispose to pneumocystis infection, it has not been uncommon to observe the onset of symptoms when these medications are being withdrawn or reduced in dosage. This suggests that steroids exert an antiinflammatory effect that leads to symptomatic disease if they are withdrawn.

No laboratory findings are specific for pneumocystis infection. However, an elevated serum LDH can be a suggestive finding in a patient with interstitial pneumonia. Mild early cases of pulmonary pneumocystis can manifest normal oxygen saturation values but they desaturate with mild exercise and have an increased alveolar/arterial oxygen gradient. Radiologically, the great majority of patients with pneumocystis infection have diffuse interstitial-alveolar infiltrates. Typical infiltrates appear either in the perihilar or basilar region and progress to form a "butterfly" pattern. Infiltrates can coalesce with progressive infection leading to lobar consolidation. There are, however, many exceptions to the "classic" roentgenologic pattern. Some individuals have had normal chest x-rays but severe dyspnea. In some documented cases abnormal gallium scans of the lung have considerably antedated the appearance of gross infiltrates (43). So-called atypical manifestations include a miliary pattern (which can be more common if patients are studied early), nodular lesions, lobar consolidation, pneumatocoeles, and lung abscess. The finding of a mediastinal mass (often occurring in a patient with a neoplasm) does not exclude the diagnosis of pneumocystis. Although no radiologic finding excludes the diagnosis of pneumocystis, the process most commonly occurs in individuals with diffuse, patchy infiltrates rather than dense lobar consolidation. Pleural effusions are uncommon.

DIAGNOSTIC APPROACHES

Progress has been made in applying the polymerase chain reaction (PCR) to diagnose pneumocystis disease (38). However, until this approach becomes widely available and standardized, no laboratory or clinical findings short of histologic identification should be used to diagnose pneumocystis disease. Many other infectious processes can mimic or be present simultaneously, such as cytomegalovirus pneumonia, nocardiosis, aspergillosis, zygomycosis, mycoplasma or chlamydia pneumonia, viral pneumonia, bacterial pneumonia, mycobacterial infection, drug reactions, metastatic neoplasm, and postradiation fibrosis.

The only widely available conventional method by which pneumocystis infection is diagnosed with confidence is to demonstrate the pathogen in lung tissue or respiratory secretions. Definitive diagnosis usually includes some method for securing lung tissue or pulmonary secretions. This can be difficult in severely ill patients. Several diagnostic approaches in varying degrees of invasiveness have been suggested, but open lung biopsy remains the standard against which all other procedures must be compared. Examination of expectorated or induced sputum, transtracheal aspiration, fiberoptic bronchoscopy with direct brushing or transbronchial biopsy, bronchoalveolar lavage, and percutaneous transthoracic needle biopsy have all been used with varying degrees of success. Invasive procedures share with open lung biopsy the risk of bleeding and pneumothorax. Hemorrhage and pneumothorax have been particularly difficult problems to control in the elderly patient subjected to "blind" needle biopsy or transbronchial biopsies because the lung might not seal adequately following the procedure. Thrombocytopenia and clotting abnormalities are relative contraindications that can be obviated by appropriate transfusions. The cardinal operative rule is that if adequate specimens are not obtained by one of the less invasive techniques, e.g., sputum examination, transtracheal aspiration, or fiberoptic bronchoscopy, then an open lung biopsy (if needed) should be expeditiously carried out.

Following an invasive procedure, prompt staining of imprints of fresh lung ("touch preparations") can yield a diagnosis within a very short period of time. Even with the hematoxylin and eosin stain there can be some valuable clues to the presence of pneumocystis infection: the "honeycombing" that is present in the intraalveolar spaces.

Noteworthy developments have occurred in the diagnosis of pneumocystis infection in patients with AIDS. Many patients with AIDS appear to have large numbers of organisms in sputum, certainly far more cysts in expectorated sputum than patients with more classical types of immune deficiency and pneumocystis infection. Although sputum might not be spontaneously produced, induced sputum and the examination of such samples by skilled observers has led to the detection of pneumocystis in 70 to 80% of patients with underlying AIDS (27,33). Caution must be exercised in extrapolating these findings to other individuals, e.g., cancer patients and recipients of transplants. In these latter patients, more conventional diagnostic techniques might be required. The one approach that has achieved considerable popularity in the last few years is the technique of bronchoalveolar lavage. By this approach, an endotracheal bronchoscopic catheter is wedged into a respiratory passage and multiple aliquots of sterile saline are rapidly introduced and then aspirated. Lavaged fluids are pooled, concentrated, and examined for a variety of pathogens, including pneumocysts (43).

A major issue that has arisen since the advent of effective chemotherapy for pneumocystis infection is whether or not patients who present with diffuse lung infiltrates should be treated empirically with trimethoprim/sulfamethoxazole and only those who fail to respond then be subjected to a lung biopsy. If AIDS can be confidently excluded, pneumocystis accounts for no more than one-third of diffuse interstitial pulmonary infection (13), and diseases treatable with alternative therapeutic approaches might be missed with empiric initiation of antipneumocystis therapy. Several studies have shown that in patients who have an underlying neoplastic process, the infiltrates are more likely to be neoplastic than the result of pneumocystis infection (36). Empiric therapy is justified if a biopsy procedure is contraindicated because of a remitting bleeding diathesis. Nonetheless, the major justification for open lung biopsy or a reasonably comparative invasive procedure is to rule out diseases other than pneumocystis infection.

There have been alternative methods to the diagnosis of pneumocystis infection, such as measurement of humoral antibodies against cyst antigen. Such studies are still investigational, however, and they can be valuable in retrospective "recouping" of the diagnosis of pneumocystis infection. Our experience strongly suggests that pneumocystis antibody measurements are helpful only when positive, and a negative titer clearly does not exclude the diagnosis. An alternative to the quantitation of the antibody response against the pneumocyst antigen is the detection of circulating pneumocyst antigens. Although detection of pneumocystis antigen has been claimed to be reliable by some investigators, others have not confirmed this result, and test results remain controversial.

TREATMENT OF PNEUMOCYSTIS INFECTION (Table 33-1)

Two types of agents have been repeatedly shown to be effective against pneumocystis infection: pentamidine or folate antagonists alone or usually paired with a sulfonamide. Pentamidine was first reported effective for the treatment of "interstitial plasma cell pneumonia" in 1958 (21). With the advent of this therapy, the mortality in infected children declined from approximately 50% to less than 5%. Of 163 biopsy confirmed cases reviewed by Walzer and colleagues in 1974 (45), mortality was 43%. Most of the patients were immunocompromised and would be expected to die if untreated. Hughes and collaborators (20) found mortality to be approximately 25% in leukemic children with pneumocystis pneumonia treated with pentamidine. The recommended therapeutic dose is 4 mg/kg/day which is administered as a single intramuscular dose. In large patients, two sites should be used to avoid the common complication of sterile abscesses. Intravenous administration of the drug is now commonly given, but care must be observed during administration in intensive care unit settings with constant monitoring of blood pressure. Complications include hypotension, hypoglycemia, tachycardia, erythema, nausea, vomiting, renal failure, and hepatotoxicity. It has long been recognized that the major problem with pentamidine is a high incidence of adverse side effects. Almost 50% of patients reviewed by the Centers for Disease Control had one or more serious adverse reactions. These complications can seriously impair the management of already seriously ill patients.

Almost two decades ago anecdotal reports began to appear of the efficacy of folate antagonists with sulfonamides in the therapy or prophylaxis of pneumocystis infection (47). In fact, the regimen of pyrimethamine and sulfidoxine was successfully used by Post and collaborators to prevent pneumocystis epidemics in Middle Eastern orphanages (34). This was followed by reports of the successful therapeutic use of a combination of pyrimethamine and sulfadiazine (9). Small studies suggested that regimen was as successful as pentamidine (49). The usual dose of pyrimethamine, which is available only in oral form, is 1 mg/kg given as a single dose. The sulfonamide can be either in the form of sulfadiazine or a triple sulfa preparation (trisulfa pyrimidine), 70 to 100 mg/kg divided into four equal portions.

For much of the last decade the preferred initial therapy of documented pneumocystis infection has been the fixed 1:5 combination of trimethoprim/sulfamethoxazole. The recommended dose of either the oral or the intravenous preparation is 15 mg/kg of trimethoprim with 75 mg of sulfamethoxazole/kg divided into three equal portions. Failures have been observed with orally administered trimethoprim/sulfamethoxazole, and the parenteral route is clearly preferred in any patient who has a problem with absorption of orally administered drugs. Clinical success has been associated with peak trimethoprim levels exceeding 5 µg/ml, with corresponding sulfamethoxazole levels being approximately 20 times higher. Hughes and collaborators (20) demonstrated that trimethoprim/sulfamethoxazole given orally to leukemic children was approximately as effective as pentamidine (20). Thus, although most current therapy includes the initial use of trimethoprim/sulfamethoxazole (because of ease of oral administration), some individuals might be allergic to one or more components in this fixed combination. Treatment with pentamidine is clearly indicated in trimethoprim- or sulfonamide-allergic patients. Folate antagonists can cause bone marrow depression, and neutropenia and thrombocytopenia have been observed. In such individuals concomitant treatment with folinic acid might be used without abrogating the antipneumocystis activity of the preparation.

TABLE 33–1. *Treatment of Pneumocystis carinii pneumonia (recommended adult doses)*

Antimicrobial regimen	Mild-to-moderate infection	Severe disease
Trimethoprim-sulfamethoxazole	5 mg/kg PO q8h	5 mg/kg IV q6–8h
Trimethoprim-dapsone	Trimethoprim 100 mg PO qd plus dapsone 100 mg PO qd	N/A
Clindamycin-primaquine	Clindamycin 600 mg PO q8h plus primaquine 30 mg PO qd	Clindamycin 900 mg IV q8h plus primaquine 30 mg PO qd
Pentamidine	Pentamidine 3–4 mg/kg IV qd	Pentamidine 4 mg/kg IV qd
Trimetrexate-leucovorin	Trimetrexate 45 mg/m$_2$ × 21 days plus leucovorin 30 mg/m^2 IV q6h for at least 10 days, then PO 816h for an additional 14 days	N/A
Atovaquone	750 mg PO TID	N/A
Adjunctive therapy		
Corticosteroids	Not recommended	Prednisone 40 mg PO BID × 5 days, then 40 mg PO qd × 5 days, then 20 mg PO qd × 11 days in conjunction with one of the above regimens

The duration of treatment of pneumocystis pneumonia in patients demonstrating a satisfactory clinical response should be 2 weeks, except in AIDS patients who should receive 3-week courses (see below).

It has recently been shown that at least one folate antagonist by itself, trimetrexate, has such potent antipneumocystis activity that it is therapeutically effective in both animal and human pneumocystosis (AIDS) (1). However, the hematologic toxicity of this compound must be abrogated by the simultaneous administration of large and costly doses of leucovorin. One disappointment about trimetrexate has been the high rate of recrudescence (65%) in the months immediately post treatment.

Eflornithine is an ornithine decarboxylase inhibitor that is of proven effectiveness in treating African trypanosomiasis. There is some evidence of modest activity against pneumocystosis, but the drug can trigger severe thrombocytopenia in AIDS patients (41) and remains experimental.

Combinations of the antibacterial agent clindamycin with antimalarials like primaquine have been promising in animal models, and studies in AIDS patients show efficacy approaching standard regimens in mildly to moderately severe cases (2,30). Similarly, a new antimalarial agent, atovaquone (BW 566C80), is effective in treating human pneumocystis if patients are not critically ill (18). Allergic reactions can still occur to clindamycin, primaquine, and atovaquone, and the near-term relapse rate with the latter agent is high.

Overall, our recommendations for treatment follow an order of priorities outlined in Table 33-1. If at all possible patients with pneumocystis pneumonia should receive a folate antagonist (trimethoprim-pyrimethamine) plus a sulfonamide or sulfone (25, 37). Subjects who might not have reliable gastrointestinal absorption should receive a parenteral preparation (trimethoprim-sulfamethoxazole is usually the most commonly available). Patients intolerant of this first-line regimen should receive iv pentamidine. Failing both of these therapies (which are equally effective), therapeutic options are either atovaquone or clindamycin-primaquine. Trimetrexate and eflornithine must be considered the last choices for "salvage" therapy.

Because there are several methods for treating pneumocystis pneumonia and no means for determining the antimicrobial susceptibility for this parasite, a major clinical dilemma occurs when a patient does not appear to be responding to an initial therapeutic regimen. It has been the experience of many workers that either pentamidine or trimethoprim/sulfamethoxazole might not cause clinical improvement for periods exceeding 1 week of treatment (49). In our studies, the median time to improvement on intravenous trimethoprim/sulfamethoxazole was 4 days, but time to improvement is often longer in AIDS patients. We believe that it would be prudent to treat for at least 4 days before deciding to "cross over" to pentamidine. If the patient is deteriorating at that point, change seems indicated. If the patient has not deteriorated, an additional 2 days of treatment can be given. Clearly, there have been some patients who have failed to respond to an initial regimen of pentamidine or trimethoprim/sulfamethoxazole but have responded clinically after a changeover to the alternative regimen. These experiences suggest drug failure rather than host failure, but the definitive assessment of this is not possible at this time. At present, there is no evidence that using trimethoprim/sulfamethoxazole plus pentamidine in humans offers additional therapeutic advantage. The failure to affect an infiltrative pulmonary process presumed to be due to pneumocystis could actually be the consequence of infections caused by other organisms such as the cytomegalovirus, mycobacteria, a disseminated fungal process, or an underlying neoplasm. Likewise, in patients with AIDS, multiple pulmonary processes might be present.

Supportive measures besides chemotherapy are extremely important in determining the clinical outcome. Reduction in immunosuppression, for example, in cancer treatment, can enhance the chance for recovery, as evidenced by recovery of a few documented cases without chemotherapy. The importance of good ventilatory support in an appropriate setting by trained specialists cannot be overemphasized. Patients who are markedly hypoxemic or hypercarbic might have to be intubated.

Pneumocystis in AIDS

Patients with AIDS have a very high incidence of pneumocystis infection, so much attention has been focused on clinical manifestations, diagnosis, treatment, and prophylaxis of infection (2,5,6,8,12,14–17,24–27,36,37,39).

The critical laboratory finding indicating susceptibility to clinical pneumocystis is a CD4 lymphocyte count of less than 200/mm^3 (32). Despite the debate that surrounds the value of so-called surrogate markers in HIV-infection, clinicians should unhesitatingly place their patients on some form of prophylaxis (see Table 33-2) when the CD4 lymphocyte count drops below 200. This is considered "primary prophylaxis" as opposed to "secondary prophylaxis," which should be instituted following an episode of clinical pneumocystis disease. The distinctions are moot in terms of choice of regimens. Several reviews have shown that patients with AIDS can have a far more indolent clinical course prior to the "declaration" of overt disease (23). Patients with AIDS might be suspected of having pneumocystis if they present with dyspnea and/or fever even with fairly normal chest x-rays. One of the clues might be an abnormal arterial-alveolar oxygen gradient which could be further provoked by some type of limited stress or exercise test. There are numerous reports indicating that chest x-rays can be normal, but gallium scans can be abnormal in patients with early pneumocystis infection complicating AIDS and other immunodeficiency states (6).

One of the more striking aspects of pneumocystis infection in AIDS patients is that whereas initial response rates to licensed medications are quite good (e.g., about 80% of patients treated for a first episode of pneumonia will improve, but this success rate decreases with repeated episodes), there is a high incidence of drug reactions. For trimethoprim/sulfamethoxazole, more than half and as many as 80% of patients can develop some type of dermal hypersensitivity. This is usually due to the sulfonamide component of the fixed combination. Some of these reactions can be quite severe, but others sufficiently mild so that patients can still be continued with medication. More often than not, these hypersensitivity reactions which appear by about the sixth to tenth day of treatment necessitate a crossover to an alternative treatment. In AIDS patients, pentamidine itself has been relatively less nephrotoxic and hepatotoxic than was reported for patients with cancer or an organ transplant. Nonetheless, one of the more striking aspects of pentamidine toxicity in AIDS patients has been neutropenia, which can be precipitous. Thus, patients with defects in cell-mediated immunity can actually develop opportunistic infections due to pathogens such as pseudomonas as a result of pentamidine-induced neutropenia.

TABLE 33–2. *Prophylaxis of P. carinii pneumonia in AIDS patients[a]*

Drug	Route	Dose	Interval	Comment
Trimethoprim + Sulfamethoxazole	Oral	160 mg 800 mg	3–7 d/wk	One (160 mg/800 mg) or DS table qd is basic recommendation; for those who can tolerate it, BID might be more effective, but one DS thrice weekly has some effect
Dapsone	Oral	50–100 mg	q d	
Pyrimethamine + Dapsone	Oral	25–50 mg 50–100 mg	q wk q d	
Pentamidine-isethionate Respirgard® II FISOnebs®	Aerosol Aerosol	300 mg 60 mg	q mo q 2 wks	Either is the acceptable alternative for those who cannot tolerate trimethoprim-sulfamethoxazole
Atovaquone Trimetrexate				New formulations are under study but cannot be recommended for prophylaxis

[a]Prophylaxis has been best studied in AIDS and leukemia patients.

Problems with existing treatment have resulted in experimental and clinical assessment of promising regimens such as dapsone/trimethoprim, eflornithine, trimetrexate, clindamycin/primaquine, and atovaquone. Eflornithine, dapsone alone, and aerosolized pentamidine appear to be less effective clinically and should not be used as initial therapy.

Almost every authority dealing with the AIDS crisis agrees that the attack rate and recurrence rate of pneumocystis is high, the latter exceeding 50% in the first year after diagnosis. Persistence of pneumocysts in lung tissue is common even in successfully treated patients (27). Predicted pneumocystis incidence in patients presenting with Kaposi's sarcoma is approximately 50%, and a controlled study demonstrates the efficacy of trimethoprim/sulfamethoxazole in preventing pneumocystis infection (8). Maintenance therapy directed at the underlying HIV disease using zidovudine does not prevent recrudescent pneumocystis infection. Therefore, a variety of measures have been evaluated for prophylaxis. For the patient who can continue to take sulfanomides, both trimethoprim-sulfamethoxazole and the fixed combination of pyrimethamine and sulfadoxine (Fansidar) appear to be effective (14). Interestingly, patients who are allergic to sulfamethoxazole might yet tolerate one of the other sulfonamide-containing compounds (26).

Aerosolized pentamidine (different preparations listed in Table 33-2) is not as effective as trimethoprim/sulfamethoxazole and should be considered only in patients intolerant of sulfonamides or sulfones (16,39). Prophylaxis against pneumocystis in AIDS patients must be assumed at this time to be a lifelong requirement.

The role of corticosteroids in pneumocystis infection has been evaluated in controlled trials. They may have an antiinflammatory effect (and transiently improve oxygenation), but because of their immunosuppressive effects they should be reserved for hypoxic patients (arterial $pO_2 < 70$ mm/Hg) (3,11,28).

PROGNOSIS AND PREVENTION IN NON-AIDS PATIENTS

These two aspects should be considered together because the necessity for preventative measures appears closely linked to the risk of recrudescent infection. By recrudescence, it is implied that the host never really eradicates the pneumocystis parasite. In animal models this appears to be the case because recurrent disease may follow reinstitution of immunosuppression. Prophylaxis with agents such as trimethoprim/sulfamethoxazole appears to be effective only for the duration of administration of the prophylactic agent. In some centers the recurrence rate among patients with malignancies has exceeded 5% per year.

As with patients having AIDS, the decision to give chemoprophylaxis should be related to the state of the host. In patients whose organ graft appears to be well accepted and where immunosuppression is being reduced, the chance of recurrent disease is low and long-term prophylaxis does not appear to be indicated. Prophylactic use of trimethoprim/sulfamethoxazole has been quite effective in the bone marrow transplant recipient between days 20 and 120, which corresponds to the period of maximum risk. Continuation of chemoprophylaxis beyond 4 months in the marrow transplant recipient who does not have graft-versus-host disease is rarely indicated because of successful reconstitution of immune function.

One of the really puzzling aspects of pneumocystis is that cancer treatment centers using similar or identical protocols have very different incidence rates for proven infection. If within a given population (similar type of neoplastic disease) the annual incidence rate of pneumocystis infection exceeds 5%, then general prophylaxis of patients with that type of disorder seems prudent. The daily dosage should be 4 to 6 mg/kg of trimethoprim (with corresponding 1:5 amount of sulfamethoxazole) in two divided doses. There is some evidence from treatment of leukemic children and marrow transplant recipients that this type of prophylaxis can be given for 3 consecutive days per week and still be effective (19).

Other approaches such as active immunization have not been efficacious in animal models. In patients with clear-cut immunodeficiency of the humoral type, it seems prudent to give replacement γ-globulin therapy, and this can be associated with reduced risk of pneumocystis infection.

REFERENCES

1. Allegra, C.J., Chabner, B.A., Tuazon, C.U., et al. (1987): Trimetrexate, a novel and effective agent for the treatment of *Pneumocystis carinii* pneumonia in patients with the acquired immunodeficiency syndrome. *N. Engl. J. Med.,* 317:978–985.
2. Black, J.R., Feinberg, J., Murphy, R.L., et al. (1991): Clindamycin and primaquine as primary therapy for mild and moderately severe *Pneumocystis carinii* pneumonia in patients with AIDS. *Eur. J. Clin. Microbiol.,* 10:204–207.
3. Bozette, S.A., Sattler, F., and Chui, J. (1990): A controlled trial of early adjuvant treatment with corticosteroids for *Pneumocystis carinii* pneumonia in the acquired immunodeficiency syndrome. *N. Engl. J. Med.,* 323:1451–1457.
4. Centers for Disease Control. (1976): *Pneumocystis carinii* pneumonia in Vietnamese orphans. *M.M.W.R.,* 25:15.
5. Centers for Disease Control. (1992): Recommendations for prophylaxis against *Pneumocystis carinii* pneumonia for adults and adolescents infected with human immunodeficiency virus. *M.M.W.R.,* 41(RR-4):1–11.
6. Coleman, D.L., Hattner, R.S., Luce, J.M., Dodek, P.M., Golden, J.A., and Murray, J.F. (1984): Correlation between gallium lung scans and fiberoptic bronchoscopy in patients with suspected *Pneumocystis carinii* pneumonia and the acquired immune deficiency syndrome. *Am. Rev. Respir. Dis.,* 130:1166–1169.
7. Edman, J.C., Kovacs, J.A., Masur, H., Santi, D.V., Elwood, H.J., and Sogin, M.L. (1988): Ribosomal RNA sequences show *Pneumocystis carinii* to be a member of the fungi. *Nature,* 334:519–522.
8. Fischl, M.A., Dickinson, G.M., and La Voie, L. (1988): Safety and efficacy of sulfamethoxazole and trimethoprim chemoprophylaxis for *Pneumocystis carinii* pneumonia in AIDS. *J.A.M.A.,* 259:1185–1189.
9. Frenkel, J.K., Good, J.T., and Shulta, J.A. (1966): Latent pneumocystis infection of rats, relapse, and chemotherapy. *Lab. Invest.,* 15:1559–1577.
10. Furuta, T., Ueda, K., Kyuwa, S., et al. (1984): Effect of T-cell transfer on *Pneumocystis carinii* infection in nude mice. *Jpn. J. Exp. Med.,* 54:57–64.
11. Gagnon, S., Boota, A.M., Fischl, M.A., et al. (1990): Corticosteroids as adjuvant therapy for severe *Pneumocystis carinii* pneumonia in the acquired immunodeficiency syndrome: a double-blind, placebo-controlled trial. *N. Engl. J. Med.,* 323:1444–1450.
12. Girard, P.M., Landman, R., Gaudebout, C., et al. (1993): Dapsone-pyrimethamine compared with aerosolized pentamidine as primary prophylaxis against *Pneumocystis carinii* pneumonia and toxoplasmosis in HIV infection. *N. Engl. J. Med.,* 21:1514–1520.
13. Goodell, B., Jacobs, J.B., Powell, R.D., and DeVita, V.T. (1970): *Pneumocystis carinii*: spectrum of diffuse interstitial pneumonia in patients with neoplastic disease. *Ann. Intern. Med.,* 72:337–340.
14. Gottlieb, M.S., Knight, S., Mitsuyasu, R., Weisman, J., Roth, M., and Young, L.S. (1984): Prophylaxis of *Pneumocystis carinii* in AIDS with pyrimethamine-sulfadoxine. *Lancet,* 2:398–399.
15. Gottlieb, M.S., Schroff, R., and Schanker, H.M. (1981): *Pneumocystis carinii* pneumonia and mucosal candidiasis in previously healthy homosexual men: evidence of a new acquired cellular immunodeficiency. *N. Engl. J. Med.,* 301:1425–1430.
16. Hardy, W.D., Feinberg, J., Finkelstein, D., et al. (1992): A controlled trial of trimethoprim-sulfamethoxazole or aerosolized pentamidine for secondary prophylaxis of *Pneumocystis carinii* pneumonia in patients with the acquired immunodeficiency syndrome. *N. Engl. J. Med.,* 26:1842–1848.

17. Hirschl, B., Lazzarin, A., Chopard, P., et al. (1991): A controlled study of inhaled pentamidine for primary prevention of *Pneumocystis carinii* pneumonia. *N. Engl. J. Med.,* 324:1079–1083.

18. Hughes, W., Leoung, G., Kramer, F., et al. (1993): Comparison of atovaquone (566C80) with trimethoprim-sulfamethoxazole to treat *Pneumocystis carinii* pneumonia in patients with AIDS. *N. Engl. J. Med.,* 21:1521–1527.

19. Hughes, W.T., Rivera, G.K., Schell, N.J., Thornton, D., and Lott, L. (1987): Successful intermittent chemoprophylaxis for *Pneumocystis carinii* pneumonitis. *N. Engl. J. Med.,* 316:1627–1632.

20. Hughes, W.T. (1987): *Pneumocystis carinii* pneumonitis. *N. Engl. J. Med.,* 317:1021–1024.

21. Ivady, G., and Paldy, L. (1976): Treatment of *Pneumocystis carinii* pneumonia in infancy. In: *Symposium on* Pneumocystis carinii *Infection,* edited by J.B. Robbins, V.T. DeVita, Jr., and W. Dutz, pp. 291–305. Monograph 40. National Cancer Institute, Bethesda, Md.

22. Jacobs, J.L., Libby, D.M., Winters, R.A., et al. (1991): A cluster of *Pneumocystis carinii* pneumonia in adults without predisposing illnesses. *N. Engl. J. Med.,* 324:246–250.

23. Kovacs, J.A., Hiemenz, J.W., Macher, A.M., et al. (1984): *Pneumocystis carinii* pneumonia: a comparison between patients with acquired immunodeficiency syndrome and patients with other immunodeficiencies. *Ann. Intern. Med.,* 100:663–671.

24. Leoung, G.S., Feigal, D.W., Montgomery, A.B., et al. (1990): Aerosolized pentamidine for prophylaxis against *Pneumocystis carinii* pneumonia: the San Francisco community prophylaxis trial. *N. Engl. J. Med.,* 323:769–775.

25. Leoung, G.S., Mills, J., Hopewell, P.C., Hughes, W.T., and Wofsy, C. (1986): Dapsone-trimethoprim for treatment of *Pneumocystis carinii* pneumonia in the acquired immunodeficiency syndrome. *Ann. Intern. Med.,* 105:45–48.

26. Masur, H. (1992): Drug therapy: prevention and treatment of *Pneumocystis* pneumonia. *N. Engl. J. Med.,* 26:1853–1860.

27. Murray, J.F., Garay, S.M., Hopewell, P.H., Mills, J., Snider, G.L., and Stover, D.E. (1987): Pulmonary complications of the acquired immunodeficiency syndrome: an update. *Am. Rev. Respir. Dis.,* 135:504–509.

28. National Institutes of Health–University of California Expert Panel for Corticosteroids as Adjuvant Therapy for *Pneumocystis carinii* Pneumonia. (1990): Consensus statement on the use of corticosteroids as adjuvant therapy for *Pneumocystis carinii* pneumonia in the acquired immunodeficiency syndrome. *N. Engl. J. Med.,* 323:1500–1504.

29. Ng, V.L., Virani, N.A., Chaisson, R.E., et al. (1990): Rapid detection of *Pneumocystis carinii* using a direct fluorescent monoclonal antibody stain. *J. Clin. Microbiol.,* 28:2228–2233.

30. Noskin, G.A., Murphy, R.L., Black, J.R., et al. (1992): Salvage therapy with clindamycin-primaquine for *Pneumocystis carinii* pneumonia. *Clin. Infect. Dis.,* 14:183–188.

31. Nouza, M. (1992): *Pneumocystis carinii* pneumonia after 40 years. *Infection,* (20)3:113–117.

32. Phair, J., Muñoz, A., Detels, R., et al. (1990): The risk of *Pneumocystis carinii* pneumonia among men infected with human immunodeficiency virus type 1. *N. Engl. J. Med.,* 322:161–165.

33. Pitchenik, A.E., Ganjei, P., Torres, A., et al. (1986): Sputum examination for the diagnosis of *Pneumocystis carinii* pneumonia in the acquired immunodeficiency syndrome. *Am. Rev. Respir. Dis.,* 133:226–229.

34. Post, C., FaKonghi, T., Dutz, W., Bandarizadeh, B., and Kohout, E.E. (1971): Prophylaxis of epidemic infantile pneumocytosis with a 20:1 sulfadoxine and pyrimethamine combination. *Curr. Ther. Res.,* 13:273–279.

35. Raviglione, M.C. (1990): Extrapulmonary pneumocystosis: the first 50 cases. *Rev. Infect. Dis.,* 12:1127–1138.

36. Ruskin, J. (1988): Parasitic diseases in the compromised host. In: *Clinical Approach to Infection in the Compromised Host,* edited by R.H. Rubin and L.S. Young, pp. 253–298. Plenum Press, New York.

37. Sattler, F.R., Cowan, R., Nielsen, D.M., et al. (1988): Trimethoprim-sulfamethoxazole compared with pentamidine for treatment of *Pneumocystis carinii* pneumonia in the acquired immunodeficiency syndrome: a prospective, noncross-over study. *Ann. Intern. Med.,* 109:280–287.

38. Schluger, N., Godwin, T., Sepkowitz, K., et al. (1992): Application of DNA amplification to pneumocystosis: presence of *Pneumocystis carinii* DNA during human and experimentally induced *Pneumocystis carinii* pneumonia. *J. Exp. Med.,* 176:1327–1333.

39. Schneider, M.M.E., Hoepelman, A.I.M., Schattenkerk, J.K.M.E., Nielsen, T.L., and Borleffs, I.C.C. (1992): A controlled trial of aerosolized pentamidine or trimethoprim-sulfamethoxazole as primary prophylaxis against *Pneumocystis carinii* pneumonia in patients with human immunodeficiency virus infection. *N. Engl. J. Med.,* 26:1836–1841.

40. Sepkowitz, K.A., Brown, A.E., Telzak, E.E., Gottlieb, S., and Armstrong, D. (1992): *Pneumocystis carinii* pneumonia among patients without AIDS at a cancer hospital. *J.A.M.A.,* 6:832–837.

41. Smith, D.E., Davies, S., Smithson, J., Harding, I., and Gazzard, B.G. (1992): Eflornithine versus cotrimoxazole in the treatment of *Pneumocystis carinii* pneumonia in AIDS patients. *AIDS* 12:1489–1493.

42. Stringer, S.L., Hudson, K., Blase, M.A., Walzer, P.D., Cushion, M.T., and Stringer, J.R. (1989): Sequence from ribosomal RNA of *Pneumocystis carinii* compared to those of four fungi suggests an asomycetous affinity. *J. Protozool.*, 36:14S–16S.

43. Tuazon, C.U., Delaney, M.D., Simon, G.L., et al. (1985): Utility of gallium 67 scintigraphy and bronchial washings in the diagnosis and treatment of *Pneumocystis carinii* pneumonia in patients with the acquired immunodeficiency syndrome. *Am. Rev. Respir. Dis.*, 132:1087–1092.

44. Walzer, P.D. (Editor). (1994): Pneumocystis carinii *Pneumonia,* 2nd Edition. Marcel Dekker, New York.

45. Walzer, P.D., Perl, D.P., Krogstad, D.J., Rawson, P.G., and Schultz, M.G. (1976): *Pneumocystis carinii* pneumonia in the United States: epidemiologic, diagnostic, and clinical features. In: *Symposium on* Pneumocystis carinii *Infection,* edited by J.B. Robbins, V.T. DeVita, Jr., and W. Dutz, pp. 55–63. Monograph 43. National Cancer Institute, Bethesda, Md.

46. Walzer, P.D. (1984): Experimental models of *Pneumocystis carinii* pneumonia. In: Pneumocystis carinii *Pneumonia: Pathogenesis, Diagnosis and Treatment.* edited by L.S. Young, pp. 7–76. Marcel Dekker, New York.

47. Whisant, J.K., and Buckley, R.H. (1976): Successful pyrimethamine-sulfadoxine therapy of pneumocystis pneumonia in infants with X-linked immunodeficiency with hyper IgM. In: *Symposium on* Pneumocystis carinii *Infection,* edited by J.B. Robbins, V.T. DeVita, Jr., and W. Dutz, pp. 211–216. Monograph 43. National Cancer Institute, Bethesda, Md.

48. Young, L.S. (1984): Introduction and historical perspective. In: Pneumocystis carinii *Pneumonia: Pathogenesis, Diagnosis, and Treatment,* edited by L.S. Young, pp. 1–6. Marcel Dekker, New York.

49. Young, L.S. (1982): Trimethoprim-sulfamethoxazole in the treatment of adults with pneumonia due to *Pneumocystis carinii. Rev. Infect. Dis.*, 4:608–613.

Respiratory Infections: Diagnosis and Management, 3d ed., edited by James E. Pennington. Raven Press, Ltd., New York © 1994

34

Parasitic Pneumonias

Peter F. Weller

Harvard Medical School and Beth Israel Hospital, 330 Brookline Avenue, Boston, Massachusetts 02215

Infections with the varied helminthic and protozoan parasites that infect humans can produce a wide range of inflammatory reactions in pulmonary tissues. The nature of the respiratory involvement depends both on the pathobiology of the parasite and on the human immunologic responses to the parasite. Pneumonitis caused by *Pneumocystis carinii* is considered elsewhere; the principal metazoan and protozoan parasites that affect human pulmonary tissues are considered in this chapter.

METAZOAN PARASITES

Ascariasis

The roundworm, *Ascaris lumbricoides,* globally one of the most prevalent helminthic parasites of humans, infrequently produces symptomatic disease. Ascariasis can be considered in three stages: (i) the pulmonary phase, (ii) the intestinal phase, and (iii) complications arising from the intestinal phase. Respiratory involvement develops primarily in the first stage and rarely as a complication of the intestinal phase.

Infection is acquired by ingesting embryonated eggs of *A. lumbricoides,* which were passed in the feces of other infected humans and may remain infectious in the soil for up to 6 years. Although infection is more common in rural areas with poor sanitation, it can occur whenever the opportunity exists for the consumption of fecally passed eggs, that is, by means of fecally contaminated agricultural products or other foodstuffs, dirty hands, or geophagy. From the swallowed eggs, larvae hatch in the intestine within 1 to 2 days and molt into second-stage larvae, which are carried hematogenously to the liver and lungs. In the lungs, roughly 1 to 2 weeks after infection, the larvae penetrate from the capillary bed into alveoli and molt again into third-stage larvae, which ascend the tracheobronchial tree, to be swallowed and to return to the intestine. In the intestine, they mature into large, 10-to-30-cm-long, adult male and female worms, which begin producing eggs 2 to 3 months after initial infection.

The principal pulmonary manifestations of *Ascaris* infection develop during the transpulmonary passage of *Ascaris* larvae and produce a syndrome of transient eosinophilic pulmonary infiltrates, commonly referred to as Loeffler's syndrome. *As-*

caris infection was retrospectively implicated as the cause of the syndrome of eosinophilic pneumonitis in the patients initially reported by Loeffler (62) and continues to be the most common cause of Loeffler's syndrome worldwide (130).

From accounts of experimental (61,127) and mischievously induced (88) human infections and the descriptions of *Ascaris* pneumonia in areas with seasonal transmission (40,41), the natural history of the clinical syndrome of pulmonary ascariasis has been delineated. Symptoms develop about 9 to 12 days after ingestion of *Ascaris* eggs, at a time when larvae are within the lungs. An irritating, nonproductive cough and burning substernal discomfort, aggravated by coughing or deep breathing, are common, with dyspnea and blood-tinged sputum experienced by some. About 15% have urticaria during the first 4 to 5 days of illness. Fever, occurring in many patients, infrequently exceeds 101°F. Over half have rales and wheezing, but signs of consolidation are absent. Hepatomegaly can develop but lymphadenopathy does not. The acute symptoms generally subside within 5 to 10 days, depending on the severity of the illness.

Radiographically round or oval infiltrates ranging in size from several millimeters to several centimeters in both lung fields are more likely to be present when blood eosinophilia exceeds 10%. These infiltrates, which are migratory and can become confluent in perihilar areas, usually clear completely after several weeks (10,40,88). Eosinophilia, the most common laboratory finding, can be absent in the early symptomatic period, but increases in magnitude after several days of symptoms and resolves over many weeks (40). In the sputum, eosinophils and Charcot-Leyden crystals, composed of the eosinophil-derived enzyme lysophospholipase (134,135), are found. Serum IgE levels and antibody titers to *Ascaris* will be elevated (88).

Because of the benignity of *Ascaris* pneumonia, pathologic studies of human infections are limited (11,89) but have documented focal areas of fibrinous and eosinophilic exudative bronchopneumonia (11,41,89). This eosinophilic cellular infiltrate probably accounts for the self-limited decreases in vital capacity observed in some patients (41). In contrast, other patients experience primarily obstructive alterations in pulmonary function (88), consistent with the experimental induction of asthmatiform airway hyperreactivity by infection of animals with *Ascaris* (15) or airway challenge of sensitized animals with *Ascaris* antigen (46,86). *Ascaris* pneumonia can be diagnosed at the time of pneumonic involvement with certainty only by detecting *Ascaris* larvae either in respiratory secretions or in gastric aspirates (41,93). At least 40 days must elapse before the intrapulmonary larvae responsible for *Ascaris* pneumonia have matured sufficiently to produce eggs detectable in the stool. Negative stool exams during or soon after an episode of pneumonitis will not exclude *Ascaris* as an etiology of the pneumonia, nor would positive stool exams for *Ascaris* eggs during the stage of pulmonary involvement establish the etiology, as these observed eggs reflect infection acquired 2 to 12 months earlier. The findings that stools are free of eggs during the pneumonic involvement and contain *Ascaris* eggs 2 to 3 months later would support *Ascaris* as the etiologic agent of the pneumonitis.

Ascaris pneumonia is self-limited and only very rarely fatal, and so specific therapy usually is not necessary. The bronchospasm can be managed with conventional medical therapy. If the pneumonia is severe, systemic corticosteroids will dramatically diminish the symptoms and the blood eosinophilia (41). Antihelminthic therapy is indicated to eradicate the *Ascaris* infection to prevent the unusual, but potentially devastating, complications of intestinal infections such as intestinal obstruction by the large adult worms or migration of adult worms into aberrant sites such as the pancreatic or biliary ducts. Very rarely, adult worms, as a result of vomiting and aspiration or of migration up the esophagus into the trachea, can incite the development of bronchopneumonia (93). The drugs of choice for *Ascaris* infections are mebendazole (100 mg twice daily for 3 days), pyrantel pamoate (a single dose of 11 mg/kg, not to exceed 1 g), or albendazole (400 mg once) (4).

Hookworm Infection

Hookworm infections, caused either by *Ancylostoma duodenale* (in Mediterranean countries, parts of Iran, India, Pakistan, and the Far East) or by *Necator americanus* (in North and South America, parts of India, Central Africa, Indonesia, and the South Pacific), are more common where sanitary practices allow for human fecal contamination of the soil. From fecal excrement hookworm eggs release larvae that mature in the soil into infective larvae. Percutaneous larval penetration constitutes the principal mode of human infection, although infections with *A. duodenale* can also be acquired by the oral route (8). In traversing the skin, larvae can induce an erythematous, pruritic, maculopapular dermatitis at their penetration sites. From the skin larvae pass hematogenously to the lungs and, like the larvae of *Ascaris,* enter the alveoli, ascend the bronchotracheal tree to the pharynx, and are swallowed. In the intestinal tract, the larvae mature into adult worms.

Respiratory involvement occurs during the transpulmonary migration of hookworm larvae. Symptoms, which are not frequently noted with naturally acquired infection (8), can develop within days of infection and include a nonproductive cough and wheezing (76). The transient, fleeting infiltrates, which can be noted radiographically, and the blood eosinophilia, which usually develops during the second or third week of infection, constitute Loeffler's syndrome. This respiratory involvement is benign and self-limited; as a consequence, the histopathology of the involvement in the human has not been examined.

The establishment of hookworm infection as the etiology of a Loeffler's-like pneumonitis requires observation of larvae in either respiratory secretions or gastric or duodenal fluid. The diagnosis is supported by a history of dermal exposure to potentially contaminated soil, by a history of an antecedent hookworm dermatitis, and by finding blood eosinophilia. Stool examinations for the eggs of *N. americanus* or *A. duodenale,* the diagnostic test for mature intestinal hookworm infections, are not helpful during the early time period when pneumonitis can occur. About 2 months for *N. americanus* and up to 38 weeks for *A. duodenale* must elapse after dermal acquisition of infection before fecal egg excretion is detectable (76). Negative stool exams would be expected during this stage of pneumonitis; positive stool exams would reflect fully established intestinal tract infections. Reliable serologic tests are not available. The other manifestations of hookworm infection, iron-deficiency anemia, gastrointestinal symptoms, and impairment of nutrition, generally occur only with heavy infections and develop after the stage of pulmonary involvement.

Hookworm infections are treated with either mebendazole (100 mg orally twice daily for 3 days), a single dose of pyrantel pamoate (11 mg/kg, not to exceed 1 g), or a single dose of albendazole (400 mg once) (4). Although rarely necessary, corticosteroids would ameliorate the pulmonary involvement.

Cutaneous Larva Migrans

Cutaneous larva migrans develops when the infective-stage larvae of the dog or cat hookworm, *Ancylostoma braziliense,* penetrate and migrate in human skin to produce an inflammatory reaction along the cutaneous tract of their migration. Infection, requiring dermal contact with soil containing infective larvae that have hatched from eggs passed in canine or feline feces, is acquired more frequently on sandy beaches, sand boxes, and under dwellings, and is more common in warmer climates such as the southeastern parts of the United States. Those at greatest risk include children, swimmers, and laborers whose activities bring their skin in contact with contaminated soil.

Pruritic, elevated, serpiginous, reddish-brown dermal lesions are the cardinal manifestations of this entity. Less commonly, larvae are carried hematogenously to the lungs. A dry cough, starting about 1 week after dermal invasion and lasting usually for 1 to 2 weeks (139) and, rarely, for 9 months, is sometimes experienced (57). Chest x-ray films can reveal transient migratory infiltrates (20,45,57,74,139). Blood eosinophilia is common and bronchoalveolar lavage can reveal eosinophils if there is pneumonia (101). A presumptive diagnosis is made from the typical dermatologic lesions; a definitive diagnosis requires recovery of larvae from respiratory secretions. Stool examinations and serologic tests are not helpful. The pulmonary involvement is mild and self-limited; therefore, specific therapy is not utilized. Either ethyl chloride or thiabendazole applied topically is employed for the skin lesions (4). Albendazole (200 mg bid for 3 days) is also effective (4).

Visceral Larva Migrans

Infection with the dog ascarid, *Toxocara canis,* or, less commonly, the cat ascarid, *Toxocara catis,* produces a syndrome in humans termed "visceral larva migrans," which can be subclinical or can present primarily as an ocular form or a visceral form. In the visceral form, pulmonary involvement is common.

Human infections are acquired by ingesting *Toxocara* eggs. These eggs, when initially shed in the feces of dogs and cats, are not infectious, but after about 3 weeks in the soil the larvae become infectious. People at risk for developing infection are not those who handle dogs or cats but rather those who ingest soil containing the embryonated eggs (42). Hence, visceral larval migrans is principally a disease of children 1 to 5 years old, especially those with a history of geophagus pica (72). *Toxocara canis* is common in North America (about 20% of adult dogs and 80% of puppies are infected), and areas where dogs defecate, including public playgrounds, quite frequently harbor potentially infectious ova (111).

After ingestion of infectious *Toxocara* eggs, larvae penetrate the gastrointestinal mucosa and are carried in the portal circulation to the liver and then into the systemic circulation. When larvae encounter vessels too small to allow their passage, they exit into surrounding tissues. The manifestations of visceral larva migrans are a consequence of both the damage produced by migrating larvae and the evoked eosinophilic granulomatous host response. Mild infections are notable only by an elevated blood eosinophilia. In heavier infections, malaise, irritability, fever, hepatomegaly, and pruritic cutaneous lesions are common. Respiratory symptoms, including dyspnea, wheezing, and a chronic, nonproductive cough, are experienced by 20 to 86% of children (51,122), and rales and wheezes are frequent. Abnormalities on chest x-ray film, demonstrable in 40% or more with symptomatic illness, include, most commonly, bilateral peribronchial infiltration and, less frequently, prominent infiltrates (51,114,122). Uncommonly, more severe respiratory tract involvement can develop with very heavy infections (14). Laboratory abnormalities include elevated serum levels of IgG, IgM, and IgE, a leukocytosis with an eosinophilia usually in excess of 30%, and, in about 50%, elevated titers of anti-A and/or anti-B isohemagglutinins. Pulmonary pathology has not been detailed, but in other tissues eosinophilic granulomas develop around the larvae.

Definitive diagnosis of visceral larva migrans would require detection of larvae in biopsied tissue, but this is rarely indicated. Often, the diagnosis is made based on a compatible clinical presentation in a patient with eosinophilia and hypergammaglobulinemia. A sensitive and specific enzyme-linked immunosorbent assay (ELISA) for antibodies can provide serologic confirmation of the diagnosis as well as detect subclinical or mild infections (29,56). Stool examinations are unrewarding because the parasite does not reach reproductive maturity.

Although rarely have deaths from myocardial or central nervous system involvement occurred, in the absence of continuing reinfection the syndrome of visceral larva migrans is self-limited and requires no therapy. For severe respiratory, myocardial, or central nervous system involvement, corticosteroids can be utilized. The antihelminthic drugs, thiabendazole and diethylcarbamazine, which are sometimes employed are of uncertain efficacy.

Strongyloidiasis

Strongyloides stercoralis, the causative agent of strongyloidiasis, is unique among the various helminthic parasites of humans in that it can proliferate to complete a life cycle entirely within the human body. As a result, the burden of adult worms can increase in the human in the absence of exogenous reinfection, as is required for other helminthic parasites. If the normal immune response is intact, the autoinfection cycle is contained; but abrogation of cell-mediated immunity unbridles this cycle, allowing for frequently fatal disseminated strongyloidiasis (63). This potential for disseminated hyperinfection, combined with the ability of the parasite to persist clinically inapparent for decades (25), endows this organism with the opportunity to produce serious disease of unsuspected etiology.

Initial infection with *S. stercoralis* occurs when filariform larvae, present in fecally contaminated soil, penetrate human skin and sequentially pass hematogenously to the lungs, penetrate into alveolar air sacs, and ascend the tracheobronchial tree to be swallowed. In the gastrointestinal tract adult worms develop in the duodenojejunal mucosa. At that site eggs are produced which hatch within the lumen of the gut to release rhabditiform larvae, which can be passed in the feces. Rhabditiform larvae can transform directly in the intestines into filariform larvae which penetrate perianal skin or colonic mucosa to reinfect the human host directly. This latter route of larval transformation is responsible for hyperinfection strongyloidiasis and disseminated disease.

Patients with *Strongyloides* infection can experience cutaneous reactions, when larvae penetrate the skin, as well as gastrointestinal symptoms, especially upper abdominal pains from the duodenitis induced by the adult worms in the small bowel (13,112). Many who harbor *Strongyloides* in their gastrointestinal tracts, however, remain free of symptoms, although they can have a mild eosinophilia. Although the transpulmonary migration of larvae could produce a Loeffler's-like syndrome as is found with *Ascaris* and hookworm, this is infrequently noted. In contrast, some patients with chronic strongyloidiasis experience repeated episodes of fever and mild pneumonitis. Eosinophilia is often absent when such patients present, but can be manifest during intercurrent periods. This pattern of symptomatic pulmonary involvement has not been well studied and can resemble repeated episodes of bacterial pneumonia. Treatment of the strongyloidiasis terminates the repeated episodes of pneumonia.

Pulmonary manifestations usually are limited to patients with the hyperinfection syndrome. Whereas hyperinfection strongyloidiasis has been noted in patients with AIDS (43), disseminated strongyloidiasis is uncommon in patients with HIV-1. Because cyclosporin is active against *Strongyloides* (109), it is possible that disseminated strongyloidiasis will not be encountered in those receiving cyclosporin therapy. Whether or not cyclosporin can eliminate human infections with *S. stercoralis* in immunosuppressed patients, and whether this or analogous immunosuppressive agents when given in concert with other immunosuppressive regimens will or will not be complicated by the development of hyperinfection strongyloidiasis await further clinical experience. By contrast, if cell-mediated immunity is impaired as a result of corticosteroid or cytotoxic drug administration, underlying malignancy, malnutrition, or alcoholism (1,28,31,49,63,95,121,123), increased numbers of rhabditiform larvae transform into filariform larvae, which penetrate the intestinal wall to enter the bloodstream. The gravity of the resultant hyperinfection syndrome derives not only from the enhanced numbers of parasites but also from their larval invasions into multiple organs and from the frequently concomitant gram-negative bacillary bacteremia in a host already immunocompromised. The increasing numbers of larvae passing through the lungs and developing in the gastrointestinal tract account for the respiratory (dyspnea, wheezing, hemoptysis, and cough) and/or gastrointestinal (nausea, vomiting, anorexia, diarrhea, abdominal pain) symptoms experienced (63,112). Larval penetrations through such organs as liver, heart, central nervous system, and endocrine glands produce signs and symptoms referable to damage in those organs. Bacteremia with intestinal gram-negative flora is often sustained and persistent. Rarely, adult parasites can develop and localize in the bronchial tree and in that site lay eggs which hatch to liberate larvae. Bronchospasm frequently accompanies this localization (80). Asthma can also be prominent with hyperinfection strongyloidiasis (124).

With hyperinfection strongyloidiasis, pulmonary infiltrates are usually notable on chest x-ray film and consist of foci of hemorrhage, pneumonitis, and edema. In addition, bacteremia can produce a superimposed bacterial pneumonia, and sputum cultures can reflect the bacterial infection.

The diagnosis of uncomplicated strongyloidiasis usually is made by detecting rhabditiform larvae in concentrates of multiple stools. A mild eosinophilia might be the only clue that the patient harbors the parasite. About 25% of those harboring the parasite have negative stool examinations, and aspiration of duodenojejunal fluid or the use of a string test is required to detect *Strongyloides* larvae (9). For *Strongyloides,* an ELISA serology has proved valuable in detecting strongyloidiasis (22,77), even when aggressive examinations of stool samples have been unrevealing (78). In disseminated strongyloidiasis, filariform larvae can be found in stool as well as sputum, bronchoalveolar lavage fluid, pleural fluid, peritoneal fluid, and surgical drainage fluid (35,110,119,121,136). In cases of suspected disseminated strongyloidiasis, sputum should be examined for larvae (47,119). The eosinophilia of strongyloidiasis can be suppressed and absent in disseminated disease because of concomitant pyogenic infection or steroid administration.

Strongyloidiasis is treated with thiabendazole (25 mg/kg orally twice daily) for 2 days in uncomplicated infection, and for 5 to 7 days in disseminated disease (4). The efficacy of therapy, in either case, should be documented with negative stool or upper small bowel fluid examinations. Treatment failures and subsequent relapses are not infrequent (112). In patients with the hyperinfection syndrome, case fatality rates are high despite appropriate antihelminthic therapy because of the concomitant immunosuppression and bacteremia. Therefore, detection and eradication of *Strongyloides* infection prior to initiation of immunosuppressive therapies is important to prevent the occurrence of the frequently fatal syndrome of disseminated strongyloidiasis. An unexplained eosinophilia, a history of serpiginous, pruritic cutaneous lesions, or a history of exposure in locales where the parasite could be present in fecally contaminated soil environments, even decades before, should prompt examination of stool and small bowel aspirates for the diagnostic larvae of *S. stercoralis*.

Paragonimiasis

Paragonimiasis results from infection with one of several species of the lung fluke, *Paragonimus*. *Paragonimus westermani* is endemic in parts of China, Korea, Japan, the Philippines, and Taiwan, whereas in West Africa and in Central and South America other, less defined, species of *Paragonimus* are responsible for human infections. Paragonimiasis due to *P. kellicotti* has been acquired within the United States (68,85).

Humans acquire the infection by ingesting raw, salted, or wine-soaked fresh water crabs or crayfish that harbor the metacercarial stage of the parasite. After human ingestion, the metacercariae excyst in the duodenum, penetrate the gastrointestinal wall, and migrate within the peritoneal cavity. Although some young flukes migrate to extrapulmonary sites, most of the developing flukes penetrate the diaphragm to migrate within the pulmonary parenchyma. The flukes become surrounded by an infiltrate of eosinophils and neutrophils, and then mononuclear leukocytes. Local necrosis of pulmonary parenchyma and then a fibrous capsule develop around the maturing flukes. By the seventh or eighth week of infection, the completely matured flukes begin egg production within the capsule, which, in turn, can enlarge and rupture, often into a bronchiole.

The manifestations of paragonimiasis differ for the early and later phases of infection. The early phase occurs between time of infection and time of the first egg production (140). During the period of larval migration within the peritoneal cavity, some patients experience abdominal pains or epigastralgia. As larvae penetrate the diaphragm and migrate within the pleural cavity, pleurisy, often bilateral, can develop. The chest x-ray film at this time, about 1 month after infection or later, can reveal a pneumothorax or pleural effusions, which are exudative and laden with eosinophils. As larval migration within the lung parenchyma increases, the patient often experiences an irritating cough, chest pain, and malaise and can have a low-grade fever and produce blood-streaked sputum. The roentgenographic findings associated with the pulmonary parenchymal migrations are those of transient, migratory, soft pulmonary infiltrates (140). A leukocytosis and very prominent blood eosinophilia occur during this time, so the clinical presentation can resemble Loeffler's syndrome. Diagnosis of paragonimiasis in this first phase before egg production starts is difficult and can be made only presumptively on the basis of compatible pulmonary signs and symptoms in a patient with eosinophilia and a history of exposure in an area endemic for paragonimiasis.

The second phase of infection, when mature flukes inhabit the lungs, can last for a decade before the flukes gradually die off. During this phase, the most common symptom is recurrent hemoptysis (79,140). The expectorated material, usually with a characteristic chocolate color, is composed of an admixture of blood, inflammatory cells, and *Paragonimus* eggs released when the capsule around mature flukes ruptures into a bronchiole. Although the patient can experience some malaise, fever is generally absent (140). The patient often does not feel or appear ill despite the recurrent hemoptytic episodes. Blood eosinophilia is minimal or absent during this phase. On chest x-ray, although no abnormalities are detected in about 20% of cases of established paragonimiasis (81), generally one or more lesions at the sites of localized encysted flukes or their burrowing tracts are recognized (79,125,140). On plain film or with tomography some of these show typical ring shadow lesions resulting from the relative lucency of the contents of the cystic cavities (52,116,117). Air fluid levels are rare. Linear streaks, often adjacent to the ring shadows, represent burrowing tracts of the flukes (52). The various pulmonary findings can resolve spontaneously and new lesions appear slowly over months. Pleural thickening can be evident. These radiographic features are sometimes attributed erroneously to tuberculosis (75). Pleural effusions, at times massive, can develop and constitute the presenting manifestation of the disease without radiologically evident parenchymal involvement (54,103). A bronchopleural fistula is an uncommon complication.

In this second phase of infection, the diagnosis, suggested by the history of recurrent hemoptysis in someone from an endemic area (141), is usually easily established by finding the characteristic eggs of *Paragonimus* in the sputum. A 24-hour collection of sputum enhances the sensitivity of detecting eggs (55). Swallowed eggs will be found in the stool, and, especially in children, the diagnostic yield is increased by examining stool samples as well as sputum. Diagnosis can also be made by fine-needle aspiration (96). ELISA and immunoblot serologic tests are available (118).

Therapy consists of praziquantel administered at a dose of 25 mg/tid for 2 days (4,55).

Schistosomiasis

Schistosomiasis, one of the major helminthic infections of humans worldwide, can be caused by one of three major species of the parasite. *Schistosoma mansoni* is found in Africa, Arabia, South America, and parts of the Caribbean; *S. haematobium* in Africa and the Middle East; and *S. japonicum* in Japan, China, and parts of the Philippines.

Schistosome eggs, passed in human excrement, hatch in fresh water into miracidia which then develop further in specific species of snails. The cercerial form, released into water from snails, can rapidly penetrate human skin to infect humans. Subsequently, mature adults localize in the mesenteric (*S. mansoni, S. japonicum*) or vesical venules (*S. haematobium*), and eggs are deposited in the wall of the intestine or bladder, respectively. Eggs can be carried in the portal circulation to the liver or passed in the feces or urine.

Pulmonary involvement with schistosomiasis can occur in three settings: (i) with acute schistosomiasis; (ii) as a complication of chronic hepatosplenic disease; or (iii) as a result of antischistosomal therapy. The syndrome of acute schistosomiasis (27,33), which occurs rarely with *S. haematobium,* is encountered principally in previously unexposed individuals and those exposed to sudden intense infection. Two to eight weeks after infection patients can experience fever, chills, anorexia, weight loss, abdominal pain, diarrhea, urticaria, myalgias, and a dry cough. Hepatosplenomegaly and lymphadenopathy develop. Blood eosinophilia becomes prominent during this phase. In addition to the frequent dry cough, bronchospasm can be experienced. Chest x-ray films have recorded basilar and midzone infiltrates (33,39) and military mottling (99) during acute schistosomiasis. Although the etiology of this syndrome is uncertain, the severity of symptoms reflects the intensity of infection (48). Antischistosomal antibodies develop and schistosome eggs become detectable in stool, rectal mucosa, or urine in the later stage of the syndrome, which is self-limited, resolving over 1 to 2 months (48). The course of acute schistosomiasis can be abbreviated by treatment with corticosteroids, followed by specific antischistosomal therapy (4).

The second form of pulmonary involvement in schistosomiasis results from chronic infection and develops in those with hepatosplenic disease (30,107). In heavy infections, embolization of eggs, principally of *S. mansoni* and *S. japonicum* in the portal circulation, results in the development of hepatic granulomata and fibrosis. The resultant presinusoidal portal hypertension fosters the development of portosystemic collateral vessels that allow schistosome eggs to embolize into the pulmonary circulation. Eggs lodge in pulmonary arterioles of 50 to 100 μm diameter and produce a granulomatous pulmonary endarteritis (3,69). Pulmonary hypertension and cor pulmonale ensue gradually. Dyspnea is the principal symptom attributable to this pulmonary process (36). The chest x-ray film will initially show fine miliary nodules; with evolution the heart enlarges and the pulmonary arteries dilate to aneurysmal proportions (36). Diagnosis can be confirmed by liver biopsy demonstrating the characteristic Symmer's pipestem fibrosis, because severe cardiopulmonary schistosomiasis does not develop in those without marked hepatic involvement (69). Detection of eggs in bronchoscopic washings or transbronchial biopsies can also establish the diagnosis (108,113). These pulmonary changes represent end-stage alterations and can be only minimally reversible with antischistosomal therapy.

Following initiation of antischistosomal therapy of established infections, adult worms can embolize to the liver or lungs (69). As a consequence, respiratory symptoms of coughing and wheezing can develop, the chest x-ray film can reveal new infiltrates, and a rise in eosinophilia can occur (87). These changes are self-limited, do not necessitate cessation of antischistosomal therapy, and probably reflect immunologic responses to exposed or released antigens from dead worms (84).

Trichinosis

Trichinosis, caused by the nematode *Trichinella spiralis,* is acquired by ingesting *Trichinella* cysts found in meat of carnivores. Most human cases derive from inadequately cooked pork, although walrus, bear, and some other meats are occasional causes of outbreaks of trichinosis. The course of the infection can be divided into three stages (44). The first stage, the intestinal stage, occurs between about the second and seventh days after infection, when encysted larvae are liberated from the meat and burrow into the intestinal mucosa. This stage can be asymptomatic or can be accompanied by intestinal symptoms. The second stage, that of muscular invasion, begins about the first week after infection and lasts for 1 to 5 weeks, depending on severity of infection. This stage is frequently characterized by periorbital edema, muscle pain, fever, leukocytosis, and eosinophilia as newly produced larvae leave the bloodstream to encyst in striated muscles. The final stage is that of convalescence. Many light infections have minimal symptoms, but ingestion of large numbers of infective cysts can produce intense and occasionally fatal infections.

Serious pulmonary involvement in trichinosis is infrequent, being recorded in only 6.5% of 856 hospitalized patients (53). Respiratory symptoms can result from larvae in pulmonary tissues, from myositis in respiratory muscles, or as a consequence of trichinous cardiomyopathy, from pulmonary congestion, or from secondary pyogenic pneumonia. Early in the stage of muscle invasion, when intravascular larvae are passing through the lungs, a dry, nonproductive cough is a common symptom. Occasionally during this period, in the early weeks of infection, patchy basilar infiltrates, small micronodular lesions, and pleural effusions are found on chest x-ray. These resolve spontaneously over 1 to 2 weeks. Between the third and fifth weeks of infection bronchitis is common, having developed in 40% in one epidemic (44). Mucoid sputum can contain many eosinophils.

As larvae encyst in muscle an attendant myositis develops. Involvement of laryngeal muscles and muscles of deglutition can result in hoarseness and dysphagia, respectively. Muscles of the diaphragm usually have one of the highest densities of encysted larvae. This diaphragmatic involvement can result in lower thoracic or epigastric pain and is often greatest in the second and third weeks of severe infection. Analogously, painful intercostal myositis can further impair respiratory function (100). In the very ill, hospitalized patient, prolonged bedrest and impaired pulmonary toilet favor the development of superimposed bacterial pneumonia in the later weeks of infection. In one large series of hospitalized patients, this late bronchopneumonia occurred in about 1% of patients (53). In severely ill patients, congestive heart failure attributable to either cardiomyositis and/or hypoalbuminemia can further compromise respiratory function (44).

The diagnosis of trichinosis is suggested by the more usual manifestations of periorbital edema, myositis, and fever and is facilitated by obtaining a history of ingestion of a suspect meat, especially inadequately cooked pork, or an epidemiologic history of others developing similar signs and symptoms after common meat ingestion. Eosinophilia can disappear—a poor prognostic sign. Serologic tests are available and reliable; however, antibody levels are not detectable until after 3 or more weeks of infection. The definitive diagnosis is made by finding larvae in biopsied muscle. The yield will be greatest in biopsying muscles that are symptomatically involved and biopsying near a tendinous insertion. In addition to routine histopathologic exam, muscle should be digested to free larvae and also examined undigested in a preparation of unfixed muscle compressed between microscope slides.

For most trichinella infections, the clinical course is uncomplicated; and because the disease is self-limited, no specific therapy is indicated. For serious disease, especially with central nervous system, myocarditis, or severe respiratory involvement, corticosteroids with mebendazole or albendazole are used (4).

Tropical Filarial Pulmonary Eosinophilia

A clinical syndrome characterized by marked blood eosinophilia, paroxysmal non-productive cough, wheezing, occasionally weight loss, lymphadenopathy, and low-grade fevers was initially described in tropical areas early in this century and more fully documented about 40 years ago (38,133). The syndrome, variously termed *tropical eosinophilia, tropical pulmonary eosinophilia,* or *tropical filarial pulmonary eosinophilia,* represents a distinct immunologic reaction to infection with the human lymphatic filarial parasites *Wuchereria bancrofti* or *Brugia malayi* (83,91).

Clinically, the onset of the syndrome is usually gradual. Prominent symptoms include a dry, hacking, nonproductive cough which often becomes paroxysmal and nocturnal, breathlessness, and wheezing, resulting from asthmatiform attacks. Dyspnea on exertion is less common. Extrarespiratory symptoms of weight loss, lassitude, and fatiguability are frequent. On physical examination, chest findings are minimal or absent in most. Rhonchi and crepitations—especially over the midzones and bases—and wheezing are audible in some. About 15% of patients have lymphadenopathy, hepatomegaly, and/or splenomegaly (130).

On chest x-ray film, increased bronchovesicular markings, diffuse interstitial lesions 1 to 3 mm in diameter, or mottled opacities, usually more prominent in lower lung fields, are common. Hilar lymphadenopathy is not common, and pleural effusions are rare. The fine miliary lesions can be subtle and overlooked; 20 to 30% have normal chest x-rays (130). Bronchoalveolar lavage reveals an intense eosinophilic alveolitis in active disease (91).

The cardinal laboratory finding is an elevation in blood eosinophilia, usually above $3,000/\mu l$. Total serum IgE levels are elevated, often above 1,000 units/ml. Characteristically, filarial antibody levels are detectable in high titers and microfilariae cannot be found circulating in peripheral blood. Pulmonary function tests reveal two main patterns: (i) 70% have a predominant restrictive pattern together with mild-to-moderate airway obstruction; and (ii) 30% have a predominant obstructive pattern with a mild restrictive component (130). The airway obstruction is reversible with bronchodilators. If the antifilarial agent diethylcarbamazine is given in the first couple of years of disease, both the restrictive and obstructive defects return toward normal, but a persisting low-grade eosinophilic alveolitis can continue (102,132). If therapy is not given in the early years of disease, or if patients suffer relapses after diethylcarbamazine, progressive interstitial fibrosis and irreversible impairments in pulmonary function develop.

From biopsied lung tissue obtained at open biopsies of patients with different durations of tropical filarial pulmonary eosinophilia, the evolution of the pulmonary histopathology in this disease has been elucidated (130). The earliest change is a histocytic infiltration. After a month of disease an eosinophilic interstitial infiltrate develops; and in severer cases, eosinophilic abscesses, eosinophilic bronchopneumonia, and eosinophilic granulomas become prominent. With chronicity, there is increasing pulmonary fibrosis. Microfilarial fragments are occasionally identifiable in the biopsied tissues.

The factors that cause only a small percentage of patients infected with lymphatic filarial parasites to develop this pulmonary presentation of filariasis are unresolved. Men, especially young adults, experience the disease four- to sevenfold more commonly than do women. The disease can occur in any tropical area where filariasis occurs, and it occurs more frequently in peoples from the Indian subcontinent. Available evidence suggests that this disease arises as a consequence of a prominent immunologic response against normally blood-borne microfilariae that become opsonized and trapped within the lung and reticuloendothelial organs (83).

The diagnosis is suggested by elevations of blood eosinophilia and serum IgE in a patient from a filarial endemic tropical area who is experiencing symptoms of cough, wheezing, and breathlessness. Elevations in filarial antibody titers corroborate the diagnosis. A therapeutic response to diethylcarbamazine therapy (5 to 6 mg/kg/day given for 2 to 4 weeks) confirms the diagnosis. Relapses can occur and are treated with another course of diethylcarbamazine. The eosinophili-rich alveolitis improves with diethylcarbamzine, but might not resolve completely (132). Bronchodilators can be used to manage the bronchospastic component pending response to diethylcarbamazine.

Other Metazoan Parasites

Other metazoan parasites can cause pulmonary involvement. Cysticercosis infrequently localizes in the pleura or parenchyma (24). Echinococcosis, caused either by *Echinococcus granulosus* or *E. multilocularis,* can produce cystic lesions in the lungs. Leakage of the contents of these cysts can produce a pneumonitis and allergic manifestations. The pulmonary effects of these two distinct *Echinococcal* species are well documented (7,12,58,90,106,129,138).

An eosinophilic pleural effusion has been reported in a patient with *Loa loa* infection (60). Zoonotic infections with the dog filarial heartworm, *Dirofilaria immitis,* arise when mosquito-borne infective larvae are transmitted to humans and develop into one or more adult worms which localize in the pulmonary arterial circulation. These infections are usually asymptomatic and are detected radiographically as single and ocassionally bilateral pulmonary coin lesions (5,6,17,26,98), but early can present as focal areas of pneumonitis (120). Serologic tests lack adequate specificity to detect these infections. Excisional biopsy is both diagnostic and curative.

PROTOZOAN PARASITES

Amebiasis

The protozoa causing human amebiasis, *Entamoeba histolytica,* is not principally a respiratory tract parasite; but pleuropulmonary involvement can arise as a complication of amebic intestinal or extraintestinal disease. Humans acquire amebiasis by ingesting the cyst form of *E. histolytica.* Amebae parasitize the large colon and proliferate in that site to form trophozoites and cysts. Patients can experience symptomatic intestinal disease of variable severity or can be asymptomatic. In addition to symptomatic and asymptomatic intestinal disease, infection can spread from the bowel to localize in extraintestinal sites, the most common of which is the liver, where amebic abscesses can develop.

Amebic pulmonary disease can develop by means of (i) rupture of an amebic hepatic abscess through the diaphragm, (ii) lymphatic spread from the liver through the diaphragm, or (iii) hematogenous embolic spread from the liver or from the colon. Hematogenous dissemination, as evidenced by pulmonary amebiasis without hepatic disease or by noncontiguous pulmonary and hepatic disease, is unusual (126). The most common mechanism for pulmonary disease is direct spread from the liver, usually with evidence of rupture of an amebic abscess through the liver. Because of the proximate location of the thorax to the liver, pleuropulmonary amebiasis is the second most common form of extraintestinal amebiasis after hepatic disease (2,65).

Amebic abscess in the liver usually develops insidiously and is significantly more common in men than in women. A history of coincident or antecedent diarrheal illness is reported by only a minority of patients. Pain is the most common presenting symptom and can be referable to the right upper quadrant of the abdomen, the epigastrium, the right chest, or the right shoulder. The pain is usually dull but can be pleuritic or aching. Other symptoms can include cough, sweating, malaise, weight loss, anorexia, and hiccough. On examination, enlargement of the liver is the most common finding, often associated with a focal area of tenderness. A leukocytosis is often present with an anemia of chronic infection. Blood eosinophilia is unusual, as is jaundice. The chest x-ray film can demonstrate an elevated right hemidiaphragm. Ultrasound examination usually detects a cystic intrahepatic cavity. On gallium citrate and technetium-labeled sulfur colloid radionuclide liver scans, the amebic abscess presents as a "cold area." Confirmation of the diagnosis can be made using amebic serologic tests such as indirect hemagglutination inhibition or gel diffusion assays which are positive in greater than 95% of those with hepatic amebic disease (2).

Although rupture of liver abscess could occur into any adjoining space or organ, extension into the chest occurs almost four times as often as extension into the peritoneal cavity. Ninety percent of amebic hepatic abscesses are found in the right lobe of the liver. Localization in the left lobe, however, predisposes to infrequent but often fatal extension into the pericardial sac. Prior to rupture, an amebic hepatic abscess can cause pleural effusion. When rupture occurs into the thorax, four types of pleuropulmonary involvement can ensue. Rupture into the pleural space results in an amebic empyema. Rupture into the lung can eventuate in consolidation, abscess formation, or a hepatobronchial fistula. Empyema and fistula formation usually account for the majority of presentations (2,18). Symptoms can include pain, cough, hemoptysis, or dyspnea (59). The pain can be pleuritic or localized to the right upper quadrant. Cough can be nonproductive, but more often is associated with expectoration of material ranging from small amounts of sputum to large amounts of amebic pus. The physical signs are those of the underlying pleuropulmonary lesion. The liver might not be palpably enlarged if the original abscess is high up in the right lobe or if it has been decompressed by rupture. Consolidation is more common in the right lower and middle lobes (2,137).

The diagnosis of amebic pleuropulmonary disease can be established by the same tests utilized to diagnose hepatic amebic abscesses. Amebic serology will be positive in over 90%. Because most pleuropulmonary disease develops from a liver abscess, the tests mentioned above to document a liver abscess are pertinent in a patient with a suspected intrathoracic amebic infection. If a hepatobronchial fistula develops, the patient can produce copious amounts of material with a reddish-brown or "anchovy sauce" appearance which strongly suggests an amebic etiology. In the era before the introduction of effective amebic chemotherapy, such expectoration of cyst contents was usually associated with a favorable response.

Therapy of amebic pleuropulmonary disease is with metronidazole (750 mg po tid for 10 days) (4). Amebic pleural effusions should be aspirated.

Cryptosporidiosis

Infections with *Cryptosporidium* species of coccidian parasites have been recognized as a cause of intestinal disease in both immunocompetent and immunocompromised patients. In the latter group, especially patients with AIDS, diarrheal illness can be profound and unremitting. In some patients with AIDS and pneumonia, oocysts of cryptosporidia have been recovered from the respiratory tract (66,73). Whether this endobronchial recovery of oocysts represents aspiration of esophageal or gastrointestinal parasites or true infection of the bronchial epithelium, as occurs with cryptosporidia in poultry, is unsettled. At present, no effective therapy has been found for cryptosporidiosis in immunoincompetent patients.

Toxoplasmosis

Toxoplasma gondii, an obligate intracellular parasite that can reproduce in any nucleated cell in the body, exists in three forms: the tachyzoite, cyst, and oocyst. The tachyzoite, the cell-invasive form responsible for acute illness in humans, multiplies intracellularly by a distinctive process termed *endodyogeny,* whereby two daughter cells arise simultaneously from one parent cell, which disintegrates when the progeny are released. After various numbers of cycles of division within the host cell, the tachyzoites can form cysts, the second form. Oocysts, the final form, occur only in infected cats. The cat has a unique enteroepithelial cycle of the organism that eventuates in oocytes that are shed in the intestine (37). Once the oocyst is excreted in the feces it must mature by sporulation, a temperature-dependent process requiring up to 3 weeks, in order to become infective. The mature oocyst thus plays a role in the transmission of disease to humans, particularly children who might ingest cat excrement. Usually, infection in humans or animals develops by ingestion of cysts, especially in rare or uncooked meat. Toxoplasmosis can also be acquired transplacentally when a mother becomes infected acutely during pregnancy. Toxoplasmosis can be transmitted from donor to recipient after organ transplantation (105) and by leukocyte transfusions (115) in immunocompromised hosts.

Although there are three major clinical forms of infection with *T. gondii*—congenital infection, a syndrome of lymphadenitis in adults, and disseminated disease—pulmonary involvement is prominent only in the last of these (34,92). The overwhelming majority of disseminated cases are in patients with defects in cell-mediated immunity, including those with AIDS (70) and those with lymphoproliferative neoplasias, particularly Hodgkin's disease, being treated with immunosuppressing doses of corticosteroids, antimetabolites, and local radiation therapy (21,104,131). Disseminated toxoplasmosis can also occur in renal and cardiac transplant recipients, patients with systemic lupus erythematosus, and patients with metastatic solid tumors undergoing chemo- and radiotherapy (97). Less commonly, pulmonary toxoplasmosis has developed in those receiving chemotherapy for leukemia (19). In disseminated toxoplasmosis the organs most frequently involved are the brain, the lungs, and the heart. Autopsy studies have demonstrated a high frequency of pulmonary infection (23). The pulmonary involvement, however, might not be solely due to *T. gondii,* and concomitant infections with other agents, including cytomegalovirus and *Pneumocystis carinii,* could be present. Despite the findings from postmortem studies, recognition of pulmonary toxoplasmosis antemortem in immunocompromised patients has been infrequent (92). The clinical and radiographic presentations of pneumonia due to *T. gondii* are not specific (23,92). Chest x-rays often show bilateral diffuse infiltrates, but small multinodal densities, isolated cavitary disease, and lobar pneumonia have also been described (82,92,94,128).

Cysts of *T. gondii* persist in tissues long after initial infection, so the diagnosis of toxoplasmosis cannot simply rest on the identification of this form of the parasite. Ideally, tachyzoites should be demonstrated within biopsied tissue. These forms can be missed on routine pathology and are best detected with immunochemical techniques such as the peroxidase-antiperoxidase method (64). As yet, most experience in tissue diagnosis has been obtained with neurotoxoplasmosis. In the brain, biopsies of inflamed tissue that contain multiple cysts can be accepted as presumptive evidence of the diagnosis, even if tachyzoites are not demonstrated (64), and the same can be pertinent for lung disease. Tachyzoites can be detected by mouse inoculation and by tissue culture (50). Until recently, the diagnosis of pulmonary toxoplasmosis has not been based on isolation of parasites from lung tissue or respiratory secretions. Some reports, however, have appeared documenting the ability to detect the parasite in bronchoalveolar lavage fluid or lung biopsy specimens (16,32,34,67,92).

Serologic criteria are considered adequate for instituting therapy, but serodiagnosis is hampered by several problems. Thirty-five to 70% of all adults in the United States have positive Sabin-Feldman dye or IgG indirect immunofluorescent tests, many at titers greater than 1:1,000 (71,131). Because the antibody titers are frequently maximal when the diagnosis of disseminated disease is first considered, rising titers might not be identified. Some patients, especially those with AIDS, can fail to develop an antibody response to disseminated toxoplasmosis.

Treatment of toxoplasmosis employs a combination of pyrimethamine and sulfadiazine (4). Pyrimethamine is given at a dose of 25 to 100 mg daily in adults after an initial loading dose of 100 to 200 mg. Sulfadiazine is given generally at a dose of 1 to 4 g four times daily, after an initial 4 g loading dose. Combination therapy is usually continued for 3 to 4 weeks. The combination frequently produces marrow suppression, and blood counts must be monitored frequently. Folinic acid can be administered to help counteract the marrow suppression. Continued suppressive therapy is needed to prevent relapses in those with AIDS.

REFERENCES

1. Adam, M., Morgan, O., Persaud, C., and Gibbs, W.N. (1973): Hyperinfection syndrome with *Strongyloides stercoralis* in malignant lymphoma. *Br. Med. J.,* 1:264–266.
2. Adams, E.B., and MacLeod, I.N. (1977): Invasive amebiasis: II. Amebic liver abscess and its complications. *Medicine* 56:325–334.
3. Andrade, Z.A., and Andrade, S.G. (1970): Pathogenesis of schistosomal pulmonary arteritis. *Am. J. Trop. Med. Hyg.,* 19:305–310.
4. Anonymous. (1992): Drugs for parasitic infections. *Med. Lett. Drugs Ther.,* 34:17–26.
5. Asimacopoulos, P.J., Katras, A., and Christie, B. (1992): Pulmonary dirofilariasis: the largest single-hospital experience. *Chest,* 102:851–855.
6. Bailey, T.S., Sohrabi, A., and Roberts, S.S. (1990): Pulmonary coin lesions caused by *Dirofilaria immitis. J. Surg. Oncol.,* 44:268–272.
7. Balikan, J.B., and Mudarris, F.F. (1975): Hydatid disease of the lungs. *Am. J. Roentgenol. Rad. Ther. Nucl. Med.,* 122:692–707.
8. Banwell, J.G., and Schad, G.A. (1978): Hookworm. *Clin. Gastroenterol.,* 7:129–156.

9. Beal, C.B., Viens, P., Grant, R.G., and Hughes, J.M. (1970): A new technique for sampling duodenal contents: demonstration of upper small-bowel pathogens. *Am. J. Trop. Med. Hyg.,* 19:349–352.
10. Bean, W.J. (1965): Recognition of ascariasis by routine chest or abdomen roentgenograms. *Am. J. Roentgenol. Rad. Ther. Nucl. Med.,* 94:379–384.
11. Beaver, P.C., and Danaraj, T.J. (1958): Pulmonary ascariasis resembling eosinophilic lung: autopsy report with description of larvae in the bronchiole. *Am. J. Trop. Med. Hyg.,* 7:100–111.
12. Beggs, I. (1985): The radiology of hydatid disease. *Am. J. Roentgenol.,* 145:639–648.
13. Berkman, Y.M., and Rabinowitz, J. (1972): The gastrointestinal manifestations of strongyloidiasis. *Am. J. Roentgenol. Rad. Ther. Nucl. Med.,* 115:306–311.
14. Beshear, J.R., and Hendley, J.O. (1973): Severe pulmonary involvement in visceral larva migrans. *Am. J. Dis. Child.,* 125:599–600.
15. Booth, B.H., Patterson, R., and Talbot, C.H. (1970): Immediate-type hypersensitivity in dogs: cutaneous, anaphylactic and respiratory responses to *Ascaris. J. Lab. Clin. Med.,* 76:181–189.
16. Bottone, E.J. (1991): Diagnosis of acute pulmonary toxoplasmosis by visualization of invasive and intracellular tachyzoites in Giemsa-stained smears of bronchoalveolar lavage fluid. *J. Clin. Microbiol.,* 29:2626–2627.
17. Bradham, R.R., Locklair, P.R.J., and Grimball, A. (1990): Bilateral pulmonary nodules caused by *Dirofilaria immitis. Ann. Thorac. Surg.,* 50:312–313.
18. Brandt, H., and Tamayo, R.P. (1970): Pathology of human amebiasis. *Human Pathol.,* 1:351–385.
19. Brown, N.J., and McKenzie, S. (1991): Decker, M.D. Case report: fatal pulmonary toxoplasmosis following chemotherapy. *Am. J. Med. Sci.,* 302:152–154.
20. Butland, R.J., and Coulson, I.H. (1985): Pulmonary eosinophilia associated with cutaneous larva migrans. *Thorax,* 40:76–77.
21. Carey, R.M., Kimball, A.C., Armstrong, D., and Lieberman, P.H. (1973): Toxoplasmosis: clinical experiences in a cancer hospital. *Am. J. Med.,* 54:30–38.
22. Carroll, S.M., Karthigasu, K.T., and Grove, D.I. (1981): Serodiagnosis of human strongyloidiasis by an enzyme-linked immunosorbent assay. *Trans. R. Soc. Trop. Med. Hyg.,* 75:706–709.
23. Catterall, J.R., Hofflin, J.M., and Remington, J.S. (1986): Pulmonary toxoplasmosis. *Am. Rev. Respir. Dis.,* 133:704–705.
24. Choi, J.H., Chung, S.I., Whang, Y.S., et al. (1991): A case of pulmonary cysticercosis. *Korean J. Intern. Med.,* 6:38–43.
25. Chu, E., Whitlock, W.L., and Dietrich, R.A. (1990): Pulmonary hyperinfection syndrome with *Strongyloides stercoralis. Chest,* 97:1475–1477.
26. Ciferri, F. (1982): Human pulmonary dirofilariasis in the United States: a critical review. *Am. J. Trop. Med. Hyg.,* 31:302–308.
27. Clark, W.D., Cox, P.M., Ratner, L.H., and Carrera-Coronas, R. (1970): Acute schistosomiasis mansoni in 10 boys. *Ann. Intern. Med.,* 73:379–385.
28. Cruz, T., Reboucas, G., and Rocha, H. (1966): Fatal strongyloidiasis in patients receiving corticosteroids. *N. Engl. J. Med.,* 275:1093–1096.
29. Cypess, R.H., Karol, M.H., Zidian, J.L., Glickman, L.T., and Gitlin, D. (1977): Larva-specific antibodies in patients with visceral larva migrans. *J. Infect. Dis.,* 135:633–640.
30. Da Silva, L.C., and Carrilho, F.J. (1992): Hepatosplenic schistosomiasis: pathophysiology and treatment. *Gastroenterol. Clin. No. Amer.,* 21:163–177.
31. Davidson, R.A. (1992): Infection due to *Strongyloides stercoralis* in patients with pulmonary disease. *South. Med. J.,* 85:28–31.
32. Derouin, F., Sarfati, C., Beauvais, B., Iliou, M.C., Dehen, L., and Lariviere, M. (1989): Laboratory diagnosis of pulmonary toxoplasmosis in patients with acquired immunodeficiency syndrome. *J. Clin. Microbiol.,* 27:1661–1663.
33. Diaz-Rivera, R.S., Ramos-Morales, F., Koppisch, E., et al. (1956): Acute Manson's schistosomiasis. *Am. J. Med.,* 21:918–943.
34. Evans, T.G., and Schwartzman, J.D. (1991): Pulmonary toxoplasmosis. *Sem. Respir. Infect.,* 6:51–57.
35. Eveland, L.K., Kenney, M., and Yermakov, U. (1975): Laboratory diagnosis of autoinfection in strongyloidiasis. *Am. J. Clin. Pathol.,* 63:421–425.
36. Farid, Z., Greer, J.W., Ishak, K.G., el Nagah, A.M., LeGolvan, P.C., and Mousa, A.H. (1959): Chronic pulmonary schistosomiasis. *Am. Rev. Tuber. Pulm. Dis.,* 79:119–133.
37. Frenkel, J.K., and Dubey, J.P. (1972): Toxoplasmosis and its prevention in cats and man. *J. Infect. Dis.,* 126:664–673.
38. Frimodt-Moller, C., and Barton, R.M. (1940): Pseudo-tuberculosis condition associated with eosinophilia. *Indian Med. Gaz.,* 75:607–613.
39. Gelfand, M. (1966): Pulmonary schistosomiasis in the early "Katayama" phase of the disease. *J. Trop. Med. Hyg.,* 69:143–144.

40. Gelpi, A.P., and Mustafa, A. (1967): Seasonal pneumonitis with eosinophilia: a study of larval ascariasis in Saudi Arabia. *Am. J. Trop. Med. Hyg.*, 16:646–657.
41. Gelpi, A.P., and Mustafa, A. (1968): *Ascaris* pneumonia. *Am. J. Med.*, 44:377–389.
42. Glickman, L.T., and Cypess, R.H. (1977): *Toxocara* infection in animal hospital employees. *Am. J. Publ. Health*, 67:1193–1195.
43. Gompels, M.M., Todd, J., Peters, B.S., Main, J., and Pinching, A.J. (1991): Disseminated strongyloidiasis in AIDS: uncommon but important. *AIDS*, 5:329–332.
44. Gould, S.E. (1970): Clinical manifestations. In: *Trichinosis in Man and Animals*, edited by S.E. Gould, pp. 269–328. Charles C. Thomas, Springfield, Ill.
45. Guill, M.A., and Odom, R.B. (1978): Larva migrans complicated by Loeffler's syndrome. *Arch. Dermatol.*, 114:1525–1526.
46. Gundel, R.H., Gerritsen, M.E., Gleich, G.J., and Wegner, C.D. (1990): Repeated antigen inhalation results in a prolonged airway eosinophilia and airway hyperresponsiveness in primates. *J. Appl. Physiol.*, 68:779–786.
47. Harris, R.A.J., Musher, D.M., Fainstein, V., Young, E.J., and Clarridge, J. (1980): Disseminated strongyloidiasis: diagnosis by sputum examination. *J.A.M.A.*, 244:65–66.
48. Hiatt, R.A., Sotomayor, Z.R., Sanchez, G., Zambrana, M., and Knight, W.B. (1979): Factors in the pathogenesis of acute *Schistosomiasis mansoni*. *J. Infect. Dis.*, 139:659–666.
49. Higenbottam, T.W., and Heard, B.E. (1976): Opportunistic pulmonary strongyloidiasis complicating asthma treated with steroids. *Thorax*, 31:226–233.
50. Hofflin, J.M., and Remington, J.S. (1985): Tissue culture isolation of Toxoplasma from blood of a patient with AIDS. *Arch. Intern. Med.*, 145:925–926.
51. Huntley, C.C., Costas, M.C., and Lyerly, A. (1965): Visceral larva migrans syndrome: clinical characteristics and immunologic studies in 51 patients. *Pediatrics*, 36:523–536.
52. Im, J.G., Whang, H.Y., Kim, W.S., Han, M.C., Shim, Y.S., and Cho, S.Y. (1992): Pleuropulmonary paragonimiasis: radiologic findings in 71 patients. *Am. J. Roentgenol. Rad. Ther. Nucl. Med.*, 159:39–43.
53. Januszkiewicz, J. (1967): Participation of the respiratory system in trichinosis. *Epidemiol. Rev.*, 21:169–178.
54. Johnson, R.J., and Johnson, J.R. (1983): Paragoniamiasis in Indochinese refugees: roentgenographic findings with clinical correlations. *Am. Rev. Respir. Dis.*, 128:534–538.
55. Johnson, R.J., Jong, E.C., Dunning, S.B., Carberry, W.L., and Minshew, B.H. (1985): Paragoniamiasis: diagnosis and the use of praziquantel in treatment. *Rev. Infect. Dis.*, 7:200–206.
56. Jones, W.E., Schnatz, P.M., Foreman, K., et al. (1980): Human toxocariasis in a rural community. *Am. J. Dis. Child.*, 134:965–967.
57. Kalman, E.H. (1954): Creeping eruption with transient pulmonary infiltration. *Radiology*, 62:222–226.
58. Katz, R., Murphy, S., and Kosloske, A. (1980): Pulmonary echinococcosis: a pediatric disease of the southwestern United States. *Pediatrics*, 65:1003–1006.
59. Kennedy, D., and Sharma, O.P. (1990): Hemoptysis in a 49-year-old man: an unusual presentation of a sporadic disease. *Chest*, 98:1275–1278.
60. Klion, A.D., Eisenstein, E.M., Smirniotopoulos, T.T., Neumann, M.P., and Nutman, T.B. (1992): Pulmonary involvement in loiasis. *Am. Rev. Respir. Dis.*, 145:961–963.
61. Koino, S. (1922): Experimental infections on human body with ascarides. *Jpn. Med. World*, 2:317–320.
62. Loeffler, W. (1956): Transient lung infiltrations with blood eosinophilia. *Int. Arch. Allergy Appl. Immunol.*, 8:54–59.
63. Longworth, D.L., and Weller, P.F. (1986): Hyperinfection syndrome with strongyloidiasis. In: *Current Clinical Topics in Infectious Diseases*, edited by J. S. Remington, M.N. Swartz. pp. 1–26. McGraw-Hill, New York.
64. Luft, B.J., and Remington, J.S. (1985): Toxoplasmosis of the central nervous system. In: *Current Clinical Topics in Infectious Diseases*, edited by J. S. Remington, M.N. Swartz. pp. 315–358. McGraw-Hill, New York.
65. Lyche, K.D., Jensen, W.A., Kirsch, C.M., Yenokida, G.G., Maltz, G.S., and Knauer, C.M. (1990): Pleuropulmonary manifestations of hepatic amebiasis. *West. J. Med.*, 153:275–278.
66. Ma, P., Villanueva, T.G., Kaufman, D., and Gillooley, J.F. (1984): Respiratory cryptosporidiosis in the acquired immune deficiency syndrome: use of modified cold Kinyoun and Hemacolor stains for rapid diagnoses. *J.A.M.A.*, 252:1298–1301.
67. Maguire, G.P., Tatz, J., Giosa, R., and Ahmed, T. (1986): Diagnosis of pulmonary toxoplasmosis by bronchoalveolar lavage. *NY State J. Med.*, 86:204–205.
68. Mariano, E.G., Borja, S.R., and Vruno, M.J. (1986): A human infection with *Paragonimus kellicotti* (lung fluke) in the United States. *Am. J. Clin. Pathol.*, 86:685–687.
69. McCully, R.M., Barron, C.N., and Cheever, A.W. (1976): Schistosomiasis. In: *Pathology of Tropical and Extraordinary Diseases*, edited by C.H. Binford, and D.J. Connor. Armed Forces Institute of Pathology, Washington, D.C.

70. Mills, J. (1986): *Pneumocystis carinii* and *Toxoplasma gondii* infections in patients with AIDS. *Rev. Infect. Dis.*, 8:1001–1011.
71. Mineo, J.R., Camargo, M.E., and Ferreira, A.W. (1980): Enzyme-linked immunosorbent assay for antibodies to *Toxoplasma gondii* polysaccharides in human toxoplasmosis. *Infect. Immun.*, 27:203–287.
72. Mok, C.H. (1968): Visceral larva migrans. *Clin. Pediatr.*, 7:565–573.
73. Moore, J.A., and Frenkel, J.K. (1991): Respiratory and enteric cryptosporidiosis in humans. *Arch. Pathol. Lab. Med.*, 115:1160–1162.
74. Muhleisen, J.P. (1953): Demonstration of pulmonary migration of the causative organism of creeping eruption. *Ann. Intern. Med.*, 38:595–600.
75. Mukerjee, C.M., Simpson, S.E., Bell, R.J., and Walker, J.C. (1992): Pleuropulmonary paragonimiasis in a Laotian immigrant to Australia. *Chest*, 101:849–851.
76. Nawalinski, T.A., and Schad, G.A. (1974): Arrested development in *Ancylostoma duodenale*: course of a self-induced infection in man. *Am. J. Trop. Med. Hyg.*, 23:895–898.
77. Neva, F.A., Gam, A.A., and Burke, J. (1981): Comparison of larval antigens in an enzyme-linked immunosorbent assay for strongyloidiasis in humans. *J. Infect. Dis.*, 144:427–432.
78. Nutman, T.B., Ottesen, E.A., Ieng, S., et al. (1987): Eosinophilia in Southeast Asian refugees: evaluation at a referral center. *J. Infect. Dis.*, 155:309–313.
79. Nwokolo, C. (1972): Endemic paragoniamiasis in Eastern Nigeria. *Trop. Georg. Med.*, 24:138–147.
80. Nwokolo, C., and Imohiosen, E.A.E. (1973): Strongyloidiasis of the respiratory tract presenting as "asthma." *Br. Med. J.*, 2:153.
81. Ogakwu, M., and Nwokolo, C. (1973): Radiological findings in pulmonary paragoniamiasis as seen in Nigeria: a review based on one hundred cases. *Br. J. Radiol.*, 46:699–705.
82. Oksenhendler, E., Cadranel, J. Sarfati, C., et al. (1990): *Toxoplasma gondii* pneumonia in patients with the acquired immunodeficiency syndrome. *Am. J. Med.*, 88:18N–21N.
83. Ottesen, E.A., and Nutman, T.B. (1992): Tropical pulmonary eosinophilia. *Ann. Rev. Med.*, 43:417–424.
84. Ottesen, E.A., and Weller, P.F. (1979): Eosinophilia following treatment of patients with *Schistosomiasis mansoni* and Bancroft's filariasis. *J. Infect. Dis.*, 139:343–347.
85. Pachucki, C.T., Levandowski, R.A., Brown, V.A., Sonnenkalb, B.H., and Vruno, M.J. (1984): American paragoniamiasis treated with praziquantel. *N. Engl. J. Med.*, 311:582–584.
86. Pare, P.D., Michound, M.C., and Hogg, J.C. (1976): Lung mechanics following antigen challenge of *Ascaris suum*–sensitive rhesus monkeys. *J. Appl. Physiol.*, 41:668–676.
87. Pedroso, E.R.P., Lambertucci, J.R., Greco, D.B., et al. (1987): Pulmonary *Schistosomiasis mansoni*: post-treatment pulmonary clinical-radiological alterations in patients in the chronic phase: a double-blind study. *Trans. Royal Soc. Trop. Med. Hyg.*, 81:778–781.
88. Phills, J.A., Harrold, A.J., Whiteman, G.V., and Perlmutter, L. (1972): Pulmonary infiltrates, asthma and eosinophilia due to *Ascaris suum* infestation in man. *N. Engl. J. Med.*, 286:965–970.
89. Piggott, J., Hansberger, E.A., and Neafie, R.C. (1970): Human ascariasis. *Am. J. Clin. Pathol.*, 53:223–234.
90. Pineyro, J.R. (1982): Hydatid disease of the lung. *Proc. Pediatr. Surg.*, 15:113–118.
91. Pinkston, P., Vijayan, V.K., Nutman, T.B., et al. (1987): Acute tropical pulmonary eosinophilia: characterization of the lower respiratory tract inflammation and its response to therapy. *J. Clin. Invest.*, 80:216–225.
92. Pomeroy, C., and Filice, G.A. (1992): Pulmonary toxoplasmosis: a review. *Clin. Infect. Dis.*, 14:863–870.
93. Proffitt, R.D., and Walton, B.C. (1962): *Ascaris* pneumonia in a two-year-old girl. *N. Engl. J. Med.*, 266:931–934.
94. Prosmanne, D., Chalaoui, J., Sylvestre, J., and Lefebvre, R. (1984): Small nodular pattern in the lungs due to opportunistic toxoplamosis. *J. Can. Assoc. Radiol.*, 35:186–188.
95. Purtilo, D.T., Meyers, W.M., and Connor, D.H. (1974): Fatal strongyloidiasis in immunocompromised patients. *Am. J. Med.*, 56:488–493.
96. Rangdaeng, S., Alpert, L.C., Khiyami, A., Cottingham, K., and Ramzy, I. (1992): Pulmonary paragonimiasis: report of a case with diagnosis by fine-needle aspiration cytology. *Acta Cytol.*, 36:31–36.
97. Remington, J.S., Jacobs, L., and Kaufman, H.E. (1960): Toxoplasmosis in the adult. *N. Engl. J. Med.*, 262:180–186, 237–241.
98. Risher, W.H., Crocker, E.F.J., Beckman, E.N., Blalock, J.B., and Ochsner, J.L. (1989): Pulmonary dirofilariasis: the largest single-institution experience. *J. Thorac. Cardiovasc. Surg.*, 97:303–308.
99. Ritchken, J., and Gelfand, M. (1954): Katayama disease, early toxaemic stage of biharziasis. *Br. Med. J.*, 1:1419–1420.
100. Robin, E.D., Crump, C.H., and Wagman, R.J. (1960): Low sedimentation rate, hypofibrinogenemia and restrictive pseudo-obstructive pulmonary disease associated with trichinosis. *N. Engl. J. Med.*, 262:758–763.

101. Roig, J., Romeu, J., Riera, C., Texido, A., Domingo, C., and Morera, J. (1992): Acute eosinophilic pneumonia due to toxocariasis with bronchoalveolar lavage findings. *Chest*, 102:294–296.
102. Rom, W.N., Vijayan, V.K., Cornelius, M.J., et al. (1990): Persistent lower respiratory tract inflammation associated with interstitial lung disease in patients with tropical pulmonary eosinophilia following conventional treatment with diethylcarbamazine. *Am. Rev. Respir. Dis.*, 142:1088–1092.
103. Romeo, D.P., and Pollock, J.J. (1986): Pulmonary paragoniamiasis: diagnostic value of pleural fluid analysis. *South. Med. J.*, 79:241–243.
104. Ruskin, J., and Remington, J.S. (1978): Toxoplasmosis in the compromised host. *Ann. Intern. Med.*, 84:193–199.
105. Ryning, F.W., McLeod, R., Maddox, J.C., et al. (1979): Probable transmission of *Toxoplasma gondii* by organ transplantation. *Ann. Intern. Med.*, 90:47–49.
106. Saksouk, F.A., Fahl, M.H., and Rizk, G.K. (1986): Computed tomography of pulmonary hydatid disease. *J. Comput. Assist. Tomogr.*, 10:226–232.
107. Sarwat, A.K., Tag el Din, M.A., Bassiouni, M., and Ashmawi, S.S. (1986): Schistosomiasis of the lung. *J. Egypt. Soc. Parasitol.*, 16:359–366.
108. Schaberg, T., Rahn, W., Racz, P., and Lode, H. (1991): Pulmonary schistosomiasis resembling acute pulmonary tuberculosis. *Eur. Respir. J.*, 4:1023–1026.
109. Schad, G.A. (1986): Cyclosporine may eliminate the threat of overwhelming strongyloidiasis in immunosuppressed patients. [Letter]. *J. Infect. Dis.*, 153:178.
110. Schainberg, L., and Scheinberg, M.A. (1989): Recovery of *Strongyloides stercoralis* by bronchoalveolar lavage in a patient with acquired immunodeficiency syndrome. *Am. J. Med.*, 87:486.
111. Schantz, P.M., and Glickman, L.T. (1978): Toxocaral visceral larval migrans. *N. Engl. J. Med.*, 298:436–439.
112. Scowden, E.B., Schaffner, W., and Stone, W.J. (1978): Overwhelming strongyloidiasis: an unappreciated opportunistic infection. *Medicine*, 57:527–544.
113. Shimazu, C., Pien, F.D., and Parnell, D. (1991): Bronchoscopic diagnosis of *Schistosoma japonicum* in a patient with hemoptysis. *Respir. Med.*, 85:331–332.
114. Shrand, H. (1964): Visceral larva migrans: *Toxocara canis* infection. *Lancet*, 1:1357–1359.
115. Siegel, S.E., Lunde, M.N., Gelderman, A.H., et al. (1971): Transmission of toxoplasmosis by leukocyte transfusion. *Blood*, 37:388–394.
116. Singcharoen, T., Rawd-Aree, P., and Baddeley, H. (1988): Computed tomography findings in disseminated paragonimiasis. *Br. J. Radio.*, 61:83–86.
117. Singcharoen, T., and Silprasert, W. (1987): CT findings in pulmonary paragonimiasis. *J. Comput. Assist. Tomogr.*, 11:1101–1102.
118. Slemenda, S.B., Maddison, S.E., Jong, E.C., and Moore, D.D. (1988): Diagnosis of paragonimiasis by immunoblot. *Am. J. Trop. Med. Hyg.*, 39:469–471.
119. Smith, B., Verghese, A., Guiterrez, C., Dralle, W., and Berk, S.L. (1985): Pulmonary strongyloidiasis: diagnosis by sputum gram stain. *Am. J. Med.*, 79:663–666.
120. Smith, L.S., and Schillaci, R.F. (1986): Pulmonary dirofilariasis in humans: pneumonitis that evolved to a lung nodule. *West. J. Med.*, 145:1516–1519.
121. Smith, S.B., Schwartzman, M., Mencia, F., et al. (1977): Fatal disseminated strongyloidiasis presenting as acute abdominal distress in an urban child. *J. Pediatr.*, 91:607–609.
122. Snyder, C. (1961): Visceral larva migrans: ten years' experience. *Pediatrics*, 28:85–91.
123. Stemmerman, G.N. (1967): Strongyloidiasis in immigrants. *Gastroenterology*, 53:59–70.
124. Strazzella, W.D., and Safirstein, B.H. (1989): Asthma due to parasitic infestation. *N. J. Med.*, 86:947–949.
125. Suwanik, R., and Harinsuta, C. (1959): Pulmonary paragoniamiasis: an evaluation of roentgen findings in 38 positive sputum patients in an endemic area in Thailand. *Am. J. Roentgenol. Rad. Ther. Nucl. Med.*, 81:236–244.
126. Takaro, T., and Bond, W.M. (1958): Pleuropulmonary, pericardial, and cerebral complications of amebiasis. *Int. Abstr. Surg.*, 107:209–229.
127. Takata, I. (1951): Experimental infections of man with *Ascaris* of man and the pig. *Kitasato Arch. Exp. Med.*, 23:49–59.
128. Tawney, S., Masci, J., Berger, H.W., and Subietas, A. (1986): Pulmonary toxoplasmosis: an unusual nodular radiographic pattern in a patient with AIDS. *Mt Sinai J. Med.* (NY), 53:683–685.
129. Thompson, W.M., Chisholm, D.P., and Tank, R. (1972): Plain film roentgenographic findings in alveolar hydatid disease: *Echinococcus multilocularis*. *Am. J. Roentgenol. Rad. Ther. Nucl. Med.*, 116:345–358.
130. Udwadia, F.E. (1975): Tropical eosinophilia. In: *Progress in Respiration Research: Pulmonary Eosinophilia*, edited by F.E. Udwadia, pp. 35–155. Karger, New York.
131. Vietzke, W.M., Gelderman, A.H., Grimley, P.M., and Valsamis, M.P. (1968): Toxoplasmosis complicating malignancy. *Cancer*, 21:816–827.
132. Vijayan, V.K., Sankaran, K., Venkatesan, P., and Prabhakar, R. (1991): Effect of diethylcarbamazine on the alveolitis of tropical eosinophilia. *Respiration*, 58:255–259.

133. Weingarten, R.J. (1943): Tropical eosinophilia. *Lancet,* 1:103–105.
134. Weller, P.F., Bach, D.S., and Austen, K.F. (1984): Biochemical characterization of human eosinophil Charcot-Leyden crystal protein (lysophospholipase). *J. Biol. Chem.,* 259:15100–15105.
135. Weller, P.F., Goetzl, E.J., and Austen, K.F. (1980): Identification of human eosinophil lysophospholipase as the constituent of Charcot-Leyden crystals. *Proc. Natl. Acad. Sci.* (USA), 77:7440–7443.
136. Williams, J., Nunley, D., Dralle, W., Berk, S.L., and Verghese, A. (1988): Diagnosis of pulmonary strongyloidiasis by bronchoalveolar lavage. *Chest,* 94:643–644.
137. Wilson, E.S. (1971): Pleuropulmonary amebiasis. *Am. J. Roentgenol. Rad. Ther. Nucl. Med.* 111:518–524.
138. Wilson, J.F., Diddams, A.C., and Rausch, R.L. (1968): Cystic hydatid disease in Alaska: a review of 101 autochthonous cases of *Echinococcus granulosus* infection. *Am. Rev. Respir. Dis.,* 98:1–15.
139. Wright, D.O., and Gold, E.M. (1946): Loeffler's syndrome associated with creeping eruption (cutaneous helminthiasis): report of 26 cases. *Arch. Intern. Med.,* 78:303–312.
140. Yang, S.P., Huang, C.T., Cheng, C.S., and Chiang, L.C. (1959): The clinical and roentgenologic courses of pulmonary paragonimiasis. *Dis. Chest,* 36:494–508.
141. Yee, B., Hsu, J.I., Favour, C.B., and Lohne, E. (1992): Pulmonary paragonimiasis in Southeast Asians living in the central San Joaquin Valley. *West. J. Med.,* 156:423–425.

Respiratory Infections: Diagnosis and Management, 3d ed.,
edited by James E. Pennington.
Raven Press, Ltd., New York © 1994

35

Pharmacokinetics of Antibiotics in Respiratory Tissues and Fluids

Eugénie Bergogne-Bérézin and Eric Vallée

*Bichat-Claude Bernard Hospital, 46 Rue Henri-Huchard,
Paris 75877, Cedex 18, France*

Serum pharmacokinetics of antibiotics constitute the first available approach of their potential *in vivo* efficacy against infecting pathogens, and pharmacokinetic properties of antibiotics, well established for most antimicrobial agents (30,42,82), are often considered good predictors of extravascular distribution of the drug. The volume of distribution calculated as the dosage divided by the peak concentration is used to express the potential antibiotic distribution in the body, with an assumed homogeneous distribution. In fact, most classes of antibiotics are unevenly distributed in tissues, and the concentrations likely to be achieved in a given tissue area cannot be accurately predicted from serum pharmacokinetic data (6,94,110). With newer macrolides (dirithromycin, azithromycin) extremely low serum levels and unusually prolonged half-lives do not allow us to establish consistent serum pharmacokinetic parameters. Thus, extravascular distribution and tissue penetration studies have become important aspects of the assessment of antimicrobials (5,6,83,84,116): the amount of drug reaching the extravascular infection site is probably of greater therapeutic relevance than intravascular levels. Many models have been used to study the distribution of antibiotics in the respiratory tract in humans; various specimens collected from the respiratory tract, obtained in surgical or exploratory conditions, have been analyzed for local concentrations of antibiotics thanks to the development of endoscopy and bronchoalveolar lavage techniques, as well as intubation or tracheostomy in intensive care patients. The concentrations of antibiotics achieved in respiratory tissues and fluids are the result of a series of events including the local transfer of antibiotics through membranes of the respiratory tract, as well as the general pharmacokinetics of drugs that govern their disposition and fate in the human body (5,6,26). Various host and drug factors affecting plasma concentrations and tissue distribution of drugs diversely influence the penetration of antibiotics into the respiratory tract. This chapter considers the pharmacokinetics of antibiotics in respiratory tissues and secretions and describes relevant data obtained from experiments in animal models and in studies in humans.

THEORETICAL BASIS: PHARMACOKINETICS OF TISSUE PENETRATION OF ANTIBIOTICS

Proper antibacterial therapy demands appropriate concentrations of antibacterial agents at the foci of infection. The drug's absorption, dilution into various volumes of distribution, binding to plasma proteins, biotransformation, and excretion in the urine or bile are dependent on pharmacokinetic laws that govern the fate of the drug in the human body (26,42). The rate of transport of a drug across the membrane barriers between "compartments" of the body is a function of the concentrations in these compartments, and passive diffusion follows a concentration gradient (26,42, 106,110); in experimental studies, if increased dosages indicate that this posulate is not valid, saturable transport or metabolic processes across membranes might be postulated. These concepts are applicable to the respiratory compartment.

A Model for the Transport of Antibiotic between Plasma and Respiratory Compartment

A simplified compartmental model is proposed to assess the magnitude of transport parameters between plasma and the respiratory compartment (see Fig. 35-1). Assuming the drug is distributed in the respiratory compartment (volume Vr), active

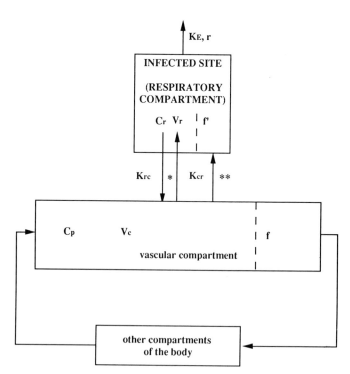

FIG. 35–1. Schematic representation of a pharmacokinetic model of an infected site, e.g., respiratory compartment in relation to the central compartment (blood).; C, concentration; V, distribution volume; Cr, unbound and nonionized drug in the respiratory compartment; Vr, volume of the extravascular compartment; Cp, unbound and nonionized drug in the plasma; Vc, volume of central compartment; f and f', protein-bound fraction of the drug; **, active transport processes; *, passive diffusion; Kcr, rate of transport of drug from central to the respiratory compartment; Krc, rate of transport in the opposite direction; $K_{E,r}$, elimination rate constant through expectoration.

transport, passive diffusion, and removal of drug by bulk flow or sputum can occur. Plasma kinetics can be simulated by a pharmacokinetic model or obtained from experimental measurements (6,26,42). A mass balance for the respiratory compartment can be defined by a quantitative mathematical equation:

$$V_r \, DC_r/dt = R + PA[C_p - C_r] - Q_r C_r - K_{E,r} C_r V_r \qquad [1]$$

where R is the rate of transport by active processes; PA = permeability × area, product for passive transport from plasma to respiratory compartment; Q_r, the flow rate through the organ; $K_{E,r}$, the elimination rate constant through expectoration; C_p and C_r, the concentrations in plasma and in the respiratory compartment, referring to the unbound and nonionized drug, which can be calculated from the total concentration if one knows the fraction bound to proteins and the pH of the media (the pK_a of the molecule should be known).

At steady state $DC_r/dt = 0$; if it is assumed that there is no active transport (R=0):

$$PA[C_p - C_r] = (Q_r + K_{E,r} V_r)C_r \qquad [2]$$

$$\rightarrow C_r = \frac{PA \, C_p}{PA + Q_r + K_{E,r} V_r} \qquad [3]$$

concentration C_r in the respiratory compartment is directly proportional to the concentration in plasma, C_p, and should be calculated from equation [3]. In practice, the respiratory tract is pharmacokinetically not homogeneous, is a slowly permeable tissue (a "deep" compartment) (5,42), and therefore does not equilibrate with the central compartment. The practical application of this mathematical expression of kinetics of antibiotics in the respiratory system can result in the design of antibiotic dosage in the treatment of respiratory infections. Actually, more clinically relevant experimental models are used for the study of disposition of antibiotics in the respiratory tract.

Transport of Antibiotics from Blood into the Respiratory Tract

Fate of Antibiotics in the Respiratory Compartment

The main biologic processes that determine the fate of antibiotics in a given compartment are transfer processes: the levels of free (unbound) antibiotic in bronchopulmonary tissues are dependent on serum levels of free drug and are achieved after the drug has passed from capillary bed to the airway lumen across a series of membranes and diffusional paths. The respiratory tract, which is a "specialized site" (5), is surrounded by blood-bronchoalveolar barriers. In parenchymal consolidation the antibiotic crossing the alveolar-capillary membrane must reach the alveolar lining fluid and parenchymal interstitium, whereas, for endobronchial infections, the antibiotic must reach the bronchial wall and lumen across the blood-bronchus barrier (3,94,106). With intracellular parthogens (*Chlamydia* sp, *Legionella* sp), the antibiotic has to concentrate within macrophagic cells of the lung (3,54,58,104).

Anatomical Lung Factors of Transfer

The distribution of a drug from blood to a tissue depends upon volume, surface area, and vascularization of the organ (110): the large alveolar surface area (30 to 100 m^2) and its rich blood supply (31) confer on the respiratory tract a major role in the exchange, absorption (19), and excretion (41) of most biologically active drugs and of antibiotics as well.

Transcapillary Movement of Antibiotics

From the blood compartment, antibiotics of molecular weight up to 1,000 cross the capillary wall easily through pores (fenestrated endothelium) (95). In response to local inflammation, additional transport pathways for large molecules can be opened and existing endothelial pathways made less restrictive (95); epithelial cells of the alveoli, separated by tight junctions (31,41) that are presumed not to allow the passage of antibiotic molecules, are well penetrated only by highly lipid soluble drugs such as macrolides or tetracyclines. However, fluoroquinolones, which are variably lipophilic (27,30) (ciprofloxacin and temafloxacin are hydrophilic), are highly concentrated intracellularly. Certain types of cells (Clara cells) of the blood-bronchoalveolar barrier have a specific metabolic function and can be responsible for metabolization and local degradation of the drugs (31,41).

Mechanisms of Transfer

By analogy with blood-brain barrier, or placental membrane, transfer of antibiotics across membranes of the respiratory tissues occurs by means of one or more of four possible mechanisms. *Passive* diffusion through membranes is not saturable, and thus local concentrations are dependent on serum levels (26). This mechanism is a function of the concentration gradient across the barrier, the transfer surface, and the thickness of the membrane (110). If increased serum levels are produced by raising the dose of antibiotic, higher local concentrations are obtained, and if the drug diffuses freely across the membrane barrier, the concentrations on each side of the membrane tend to create an equilibrium between the vascular and the extravascular compartments. However, equilibrium conditions occur only *in vitro* and in death, whereas in dynamic processes *in vivo* the drug is continually being influenced by binding, fluid flow, metabolism, degradation, and excretion (26). *Active* transport, involving carrier processes and requiring energy, is a saturable system with an independent relationship between serum and extravascular concentrations of an antibiotic. Such a transfer system occurs in a few "specialized sites" with barriers (placental barrier, blood-brain barrier [choroid plexus]) but is hypothetical in the respiratory tract (54,106), as is *filtration* and *pinocytosis*. Of these mechanisms, diffusion is by far the most important process by which antibiotics are transported within body tissues and fluids.

Physicochemical Factors of Transfer (Table 35-1)

Among drug factors influencing the antibiotic penetration into the respiratory tract, the role of protein binding (in serum and tissues) (25,68,87,101,116), lipid solubility, and degree of ionization has been well documented (5,26,87).

Host-Related Factors Influencing Drug Penetration in the Respiratory Tract (Table 35-1)

In pathologic conditions, local characteristics of the tissues, such as vascularization, inflammatory conditions, purulence, fibrosis, and edema, can enhance or reduce permeability of the barrier to antibiotic molecules (5,7,10). Correlation of local concentrations of antibiotics with the route and mode of administration is an important consideration. The effect of different routes of administration of the same drug has been studied in a dog model (87,88): in comparing the effective gentamicin levels in bronchial secretions after administration of full dose intravenously (i.v.), intramuscularly (i.m.), and divided dose i.m., only i.v. bolus method resulted in inhibitory levels in the bronchi. Similar studies were performed in humans with comparable results (66).

TABLE 35–1. *Host-related and drug-related factors influencing the transport of antibiotics into respiratory tissues and fluids*
(ref. no(s).)

1. Penetration
   Physiochemical properties of drugs
      Lipid solubility (5,26,87,106)
      Degree of ionization (5,26,87,106)
   Molecular weight
   Serum protein binding (116)
   Other binding sites
      Noninfected tissues (25,68)
      Purulent exudates (111)
   Subcellular structures (leukocytic chromatin) (68,101,111)
2. Site of infection
   Intramacrophagic pathogens (atypical pneumonia) (104)
   Parenchymal consolidation (106)
   Endobronchial infections (106)
   Degree of inflammation (10,87,88,106)
   Mechanical injury, bleeding (10,87,88,106)
   Role of respiratory secretions, variable in volume and composition (41)
   Binding and/or inactivation of antibiotics in variable degrees depending on amounts of:
      Proteins (59,68)
      Nucleic acids (59,68)
      Cellular membranes (59,68)
      Mucopolysaccharides of the mucus (59,68)
   Endotracheal pH (12)
3. Accumulation and elimination of antibiotics (59,87)
   Accumulation in cells, in mucus (87)
   Reabsorption across blood-bronchus barrier (87)
   Intrabronchial metabolism, degradation (31,41)
   Mechanical excretion (cough, mucociliary movement); fluidifying agents (9)
   Inactivation (local β-lactamase production, leucocytic enzymes) (15,106)

Modified from Pennington (87).

MODELS OF STUDIES OF ANTIBIOTIC DISPOSITION IN THE RESPIRATORY TRACT

Animal Models

There is an increasing development of animal models, even though kinetics of antimicrobial agents can differ significantly between humans and animals, with dissimilarities in (i) bioavailability of the administered dose, serum protein binding, and volumes of distribution of the drug in different species; (ii) predominant mechanisms of clearance and metabolization of drugs in laboratory animals; and (iii) elimination rate known to be faster in small animals (14,119). Animal models have proved useful in the evaluation of pharmacokinetics of antibiotics in well-defined, comparative, and reproducible conditions not achievable in human studies. Experimental studies in animals focus on (i) kinetic properties of new drugs, compared to reference compounds in preclinical studies (81,107); (ii) disposition of antibiotics at specific sites of infection, including the lung (91,92), and the possible role of infection in their disposition (17,18,45,107,109,112); and (iii) the suitability of specific routes of administration in delivering higher amounts of antibiotics at sites of infection (targeted delivery) and in reducing their systemic toxicity.

Aminoglycosides

Pennington utilized a canine model to study pharmacokinetics of anti-*Pseudomonas* antibiotics in bronchial secretions (90,91). The studies were carried out in noninfected dogs; correlation between dog and human bronchial levels (85,100) were observed, along with a slow disappearance of gentamicin and tobramycin as compared with serum, probably the result of accumulation of drugs in bronchial secretions. In a model of experimental *Pseudomonas* pneumonia (91), penetration studies were performed in guinea pigs receiving comparative regimens with tobramycin, gentamicin, carbenicillin, and ticarcillin used as single and combined therapy. This model documented the penetration of drugs into bronchial space and the therapeutic efficacy of several antibiotic regimens, showing superiority of aminoglycosides over penicillins. The effects of infection on disposition of gentamicin were studied in calves with experimental pneumonic pasteurellosis (17). After multiple i.m. dosing (5 mg/kg), significantly greater concentrations of gentamicin were observed in pneumonic lungs compared with noninfected tissue (tissue/serum ratios were 0.5 ± 0.04 for pneumonic lung vs. 0.22 ± 0.07 for nonpneumonic lung, $p < 0.05$). These data could result from ion-trapping of a basic drug in an inflammatory area with reduced pH; a possible decreased antimicrobial activity can be associated with such an environment (12,111).

Fluoroquinolones

Fluoroquinolones exhibit the same lung tissue penetration in animals (107,108) as in humans (27,30) and a greater efficacy in treating mouse *Hemophilus* pneumonia than other antimicrobial agents (65). Differences between pharmacokinetics of fluoroquinolones observed in humans (30) are observed in mice as well (108), with a faster elimination rate in small animals. The efficacy of temafloxacin and sparfloxacin was probably favored by the marked prolongation of their residence time at bactericidal levels in the presence of infection, as compared to noninfected mice (108). However, comparison between antibiotic levels and bactericidal effect in lungs and time indicated that serum levels were better correlated to pulmonary bacterial clearance; they probably reflected more effective concentrations in interstitial fluid, more relevant to pneumococcal infection, than in lung homogenates (intracellular accumulation of the drugs) (107).

Macrolides

Concentrations in lung tissue are far higher than in serum, as a result of intracellular accumulation of macrolides (104). Differences in tissue penetration and elimination rates between macrolides correlate with intracellular uptake and release from cells, as shown *in vivo* with spiramycin compared to erythromycin in rat lungs (92). In mice (see Table 35-2), azithromycin and spiramycin, highly concentrated and slowly released from cells, exhibited the highest penetration and the longest elimination rates from lung tissue (much longer than in serum). The elimination rate from tissue of erythromycin, roxithromycin, and clarithromycin (quickly released from cells) was markedly shorter and paralleled that in serum (112). Inflammatory cells play a major role in the local delivery of macrolides at sites of infection. In hemophilus otitis in gerbils (45), only erratic levels of azithromycin were found in bulla washes when inflammation was absent; inflammation resulted in sevenfold higher concentrations, and more than 70% of drug was associated with phagocytes. In mice infected with *H. influenzae,* concentrations of azithromycin in lungs closely paralleled phagocytic infiltration, and antibiotic persisted at infection sites for more than 24 hours, whereas serum levels decreased 1 hour after drug administration (109).

β-Lactams

In the canine model, infusion of a large dose (125 mg/kg i.v.) of carbenicillin resulted in bronchial levels that were 25% of serum levels (90). The entry into the ovine lungs of four cephalosporins has been evaluated in using cannulation of the principal channel for lymph efferent from lungs, supposed to reflect the interstitial milieu (22). All drugs appeared in the pulmonary lymph during the i.v. infusion (30 min). Peak concentration of moxalactam was significantly delayed as compared with cefazolin, cefoperazone, and ceftriaxone; cefazolin and cefoperazone penetrated better than ceftriaxone and moxalactam, which declined more gradually, and were bound twice higher to plasma proteins so that their penetration was significantly lower. The effects of serum protein binding on extravascular penetration of antimicrobials provided contradictory results in animals and in humans, questioning their affinity to proteins rather than their binding rate.

Models for Studies in Human Respiratory Tissues and Fluids

Many studies in human respiratory tissues have been carried out. The design of these studies must take into account ethical and technical limitations which do not allow kinetic studies with tissue samples collected at surgery; only in selected conditions can consecutive samples of bronchial secretions be taken and pharmacoki-

TABLE 35–2. *Lung pharmacokinetics of antibiotics in experimental mouse models of pneumococcal pneumonia*

Drugs (mg/kg)	Mice	Cmax (mg/kg)	T½β (h)	AUC (mg.h/l)	Tissue penetr. ratio	ΔtMIC(h) [MIC:mg/l]
Fluoroquinolones						
Tmfx 100	NI	90.7 ± 16.7	1.4 ± 0.1	250.7 ± 51.1	3.4 ± 0.1	8 [1]
	–	133.8 ± 14.0	10.0 ± 5.3	470.2 ± 28.2	3.3 ± 0.1	>24
Cpfx 100	NI	37.7 ± 5.9	1.1 ± 0.1	83.0 ± 29.9	2.1 ± 0.5	6 [1]
	–	45.9 ± 5.6	1.6 ± 0.2	125.1 ± 14.8	2.1 ± 0.4	6
Ofx 100	NI	24.4	0.9	47	1.7	3 [2]
	–	30.0	1.8	61	1.4	3
Cpfx 50	NI					
Spfx 50	–	20.4	1.2	42.0	1.8	5 [1]
	NI	18.5	2.9	38.0	2.1	24 [0.25]
	–	27.0	5.7	64	2.6	>24
Macrolide antibiotics						
Ery 50	NI	20.0	0.6	32.2	2.0	
	–	16.1	1.2	32.0	2.9	
Roxi 50	NI	32.8	1.7	140.0	6.8	6 [0.06]
	–	44.6	1.7	160.0	4.6	8 [0.125]
Clari 50	NI	87.5	1.7	324.0	15.4	
	–	70.4	1.6	262.0	15.9	8 [0.015]
Spira 50	NI	19.4	10.0	185.0	29.8	
	–	19.2	9.6	211.0	49.0	24 [0.5]
Azi 50	NI	36.3	17.1	676.0	21.1	
	–	58.1	18.6	1041.0	34.7	96 [0.125]
Azi 50		16.4	16.5	214.0	39.9	
(leukopenic)						

Pharmacokinetic parameters were determined after a single s.c. injection of the drugs.
Cmax, peak concentration; T½β, elimination half-life; AUC, area under the curve; ΔtMIC, time during which concentrations exceeded MICs.
NI, noninfected mice; I, infected mice; Tmfx, temafloxacin; Cpfx, ciprofloxacin; Ofx, ofloxacin; Spfx, sparfloxacin; Ery, erythromycin; Roxi, roxithromycin; Clari, clarithromycin; Spira, spiramycin; Azi, azithromycin.
From Vallée et al. (107–109) and Veber et al. (112).

netic parameters calculated. In early studies, expectorated material was used (48, 56,69,72,74,98), but, as has been pointed out (88), dilution of sputum with saliva could be responsible for experimental errors and for underestimation of antibiotic levels. Improvement in studies on sputum was obtained by using pooled sputa collected for 24 hours and measurement of average antibiotic levels. The major drawbacks of this technique were the lack of a kinetic approach to antibiotic penetration and a poor correlation between serum and pooled sputa (74,94,96). Specimens of bronchial secretions obtained from the lower respiratory tract and collected through endotracheal tube, tracheostomy cannula, or fiberoptic bronchoscope appeared more suitable for clinical studies (7,11,80). Antibiotic concentrations measured in bronchial samples were interpreted as the final net effective level of free drug, the product of the rates of penetration, metabolism in the lung, and clearance from bronchial secretions; it must be also taken into account that bronchial secretions are constantly produced and constantly diluted in a dynamic process (106). Samples of lung parenchyma taken during thoracotomy (16,28,79), bronchial mucosa (29,117) collected by fiberoptic bronchoscopy, alveolar (epithelial) lining fluid, and alveolar macrophages (3,4,54,94) collected by using bronchoalveolar lavage have increasingly allowed for studies of antibiotic concentrations at sites of potential respiratory infections.

STUDIES IN HUMAN RESPIRATORY TRACT: SPECIFIC DRUGS

Penetration of β-Lactams into Respiratory Tissues and Fluids (Table 35-3)

β-lactams are hydrophilic drugs which achieve relatively low concentrations in respiratory tissues and fluids.

Aminopenicillins

Early studies using sputum (69,74) provided convergent results: sputum concentrations of ampicillin varied from patient to patient but never exceeded 0.5 mg/l. Related to higher serum levels, higher concentrations of amoxycillin were measured in sputum (56,75,98) and in bronchial secretions (7,16,100); the same advantage was noted with bacampicillin (7,71), due certainly to a better gastrointestinal absorption. A sputum/serum ratio of 13 to 20% expressed a dose-dependent effect with clinical outcome related to the length of time over which ampicillin sputum levels were superior to the minimal inhibitory concentrations (MICs) for *H. influenzae* (71). The mean lung tissue (16) and bronchial mucosa (117) concentrations of amoxycillin were 3.05 ± 1.75 and 2.7 ± 1.2 mg/kg, respectively; these values were in a ratio to serum below 1. The tissue concentrations of amoxycillin appeared much higher than those in secretions as the result of contribution of different compartments of lungs and mucosa: extracellular fluids, interstitium, and capillary blood which contains variable antibiotic levels (106). All of the above-mentioned studies were carried out with aminopenicillins administered orally at usual doses (500 or 1,000 mg). After i.v. administration of 2 g amoxycillin plus 200 mg clavulanate in ten surgical patients, mean lung tissue concentrations were 28.5 ± 10.7 and 1.8 ± 0.2 mg/kg, respectively, as measured by bioassay (23). After 500 mg amoxycillin + 250 mg clavulanate in bronchial secretions (50), clavulanate level was only 0.23 ± 0.4 mg/l, which is about

TABLE 35–3. *Antibiotic concentrations in human lung parenchyma, bronchial mucosa, and secretions (peak concentrations)*

Antibiotic	Route & dose	Serum level (mg/l)	Parenchyma (mg/kg)	Bronchial mucosa (mg/kg)	Bronchial secretion (mg/l)	Ref. no(s).
β-lactams						
amoxycillin (SD)	1 g i.v. p.o.	6.9	4.4–5.6	2.7 ± 1.2	0.52 (0.23–0.98)	(7,75,98,100,117)
carbenicillin (MD)	20 g iv.	130	45–75	–	15–49	(100)
mezlocillin (SD)	5 g iv.	140	25–35	–	10.0 (1.0–22.0)	(7,100)
piperacillin (MD)	4 g i.v.	196.3	–	55.2	12.2 ± 8.5	(7,73,100)
cephalexin (MD)	500 mg p.o.	3–4	–	–	0.32 (0.3–3.42)	(7,48)
cephalothin (MD)	12 g i.v.	40–60	12–25	–	–	(100)
cefoxitin (SD)	2 g i.v.	11.3 (2.15–23.5)	5.6–18.5	–	2.8 (1.4–3.6)	(7,100)
cefuroxime (SD)	0.75 g i.m.	10.6 (7.6–15.5)	–	–	1.95 (0.4–3.5)	(7,100)
cefuroxime-axetil	500 mg p.o.	3.4 ± 2.4	–	3.8 ± 1.6	1.0–3.5	(113,117)
cefotaxime (SD)	2 g i.v.	40	5.0–14.0	–	1.45 (0.12–1.6)	(7,100)
moxalactam (MD)	1 g i.m.	54.9 (24–99)	–	–	5.0 (1.4–6.2)	(77)
ceftriaxone (SD)	2 g i.v.	127 ± 17.6	57.4 ± 13.3	–	–	(61)
cefepime (SD)	2 g i.v.	40.4 ± 28.1	–	24.1 ± 17.8	–	(117)
cefpirome (SD)	1 g i.v.	55.6 ± 15.7	–	33.0 ± 11.1	–	(117)
cefpodoxime-proxetil (SD)	260 mg p.o.	1.05 ± 0.74	0.89 ± 0.8	–	–	(79)
imipenem (SD)	1 g i.v.	69 (33–100.5)	6.6 (0.9–18.8)	–	0.94 ± 0.12	(70,80)
Aminoglycosides						
gentamicin (MD)	5 mg/kg	5.0–6.0	5.0–7.0	–	1.83 (0.10–4.3)	(72,85,115)
amikacin (SD)	500 mg i.v.	11–20	6.0–9.0	–	6.7 (5.0–8.4)	(7,34,100)
tobramycin	1.7 mg/kg	6.0–8.0	6.0–9.0	–	2.68 (1.2–5.9)	(1,7,47)

	Dose					References
Macrolides						
erythromycin (SD)	270 mg i.v.		5.52 ± 2.16	7.2 ± 4.3	–	(118)
erythromycin (MD)	500 mg i.v.	3.05 ± 0.97	6.53 ± 3.18		1.28 (0.5–2.5)	(8,16,54)
erythromycin (SD)	1 g p.o.	1.37 ± 0.89	4.23 ± 2.14		0.59 (0.125–2.49)	(7,8,16)
roxithromycin (MD)	150 mg p.o.	6.26 ± 0.7	5.64 ± 0.53		3.1 ± 0.77	(103)
clarithromycin (MD)	500 mg p.o.	2.51 ± 0.87	17.47 ± 3.29 (24h)	3.89 ± 1.2	–	(40)
azithromycin (SD)	500 mg p.o.	0.2–0.4	0.8–7.2 (72h) 1.3–4.8 (72h) 2.3–8.1 (96h)		0.23–9.5	(39,117)
spiramycin (MD)	2–3 g p.o.	2.4 (0.7–4)	19.25 ± 7.5	13–36	7.3 (1.0–18)	(4,7,8)
Quinolones						
ciprofloxacin (SD)	500 mg p.o.	1.64 ± 0.42	2.2–4.5	4.4 ± 3.3	1.3–2.33	(27,117)
	200 mg i.v.	0.6 ± 0.49	4.71 ± 3.12	2.53 ± 0.68	–	
ofloxacin (SD)	200 mg p.o.	4.8–4.9		6.0–9.8	1.51 ± 0.7	(29,30)
ofloxacin (MD)	200 mg p.o.	1.90–5.18	6.7–7.3	10.2–12.9	–	
temafloxacin (MD)	600 mg p.o.	6.05 ± 2.19	27.97 ± 17.02	12.2 ± 4.0	2.78 ± 3.64 (SD)	(27,30,117)
lomefloxacin (MD)	400 mg p.o.	2.8 ± 1.0		5.8 ± 3.7		(11,117)
sparfloxacin (SD)	400 mg p.o.	1.2		2.5	1.80 ± 1.03	(4,54)
Tetracyclines						
doxycycline (SD)	100 mg p.o.	2.74	5.4–23		1.05 (0.12–3.27)	(43,100)
minocycline (SD)	200 mg p.o.	4.6 (1.2–5.3)			1.7 (0.4–5.4)	(7)
Miscellaneous						
thiamphenicol (SD)	750 mg p.o.	5.8 (1.5–15.5)			3.4 (2.4–6.4)	(7)
co-trimoxazole						
TMP (SD)	800 mg p.o.	47.4			8.7	(7,55)
SMZ (SD)	160 mg	1.58			2.2	
clindamycin (SD)	300 mg p.o.	2.6 (2.2–14.4)			1.6 (0.3–4.8)	(7)
vancomycin (SD)	1 g i.m.	5.3	13.0			(100)

SD, single dose; MD, multiple dose; i.v., intravenous administration; i.m., intramuscular administration; p.o., *per os*.

10% of serum level (2.59±2.5 mg/l) and equal to amoxycillin bronchial level (0.26±0.28 mg/l). Despite low local levels of clavulanic acid, its addition to amoxycillin is supposed to better control pneumonia due to β-lactamase producers.

Carbenicillin/Anti-Pseudomonas Penicillins

Carbenicillin penetration in bronchial secretions has been studied in the canine model (90) and in patients with cystic fibrosis (72). It was shown that optimal concentrations of carbenicillin were not achieved in bronchial secretions; a bronchial peak of 7.8 mg/l in sputum of children with cystic fibrosis was higher than the MICs of only 75% of *P. aeruginosa* isolates. Bronchial levels were less than 20% of those in serum, and resistance to carbenicillin emerged in 6 of 11 patients (72). In order to achieve a maximal gradient between serum and bronchial fluid in humans, carbenicillin or ticarcillin should be infused over shorter periods of time to achieve a higher peak in serum (90). The penetration of ureidopenicillins, mezlocillin and azlocillin, was of the same order as that of carbenicillin, with a ratio of bronchial peak to serum level of 10 to 20% (7,100). In bronchial mucosa, tissue level of piperacillin was 55.2 mg/kg, in a 28% ratio to serum concentration (73). These moderate concentrations suggest that treatment of *Pseudomonas* pneumonia should be optimal if these penicillins are associated with an aminoglycoside (13) or a fluoroquinolone. However, subinhibitory local levels (102) can have an impact on colonization and adherence of *Pseudomonas* to epithelial cells of the respiratory tract (57,93).

Cephalosporins

In early studies, low concentrations (≤15% of corresponding serum levels) of first-generation cephalosporins were found in respiratory secretions (7,10,48,100,106), and their place in the treatment of pneumonia remained controversial. Improvement in pharmacokinetic properties was obtained with more recent molecules, and several studies (7,54,61,77,105) showed that the penetration of cefamandole, cefuroxime, cefotaxime, ceftazidime, and moxalactam into respiratory tissues and fluids was significantly increased (25 to 30% of serum levels); the peak of bronchial concentrations was attained generally at the second hour after the last dose, irrespective of the route of administration. There was no accumulation of these drugs in bronchial tissues and secretions, which suggests that repeated doses at frequent intervals might be given to create successive peak serum concentrations so that high-enough antibiotic local levels could be maintained. However, with ceftriaxone, early lung tissue levels (57.4±13.3 mg/kg [1–2 hrs after 2 g i.v.]) were followed by a slow decrease; and late, sustained parenchymal concentrations (31.8±22.9 mg/kg at 6 hrs) certainly were related to its prolonged serum half-life (6–8 hours) (61). Newer cephalosporins achieved bronchial mucosal concentrations about half of the corresponding serum levels (3,117): cefepime reached 24.1±17.8 mg/kg (after a 2 g i.v. dose); cefpirome: 33.0±11.1 mg/kg (after 1 g i.v.). Among orally administered cephalosporins, cefpodoxime-proxetil (79) achieved lung concentration of 0.89±0.8 mg/kg, which was 84% of the serum level. In bronchial mucosa, cefixime reached 1.5 mg/kg after a 200 mg oral dose; with cefuroxime-axetil (500 mg p.o.), the mean mucosal concentration of cefuroxime (3.8 ± 1.6 mg/kg) was equal to that in serum (3.4 ± 2.4 mg/l) (3,113,117). New cephalosporins are increasingly used in the treatment of respiratory infections, as a result of improved tolerance, diffusibility, and spectrum as well as β-lactamase stability.

Carbapenems

Imipenem has been studied in ICU patients (80): 2 hours after 1 g i.v. infusion of imipenem/cilastatin, appreciable bronchial levels of 2.1 ± 1.03 mg/l were reached, representing 20% of serum levels. Much higher concentrations of imipenem were measured in bronchoalveolar epithelial lining fluid, reaching up to 24.1–51.4 mg/l, exceeding plasma levels (serum peak: 28.4 ± 1.3 mg/l) (70). With meropenem, a newer carbapenem, bronchial secretion levels were in a ratio of 20% of serum concentrations (personal unpublished data). Carbapenems have proved to be extremely useful in treating nosocomial pneumonia, especially those cases involving *Pseudomonas* sp, *Acinetobacter* sp, and *Pseudomonas* superinfections in cystic fibrosis patients.

Penetration of Aminoglycosides into Respiratory Tissues and Fluids (Table 35-3)

Despite *in vitro* susceptibility of causative organisms, infected bronchiectasis or *Pseudomonas* pneumonia can be resistant to aminoglycoside therapy. Factors that determine these failures probably include inability to achieve proper tissue concentrations. In clinical studies, intramuscularly administered gentamicin (100), netilmicin (66), tobramycin (1,47), and amikacin (7,34) resulted in bronchial concentrations ranging from 1 to 5 mg/l, 2 to 4 hours after administration, and a bronchial/serum ratio of about 30%. The reported parenchymal concentrations of aminoglycosides never exceeded 5–6 mg/kg (100). Peripheral inactivation of aminoglycosides has been analyzed (69,76,101,111); the role played by lysed polymorphonuclear leucocytes, purified chromatin, or DNA from purulent exudates resulted in a decrease of the concentration of the free bio-active drug; the endobronchial pH (12) and the presence of mucopolysaccharides might cooperate in the inactivation of aminoglycosides within infected areas. On the whole, aminoglycosides are known as poorly lipophilic drugs which never exceed a 0.5 ratio of site-of-infection to serum (3); they accumulate extremely slowly in phagocytic cells, with a limited intracellular antibacterial activity due to acidic local pH (58,104). This limited diffusion of aminoglycosides into the tracheobronchial tree results in concentrations insufficient to inhibit the growth of *P. aeruginosa* in cystic fibrosis patients (47,72,96).

Penetration of Macrolides into Respiratory Tissues and Fluids (Table 35-3)

With many indications in the treatment of respiratory infections, including Legionnaires' disease and *Chlamydia* pneumonia, macrolides have been studied for their penetration into respiratory tissues and fluids. Higher erythromycin concentrations in lung parenchyma were found after administration of erythromycin i.v. (500 mg) (6.53 ± 3.18 mg/kg) (16) than after oral administration of ethylsuccinate of erythromycin (1 g) (4.23 ± 2.14 mg/kg). Newer macrolides such as clarithromycin and its major metabolite, 14-hydroxy-6-0-methyl erythromycin, reached much higher lung concentrations than erythromycin (17.47 ± 3.29 mg/kg) (40). Dirithromycin and the newer, 15-membered azithromycin (39) behaved similarly, characterized by hardly detectable serum concentrations, and high and stable lung tissue concentrations persistent at 24th and 96th hours, respectively. In the bronchial mucosa, a recent study showed a mean tissue level of erythromycin of 7.20 ± 4.30 mg/kg and a penetration ratio of 171 ± 70%, 4.28 hours after multiple 500 mg oral doses (54). In the same study, the disposition of azithromycin in the respiratory tree showed significantly higher concentrations in bronchial mucosa (3.89 mg/kg) than in serum and epithelial lining fluid. After multiple oral doses of 2 or 3 g of spiramycin, concentrations in the bronchial mucosa (16 to 36 mg/kg) were 6 to 15 times higher than peak serum concentrations. In bronchial secretions (8), the penetration of spiramycin was found excellent, reaching rapidly higher bronchial levels than simultaneous serum levels. These data suggest a nonsaturable diffusion of macrolides across membranes. In studies of tissue concentrations the contribution of the intracellular antibiotic is certainly of major importance in the apparent disposition of macrolides in the respiratory tract (3,54,92,104). Otherwise, the concentrations of macrolides achieved in respiratory tissues and intracellularly are high enough to inhibit most susceptible respiratory pathogens including the intramacrophagic obligate bacteria such as *Legionella pneumophila*. Macrolides seem not to be affected by the low endobronchial pH associated with infection (12,32) and achieved notable local levels in all studies.

Penetration of Fluoroquinolones into Respiratory Tissues and Fluids (Table 35-3)

This new class of antibiotics has become important in the treatment of respiratory infections; distribution of quinolones has been investigated in various sites of potential infection of the respiratory tract (3,11,27,29,30). Fluoroquinolones reached high parenchymal concentrations ranging from 2.2 to 4.5 mg/kg for ciprofloxacin (500 mg), 6.7 to 7.3 mg/kg for ofloxacin (400 mg), and 27.9 ± 17.0 mg/kg for temafloxacin (600 mg) (27,30). Quinolone concentrations were measured also in small volumes of mucosal samples. Several studies used i.v. route and doses of 100 or 200 mg of ofloxacin (29) and ciprofloxacin (28) or oral 500 mg single or multiple doses of ciprofloxacin (27,117); lomefloxacin, temafloxacin, and sparfloxacin, measured after 400 mg (single or multiple doses) (54,117), reached high mucosal concentrations varying from 2.5 mg/kg for sparfloxacin to 10–12 mg/kg for ofloxacin and temafloxacin, all mucosal values being twice higher than corresponding serum levels. In bronchial secretions a high rate of penetration of fluoroquinolones was also found, and therapeutically relevant bronchial levels were measured (3,11,30). High intracellular concentrations of quinolones (104) are considered good predictors of their potential activity against intracellular pathogens. All fluoroquinolones seem to behave similarly in various models, and this should be related to their non-ionized state in serum, small molecular size, and low protein binding, which allow a rapid distribution in extravascular and intracellular sites (27,30).

Penetration of Other Antibiotics into Respiratory Tissues and Fluids (Table 35-3)

Tetracyclines

Tetracyclines, thanks to their lipid solubility and good tissue penetration, were widely used in the treatment of lung infections (*Mycoplasma*) or purulent exacerbations of chronic bronchitis. Their penetration into respiratory tissues (43,100) and secretions (7,20,49) has been evaluated. Notable bronchial penetration was found for minocycline and doxycycline and was higher for rolitetracycline administered intravenously (7). Bronchial concentrations generally were 1.5–2 mg/l, about 30 to 60% of corresponding serum levels. Bronchial wall and lung tissue levels of doxycycline (43) were higher than the MICs of most common pathogenic bacteria, repeated dosing resulted in increasing tissue concentrations.

Co-Trimoxazole

Penetration of co-trimoxazole (trimethoprim [TMP]-sulfamethoxazole [SMZ]) has been studied in bronchial secretions (7,55,60) and in lung tissues (24). The results of experimental and clinical studies are in good agreement, showing a poor penetration of SMZ in contrast with TMP, which quickly reaches concentrations equal to or higher than the corresponding serum level. The ratio TMP/SMZ between both components of the combination was 5% in the serum and 20% in bronchial secretions (7), but synergistic *in vitro* activity was maintained in the latter ratio. The difference in penetration of TMP and of SMZ is attributable to the highly protein-bound sulfonamide. Clinical experiences (55) were generally favorable in most cases of pneumonia, lung abscess, and bronchiectasis involving *H. influenzae* and *S. pneumoniae*.

Fosfomycin

This underestimated drug is completely different in structure from all classes of available antibiotics. Its *in vitro* characteristics suggest its use in severe infections (62) due to *Staph. aureus* and most resistant gram-negative bacilli. The high rate of extravascular diffusion of fosfomycin was confirmed in a study of its penetration into bronchial secretions. After 4 g of i.v. infusion (4 hrs), the bronchial peak levels ranged from 5 to 31 mg/l, with a penetration ratio of about 13%. Clinical evaluation showed a successful use in treating severe respiratory infections; its major drawback is the prolonged i.v. route which restricts its use in hospitals.

Metronidazole

The study of penetration of metronidazole into bronchial secretions is of potential value in lung abscesses and severe aspiration pneumonia mainly caused by anaerobes, especially *Bacteroides fragilis*. Metronidazole rapidly achieves and maintains concentrations much higher than the MICs for susceptible anaerobes. Sputum levels were as high as those in serum and ranged from 5.0 to 38.0 mg/l (97) in patients receiving 400 mg of metronidazole 3 times daily for 7 days; these values are well within the therapeutic range for the treatment of anaerobic pneumonia.

Antifungal Drugs

In the canine model (89), the penetration of amphotericin-B and 5-fluorocytosine has been evaluated. Amphotericin-B was not measurable in bronchial secretions even after maximum i.v. dosage. In human pulmonary aspergilloma, it is controversial whether or not the drug reaches a fungus ball existing in a free state within a cavity, in adequate concentrations. In contrast, 5-fluorocytosine (5-FC) exhibited a good penetration, achieving bronchial concentrations above 20 mg/l after administration of 35 mg/kg; this exceeds the MICs for most *Candida* species and suggests an effective role for 5-FC in treating tracheobronchial candidosis. More-recent drugs, such as ketoconazole, are available for treatment of pulmonary mycoses, but no data on their penetration into the respiratory fluids are found in the literature.

Pulmonary Disposition of Antituberculous Drugs

There is a current revival of tuberculosis and an increasing role of atypical mycobacteria in pulmonary as well as extrapulmonary pathological processes in immunodepressed patients (AIDS). Few publications deal with the pulmonary distribution of antituberculous drugs. In one study with isoniazid (114), high concentrations of isoniazid were found in the lung, and the drug penetrated in caseous tissues with retention of amounts well above bacteriostatic levels. The diffusion of rifampicin in bronchial secretions (86) was more rapid in hypersecretory bronchopathies than in nonhypersecretory ones. After administration of 600 mg, the bronchial concentrations reached a mean bronchial peak higher than 5 mg/l, followed by a slow decrease and concentrations still measurable 12 hours after absorption (0.5 to 1 mg/l). The levels of rifampicin in healthy lung parenchyma (21) and in cavity wall (10 to 12 mg/l 3 hours after 600 mg) were higher than in caseous lesions where the amount did not exceed 2 mg/kg. Rifampicin reached tissue concentrations higher than simultaneous serum levels, due to its liposolubility, and was also concentrated in macrophages (58,104). Early studies showed the superiority of ethionamide to streptomycin, rifampicin, and isoniazid in penetration into caseous lesion (21).

Newer antituberculous drugs are being developed. Rifapentine, a new semi-synthetic rifamycin, reached high concentrations (9.49 mg/kg) in rat lungs after an oral dose of 10 mg/kg. The parenchymal concentrations were higher than serum levels and persisted for 72 hours, with values exceeding MICs for *M. tuberculosis* var. *hominis* (2). Rifabutine is also a new rifamycin derivative, with much lower MICs than rifampicin for mycobacteria, increasingly used in therapy, especially against *M. avium* (MAC) (in combination with other antimycobacterial drugs and even with clarithromycin). In man, after administration of multiple oral doses (300 mg), the parenchymal concentration was 1.39 mg/kg, exceeding by far (7 to 10 times) the plasma level (78) and persisting at significant level until the 48th hour. High intramacrophagic concentrations of rifabutine have also been measured. Clofazimine has been used since 1962 against leprosy and more recently against atypical mycobacteria in immunodeficiency viral infections; its pharmacokinetics have been reassessed (52). This highly lipophilic drug demonstrates an extremely prolonged half-life (70 days) and significant distribution in human tissues including lung parenchyma (0.17–1.4 mg/kg after a 200 or 300 mg daily dose). Combined with ethambutol, rifabutine, and ciprofloxacin, clofazimine should contribute to control disseminated MAC infection.

NEW MODELS OF HUMAN STUDIES OF ANTIBIOTIC DISTRIBUTION IN LUNGS (TABLE 35-4)

Epithelial Lining Fluid (ELF)

New approaches of antibiotic disposition in human lungs have been developed recently, thanks to the increasing use of bronchoalveolar lavage (BAL) in pneumology. ELF and human alveolar macrophages are collected by using BAL (3,4,54,79). ELF concentrations of a few quinolones, macrolides, and β-lactams have been measured; with β-lactams local levels were equal or higher than those in bronchoscopically aspirated secretions (3). ELF levels of macrolides were lower than those measured in bronchial mucosa (Table 35-4). Concentrations of quinolones in ELF ranged from 4 mg/l for ciprofloxacin to 26.5 mg/l for temafloxacin (54). Data on ELF concentrations, although still limited, should be considered good predictors of antibiotic efficacy in the lung acinus, which is the site of the pneumonic process, as in pneumococcal pneumonia (3). Azithromycin reaches 2.2 mg/kg in ELF (after a single 500 mg single dose), a value 17.5 times higher than the MIC_{90} for pneumococci (0.125 mg/l). Two new fluoroquinolones, temafloxacin and sparfloxacin, are highly concentrated in ELF (26.5 ± 3.6 and 15.0 ± 8.3 mg/kg, respectively), with otherwise low MIC_{90} for pneumococci (0.5–1.0 and 0.25 mg/l, respectively), so that both drugs might be expected to be potentially more useful for treatment of pneumococcal pneumonia than the earlier fluoroquinolones (4,54).

Alveolar Macrophages (AM)

In order to control typical obligatory intracellular pathogens responsible for atypical pneumonias, like *Legionella* sp and *Chlamydiae* sp, intracellularly achievable antibiotic concentrations are needed. The uptake, intracellular disposition, and subcellular localization of several antibiotic classes have been studied (4,58,104). By using alveolar macrophages collected from BAL, or in an *in vitro* model (104), concentrations of fluoroquinolones and of macrolides have been investigated (Table 35-4). Erythromycin and josamycin have been shown to concentrate and accumulate intracellularly at levels 17 and 25 times, respectively, higher than extracellular levels. Newer compounds such as roxithromycin and azithromycin show even much greater accumulation (3,54); the uptake of macrolides is rapid (15–20 min); the new azalide azithromycin behaves differently: its uptake by cells is much slower, is completed after 24 hours, with a sudden rise in concentrations at 48 hours (104). The lysosomal localization of macrolides has been demonstrated. Fluoroquinolones accumulate in macrophages at concentrations 5 to 8 times higher than in extracellular fluid, but their subcellular localization has not yet been established. In other models (104), the intracellular concentration of quinolones was 4.6 to 8.0-fold that in extracellular environment; in human polymorphonuclear neutrophils or in guinea pig macrophages, the intracellular concentrations clearly related to intracellular activity of quinolones. Thus, their role in treating respiratory infections is extremely interesting, due also to their wide spectrum of antibacterial activity, including *Pseudomonas* sp, *Legionella pneumophila,* and *Mycoplasma pneumoniae,* all of which are susceptible to new quinolones (28,30).

TABLE 35–4. *Concentrations of antibiotics in alveolar macrophages and in epithelial lining fluid*

Antibiotics	Doses (mg) & route	No. patients	Serum (mg/l)	ELF[a] (mg/l)	Intra-macrophagic concentrations (mg/kg)	Ratio intra/extra-cellular concentrations	Ref. no.
β-Lactams							
amoxycillin	500 (MD), p.o.	9	—	2.56 ± 1.41	2.0	—	(4)
clavulanic acid	250 (MD), p.o.	—	—	1.33 ± 0.65	—	—	(4)
cefuroxime-axetil	613 (MD), p.o.	8	—	1.04 ± 0.66	1.20	—	(4)
cefpodoxime-proxetil	260 (SD), p.o.	6	1.85 ± 0.82	0.22 ± 0.13	—	—	(79)
cefpirome	1 g i.v. (SD)	37	3.45 ± 3.3	7.1 ± 1.1	—	—	(4)
imipenem	1 g i.v. (SD)	20	19.0 ± 1.1	24.1–51.4	—	—	(70)
Macrolides							
erythromycin	500 (MD), p.o.	—	—	—	22	17	(54)
josamycin	1000 (MD), i.v.	—	—	—	44 (88)	25	(3)
azithromycin	500 (MD), p.o.	22	0.13 ± 0.05	1.4	23	96–225	(54)
roxithromycin	300 (MD), p.o.	8	—	2.0 ± 1.7	21	61	(54)
clarithromycin	250 (MD), p.o.	—	1.2 ± 0.04	10.4 ± 0.7	86.5 ± 3.6	—	(54)
Quinolones							
ciprofloxacin[b]	10 mg/l	—	—	4	45.2 ± 6.5[b]	5.5	(4)
temafloxacin	600 (MD)	14	9.6 ± 1.2	26.5 ± 3.6	83 ± 11.5	7.9 (4.6–43)	(54)
sparfloxacin	400 (SD)	21	0.72 ± 0.65	8.65 ± 8.44	42.7 ± 34.0	—	(54)
	400 (MD)	10	1.2 ± 0.41	15 ± 8.3	53.7 ± 38.4	—	

SD, single dose; MD, multiple dose.
i.v., intravenous admin.; p.o., per os.
[a]Epithelial lining fluid.
[b]Studies in *in vitro* phagocytic cell systems (104).

ANTIBIOTIC PENETRATION INTO UPPER RESPIRATORY TISSUES AND FLUIDS

The ability of antimicrobial agents to achieve significant concentrations in infection sites of the upper respiratory tract, sinus mucosa and fluid, otitis media, and tonsils responds to the same pharmacokinetic rules as it does in the lower respiratory tract.

Tonsils

In 1–3% of patients receiving benzathine-penicillin and in 15% of those receiving penicillin V orally, relapses of streptococcal pharyngitis occur (64). This suggests that foci of β-hemolytic streptococcal tonsillar infections persist because of inadequate antibiotic levels in tonsils. The presence of β-lactamase producing strains in the throat (15) could also explain relapses even if notable tissue levels of β-lactams are achieved. Tonsillar penicillin activity was found to be higher than 0.2 mg/kg, with a decrease to less than 0.2 mg/kg after 3–4 hours, after one single i.m. dose of 5,000 units/kg of potassium penicillin G. After oral administration of 0.8 g of penicillin V 3 times a day, or cefadroxil (1g × 2), the mean antibiotic tissue levels reached 0.5 and 2 mg/kg, respectively, exceeding the MIC for β-hemolytic streptococci (53). Concentrations of erythromycin in tonsils 4 to 7 hours after oral administration of 125 mg (64) were similar to those reported for the lower respiratory tract (8), ranging from 0.34 to 1.20 mg/l after multiple doses; they exceeded the highest MIC of erythromycin for group A streptococci (0.02 to 0.2 mg/l). Other macrolides, clarithromycin and roxithromycin (40), reached tonsillar concentrations up to 5.4 or 6.7 mg/kg, respectively, at the usual dosages (multiple doses) of these drugs in pediatrics (5 mg/kg and 250 mg, respectively); these local values exceeded by far the contemporaneous serum levels. Azithromycin tonsillar concentration was 4.5 mg/kg and persisted for 8 days after a single 50 mg dose (39).

Sinusitis

In acute or chronic sinusitis, in order to reduce the number of bacteria (*S. pneumoniae, H. influenzae,* and anaerobes) so that host defenses can re-establish a normal flora, it is important to obtain adequate antibiotic concentrations in sinus secretions and mucosa. In several studies (36,63), the local levels of penicillin V, ampicillin, tetracyclines, erythromycin, and newer macrolides such as roxithromycin (40) were higher than the MIC for most sinusitis-inducing bacteria. When bacteria persist in the presence of adequate antibiotic levels, local host factors can explain the failures.

Otitis Media

In acute purulent or chronic otitis media, ear fluid antibiotic concentrations have been reviewed (67,99); it is not yet established whether rapid clearing of bacteria depends on high antibiotic levels in the middle ear. Clinical studies have shown that ampicillin or erythromycin plus sulfonamide are excellent agents for *H. influenzae* and pneumococcal otitis media. The clinical results correlate with the concentrations of these drugs in middle ear fluid. However, the increasing frequency of isolation of ampicillin-resistant *H. influenzae* can lead to the use of a combination of erythromycin and sulfonamides or cefaclor (67); newer β-lactamase stable cephalosporins would be effective as well in such a situation. Local anatomical factors, inflammatory conditions, and eustachian tube–associated dysfunction leading to obstruction can result in an unsatisfactory response to antimicrobial therapy, even when adequate antibiotic levels are achieved in the middle ear fluid. More recent problems related to the increasing incidence of penicillin-resistant pneumocci impose better knowledge of antibiotic penetration into middle ear in order to improve therapeutic strategies.

Chemoprophylaxis of the Nasopharyngeal Carriage of Neisseria meningitidis

A positive correlation between the concentration of an antibiotic in saliva and its efficacy in eliminating meningococcal carriage has been assessed (33,38,51). In spite of the good *in vitro* activity of many antimicrobials against *N. meningitidis,* and the ineffectiveness of β-lactams, erythromycin or doxycyclin has been attributed to low salivary concentrations (46,48,74,98). Antimicrobials that attain significant concentration in saliva showed efficacy in eradicating carrier state *N. meningitidis* from the nasopharynx. Despite high salivary concentrations, spiramycin was less effective than rifampicin due to a moderate *in vitro* activity against meningococci (MICs: 0.12 to 4 mg/l) (37). Factors influencing saliva concentrations appeared to be serum-protein binding, plasma and saliva pH, pKa of the drugs, and buccal partitioning (35). Concentrations of SMZ and TMP in saliva achieved the same ratios of local to serum concentrations as that in bronchial secretions (7,60) with a better penetration of TMP than SMZ. However, the synergistic *in vitro* effect of TMP-SMZ combination for *Neisseria* sp has not been confirmed *in vivo* (38); this has led to use of different alternative antibiotics such as ciprofloxacin, providing promising results in eradicating nasopharyngeal carriage of *N. meningitidis* in 100% of cases (44).

TECHNICAL PROBLEMS

Methodological and Interpretive

Methodological and interpretive problems are associated with the results of studies like those reported above. No single model could be considered the "ideal" model for tissue pharmacokinetic studies. The design of the study is important in the assessment of drug concentrations in respiratory tissues and fluids (3,7,87,88,117). The correlation of local levels of antibiotics with the dose, the route, and the mode of administration has been established (66,87,106). The oral route of administration used for aminopenicillins (7,16,71), oral cephalosporins (7,54,79,113,117), or fluoroquinolones (11,27,29,117) resulted in slower increase of antibiotic concentrations, lower peaks, and longer tissue half-lives than the parenteral preparations of these drugs when available. The number of patients included in study groups and the number of consecutive samples collected in patients have an impact on the results. In human studies it is quite impossible to obtain consecutive samples from the same individual in varying conditions of drug administration; tissue pharmacokinetics must be deduced from single measurements in groups of patients with unavoidable interindividual variation (4,27,106).

Assay Methods

The choice of assay methods can provide results of different significance. Antibiotic concentrations measured by microbiological assays (32) reflect the actual antibacterial activity of free drug; nonmicrobiological assays (radioimmunoassay [34], radioenzymatic assays [76], high-performance liquid chromatography (HPLC) [28, 29]), which require specific preparation of samples and extractions of the drug, can include inactive metabolites in the final results of the assay and thus can result in an overestimation of the antibiotic levels. Measured by HPLC in human lung tissue after a 250 mg dose, ciprofloxacin concentrations, ranging from 1.2 to 3 mg/kg, were associated with low levels of metabolites desethyl-ciprofloxacin (M1), sulfonylciprofloxacin (M2), and oxociprofloxacin (M3), which are not detected by using bioassay (27). In a study using a single oral dose of 200 mg of ofloxacin (29), the mucosal concentrations, measured by HPLC, ranged from 6.0 to 9.8 mg/kg, exceeding by 1.5 times the similtaneous serum concentrations. The authors assumed that higher concentrations obtained from HPLC analysis than from bioassay (30) resulted from the sonification procedure which might have released fractions of the drug bound to DNA within the cells, or to other sites on cell surface. In fact, comparing the results obtained with different procedures, similar levels were generally obtained in studies of diffusion of most antibiotics in respiratory tissues and fluids. A unique study using positron tomography for determining erythromycin concentrations in patients (118) resulted in parenchymal levels very similar to values measured by bioassay (16). In tissue samples the final level of the antibiotic is measured in a homogenate containing unknown amounts of blood, body fluids, and intracellular contents. Thus, it is mandatory to express the concentration of the drug in the blood-free fraction of the tissue by correction of the blood factor by an assay of the hemoglobin content of the tissue (16,27,32,79).

CLINICAL SIGNIFICANCE

Despite methodological and interpretive problems associated with studies of antibiotic levels in tissues, it is of major interest to confirm the presence of the drug at significant concentrations in respiratory tissues and fluids for prediction of therapeutic efficacy of an antibiotic. Clinicians have at their disposal reliable information on tissue distribution of most antibiotics in sites of potential infection in the respiratory tree. All the models as described above have their uses and all have their limitations. Measurement of concentrations of antibiotics achieved in lung parenchyma, ELF, bronchial mucosa, or bronchial secretions have provided a trend toward approximately similar figures for the same drug. Among antibiotic classes as examined above, three schematic groups behave differently:

1. *β-lactams and aminoglycosides* reach tissue concentrations lower than serum levels, do not penetrate cells, but establish a rapid equilibrium between intravascular space and pulmonary interstitium; they reach significant concentrations in alveolar space and in bronchial mucosa and secretions. Studies in *P. aeruginosa* and other gram-negative pneumonias have demonstrated the importance of maintaining effective concentrations of gentamicin or tobramycin for a long-enough time. In acute exacerbations of chronic bronchitis, the site of infection in the epithelial areas is

reached by β-lactams (bronchial mucosa and secretions), and in practice, response to treatment has been related in many cases to the bronchial levels of β-lactams.

2. *Fluoroquinolones* diffuse freely and quickly in all tissues in the interstitium and inside cells so that tissue levels exceed that in serum and are predictive of their therapeutic efficacy. Animal models of severe pneumonia and studies in patients with nosocomial pneumonia have provided correlation between clinical outcomes and high lung tissue and intramacrophagic concentrations of fluoroquinolones.

3. *Macrolides* have an extremely large pulmonary volume of distribution in relation to their high intracellular concentrations and lysosomal fixation; exchange between respiratory compartments is extremely rapid, and intracellular kinetics parallel that in serum. Many respiratory infections are caused by obligate or facultative intracellular pathogens, which might be eradicated thanks to intracellular penetration and accumulation of macrolides and to their intracellular antibacterial activities.

Convergent data on the major antibiotic classes would be valuable to predict their potential for treatment of respiratory infections.

ACKNOWLEDGMENTS

We are extremely grateful to Edward R. Garrett (Gainesville, Florida) for his kind advice, comments, and critiques of our personal studies; to Alan Gouyette (Villejuif) for his help in the interpretation of our personal results and his proposed pharmacokinetic model of the respiratory compartment; and to Professor J.M. Brogard (Strasbourg) for the revision of the pharmacokinetic data in the chapter. We also wish to thank Marie-Jeanne Julliard for her careful secretarial assistance.

REFERENCES

1. Alexander, M.R., Schoell, J., Hicklin, G., Kasik, J.E., and Coleman, D. (1982): Bronchial secretions concentrations of tobramycin. *Am. Rev. Respir. Dis.*, 125:208–209.
2. Assandri, A., Ratti, B., and Cristina, T. (1984): Pharmacokinetics of rifapentine, a new long-lasting rifamycin in the rat, the mouse and the rabbit. *J. Antibiotics*, 37:1066–1075.
3. Baldwin, D.R., Honeybourne, D., and Wise, R. (1992): Pulmonary disposition of antimicrobial agents: *in vivo* observations and clinical relevance. *Antimicrob. Agents Chemother.*, 36:1176–1180.
4. Baldwin, D.R., Wise, R., Andrews, J.M., and Honeybourne, D. (1990): Concentrations of antimicrobials in the pulmonary alveolar epithelial lining. *Res. Clin. Forums*, 12:103–113.
5. Barza, M. (1981): Principles of tissue penetration of antibiotics. *J. Antimicrob. Chemother.*, 8(Suppl. C):7–28.
6. Bergan, T. (1981): Pharmacokinetics of tissue penetration of antibiotics. *Rev. Infect. Dis.*, 3:45–65.
7. Bergogne-Bérézin, E. (1981): Penetration of antibiotics into the respiratory tree. *J. Antimicrob. Chemother.*, 8:171–174.
8. Bergogne-Bérézin, E. (1986): The tissue penetration of macrolides with particular reference to the respiratory tract. In: *Macrolides: A Review with an Outlook on Future Developments*, edited by J.P. Butzler and H. Kobayashi, pp. 43–53. Excerpta Medica, Amsterdam.
9. Bergogne-Bérézin, E., Berthelot, G., Kafé, H., Pierre, J., and Dournovo, P. (1985): Influence of a fluidifying agent (bromhexine) on the penetration of antibiotics into the respiratory secretions. *Int. J. Clin. Pharm. Res.*, 5:341–344.
10. Bergogne-Bérézin, E., Morel, C., Benard, Y., and Berthelot, G. (1978): Etude de deux critères d'inflammation bronchique et de leurs corrélations avec la pénétration des antibiotiques dans les sécrétions bronchiques. *Rev. Fr. Mal. Resp.*, 6:507–514.
11. Bergogne-Bérézin, E., Muller-Serieys, C., and Kafé, H. (1992): Penetration of lomefloxacin into

bronchial secretions following single and multiple oral administration. *Am. J. Med.*, 92(Suppl. 4A):8S–11S.

12. Bodem, C.R., Lampton, L.M., Miller, D.P., Tarka, E.F., and Everett, E.D. (1983): Endobronchial pH: relevance to aminoglycoside activity in gram-negative bacillary pneumonia. *Am. Rev. Respir. Dis.*, 127:39–41.

13. Bodey, G.P., Ketchel, S.J., and Rodriguez, V.A. (1979): A randomized study of carbenicillin plus cefamandole or tobramycin in the treatment of febrile episodes in cancer patients. *Am. J. Med.*, 67:608–616.

14. Boxenbaum, H. (1982): Interspecies scaling, allometry, physiological time, and the ground plan of pharmacokinetics. *J. Pharmacokinet. Biopharm.*, 10:210–227.

15. Brook, I. (1989): The concept of indirect pathogenicity by β-lactamase production, especially in ear, nose and throat infection. *J. Antimicrob. Chemother.*, 24(Suppl. B):63–72.

16. Brun, Y., Forey, F., Gamondes, J.P., Tebib, A., Brune, J., and Fleurette, J. (1981): Levels of erythromycin in pulmonary tissue and bronchial mucus compared to those of amoxycillin. *J. Antimicrob. Chemother.*, 8:459–466.

17. Burrows, G.E., Barto, P.B., and Martin, B. (1986): Antibiotic disposition in experimental pneumonic pasteurellosis: gentamicin and tylosin. *Can. J. Vet. Res.*, 50:193–199.

18. Burrows, G.E., Gentry, M., and Ewing, P. (1989): Serum and tissue concentrations of erythromycin in calves with induced pneumonic pasteurellosis. *Am. J. Vet. Res.*, 50:1166–1169.

19. Burton, J.A., and Schanker, L.S. (1974): Absorption of antibiotics from the rat lung. *Proc. Soc. Exp. Biol. Med.*, 145:752–756.

20. Campbell, M.J. (1980): Tetracycline levels in bronchial secretions. *J. Clin. Pathol.*, 23:427–434.

21. Canetti, G., Parrot, R., Porven, G., and Le Lirzin, M. (1969): Les taux de rifampicine dans le poumon et dans les lésions tuberculeuses de l'homme. *Acta Tuberc. Pneumol. Belg.*, 60: 315–322.

22. Cohen, S.H., Hoeprich, P.D., Demling, R., Gunther, R., Merry, J.M., Franti, C.E., and Miner, D.J. (1984): Entry of four cephalosporins into the ovine lung. *J. Infect. Dis.*, 149:264–270.

23. Cox, A.L., Meewis, J.M., and Horton, R. (1989): Penetration into lung tissue after intravenous administration of amoxycillin/clavulanate. *J. Antimicrob. Chemother.*, 24(Suppl. B):87–91.

24. Craig, W.A., and Kunin, C.M. (1973): Distribution of trimethoprim-sulfamethoxazole in tissues of rhesus monkeys. *J. Infect. Dis.*, 128:S575–S579.

25. Craig, W.A., and Kunin, C.M. (1976): Significance of serum protein and tissue binding of antimicrobial agents. *Ann. Rev. Med.*, 27:287–300.

26. Curry, S.H. (1980): *Drug Disposition and Pharmacokinetics with a Consideration of Pharmacological and Clinical Relationships*, 3rd Edition. Blackwell Scientific Publications, Oxford.

27. Dalhoff, A. (1989): A review of quinolone tissue pharmacokinetics. In: *Quinolones*, edited by P.B. Fernandes. pp. 277–312. JR Prous Science SA, Barcelona.

28. Dan, M., Torossian, K., Weissberg, D., and Kitzes, R. (1990): Penetration of ciprofloxacin into bronchial mucosa, lung parenchyma and pleural tissue following intravenous administration. [Abstract 346]. 3rd Intern. Symp. on New Quinolones, Vancouver, 12–14 July.

29. Davey, P.G., Precious, E., and Winter, J. (1991): Bronchial penetration of ofloxacin after single and multiple oral dosage. *J. Antimicrob. Chemother.*, 27:335–341.

30. Decré, D., and Bergogne-Bérézin, E. (1993): Pharmacokinetics of quinolones with special reference to the respiratory tree: an update. *J. Antimicrob. Chemother.* 31:331–343.

31. Deffebach, M.E., Charan, N.B., Lakshminarayan, S.A., and Butler, J. (1977): The bronchial circulation: small but a vital attribute of the lung. *Am. Rev. Respir. Dis.*, 135:463–481.

32. De Louvois, J. (1982): Factors influencing the assay of antimicrobial drugs in clinical samples by the agar plate diffusion method. *J. Antimicrob. Chemother.*, 9:253–265.

33. Devine, L.F., Johnson, D.P., Hagerman, C.R., Pierce, W.E., Rhode, S.L., and Peckinpaugh, R.O. (1970): Rifampicin: level in serum and saliva and effect on the meningococcal carrier state. *J.A.M.A.*, 214:1055–1059.

34. Dull, W.L., Alexander, M.R., and Kasik, J.E. (1979): Bronchial secretion levels of amikacin. *Antimicrob. Agents Chemother.*, 16:767–771.

35. Eatman, F.B., Maggio, A.C., Pocelinko, R., et al. (1977): Blood and salivary concentrations of sulfamethoxazole and trimethoprim in man. *J. Pharmacokin. Biopharmacol.*, 5:615–624.

36. Ekedhal, C., Holm, S.E., and Bergholm, A.M. (1978): Penetration of antibiotics into the normal and diseased maxillary sinus mucosa. *Scand. J. Infect. Dis.*, 14(Suppl.):279–284.

37. Engelen, F., Vandepitte, L., and De Maeyer-Cleempoel, S. (1981): Effect of spiramycin on the nasopharyngeal carriage of *Nesseria meningitidis*. *Chemotherapy*, 27:325–333.

38. Feldman, H.A. (1973): Effects of trimethoprim and sulfisoxazole, alone and in combination, on growth and carriage of *Neisseria meningitidis*. *J. Infect. Dis.*, 128(Suppl.):723–728.

39. Foulds, G., Shepard, R.M., and Johnson, R.B. (1990): The pharmacokinetics of azithromycin in human serum and tissues. *J. Antimicrob. Chemother.*, 25(Suppl. A):73–82.

40. Fraschini, F., Scaglione, F., Pintucci, G., Maccarinelli, G., Dugnani, S., and Demartini, G. (1991): The diffusion of clarithromycin and roxithromycin into nasal mucosa, tonsil and lung in humans. *J. Antimicrob. Chemother.*, 27(Suppl. A):61–65.

41. Gail, D.B., and Lenfant, C.J. (1983): Cells of the lung: biology and clinical implications. *Am. Rev. Respir. Dis.,* 127:366–387.
42. Garrett, E.R., and Hinderling, P.H. (1973): Clinical relevance of pharmacokinetics in antibiotic treatment. *Med. Sci. Donat.,* 15:3–14.
43. Gartmann, J. (1975): Doxycycline concentrations in lung tissue, bronchial wall, bronchial secretions. *Chemotherapy,* 21:19–26.
44. Gaunt, P.N., and Lambert, B.E. (1988): Single dose ciprofloxacin for the eradication of pharyngeal carriage of *Neisseria meningitidis. J. Antimicrob. Chemother.,* 21;489–496.
45. Girard, A.E., Cimochowski, C.R., Faiella, J.A., and Girard, D. (1990): Correlation and increased azithromycin levels with phagocyte infiltration into sites of infections. In: *Program and Abstracts of the 30th Interscience Conference on Antimicrobial Agents Chemotherapy,* Atlanta. [Abstract 762]. American Society for Microbiology. Washington, D.C.
46. Hafez, F.F., Stewart, S.M., and Burnet, M.E. (1965): Penicillin levels in sputum. *Thorax,* 20: 219–225.
47. Hall, W.H., Gerding, D.N., and Schierl, E.A. (1977): Penetration of tobramycin into infected extravascular fluids and its therapeutic effectiveness. *J. Infect. Dis.,* 135:457–461.
48. Halprin, G.M., and McMahon, S.M. (1973): Cephalexin concentration in sputum during acute respiratory infections. *Antimicrob. Agents Chemother.,* 3:703–707.
49. Harnett, B.J.S., and Martin, G.E. (1976): Doxycycline in serum and in bronchial secretions. *Thorax,* 34:144–148.
50. Havard, C.W.H., Fernando, A., Brumfitt, W., and Hamilton-Miller, J.M.T. (1982): A pilot study of "augmentin" in lower respiratory tract infections: pharmacokinetic and clinical results. *Br. J. Dis. Chest,* 76:255–260.
51. Hoeprich, P.D. (1971): Prediction of antimeningococcic chemoprophylactic efficacy. *J. Infect. Dis.,* 123:125–133.
52. Holdiness, M.R. (1989): Clinical pharmacokinetics of clofazimine: a review. *Clin. Pharmacokin.,* 16:74–85.
53. Holm, S.E., and Ekedhal, C. (1982): Comparative study of the penetration of penicillin V and cefadroxil into tonsils in man. *J. Antimicrob. Chemother.,* 10(Suppl. B):121–123.
54. Honeybourne, D., and Baldwin, D.R. (1992): The site concentrations of antimicrobial agents in the lung. *J. Antimicrob. Chemother.,* 30:249–260.
55. Hughes, D.T.D. (1983): The use of combinations of trimethoprim and sulphonamides in the treatment of chest infections. *J. Antimicrob. Chemother.,* 12:423–434.
56. Ingold, A. (1975): Sputum and serum levels of amoxycillin in chronic bronchial infections. *Br. J. Dis. Chest,* 69:211–216.
57. Johanson, W.G., Woods, D.E., Jr., Chaudhvri, T. (1979): Association of respiratory tract colonization with adherence of gram-negative bacilli to epithelial cells. *J. Infect. Dis.,* 139:667–673.
58. Johnson, J.D., Hand, W.L., Francis, J.B., King-Thompson, N., and Corwin, R.W. (1980): Antibiotic uptake by alveolar macrophages. *J. Lab. Clin. Med.,* 95:429–439.
59. Jones, R. (1978): The glycoproteins of secretory cells in airway epithelium. In: *Respiratory Tract Mucus,* pp. 175–193. Ciba Foundation Symposium. Elsevier-Excerpta Medica, North Holland.
60. Jordan, G.W., Krajden, S.F., Hoeprich, P.D., Wong, G.A., Pierce, T.H., and Rausch, D.C. (1975): Trimethoprim-sulfamethoxazole in chronic bronchitis. *CMA J.,* 112:91S–95S.
61. Just, H.M., Frank, U., Simon, A., Kaiser, D., and Daschner, F.D. (1984): Concentrations of ceftriaxone in serum and lung tissue. *Chemotherapy,* 30:81–83.
62. Kafé, H., Berthelot, G., Daumal, M., Gillon, J.C., and Bergogne-Bérézin, E. (1983): A study of the penetration of fosfomycin into respiratory secretions. *Proc. 13th Intern. Congress Chemother.,* Vienna.
63. Kalm, O. (1981): Penetration of various antibiotics into sinus cavities. In: *Developments in Antibiotic Treatment of Respiratory Infections* (New Perspectives in Clinical Microbiology), edited by R. Van Furth, pp. 116–128. Martinus Nijhoff, The Hague.
64. Kaplan, J.M., McCracken, G.H., Jr., Culberston, M.C., and Dallas, M.D. (1974): Penicillin and erythromycin concentrations in tonsils: relevance to treatment failures in streptococcal pharyngitis. *Am. J. Dis. Child.,* 127:206–211.
65. Kemmerich, B., Borner, K., and Pennington, J.E. (1987): Comparative evaluation of enoxacin, ofloxacin, ampicillin and chloramphenicol for treatment of experimental *Hemophilus influenzae* pneumonia. *Antimicrob. Agents Chemother.,* 31:417–420.
66. Klastersky, J., Thys, J.P., and Mombelli, G. (1981): Comparative studies of intermittent and continuous administration of aminoglycosides in the treatment of bronchopulmonary infections due to gram-negative bacteria. *Rev. Infect. Dis.,* 3:74–83.
67. Krause, P.J., Owens, N.J., Nightingale, C.H., Klimek, J.J., Lehmann, W.B., and Quintiliani, R. (1982): Penetration of amoxycillin, cefaclor, erythromycin-sulfisoxazole, and trimethoprim-sulfamethoxazole into the middle ear fluid of patients with chronic serous otitis media. *J. Infect. Dis.,* 145:815–821.

68. Kunin, C.M. (1970): Binding of antibiotics to tissue homogenates. *J. Infect. Dis.*, 121:55–64.
69. Levy, J. (1986): Antibiotic activity in sputum. *J. Pediatr.*, 108:841–846.
70. Loos, U., Friess, D., and Springmann, K. (1991): Pulmonary penetration of imipenem. [Abstract 974]. *17th Intern. Congress Chemother.*, Berlin.
71. Maesen, F.P.V., Beenwkes, H., Davies, B.I., Buytendijk, H., Brombacher, P.J., and Weesman, J. (1976): Bacampicillin in acute exacerbation of chronic bronchitis: a dose range study. *J. Antimicrob. Chemother.*, 2:279–285.
72. Marks, M.I., Prentice, R., Swarson, R., Cotton, E.K., and Eichkoff, T.C. (1971): Carbenicillin and gentamicin: pharmacologic studies in patients with cystic fibrosis and pseudomonas pulmonary infections. *J. Pediatr.*, 79:822–828.
73. Marlin, G.E., Burgess, K.R., Burgoyne, J., Funnell, G.R., and Guinness, M.D.G. (1981): Penetration of piperacillin into bronchial mucosa and sputum. *Thorax*, 36:774–780.
74. May, J.R., and Delves, D.M. (1965): Treatment of chronic bronchitis with ampicillin: some pharmacological observations. *Lancet*, i:929–933.
75. May, J.R., and Ingold, A. (1972): Amoxycillin in the treatment of chronic non-tuberculous bronchial infections. *Br. J. Dis. Chest*, 66:185–191.
76. Mendelman, P.M., Smith, A.L., Levy, J., Weber, A., Ramsey, B., and Davis, R.L. (1985): Aminoglycoside penetration, inactivation, and efficacy in cystic fibrosis sputum. *Am. Rev. Respir. Dis.*, 132:761–765.
77. Mouton, Y., Caillaux, M., Beaucaire, G., and Fourrier, A. (1981): Penetration of moxalactam in bronchial secretions and clinical evaluation in intensive care units. [Abstract 732]. (21st ICAAC) (Chicago).
78. Mozzi, E., Germiniani, R., Cantaluppi, G., Marchetti, V., Vettaro, M.P., and Sardi, A. (1983): Human pharmacokinetics of LM 427, a new antimycobacterial agent: tissue distribution and excretion. *Proc. 13th ICC*, 45413–45419.
79. Muller-Serieys, C., Bancal, C., Dombret, M.C., et al. (1992): Penetration of cefpodoxime-proxetil in lung parenchyma and epithelial lining fluid of noninfected patients. *Antimicrob. Agents Chemother.*, 36:2099–2103.
80. Muller-Serieys, C., Bergogne-Bérézin, E., Rowan, C., and Dombret, M.C. (1987): Imipenem penetration into bronchial secretions. *J. Antimicrob. Chemother.*, 20:618–619.
81. Nakamura, S., Jurobe, N., Kashimoto, S., Ohue, T., Takase, Y., and Shimizu, M. (1983): Pharmacokinetics of AT-2266 administered orally to mice, rats, dogs and monkeys. *Antimicrob. Agents Chemother.*, 24:54–60.
82. Nilsen, O.G. (1987): Comparative pharmacokinetics of macrolides. *J. Antimicrob. Chemother.*, 20(Suppl. B):81–88.
83. Nix, D.E., Goodwin, S.D., Peloquin, C.A., Rotella, D.L., and Schentag, J.J. (1991): Antibiotic tissue penetration and its relevance: models of tissue penetration and their meaning. *Antimicrob. Agents Chemother.*, 35:1947–1952.
84. Nix, D.E., Goodwin, S.D., Peloquin, C.A., Rotella, D.L., and Schentag, J.J. (1991): Antibiotic tissue penetration and its relevance: impact of tissue penetration on infections response. *Antimicrob. Agents Chemother.*, 35:1953–1959.
85. Odio, W., Vanlaer, E., and Klastersky, J. (1975): Concentrations of gentamicin in bronchial secretions after intramuscular and endotracheal administration. *J. Clin. Pharmacol.*, 15:518–524.
86. Olivieri, D. (1971): Modalita di diffusione della rifampicina nella secrezioni bronchiali. *Arch. Tisiol. Mal. App. Resp.*, 25:422–432.
87. Pennington, J.E. (1976): Kinetics of penetration and clearance of antibiotics in respiratory secretions. In: *Immunologic and Infectious Reactions in the Lung*, edited by G.H. Kirkpatrick and H.Y. Reynolds, pp. 355–374. Marcel Dekker, New York.
88. Pennington, J.E. (1981): Penetration of antibiotics into respiratory secretions. *Rev. Infect. Dis.*, 3:67–73.
89. Pennington, J.E., Block, E.R., and Reynolds, H.Y. (1973): Five-fluorocytosine and amphotericine B in bronchial secretions. *Antimicrob. Agents Chemother.*, 61:324–326.
90. Pennington, J.E., and Reynolds, H.Y. (1973): Concentration of gentamicin and carbenicillin in bronchial secretions. *J. Infect. Dis.*, 128:63–68.
91. Pennington, J.E., and Stone, R.M. (1979): Comparison of antibiotic regimens for treatment of experimental pneumonia due to *Pseudomonas*. *J. Infect. Dis.*, 140:881–889.
92. Pocidalo, J.J., Albert, F., Desnottes, J.F., and Kernbaum, S. (1985): Intraphagocytic penetration of macrolides: *in vivo* comparison of erythromycin and spiramycin. *J. Antimicrob. Chemother.*, 16(Suppl. A):167–173.
93. Ramphal, R., Guay, C., and Pier, G.B. (1987): *Pseudomonas aeruginosa* adhesins for tracheobronchial mucin. *Infect. Immun.*, 55:600–603.
94. Rebuck, A.S., and Braude, A.C. (1984): Assessment of drug disposition in the lung. *Drugs*, 28:544–553.
95. Renkin, E.M. (1992): Cellular and intercellular transport pathways in exchange vessels. *Am. Rev. Respir. Dis.*, 146:S28–S31.

96. Saggers, B.A., and Lawson, D. (1968): *In vivo* penetration of antibiotics into sputum in cystic fibrosis. *Arch. Dis. Child,* 43:404–409.

97. Siegler, D., Kaye, C.M., Reilly, S., Willis, A.I., and Sankey, M.G. (1981): Serum saliva and sputum levels of metronidazole in acute exacerbations of chronic bronchitis. *Thorax,* 36:781–783.

98. Stewart, S.M., Anderson, I.M.E., Jones, G.R., and Galder, M.A. (1974): Amoxycillin levels in sputum, serum and saliva. *Thorax,* 29:110–114.

99. Sundberg, L., and Ernston, S. (1981): Penetration of various antibiotics into the middle ear. In: *Developments in Antibiotic Treatment of Respiratory Infections* (New Perspectives in Clinical Microbiology), edited by R. Van Furth, pp. 98–115. Martinus Nijhoff Publishers, The Hague.

100. Thadepalli, H. (1984): Lower respiratory tract. In: *Antimicrobial Therapy,* edited by A.M. Ristuccia and B.A. Cunha, pp. 439–454. Raven Press, New York.

101. Thys, J.P., Husson, M., and Klastersky, J. (1984): Inactivation of netilmicin and amikacin by intact or disrupted leucocytes. *J. Antimicrob. Chemother.,* 14:435–438.

102. Tornqvist, I.O., Holm, S.E., and Cars, O. (1991): Pharmacodynamic effects of subinhibitory antibiotic concentrations. *Scand. J. Infect. Dis.,* 74(Suppl.):94–101.

103. Tremblay, D., Mignot, A., Couraud, L., Saux, M.C., and Manuel, C. (1988): Concentrations of roxithromycin in lung tissue after repeat dosing. *Brit. J. Clin. Pract.,* 42(Suppl. 55):73

104. Tulkens, P.M. (1991): Intracellular pharmacokinetics and localization of antibiotics as predictors of their efficacy against imtraphagocytic infections. *Scand. J. Infect. Dis.,* 74(Suppl.):209–217.

105. Turner, A., Pedler, S.J., Carswell, F., Spencer, G.R., and Speller, D.C.E. (1984): Serum and sputum concentrations of ceftazidime in patients with cystic fibrosis. *J. Antimicrob. Chemother.,* 14:521–527.

106. Valcke, Y., Pauwels, R., and Van der Streten, M. (1990): Pharmacokinetics of antibiotics in the lungs. *Eur. Respir. J.,* 3:715–722.

107. Vallée, E., Azoulay-Dupuis, E., Bauchet, J., and Pocidalo, J.J. (1992): Kinetic disposition of temafloxacin and ciprofloxacin in a murine model of pneumococcal pneumonia: relevance for drug efficacy. *J. Pharm. Exp. Therap.,* 263:1203–1208.

108. Vallée, E., Azoulay-Dupuis, E., Pocidalo, J.J., and Bergogne-Bérézin, E. (1991): Pharmacokinetics of four fluoroquinolones in a mouse model of infected lung. *J. Antimicrob. Chemother.,* 28(Suppl. C):39–44.

109. Vallée, E., Azoulay-Dupuis, E., Pocidalo, J.J., and Bergogne-Bérézin, E. (1992): Activity and local delivery of azithromycin in a mouse model of *Hemophilus influenzae* lung infection. *Antimicrob. Agents Chemother.,* 36:1412–1417.

110. Van Etta, L.L., Peterson, L.R., Fashing, C.E., and Gerding, D.N. (1982): Effect of the ratio of surface area to volume on the penetration of antibiotics into extravascular spaces in an *in vitro* model. *J. Infect. Dis.,* 146:423–428.

111. Vaudaux, P. (1981): Peripheral inactivation of gentamicin. *J. Antimicrob. Chemother.,* 8(Suppl. A):17–25.

112. Veber, B., Azoulay-Dupuis, E., Vallée, E., and Pocidalo, J.J. (1991): Correlation between efficacy and pharmacokinetics of macrolides in infected lung: elimination half-life as a predictor of drug efficacy. In: *Program and Abstracts of the 31th Interscience Conference on Antimicrobial Agents Chemotherapy.* Chicago. [Abstract 508]. American Society for Microbiology, Washington, D.C.

113. Walstad, R., Thurmann-Nielsen, E., Vilsvik, J., Griggs, J., and Brown, G. (1988): Pharmacokinetics of cefuroxime-axetil in patients with LRTI. In: *Proc. One-Day Symp.: A Profile of Cefuroxime-Axetil,* pp. 65–67. *The Practitioner* (Editorial). Royal College of Physicians, London.

114. Weber, W.W., and Hein, D.W. (1979): Clinical pharmacokinetics of isoniazid. *Clin. Pharmacokinet.,* 4:401–422.

115. Weiser, O., Reguea, H., and Wundt, W. (1971): Die Ausscheidung von Gentamicin über den Bronchialbaum. *Deutsch Med. Wochenschr.,* 96:870–972.

116. Wise, R. (1986): The clinical relevance of protein binding and tissue concentrations in antimicrobial therapy. *Clin. Pharmacokinet.,* 11:470–482.

117. Wise, R., Baldwin, D.R., Honeybourne, D., and Andrews, J.M. (1990): Penetration of antibiotics into the bronchial mucosa: a review. *Res. Clin. Forums,* 12:95–100.

118. Wollmer, P., Rhodes, C.G., Pike, V.W., et al. (1982): Measurement of pulmonary erythromycin concentration in patients with lobar pneumoniae by means of positron tomography. *Lancet* (December 18):1361–1364.

119. Zak, O., and O'Reilly, T. (1991): Animal models in the evaluation of antimicrobial agents. *Antimicrob. Agents Chemother.,* 35:1527–1531.

Respiratory Infections: Diagnosis and Management, 3d ed.,
edited by James E. Pennington.
Raven Press, Ltd., New York © 1994

36

Local Antibiotic Therapy for Bronchopulmonary Infections

*Jean-Pierre Thys, †Mickael Aoun, and †Jean Klastersky

*Infectious Diseases Clinic, Erasme University Hospital,
Route Lennik 808, Brussels, Belgium; and
†Infectious Disease Department, Institute Jules Bordet,
Rue Heger-Bordet 1, Brussels, Belgium

The distribution of an anti-infectious agent within the body is a critical factor in determining its therapeutic efficacy. If the site of infection is inaccessible to the agent, growth of the pathogen and the infectious process will continue despite *in vitro* sensitivity. Pharmacologic studies suggest that penetration of many antibiotics into the bronchial secretions is relatively poor, frequently resulting in local levels that are lower than those achieved in the serum. Consequently, minimal antibacterial activity is attained at the presumed site of the infection. In addition, many antibiotics are inhibited in purulent bronchial secretions as a result of local conditions existing in the inflamed and infected bronchi. Enzymatic inactivation of antibiotics by pathogens present in bronchial secretions has been described (81). Moreover, the aminoglycosides can be partially inactivated in purulent bronchial secretions by acid pH and by the high ionic content of the exudate; their activity might also be reduced by a binding of these drugs to the nucleoproteins that are abundant in these secretions (75). These inhibitions can probably be overcome by high concentrations of antibiotics. To increase the concentrations of anti-infectious agents in the bronchial tree, while reducing systemic toxicity due to limited absorption, topical administration of drugs by aerosolization or direct instillation appears attractive. In this chapter, the role of the local administration of anti-infectious agents for the prophylaxis and the treatment of bronchopulmonary infections due to bacteria, fungi, virus, and protozoan agents will be discussed.

BACTERIAL INFECTIONS

Clinical Significance of the Concentration of Antibiotics within Bronchial Secretions

The rational goal of an effective antimicrobial drug therapy is to induce, at the site of infection, a concentration-time profile such that free drug concentration exceeds the minimal inhibitory concentration (MIC) of the offending pathogen. It seems therefore logical to assume that the efficacy of antibiotic treatment of pulmonary or bronchial infections will greatly depend upon the drug level at the presumed site of infection. In the lung, the epithelial lining fluid and alveolar macrophages should be considered to be important sites of infection. In exacerbations of chronic bronchitis, pathogens are principally found in sputum and bronchial mucosa (7).

As far as bronchial infections are concerned, the relationship between clinical outcome of acute exacerbations of chronic bronchitis and concentrations of antimicrobials within the bronchial secretions remains controversial. In a series of patients with purulent bronchitis or pneumonia, a positive correlation between clinical outcome and the levels of amoxicillin in bronchial secretions has been reported. A significantly higher number of patients showed a good response to the treatment when sputum levels were 0.25 µg/ml or more, although there was a tendency of higher serum levels to be associated with more clinical responses (117). Maesen et al. (82) studied three groups of seven patients with acute exacerbation of chronic bronchitis who received 600, 1,200 and 2,400 mg of bacampicillin per day. In that study, clinical improvement and the bronchial levels of the drug were related to the dose administered. In addition, the pathogenic organisms (pneumococci and *Hemophilus* sp) that were present in the sputum of all the patients before therapy were eradicated in all the patients receiving the higher dosages, but only in a few of those receiving 600 mg per day. It must be noted, however, that, as in the previous study (117), higher sputum levels were associated with higher serum levels. The respective role of the antibiotic levels in these two fluids is thus difficult to interpret. In a trial of treatment of acute exacerbations of chronic bronchitis with azithromycin, poor clinical results and persistence of *H. influenzae* in sputum were noted; this might be explained by the relatively high MIC of this pathogen, compared to the sputum level of this drug (31). Moreover, the relatively poor clinical outcome of pulmonary infections in cystic fibrosis patients, associated with the persistence of *P. aeruginosa* in the sputum, might be, among other factors, due to the low antipseudomonal drug levels and bioactivity in this exudate (84). The efficacy of inhaled amikacin as an adjunct to intravenous therapy in cystic fibrosis patients has been studied (107). The aerosolized aminoglycoside produced a higher, but transient, eradication of *P. aeruginosa* in the sputum than was observed in the control group. Suppression of the pathogens was associated with high concentrations of amikacin in the sputum. However, no correlation between clinical outcome and transient eradication of the pathogen was observed.

By contrast, the role of very high antibiotic levels in bronchial secretions obtained by endotracheal instillation has been studied in the treatment of gram-negative bronchopneumonia in tracheotomized patients. Such topical treatment reduced the morbidity and mortality of the patients (61). In this study, which will be discussed in detail later, the level of sisomicin and the bactericidal activity of the bronchial secretions were very high, contrasting with corresponding low values in the control group. However, serum levels were similarly low in the two groups. This study is the only one that suggests a clear relationship between the clinical outcome and the level of antimicrobials in the bronchial secretions.

Theoretically, bronchial mucosa antibiotic concentrations should be important in the treatment of bronchial infections. Higher antibiotic concentrations have been found in the mucosa than in the sputum, particularly for fluoroquinolones (132). To explain the unclear correlation between sputum antibiotic levels and clinical outcome of patients with chronic bronchitis, it might be speculated that the drug concentration in the bronchial mucosa might be even more relevant than that achieved in the bronchial secretions. In addition, other studies suggest that sub-MIC levels of antibiotics in the bronchial secretions might still be useful in the treatment of tracheobronchial infections, reducing the adherence of *P. aeruginosa* to bronchial mucin or inhibiting the release of toxic substances by the invading bacteria (42,127). These studies might partially explain the clinical efficacy of several drugs despite their variable and often poor levels in the bronchial secretions.

Despite these conflicting data concerning the relationship between clinical outcome of bronchopulmonary infections and levels of antibiotics in bronchial secretions, achieving a very high level of these drugs in the exudate could be useful in the treatment of these infections (61). If the level of antimicrobial activity cannot be increased significantly by increasing the systemic dosage, local administration of antibiotics is thus a logical alternative to achieve sufficient antimicrobial activity within the bronchial secretions.

Pharmacokinetics of Endotracheally Administered Antibiotics

Techniques for Endotracheal Administration of Antibiotics

The administration of antibiotics into the tracheobronchial tree can be performed by two techniques: either by direct injection of the material within the bronchial lumen, or by aerosolization. The direct instillation of antibiotics into the tracheobronchial tree can be achieved with a catheter inserted into the trachea through a tracheostomy or an intubation prosthesis. The dose of the antibiotic, dissolved in 2 ml saline or more, can be injected 3 to 6 times daily, or given as a continuous endotracheal infusion via the catheter into the bronchial tree (2,16,62).

Pharmacokinetics of Endobronchially Administered Antibiotics

During antibiotic aerosolization, the dose and pattern of pulmonary deposition depend on the type of nebulizer, size of the inhaled particles, and the patient's inhalation technique. Moreover, penetration of the aerosol into the respiratory tract is also influenced by altered breathing pattern and airway obstruction (3,57,58). Ilowite et al. (57) have recently studied the pulmonary pharmacokinetics of aerosolized gentamicin in cystic fibrosis patients. Less than 10% of the drug placed in the nebulizer had reached the lung, the rest of gentamicin being lost to the environment, swallowed, or left as a residuum in the nebulizer. A wide interpatient variation was observed. Sputum levels were found to correlate with the regional distribution of the aerosol (i.e., the more centrally the aerosol was deposited, as in patients with the worst pulmonary function, the higher the sputum level obtained). Furthermore, an inverse relationship was found between the regional distribution of the aerosol and the pulmonary function of the subjects. Finally, the dose reaching the lungs was largely dependent on the patient's breathing pattern (57). A previous study showed that in patients with cystic fibrosis there is a marked heterogenicity in the pattern of the deposition of particles within the lungs. Deposition appeared to be the least in areas of atelectasis and consolidation where airflow was minimal and the sites of infection presumably greatest. This constraint might limit the therapeutic effectiveness of inhaled antibiotics, particularly in patients with advanced lung diseases (3). In patients with chronic obstructive pulmonary diseases, deposition of aerosol is reduced in peripheral areas of the lung and increased in central airways (58). Pulmonary distribution of antibiotics after endotracheal instillation is very poorly known; results from a preliminary study seem to suggest an extensive bronchial distribution of the instilled drug (101). On the other hand, liposome aerosols can facilitate the nebulization of substances that are poorly water soluble and broaden the array of topical antibiotic administration. With their potential for slow drug release, liposomes can serve as a reservoir for pulmonary drug delivery. Furthermore, liposomes could target the antibiotic specifically to the alveolar macrophages. This can be an important issue for facultative intracellular parasites such as mycobacteria, viruses, and fungi. These therapeutic opportunities need to be confirmed during the next few years (109).

The endobronchial concentrations of gentamicin in bronchial secretions and in sputum after either direct endotracheal instillation or aerosolization have been compared in children with cystic fibrosis or in tracheotomized children with neurologic diseases (8). After the administration of 40 mg of gentamicin by the two techniques, the bronchial levels of gentamicin were in the range of 700 μg/ml after the endotracheal instillation and 55 μg/ml after aerosolization. In another study, Odio et al. (93) have also compared these two modes of administration in tracheotomized adults. The mean concentration in the bronchial secretions was 480 μg/ml, 30 min. after the endotracheal insillation of 2 mg/kg of gentamicin; after 4 to 6 hours, the mean concentrations were 43 and 14 μg/ml, respectively. When the same dosages of gentamicin were administered to nontracheotomized patients by aerosolization, the mean level of the antibiotic in the bronchial secretions, obtained by transtracheal aspiration, was in the range of 22 μg/ml; in the spontaneously expectorated sputum, the level of gentamicin was similar. However, Ilowite et al. (57) have observed higher sputum levels (>300 μg/ml) of gentamicin after aerosolization of 160 mg of the drug in cystic fibrosis patients. After endotracheal instillation of sisomicin (0.70 mg/kg), peak bronchial secretions levels reached 1300 μg/ml (121).

Thus, it is clear that direct endotracheal instillation of aminoglycosides or aerosol administration of these drugs can result in elevated and persistent concentrations of these antibiotics within the bronchial secretions. The levels that can be obtained with these modes of administration usually exceed several times the minimal bactericidal activity of most bacteria responsible for severe bronchial infections in tracheotomized patients or in children with cystic fibrosis.

Because aminoglycosides are potent bactericidal agents but have a narrow therapeutic ratio, these drugs have been administered locally into the tracheobronchial tree in order to avoid systemic toxicity while achieving high local levels. Accordingly, most of the following considerations about pharmacology or clinical effectiveness will deal with the administration of aminoglycosides. Polymyxins have also been used as a local therapy by aerosol or direct instillation into the bronchial tract. Besides these two groups of antimicrobial agents, drugs such as chloramphenicol analogues, amoxicillin, carbenicillin, cephaloridine, and ceftazidime have been used in the local therapy of patients with acute exacerbation of chronic bronchitis (97,99,118) and with cystic fibrosis (24,56,59,92,114,129). The kinetics of these endotracheally administered antibiotics in bronchial secretions was poorly studied. However, pharmacokinetic parameters of ceftazidime after endotracheal instillation and aerosolization have been recently compared in mechanically ventilated patients with nosocomial pneumonia. After instillation of 1 g of the drug, the mean peak bronchial concentration was 1300 μg/ml; 24 hours later, the mean concentration was still 57 μg/ml. After aerosolization of the same dose, the corresponding values (determined in only two patients, however) was in the same range (16).

On the other hand, concentrations of tobramycin in the epithelial lining fluid obtained by bronchoalveolar lavage have been studied in rats after endotracheal instillation or aerosolization. Very high and long-persisting concentrations of the drug were reached in this fluid with both modes of administration (124). In humans, a preliminary study suggested that aerosolization of 80 mg of tobramycin produced concentrations of the drug in the range of 2 μg/ml (9).

Adverse Effects of Locally Administered Antibiotics

Potential adverse effects of endotracheally administered antibiotics are bronchial irritation, resorption of the drug with resultant systemic toxicity, and emergence of resistant germs.

Bronchial Tolerance of Topically Administered Antibiotics

Endobronchial administration of antibiotics can cause cough and irritation with bronchospasm of the bronchi. This intolerance to the local administration of antibiotics has been reported chiefly for polymyxin in patients who presented a chronic obstructive bronchopathy. Some aggravation of parameters of ventilatory function has been observed in patients treated with aerosolized polymyxin (33,131), although aerosolized colistin methansulfate did not cause bronchospasm in a group of 20 cystic fibrosis patients (59). Moreover, no bronchial intolerance to topical polymyxin B was noted in a large study in which such treatment was given to 292 patients (37). On the other hand, the endotracheal administration of aminoglycosides, by direct instillation and/or by aerosolization, was usually very well tolerated and did not cause untoward reactions detectable from the clinical point of view. In some studies in which parameters of lung function have been closely monitored during aerosolization of aminoglycosides, some reduction of the maximum expired volume per second has occasionally been observed as well as minimal bronchospasm (29,33). Excellent clinical tolerance has been reported for kanamycin (5,13,76), gentamicin (56,62,63,64,70,93,114), sisomicin (54,62,121), tobramycin (17,24,79,115,116,129), and amikacin (107). Amoxicillin (118), carbenicillin (24,56,114,129), cephaloridine (92), and ceftazidime (16,114) were also well tolerated, although some bronchostriction has been observed after ticarcillin nebulization in cystic fibrosis patients (20).

Resorption of Aminoglycosides from the Bronchial Lumen to the Blood

It might be feared that endotracheally administered, potentially nephrotoxic and ototoxic antibiotics, such as aminoglycosides and polymyxins, could have some systemic toxicity, especially if local therapy is associated with systemic administration of the same or other potentially nephrotoxic drugs. In fact, the serum levels of aminoglycosides observed after endotracheal instillation in patients with normal renal function are very low and most often less than 1 μg/ml (8,27,29,54,61,62,70,93). Under these circumstances, the local administration of aminoglycosides should not interfere with the dosage of systematically administered antibiotics. As an example, the serum levels of gentamicin after the endotracheal instillation of 2 mg/kg or of tobramycin (multiple doses of 40 mg every 4 hrs) do not exceed 1 μg/ml (27,93).

After the instillation of sisomicin at two different dosages (0.35 and 0.70 mg/kg), the peak levels in the serum were less than 0.4 µg/ml (121). Nevertheless, the urinary excretion of these aminoglycosides after endotracheal administration is not neglible. After the instillation of sisomicin, at the dosage indicated above, the urinary excretion of sisomicin over the 24 hours following injection was up to 15% of the total dose administered locally to the tracheobronchial tree (121). In another study (27), 17% of the endotracheally instilled tobramycin was recovered in urine. This urinary excretion is obviously an indication of significant systemic absorption of the aminoglycosides from the bronchial lumen into the blood. It is not surprising, therefore, that potentially toxic levels of these aminoglycosides in the blood can be detected in patients who present with an impairment of renal function. Significant serum levels of aminoglycosides have been observed after endotracheal administration in patients with renal failure (70,96,128). Therefore, in patients with severe renal insufficiency, especially when aminoglycosides are also given by the systemic route, close monitoring of the serum levels is mandatory to avoid exceesive blood levels and subsequent toxicity.

On the other hand, systemic absorption of aminoglycosides aerosolized into the bronchi appears to be significantly lower than after direct endotracheal instillation. The blood levels after aerosolization are negligible in most instances (5,8,10,57,70, 76,93,98,103,115). The urinary excretion of aminoglycosides administered by aerosol is in the range of 1 to 5% after administration of 80 mg of gentamicin and 250 mg of kanamycin (76,103). It is understandable that systemic toxic effects are less likely after aerosol administration than after direct endotracheal instillation, even in patients with impairment of renal function.

Emergence of Resistant Germs

A major adverse effect of the local administration of antibiotics to the tracheobronchial tree is the selection of antibiotic-resistant strains which might be responsible subsequently for serious infections. This has occurred predominantly in the setting of prophylactic rather than therapeutic local administration. Feeley et al. (37) have used polymyxin B in a continuous fashion to prevent *P. aeruginosa* pneumonia in tracheotomized patients. In this study, efficacy of the endotracheal administration in the prevention of such infection could be demonstrated, as will be discussed later, but tracheal colonization and severe pneumonias due to other germs resistant to the locally administered drugs occurred. However, if placebo and polymyxin were given to the patient in alternating 2-month cycles, polymyxin-resistant germs were not significantly increased (65). Similarly, in trials using endotracheally administered gentamicin to prevent colonization and infection by gram-negative bacteria in tracheotomized patients, emergence of resistant germs—such as *Providencia* and *Pseudomonas*—has been observed (64,74). In order to reduce this emergence of resistance, Klastersky et al. (63) compared treatment with topical gentamicin alone and a combination of polymyxin and aminosidin. Some reduction of the emergence of resistance with the combination has been noted. The mean MIC of gentamicin for the Enterobacteriaceae and *P. aeruginosa* was 6.0 µg/ml in the gentamicin-treated group vs. 1.5 µg/ml in the other group (63).

On the other hand, during long-term aerosol suppressive treatment in cystic fibrosis patients, resistance to antipseudomonal drugs such as colistin or aminoglycosides seems of minor importance; in most of the studies, resistant *P. aeruginosa* colonization was a rare and transient event, occurring after many months of continuous prophylaxis and without clinical consequences (56,59,69,114,115,129). In another study, however, incidence of emergence of bacterial resistance was higher but not detrimental to the patient (79).

Clinical Studies Using Topically Administered Antibiotics in the Treatment of Bacterial Bronchopulmonary Infections

Prophylactic Therapy: Non–Cystic Fibrosis Patients

Prophylatic therapy with endotracheal administration of antibiotics by aerosol or instillation. The tracheobronchial tree of hospitalized patients, especially those who are admitted to intensive care units (ICU) and need respiratory support, and those with underlying bronchial diseases such as chronic bronchitis and cystic fibrosis, are frequently colonized by gram-negative bacilli. Colonization by these bacteria is frequently associated with the development of pneumonia. Therefore, reducing colonization of the respiratory tract by administering antibiotics via the endotracheal route should theoretically decrease the incidence of nosocomial lung infections.

Attempts have been made to reduce with aerosols of colistin the colonization of the bronchial tract in patients with chronic bronchitis (106). Effective prevention of colonization was achieved, but colistin-resistant strains emerged. Aerosolized gentamicin has been used in a study of burn patients with pulmonary injury. Pulmonary and septic complications were not reduced with this topical therapy (74). A group from Boston has reported their experience in the prevention of *P. aeruginosa* pneumonia in ICU patients with or without endotracheal intubation (37,47,65). In a first randomized control trial (47), polymyxin B was aerosolized either in the pharynx or down the endotracheal tube. A significant reduction of the gram-negative tracheal colonization was observed (21 vs. 68% in the placebo group). In a subsequent trial (65), polymyxin and placebo were given in alternating 2-month cycles to all patients admitted to the ICU. Polymyxin reduced rates of both gram-negative oropharyngeal colonization and nosocomial pneumonia, especially those due to *P. aeruginosa*. However, overall mortality was not decreased by the topical treatment. In a last study (37), polymyxin was applied in a continuous fashion to all patients admitted in the ICU during 7 months. Once again, the overall incidence of pneumonia, especially *Pseudomonas* pneumonia, decreased. However, a very high pneumonia-associated mortality due to polymyxin-resistant organisms was noted, and the overall mortality remained unchanged.

To reduce the colonization of the upper respiratory tract by gram-negative bacilli, Klastersky et al. (64) studied the role of endotracheal instillation of gentamicin (80 mg, 3 times daily) in a double-blind placebo-controlled study with 85 tracheotomized neurosurgical patients. A significant reduction of the tracheal gram-negative bacilli colonization was observed in the patients treated with gentamicin (79 vs. 56%). Pulmonary infections requiring antibiotics were statistically less frequent in the antibiotic-treated patients than in controls. The mortality rate due to pulmonary infection was higher among the controls as compared with the patients receiving endotracheal gentamicin; however, the difference was not significant. In another study (63), the combination of aminosidin and polymyxin was as effective as gentamicin alone in decreasing colonization of bronchial secretions and tracheobronchial infections. More recently, a prospective double-blind, randomized, multicentric study was performed to investigate the role of endotracheal gentamicin in colonization, infection, and mortality in 162 ventilated ICU patients (77). Significant reduction in colonization has been shown in the gentamicin vs. the placebo group. Emergence of resistant strains was not stated. However, no significant reduction in the incidence of pneumonia or in death rate could be demonstrated in the two groups of patients (77).

These last studies strongly suggest that prophylaxis of bronchopulmonary infections with endobronchial antibiotics should not be applied as a routine procedure for ICU patients because of the lack of efficacy of the treatment on death rate and the fear of selecting antibiotic-resistant strains among these patients (37,63–65,77).

Prophylactic treatment with selective digestive decontamination. The rationale for use of selective digestive decontamination (SDD) in ICU patients is to prevent colonization of the oropharynx and the gut by potentially pathogenic germs that can lead to a variety of infections, particularly pneumonia due to gram-negative bacteria. SDD is a particular strategy of topical chemoprophylaxis in which nonabsorbable antibiotics (more often, polymyxin E, tobramycin, and amphotericin) are applied to the oral mucosa in a sticky paste and injected enterally in the nasogastric tube. In some studies, this regimen was further supplemented by intravenous cefotaxime during the first few days in order to treat infection incubating or present on admission.

Excellent reviews and editorials concerning SDD have been recently published (26,38,46,78,104,125,126). The main recent controlled trials are presented in Table 36-1. It must be noted that the SDD trials are somewhat difficult to compare. The study designs have varied; the first studies were consecutive or used retrospective controls. Subsequent trials were prospective with concurrent control groups, and the more recent studies were randomized, placebo-controlled, and double-blind (Table 36-1) (41,51,100). Very heterogeneous populations were included, particularly with respect to their risk of acquiring nosocomial pneumonias. For example, most of the studies assessed only patients who required ventilation of 2 to 7 days, but others analyzed all the patients admitted to the ICU. Oral regimens were somewhat variable, as was the addition of a parenteral agent. Finally, the difficulty in separating true bacterial pneumonias from other "febrile lung infiltrates" cannot be overemphasized. The lack of clear consensus of clinical and microbiological definitions of bacterial pneumonia complicates comparison between the studies.

With these reservations in mind, studies on the role of SDD in preventing pneumonias and other nosocomial infections and subsequent death can be briefly summarized as follows:

1. *Reduction of respiratory colonization rates.* SDD achieved, after 5 to 10 days of treatment, a constant reduction in gram-negative bacilli colonization of oropharynx and/or of the lower respiratory tract to less than 5 to 40%, compared to 51 to 100% in the control group (1,14,21,39,51,60,100,120,122,123,133).

2. *Role of SDD in decreasing the rate of nosocomial infections, particularly pneumonias.* Twelve of 13 controlled trials listed in Table 36-1 showed a reduction in overall acquired infections. In most cases, the reduction was significant, to 8 to 52% in the SDD-treated patients compared to 27 to 81% in untreated patients (1,6,14,21, 39,45,51,60,94,120,122,133). Moreover, 10 of 17 of these studies mentioned a significant decrease in nosocomial lower respiratory tract infections, mainly pneumonias (1,14,45,60,94,100,105,120,122,123) (Table 36-1). Vandenbroucke (125) carried out a meta-analysis of clinical studies comparing patients treated with SDD and untreated controls. Based upon 11 trials (1,489 patients), SDD has a significant protective effect on the frequency of respiratory tract infections. Similar results were obtained in

studies with historical controls and randomized trials. For these last studies, odds ratio was 0.12 (95% confidence limits 0.08 to 0.19, p < 0.05). In a recent study, however, the rates of pneumonia occurring in the two groups of patients were similar, but gram-negative lung infections were significantly less in the treated group (41).

3. *Influence of SDD on mortality rates.* Despite a clear improvement in colonization and infection rates (particularly with pneumonias) among SDD-treated patients, all the mentioned studies except one (122) showed that the overall mortality was not statistically different between treated and control groups of patients (1,6,14,18,21, 39,41,45,51,60,94,100,105,120,123,133) (Table 36-2). Moreover, only 2 of 15 studies showed a significant reduction of the death rate due to infection (60,122). The very limited effect on survival of treated patients was confirmed by meta-analysis (125). The role of SDD in decreasing mortality in selected subsets of patients has been insufficiently studied. Some beneficial effect on mortality rate has been claimed in patients with "curable diseases" such as trauma. SDD might induce a significant reduction in mortality in "moderately ill" patients with mid-range physiologic scores (APACHE or SAPS) (14,45). However, a well-designed recent study did not show any significant difference in the mortality rates of any specific subgroup of patients (41).

The apparent failure of SDD to reduce overall ICU mortality might be a consequence of several factors, including the high mortality of patients with severe underlying diseases associated with a nosocomial pneumonia. In fact, it is likely that the severity of the associated clinical conditions is the principal determinant of outcome in critically ill patients; it should thus be logical that the cure of pneumonias does not substantially improve the final outcome of the patient. Therefore, it appears reasonable in future studies to consider SDD for patients who are likely to die primarily from infection and not from underlying diseases. It must be noted that clinical trials to test this hypothesis should include a large number of patients to achieve a statistically significant difference in mortality rates. In published studies, the number of deaths is frequently low; these trials are probably lacking of statistical power to detect a possible benefit of SDD on mortality, particularly on mortality due to infection.

4. *Role of SDD in duration of ICU and hospital stay. Cost-effectiveness of SDD.* Several recent trials failed to document a significant shortening of ICU or hospital stay, duration of mechanical ventilation, or a significant decrease in the use of antibiotics (21,41,51). Moreover, cost of SDD appears high because of the expenses of prophylactic antibiotics and microbiological surveillance (41,51). In the study by Gastinne et al. (41), the total cost of antibiotics was 2.2 times higher in the treatment groups.

5. *Role of SDD in the emergence of resistance.* In the first studies, emergence of resistant germs during SDD has been reported as negligible. More recently, overgrowth and emergence of resistant gram-positive cocci, such as aminoglycoside-resistant enterococci, or methicillin-resistant coagulase-negative staphylococci, have been reported (30,130). SDD-induced selection of resistant gram-negative bacilli is also a major concern. Although the epidemiological and clinical consequences of such emergence seem up to now minor, careful and long-term bacteriological monitoring of SDD-treated patients is mandatory to strictly control the sensitivity pattern of ICU flora.

In conclusion, the available data do not permit an unequivocal recommendation for the use of SDD in any particular population of patients. Long-term, well-designed trials of sufficient statistical power are urgently required. The studies should

TABLE 36–1. *Controlled trials of selective digestive decontamination (SDD)*

| | | | Drug regimen | | Acquired infections | | | | Mortality | | |
| | | | | | Respiratory | | Total infections | | | | |
Reference	Study design	No. of evaluable patients	Topical agents	Systemic agents	SDD [N°(%)]	Controls [N°(%)]	SDD [N°(%)]	Controls [N°(%)]	SDD [N°(%)]	Controls [N°(%)]	Comments
Unertl et al. (123)	randomized, controlled trial	39	polymyxin B gentamicin amphotericin	none	4 (21)	14 (70)[b]	NA	NA	5 (26)	6 (30)	
Kerver et al. (60)	randomized, controlled trial	96	polymyxin E tobramycin amphotericin	cefotaxime	6	40[*c]	19 (39)	38 (81)[*c]	14(29)	15 (32)	Deaths due to an acquired infection: 2 patients in SDD group (p < 0.05)
Brun-Buisson et al. (18)	randomized, controlled trial	86	polymyxin E neomycin nalidixic acid	none	7	11[*]	12 (33)	17 (34)	8 (22)	12 (24)	Trial to study the efficacy of SDD to control outbreak of infections due to multiresistant Enterobacteriaceae
Ulrich et al. (122)	randomized, controlled trial	100	polymyxin E norfloxacin amphotericin	trimethoprim	7 (15)	26 (50)[c]	25 (52)	40 (77)[b]	15 (31)	28 (54)[a]	Deaths due to an acquired infection: 0 patient in SDD group vs. 8 in control group (p < 0.004)
Flaherty et al. (39)	randomized controlled trial	107	polymyxin E gentamicin nystatin	cefazolin	1 (2)	5 (9)	6 (12)	15 (27)[a]	0 (0)	1 (2)	Control group patients given sucralfate
Godart et al. (45)	consecutive cross-over, double-blind, placebo-controlled	181	polymyxin E tobramycin	none	2 (2)	13 (15)[b]	24 (26)	29 (35)	12 (12)	15 (18)	All patients given oral amphotericin

Study	Design	N	SDD regimen	Control							Comments
Tetteroo et al. (120)	randomized, controlled trial	114	polymyxin E tobramycin amphotericin	cefotaxime metronidazole	1	8*a	12 (21)	32 (55)c	3 (5)	2 (3)	Perioperative antibioprophylaxis was cefamandole and metronidazole in control group (all patients undergoing resection of the eosophagus). Mortality reduced for patients with mid-range SAPS (p < 0.05)
Rodriguez-Roldan et al. (105)	randomized, controlled trial	28	polymyxin E tobramycin amphotericin	none	3 (23)	14 (73)c	NA	NA	4 (30)	5 (33)	
Aerdts et al. (1)	randomized, controlled, blinded	56	polymyxin E norfloxacin amphotericin	cefotaxime	1 (6)	27 (69)	11	102*c	2 (12)	6 (15)	
Pugin et al. (100)	randomized, placebo-controlled, double-blind	52	polymyxin B neomycin vancomycin	none	4 (16)	21 (78)c	NA	NA	7 (28)	7 (26)	
Blair et al. (14)	randomized, controlled	256	polymyxin tobramycin amphotericin	cefotaxime	12	45*b	21 (17)	40 (31)b	17 (14)	22 (17)	Patients stratified by APACHE II score prior to randomization: most significant reduction of infection and mortality observed in patients with mid-range, APACHE group (10 to 19)
Palomar (94)	randomized, controlled	88	polymyxin E tobramycin amphotericin	cefotaxime	15 (26)	18 (60)b	58	27*	"no difference"		33 of 58 patients randomized to SDD also given sucralfate

continued

TABLE 36-1. *Continued*

Reference	Study design	No. of evaluable patients	Drug regimen Topical agents	Drug regimen Systemic agents	Acquired infections Respiratory SDD [N°(%)]	Acquired infections Respiratory Controls [N°(%)]	Acquired infections Total infections SDD [N°(%)]	Acquired infections Total infections Controls [N°(%)]	Mortality SDD [N°(%)]	Mortality Controls [N°(%)]	Comments
Badger et al. (6)	randomized, controlled	30	polymyxin E tobramycin amphotericin	(see comments)	0	4*	2 (14)	8 (50)	3 (21)	3 (19)	All patients were liver transplant recipients. All patients received cefotaxime and ampicillin as perioperative prophylaxis. Control patients were given oral nystatin
Zobel et al. (133)	randomized, controlled	50	polymyxin E gentamicin amphotericin	cefotaxime	1 (4)	5 (20)	2 (8)	9 (36)[a]	3 (12)	2 (8)	
Cockerill et al. (21)	randomized, controlled	150	polymyxin B gentamicin nystatin	cefotaxime	4 (5)	12 (16)	10 (13)	19 (25)	8 (11)	14 (19)	After dismissal from ICU and discontinuing SDD, colonization and infection rates similar in the 2 groups during in-hospital follow-up period
Hammond et al. (51)	randomized, placebo-controlled, double-blind	239	polymyxin E tobramycin amphotericin	cefotaxime	25 (22)	28 (23)	30 (26)	43 (34)	21 (18)	21 (17)	Incidence of infection lowered by SDD for patients in mid-range APACHE II (p < 0.01)
Gastinne et al. (41)	randomized, placebo-controlled, double-blind	445	polymyxin E tobramycin amphotericin	none	26 (12)	33 (15)	NA	NA	88 (40)	82 (36)	Pneumonia due to gram-negative bacilli were less frequent in SDD than in placebo group (p = 0.01). A trend toward increase in the rate of staphylococcal pneumonia noted in the SDD group. Mortality within 60 days of randomization similar in the 2 groups

*In these studies, results for acquired infections are presented as N° of infectious episodes and not as N° of infected patients.

[a]p < 0.05; [b]p < 0.01; [c]p < 0.001; NA, not available.

be performed in homogeneous subsets of patients, who must be stratified according to appropriate scoring systems. Careful surveillance of emergence of resistant germs is necessary. Based upon current information, routine use of SDD in a multidisciplinary ICU cannot be recommended.

Prophylactic Therapy: Cystic Fibrosis Patients

Long-term aerosolized antipseudomonal antibiotics have been proposed for the prophylaxis of pulmonary infections in cystic fibrosis patients. The main studies concerning such chronic suppressive treatment are presented in Table 36-2. It must be noted that the study design of the trials, such as cross-over or prospective comparative studies, as well as the antibiotics used, are variable; thus, direct comparison of the studies is sometimes difficult. Moreover, criteria to evaluate the efficacy of such topical treatment are somewhat variable. In a randomized, double-blind, cross-over study, 20 patients who were chronically colonized by *P. aeruginosa* were given 6 months of aerosolized carbenicillin 1 g and gentamicin 80 mg twice daily, or a placebo. A significant improvement in subjective signs and pulmonary function as well as fewer hospitalizations were found during the active treatment period (56). By contrast, 47 cystic fibrosis patients were studied in a prospective study during 2 years. One group received inhaled cephaloridine and the other no topical drugs, both groups receiving cloxacillin orally. No differences were observed in clinical or radiological status or in the rate of changes in pulmonary function, or in the incidence of hospital admissions in the two groups (92). In this last study, however, it might be speculated that antipseudomonal antibiotics would have been more efficient than the used drugs in these patients heavily colonized by *P. aeruginosa*. Overall, the studies suggest that prophylaxis with aerosolized antipseudomonal drugs seems effective. Better clinical scores, slower rate of loss of pulmonary function, and decreased hospitalization are often noted. Moreover, rare and transient emergence of bacterial resistance are without clinical consequences. Criteria to start this topical treatment are not clearly defined. However, most authorities would recommend prophylactic aerosolized antibiotics only in patients who have moderate-to-severe lung disease with chronic pseudomonal colonization and who are deteriorating despite all other conventional treatment or who require frequent hospital admission for intravenous therapy (56,80).

Curative Therapy: Non–Cystic Fibrosis Patients

Patients with chronic bronchitis presenting with superinfection by Enterobacteriaceae or *P. aeruginosa* were treated by Pines et al. (98,99) with gentamicin administered by aerosol. However, in these studies, endotracheal therapy with the aminoglycoside was often associated with endotracheal carbenicillin or colistin and, sometimes, with systemic carbenicillin, colistin, or gentamicin. It is therefore difficult to evaluate the clinical effectiveness of the endotracheal regimen, which, however, seems limited. Stockley et al. (118) reported on six patients with purulent bronchiectasis who failed to improve clinically on oral amoxicillin; four of them responded with aerosolized amoxicillin (500 mg bid). According to these limited investigations, the role of aerosolized antibiotics in the treatment of chronic bronchial infections remains to be established in more appropriately designed and larger trials.

TABLE 36–2. *Prophylaxis of pulmonary infections in cystic fibrosis patients with aerosolized antibiotics*

Reference	Study design	N° of evaluable patients	Aerosolized antibiotics	Results
Hodson et al. (56)	randomized, double-blind, cross-over (6 months)	17	carbenicillin 1 g bid and gentamicin 80 mg bid vs. placebo	subjective improvement lung function tests improvement (S) fewer hospitalizations (NS)
Nolan et al. (92)	open, randomized (2 years)	47	cephaloridine 500 mg bid or tid vs. placebo (all patients on oral cloxacillin)	clinical scores lung function tests radiological scores } unchanged
Wall et al. (129)	open, comparative before and after treatment (5–15 months)	9	ticarcillin 1 g bid and tobramycin 80 mg bid	In 89 patients/months: 5 vs. 31 hospital admissions (S) increase of weight (9%) lung function tests unchanged
Nathanson et al. (90)	randomized, placebo-controlled, double-blind, cross-over (3 months)	7	gentamicin 80 mg tid vs. placebo	clinical scores lung function tests sputum bacterial density } unchanged
Kun et al. (69)	randomized, placebo-controlled, single-blind, cross-over (12 months)	29	gentamicin 20 mg bid vs. placebo	clinical scores antibiotic usage days in hospital } unchanged lung function tests improvement (S)

Study	N	Treatment	Design	Results
Stead et al. (114)	13	ceftazidime 1 g bid vs. carbenicillin 1 g bid and gentamicin 80 mg bid vs. placebo	randomized, placebo-controlled, single-blind, cross-over (4 months)	antibiotics vs. placebo: fewer hospitalizations (S), weight gain (S), lung function tests improvement (S); antibiotics regimens: no difference
Jensen et al. (59)	29	colistin 1 Mu bid vs. placebo	randomized, placebo-controlled, double-blind (3 months)	clinical scores, lung function tests, inflammmatory parameters } improved (S)
Steinkamp et al. (115)	14	tobramycin 80 mg bid	open, comparative before and after treatment (20 months)	clinical scores, radiologic scores, lung function tests } improved (S); fewer hospitalizations
McLusky et al. (79)	27	tobramycin 80 mg tid vs. saline (all patients on cloxacillin or cephalexin)	randomized, single-blind (32 months)	clinical scores and lung function tests stabilized (or improved) (S); hospital admissions: unchanged

S, significant; NS, not significant.

Klastersky et al. (62) studied the efficacy of endotracheally administered gentamicin (80 mg, 3 times daily) compared with the same dosage administered intramuscularly for tracheotomized patients with bronchial infections due to gram-negative
germs. All endobronchially treated patients had a favorable clinical response,
whereas only a few patients treated by the systemic route could be considered as
clinically and bacteriologically improved. The same group of investigators compared, in a randomized double-blind study, the efficacy of endotracheally administered sisomicin (25 mg every 8 hr) with that of placebo in 38 patients with tracheostomy and severe gram-negative bacillary bronchopneumonia (61). All of these
patients were treated with systemic carbenicillin and sisomicin. Favorable clinical
results were observed in 14 (77%) of the patients receiving endotracheal sisomicin
and in only nine (45%) of those receiving the placebo; the difference was statistically
significant. No death due to infection occurred in the sisomicin-treated group,
whereas four patients died primarily from a lung infection in the placebo group. If
the pathogenic organisms were sensitive to both carbenicillin and sisomicin, the endotracheal administration of sisomicin was more effective than that of the placebo;
clinical cure was observed in 11 of 14 (79%) and 7 of 13 (54%) of the cases, respectively. If the pathogens were sensitive to only sisomicin, the efficacy of the local
therapy with sisomicin was even more clear, in a limited number of cases, however.
In that study, it was shown that the administration of endotracheal sisomicin resulted
in bronchial concentrations of the aminoglycoside that were considerably higher than
those observed in patients who received sisomicin and carbenicillin systemically and
the placebo endotracheally (1051 and 0.45 µg/ml, respectively). In addition, no bactericidal activity could be detected in the bronchial secretions of the patients who
received only the endotracheal placebo, whereas the antimicrobial activity within
the bronchial secretions of patients receiving endotracheal sisomicin was 1 : 256.
This latter value was not modified by the addition of penicillinase to the bronchial
secretions, demonstrating that the high antimicrobial activity found in the bronchial
secretions after administration of endotracheal sisomicin was related to the presence
of the aminoglycoside. On the other hand, it was shown that the antimicrobial activity in the serum in both groups of patients was similar. This study suggested that
endotracheally administered aminoglycosides might be an important adjunct to systematically administered antibiotic in the treatment of severe gram-negative bronchopneumonias. Sculier et al. (110) has compared two groups of 10 patients with
gram-negative bronchopneumonias treated with systemic mezlocillin and endotracheally administered sisomicin, with or without systemic administration of the aminoglycoside. A similar clinical effectiveness was observed in both groups, which
might suggest that, provided endotracheal aminoglycoside is given to non-bacteremic patients, the parenteral treatment with this drug might not be necessary. By
contrast, a recent double-blind study examined endotracheal administration of
tobramycin vs. placebo as an adjunct to systemic antibiotics in 41 patients with
gram-negative pneumonia. The causative pathogens were eradicated from sputum
significantly more frequently in the tobramycin than in the placebo group. However,
clinical outcomes were similar in the two groups (17).

From these studies, it could be concluded that the role of endotracheally administered antibiotics in the treatment of nosocomial lung infection has not been fully
assessed. Moreover, colonization with resistant pathogens to the topical drug has
been noted (61,62,110). Therefore, indications for such topical treatment might be
restricted to documented severe gram-negative pneumonias, especially due to "dif-

ficult-to-treat" bacilli. Careful surveillance of the emergence of resistance is mandatory.

Curative Therapy: Cystic Fibrosis Patients

Aerosol antibiotic therapy as an adjunct to systemic treatment of acute exacerbations in cystic fibrosis has been considered. In a total group of 18 patients, aerosolized tobramycin (80 mg) and carbenicillin (1 g) twice daily was considered as effective as an intravenous treatment with the same drugs when evaluated in terms of clinical and pulmonary function tests improvement (24). By contrast, no different clinical course was observed in 28 cystic fibrosis patients who received aerosolized tobramycin (80 mg tid) in conjunction with a parenteral treatment, when compared with patients who were given only parenteral therapy; however, inhaled tobramycin produced a significantly greater suppression of colonization by *P. aeruginosa* (63 vs. 25%) (116). In another study (107), 87 patients with an acute exacerbation of pulmonary symptoms were randomly allocated to intravenous ceftazidime and amikacin alone, or with inhaled amikacin (100 mg bid). Both regimens resulted in similar improvements in clinical, radiological, laboratory, and pulmonary function evaluation. However, aerosolized amikacin did produce a significantly higher, but transient, eradication of *P. aeruginosa* (70 vs. 41%); no emergence of resistance was noted. In conclusion, the role of aerosolized antibiotics as an adjunct, or in place of a parenteral treatment in acute exacerbation of cystic fibrosis, has been insufficiently studied. Presently, this topical treatment in this clinical setting seems of minor importance.

FUNGAL INFECTIONS

Intracavitary instillation of antifungal agents has been applied to patients with symptomatic aspergilloma and who are inoperable. Twenty-three patients with aspergilloma received either nystatin or amphotericin B paste, by intracavitary needlings through the chest wall (68). More recently, Hargis et al. (53) reported clinical and radiological improvement in four out of six patients with symptomatic aspergilloma and treated with percutaneous intracavitary instillation of amphotericin B; single daily doses up to 50 mg and a total cumulative dose of 500 mg have been well tolerated. Despite these encouraging data, the small number of patients treated and the lack of controlled studies do not allow definitive conclusions to be made about the precise value of this form of therapy. However, it should be considered for a symptomatic aspergilloma with severe hemoptysis whenever surgery is contraindicated (71). Schmitt et al. (108) used a rat model of pulmonary aspergillosis to demonstrate that amphotericin B delivered as an aerosol was biologically available, and active as prophylaxis and therapy. Eisenberg (34) reported four cases of coccidioidomycosis where the patients received a daily dose of aerosolized amphotericin B of 40 mg; clinical improvement of infection without significant toxicity was observed. Attempts to reduce the risk of *Aspergillus* infections in immunocompromised patients have included local administration of amphotericin B to the airways. Amphotericin B nose spray has been well tolerated and decreased the nasopharyngeal colonization with *Aspergillus* in granulocytopenic patients. In one study comparing amphotericin B nose spray with a placebo, the incidence of invasive aspergillosis was reduced significantly by the nose spray (86). By contrast, another similar study with a larger number of patients failed to demonstrate a reduction of invasive aspergillosis, probably because *Aspergillus* colonized the lower respiratory tract which is not reached by the nose spray (28). Aerosol amphotericin B, which allows delivery of the drug to the bronchioles and alveolar spaces, has the potential to inhibit the germination of the inhaled spores. Conneally et al. (22), in a non-comparative trial of nebulized amphotericin B given prophylactically to all granulocytopenic patients, found a marked reduction in the incidence of invasive aspergillosis in comparison with historical controls. The tolerance was excellent except for mild nausea during the procedure. No renal toxicity was observed.

The role of aerosolized amphotericin B in the prevention of aspergillosis should be further studied in large controlled trials.

VIRAL INFECTIONS

Ribavirin is active *in vitro* against a wide variety of viruses including respiratory syncytial virus (RSV) and influenza A and B viruses. In bronchopulmonary RSV infections, the efficacy of nebulized ribavirin has been studied mostly in double-blind trials involving normal children and those with underlying diseases (11,35,43, 48–50,112,119). Clinical improvements were greater or more rapid on ribavirin than on placebo treatment, including in infants on mechanical ventilation. The effect on viral shedding was variably reported (11,49,50,119). No clinical or laboratory evidence of toxicity was observed (11,35,48–50,67,112,119). Serious RSV pneumonia that occurred in a healthy adult patient (4) and in a renal transplant recipient (95) has been treated successfully with ribavirin aerosol. On the other hand, the efficacy of ribavirin aerosol on symptoms from influenza A and B in young adults is variably appreciated (12,44); there are reports of isolated cases of influenza A and parainfluenza pneumonia that responded to this therapy. Diluted ribavirin can be nebulized by a small-particle aerosol generator and delivered to patients via face mask, oxygen hood, or ventilator. Because of possible precipitation of the drug in valves and ventilation tubings, careful surveillance of the mechanical ventilator must be ensured if the aerosol is given during assisted respiration (131). A new vacuum exhaust hood for aerosol delivery has lowered the leakage of ribavirin during inhalation and limited the exposure of health care workers (15,83). Ribavirin aerosol therapy, at a dose of 10 to 16 mg/kg per day, has been administered safely over a period of 12 to 18–20 hours a day, for at least 3 to 6 days. More recently, higher doses up to 3 times the usual doses were administered over a short period of 2 hours a day, for up to 5 days without significant toxicity. This modification of dosage results in high respiratory secretion concentrations that can improve the therapeutic results and offers easier accessibility for patient care (66).

Today, ribavirin aerosol treatment should be considered for infants with severe bronchiolitis or pneumonia and for high-risk patients with underlying cardiopulmonary disorders or immunodeficiency with probable RSV or influenza infections (72,112).

PROTOZOAL INFECTIONS

Aerosolized administration of pentamidine has been used to deliver high concentrations of the drug to the alveolar airspaces which are the primary sites of *Pneu-*

mocystis carinii pneumonia (PCP). Debs et al. (32) demonstrated in an animal model that aerosol delivery of pentamidine produced higher concentrations in the alveolar space than was obtained with intravenous pentamidine administration. Extrapulmonary drug levels were negligible, suggesting a poor systemic absorption from the lungs. Human studies reported higher levels of pentamidine in BAL fluid sediment (705 ± 242 vs. 9.3 ± 1.7 ng/ml) and lower systemic levels (5.9 ± 0.9 vs. 60.5 ± 15.0 ng/ml) in patients receiving aerosol pentamidine (AP), when compared with patients receiving the intravenous drug (23,88,113).

Three controlled trials have assessed the effectiveness of AP in PCP prophylaxis. A prospective double-blind, placebo-controlled study (55) showed a benefit from AP as primary prophylaxis in 223 patients who had AIDS, AIDS-related complex, or less than 200 CD4+ T cells/mm^3, but no previous episode of PCP. Three hundred mg of AP were delivered via the Respirgard II jet nebulizer, once monthly, in comparison to a placebo. The PCP breakthrough rates were 8.6% and 27.6% per patient-year, respectively. Two other controlled trials explored the effectiveness of AP as secondary prophylaxis, delivered via the Fisoneb ultrasonic nebulizer. In the Canadian cooperative trial (87), 84 patients received 60 mg of AP bimonthly and were compared to 78 patients receiving placebo. The PCP breakthrough rates after a 6-month follow-up period were 9% and 50%, respectively. Similar results were obtained in the U.S. study (89) comparing 60 and 120 mg of AP biweekly. These two studies demonstrated that other regimens of AP, and other nebulizers, can be used safely, with similar results to the San Francisco dose comparison study (73). In this latter study, the patients were randomized to receive either 30 mg bimonthly, or 300 mg monthly. AP was administered via Respirgard II nebulizer system. The study was conducted for 18 months, with a mean follow-up time of 10 months. The recurrence rate of PCP was the lowest for the patients receiving 300 mg monthly (6.2%), in comparison to 13.3% and 18.8% for the 150 mg bimonthly and 30 mg bimonthly regimens, respectively. Consequently, the Food and Drug Administration approved 300 mg monthly delivered via the Respirgard II nebulizer for PCP prophylaxis. More recently, it has been suggested that higher doses of AP could result in a high degree of protection (40).

The tolerance of AP is good. Airway irritation with coughing occurs in 10 to 20% and bronchospasm in 1 to 2% of the patients (25). Pretreatment with bronchodilators can prevent or ameliorate these two events (113). Dysgeusia associated with inhaled pentamidine was brief and only noted during treatment. Surprisingly, hypoglycemia occurred in 27% of patients during inhaled pentamidine (113).

Once popularized and used extensively, limitations to AP prophylaxis became apparent. Pneumothoraces, extrapulmonary infections, atypical presentations of PCP, and difficulties in the diagnosis of PCP in patients under AP prophylaxis have been well documented (19,36,85,91,102).

Many factors influence the alveolar deposition of AP. A nebulizer system with a high output, and generating 1 to 2 μm particles, seems to be the best suited. Particles more than 2 μm are more likely to deposit on large airways (111). The patient's pulmonary function is important. Patients with tachypnea, emphysema, bronchospasm, chronic obstructive lung disease, or prior lung damage can have a decreased alveolar deposition of AP (25). Consolidation areas of the lungs have impaired alveolar deposition. Supine position of the patient during inhalation is supposed to increase the delivery to the apex.

A prospective randomized study (52) compared oral trimethoprim-sulfamethoxazole (TMP-SMX), one double-strength tablet daily, with AP 300 mg monthly through a Respirgard II nebulizer as secondary prophylaxis for PCP in high-risk HIV-infected patients. The recurrence rates were 11.1% and 27.6% per patient-year, respectively (p < 0.001). Another controlled trial (109) compared three regimens for primary prophylaxis of PCP in HIV patients with CD4 cell counts below 200 per cubic millimeter: 300 mg of AP monthly, low-dose TMP-SMX (80 mg–400 mg) given orally once a day, and high-dose TMP-SMX (160 mg–800 mg) given orally once a day. PCP occurred in 11% of patients receiving AP, in comparison to 0% in patients receiving TMP-SMX (p = 0.002). Based on these data, the greater cost-effectiveness of TMP-SMX, and its potential for protection against other major opportunistic infections such as toxoplasmosis and nocardiosis has caused TMP-SMX to be recommended as the first-line choice for PCP prophylaxis. AP is an alternative for patients who do not tolerate or who are known to be hypersensitive to sulfonamides.

CONCLUSION

Experimental and clinical data support the thesis that local administration of anti-infectious agents to the respiratory tract can be beneficial to bronchopulmonary infections due to various pathogens.

As far as bacterial infections are concerned, initial studies suggest that the endotracheal administration of antibiotics can be used to prevent the colonization of the respiratory tract. However, selection of resistant pathogens has been observed, sometimes associated with the development of severe pneumonias; therefore, prophylaxis of bronchopulmonary infections with endotracheal antibiotics in non–cystic fibrosis patients should not be applied because of the fear of selection of antibiotic-resistant strains and the lack of efficacy of this treatment on death rate. Selective digestive decontamination is effective, in most studies, in decreasing the rate of nosocomial lower respiratory rates of infections. However, mortality rate of the patients treated with this topical prophylaxis remains unchanged; moreover, emergence of resistant pathogens has been recently described. Therefore, the routine use of selective digestive decontamination is not recommended, and awaits future well-designed studies. On the other hand, long-term aerosolized antipseudomonal drugs are very probably useful in preventing acute pulmonary infections in cystic fibrosis patients. If the therapeutic role of locally administered antibiotics in the treatment of bacterial lower respiratory tract infections in non–cystic fibrosis patients is considered, it appears that this topical treatment should be restricted to severe, documented gram-negative pneumonias.

The role of aerosolized amphotericin B in the prevention of aspergillosis seems promising, but further trials are needed in this field.

Treatment with aerosolized ribavirin should be considered for infants with RSV bronchiolitis and for high-risk patients with probable RSV or influenza infections.

Recent studies demonstrated that aerosolized pentamidine is efficient in the prophylaxis of *Pneumocystis* pneumonia; however, in comparative trials, trimethoprim-sulfamethoxazole appears superior to this topical treatment in the prevention of this pulmonary disease.

ACKNOWLEDGMENTS

We should like to acknowledge the great help of Ms. L. Zech and I. Hagon for preparing the manuscript. The help of B. Delaere, M.D., was greatly appreciated.

REFERENCES

1. Aerdts, S.J., van Dalen, R., Clasener, H.A., Festen, J., van Lier, H.J.J., and Vollard, E.J. (1991): Antibiotic prophylaxis of respiratory tract infection in mechanically ventilated patients: a prospective, blinded, randomized trial of the effect of a novel regimen. *Chest,* 100:783–791.
2. Aguilera, D., Coupry, A., Karlin, P., Carrère-Debat, D., Giudicelli, D.P., and Gontier, D. (1986): Etude des concentrations sériques et bronchiques au cours de l'administration continue de né-tilmicine intratrachéale. *Path. Biol.,* 34:657–662.
3. Alderson, P.O., Secker-Walker, R.H., Strominger, D.B., Markham, J., and Hill, R.L. (1974): Pulmonary deposition of aerosols in children with cystic fibrosis. *J. Pediatr.,* 84:479–484.
4. Aylward, R.B., and Burdge, D.R. (1991): Ribavirin therapy of adult respiratory syncytial virus pneumonitis. *Arch. Intern. Med.,* 151:2303–2304.
5. Ayres, S.M., Griesbach, J., and Gianneli, S., Jr. (1972): A study of bronchial irritation and systemic absorption of aerosolized kanamycin. *Curr. Ther. Res.,* 14:153–157.
6. Badger, I.L., Crosby, H.A., Kong, K.L., et al. (1991): Is selective decontamination of the digestive tract beneficial in liver transplant patients? Interim results of a prospective, randomized trial. *Transplant. Proc.,* 23:1460–1461.
7. Baldwin, D.R., Honeybourne, D., and Wise, R. (1992): Pulmonary disposition of antimicrobial agents: methodological considerations. *Antimicrob. Agents Chemother.,* 36:1171–1175.
8. Baran, D., Dachy, A., and Klastersky, J. (1975): Concentration of gentamicin in bronchial secretions of children with cystic fibrosis or tracheotomy. *Int. Clin. Pharmacol.,* 12:336–341.
9. Baran, D., de Vuyst, P., and Ooms, H.A. (1990): Concentration of tobramycin given by aerosol in the fluid obtained by bronchoalveolar lavage. *Respir. Med.,* 84:203–204.
10. Barnes, P., and Waterworth, P.M. (1977): New cause of penicillin treatment failure. *Br. Med. J.,* 1:991–993.
11. Barry, W., Cockburn, F., Cornall, R., Price, J.F., Sutherland, G., and Vardag, A. (1986): Ribavirin aerosol for acute bronchiolitis. *Arch. Dis. Child.,* 61:593–597.
12. Bernstein, D.I., Reuman, P.D., Sherwood, J.R., Young, E.C., and Schiff, G.M. (1988): Ribavirin small-particle-aerosol treatment of influenza B virus infection. *Antimicrob. Agents Chemother.,* 32:761–764.
13. Bilodeau, M., Roy, H.C., and Giroux, M. (1966): Studies of absorption of kanamycin by aerosolization. *Ann. NY Acad. Sci.,* 132:870–878.
14. Blair, P., Rowlands, B.J., Lowry, K., Hugh, W., Armstrong, P., and Smilie, J. (1991): Selective decontamination of the digestive tract: a stratified, randomized, prospective study in a mixed intensive care unit. *Surgery,* 110:303–310.
15. Bradley, J.S., Connor, J.D., Compogiannis, L.S., and Eiger, L.L. (1990): Exposure of health care workers to ribavirin during therapy for respiratory syncytial virus infections. *Antimicrob. Agents Chemother.,* 34:668–670.
16. Bressolle, F., de la Coussaye, J.-E., Ayoub, R., et al. (1992): Endotracheal and aerosol administrations of ceftazidime in patients with nosocomial pneumonia: pharmacokinetics and absolute bioavailability. *Antimicrob. Agents Chemother.,* 36:1404–1411.
17. Brown, R.B., Kruse, J.A., Counts, G.W., Russell, J.A., Christou, N.V., Sands, M.L., and the Endotracheal Tobramycin Study Group (1990): Double-blind study of endotracheal tobramycin in the treatment of gram-negative bacterial pneumonia. *Antimicrob. Agents Chemother.,* 34:269–272.
18. Brun-Buisson, C., Legrand, P., Rauss, A., et al. (1989): Intestinal decontamination for control of nosocomial multiresistant gram-negative bacilli. *Ann. Intern. Med.,* 110:873–881.
19. Chaffey, M.H., Klein, J.S., Gamsu, G., Blanc, P., and Golden, J.A. (1990): Radiographic distribution of *Pneumocystis carinii* pneumonia in patients with AIDS treated with prophylactic inhaled pentamidine. *Radiology,* 175:715–719.
20. Chua, H.L., Collis, G.G., and Le Souëf, P.N. (1990): Bronchial response to nebulized antibiotics in children with cystic fibrosis. *Eur. Respir. J.,* 3:1114–1116.
21. Cockerill, F.R., Muller, S.R., Anhalt, J.P., et al. (1992): Prevention of infection in critically ill patients by selective decontamination of the digestive tract. *Ann. Intern. Med.,* 117:545–553.
22. Conneally, E., Cafferkey, M.T., Daly, P.A., Kearne, C.T., and McCann, S.R. (1990): Nebulized amphotericin B as prophylaxis against invasive aspergillosis in granulcytopenic patients. *Bone Marrow Transplant.,* 5:403–406.
23. Conte, J.E., Jr., Hollander, H., and Golden, J.A. (1987): Inhaled or reduced-dose intravenous pentamidine for *Pneumocystis carinii* pneumonia. *Ann. Intern. Med.,* 107:495–498.
24. Cooper, D.M., Harris, M., and Mitchell, I. (1985): Comparison of intravenous and inhalation antibiotic therapy in acute pulmonary deterioration in cystic fibrosis. *Am. Rev. Respir. Dis.,* 131:A242.
25. Corkery, K.J., Luce, J.M., and Montgomery, A.B. (1988): Aerosolized pentamidine for treatment and prophylaxis of *Pneumocystis carinii* pneumonia: an update. *Respir. Care,* 33:676–685.
26. Craven, D.E. (1992): Use of selective decontamination of the digestive tract. *Ann. Intern. Med.,* 117:609–611.

27. Crosby, S.S., Edwards, W.A., Brennan, C., Dellinger, P., and Bauer, L.A. (1987): Systemic absorption of endotracheally administered aminoglycosides in seriously ill patients with pneumonia. *Antimicrob. Agents Chemother.*, 31:850–853.
28. Cushing, D., Bustamante, C., Devlin, A., Finley, R., and Wade, J. (1991): Aspergillus infection prophylaxis: amphotericin-B (AB) nose spray, a double-blind trial. [Abstract 737]. In: *Program and Abstracts of the 31st ICAAC.* American Society for Microbiology, New York.
29. Dally, M.B., Kurrle, S., and Breslin, A.B.X. (1978): Ventilatory effects of aerosol gentamicin. *Thorax,* 33:54–56.
30. Daschner, F. (1992): Emergence of resistance during selective decontamination of the digestive tract. *Eur. J. Clin. Microbiol. Infect. Dis.,* 11:1–3.
31. Davies, B.I., Maesen, F.P.V., and Gubbelmans, R. (1989): Azithromycin (CP-62,993) in acute exacerbations of chronic bronchitis: an open clincal, microbiological and pharmacokinetic study. *J. Antimicrob. Chemother.,* 23:743–751.
32. Debs, R.J., Straubinger, R.M., Brunette, E.N., et al. (1987): Selective enhancement of pentamidine uptake in the lung by aerosolization and delivery in liposomes. *Am. Rev. Respir. Dis.,* 135:731–737.
33. Dickie, K.J., and De Groot, W.J. (1973): Ventilatory effects of aerosolized kanamcyin and polymyxin. *Chest,* 63:694–697.
34. Eisenberg, R.S., and Oatway, W.H. (1971): Nebulization of amphotericin B. *Am. Rev. Respir. Dis.,* 103:289–292.
35. Englund, J.A., Piedra, P.A., Jefferson, L.S., Wilson, S.Z., Taber, L.H., and Gilbert, B.E. (1990): High-dose, short duration ribavirin aerosol therapy in children with suspected respiratory syncytial virus infection. *J. Pediatr.,* 117:313–320.
36. Fahy, J.V., Chin, D.P., Schnapp, L.M., et al. (1992): Effect of aerosolized pentamidine prophylaxis on the clinical severity and diagnosis of *Pneumocystis carinii* pneumonia. *Am. Rev. Respir. Dis.,* 146:844–848.
37. Feeley, T.W., Dumoulin, G.C., Hedley-Whyte, J., Bushnell, L.S., Gilbert, J.P., and Feingold, D.S. (1975): Aerosol polymyxin and pneumonia in seriously ill patients. *N. Engl. J. Med.,* 293:471–475.
38. Fink, M.P. (1992): Selective digestive decontamination: a gut tissue for the nineties. *Crit. Care Med.,* 20:559–561.
39. Flaherty, J., Nathan, C., Kabins, S.A., and Weinstein, R.A. (1990): Pilot trial of selective decontamination for prevention of bacterial infection in an intensive care unit. *J. Infect. Dis.,* 162:1393–1397.
40. Flamhole, L., Haidl, S., Westin, E., Borgdalen, L., and Prellner, T. (1992): High dose aerosol pentamidine for secondary *Pneumocystis carinii* pneumonia prophylaxis in AIDS patients. *Infection,* 20:309–312.
41. Gastinne, H., Wolff, M., Delatour, F., et al. (1992): A controlled trial in intensive care units of selective decontamination of the digestive tract with nonabsorbable antibiotics. *N. Engl. J. Med.,* 326:594–599.
42. Geers, T.A., and Baker, N.R. (1987): The effect of sublethal levels of antibiotics on the pathogenicity of *Pseudomonas aeruginosa* for tracheal tissue. *J. Antimicrob. Chemother.,* 19:569–578.
43. Gelfand, E.W., McCurdy, D., Pandu Rao, C., and Middleton, P.J. (1983): Ribavirin treatment of viral pneumonitis in severe combined immunodeficiency disease. *Lancet,* II:732–733.
44. Gilbert, B.E., Wilson, S.Z., Knight, V., et al. (1985): Ribavirin small-particle aerosol treatment of infections caused by influenza virus strains A/Victoria/7/83 (H1N1) and B/Texas/1/84. *Antimicrob. Agents Chemother.,* 27:309–313.
45. Godart, J., Guillaume, C., Reverdy, M.E., et al. (1990): Intestinal decontamination in a polyvalent ICU: a double-blind study. *Intensive Care Med.,* 16:307–311.
46. Gomez, E.C., Markowsky, S.J., and Rotschafer, J.C. (1992): Selective decontamination of the digestive tract in intensive care patients: review and commentary. *Ann. Pharmcother.,* 26:963–976.
47. Greenfield, S., Teres, D., Bushnell, L.S., Hedley-White, J., and Feingold, D.S. (1973): Prevention of gram-negative bacillary pneumonia using aerosol polymyxin as prophylaxis: I. Effect on the colonization pattern of the upper respiratory tract of seriously ill patients. *J. Clin. Invest.,* 52:2935–2940.
48. Groothuis, J.R., Woodin, K.A., Katz, R., et al. (1990): Early ribavirin treatment of respiratory syncytial viral infection in high-risk children. *J. Pediatr.,* 117:792–798.
49. Hall, C.B., McBride, J.T., Gala, C.L., Hildrets, S., and Schnabel, K.C. (1985): Ribavirin treatment of respiratory syncytial viral infection in infants with underlying cardiopulmonary disease. *J.A.M.A.,* 254:3047–3051.
50. Hall, C.B., McBride, J.T., Walsh, E.E., et al. (1983): Aerosolized ribavirin treatment of infants with respiratory syncytial viral infection: a randomized double-blind study. *N. Engl. J. Med.,* 308:1443–1447.
51. Hammond, J.M., Potgieter, P.D., Saunders, G.L., and Forder, A.A. (1992): Double-blind study of selective decontamination of the digestive tract in intensive care. *Lancet,* 340:5–9.

52. Hardy, W.D., Holzman, R.S., Feinberg, J., et al. (1992): A controlled study of trimethoprim-sulfamethoxazole or aerosolized pentamidine for secondary prophylaxis of *Pneumocystis carinii* pneumonia in patients with the acquired immunodeficiency syndrome. *N. Engl. J. Med.*, 327:1842–1848.

53. Hargis, J.L., Bone, R.C., Stewart, J., Rector, N., and Hiller, F.C. (1980): Intracavitary amphotericin B in the treatment of symptomatic pulmonary aspergillomas. *Am. J. Med.*, 68:389–394.

54. Hellstrom, P.E., Gruenwaldt, G., and Scheer, M. (1979): A preliminary report on serum concentrations of sisomicin following aerosol inhalation and intravenous injection. *Infection*, 7(Suppl. 3):283–284.

55. Hirschel, B., Lazzarin, A., Chopard, P., and the Swiss Group for Clinical Studies on AIDS. (1991): A controlled study of inhaled pentamidine for primary prevention of *Pneumocystis carinii* pneumonia. *N. Engl. J. Med.*, 324:1079–1083.

56. Hodson, M.E., Penketh, A.R., and Batten, J.C. (1981): Aerosol carbenicillin and gentamicin treatment of *Pseudomonas aeruginosa* infection in patients with cystic fibrosis. *Lancet*, 2:1137–1139.

57. Ilowite, J.S., Gorvoy, J.D., and Smaldone, G.C. (1987): Quantitative deposition of aerosolized gentamicin in cystic fibrosis. *Am. Rev. Respir. Dis.*, 136:1445–1449.

58. Itoh, H., Ishii, Y., Maeda, H., Todo, G., Torizuka, K., and Smaldone, G.C. (1981): Clinical observations of aerosol deposition in patients with airways obstruction. *Chest*, 80(Suppl.):837–840.

59. Jensen, T., Pedersen, S.S., Garne, S., Heilmann, C., Hoiby, N., and Koch, C. (1987): Colistin inhalation therapy in cystic fibrosis patients with chronic *Pseudomonas aeruginosa* lung infection. *J. Antimicrob. Chemother.*, 19:831–838.

60. Kerver, A., Rommes, J.H., Mevissen-Verhage, E., et al. (1988): Prevention of colonization and infection in critically ill patients: a prospective randomized study. *Crit. Care Med.*, 16:1087–1093.

61. Klastersky, J., Carpentier-Meunier, F., Kahan-Coppens, L., and Thys, J.P. (1979): Endotracheally administered antibiotics for gram-negative bronchopneumonia. *Chest*, 75:586–591.

62. Klastersky, J., Geuning, C, Mouawad, E., and Daneau, D. (1972): Endotracheal gentamicin in bronchial infections in patients with tracheostomy. *Chest*, 61:117–120.

63. Klastersky, J., Hensgens, C., Noterman, J., Mouawad, E., and Meunier, F. (1975): Endotracheal antibiotics for the prevention of tracheobronchial infections in tracheotomized unconscious patients. A comparative study of gentamicin and aminosidin-polymixin B combination. *Chest*, 68:302–306.

64. Klastersky, J., Huysmans, E., Weerts, D., Hensgens, C., and Daneau, D. (1974): Endotracheally administered gentamicin for the prevention of infection of the respiratory tract in patients with tracheostomy: a double-blind study. *Chest*, 65:650–654.

65. Klick, J.M., du Moulin, G.C., Hedley-Whyte, J., Teres, D., Busnell, L.S., and Feingold, D.S. (1975): Prevention of gram-negative bacillary pneumonia using polymyxin aerosol as prophylaxis: II. Effect on the incidence of pneumonia in seriously ill patients. *J. Clin. Invest.*, 55:514–519.

66. Knight, V., and Gilbert, B.E. (1990): Aerosol treatment of respiratory viral disease. *Lung*, 168:406–413.

67. Knight, V., Wilson, S.Z., Quarles, J.M., et al. (1981): Ribavirin small-particle aerosol treatment of influenza. *Lancet*, II:945–949.

68. Krakowka, P., Traczyk, K., Walczak, J., Halweg, H., Elsner, Z., and Pawlicka, L. (1970): Local treatment of aspergilloma of the lung with a paste containing nystatin or amphotericin B. *Tubercle*, 51:184–191.

69. Kun, P., Landau, L.I., and Phelan, P.D. (1984): Nebulized gentamicin in children and adolescents with cystic fibrosis. *Aust. Paediatr. J.*, 20:43–45.

70. Lake, K.B., Van Dijke, J.J., and Rumsfeld, J.A. (1975): Combined topical pulmonary and systemic gentamicin: the question of safety. *Chest*, 68:62–64.

71. *Lancet II* (1983): Aspergillomas, II:1066–1067. (Editorial).

72. *Lancet I* (1986): Ribavirin and respiratory syncytial virus, 392–393. (Editorial).

73. Leoung, G.S., Feigal, D.W., Montgomery, A.B., and the San Francisco County Consortium (1990): Aerosolized pentamidine for prophylaxis against *Pneumocystis carinii* pneumonia. *N. Engl. J. Med.*, 323:769–775.

74. Levine, B.A., Petroff, P.A., Slade, C.L., and Pruitt, B.A. (1978): Prospective trials of dexamethasone and aerosolized gentamicin in the treatment of inhalation injury in the burned patient. *J. Trauma*, 18:188–193.

75. Levy, J. (1986): Antibiotic activity in sputum. *J. Pediatr.*, 108:841–846.

76. Lifschitz, M.I., and Denning, C.R. (1971): Safety of kanamycin aerosol. *Clin. Pharmacol. Ther.*, 12:91–95.

77. Lode, H., and Goecke, J.: Endotracheal application of gentamicin: a randomized placebo controlled double-blind study in ventilated patients. *Chemother. J.* (In press).

78. Loirat, Ph. (1992): Selective digestive decontamination in intensive care unit patients. *Intensive Care Med.*, 18:182–188.
79. MacLusky, I.B., Gold, R., Corey, M., and Levison, H. (1989): Long-term effects of inhaled tobramycin in patients with cystic fibrosis colonized with *Pseudomonas aeruginosa*. *Pediatric. Pulmonol.*, 7:42–48.
80. MacLusky, I.B., Levison, H., Gold, R., and McLaughlin, F. (1986): Inhaled antibiotics in cystic fibrosis: Is there a therapeutic effect? *J. Pediatr.*, 108:861–865.
81. Maddocks, J.L., and May, F.R. (1969): "Indirect pathogenicity" of penicillinase-producing enterobacteria in chronic bronchial infections. *Lancet*, 1:793–795.
82. Maesen, F.P.V., Beeuwkes, H., Davies, B.I., Buytendijk, H.J., Brombacher, P.J., and Wessman, J. (1976): Bacampicillin in acute exacerbations of chronic bronchitis: a dose-range study. *J. Antimicrob. Chemother.*, 2:279–285.
83. Marlock, D., Buchan, R.M., and Tillery, M. (1991): A local exhaust ventilation system to reduce airborne ribavirin concentrations. *Am. Ind. Hyg. Assoc. J.*, 52:428–432.
84. Mendelman, P.M., Smith, A.L., Lévy, J., Weber, A., Ramsey, B., and Davis, R.L. (1985): Aminoglycoside penetration, inactivation, and efficacy in cystic fibrosis sputum. *Am. Rev. Respir. Dis.*, 132:761–765.
85. Metersky, M.I., and Catanzaro, A. (1991): Diagnostic approach to *Pneumocystis carinii* pneumonia in the setting of prophylactic aerosolized pentamidine. *Chest*, 100:1345–1349.
86. Meunier-Carpentier, F., Snoeck, R., Gérain, J., Muller, C., and Klastersky, J. (1984): Amphotericin B nasal spray as prophylaxis against aspergillosis in patients with neutropenia. *N. Engl. J. Med.*, 311:1056.
87. Montaner, J.S.G., Lawson, L.M., Gervais, A., et al. (1991): Aerosol pentamide for secondary prophylaxis of AIDS-related *Pneumocystis carinii* pneumonia: a randomized, placebo-controlled study. *Ann. Intern. Med.*, 114:948–953.
88. Montgomery, A.B., Debs, R.J., Luce, J.M., Corkery, K.J., Turner, J., and Hopewell, P.C. (1987): Aerosolized pentamidine as sole therapy for *Pneumocystis carinii* pneumonia in patients with the acquired immunodeficiency syndrome. *Lancet*, 2:480–483.
89. Murphy, R.L., Lavelle, J.P., Allan, J.D., et al. (1991): Aerosol pentamidine prophylaxis following *Pneumocystis carinii* pneumonia in AIDS patients: results of a blinded dose-comparison study using an ultrasonic nebulizer. *Am. J. Med.*, 90:418–426.
90. Nathanson, I., Cropp, G.J.A., and Li, P. (1985): Effectiveness of aerosolized gentamicin in cystic fibrosis. *Cystic Fibrosis Club Abstracts*, 26:145.
91. Newsome, G.S., Ward, D.J., and Pierce, P.F. (1990): Spontaneous pneumothorax in patients with acquired immunodeficiency syndrome treated with prophylactic aerosolized pentamidine. *Arch. Intern. Med.*, 150:2167–2168.
92. Nolan, G., McIvor, P., Levison, H., Fleming, P.C., Corey, M., and Gold, R. (1982): Antibiotic prophylaxis in cystic fibrosis: inhaled cephaloridine as an adjunct to oral cloxacillin. *J. Pediatr.*, 101:626–630.
93. Odio, W., Van Laer, E., and Klastersky, J. (1975): Concentrations of gentamicin in bronchial secretions after intramuscular and endotracheal administration. *Int. Clin. Pharmacol.*, 15:518–524.
94. Palomar, M. (1991): Prevention of nosocomial pneumonia in ventilated patients using cefotaxime and SDD. [Abstract 505]. In: *Proceedings of the 17th International Congress of Chemotherapy*, Berlin.
95. Peigue-Lafeuille, H., Gazuy, N., Mignot, P., Deteix, R., Beytout, D., and Baguet, J.C. (1990): Severe respiratory syncytial virus pneumonia in an adult renal transplant recipient: successful treatment with ribavirin. *Scand. J. Infect. Dis.*, 22:87–89.
96. Peromet, M., Schoutens, E., and Yourassowsky, E. (1973): Endotracheal administration of gentamicin: relationship between obtained serum levels and creatininemia. *Chemotherapy*, 19:211–214.
97. Pines, A., Bundi, R.S., and Greenfield, J.S.B. (1965): Chloramphenicol analogues in the intrabronchial treatment of severe chronic chest infections. *Br. J. Dis. Chest*, 59:81–89.
98. Pines, A., Raafat, H., and Plucinsky, K. (1967): Gentamicin and colistin in chronic purulent bronchial infections. *Br. Med. J.*, 2:543–545.
99. Pines, A., Raafat, H., Siddiqui, G.M., and Greenfield, J.S.B. (1970): Treatment of severe *Pseudomonas* infections of the bronchi. *Br. Med. J.*, 1:663–665.
100. Pugin, J., Auckenthaler, R., Lew, D.P., and Suter, P.M. (1991): Oropharyngeal decontamination decreases incidence of ventilator-associated pneumonia. *J.A.M.A.*, 265:2704–2710.
101. Ramirez, J., and O'Neil, E.F. (1970): Endobronchial polymyxin B: experimental observations in chronic bronchitis. *Chest*, 58:352–357.
102. Raviglione, M.C. (1990): Extrapulmonary pneumocystosis: the first 50 cases. *Rev. Infect. Dis.*, 12:1127–1138.
103. Regula, H., Wieser, O., and Naumann, P. (1973): Pharmakokinetische Untersuchungen über Sputum, Serum und Urinkonzentration von Gentamicin nach aerosol-Inhalation. *Int. J. Clin. Pharmacol.*, 7:95–100.

104. Reidy, J.J., and Ramsay, G. (1990): Clinical trials of selective decontamination of the digestive tract: review. *Crit. Care Med.*, 18:1449–1456.
105. Rodriguez-Roldan, J.M., Altuna-Cuesta, A., Lopez, A., et al. (1990): Prevention of nosocomial lung infection in ventilated patients: use of an antimicrobial pharyngeal nonabsorbable paste. *Crit. Care Med.*, 18:1239–1242.
106. Rose, H.D., Pendharker, M.B., Snider, G.L., and Kory, R.C. (1970): Evaluation of sodium colistemethate aerosol in gram-negative infections of the respiratory tract. *J. Clin. Pharmacol.*, 10:274–281.
107. Schaad, U.B., Wedgwood-Krucko, J., Suter, S., and Kraemer, R. (1987): Efficacy of inhaled amikacin as adjunct to intravenous combination therapy (ceftazidime and amikacin) in cystic fibrosis. *J. Pediatr.*, 111:599–605.
108. Schmitt, H.J., Bernard, E.M., Hauser, M., and Armstrong, D. (1988): Aerosol amphotericin B is effective for prophylaxis and therapy in a rat model of pulmonary aspergillosis. *Antimicrob. Agents Chemother.*, 32:1676–1679.
109. Schreier, H. (1992): Liposome aerosols. *J. Liposome Res.*, 2:145–184.
110. Sculier, J.P., Coppens, L., and Klastersky, J. (1982): Effectiveness of mezlocillin and endotracheally administered sisomicin with or without parenteral sisomicin in the treatment of gram-negative bronchopneumonia. *J. Antimicrob. Chemother.*, 9:63–68.
111. Simonds, A.K., Newman, S.P., Johnson, M.A., Talaee, N., Lee, C.A., and Clarke, S.W. (1990): Alveolar targeting of aerosol pentamidine: toward a rational delivery system. *Am. Rev. Respir. Dis.*, 141:827–829.
112. Smith, D.W., Frankel, C.B., Mathers, L.H., et al. (1991): A controlled trial of aerosolized ribavirin in infants receiving mechanical ventilation for severe respiratory syncytial virus infection. *N. Engl. J. Med.*, 325:24–29.
113. Soo Hoo, G.W., Mohsenifar, Z., and Meyer, R.D. (1990): Inhaled or intravenous pentamidine therapy for *Pneumocystis carinii* pneumonia in AIDS: a randomized trial. *Ann. Intern. Med.*, 113:195–202.
114. Stead, R.J., Hodson, M.E., and Batten, J.C. (1987): Inhaled ceftazidime compared with gentamicin and carbenicillin in older patients with cystic fibrosis infected with *Pseudomonas aeruginosa*. *Br. J. Dis. Chest*, 81:272–279.
115. Steinkamp, G., Tümmler, B., Gappa, M., et al. (1989): Long-term tobramycin aerosol therapy in cystic fibrosis. *Pediatr. Pulmonol.*, 6:91–98.
116. Stephens, D., Garey, N., Isles, A., Levison, H., and Gold, R. (1983): Efficacy of inhaled tobramycin in the treatment of pulmonary exacerbations in children with cystic fibrosis. *Pediatr. Infect. Dis.*, 2:209–211.
117. Stewart, S.M., Anderson, I.M.E., Jones, G.R., and Calder, M.A. (1974): Amoxycillin levels in sputum, serum and saliva. *Thorax*, 29:110–114.
118. Stockley, R.A., Hill, S.L., and Burnett, D. (1985): Nebulized amoxicillin in chronic purulent bronchiectasis. *Clin. Ther.*, 7:593–599.
119. Taber, L.H., Knight, V., Gilbert, B.E., et al. (1983). Ribavirin aerosol treatment of bronchiolitis associated with respiratory syncytial virus infection in infants. *Pediatrics*, 72:613–618.
120. Tetteroo, G.W., Wagenvoort, J.H., Castelein, A., Tilanus, H.W., Ince, C., and Bruining, H.A. (1990): Selective decontamination to reduce gram-negative colonization and infections after oesophageal resection. *Lancet*, 335:704–707.
121. Thys, J.P., and Klastersky, J. (1978): Concentrations of sisomicin in serum and in bronchial secretions after intratracheal administration. In: *Current Chemotherapy and Infectious Diseases*, pp. 920–921. Edited by Siegenthäler and Lüthy. American Society for Microbiology, Washington, D.C.
122. Ulrich, C., Harinck-de Weerd, J.E., Bakker, N.C., Jacz, K., Doornbos, L., and de Ridder, V.A. (1989): Selective decontamination of the digestive tract with norfloxacin in the prevention of ICU-acquired infections: a prospective randomized study. *Intensive Care Med.*, 15:424–431.
123. Unertl, K., Ruckdeschel, G., Selbmann, H.K., et al. (1987): Prevention of colonization and respiratory infections in long-term ventilated patients by local antimicrobial prophylaxis. *Intensive Care Med.*, 13:106–113.
124. Valcke, Y.J., and Pauwels, R.A. (1991): Pharmacokinetic evaluation of tobramycin in the alveolar lining fluid of the rat after endotracheal administration. *Am. Rev. Respir. Dis.*, 144:1199–1201.
125. Vandenbroucke-Grauls, C.M.J.E., and Vandenbroucke, J.P. (1991): Effect of selective decontamination of the digestive tract on respiratory tract infections and mortality in the intensive care unit. *Lancet*, 338:859–862.
126. van Saene, H., Stoutenbeek, C.C., and Stoller, J.K. (1992): Selective decontamination of the digestive tract in the intensive care unit: current status and future prospects. *Crit. Care Med.*, 20:691–703.
127. Vishwanath, S, Guay, C.M., and Ramphal, R. (1987): Effects of subminimal inhibitory concentrations of antibiotics on the adherence of *Pseudomonas aeruginosa* to tracheobronchial mucin. *J. Antimicrob. Chemother.*, 19:579–583.

128. Vogel, F., Exner, H., Lilienfeld-Toal, H.V., Cattelaens, N., and Eichelbaum, M. (1984): Serum gentamicin concentrations during intratracheal administration. *Klin. Wochenschr.,* 62:394–398.
129. Wall, M.A., Terry, A.B., Eisenberg, J., McNamara, M., and Cohen, R. (1983): Inhaled antibiotics in cystic fibrosis. *Lancet I,* 1325.
130. Webb, C.H. (1992): Antibiotic resistance associated with selective decontamination of the digestive tract. *J. Hosp. Infect.,* 22:1–5.
131. Wilson, F.E. (1981): Acute respiratory failure secondary to polymyxin-B inhalation. *Chest,* 79:237–239.
132. Wise, R., Baldwin, D.R., and Honeybourne, D. (1990): Penetration of antibiotics into the bronchial mucosa: a review. *Res. Clin. Forums,* 12:95–102.
133. Zobel, G., Kuttnig, M., Grubbauer, H.-M., Semmelrock, H.-J., and Thiel, W. (1991): Reduction of colonization and infection rate during pediatric intensive care by selective decontamination of the digestive tract. *Crit. Care Med.,* 19:1242–1246.

Respiratory Infections: Diagnosis and Management, 3d ed.,
edited by James E. Pennington.
Raven Press, Ltd., New York © 1994

37

Rational Use of New Antibiotics in Respiratory Infections

Hartmut Lode and Berndt Kemmerich

*Free University of Berlin and City Hospital Zehlendorf/Hecheshörn,
Zum Hecheshom 33, Berlin, Germany; and Leopoldstrasse 87,
80802 Munich, Germany*

Therapeutic regimens for lower respiratory tract infections must be selected empirically for most patients based on the spectrum of pathogens expected in a specific situation. Treatment is usually initiated before culture results are available, and a definite diagnosis is complicated by the fact that potential pathogens could only contaminate culture specimens. Pneumonia, especially hospital-acquired pneumonia, is frequently caused by gram-negative organisms in which resistance against multiple antibiotics is not uncommon. The diagnostic uncertainty and the high mortality of these infections explain the preference for broad-spectrum agents or combination therapy. Only very few new antibiotics in the penicillin, cephalosporin, carbapenem groups have been introduced to clinical use in the last few years, such as cefpirome, cefepime, cefixime, and cefpodoxime. Because of limited information, a final evaluation of these antibiotics is currently not possible. This chapter mainly describes the relevant microbiological and therapeutic properties of the fluoroquinolones and macrolides.

FLUOROQUINOLONES

In Vitro Activity Against Bronchopulmonary Pathogens

Streptococcus pneumoniae accounts for the majority of cases in community-acquired pneumonia. Other pathogens that can cause outpatient episodes of pneumonia are *Legionella pneumophila* and other *Legionella* species, *Hemophilus influenzae*, *Staphylococcus aureus*, *Mycoplasma pneumoniae*, and *C. pneumoniae*. Like other streptococci, *S. pneumoniae* is only moderately susceptible to the fluoroquinolones. The most active compounds are sparfloxacin, ciprofloxacin, and ofloxacin, with MIC_{90} values between 0.5 and 2 mg/l (15,36,37). For other quinolones, such as enoxacin and pefloxacin, the MIC_{90}'s range between 8 and 16 mg/l, which is above the peak serum levels of these drugs after standard dosage. Quinolones are only moderately potent inhibitors of *S. aureus*. Again, sparfloxacin, ofloxacin, and ciprofloxacin are the most active drugs (MIC_{90}: 0.5–1 mg/l); other derivatives like enoxacin tended to be less active (36,37). Fluoroquinolones inhibit all *Legionella* species effectively *in vitro*. They are more active than erythromycin but less potent compared to rifampicin (13). *Mycoplasma pneumoniae* is less susceptible to 4-quin-olones, of which ofloxacin exhibits the greatest activity. Also, *Chlamydia* species are only moderately sensitive to fluoroquinolones; tetracyclines and macrolides are considerably more potent.

Acute bacterial exacerbation of chronic bronchitis is caused predominantly by *H. influenzae, S. pneumoniae,* and *B. catarrhalis.* Except for *S. pneumoniae,* 4-quino-lones are highly active against these organisms, including *H. influenzae,* which are resistant to ampicillin as a result of beta-lactamase production (37). The predominant pathogens of hospital-acquired pneumonia in critically ill patients are enteric bacte-ria, *P. aeruginosa,* and *S. aureus.* In chronic bronchial disease similar pathogens can be isolated from the sputum in patients with end-stage disease, bronchiectasis, and antibiotic pretreatment. Quinolones exhibit great antibacterial potency against most of these species (Table 37-1). Enterobacteriaceae are particularly susceptible to 4-quinolones; ciprofloxacin is the most active derivative. *P. aeruginosa* is the major pathogen that causes purulent episodes in patients with bronchiectasis and advanced cystic fibrosis. This organism proved less susceptible than other gram-negative bac-teria with MIC_{90} value of 0.5–1.0 mg/l for ciprofloxacin and 3.2–7.2 mg/l for enoxacin and ofloxacin (37,43).

Penetration into Lung Tissue and Bronchial Secretion

Although tissue distribution studies of antibiotics and their clinical significance are still controversial (8), modern pharmacokinetics studies include measurements of distribution into various tissues and body fluids. These fluoroquinolone tissue concentrations are generally high, as a result of excellent bioavailability of 70-95% when administered orally, low serum protein binding ranging from 10 to 30%, and isoelectric points to plasma ranging from 6.8 to 7.5, indicating the quinolones are in the least ionized state while circulating in serum. Consequently, the major fraction of the quinolones can diffuse freely from the intra- to the extravascular space (10). Liposolubility, usually advocated as a drug factor contributing to tissue distribution (17), does not seem to play a significant role for quinolones: some are hydrophilic (ciprofloxacin); others are lipophilic (pefloxacin, sparfloxacin) or intermediate (ofloxacin, fleroxacin, lomefloxacin), depending on the octanol/water partition co-

TABLE 37–1. *Susceptibility of gram-negative bacilli (MIC 90, mg/l) to fluoroquinolones*

Organism	Cipro	Oflo	Peflo	Flero	Lomeflo	Sparflo
E. coli	≤0.06	0.125	0.125	0.125	0.25	0.06
Klebsiella sp	0.125	0.5	0.5	0.5	0.5	0.25
Enterobacter sp	0.125	0.5	0.5	0.5	0.5	0.25
Serratia sp	0.25	1.0	1.0	1.0	2.0	1.0
Citrobacter sp	0.125	0.5	0.5	0.25	1.0	0.5
P. mirabilis	0.06	0.25	0.25	0.125	0.25	0.5
P. vulgaris	≤0.06	0.125	0.25	0.125		0.5
M. morganii	≤0.06	0.25	0.25	0.25	0.25	0.25
P. stuartii	0.25	1.0	4.0	1.0	4.0	2.0
Acinetobacter sp	0.5	1.0		1.0	4.0	0.25
P. aeruginosa	0.5	4.0	2.0	8.0	4.0	2.0
H. influenzae	≤0.06	≤0.06	≤0.06	0.06	0.12	≤0.06

Compiled data published by F. Modai (36), *Quinolones Bulletin* 10:6-11; 1993.

efficient which ranges from <0.1 (ciprofloxacin) to >2 (pefloxacin). In several well-designed fiberbronchoscopic studies the penetration of quinolones to the lower respiratory tract was investigated (5,6). In general, the lung dispositions of quino- lones measured by these authors were: sputum levels, ca 90% of serum concentra- tions; bronchomucosal levels, ca 1.6 × serum concentrations; epithelial lining fluid levels (ELF), ca 2–3 × serum concentrations; and alveolar macrophage levels, ca 14–18 × serum concentrations. These results with the fluoroquinolones contrast fa- vorably to the poor penetration of most beta-lactams and aminoglycosides into bron- chial secretions and lung tissue.

Clinical Evaluation in Lower Respiratory Tract Infections

In view of the antimicrobial activity and pharmacological properties, fluoroquin- olones should be suitable for the treatment of lower respiratory tract infections. These drugs have been studied extensively as a therapy for chest infections using oral or parenteral regimens. Most studies were carried out openly and were noncom- parative (8,15,21,34,47). For bacterial exacerbation of chronic bronchitis and pneu- monia, a number of well-controlled randomized studies have been published com- paring standard treatment with aminopenicillins, tetracyclines, co-trimoxazole, or oral cephalosporins. In a thorough analysis of published data, Thys et al. (47) re- ported on valid data on treatment of such chest infections and found more aban- doned information for ciprofloxacin and ofloxacin than for enoxacin and pefloxacin. With these reservations in mind, these four quinolones seem equally effective clini- cally; the rates of cure or improvement are 89% (263 of 294 patients) for enoxacin; 82% (205 of 250 patients) for pefloxacin; 88% (2,147 of 2,451 patients) for ofloxacin, and 88% (2,038 of 2,329 patients) for ciprofloxacin. The corresponding bacteriolog- ical eradication rates for the four drugs were as follows: 70% (201 of 288 pathogens) for enoxacin; 81% (160 of 197 pathogens) for pefloxacin; 81% (981 of 1,212 patho- gens) for ofloxacin; and 83% (1,232 of 1,488 pathogens) for ciprofloxacin. No differ- ences in efficacy were found when ofloxacin and ciprofloxacin were compared in a double-blind, cross-over study in cystic fibrosis patients (24). Most trials comparing these quinolones with other commonly used antibiotics for treatment of lower res- piratory tract infections suggest similar activity of the two compounds. However, some studies indicate that the quinolone is more efficacious than comparative drugs. From a clinical point of view, ofloxacin has been found to be superior to amoxicillin and cefaclor (18), and ciprofloxacin to cefaclor (30), josamycin (30), and ceftazidime (48).

The role of the new quinolones in the treatment of bronchopulmonary infection due to *Streptococcus* pneumonia has not been fully established. Doubt arises when considering the relationship between the concentrations of these antibiotics in blood and in bronchial secretions, and the MICs for the pathogens. This relationship is highly favorable for *H. influenzae* and *Moraxella catarrhalis,* but far less so for *S. pneumoniae.* In 122 patients in whom the clinical efficacy of quinolones in pneu- mococcal lower respiratory infections could be evaluated, the mean rate of clinical cure or improvement was 91% (47), whereas the mean rate of clinical success in 253 patients with *H. influenzae* infections was 90% (47). Thus, the clinical efficacy of the new quinolones in *H. influenzae* and *S. pneumoniae* lower respiratory tract in- fection seems similar and appears to be very good. However, the mean rate of bac- teriological eradication for 785 isolates of *H. influenzae* was 95%, but the same parameter for 542 *S. pneumoniae* isolates was only 73%, which is significantly lower. Thus, these drugs appear to be less effective in eliminating *S. pneumoniae* from the sputum than *H. influenzae*. For example, in a comprehensive study of 280 cases of exacerbation of chronic bronchitis treated with the 4-quinolones respectively, persistance, recurrence, or superinfection due to *S. pneumoniae*, was observed in 58 (67%) of 87 patients with primary pneumococcal infection (14). Due to the excellent *in vitro* activity against gram-negative organisms and good penetration into the respiratory tract, the new quinolones have potential in the treatment of gram-negative pneumonia, as shown in many randomized controlled prospective studies (36). However, there are some remaining problems, one of them being the development of resistance. Rising MICs have been observed during quinolone therapy of gram-negative respiratory infections in many studies, especially when the MIC of the pathogens is in the order of 1–2 g/l. The emergence of resistance to fluoroquinolones was reported (7), especially in *Pseudomonas aeruginosa* as well as *S. aureus* (especially MRSA). Several approaches might be taken to attempt to suppress emergence of quinolone resistance in this clinical setting. Drug use should be carefully targeted, and optimal dosing regimens should be used, especially in ICU patients (29). Adverse effects related to treatment with 4-quinolones predominantly involved the gastrointestinal tract or central nervous system (46). An additional problem for the tolerance of these drugs in patients with chronic bronchial disease is the possible interaction with theophyllin, a drug widely used in these patients. Increase in theophyllin serum levels has been observed in patients on a stable theophyllin medication following co-administration of enoxacin and, less frequently, ciprofloxacin (25,50). There are other possible interactions which should be considered when a fluoroquinolone treatment is instituted (Table 37-2).

In conclusion, the following indications for fluoroquinolones are proposed. For acute exacerbation of chronic bronchitis, fluoroquinolones, particularly sparfloxacin, ofloxacin, and ciprofloxacin, might be a good choice, especially if the sputum smear reveals gram-negative pathogens. However, taking into account the high efficacy of ampicillin combined with a beta-lactamase inhibitor, or of oral cephalosporins in the treatment of this condition, it should be pointed out that these drugs are equally good alternatives. In the case of gram-positive cocci in sputum, aminobenzyl derivatives or macrolides are preferable. In addition, the potential of quinolones for selecting resistant bacteria suggests that some restrictions on the use of these drugs might be necessary.

In community-acquired pneumonia, the newer quinolones should not be used for initial treatment of outpatient pneumonia. In fact, other established regimens such as beta-lactams or macrolides seem a better choice because of the limited efficacy of quinolones in the treatment of severe pneumococcal infections and because of the poor activity of these drugs against the anaerobic flora causing aspiration pneumo-

TABLE 37–2. *Potential drug interactions of fluoroquinolones*

Methylxanthines
Multivalent metal cations
Cimetidine
Probenecid
NSAIDs
Cyclosporine
Warfarin

nia. However, preliminary results with sparfloxacin are very promising, even in proven pneumococcal pneumonia. Moreover, experience in the treatment of *Mycoplasma* pneumonia infections with fluoroquinolones is still limited. Preliminary data suggest that quinolones—used with or without erythromycin and rifampicin—might be useful in the treatment of Legionnaires' disease; however, this therapeutic approach needs further clinical evaluation. Finally, the role of these drugs in the treatment of *Chlamydia* and *Rickettsiae* infections is still uncertain. In contrast, the clinical trials with quinolones in the treatment of nosocomial pneumonia caused by gram-negative bacilli are promising. In sequential therapy, these quinolones or other compounds can be given intravenously followed by an oral form of the quinolone. Fluoroquinolones are an attractive alternative to beta-lactams and aminoglycosides in treatment of gram-negative pneumonia. However, in chest infections induced by *P. aeruginosa* and *S. aureus,* the emergence of resistance to fluoroquinolones in these species is a considerable risk and must be balanced against potential benefit. The fluoroquinolones should never be used for trivial infections caused by staphylococci or *P. aeruginosa.*

MACROLIDE ANTIBIOTICS

In recent years there have been a number of 14-, 15-, and 16-membered macrolides synthesised (27,28). For the 14-membered macrolides the spirochetal activity has been blocked by modifying the C-6 hydroxy, C-9 ketone, or proton at C-8 and the diol at C-11 and C-12. These changes, in effect, prevent internal acetel formation of the C-9 carboxyl group A and the hydroxyls of the C-6 and C-12 in the lactone ring. The first agent to be investigated was an oximederivative, roxithromycin, which has been in clinical use for several years (39). Other agents have included dirithromycin, the prodrug of erythromycylamine, flurithromycin, and clarithromycin. One new 15-membered macrolide in development is azithromycin. New 16-membered macrolides are roxithromycin, miocamycin, and midecamycin (38).

In Vitro Activity Against Bronchopulmonary Pathogens

Macrolide antibiotics exhibit antimicrobial action by binding to the 50 S subunit of the 70 S ribosome, thereby inhibiting bacterial RNA-dependent protein synthesis. The concentrations necessary to inhibit 90% of the growth (MIC_{90}) values of erythromycin and the new macrolide antibiotics are given in Table 37-3 (4). In general, none of the macrolide antibiotics is active against methicillin-resistant *S. aureus, S. epidermidis,* or *Pseudomonas* sp. Azithromycin is as active as or less active than erythromycin for most gram-positive organisms but is more active against *M. pneumoniae* and gram-negative organisms such as *H. influenzae, H. parainfluenzae,* and *Moraxella catarrhalis. In vitro,* clarithromycin demonstrates equal or better activity than erythromycin against many gram-positive anaerobic organisms such as *Chlamydia trachomatis, M. catarrhalis,* and *L. pneumophila,* but alone does not improve the coverage of *H. influenzae* or *H. parainfluenzae* (27,40). The activity of clarithromycin and its 14-OH metabolite appears to be additive, however, thereby expanding the spectrum to include *H. influenzae* (40). Dirithromycin has a similar spectrum of activity to erythromycin; it does not provide adequate antimicrobial activity against *H. influenzae* or *L. pneumophila.* Roxithromycin is generally as ac-

TABLE 37–3. In vitro MIC_{90} values of erythromycin, azithromycin, clarithromycin, dirithromycin, and roxithromycin

Bacteria	MIC_{90} (mg/l)				
	Erythromycin	Azithromycin	Clarithromycin	Dirithromycin	Roxithromycin
Streptococcus pneumoniae	0.015–0.25	0.015–0.25	0.015–0.06	0.06–0.12	0.03–0.12
Streptococcus pyogenes	0.03–4.0	0.03–4.0	0.015–0.25	0.12–2.0	0.06–2.0
Corynebacterium sp	16.0	128	4.0	8.0	16.0
Listeria monocytogenes	0.5–4.0	2.0–4.0	0.25–2.0	2.0–4.0	1.0–2.0
Clostridium perfringens	1.0	0.25–0.5	0.5	4.0	2.0
Peptococcus-Peptostreptococcus	4.0–16.0	2.0–4.0	2.0–4.0	16.0–128	8.0–32.0
Propionibacterium acnes	0.03	0.03	0.03	0.5–1.0	0.06
Moraxella catarrhalis	0.25	0.06[a]	0.12–0.25	0.25	0.5–1.0
Neisseria gonorrhoeae	0.25–0.5	0.03–0.06[a]	0.25–0.5	2.0–4.0	0.5–1.0
Bordetella pertussis	0.03	0.06	0.03	0.03	0.25
Campylobacter jejuni	1.0	0.12[a]	2.0	0.25[a]	4.0
Helicobacter pylori	0.25	0.25	0.03[a]	0.5	0.25
Hemophilus influenzae	2.0–8.0	0.25–1.0[a]	2.0–8.0[b]	8.0–>16	4.0–16.0
Legionella pneumophilia	2.0	2.0	0.25[a]	16	0.5[a]
Bacteroides fragilis	4.0–8.0	2.0–4.0	2.0–8.0	>128	32
Chlamydia trachomatis	2.0	0.25[a]	0.125[a]	4.0	1.0

MIC_{90}, minimum concentration necessary to inhibit 90% of the growth.
[a]Improved activity versus erythromycin.
[b]MIC_{90} of clarithromycin alone. With 14-OH metabolite. MIC_{90} value may be lower.
From Bahal and Nahata (4).

tive as or less active than erythromycin for most of the commonly isolated gram-positive and gram-negative organisms (27).

Penetration into Lung Tissue and Bronchial Secretion

The major difference between the newer macrolide antibiotics and erythromycin is the improved pharmacokinetic profile of the new agents. New macrolides have improved and more predictable absorption. Like erythromycin, peak serum concentrations of these derivatives generally occur between 1 and 4 hours following oral administration. In comparison to erythromycin, roxithromycin achieves higher peak serum concentrations; peak concentrations of azithromycin and clarithromycin are lower than that of erythromycin. In general, macrolide antibiotics are lipophilic and consequently penetrate well into tissues, resulting in high volumes of distribution (31). This confounds the interpretation of the MIC values because adequate tissue concentrations can be achieved in the presence of low blood concentrations. An important characteristic of the newer macrolide antibiotics is the ability to achieve high intracellular concentrations. Azithromycin, clarithromycin, dirithromycin, and roxithromycin have been shown to be concentrated in macrophages and leukocytes. This is particularly beneficial against intracellular pathogens such as *L. pneumophila*, *Chlamydia* sp, and *Mycoplasma* sp. In general, these agents achieve intracellular/extracellular cell ratio of 5 : 100 in human polymorphonuclear leukocytes, and 5 : 30 intracellular/extracellular cell ratio in macrophages (49). The prolonged, high tissue concentrations of azithromycin and dirithromycin (also, its metabolite erythromycylamine) were the basis for successful short duration treatment times of lower respiratory tract infections.

Clinical Evaluation

Although many noncomparative studies and abstracts evaluating the comparative efficacy of the new macrolides against standard antibiotic regimens have been published, these results must be interpreted cautiously as many of the comparative studies were performed by nonstandardized definitions and techniques. Also, different dosage regimens were used, and sometimes the duration of therapy was not specified, which could account for lower response rates. Finally, the definition of clinical cure was often not stated.

Azithromycin

Azithromycin has proved effective in the treatment of lower respiratory tract infections. An open label–randomized multicenter study compared azithromycin 250 mg twice a day for 1 day, then 250 mg per day on days 2–5, with erythromycin 500 mg 4 times per day for 10 days for serologically proved (> fourfold increase of serological titer) pneumonia (44). Causative pathogens for azithromycin- and erythromycin-treated patients, respectively, were *M. pneumoniae* (31 and 24) and *C. Spsitaci* (8 and 8). No therapeutic failures occurred in either group. A randomized third-party blinded trial compared similar doses of azithromycin to cefaclor 500 mg 3 times per day for 10 days in patients with acute bronchitis or pneumonia (11). Of the 272 available patients, 249 had bronchitis and 23 had pneumonia. Cure or improvement was observed in 96% and 94% of azithromycin- and cefaclor-treated patients, respectively.

Although overall bacterial eradication rates were 87.8% and 86.2%, respectively, the elimination of *H. influenzae* was significantly better for azithromycin (p < 0.001).

In an open label trial, 21 patients with chronic bronchitis were given azithromycin 500 mg orally for one dose, then 250 mg per day for 5 days (16). Although *S. pneumoniae* and *B. catarrhalis* were effectively eradicated, the authors reported persistance of *H. influenzae* infections in six of nine patients and relapse after therapy in two, with increased geometric mean MICs from 1.25 mg/l before treatment to 4.87 mg/l 1 week after the end of treatment. Similar observations were made with erythromycin in a previous noncomparative, unblinded study in which clinical failures with *Hemophilus* sp were associated with an increase in MIC during therapy.

In a randomized double-blind study carried out in 28 centers, azithromycin (500 mg single dose on day 1, followed by 250 mg once daily on days 2–5) was compared with cefaclor (500 mg tid for 10 days) in the treatment of acute bacterial pneumonia (26). A total of 119 patients entered the study and of these 71 were available and included in the efficacy analysis. The overall satisfactory clinical response was 97.3% for azithromycin patients and 100% for cefaclor patients. The clinical cure rates of azithromycin and cefaclor were 46.9% and 41.0%, respectively; improvement was seen in an additional 46.9% of azithromycin-treated patients and in 50.0% of the cefaclor group. The bacteriological eradication rates were 80.4% and 92.6%, respectively.

Clarithromycin

Clarithromycin has been studied in a variety of lower respiratory tract infections. Successful treatment has been reported in *Mycoplasma pneumoniae* (9), community-acquired pneumonia (2,47), chlamydial pneumonia (38), and in 44 patients with *Legionella pneumophila* respiratory infections (38). The average dosage of clarithromycin in the pneumonia cases was 250 mg to 500 mg every 12 hours. Also, successful treatments were reported in acute bacterial exacerbations of chronic bronchitis (1,3). Clarithromycin has been compared with a variety of penicillins (e.g., ampicillin, amoxicillin, penicillin VK) as well as cefadroxil, erythromycin, and roxithromycin. Overall it appears that clarithromycin is as effective as are the currently available agents in treating the lower respiratory tract infections studied today.

Dirithromycin

Dirithromycin treatment results in lower repiratory tract infections were recently published. In a double-blind multicenter study the efficacy and safety of dirithromycin 500 mg/day given orally once daily for 10–14 days were compared with those of erythromycin 1000 mg/day given orally 2 times daily for 10–14 days in 173 evaluable patients (45). Symptomatic responses and bacteriological results were comparable in both groups. More than 1,600 patients suffering from exacerbations of chronic bronchitis or acute bacterial bronchitis were treated with dirithromycin (500 mg/day for 7 days) or erythromycin (4 × 250 mg/day for 7 days); clinical and bacteriological responses as well as safety were comparable in both treatment arms (19).

TABLE 37–4. *Improvements of the new macrolides over erythromycin*

Drug	Improvement
Azithromycin	Reduced incidence of GI adverse effects; once-daily-dosing (following loading dose); improved antimicrobial activity against selected gram-negative organisms and anaerobic organisms (i.e., *C. jejuni, H. influenzae, H. parainfluenzae, M. pneumoniae, M. catarrhalis, N. gonorrhoea, C. perfringens*); higher tissue concentrations
Clarithromycin	Reduced incidence of GI adverse effects; twice-daily-dosing; improved antimicrobial activity against *L. pneumophila, H. pylori, M. catarrhalis, C. trachomatis*; higher tissue concentrations
Dirithromycin	Once-daily dosing; higher tissue concentrations
Roxithromycin	Reduced incidence of GI adverse effects; once-daily dosing; higher serum concentrations

GI, gastrointestinal.
From Bahal and Nahata (4).

Roxithromycin

Roxithromycin has been studied *in vivo* in a variety of infections, including pneumonia and bronchitis most commonly caused by *S. pneumoniae, H. influenzae,* and, less frequently, *Mycoplasma, Chlamydia,* and *Legionella* sp (12,20,22,32,33,35,42). It has been compared with cefradin, erythromycin, or doxycycline. Standard roxithromycin dosing regimens employed were 300 mg/d or 150 to 300 mg bid. Roxithromycin was found to be similar in efficacy to the established regimen for most infections.

The most commonly reported adverse effect associated with the macrolides is gastrointestinal toxicity (nausea, vomiting, diarrhea, abdominal pain). However, in general, the incidence of side effects with the newer macrolides are significantly lower in most trials in comparison to erythromycin.

In conclusion, the potential advantages of the new macrolides over erythromycin, based on available studies, are described in Table 37-4. The newer macrolides offer several advantages over erythromycin, including greater antimicrobial activity against certain organisms and longer elimination half-life, thus allowing less frequent administration and a lower incidence of adverse gastrointestinal effects. The definitive conclusions about the therapeutic role of these drugs should await completion of ongoing clinical studies.

REFERENCES

1. Aldons, P.M. (1991): A comparison of clarithromycin with ampicillin in the treatment of patients with acute bacterial exacerbations of chronic bronchitis. *J. Antimicrob. Chemother.,* 27(Suppl. A):91–100.
2. Anderson, G., Esmonde, T.S., Coles, S., Macklin, J., and Carnegie, C. (1991): A comparative safety and efficacy study of clarithromycin and erythromycin stearate in community-acquired pneumonia. *J. Antimicrob. Chemother.,* 27(Suppl. A):117–124.
3. Bachand, R.T. (1991): Comparative study of clarithromycin and ampicillin in the treatment of patients with acute bacterial exacerbations of chronic bronchitis. *J. Antimicrob. Chemother.,* 27(Suppl. A):91–100.
4. Bahal, N., and Nahata, M.C. (1992): The new macrolide antibiotics: azithromycin, clarithromycin, dirithromycin, and roxithromycin. *Ann. Pharmacother.,* 26:46–55.

5. Baldwin, D.R., Honeybourne, D., and Wise, R. (1992): Pulmonary disposition of antimicrobial agents: in vivo observations and clinical relevance. *Antimicrob. Agents Chemother.*, 36:1176–1180.

6. Baldwin, D.R., Wise, R., Andrews, J.M., and Honeybourne, D. (1990): Concentration of antimicrobials in the pulmonary alveolar epithelial lining. *Res. A. Clin. Forums*, 12:103–113.

7. Ball, P. (1990): Emergent resistance to ciprofloxacin amongst *Pseudomonas aeruginosa* and *Staphylococcus aureus:* clinical significance and therapeutic approaches. *J. Antimicrob. Chemother.*, 26(Suppl. F):165–179.

8. Carbon, C. (1990): Significance of tissue levels for prediction of antibiotic efficacy and determination of dosage. *Eur. J. Clin. Microb. Infect. Dis.*, 9:510–516.

9. Cassell, G.H., Donec, J., Waitesk, B., Pate, M.S., Duffy, L.B., Watson, H.L., and McIntosh, J.C. (1991): Efficacy of clarithromycin against *Mycoplasma pneumoniae. J. Antimicrob. Chemother.*, 27(Suppl. A):47–60.

10. Dalhoff, A. (1989): A review of quinolone tissue pharmacokinetics. In: *International Telesymposium on Quinolones,* edited by P.G. Fernandes, pp. 277–312. J.R. Prous Science Publishers, Barcelona.

11. Dark, D. (1991): Multicenter evaluation of azithromycin and cefaclor in acute lower respiratory tract infections. *Am. J. Med.*, 91(Suppl. 3A):31S–35S.

12. Dautzenberg, B., Scheimberg, A., Brambilla, C., Camus, P., Godard, P., Guerin, J.C., Lemarie, E., Rezvani, Y., Rosembaum, M., Tuchais, E., and Wallaert, B. (1992): Comparison of two oral antibiotics, roxithromycin and amoxicillin plus clavulanic acid, in lower respiratory tract infections. *Diagn. Microb. Infect. Dis.*, (Suppl. 4):85–90.

13. Davies, B.I., and Maesen, F.P.V. (1986): Quinolones in chest infections. *J. Antimicrob. Chemother.*, 18:296–299.

14. Davies, B.I., and Maesen, F.P.V. (1987): Respiratory infections: clinical experiences with the new quinolones. *Pharmaceutisch, Weekblad*, (Suppl. 9)P:53–57.

15. Davies, B.I., Maesen, F.P.V., Baur, C., Teengs, J.P., and Cremers, H.M.H.G. (1985): Ciprofloxacin in purulent exacerbations of chronic bronchitis: a clinical, microbiological and pharmacokinetic study. In: *Recent Advances in Chemotherapy, Antimicrobial Section 2,* edited by J. Ishigami, pp. 1626–1627. *Proceedings of the 14th International Congress of Chemotherapy,* Kyoto. University of Tokyo Press, Tokyo.

16. Davies, B.I., Maesen, F.P.V., and Gubbelmans, R. (1989): Azithromycin (CP-62, 993) in acute exacerbations of chronic bronchitis: an open clinical, microbiological and pharmacokinetic study. *J. Antimicrob. Chemother.*, 23:743–751.

17. Decré, D., and Bergogne-Berezin, E. (1993): Pharmacokinetics of quinolones with special reference to the respiratory tree. *J. Antimicrob. Chemother.*, 31:331–344.

18. Fujimori, I., Kobayashi, Y., Obana, M., Saito, A., Tomizawa, M., Nakayama, I., Hiraga, Y., Kikuchi, K., Yamamoto, A., and Takebe, K. (1984): Comparative clinical study of ofloxacin and cefaclor in bacterial bronchitis. *Kansenshogaku Zasshi*, 58:832–861.

19. Gaillat, J. (1993): A multicenter study: comparing the safety and efficacy of dirithromycin with erythromycin in the treatment of bronchitis. *J. Antimicrob. Chemother.*, 31(Suppl. C):139–152.

20. Gentry, L.O. (1987): Roxithromycin, a new macrolide antibiotic, in the treatment of infections in the lower respiratory tract: an overview. *J. Antimicrob. Chemother.*, 20(Suppl. B):145–152.

21. Gleadhill, I.C., Ferguson, W.P., and Lowry, R.C. (1986): Efficacy and safety of ciprofloxacin in patients with respiratory infections in comparison with amoxycillin. *J. Antimicrob. Chemother.*, 18(Suppl. D):133–138.

22. Humbrechts, J.M., Kupperberg, A., Smets, P., Dramaix, M., Valante, F., and Vanhoof, R. (1988): Multicentre comparative study of roxithromycin and amoxycillin in the treatment of respiratory tract infections. *Br. J. Clin. Pract.*, 42(Suppl. 55):102–103.

23. Jacobson, K. (1993): Clinical efficacy of clarithromycin in pneumonia. *J. Antimicrob. Chemother.*, 31(Suppl. C):121–130.

24. Jensen, T., Pedersen, S.S., Nielsen, C.H., Hoiby, N., and Koch, C. (1987): The efficacy and safety of ciprofloxacin and ofloxacin in chronic *Pseudomonas aeruginosa* infection in cystic fibrosis. *J. Antimicrob. Chemother.*, 20:585–594.

25. Khan, F., and Raoof, S. (1986): Ciprofloxacin in the treatment of respiratory tract infections. In: *Proceedings of the 1st International Ciprofloxacin Workshop,* pp. 252–256. Excerpta Medica, Amsterdam.

26. Kinasewitz, G., and Wood, R.G. (1991): Azithromycin versus cefaclor in the treatment of acute bacterial pneumonia. *Eur. J. Clin. Microbiol. Infect. Dis.*, 10:872–876.

27. Kirst, H.A., and Sides, G.D. (1989): New directions for macrolide antibiotics: structural modifications and *in vitro* activity. *J. Antimicrob. Agents Chemother.*, 33:1413–1418.

28. Kirst, H.A., and Sides, G.D. (1989): New directions for macrolide antibiotics: pharmacokinetics and clinical efficacy. *Antimicrob. Agents Chemother.*, 33:1419–1422.

29. Kljucar, S., Heimesaat, M., von Pritzbuer, E., Timm, J., and Bauernfeind, A. (1992): A comparison of intravenous ciprofloxacin dosage regimens in severe nosocomial infections. *Infections in Medicine*, 22(Suppl.):58–72.

30. Kobayashi, H., Takamura, K., Takeda, H., Kono, K., and Saito, A. (1986): Comparative clinical study of ciprofloxacin and cefaclor in the treatment of respiratory tract infections. *Chemother.,* 34:1011–1037.
31. Lode, H., Boeck, M., Schaberg, T., Borner, K., and Koeppe, P. (1993): Pharmacology of new macrolides, azalides and streptogramins. In: *The New Macrolides, Azalides, and Streptogramins,* edited by H.C. Neu, L.S. Young, and S.H. Zinner, pp. 61–68. Marcel Dekker, New York.
32. Lousbergh, D., Jochems, G., Everaert, L., and Puttemans, M. (1991): Roxythromycin versus amoxicillin-clavulanic acid in the treatment of respiratory tract infections. *17th International Congress of Chemotherapy,* (Abstract 770), Berlin.
33. MacLoughlin, G.F.F., Lanoel, J., Stamboulian, D., and Sarachian, B. (1988): Roxithromycin in the treatment of atypical pneumonia. *Br. J. Clin. Pract.,* 42(Suppl. 55):92–93.
34. Magnani, C., Fregni, S., Valli, G., Cosentinav, R., and Bisetti, A. (1986): Comparative clinical study of ciprofloxacin and co-trimoxazole in respiratory tract infections. In: *Proceedings of the 1st International Cicprofloxacin Workshop,* pp. 260–264. Excerpta Medica, Amsterdam.
35. Marsac, J., Akoun, G., Balmes, P., Butaeye, Charpin, J., Carroler, J., et al. (1988): Multicenter comparative study of the efficacy and safety of roxithromycin and doxycycline in the treatment of lower respiratory tract infections. *Br. J. Clin. Pract.,* 42(Suppl. 55):100–101.
36. Modai, J. (1988): The role of quinolones in gram-negative pneumonia. *Quinolone Bulletin.,* 10:6–11.
37. Monk, J.P., and Campoli-Richards, D.M. (1987): Ofloxacin: a review of its antibacterial activity, pharmacokinetic properties and therapeutic use. *Drugs,* 33:346–391.
38. Neu, H.C. (1991): The development of macrolides: clarithromycin in perspective. *J. Antimicrob. Chemother.,* 27(Suppl. A):1–9.
39. Neu, H.C., and Acar, J.F. (Editors) (1989): Roxithromycin: a new antibiotic. *Br. J. Clin. Pract.,* 42(Suppl. 55):1–119.
40. Olsson-Liljequist, B., and Hoffman, B.M. (1991): In-vitro activity of clarithromycin combined with its 14-hydroxy metabolite A-62671 against *Haemophilus influenzae. J. Antimicrob. Chemother.,* 27(Suppl. A):11–18.
41. Poirier, R. (1991): Comparative study of clarithromycin and roxithromycin in the treatment of community-acquired pneumonia. *J. Antimicrob. Chemother.,* 27(Suppl. A):109–116.
42. Rahlwes, M., Wagner, J., Schuster, L., Berntsson, E., Ruckdeschel, G., Ehret, W., et al. (1988): Prospective randomized comparison of roxithromycin and amoxycillin in non-hospital-acquired pneumonia. *Br. J. Clin. Pract.,* 42(Suppl. 55):91.
43. Sanders, C.C., Sanders, W.E., and Goering, R.V. (1987): Overview of preclinical studies with ciprofloxacin. *Am. J. Med.,* 82(Suppl. 4A):2–11.
44. Schonwald, S., Gunjaca, M., Kolacny-Babie, L., et al. (1990): Comparison of azithromycin and erythromycin in the treatment of atypical pneumonias. *J. Antimicrob. Chemother.,* 25(Suppl. A):123–126.
45. Sides, G.D. (1993): Clinical efficacy of dirithromycin in acute exacerbation of chronic bronchitis. *J. Antimicrob. Chemother.,* 31(Suppl. C):131–138.
46. Stahlmann, R., and Lode, H. (1988): Safety overview: toxicity, adverse effects and drug interactions. In: *The Quinolones,* edited by V.T. Andriole, pp. 201–234. Academic Press, London.
47. Thys, J.P., Jacobs, F., Byl, B. (1991): Role of quinolones in the treatment of bronchopulmonary infections, particularly pneumococcal and community-acquired pneumonia. *Eur. J. Clin. Microbiol. Infect. Dis.,* 10:304–315.
48. Trenholme, G.M., Schmitt, B.A., Spear, J., Gvazdinskas, L.C., and Levin, S. (1989): Randomized study of intravenous/oral ciprofloxacin versus ceftazidime in the treatment of hospital and nursing home patients with lower respiratory tract infections. *Am. J. Medicine,* 87(Suppl. 5A):116–118.
49. Tulkens, P.M. (1990): The intracellular pharmacokinetics and activity of antibiotics. In: *New Antibacterial Strategies,* edited by H.C. Neu, pp. 243–259. Churchill Livingston, Edinburgh.
50. Wijnands, W.J.A., van Griethuysen, A.J.A., Vree, T.B., van Klingeren, B., and van Herwaarden, C.L.A. (1986): Enoxacin in lower respiratory tract infections. *J. Antimicrob. Chemother.,* 18:719–727.

Subject Index